KU-715-761

SURGICAL ONCOLOGY

Fundamentals, Evidence-based Approaches and New Technology

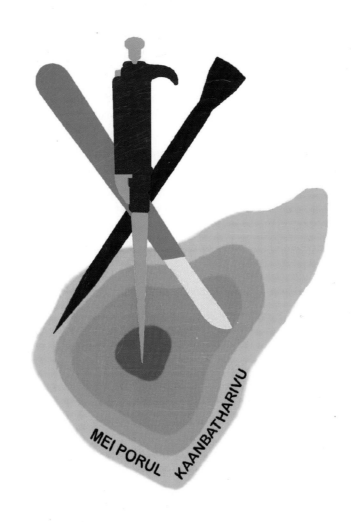

MEI PORUL KAANBATHARIVU

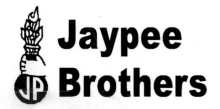

Jaypee Brothers

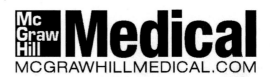

Medical

MCGRAWHILLMEDICAL.COM

Philosophy of the Emblem

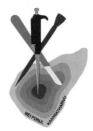

The emblem found in the cover has been conceived by the authors to represent the core aspects of surgical oncology, namely academics and literature (symbolized by the ancient writing instrument – the stylus), operative skill (symbolized by the scalpel), and research (symbolized by the pipette). The inscription *"Meiporul kaanbatharivu"* is a transliteration of the Tamil words "மெய்ப்பொருள் காண்பதறிவு". These words may be translated as *"Seeking the sterling truth is the hallmark of knowledge"*. These words appear in the famous Tamil literary classical work called the Thirukkural, which is a collection of two-liner (couplet) wise aphorisms. This inscription was selected, in order to convey the wisdom conveyed by 2 couplets, in which these words appear, for that wisdom is relevant to the practicing surgical oncologist.

Kural/Couplet # 355: "Epporul eththhanmai thaayinum apporul, meiporul kaanbatharivu". It may be translated to mean the following - Seeing the sterling truth in everything, beyond whatever quality, nature or appearance it may possess, is the hallmark of knowledge. Explanation: Any reality that is attempted to be understood may manifest a certain quality or nature or appearance or dimension. One's perception of such manifestations of the reality may render an understanding of the reality that is unrepresentative or misrepresentative of the actual reality, i.e. the 'sterling truth'. One who is knowledgeable will always seek an understanding of that sterling truth. In summary, one shall seek to realize the ultimate truth by discerning it, despite and beyond what is rendered by perception of the manifestations of reality. The surgeon-and-oncologist, shall also, under any and every circumstance, seek to discern the ultimate reality or sterling truth behind the phenomenon of cancer, and not be stranded with the understanding of the disease, rendered by perception alone

Kural/Couplet # 423: "Epporul yaryarvaik ketpinum apporul, meiporul kaanbatharivu". It may be translated to mean the following - Grasping the sterling truth in everything, in and beyond whatever is said about it by whomsoever, is the hallmark of knowledge. Explanation: Any reality that is to be understood, and/or any information pertaining to such reality may be expounded by any number of people, in any number of ways and in any number of versions. The person expounding the reality or any information pertaining to it, provide neither validity nor authenticity to what is expounded. One who is knowledgeable will always seek to acquire the sterling truth, in and beyond whatever is expounded about it, by whomsoever. The surgeon-and-oncologist is also surrounded and sometimes even overwhelmed by information from all sides - however, he or she shall not attach validity or authenticity to any of such information that is available to him/her by default, or by virtue of the source of such information. He/she shall seek for one's own self, to discern the truth and analyze its validity.

We thank artist Mr. Veera Santhanam for designing the emblem, my mother, father and brother for assistance in selecting an inscription and drafting the explanation and the famous Tamil scholar, Mr. Avvai Natarajan for his expertise in assisting the translation of the couplets.

Pragatheeshwar Thirunavukarasu, MD

SURGICAL ONCOLOGY

Fundamentals, Evidence-based Approaches and New Technology

Editors

David L Bartlett, MD
Bernard Fisher Professor of Surgery and Chief
Division of Surgical Oncology
Department of Surgery
University of Pittsburgh, USA

Pragatheeshwar Thirunavukarasu, MD
Resident, General Surgery
Department of Surgery
University of Pittsburgh, USA

Matthew D Neal, MD
Resident, General Surgery
Department of Surgery
University of Pittsburgh, USA

Special Contributing Editors

Phil Bao, MD
Assistant Professor of Surgery
Division of Surgical Oncology
Department of Surgery
SUNY Stony Brook, USA

Kothai Divya Pragatheeshwar, MBBS
University of Pittsburgh Cancer Institute
UPMC Cancer Pavilion, USA

Disclaimer: This text shall not be used as a direct and/or sole manual for clinical use. The editors, authors and the publisher shall not be responsible for any consequences due to application of information presented in the text. The editors, authors and publishers do not guarantee and/or make no warranty, expressed or implied, in regard to the completeness or accuracy of information. Doses and regimens mentioned in the text are not absolute and application in the clinical setting warrants analysis of the specific circumstances relating to the patient and practice of the physician. Any clinical decision shall be made only with critical analysis of all patient-relevant data.

© 2012, Jaypee Brothers Medical Publishers
First published in India in 2011 by

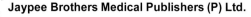

Jaypee Brothers Medical Publishers (P) Ltd.

Corporate Office
4838/24 Ansari Road, Daryaganj, **New Delhi** - 110002, India, +91-11-43574357

Registered Office
B-3 EMCA House, 23/23B Ansari Road, Daryaganj, **New Delhi** 110 002, India
Phones: +91-11-23272143, +91-11-23272703, +91-11-23282021,
+91-11-23245672, Rel: +91-11-32558559 Fax: +91-11-23276490, +91-11-23245683
e-mail: jaypee@jaypeebrothers.com, Website: www.jaypeebrothers.com

First published in USA by The McGraw-Hill Companies, 2 Penn Plaza, New York, NY 10121. Exclusively worldwide distributor except South Asia (India, Nepal, Sri Lanka, Bhutan, Pakistan, Bangladesh, Malaysia).

All rights reserved. No part of this publication may be reproduced, stored in a retrieval system, or transmitted, in any form or by any means, electronic, mechanical, photocopying, recording, or otherwise, without the prior permission of the publisher or in accordance with the provisions of the Copyright, Designs and Patents Act 1988 or under the terms of any licence permitting limited copying issued by the Copyright Licensing Agency, 90 Tottenham Court Road, London W1P 0LP.

ISBN-13: 978-0-07-178610-2
ISBN-10: 0-07-178610-4

Acknowledgments and Dedication

I acknowledge the sacrifices my family makes to my lofty goals and aspirations, and dedicate this book to Susan, Chrissy, and Chad Bartlett.

— *David L Bartlett*

I sincerely dedicate my work to my father Thirunavukarasu, my mother Chitra, my brother Nirmaleswar, all my teachers and my friends.

— *Pragatheeshwar Thirunavukarasu*

I dedicate this text to my parents, David and Kathy, brother, Jeremy, and especially my wife Donielle and son Cameron for their sacrifices and unwavering support. Also, to the patients who have inspired me through their battles, especially my grandfathers Wendell and Harold, and my friend Diane.

— *Matthew D Neal*

It is becoming increasingly difficult to balance busy clinical practices and academic endeavors, and we appreciate the sacrifice that each of the authors and their loved ones have made to complete the chapters in a timely manner. We would especially like to thank Margaret Corson for her administrative assistance throughout this mission.

— *The Editors*

Contributors

Gretchen Ahrendt MD
Associate Professor of Surgery
Division of Surgical Oncology
Department of Surgery
University of Pittsburgh, USA

Steven A Ahrendt MD
Assistant Professor of Surgery
Division of Surgical Oncology
Department of Surgery
University of Pittsburgh, USA

Marco A Alcala MD
Research Fellow, Division of Surgical Oncology
Department of Surgery
University of Pittsburgh, USA

Robert Arnold MD
Professor of Medicine
Division of General Internal Medicine
Section of Palliative Care and Medical Ethics
Department of Medicine
University of Pittsburgh, USA

Frances Austin MD
Resident, General Surgery
Department of Surgery
Penn State Milton S. Hershey
Medical Center, USA

Nathan Bahary MD, PhD
Assistant Professor of Medicine
Department of Medicine
University of Pittsburgh, USA

Farzaneh Banki MD
Assistant Professor of Cardiothoracic Surgery
University of Southern California
Visiting Surgeon; Heart, Lung and Esophageal Surgery Institute
University of Pittsburgh Medical Center, USA

Donald T Baril MD
Assistant Professor of Surgery
Division of Vascular Surgery
Department of Surgery
University of Pittsburgh, USA

Christopher J Bartels MD
Assistant Professor of Surgery
Department of Surgery
University of Pittsburgh, USA

David L Bartlett MD
Bernard Fisher Professor of Surgery and Chief
Division of Surgical Oncology
Department of Surgery
University of Pittsburgh, USA

Marguerite Bonaventura MD
Assistant Professor of Surgery
Department of Surgery
University of Pittsburgh, USA

Jason A Breaux MD
Clinical Instructor
Division of Surgical Oncology
Department of Surgery
University of Pittsburgh, USA

Au H Bui MD
Resident, General Surgery
Department of Surgery
University of Pittsburgh, USA

Evie Carchman MD
Resident, General Surgery
Department of Surgery
University of Pittsburgh, USA

Benedito A Carneiro MD
Fellow, Division of Hematology Oncology
Department of Medicine
University of Pittsburgh, USA

Sally E Carty MD
Professor of Surgery
Division of Surgical Oncology
Department of Surgery
University of Pittsburgh, USA

Rabih A Chaer MD
Assistant Professor of Surgery
Division of Vascular Surgery
Department of Surgery
University of Pittsburgh, USA

Sri Chalikonda MD
Digestive Disease Institute
Section of Surgical Oncology
Director of Robotics Program
Cleveland Clinic, USA

Edward Cheong MD
Fellow, Cardiothoracic Surgery
Heart, Lung and Esophageal Surgery Institute
University of Pittsburgh
Medical Center, USA

Julie W Childers MD
Instructor of Medicine
Division of General Internal Medicine
Section of Palliative Care and Medical Ethics
Department of Medicine
University of Pittsburgh, USA

Haroon A Choudry MD
Assistant Professor of Surgery
Division of Surgical Oncology
Department of Surgery
University of Pittsburgh, USA

Jon M Davison MD
Assistant Professor of Pathology
Department of Pathology
University of Pittsburgh, USA

Michael E de Vera MD
Assistant Professor of Surgery
Thomas E. Starzl Transplantation Surgery Institute
Department of Surgery
University of Pittsburgh, USA

Howard Edington MD
Associate Professor of Surgery
Surgical Oncology, Plastics and Reconstruction
Division of Surgical Oncology
Department of Surgery
University of Pittsburgh, USA

Robert P Edwards MD
Professor of Surgery
Division of Gynecology Oncology
Department of Surgery
University of Pittsburgh, USA

Raymond Eid MD
Resident,General Surgery
Department of Surgery
University of Pittsburgh, USA

Fateh Entabi MD
Resident, General Surgery
Department of Surgery
University of Pittsburgh, USA

Linda M Farkas MD
Assistant Professor of Surgery
Division of Surgical Oncology
Department of Surgery
University of Pittsburgh, USA

Bernard Fisher MD
Distinguished Service Professor
Founding Member and Former Director
National Surgical Adjuvant Breast and
Bowel Project (NSABP)
Department of Surgery
University of Pittsburgh, USA

Richard Fortunato MD
Fellow, Colorectal Surgery
Department of Surgery
LSU Health Science Center
Shreveport, Louisiana, USA

Jan Franko MD
Clinical Professor of Surgery
Mercy Surgical Affiliates
Department of Surgery
University of Des Moines
Des Moines, Iowa, USA

T Clark Gamblin MD
Assistant Professor of Surgery
Divisions of Surgical Oncology and Transplantation
Department of Surgery
University of Pittsburgh, USA

Joel S Greenberger MD
Professor and Chairman
Department of Radiation Oncology
University of Pittsburgh Cancer Institute, USA

A Serhat Gur MD
NCI-STSEP Scholar
Postdoctoral Research Fellow
Department of Surgery
University of Pittsburgh, USA

Daniel E Hall MD MDiv MHSc
Assistant Professor of Surgery
Department of General Surgery
University of Pittsburgh, USA

Marcus K Hoffman MD
Resident, General Surgery
Department of Surgery
University of Pittsburgh, USA

Matthew P Holtzman MD
Assistant Professor of Surgery
Division of Surgical Oncology
Department of Surgery
University of Pittsburgh, USA

Bruce O Hough MD
Fellow, Department of Medical Oncology
University of Pittsburgh, USA

Steven Hughes MD
Associate Professor of Surgery
Division of Surgical Oncology
Department of Surgery
University of Pittsburgh, USA

Kamran Idrees MD
Fellow, Division of Surgical Oncology
Department of Surgery
University of Pittsburgh, USA

Ronald Johnson MD
Associate Professor
Division of Surgical Oncology
Department of Surgery
University of Pittsburgh, USA

Pawel Kalinski MD PhD
Associate Professor of Surgery Immunology,
and Infectious Disease and Microbiology
Division of Surgical Oncology
Department of Surgery
University of Pittsburgh, USA

Linda King MD
Assistant Professor of Medicine
Division of General Internal Medicine
Section of Palliative Care and Medical Ethics
Department of Medicine
University of Pittsburgh, USA

Kenneth KW Lee MD
Associate Professor of Surgery
Department of Surgery
University of Pittsburgh, USA

Mario Lora MD
Research Fellow
Department of Surgery
University of Pittsburgh, USA

Michael T Lotze MD
Professor of Surgery and Bioengineering
Department of Surgery
Asst. Vice Chancellor, UPSHS
University of Pittsburgh, USA

Tara J Loux MD
Resident, General Surgery
Department of Surgery
University of Pittsburgh, USA

James D Luketich MD
Henry T Bahnson Professor and Chief
Division of Cardiothoracic Surgery
Heart, Lung and Esophageal Surgery Institute
University of Pittsburgh Medical Center, USA

Deepa Magge MD
Resident, General Surgery
Department of Surgery
University of Pittsburgh, USA

William C McBee MD
Fellow, Division of Gynecology Oncology
Department of Surgery
University of Pittsburgh, USA

Thomas McDonald
Medical Student
University of Pittsburgh School of Medicine, USA

Kevin P Mollen MD
Fellow, Division of Pediatric Surgery
University of Pittsburgh, USA

A James Moser MD
Associate Professor of Surgery
Division of Surgical Oncology
Department of Surgery
University of Pittsburgh, USA

Gary Nace MD
Resident, General Surgery
Department of Surgery
University of Pittsburgh, USA

Rahul Narang MD
Research Fellow, Department of Surgery
University of Pittsburgh, USA

Isam W Nasr MD
Resident, Department of Surgery
University of Pittsburgh, USA

Matthew D Neal MD
Resident, General Surgery
Department of Surgery
University of Pittsburgh, USA

Leo A Neimeier MD
Clinical Fellow, Gynecology and Breast Pathology
Department of Pathology
University of Pittsburgh Medical Center, USA

Kevin Tri Nguyen MD
Fellow, Division of Surgical Oncology
Department of Surgery
University of Pittsburgh, USA

Juan Ochoa MD
Professor of Surgery and Critical Care
Department of Surgery
University of Pittsburgh, USA

Jennifer B Ogilvie MD
Assistant Professor of Surgery
Department of Surgery
New York University Langone Medical Center, USA

Arjun Pennathur MD
Assistant Professor of Surgery
Heart, Lung and Esophageal Surgery Institute
University of Pittsburgh Medical Center, USA

James F Pingpank Jr MD
Associate Professor of Surgery
Division of Surgical Oncology
Department of Surgery
University of Pittsburgh, USA

Patricio M Polanco MD
Resident, General Surgery
Department of Surgery
University of Pittsburgh, USA

Kurian Puthenpurayil MD
Assistant Professor of Radiology
Department of Radiology
St. Margaret's Hospital and
University of Pittsburgh, USA

Scott D Richard MD
Assistant Professor of Surgery
Division of Gynecology Oncology
Department of Surgery
University of Pittsburgh, USA

David A Rodeberg MD
Assistant Professor of Surgery
Division of Pediatric General and Thoracic Surgery
Department of Surgery
University of Pittsburgh, USA

Antonio Romo de Vivar Chavez MD
Research Fellow
Division of Surgical Oncology
Department of Surgery
University of Pittsburgh, USA

Joshua T Rubin MD
Associate Professor of Surgery
Division of Surgical Oncology
Department of Surgery
University of Pittsburgh, USA

Wolfgang Schraut MD
Professor of Surgery
Division of Surgical Oncology
Department of Surgery
University of Pittsburgh, USA

Atilla Soran MD
Professor of Surgery
Division of Surgical Oncology
Department of Surgery
University of Pittsburgh, USA

Michael T Stang MD
Assistant Professor of Surgery
Division of Surgical Oncology
Department of Surgery
University of Pittsburgh, USA

Yewching Teh MD
Breast Research Fellow
Division of Surgical Oncology
Department of Surgery
University of Pittsburgh, USA

Pragatheeshwar Thirunavukarasu MD
Resident, General Surgery
Department of Surgery
University of Pittsburgh, USA

Bulent Unal MD
NCI-STSEP Scholar
Postdoctoral Research Fellow
Department of Surgery
University of Pittsburgh, USA

Tsafrir Vanounou MD
Fellow, Division of Surgical Oncology
Department of Surgery
University of Pittsburgh, USA

Gregory Vorona MD
Resident, Radiology
Department of Radiology
West Penn Allegheny Health System
Pittsburgh, USA

Andrew R Watson MD
Assistant Professor of Surgery
Division of Surgical Oncology
Department of Surgery
University of Pittsburgh, USA

Amber Wooten MD
Resident, General Surgery
Department of Surgery
University of Pittsburgh, USA

Ibrahim Yazji MD
Resident, General Surgery
Department of Surgery
University of Pittsburgh, USA

Linwah Yip MD
Assistant Professor of Surgery
Division of Surgical Oncology
Department of Surgery
University of Pittsburgh, USA

Theodore H Yuo MD
Resident, Vascular and Endovascular Surgery
Department of Vascular Surgery
University of Pittsburgh, USA

Narcis Octavian Zarnescu MD
Postdoctoral Fellow
Department of Surgery
University of Pittsburgh Medical Center, USA

Herbert J Zeh III MD
Assistant Professor
Division of Surgical Oncology
Department of Surgery
University of Pittsburgh, USA

Kent Zettel MD
Resident, General Surgery
Department of Surgery
University of Pittsburgh, USA

Preface

There has never been a more exciting time to be a surgical oncologist. The field is dynamic and rapidly evolving, with new technology constantly emerging at all levels of care, ranging from molecular diagnostics and gene therapy to minimally invasive and robotic surgery. The pace of basic science, clinical, and translational research is intense, and the amount of information generated in the cancer literature can be overwhelming for the busy clinician.

For this reason, we have embarked upon the creation of a reference for the surgical oncologist that will incorporate the basic tenets of surgical practice with the innovations of modern technology in an evidenced-based fashion. We believe that *Surgical Oncology: Fundamentals, Evidence-based Approaches and New Technology*, will serve as a guide for not only the surgeon-in-training but also for the practicing clinician who faces the challenge of summarizing the plethora of research in cancer therapy.

Our goal is to create a resource that will present the opinions of experts in the field alongside an analytical and unbiased review of the evidence. Each chapter contains not only a summary of the relevant data but also presents succinctly a list of landmark studies and a Level of Evidence table citing the most important recommendations for each disease or organ system. Although the text has abundant detail and may serve as a definitive reference, it is our hope that the tables of evidence and summarized landmark studies will present a quick, user-friendly guide for each chapter. An emphasis on the surgical management of disease is present in all chapters, however, an entire section of the book is dedicated to the principles of adjunct therapies to emphasize the need for a multidisciplinary approach. Additional chapters on Ethics, Palliative Care and Pain Management, as well as summaries of the ground-breaking work in molecular biology of cancer and immunotherapy round out a comprehensive review of the surgical management of cancer.

It is our hope that *Surgical Oncology: Fundamentals, Evidence-based Approaches and New Technology* will not only stimulate the interests of medical students, residents, and fellows in training, but will also become a key source of up-to-date information and a tool for practicing surgeons in the ongoing fight against cancer.

Editors

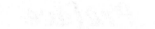

Introduction to Level of Evidence (LOE) Table

Part of the richness of academic surgery is that many of its principles and practices derive as much from tradition as from rigorous scientific research and development. The history of the surgical management of cancer is a fascinating story of personalities, technical and scientific advances, and paradigm shifts in our understanding of both cancer biology and the surgeon's role as part of a multidisciplinary approach to cancer therapy. The evolution of modern breast cancer management is a classic example. However, surgical epistemology does not lend itself easily to the current demand for evidence-based medicine in medical decision making. A randomized controlled trial may not be feasible for each problem, and the more recent, somewhat diametric, call for personalized medicine speaks to how limited our knowledge of cancer at the individual level can be. Nevertheless, in an effort to provide some justification for the practices described in this text and their general applicability, at the end of each chapter is a table highlighting some of the main diagnostic and therapeutic choices associated with each disease along with their corresponding quality of evidence, strength of recommendation and relevant citation(s). It is rare that an issue will be whether surgical resection is necessary when possible. Most controversies will instead surround the timing of surgery with respect to other treatment modalities, its extent, and the preparation of the cancer patient for surgery.

The bibliography is not meant to be comprehensive; rather, it is intended to represent some of the most current and best evidence available, to identify where the literature may be lacking, and to serve as a starting point for additional investigations. An effort has also been made to identify a few studies that had conclusions opposite the primary recommendation. Several groups including the US Preventive Services Task Force (www.ahrq.gov/clinic/), the GRADE working group (www.gradeworkinggroup.org) and the Oxford University Center for Evidence Based Medicine (www.cebm.net), have developed similar ratings to help stratify the evidence and generate clinical guidelines. The types of studies qualifying as good evidence will also depend upon the research question, as supportive data for a therapeutic intervention will differ from that needed for a diagnostic or prognostic test. We use the following schema adapted primarily from the Oxford University and US Preventive Services Task Force groups **(Tables 1 and 2).**

TABLE 1	Levels of evidence by clinical question and study design	
Level	Clinical aim	Study design or characteristics
1a	Therapy/Prevention	Systematic review (SR) of randomized controlled trials (RCTs)
	Diagnosis	SR of Level 1 diagnostic studies. Clinical decision rule (CDR) with level 1b studies from different clinical centers
	Prognosis	SR of inception cohort studies. CDR validated in different populations
	Economic and decision analyses	SR of Level 1 economic studies
1b	Therapy/Prevention	Individual RCT
	Diagnosis	Validating cohort study with good reference standards. CDR validated within one center
	Prognosis	Individual inception cohort study with good follow-up. CDR validated in a single population
	Economic and decision analyses	Analysis based on clinically sensible costs or alternative. Includes multiway sensitivity analyses. Systematic review of evidence
2a	Therapy/Prevention	SR of cohort studies
	Diagnosis	SR of Level 2 or better diagnostic studies
	Prognosis	SR of retrospective cohort studies or untreated control groups in RCTs
	Economic and decision analyses	SR of Level 2 or better economic studies

Contd...

Contd...

2b	Therapy/Prevention	Individual cohort study or low-quality RCT
	Diagnosis	Exploratory cohort study with good reference standards. Unvalidated CDR or validated only on a split sample
	Prognosis	Retrospective cohort study or follow-up of untreated control patients in an RCT. Derivation of a CDR or validated on a split sample only
	Economic and decision analyses	Limited review of evidence or single studies. Includes multiway sensitivity analysis
2c	Therapy/Prevention	Outcomes research and ecologic studies
	Prognosis	Outcomes research
	Economic and decision analyses	Outcomes research
3a	Therapy/Prevention	SR of case-control studies
	Diagnosis	SR of Level 3b and better studies
	Economic and decision analyses	SR of Level 3b and better studies
3b	Therapy/Prevention	Individual case-control study
	Diagnosis	Non-consecutive study. Reference standards not consistently applied
	Economic and decision analyses	Analysis based on limited alternatives or costs. Poor quality estimates of data. Some sensitivity analysis performed
4	Therapy/Prevention	Case-series and poor quality cohort or case-control studies (limited follow-up; poorly defined exposure or outcome comparison groups)
	Diagnosis	Case-control study. Non-independent reference standard
	Prognosis	Case-series and poor quality cohort studies (non-objective outcomes, no correction for confounding)
	Economic and decision analyses	No sensitivity analysis
5	Therapy/Prevention	Expert opinion without critical review
	Diagnosis	Expert opinion without critical review
	Prognosis	Expert opinion without critical review
	Economic and decision analyses	Expert opinion without critical review

TABLE 2	Grades of recommendation
Grade	**Study evidence, clinical risk/benefit ratio and treatment alternatives**
A	Consistent Level 1 studies or otherwise appropriate levels of scientific evidence suggest that the benefits substantially outweigh the potential risks. A responsibility exists to consider and discuss the practice with eligible patients.
B	Consistent Level 2 studies or extrapolations from Level 1 studies. At least fair scientific evidence suggests that the benefits outweigh the potential risks. Clinicians should discuss the recommendation with eligible patients.
C	Levels 3 and 4 studies or extrapolations from Level 2 studies. At least fair scientific evidence suggests that there may be benefits but a general recommendation cannot be made. Clinicians need not offer it unless there are individual considerations.
I	Level 5 studies (expert opinion) or scientific evidence that is lacking due to inconsistent or inconclusive studies of any level.

Other good resources for practice guidelines are the National Comprehensive Care Network (www.nccn.org) and various societal recommendations. In surgical oncology, most evidence will be Levels 2 and 4 (cohort studies and case series) with corresponding Grade B recommendation. However, there may also exist therapies (e.g. chemoradiation for anal cancer) for which the current standard of care is based upon low-level observational data but with overwhelming potential benefits. Whether 'higher' levels of evidence are absolutely necessary remain to be seen, and the grades of recommendation in this text reflect a combination of the formal evidence, the balance between risk and benefit to the patient, and the availability of alternatives. We encourage surgeons and all practitioners to evaluate the evidence in the contexts of their individual patients as well as overall practice, local expertise, and available resources. We also support entering patients into clinical trials or at least prospective databases such that good quality data can be generated for analysis.

Phil Bao MD

Contents

SECTION 3
PRINCIPLES AND PHILOSOPHY OF CANCER THERAPY

SECTION 4
SUPERFICIAL TISSUES

SECTION 5
ENDOCRINE ORGANS

SECTION 6
GASTROINTESTINAL TRACT

SECTION 7
HEPATOBILIARY SYSTEM

SECTION 8
SPECIAL TOPICS

Section 1

Introduction and Background

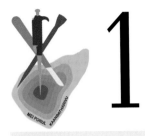

1

Surgical Oncology—Definition, History, Scope, Philosophy

Kamran Idrees, David L Bartlett, Bernard Fisher

Introduction

The history of surgical oncology dates back to the ancient times where reports of cancer and cancer therapy appeared in the Edwin Smith and Ebers Papyri between 1600 and 1700 BC. Included in these reports is a brief description of cautery destruction of cancer as a surgical approach. Hippocrates in the 5th century BC made observations about breast cancer, but he had a pessimistic view on the role of surgical management, cautioning that surgery would shorten survival. It was not until the 5th century AD when Leonidas, a Greek physician, described a formal operation for cancer, this being a mastectomy. Because of the limitations of surgical technique, surgical treatment was limited to superficial tumors of the skin and breast at that time. Surgical oncology seemed to be at a standstill through the dark ages of medicine, which lasted from the 5th till the 17th century.

John Hunter (1728–1793) is considered as the father of the modern surgery and believed that cancer was a localized process and amenable to curative surgical removal **(Figure 1-1)**. He stressed the importance of wide excision, which would include the potential areas of lymphatic spread. Many of his ideas were later expressed by Dr William Stewart Halsted in the late 1800s. The major advances in surgical oncology required the refinement of anesthesia, which was first used by Crawford Long in 1842 and was effectively demonstrated for major surgery by Morton in 1846 at Massachusetts General Hospital. Similarly, the advancement of antisepsis by Lister in 1867 was another necessary requirement for more advanced surgical oncology procedures. Once anesthesia and antisepsis were introduced, major abdominal surgery for cancer became feasible. The latter half of the 1800s, therefore, saw the development of multiple surgical procedures for cancer. The description of the optimal technique for surgical management of cancer by William Halsted of Johns Hopkins Hospital and his description of the radical mastectomy for breast cancer in 1891 defined the principles behind the surgical treatment of cancer for most of the 1900s **(Figure 1-2)**. It was not until the 1970s when, as a result of randomized clinical trials from the National Surgical Adjuvant Breast Project (NSABP) under Dr Bernard Fisher, the empiricism of Halsted was replaced with the scientific results defining cancer as a systemic disease requiring less extensive surgery combined with adjuvant radiation and/or chemotherapy.

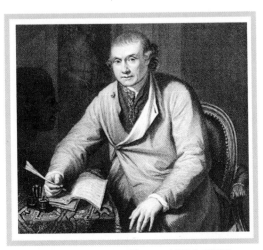

Figure 1-1: John Hunter (1728-1793)

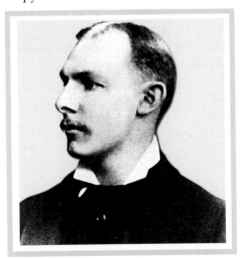

Figure 1-2: William Halsted (1852-1922)

The Society of Surgical Oncology

Dr James Ewing was appointed as Pathologist of the Memorial Hospital in New York City in 1912, and became Director of the Hospital in 1931. He was instrumental in developing the field of radiation therapy, and focusing Memorial Hospital as a cancer hospital. He developed fellowship training programs in oncology and trained numerous physicians who practiced across the world the techniques learned at Memorial Hospital. In the mid 1930s, Dr Hayes Martin and the Superintendent of Memorial Hospital, Mr George Holmes, took the initial steps to develop an alumni association for those who had trained at Memorial Hospital. This took the form of a formal society in 1940, under the chairmanship of William MacComb. Dr Ewing reluctantly approved the name of this society as "The James Ewing Society", and it was established with a constitution and by laws approved in 1941. The first James Ewing Society's Cancer Symposium was held in 1948 at Memorial Hospital, consisting of scientific sessions, clinical demonstrations and scientific displays. Eventually the decision was made to expand the membership eligibility to cancer specialists not trained at Memorial, and to hold annual meetings at locations other than Memorial Hospital.

Under the chairmanship of Edward Scanlon, in 1975, the decision was made to change the name of the society to the Society of Surgical Oncology (SSO). This was necessary to attain national recognition by the American Medical Association and other national medical organizations. The James Ewing Foundation was developed as the primary foundation associated with the SSO. The SSO has grown to a membership of 2400 in 2009, with 24 standing committees and an annual meeting that attracts 1600 attendees. The journal, Annals of Surgical Oncology, under the editorship of Charles Balch was launched as the official journal of the SSO in 1994. This journal has steadily grown in stature and reputation, and has become an important aspect of the society. The annual meeting continues to be a vibrant display of basic science and clinical studies in the field of surgical oncology. One of the original tenets in 1947 was the establishment of a subspecialty board of oncology of the American Board of Surgery. This continues to be a goal of the society today, but has not been achieved.

Clinical Trial Programs

Dr Sydney Farber, Mary Lasker and others proposed in 1955 that congress begin funding a clinical trials program. In response, congress appropriated five million dollars to the NCI for the establishment of the Chemotherapy National Service Center. By 1957, 17 institutional networks had been organized forming the seed for the cooperative group programs. These cooperative groups became organized and evolved into the 10 cooperative groups in existence today in the United States. The groups along with their founding year are listed in **Table 1-1**.

Surgeons became involved in a major way in 1957 with the initiation of the National Surgical Adjuvant Breast Project (NSABP) under the direction of Rudolph Noer. Dr Bernard Fisher took over the directorship in 1967 and performed landmark studies of breast and colon cancer, shaping the way cancer is managed today. The landmark NSABP study which changed the paradigm of surgical therapy for cancer and cemented the surgical oncologist's role in clinical research was the B-04 study in 1971 which demonstrated the equivalency of total mastectomy versus radical mastectomy. This was followed in 1976 with B-06 which demonstrated that lumpectomy, axillary dissection and radiotherapy was equivalent to mastectomy and much less disfiguring. To date, the NSABP investigators have enrolled over 110,000 patients and the program consists of over 1,000 university hospitals, major medical centers, large oncology practice groups and health maintenance organizations in the United States, Canada,

TABLE 1-1 Cooperative Groups supported by the NCI for clinical trials	
Cooperative Group	**Year**
Eastern Cooperative Oncology Group (ECOG)	1955
Cancer and Leukemia Group B (CALGB)	1956
National Surgical Adjuvant Breast and Bowel Project (NSABP)	1957
Southwest Oncology Group (SWOG)	1958
Radiation Therapy Oncology Group (RTOG)	1968
Gynecologic Oncology Group (GOG)	1970
North Central Cancer Treatment Group (NCCTG)	1977
American College of Surgeons Oncology Group (ACOSOG)	1998
American College of Radiology Imaging Network (ACRIN)	1999
Children's Oncology Group (COG)	2000

Puerto Rico, Ireland and Australia. As a result of Dr Fisher's leadership, the role of the surgical oncologist has evolved into that of being a leader in clinical trial research.

In the late 1990s, the American College of Surgeons under the leadership of Dr Samuel A Wells, Jr. formed the American College of Surgeons Oncology Group (ACOSOG). This program was designed specifically to evaluate the surgical management of patients with malignant solid tumors and has accrued thousands of patients to numerous clinical trials to date. The group was originally housed at the American College of Surgeons office in Chicago, but moved to Duke University in 2001. While this is the only group specifically focused on surgical oncology, surgical leadership plays an important role for most of the cooperative groups funded through the National Cancer Institute. The SSO has also recognized the importance of clinical trials, supporting clinical research through grants and presenting clinical trial updates at their annual meeting.

Biologic Research Leading to the Alternative Hypothesis

The significance of the change from Halsted's empiricism to Fisher's hypothesis driven scientific evidence for the surgical management of cancer deserves special consi-deration in the history of surgical oncology. For almost a century, surgical practice was dictated by the idea that cancer progressed and spread via direct extension into lymph nodes with a predictable pattern. Virchow in 1863 formulated a theory that lymph nodes could provide an effective barrier to the passage of tumor cells and perhaps based on this, Halsted formulated the theory that all tumor spread was related to lymphatics. He stated ". . . the metastases to bone, to pleura, to liver, are probably parts of the whole and that the involvements are almost invariably by process of lymphatic permeation and not embolic by way of the blood . . . It must be our endeavor to trace more definitely the routes traveled in the metastases to bone, particularly to the humerus, for it is even possible in case of involvement of this bone that amputation of the shoulder joint plus a proper removal of the soft parts might eradicate the disease. So, too, it is conceivable that, ultimately, when our knowledge of the lymphatics traversed in cases of femur involvement becomes sufficiently exact, amputation at the hip joint may seem indicated." This was an appropriate theory based on the biology and anatomy understood at the time, but surgical principles did not change and were not studied as new biology was defined. These principles ultimately led to super-radical surgery for cancers as seen in **Figure 1-3**.

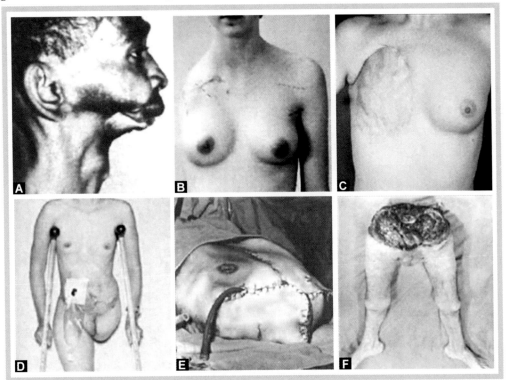

Figure 1-3: Examples of super-radical surgery: (A) radical neck dissection; (B) forequarter amputation; (C) radical mastectomy; (D) hemipelvectomy; (E and F) hemicorporectomy. (Reproduced with permission from Fisher B. Biological research in the evolution of cancer surgery: a personal perspective. Cancer Research. 2008 Dec 15;68(24):10007-20).

Dr Bernard Fisher and his brother Edwin Fisher began in 1957 to study the biology of tumor metastases **(Figure 1-4)**. Based on their experiments, they concluded that there was no orderly pattern to tumor spread and that intrinsic factors in tumor cells combined with a multiplicity of host and organ factors to result in metastases. They were also able to demonstrate that cells could traverse through a lymph node, gaining access to the bloodstream and efferent lymphatic vessels. The lymph nodes had important biologic and immunologic significance and were not simply "mechanical receptacles". Dr Fisher developed the Alternative Hypothesis **(Table 1-2)**. He then developed a series of clinical trials through the NSABP to test his hypotheses. The B-04 trial compared the outcome of almost 2,000 women comparing Halsted's radical mastectomy with lesser operations and demonstrated no difference in survival. A follow up study, B-06, compared lumpectomy, lumpectomy plus radiation and mastectomy, and demonstrated no difference in survival with 20-year follow-up. These trials effectively validated the alternative hypothesis, which changed the paradigm of surgical management for all cancers. *En bloc* radical resections were not warranted, and adjuvant chemotherapy should be considered when the risk of metastases is significant.

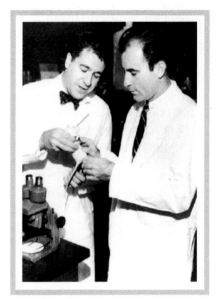

Figure 1-4: Bernard and Edwin Fisher – 1957

Historic Operations

The technical feats which set the stage for routine performance of complex surgical oncology procedures are discussed by organ site below and see **Table 1-3** for a complete review.

TABLE 1-2	Comparison of the tenets comprising the Halsted and Fisher's alternative hypothesis
Halstedian hypothesis (1894)	**Alternative hypothesis (1968)**
Tumors spread in an orderly, defined manner based on mechanical considerations	There is no orderly pattern of tumor cell dissemination.
Tumor cells traverse lymphatics to lymph nodes by direct extension, supporting *en bloc* dissection.	Tumor cells traverse lymphatics by embolization, challenging the merit of *en bloc* dissection.
The positive lymph node is an indicator of tumor spread and is the instigator of distant diseases.	The positive lymph node is an indicator of a host-tumor relationship that permits development of metastases rather than the instigator.
RLNs are barriers to the passage of tumor cells.	RLNs are ineffective as barriers to tumor cell spread.
RLNs are of anatomical importance.	RLNs are of biologic importance.
The bloodstream is of little significance as a route of tumor dissemination.	The bloodstream is of considerable importance in tumor dissemination.
A tumor is autonomous of its host.	Complex host-tumor inter-relationships affect every facet of the disease.
Operable breast cancer is a locoregional disease.	Operable breast cancer is a systemic disease.
The extent and nuances of operation are the dominant factors influencing patient outcome.	Variations in locoregional therapy are unlikely to substantially affect sruvival.
No consideration was given to tumor multicentricity in the breast.	Multicentric foci of occult tumor are not of necessity a precursor of clinically overt cancer.

Abbreviation: RLN — regional lymph node

Fisher et al, J Clin Oncol, Jan 20;28(3):366-74.Reprinted with permission. © 2008 American Society of Clinical Oncology. All rights reserved.

TABLE 1-3	Historical advances in cancer surgery according to tumor site		
Nervous System			
Craniotomy	Harvey Cushing	1910
Cordotomy for pain	E. Martin	1912
Trans-sphenoidal craniotomy	Harvey Cushing	1920
Head and Neck			
Total Laryngectomy	Theodor Billroth	1873
Thyroidectomy#	Theodore Kocher	1883
Radical neck dissection	George W Crile	1906
Functional/Modified radical neck dissection	Osvaldo Suarez	1963
Breast			
Radical mastectomy	William S Halsted	1891
Lung			
One-stage lobectomy£	Harold Brunn	1928
First one-stage pneumonectomy£	Evarts A Graham	1933
Segmental resection	Edward Churchill	1939
Thoracoscopic lobectomy	Ralph J. Lewis	1991
Esophagus			
Cervical esophagectomy	Czerny	1877
Transthoracic esophagectomy£	Franz Torek	1913
Transhiatal esophagectomy	George G Turner	1933
Two-field esophagectomy	Ivor Lewis	1946
Three-field esophagectomy	K McKeown	1962
Laparoscopic transhiatal esophagectomy	AL DePaula	1995
Stomach			
First gastrectomy	Theodor Billroth	1881
Total gastrectomy	Carl Schlatter	1897
Liver			
Hepatic resection	D Langenbuch	1888
Right hepatic lobectomy with hilar ligation	W Wendel	1911
True anatomic hepatic resection with vascular control (Right hepatic lobectomy)	J Lortat-Jacob	1952
Laparoscopic hepatic resection	W Wayand	1993
Pancreas			
Transduodenal ampullectomy	William S Halsted	1898
Two-stage pancreaticoduodenectomy£	W Kausch	1909
One-stage pancreaticoduodenectomy	Allen O Whipple	1945
Total pancreatectomy	EW Rockey	1943
Laparoscopic pancreaticoduodenectomy	M Gagner	1994
Colon and Rectum			
Rectal resection with end-colostomy	R Von Volkmann	1878
Abdomino-perineal resection (APR)*	Vincent Czerny	1884
Colectomy with end-colostomy	Robert Weir	1885

Contd...

Contd...

Trans-sacral rectal excision	P Kraske	1885
Total mesorectal excision	R Heald	1982
Laparoscopic colectomy	Moises Jacobs	1990
Laparoscopic APR	J Sackier	1992
Adrenal		
Open adrenalectomy	Sargent	1914
Open bilateral adrenalectomy	Young	1936
Laparoscopic adrenalectomy	M Gagner	1992
Prostate		
Perineal prostatectomy	George Goodfellow	1891
Radical perineal prostatectomy	JJ Young	1904
Radical retropubic prostatectomy	Millin	1945
Laparoscopic radical prostatectomy	A Raboy	1997
Gynecologic		
Oophorectomy	Ephraim McDowell	1809
Vaginal hysterectomy	Conrad Langenbeck	1813
Abdominal hysterectomy	WA Freund	1878
Radical abdominal hysterectomy $	John G Clark	1895
Laparoscopic hysterectomy	Harry Reich	1988

\# Thyroidectomy performed for goiter
£ "Successful" defined as the patient survived the postoperative period
* W Ernest Miles perfected and popularized abdominoperineal resection (APR)
$ Ernst Wertheim perfected and popularized radical hysterectomy

Breast

Breast cancer and its treatment are first described in the Edwin Smith Papyrus (3000 BC). In this era, treatment consisted of either cauterization (with fire drills or caustic agents such as sulfuric acid) or amputation of the ulcerated, locally advanced disease. Roman physicians, especially Galen, recommended surgical excision of breast cancer rather than cauterizing it and emphasized achieving clear margins with occasional removal of pectoralis muscles. Vesalius provided the first detailed anatomical description of the breast that facilitated the surgeons' dissection and control of bleeding. In this pre-anesthesia era, several instruments were developed to aid in rapid amputation of the diseased breast. In the 18th century, the French surgeon Petit and German surgeon Heister recommended *en bloc* removal of the primary tumor with surrounding normal breast tissue, the pectoralis fascia, enlarged axillary lymph nodes and pectoralis muscle or chest wall if involved.

Breast cancer has contributed greatly to our understanding of the lymphatic system and its role in the metastatic process. In the 16th century, Ambrose Pare was one of the first surgeons to observe metastatic involvement of axillary lymph nodes in patients with breast cancer, while Michael Servetus was the first to propose lymph node removal along with breast resection. Most of these findings went unnoticed till the 17th century when Jean Louis Petit, first president of the French Academy of Surgery, advocated routine removal of enlarged axillary lymph nodes along with resection of breast tumor. Joseph Pancoast is credited for describing the operative technique of axillary dissection in 1844. However, it was Charles Hewitt Moore who promoted routine complete axillary lymphadenectomy irrespective of clinically palpable lymph nodes in 1867. This change was based on his observations of high local recurrence rate at or near incision sites and that lymph nodes can harbor metastases even though they might not be clinically palpable. But the true credit for widely popularizing axillary lymphadenectomy goes to William Halsted and Willie Meyer who concurrently published, in 1894, their meticulous and systematic operative technique of in-continuity removal of the entire breast with axillary tissue. Halsted described the technique of "classical" radical mastectomy that involved the *en bloc* removal of the entire breast, axillary lymph nodes and pectoralis muscles. It is thought that Halsted was greatly influenced by the

German School of Surgery, including Volkmann, Kuster and Heidenhain and went on to incorporated their philosophy and techniques to develop the "complete" breast operation. With his technique, he reported 5-year overall survival of 45% and for patients with node-negative disease the 5-year survival of 72%. Halsted's radical mastectomy remained the classical surgical approach for breast cancer for the first three quarters of the 20th century and the Halstedian principle of *en bloc* lymphadenectomy were applied to surgery of other organ sites as discussed above.

In the mid-20th century, Taylor, Wallace, Handley, Urban and Wangensteen extended the limits of radical mastectomy by routinely performing supraclavicular, internal mammary and mediastinal lymphadenectomy along with *en bloc* chest wall resection. However, this concept of supraradical mastectomy was never widely adopted. Cushman D Haagensen of New York wrote the textbook of "Diseases of the Breast" which was regarded as the gold standard in the management of breast cancer. His criteria for inoperability are regarded as a landmark in the field of surgical oncology. He realized that surgical intervention offered little or no benefit to survival if the breast cancer involved skin (ulcerated or inflammatory), was fixed to the chest wall, or if advanced axillary lymphadenopathy (matted or fixed to chest wall) was present.

In 1912, JB Murphy in his published report argues against radical mastectomy and his approach is regarded as an early attempt at the modified radical mastectomy. However, it was DH Patey of London who coined the term "modified radical" mastectomy for an operation in which he removed the entire breast, axillary lymph nodes and pectoralis minor but preserved the pectoralis major. Later on, Auchincloss and Madden further modified this operation by saving both the pectoralis major and minor. The results of the modified radical mastectomy were comparable to that of the classic radical mastectomy and this operation became standard of care during the 1970s in North America. This transition was also partly as a result of utilization of external beam radiation as adjuvant therapy in the treatment of breast cancer.

George Crile, Jr., of Cleveland helped pave the way for breast conservation surgery. In his published reports in 1965 and 1971, he demonstrated similar 5-year survival results with local excisions compared to mastectomy in carefully selected patients. It was not until Dr Fisher carried out his landmark randomized studies through the NSABP, that lumpectomy plus radiation became the standard of care for breast cancer, as discussed above.

The management of axillary lymph nodes has evolved from the radical *en bloc* resection of all lymph nodes, to the excision of a single, sentinel lymph node for sampling. The principle of complete resection of all axillary lymph nodes to prevent recurrence has evolved into the evaluation of lymph nodes as a marker for systemic metastases and as an indication for systemic chemotherapy. The complete three level axillary dissection which was popular until the 1980s and early 1990s was replaced by axillary sampling in the late 1990s and finally the sentinel lymph node biopsy in the first decade of the 21st century. Sentinel lymph node mapping was initially utilized in melanoma, parotid and penile cancers. Krag and Guiliano introduced the concept of sentinel lymph node mapping in breast cancer in the early 1990s. This technique has evolved into the best method of assessing lymph node involvement in breast cancer resulting in a decrease in the number of axillary lymphadenectomies performed and thus a reduction in its associated morbidity.

Head and Neck Cancer

In 1847, Sims is credited for performing the first successful superior maxillectomy for a tumor and a mandibulectomy for an osteosarcoma. Theodor Billroth of Vienna not only performed the first successful gastrectomy but also pioneered total laryngectomy in 1873 **(Figure 1-5)**. Theodor Kocher received the recognition for his contributions to our understanding of the pathophysiology and surgery of the thyroid gland and was bestowed with the Nobel Prize. It was the first Nobel Prize awarded to a surgeon.

It was the seminal work of George Washington Crile, founder of the Cleveland Clinic, which established the importance of radical neck dissection in the management of patients with head and neck cancers. His meticulous surgical technique was described in a beautifully illustrated article published in Journal of the American Medical Association in 1906. Because of the functional morbidity and cosmetic deformity of radical neck

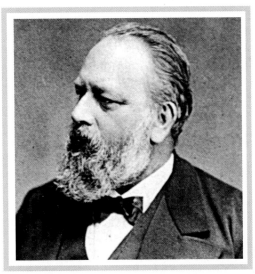

Figure 1-5: Theodor Billroth (1829-1894)

dissection, there was gradual change in the viewpoint of head and neck surgeons in the management of these cancers. Osvaldo Suarez, an Argentinean surgeon, is credited for proposing removal of all the lymphatic tissue within fascial compartments with preservation of uninvolved neck structures including the spinal accessory nerve, sternocleidomastoid muscle and internal jugular vein. This approach was known as "functional neck dissection". A better understanding of the nodal spread, the biology of the disease and improvement of adjuvant therapies led to further modification to the extent and approach to neck dissection now classified as selective and modified radical neck dissections. This approach was advocated by Jesse and colleagues from M.D. Anderson Cancer Center and has completely replaced the need for radical neck dissection without compromising the oncologic outcome.

Esophagus

Theodore Billroth performed the first cervical esophageal resection in dogs in 1871. In 1877, Czerny performed the first cervical resection with re-anastomosis in humans. Mickulicz-Radecki then performed cervical esophagectomy with reconstruction of the cervical esophagus with a skin flap in 1886. Franz Torek performed the first successful transthoracic esophagectomy for squamous cell carcinoma of thoracic esophagus in 1913. Interestingly, the gastrointestinal continuity was reestablished with a rubber tube connected externally between a cervical esophagostomy and a gastrostomy **(Figure 1-6)**. Amazingly the patient survived both the operation and the cancer for another 13 years. Yet routine esophageal surgery remained decades away because of the lack of a durable esophageal replacement.

In 1933, George Grey Turner performed the first transhiatal esophagectomy for cancer. The gastrointestinal continuity was restored with an ante-thoracic skin tube at a second stage. Ohsawa performed a similar procedure with an ante-thoracic esophagogastric anastomosis. William Adams and Dallas Phemister were the first to describe the immediate reconstruction with an esophagogastric anastomosis after distal esophagectomy in the United States in 1938. It was Richard Sweet in 1945 who described the esophagogastric anastomosis utilizing stomach as a conduit with the blood supply based on the right gastroepiploic vascular pedicle. A year later, Ivor Lewis published his technique of utilizing a laparotomy incision for gastric mobilization and a right thoracotomy incision for the resection of the esophagus and intrathoracic reconstruction. McKeown later in 1962 reported his "three stage esophagectomy" with a midline laparotomy incision, right thoracotomy and left cervical incision followed by cervical esophagogastrostomy. In 1978, Mark Orringer at University of Michigan modified

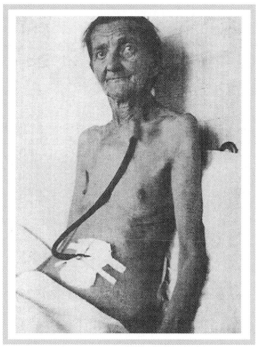

Figure 1-6: The first patient to have successful transthoracic esophagectomy for squamous cell carcinoma. Notice patient has a rubber tube as a conduit. Patient lived for 13 years

and then popularized the transhiatal esophagectomy, initially described by Turner, without the morbidity of a thoracotomy for esophageal cancer.

Lung

Hugh Davies reported the first anatomic lobectomy in 1912, however, his patient died 27 days later. Brunn published the first successful lobectomy in 1929 for lung cancer. Rudolf Nissen performed the first total pneumonectomy in 1931, but it is Evart Graham (1933) who is credited for the first successful one-stage pneumonectomy for lung cancer. In the 1940s, Oschner and DeBakey postulated the role of lymph node dissection in the treatment of lung carcinoma. Later on, Allison followed by Cahan described performing hilar and mediastinal lymphadenectomy with pneumonectomy. In 1939, Edward Churchill first reported segmental resection followed by a 20-year retrospective review of their surgical experience in the treatment of lung cancer suggesting equivalent survival results for lobectomy compared to total pneumonectomy. This was subsequently validated by the work of Watson, Johnson and Cahan.

Gastric Cancer

In 1875, Pean reported the first gastrectomy for gastric cancer, however, his patient died in the immediate postoperative period. The first reported successful gastrectomy for gastric cancer was performed in 1881 by Theodore Billroth, who is regarded as the father of gastric surgery. He reported his accomplishment of performing pylorectomy in a letter with an end-end gastroduodenostomy (known as Billroth I reconstruction to this day) a few days later. His patient survived the operation but subsequently died of gastric recurrence. He later published a variation of his previous gastric reconstruction in 1885. In this modification, he described performing a bypass between the gastric remnant and a loop of jejunum (Billroth II reconstruction) and the technique of blind duodenal stump closure. It was many years later that Carl Schlatter performed the first successful total gastrectomy in Zurich, Switzerland. Despite the significant contributions of both Billroth and Schlatter to the surgery of the gastric cancer, most of these procedures were not regularly performed because of associated high morbidity and mortality.

It was in the second quarter of the 20th century that gastric surgery was performed more commonly and safely with the introduction of antibiotics and advancement of anesthesia. Pioneering work by Balfour and Broder demonstrated that one half of all gastric ulcers are cancerous and gross appearance is misleading in establishing whether an ulcer is benign or malignant. Based on these observations, Balfour suggested wider resections for the operative management of gastric ulcers in case they turn out to be malignant. This was subsequently substantiated by Vanbrugghen. The work of Coller and his colleagues was instrumental in illustrating the increased predilection of gastric cancers to spread to lymph nodes in the perigastric and peripancreatic region. Autopsy studies on patients with previous gastrectomies validated high local recurrences in the proximal stomach and duodenal stump but also revealed a high incidence of regional lymph node disease.

McNeer and his colleagues at Memorial Hospital in New York contributed significantly to the surgical management of gastric cancer. They carefully and meticulously tabulated the operative mortality, recurrence pattern and survival in 1315 gastric resections. Because of a high local recurrence with limited resections, McNeer advocated for extended gastric resections including total gastrectomy with lesser and greater omentectomy, splenectomy and distal pancreatectomy. He also recommended *en bloc* resection of involved organs. McNeer reported improved survival in patients with distal gastric cancers but operative mortality remained high. With inability to reproduce similar results and high surgical mortality, others including Longmire and Gilbertsen questioned this approach. However, it was the collective contributions of McNeer, Pack, Longmire and Lahey that broadened the field of gastric surgery.

Pancreas

Surgery of the pancreas lagged behind other organs secondary to lack of complete understanding of the pathophysiology and difficult anatomic location. In 1878, MacBurney performed the first papillotomy via a duodenotomy for choledocholithiasis. It was roughly two decades later that Kocher described his technique of extracting gallstones through a transduodenal papillotomy after lateral mobilization of the duodenum, now known as the Kocher maneuver. Utilizing the technique described by MacBurney and Kocher, William Halstead in 1898 performed the first transduodenal ampullectomy for a periampullary neoplasm.

At the end of the 19th century, several surgeons attempted pancreatic resections but without success because of a lack of appreciation for pancreatic secretory physiology and adequate knowledge of blood supply to the head of the pancreas and duodenum. These factors along with high immediate postoperative mortality swayed the surgeons away from pancreatic resections and toward palliative bypasses such as cholecystogastrostomy, gastrojejunostomy and choledochojejunostomy. It was the knowledge acquired from the technical refinement of these bypasses combined with the better understanding of the anatomy and physiology which subsequently paved the way for pancreatic resections, especially pancreaticoduodenectomy. Codvilla, in 1898, is credited for the first true pancreaticoduodenectomy. In his procedure, he resected the common bile duct, head of the pancreas and duodenum with biliary and gastric diversion. There was no pancreatic anastomosis performed and the patient died in the immediate postoperative period. The first successful pancreaticoduodenectomy was performed in two stages by Kausch in 1909. The first stage of the procedure entailed cholecystojejunostomy (to relieve jaundice and associated coagulopathy) followed by resection 6 weeks later. However, it was Allen Whipple and his colleagues at Memorial Hospital in New York who popularized pancreaticoduodenectomy. They published their surgical experience in the treatment of ampullary carcinoma in 1935 describing various procedures including common bile duct resection, duodenectomy and a two-stage pancreaticoduodenectomy. This operation underwent numerous anatomic modifications over several years by many others surgeons including Hunt, Brunschwig and Trimble. In 1945, Whipple reported the first case of a single stage procedure for a periampullary cancer. It was the numerous noteworthy contributions of Whipple to the field of pancreatic surgery that pancreaticoduodenectomy is still known as the "Whipple procedure". Rockey, in 1943, reported the first total pancreatectomy for pancreatic cancer obviating the morbidity of a pancreatic leak and the possibility of recurrence by removing the entire pancreas. Although Whipple in his original description of pancreatico-duodenectomy preserved the pylorus, it was Traverso and Longmire, in 1978, who reintroduced the concept of pylorus-preserving pancreaticoduodenectomy to decrease the morbidity from marginal ulcers.

Colon and Rectum

In the late 18th century, fecal diversion was preformed for an obstructing rectal cancer with a cecostomy by Pillore. Most of colorectal cancers at that time (late 1800s and early 1900s) were treated with a two staged procedure consisting of fecal diversion with a colostomy initially followed by resection of tumor a few weeks later. The first transrectal removal of rectal tumor was performed by Kraske in 1885. However, these procedures were extremely morbid and associated with a high recurrence rate. Czerny is credited with the first combined abdominal and perineal resection (APR) of a rectal cancer. He performed this procedure out of necessity after failing to remove the rectal tumor through a perineal approach. Subsequently, two French surgeons Chalot and Quenu reported planned APR in late 19th century while Charles Mayo published his series in early 20th century. Unfortunately, because of the high morbidity and mortality of this procedure, this approach was not commonly practiced.

In 1908, Ernest Miles reported his technique of abdominoperineal resection in a landmark paper which popularized this approach for the carcinoma of the rectum that is still being performed to this date for low rectal tumors in which sphincter salvage is not possible. However, Dr Miles realized the high local recurrence rate (~95%) in his patients which he largely thought were because of incomplete lymph node removal. He subsequently modified his technique to incorporate more radical lymphadenectomy (from the origin of the IMA proximally to the ischiorectal fat below the levator ani distally). He reported three patients surviving beyond three years without local recurrence with this approach.

In the ensuing years, the clinical capability of whole blood transfusions and the two-team approach in Lithotomy-Trendelenburg position, as described by Llyod-Davies, were instrumental in decreasing the high mortality rate. In the 1960s, Turell pioneered the use of endoscopy for evaluation of the colon and rectum. In 1966, Mark Ravitch at the University of Pittsburgh introduced the use of surgical staplers for intestinal anastomosis in the United States.

During the 1970s and 1980s, the advent of doubled-stapled technique for low anterior resection and the development of the coloanal anastomosis paved the way for sphincter preservation. In 1972, Parks reported the technique of hand-sewn coloanal anastomosis while Griffen and Knight described the use of an EEA stapler for a low anterior resection in 1980. This led to an increase in the number of sphincter preservation procedures for rectal cancer patients who would otherwise undergo permanent colostomies. The local pelvic recurrence rates after resection of rectal cancer remained high (35-38%) during 1950s to early 1980s. However, this changed dramatically when Heald and his colleagues described the concept of total mesorectal excision (TME) in 1982. The total mesorectal excision resulted in significant reduction in positive lateral (circumferential resection) margins reducing local failure rates to 5-7% after rectal resection.

Uterus, Cervix and Ovaries

The first Oophorectomy was performed by Ephraim McDowell for a massive ovarian tumor in the patient's home in 1809. Conrad Langenbeck, Surgeon-General to the Hanoverian army, performed the first vaginal hysterectomy for endometrial cancer in 1913 while Sauter performed this procedure for cervical cancer in 1821. In 1895, John G Clark performed the first hysterectomy for cancer at Johns Hopkins Hospital. Although Ernest Wertheim was not the first to describe the procedure, his significant contributions to the field resulted in his name being virtually synonymous with the procedure of radical hysterectomy.

Alexander Brunschwig, a professor of Surgery at the University of Chicago, performed the first pelvic exenteration for cervical carcinoma in 1946. Subsequently, as a chief of gynecological service he continued to perform these radical operations for uterine and cervical carcinomas. In 1950, Eugene M Bricker at Ellis Fischel State Cancer Hospital in Missouri described the ileal conduit for urinary diversion—a major advancement in the field of pelvic surgery. Brunschwig in New York, Meigs in Boston, Bricker in St. Louis and Appleby in Vancouver continued these radical surgeries for these otherwise incurable advanced gynecological cancers with the possibility of cure in selected patients.

Soft Tissue Sarcoma

The surgical management of extremity sarcoma was the epitome of "radical surgery" in the late 19th and first three quarters of the 20th century. The first successful forequarter amputation was performed by Grosby in 1836. The first hemipelvectomy was performed by Theodore Billroth in 1891, but unlike his other successful endeavors such as the first total laryngectomy, the first gastrectomy, the first prostatectomy and the first suprapubic cystectomy, his hemipelvectomy patient died in the immediate postoperative period. The first successful hemipelvectomy was detailed by a Frenchman, Charles Girard, in 1895. Both these procedures were performed for osteosarcoma. The most "radical" of all surgeries, the hemicorporectomy, was proposed by Frederick Kredel. However, the first successful operation of this kind was performed by Aust and Absolon in 1961. It was Bowden and Booher, in 1958 who challenged the need for amputation for all cases of soft tissue sarcomas. This was further validated the work of Shiu and his colleagues. It was the seminal work at the National Cancer Institute Surgical branch by Rosenberg and his colleagues who demonstrated equivalent results between amputations and limb-sparing surgery in a prospective randomized trial. This laid the foundation for the role of limb sparing surgery in the treatment of soft tissue sarcoma in combination with radiation and chemotherapy.

Liver

The first liver resection was performed by Berta who removed part of the liver in a trauma patient. The first planned liver resection was a left lobectomy in a patient presenting with a liver mass, performed by D Langenbuch in 1888 in Germany.

L Tiffany performed the first hepatic resection for cancer in the United States in 1890. The largest series of hepatic resections in the 19th century was reported by William W Keen, Professor of Surgery at the Jefferson Medical College, when he described 76 liver resections of which 37 were for benign or malignant tumors with a mortality of 17%. In 1908, J Hogarth Pringle described the technique of compression of the portal triad to decrease bleeding from the liver. Interestingly, in his original description of eight patients, all of them died either during or in the immediate postoperative period. However, Pringle was able to successfully utilize this maneuver later on—which now bears his name. Despite these developments, most of the surgeons were hesitant to perform liver operations because of its friability and high propensity to bleed.

It was the improved understanding of surgical anatomy of the liver which contributed greatly to the advent of liver surgery. Initial anatomic studies were performed by Rex and Cantlie but it was the seminal work of Claude Couinaud who introduced the concept of segmental hepatic anatomy—the basis for segment-oriented hepatic resections. Wendel, in 1911, performed the first true anatomic right hepatic lobectomy using hilar ligation along the Cantlie's line. But the true credit goes to the French surgeon, Jean Louis

Lortat-Jacob, who in 1952 performed a successful anatomic liver resection with vascular inflow and outflow control (right hepatic lobectomy) through a thoraco-abdominal incision. He performed this procedure on a patient with metastatic colorectal cancer without any blood transfusion. Around the same time, JK Quattlebaum from Savannah, Georgia, reported his case of right lobectomy for a hepatoma at the Southern Surgical Association's meeting, likely unaware of Lortat-Jacob's procedure.

Nonsurgical Advances

It is also important to mention some of the nonsurgical advances that made it possible to perform some of these radical surgeries for various cancers at the end of the 19th century and in the first half of the 20th century. The importance of the discovery of ether in the 1840s as an anesthetic to perform various operations cannot be understated. Subsequent advancements in anesthetic drugs and monitoring made it possible to perform more and more extensive surgeries safely. Utilizing carbolic acid in 1867, John Lister applied the concepts of Louis Pasteur to surgery and subsequently described the principles of antisepsis. This greatly improved the safety of all operations.

The discovery of blood types by Karl Landsteiner led to the ability to transfuse blood during and after surgery. This made radical cancer surgery feasible by reducing intraoperative and postoperative mortality. The work of John Scudder and Charles Drew further advanced the field of transfusion medicine. Further important advances after World War II included antibiotic therapy, anesthesia, blood transfusion, nutritional support and intensive cardiopulmonary monitoring reducing the perioperative morbidity and mortality associated with radical procedures such as the radical mastectomy, pelvic exenteration, pancreaticoduodenectomy, forequarter amputations, hemipelvectomy and even hemicorporectomy.

The development of the pressure-differential chamber for the management of pneumothorax was an essential factor in allowing lung resections. The device was invented by Ferdinand Sauerbruch in 1908, followed shortly by the development of insufflation for intratracheal anesthesia by Samuel Meltzer. These developments allowed the expansion of the lung after a thoracotomy.

Other important non-surgical advances included the discovery of insulin, allowing safe resection of the pancreas and the discovery of thyroid hormones for replacement therapy after thyroidectomy. While Theodore Kocher had mastered the technical aspects of thyroidectomy, his patients had "turned to cretins, saved for a life not worth living". Only after replacement therapy was identified, and could a total thyroidectomy be performed.

All of these nonsurgical milestones made it possible to extend the horizon of surgery which otherwise would have become dormant despite better anatomical understanding and the exceptional technical skills of the surgeons.

Summary and Recent Advances

The practice of cancer surgery is as old as medicine itself, dating back to 1700 BC. The evolution of the field required advances in anesthesia, antisepsis, blood transfusions, insulin therapy, ventilator management and more. **Figure 1-7** provides a timeline of important advances in surgical oncology. Surgeons began attempting bigger and better surgeries as patients were able to survive them and the technical prowess of the surgeon improved. The culmination of this was the successful pancreaticoduo-

denectomy for pancreas cancer described by Kausch in 1909 and major hepatectomies and pneumonectomies, described by Wendel in 1911 and Graham in 1933. A preliminary understanding of the biology of cancer led to Halsted's recommendation of *en bloc* resection of draining lymph nodes with the primary tumor, leading to the description of the radical mastectomy in 1891. The trend continued with wider resections of all primary cancers.

Dr Bernard Fisher shifted the paradigm of increasing radicalism and through hypothesis driven randomized cooperative group clinical trials established that cancer is

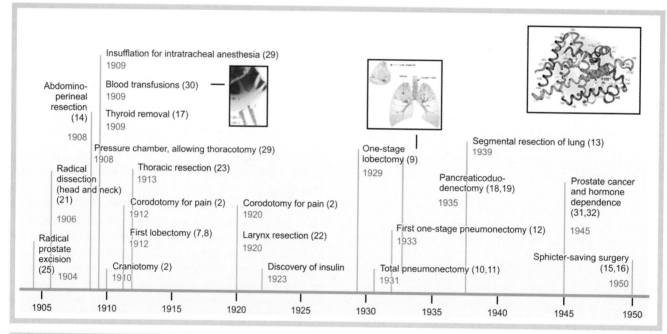

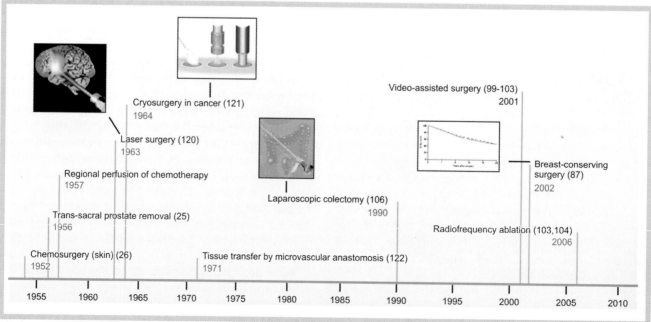

Figure 1-7: Timeline of advances in surgery. (Reproduced with permission from Fisher B. Biological research in the evolution of cancer surgery: a personal perspective. Cancer Research. 2008 Dec 15;68(24):10007-20.

a systemic disease and that survival equivalence could be obtained with lesser operations. The advantage associated with postoperative adjuvant radiation therapy and chemotherapy became established for breast cancer therapy with landmark trials from the NSABP. This principle has been applied to other cancers where effective chemotherapy has been defined.

As surgeons refined the techniques for the management of the primary tumors, they turned their technical expertise onto the management of metastatic tumors, including hepatic and pulmonary metastasectomy for colorectal cancer and sarcoma and the regional delivery of chemotherapy for regionally confined metastatic cancers. This includes isolated limb perfusion described by Creech and Krementz in 1958 and hepatic arterial infusion therapy described by Sullivan in 1964. The field of intraperitoneal chemotherapy and the treatment of peritoneal carcinomatosis has been developed by many, but perhaps Paul Sugarbaker has been most instrumental in developing this field over the last three decades, with a focus on combined surgical cytoreduction and regional chemotherapy for pseudomyxoma peritonei, colon carcinomatosis and peritoneal mesothelioma. He published his first randomized trial of intraperitoneal 5-FU versus intravenous 5-FU in 1985.

Technological advances have led to new options for the surgical treatment of cancer. For instance, cryotherapy had been explored as a means of treating superficial skin tumors since the 1960s, but with the development of cryoprobe technology this technique could be applied to liver tumors as described by Morris in 1989. Radiofrequency ablation was developed as an alternative to cryotherapy for liver tumors, with the advantage of using smaller probes and increasing the size of safe ablations. These techniques improved the safety and minimized the physical insult to the patient, expanding the patient population that could undergo surgical management of cancer.

The current trend is to move toward minimally invasive and robotic approaches to cancer surgery, minimizing the nutritional and immunologic insult to the patient while maintaining the principles of margin negative resection of tumors. The patient with cancer often requires adjuvant therapy and may be of advanced age. Minimally invasive approaches minimize the insult to the patient, expand the eligibility and help lessen the time to initiation of adjuvant therapy. An important survival equivalency study was performed in colon cancer by Nelson et al in 2004. This study demonstrated that minimally invasive cancer surgery could be performed with equivalent cancer related survival to open surgery, with many advantages in terms of quality of life. This has opened the door leading to complex minimally invasive procedures, such as robotic pancreaticoduodenectomies, representing the ultimate fusion of technology and advanced surgical cancer care.

The importance of studying the history of surgical oncology lies in learning from our predecessors and not repeating past mistakes. The most striking lesson is that we must not base our practice on empiricism or anecdotes. We should use the anecdotes to develop hypotheses and use the basic science laboratory and the clinical trial "laboratory" to test our hypotheses. The cooperative group clinical trial programs must be well supported and utilized to definitively answer questions with regards to surgical procedures in the future.

Landmark Papers

1. Ellis H. A History of Surgery. Cambridge: Cambridge University Press; 2001.
2. Fisher B. Biological research in the evolution of cancer surgery: A personal perspective. Cancer Res 2008; 68: 10007-20.
3. Fisher B. The evolution of paradigms for the management of breast cancer: A personal perspective. Cancer Res 1992; 52:2371-83.
4. Lawrence WJr. History of Surgical Oncology. In: Norton (Ed). Surgery: Basic Science and Clinical Evidence. New York: Springer; 2008:1889-1900.
5. Lopez M. The evolution of radical cancer surgery. Surg Oncol Clin N Am 2005; 14:441-649.

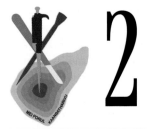

2 *Multidisciplinary Approach*

Haroon A Choudry, David L Bartlett

Introduction

The concept of a multidisciplinary approach to cancer care is not new. In 1977, Bernard Fisher quite rightly stressed the role of surgery as just one aspect of comprehensive cancer care when he stated that "Surgery makes its contribution to cancer treatment in concert with other modalities. Advances in the treatment of cancer will derive from improved orchestration with the other modalities rather than from improved operative technique alone." The tremendous advancements in technology along with a better understanding of the molecular basis of cancer have exposed a myriad array of new possibilities in cancer prevention, diagnosis and therapy, blurring the lines between medical disciplines and making multidisciplinary collaboration vital.

Despite significant advances in cancer care over the last few decades, the prognosis for most solid cancers remains quite poor. At present most solid cancers are diagnosed at a late stage, when they are locally advanced or metastatic. Contemporary maximal multimodality "curative" therapy, including surgery, radiation, conventional chemotherapy and limited biological therapy, is suboptimal with high rates of relapse, metastasis and death, even occurring many years after the index therapy. This suggests the presence of minimal residual disease that is not detected and treated by current conventional therapies.

The surgical perspective of cancer evolved from the Halstedian view of cancer as a loco-regional disease with predictable centrifugal progression to the contemporary view of cancer as a systemic disease. The Halstedian approach led to more and more radical surgical resections to achieve loco-regional "cure." However, failure to prevent cancer relapse and metastatic disease and the discovery of circulating tumor cells and disseminated tumor cells in organs and lymph nodes early on in the tumorigenic process emphasized the systemic nature of cancer and inadequacy of locoregional therapy alone. The current surgical approach to cancer therapy relies on less radical resections to achieve R0 resections, while preserving the principles of cancer surgery, in conjunction with adjuvant and neoadjuvant non-surgical therapies. At the same time emphasis is also placed on meticulous surgical technique, minimally invasive approaches, minimizing morbidity and mortality, improving function and quality of life.

A paradigm shift in the perception and approach has emerged in an attempt to cure and preferably prevent cancer from arising. A pre-requisite to this is a comprehensive understanding of the molecular basis of cancer leading to new and innovative multimodality preventative and therapeutic interventions. The success of this complex task lies in multidisciplinary collaboration from pre-clinical to clinical arenas including basic science researchers, biomedical research and development, transitional research, multi-institutional clinic trials, medical oncologists, radiation oncologists, diagnostic and interventional radiologists, pathologists, reconstructive and transplant surgeons, as well as medical sub-specialists like gastroenterologists. In addition, close collaboration with primary care providers, psycho-oncologists, rehabilitation specialists, oncology nurses, oncology pharmacists, family and social networks is crucial to comprehensive care. Such a symbiotic multidisciplinary relationship will lead to comprehensive, evidence-based, unbiased treatment plans. However, this requires all cancer specialists, regardless of subspecialty, to be well-versed in all aspects of cancer care to allow meaningful discussion and application of knowledge. The surgical oncologist must be an active participant in all aspects of cancer care, surgical and non-surgical, to be truly effective. This flux in the role of the surgical oncologist is an opportunity that must be seized and actively directed toward an integrated, multidisciplinary approach to cancer care.

The rapid advances in technology, in concert with a better understanding of cancer biology, cancer genetics, cancer immunology and cancer biomarkers have led to a plethora of innovative surgical and non-surgical approaches to cancer care. From a technical point of view, the role of a surgical oncologist includes prevention, diagnosis, staging, cure, palliation, cytoreduction, reconstruction, vascular access as well as management of surgical complications and emergencies. Some of the contemporary issues include feasibility of pre-emptive surgery in patients with hereditary predisposition to cancer, minimally invasive and robotic surgery and transplantation related to tissue-engineering. Major advances in molecular imaging technologies and molecular biomarker assays, endoscopic and percutaneous modalities, chemotherapy and biological therapies, radiotherapy, cancer vaccines, immunotherapy and gene therapy provide a whole range of opportunities available to cancer care specialists.

The aim of surgical oncology training programs is therefore to train not only a technically capable cancer surgeon but also to develop an oncologist with broad based training in all aspects of cancer care. Trainees are therefore exposed to various oncologic subspecialties, multidisciplinary conferences and cancer research opportunities, since surgical oncologists must be comfortable with theoretical and practical aspects of surgical and non-surgical cancer care modalities. Only through a holistic and in-depth understanding of molecular and clinical oncology can we hope to find a cure for cancer and provide optimal care.

Multidisciplinary Care Models

The organizational structure of comprehensive cancer care programs may vary depending on the disease entity, available resources, expertise and infrastructure. However, the aim of developing such programs is to deliver optimal patient-centered, evidence-based cancer care efficiently while minimizing delays and patient-anxiety. There are five main multidisciplinary care models: Coordinated Referral Intake model, which involves referral of cancer patients by a central contact person to free standing subspecialties based on disease-specific requirement for work-up, diagnosis and treatment; Coordinated Group model has common services but does not operate within the confines of a single physical structure; the Multidisciplinary Intake model is one in which the patient is seen by all the specialties at one location during their first visit and then seen at different locations for further management; an Integrated Care model is patient-centered with all specialties working in a single building; finally, a Totally Integrated model shares services and works in a single building.

The success of such integrated multidisciplinary comprehensive care models is dependent on a number of vital elements; a good working relationship among the various subspecialties based on trust, respect and collegiality; well organized multidisciplinary conferences where the various sub-specialists can develop optimal diagnostic and management strategies, make relevant

referrals or discuss eligibility for clinical trials in a real-time case-based manner; and meticulous documentation, data-collection and quality control to assure optimal care. This kind of communication improves patient care and minimizes confusion among the care-givers and the patient.

Multidisciplinary Approach: Understanding the Molecular Basis of Cancer

Understanding the molecular biology of cancer is the basis for a logical application of the various cancer care modalities. Cancer is a complex, multi-factorial disease that evolves as a consequence of genetic and environmental pressures. The molecular predisposition to cancer lies in genetic or epigenetic modifications leading to tumor initiation and progression, influenced to variable degrees by hereditary, sporadic, environmental and viral factors. These genotypic alteration lead to phenotypic characteristics that encompass the six hallmarks of cancer, including self-sustaining growth signals, insensitivity to growth-inhibiting signals, avoidance of apoptosis, unregulated replication, angiogenesis and invasion. More recently, with the conceptual evolution in tumor immunology, immuno-editing has been proposed as the seventh phenotypic hallmark of cancer. The concept of tumor elimination through immune-surveillance; tumor equilibrium through immunosculpting, with survival of resistant tumor clones similar to Darwin's theory of "survival of the fittest"; and ultimately tumor escape though immune-suppression and immune-evasion may hold the keys to future successes in cancer therapy. The development of new biological therapies, including immunotherapy, gene-therapy, cancer-vaccines and anti-angiogenic agents to name a few, as a result of molecular research in cancer, illustrates the importance of multidisciplinary collaboration in cancer care.

Some important areas of research including cancer stem cells, disseminated tumor cells and mechanisms of chemo-radiotherapy resistance are rich with academic and therapeutic potential. Stem cells are undifferentiated cells that have the ability to self-renew, replicate as well as differentiate. They may represent a Darwinian clonal selection of cells by successive advantageous mutations as a result of microenvironmental factors. However, current understanding is still somewhat controversial with various theories regarding their existence, location, characteristics and functional implications. Cancer stem cells tend to be more resistant to conventional adjuvant therapies; they tend to remain dormant in a quiescent G0 phase, have limitless self-replication abilities, self-protection capabilities with well developed drug-efflux mechanisms and may reside in protective niches. Failure to eradicate this sub-population may explain the relapse and metastatic potential of solid cancers despite current maximal surgical and adjuvant therapies. However, these survival characteristics may be exploited in order to develop cancer stem cell targeted adjuvant therapies.

The presence of disseminated tumor cells has been correlated with cancer relapse and metastasis suggesting that these disseminated cells represent the metastatic tumor initiating cells. Gene expression profiling of primary tumors and the detection of large numbers of circulating and disseminated tumor cells seems to suggest that metastatic potential is conferred to the majority of cancer cells and not a small subclone and this occurs early on in tumorigenesis. However, only a small proportion of these disseminated cells give rise to overt metastasis. Additionally, these disseminated tumor cells have been found to be more resistant to conventional adjuvant therapies and have been found to persist for years in a dormant state. The relationship between disseminated tumor cells and cancer stem cells is still under investigation. Cancer biology has shed some light on cancer resistance mechanisms to chemotherapy and radiation therapy. Pharmacological-Physiological factors include drug metabolism, excretion, delivery, rate of infusion and infusion route. Cell or tissue specific factors include alteration in drug-activation/degradation enzymes, DNA repair mechanisms, evasion of apoptosis, senescence and alteration in membrane proteins like carriers or channels. Recent data suggests that the ability to acquire drug resistance is not a late event, as previously thought, but occurs early on, even before full transformation has occurred. This supports a possible connection between cancer stem cells and drug resistance with the selection of unaffected, drug resistant cancer stem cell clones after chemo-radiotherapy.

This brief glimpse at the complicated nature of cancer emphasizes the inadequacy of unimodal cancer therapy and the unprecedented need for collaboration across specialties.

Multidisciplinary Approach: Progress in Molecular Imaging

Advancements in anatomic and functional imaging technology and techniques have had a major impact in the field of oncology affecting the clinician's ability to detect, diagnose, prognosticate and predict therapeutic response of cancers. Strategic planning of cancer care is increasingly dependent on the relationship between the diagnostic radiologist and surgical oncologist.

Although anatomic imaging has vastly improved with higher resolution in CT, MRI and Ultrasound capabilities, molecular imaging technology is revolutionizing the field. Much of this technology is still in experimental and early clinical phases but shows great potential. Molecular imaging may include assessment of gene expression,

receptors, enzyme and protein abnormalities, protein-protein interactions, pathway regulation, signalling transduction abnormalities, altered cell metabolism, hypoxia, angiogenesis, apoptosis, blood flow, oxygen consumption, proliferation and many other such biological features as they take place in living cells and tissues. This has been possible through better understanding and characterization of the molecular basis of disease processes; technological advancements in imaging modalities including in MR-imaging, PET-imaging and Optical imaging; miniaturization for minimally invasive application of these imaging techniques; and the use of innovative image-enhancers including probes, ligands, pharmaceutical agents and nano-particles that allow targeted disease-specific visualization and quantitation.

The clinical applicability of molecular imaging techniques includes early detection, diagnosis, staging, response to treatment and determination of disease-prognosis. Combining the various molecular imaging technologies will make it possible to visualize and quantitate the intracellular changes as the cell transforms from normal to diseased, evaluate high-risk patient populations earlier in the disease process and even identify the actual molecular signature of disease processes *in situ*. Contrast-enhanced MRI is more sensitive for the detection of breast cancers and specificity has improved with algorithms using morphologic and kinetic data. As ablative procedures become more standardized in breast cancer care the accuracy of MRI for assessment of tumor size and margins will be increasingly vital. Initial trials using breast tomosynthesis to reconstruct 2-dimensional digital mammograms into 3-dimensional images have shown improved accuracy. Molecular and optical imaging techniques are being used in conventional and experimental endoscopic surveillance programs for early detection of pre-malignant changes in patients with Barrett's disease or inflammatory bowel disease including high magnification endoscopy, chromoendoscopy, laser-induced fluorescence endoscopy, reflectance spectroscopy, light-scattering spectroscopy, tri-modal spectroscopy, Raman spectroscopy, optical coherence tomography and endoscopic confocal microscopy. PET is currently approved in the United States for lung, melanoma, breast, esophageal, colorectal and thyroid cancers in varying capacities for diagnosis, staging, surveillance or response to therapy. PET scans improve accuracy of staging thereby preventing unnecessary operations and have shown the capability of predicting responders to neoadjuvant therapies in a number of cancers. Positron emission mammography (PEM) is a modification of whole-body PET to focus on the breast and shows promising results for detection of small *in situ* and invasive malignancies. Hand-held positron emitter probe for intraoperative detection of F[18]-FDG-avid structures and integrated PET/MRI machines are being developed. In addition, molecular imaging will also be an integral part of directed drug therapy development process through more direct measurement of drug effects in the body.

Multidisciplinary Approach: Progress in Molecular Biomarker Assays and Targeted-agent Therapy

Traditional pathological cancer diagnosis and classification involves histological and morphological analysis of tumor type, grade, stage and completeness of resection, with limited use of molecular markers. However, cancers are complex, heterogenous processes involving interaction of many different molecular biomarkers and pathways that are inadequately assessed by histopathological examination and limited individual marker studies. Each individual cancer has its own gene expression profile or gene signature such that prognosis or response to therapy of two phenotypically similar cancers varies. The surgical oncologist must rely more and more on the molecular pathologic profiling of cancers to optimize patient care, once again emphasizing the importance of co-ordination and communication across subspecialties.

Recent advances in biomarker assay technology have revealed tremendous heterogeneity between and within cancers. Single-gene biomarker assays lack predictive value since most cancers involves multiple genetic abnormalities. Multiple gene assays combine multiple cancer-specific biomarkers into an index that are more predictive of cancer-prognosis and treatment response. Quality control and validation of these assays is essential for clinical use. Advances in high-throughput mutational analysis at the protein level (Protein arrays) or at the gene level using (DNA arrays, Comparative genomic hybridization and DNA sequencing) have allowed the identification of genotypically heterogeneous subtypes within morphologically homogeneous cancers based on expression profiles that have different prognoses.

Biomarkers may assist with risk factor control (CYP2A6 gene polymorphisms affect susceptibility to smoking-induced squamous cell cancer of the esophagus), cancer diagnosis and early screening (Fecal DNA assay for colon cancer shows sensitivity of 71-91% using multi-panel mutation detection with target markers like *k*-ras, APC, TP53, BAT-26), cancer prediction (BRCA-assay for breast cancer), cancer prognosis (Oncotype DX), response to therapy (Her2/neu expression and Herceptin therapy, Estrogen receptor expression and Tamoxifen therapy, KIT-mutation and Gleevec therapy) or drug toxicity prediction (UTG1A1 gene polymorphisms effecting Irinotecan toxicity profile). More and more biomarkers are being discovered and characterized that will further enhance diagnosis, prognosis and prediction, for example, markers associated with poor survival in patients with esophageal

cancer include over-expression of cyclin D1, *c*-erbB2, COX2, EGFR, VEGF and APC levels. Similarly, squamous cell carcinomas of the esophagus with over-expression of p53 show decreased sensitivity to radiotherapy.

These unique biomarkers may also be used to develop therapeutic targeted-agents. For example, since 30-70% of esophageal and gastric cancers express EGFR and 50% of esophageal cancers express VEGF, monoclonal antibodies (Cetuximab against EGFR and Bevacizumab against VEGF) and small molecule Tyrosine Kinase inhibitors (Erlotinib against EGFR) have been tested alone or as components of combination therapies. EGFR inhibitor Erlotinib in combination with gemcitabine-based chemotherapy has shown good results in metastatic pancreatic cancer. Since most cancers have polygenic defects, they are driven by and are dependent on multiple aberrant signalling-pathways (redundancy), therefore, "single-hit" targeted-agents may be insufficient. Multiple, different targeted-agents or drugs that target generic, fundamental tumor processes such as angiogenesis, apoptosis and cell proliferation, or drugs that target critical transforming-defects may be more successful.

Multidisciplinary Approach: Progress in Pre-emptive Diagnosis and Therapy

The pre-emptive diagnosis of cancer in certain high-risk patients relies on vigilance among physicians from all disciplines, meticulous exploration for familial clustering of cancers and the use of molecular biomarker testing. This vital collaboration allows for implementation of intensive surveillance programs and preventative non-surgical or surgical options.

The genetic predisposition to most cancers occurs as a result of multiple, sequential low-risk (low-penetrance) gene mutations resulting in a phenotypic progression from hyperplastic to dysplastic and finally malignant lesions. However, less common hereditary cancers like hereditary breast-ovarian cancer syndromes (BRCA gene), hereditary colon cancer syndromes (APC, MSH2, MLH1, PMS1, PMS2 genes), hereditary MEN2-associated medullary thyroid cancer syndromes (RET gene) and hereditary gastric cancer syndromes (E-CAD gene) to name a few occur due to high-risk (high-penetrance) mutations in key cancer forming pathways. Evolution in DNA analysis technology has led to the identification of these specific high-risk genetic mutations responsible for familial clustering of hereditary cancers.

The clinical implications include prediction of future risk of cancer development and assessment of prognostic behavior of cancers and predictive response to specific therapies, from which pre-emptive therapeutic strategies and tailored treatment strategies may be developed. However, such predictive information is fraught with challenges; genetic testing is not 100% accurate or predictive, pre-emptive surgeries may not always be curative especially when dealing with cancer syndromes, surgical complications may occur and long-term consequences of pre-emptive organ removal or synthetic supplementation are unknown. In addition, issues surrounding medicolegal and ethical consequences, medical insurance coverage, cost-effectiveness, informed consent especially when dealing with children and prenatal diagnosis must also be considered. Moreover, guidelines for surveillance, pre-emptive or treatment strategies in patients with cumulative low-penetrance (low-risk) genetic mutations are even less clear.

Such sensitive and complex issues underline the importance of multidisciplinary collaboration for early identification of high-risk individuals, expert genetic counseling and optimal multimodality therapy.

Multidisciplinary Approach: Progress in Minimally Invasive Approaches

Evolution in minimally invasive techniques has influenced cancer management in many aspects including screening, diagnosis, staging and therapy. At the same time, this evolution epitomizes the need for a multidisciplinary approach to the care of cancer patients since these technical abilities span multiple subspecialties.

Meticulous surveillance programs like the Seattle protocol in patients with Barrett's disease or surveillance of patients with inflammatory bowel disease are essential for diagnosing pre-malignant changes. In addition endoscopic curative therapies are showing promising potential in cancer treatment. Techniques like endoscopic mucosal resection, endoscopic mucosal dissection, photodynamic therapy, argon plasma coagulation, high dose rate endobrachytherapy and radiofrequency ablation are being used as curative therapies for early esophageal and gastric cancers. Similarly endoscopic polypectomy is used for diagnosis and pre-emptive resection of premalignant adenomatous polyps. Endoscopic ultrasound is now an essential component in the staging cancers of the esophagus and rectum and the addition of endoscopic ultrasound guided fine-needle aspiration of suspicious lymph nodes has improved accuracy of locoregional staging and influenced further therapy. Endoscopy has also been used for procuring cytology specimens as in pancreatic masses, provide minimally invasive feeding access and for palliative procedures like stent deployment, dilation and ablation. Endoscopic ultrasound based fine needle injection of cytokines and introduction of ONYX-015 virus for gene therapy directly into pancreatic cancer masses are just some examples of the application of endoscopy.

Percutaneous approaches to diagnostic biopsies, therapy (percutaneous ethanol injection, radiofrequency

ablation, cryotherapy), palliation and management of complications are changing the face of cancer care. Use of thoracoscopic and laparoscopic techniques may avoid unnecessary laparotomy in 20% of patients through improved staging accuracy, allow therapeutic resections with less morbidity and facilitate placement of feeding access or palliative procedures. For example, laparoscopic surgical resections for colorectal cancer have demonstrated better short-term outcomes, lower morbidity and equivalent survival. Sentinel lymph node biopsy techniques have made a large impact on the care of breast and melanoma cancer patients.

Multidisciplinary Approach: Progress in Conventional Chemo-Radiotherapy

Significant advancements have been made in cancer radiotherapy technology and techniques as well as cancer chemotherapy through newer cytotoxic drugs, novel targeted-agents and dosing schedules. Optimal utilization of such modalities in the neoadjuvant, adjuvant, perioperative, intraoperative setting for improved patient outcome requires close communication among care givers.

Neoadjuvant combination chemoradiation strategies are rapidly becoming the method of choice based on success in certain solid cancers and sound theoretical principles. There are three main drives for concomitant chemoradiation; definitive primary chemoradiotherapy may avoid the need for surgery altogether; chemotherapy can be used as a chemosensitizer to boost the effect of radiotherapy; and concomitant chemotherapy can have a synergistic locoregional effect with radiation as well as potentially eliminate systemic disseminated cancer cells. Molecular targeted therapies have been even more successful than conventional chemotherapeutic agents as chemosensitizers for radiation therapy since they are more specific for the target and inhibit radioresistance pathways. Close collaboration with radiation oncologists can optimize patient selection for intraoperative radiation therapy and brachytherapy. Intensity-Modulated Radiation Therapy (IMRT), image-guided radiotherapy via linear accelerator based techniques and gating radiation delivery with the respiratory cycle allow better targeted delivery of radiation while minimizing toxicity to surrounding normal cells.

Multidisciplinary Approach: Progress in Biological Therapy

There has been a vast increase in the development and utilization of biological therapies to combat cancer in concert with increased understanding of biologic processes and pathways involved in cancer and identification of biomarkers. This has been the result of collaboration between multiple disciplines with an emphasis on translational research.

Cancer vaccines are being extensively studied. They act through two main routes; one approach harnesses the immune system as in immunotherapy and the other approach involves gene transfer therapy. Prophylactic cancer vaccines have shown impressive results in "preventing" tumors in animal models however, efficacy has been inconsistent and modest when used in a "therapeutic" capacity against advanced tumors in both animal models and human trials. At this stage of advanced tumorigenesis extensive genetic heterogeneity and well-developed immune-evasion mechanisms exist which present numerous challenges in cancer vaccine development and efficacy. Therapeutic vaccines should be targeted at patients with minimal early stage disease or post-resection and ideally vaccines should be used prophylactically when minimal heterogeneity and evasion/suppression mechanisms exist. The use of vaccines to prevent cancer by targeting high-risk patients like BRCA mutation carriers or those with pre-malignant lesions like PanIN or high risk polyps with MUC-1 mutation may hold the key to future successes.

The extent of involvement of the immune system in cancer biology as well as the potential of immunotherapy has been a source of great controversy. Immunotherapy approaches to date have included passive and active humoral and cellular strategies including cytokine administration, antibody therapy, adoptive transfer of T-cells and tumor vaccines. Immunotherapy-based cancer vaccines involve the use of vaccination to actively boost the immune system against cancer cells in order to overcome the immune-suppressive and immune-evasive cancer mechanisms in favor of cancer elimination. The tumor micro-environment plays an important role in the immune-mediated eradication of cancer. Vaccination deems the tumor cells more immunogenic thus allowing a more robust inflammatory reaction which is conducive to optimal dendritic cell activation for antigen presentation. The development of cancer vaccines with respect to immunotherapy involves the identification of potent tumor-rejection antigens, effectively stimulating an anti-tumor immune response, avoiding autoimmunity or tolerance and preventing immune-evasion or suppression. There are various options for tumor antigen presentation via cancer vaccines including administration of intact, non-modified or genetically modified whole tumor cell with or without co-stimulatory molecules, tumor antigen or peptide vaccine (e.g. MART-1, gp-100, heat shock proteins), recombinant bacterial or viral vaccines transfected with tumor antigen, naked DNA vaccines encoding for tumor antigen and dendritic cell vaccines after *ex vivo* priming of dendritic cells using tumor cell, antigen or peptide exposure. The application of gene therapy to immunotherapy involves boosting the immune system to target and destroy cancer cells by presenting it with genetically engineered highly antigenic and immune-stimulatory cancer cells. Autologous or allogeneic cancer cells are genetically modified *in vitro* or *in vivo* with genes expressing highly antigenic proteins (PANVAC-VF vaccine expressing CEA, MUC-1 genes) or immune-stimulatory cytokines (GVAX vaccine expressing GM-CSF gene) or co-stimulatory molecules using viral vectors which leads to immune-mediated cancer eradication.

Gene therapy is a broad term that involves the *in vivo* or *in vitro* genetic manipulation of cells to combat cancer. There are three main areas where gene therapy has been applied; immunotherapy as discussed previously, oncoviral therapy and gene transfer therapy. Gene therapies have shown encouraging results in pre-clinical animal models of various solid tumors and currently there are a number of human clinical trials in various phases of investigation. In addition, they have minimal side effects as compared to conventional chemotherapy. Gene therapy based oncolytic virotherapy involves genetically engineering replication-competent viruses to specifically target cancer cells and then destroy them by propagation and expression of cytotoxic proteins. ONYX-015 is an adenovirus that has been genetically modified to lack E1B viral protein allowing it to only replicate in cells with an abnormal p53 pathway, common to cancerous cells. It has shown encouraging results in squamous cell cancer of the head and neck. Similarly G207 and NV1020 are genetically engineered HSV1 viruses that cannot replicate in non-dividing cells and have been successfully used in malignant glioma and colorectal cancer trials respectively. Gene transfer therapy is a relatively new technique of introducing a foreign gene into cancer cells or surrounding tissue using viral or non-viral vectors like naked-DNA transfer, nano-vectors or liposomes to induce apoptosis, cell-stasis, anti-angiogenesis or other cell-death mechanisms. Gene therapy targets may involve inactivation of oncogenes using direct targeting of aberrant mRNA transcripts with synthetic DNA sequences, siRNA or small molecule inhibitors (Imatinib). Restoration of tumor suppressor genes like p53 via gene transfer (INGN-201/Gendicine vaccine for p53 gene transfer) may directly induce cancer cell apoptosis or destroy cancers via a by-stander effect by down-regulating VEGF or activating IGF-1BP. Suicide genes may also be introduced as in the case of HSV-tk gene insertion which metabolizes gancyclovir pro-drug to its active form to inhibit DNA synthesis. Some human trial vaccines include TNFerade (GenVec) an adenovirus that introduces TNFα gene in soft tissue sarcoma and Rexin-G which involves a retroviral vector that incorporates in DNA and interferes with Cyclin G1 gene in pancreatic cancer patients.

All cancer care specialists, including surgical oncologists must remain at the forefront of such scientific research and clinical trials in order to integrate these potential therapeutic options into everyday patient care and improve outcomes.

UHB TRUST LIBRARY QEHB

Multidisciplinary Approach: The Extended Team

Any attempt at optimal care requires a comprehensive, integrated team approach at many levels. This includes well trained clinical nurse coordinators and specialists, who are a vital component of the day-to-day care of cancer patients and coordinate the complex care pathways. Management of cancer patients requires an aggressive approach to nutritional care given the inherent issues with cancer cachexia and frequent need for alternate routes or supplementation of nutrition. Pain control is often inadequately addressed and must be optimally managed to minimize patient suffering during an already difficult situation; close collaboration with anesthesiologists and interventional radiologists can provide targeted pain control options. Palliative care specialists are an essential part of the cancer care team and can help tackle a multitude of difficult issues including adequate pain control, patient comfort, facilitating home-care needs, hospice care and family support. Cancer patients require meticulously organized extended follow-up and surveillance; this process can be tremendously facilitated through close collaboration with primary care physicians and other first-line care providers. Management of side-effects and complications related to non-surgical and surgical interventions as well as oncologic emergencies must be dealt with in a timely comprehensive manner through good communication among the many specialists involved in the care of cancer patients. The vital importance of psychological and emotional support, rehabilitation facilities, social and financial support to maximize quality of life must never be under-estimated. Clinical nurse coordinators often form the backbone of such team approaches by organizing the complex issues, referrals and care pathways involved in management of cancer patients.

Multidisciplinary Approach: Research

Dedicated research lies at the heart of the progress achieved in cancer care so far and the opportunities that lie ahead. Integrated research programs with multi-disciplinary collaboration achieve the greatest success through optimal utilization of expertise and resources. Clinical trials require a high degree of coordination and dedication among physicians and non-physicians in various fields to ensure adequate patient accrual and meticulous conduct while preserving patient rights and welfare through coordination with institutional review boards. The tremendous advancements in the under-standing of the molecular basis of cancer through basic science research have increased the need to focus on translational research to transition these successes into the clinical arena efficiently and safely.

Summary

The convergence of the rapidly expanding knowledge regarding the molecular biology of cancer and the tremendous technological advancements in medicine have provided clinicians from multiple subspecialties with new tools and innovative ways to combat cancer. Cancer is a complex disease that requires a cognitive, multi-faceted, strategic approach which transcends the artificial boundaries between the various medical and surgical disciplines.

Landmark Papers

1. Pollock RE. Surgical oncology: Training for multidisciplinary cancer care. Journal of Surgical Oncology 2008; 97:3-4.
2. Eberlein TJ. Assessing the state of surgical oncology: The future is now. Annals of Surgical Oncology 2006; 13(11):1345-53.
3. Kolb GR. Integrate, innovate, imitate: Surviving and thriving in the world of breast cancer economics. The Breast Journal 2005; 11(Suppl 1):S20-S23.
4. Ponder BAJ. Cancer genetics. Nature 2001; 411:336-41.
5. Zitvogel L, Tesniere A, Kroemer G. Cancer despite immu-nosurveillance: Immunoselection and immunosubversion. Nature Reviews. Immunology 2006; 6:715-27.
6. Chumsri S, Burger AM. Cancer stem cell targeted agents: Therapeutic approaches and consequences. Current Opinion in Molecular Therapeutics 2008; 10(4):323-33.
7. Riethdorf S, Wikman H, Pantel K. Review: Biological relevance of disseminated tumor cells in cancer patients. International Journal of Cancer 2008; 123:1991-2006.
8. Margolis DJA, Hoffman JM, Herfkens JA, et al. Molecular imaging techniques in body imaging. Radiology 2007; 245(2):333-56.
9. Pierce MC, Javier DJ, Richards-Kortum R. Optical contrast agents and imaging systems for detection and diagnosis of cancer. International Journal of Cancer 2008; 123:1979-90.
10. Lakhani SR, Ashworth A. Microarray and histopathological analysis of tumors: The future and the past. Nature Reviews. Cancer 2001; 1(2):151-7.
11. Lea P, Ling M. New molecular assays for cancer diagnosis and targeted therapy. Current Opinion in Molecular Therapeutics 2008; 10(3):251-9.
12. You YN, Lakhani VT, Wells SA. The role of prophylactic surgery in cancer prevention. World Journal of Surgery 2007; 31:450-64.
13. Anderlik MR, Lisko EA. Medicolegal and ethical issues in genetic cancer syndromes. Seminars in Surgical Oncology 2000; 18:339-46.
14. Seiwert TY, Salama JK, Vokes EE. The concurrent chemoradiation paradigm—General principles. Nature Clinical Practice Oncology 2007; 4(2):86-100.
15. Finn OJ. Cancer vaccines: Between the idea and the reality. Nature Reviews. Immunology 2003; 3:630-41.
16. Cross D, Burmester JK. Gene therapy for cancer treatment: past, present and future. Clinical Medicine and Research 2006; 4(3):218-27.
17. McCormick F. Cancer gene therapy: Fringe or cutting edge? Nature Reviews. Cancer 2001; 1(2):130-41.

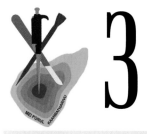

3

Ethical Considerations in Surgical Oncology

Thomas McDonald, Daniel E Hall

Introduction to Surgical Oncology as Applied Ethics

To practice surgical oncology is to practice applied ethics. This chapter aims to explain why the practice of surgical oncology is inseparable from the practice of applied ethics and it seeks to provide an orientation to some of the key ethical issues that are relevant to the daily practice of surgical oncology. Throughout the chapter we will refer to a single clinical case that brings the ethical dimensions of surgical oncology to the surface. The case begins as follows:

> An 83-year-old man is diagnosed with Stage III rectal cancer. His surgeon tells him that he has three treatment options. After learning about these options, he turns to the surgeon and says "I understand the three options you describe for treating my cancer, but I can't make this decision on my own. What should I do, doc?"

Science alone cannot determine how surgeons should answer this question, yet answer it they must. The patient is asking for guidance and although science will surely inform the surgeon's advice, there is no conceivable randomized controlled trial that can tell the surgeon what should or should not be done. Science informs the surgeon regarding the likely outcomes of certain procedures under specific conditions (e.g. the 5-year-survival rate after neoadjuvant chemoradiation and resection for stage III rectal cancer), but surgical science is only a tool. The surgeon and patient together must choose how best to use the tools that they have and this requires that both the surgeon and the patient share a clear understanding about the goals they hope to achieve through their collaboration. The ethical deliberation required to articulate and understand the goals of surgical practice is at the very heart of what surgical oncologists do.

Consciously or subconsciously, each decision made by surgeons regarding the care of patients has moral content. In other words, surgeons choose among the available

options because they have particular opinions regarding what would be good (or bad) for their patients. Although surgeons frequently make their decisions according to the relatively narrow "good" of disease free survival or physiological homeostasis, a fully articulated notion of health as human flourishing requires surgeons to consider many psychological, social and spiritual factors that also properly guide clinical decision making.

Deciding how best to help patients flourish requires good judgment. The precise kind of judgment required is sometimes called "practical wisdom", a technical term first developed by Aristotle. Practical wisdom is the capacity to choose the best option among several imperfect alternatives. Such choice and the capacity to choose wisely, are the precise foci of medical and surgical practice. However, unlike factual knowledge that can be learned from books and taught in classes, practical wisdom is developed only through experience. Without the practical wisdom acquired through experience, well motivated efforts often fail to achieve the good they intend. For example, consider the child who expresses love for his mother by creating a magnificent crayon drawing of his happy family, but foolishly chooses the bedroom wall for his canvas. The good token of affection that the child intends is thwarted because he does not yet know that drawings on the wall cause more anguish than joy. Practical wisdom is the capacity to actually achieve the intended goal.

Acquiring the practical wisdom to make good decisions is usually accomplished gradually over many years through the apprenticeship surgeons call residency. By working alongside surgeons who embody proven practical wisdom, the resident progressively acquires the ability to discern what is good (and bad) for a patient. Indeed, in his seminal text describing surgical training, the sociologist Charles Bosk argues that the "postgraduate training of surgeons is above all things an ethical training". Practical wisdom, it should be emphasized, is embodied by individuals, but it is transmitted through a community of wise and experienced people.

Given the central role of ethical deliberation in surgical practice, it is possible to think of surgical oncologists as applied ethicists. However, despite the many similarities between applied ethics and surgery, most surgeons do not think of themselves as ethicists and, generally speaking, they are not well-versed in the bioethics literature. There are several reasons for this incongruity. Few surgeons obtain advanced training in philosophy and they are thereby ill-equipped to join the professional discourse of ethicists. Furthermore, given all the other things to learn and master, there is little space in medical school and residency for explicit instruction in ethical analysis. Finally, the conditions of a busy clinical practice demand quick solutions to difficult problems.

The end result of these three factors is frequently a rough-and-ready approach that simplistically uses patient autonomy to trump all other ethical considerations, such that the right course of action is merely to follow the wishes of the patient. Autonomy, beneficence and justice are all considered to be important principles, but autonomy frequently trumps the others if there is a conflict among them. Such an approach seemingly satisfies the need for an efficient technique to resolve urgent questions, but in the final analysis, however, we agree with the many ethicists who maintain that this approach is unsound. In addition, we believe that most surgeons do not find such an approach to be particularly useful in the clinical setting and we doubt that many surgeons actually follow this kind of ethics.

Instead of capitulating to patient autonomy, many surgeons use the trustworthy rule of thumb that frames ethical deliberation in terms of the question, "What would I do if this patient were my mother, grandmother or child?" This question appeals to the surgeon's own ethical tradition, but note that it does so silently, effectively driving the normative assumptions of what is and is not good beneath the surface of the conversation. The rule of thumb essentially assumes that the surgeon is, in fact, an ethical person who shares similar values with the patient. Although it is sometimes safe to make this assumption, the assumption is rarely examined explicitly by either the surgeon or the patient.

Rather than searching for an ethical principle that can be applied in all cases, it is perhaps helpful to approach ethical analysis as a way to test and clarify the ethical assumptions that surgical oncologists make while caring for patients. The field of medical ethics is vast and complex and although there are broad areas of consensus, it is often true that wise people disagree regarding the best course of action. Although some approaches to ethical analysis are more widely employed than others, it is not possible to speak of a unified bioethic, but only of a plurality of bioethics as diverse as the patients, physicians and ethicists who try to make wise choices in the context of clinical care. As such, the goal of ethical analysis is not so much to find the "right" answer as it is to make explicit the

reasons why a particular course of action seems best. By making the reasons explicit, the ethical assumptions can be tested by all those who hold a stake in the decision (e.g. clinicians, patients, researchers, nurses, families, insurers, etc.).

Establishing the Goals of Care

Returning to the case, the patient had just said: "I understand the three options you describe for treating my cancer, but I can't make this decision on my own. What should I do, doc?"

The surgeon replies, "Well, the data suggest that we'll get the best results if we give you some chemotherapy and radiation for a few weeks and then cut out the cancer." To which the patient responds, "But that means that I have to wait to get this cancer out of my body. I'm not sure if I can wait that long. Can't you just cut it out tomorrow?"

The surgeon then says, "Let's back up a minute. I'm going to help you decide what to do and I'm going to give you my best advice. But before I can do that we need to talk about some bigger issues that can put my advice into the context of *your* life. Can you tell me something about what you are afraid of? And for that matter, can you tell me what you are hoping we can accomplish as we treat this cancer?"

Discerning the best course of action in the context of treating cancer requires that the patient and the surgeon share a concrete understanding of the goals of care. This requires deliberate and open discussion throughout the course of treatment. Surgeons should initiate this discussion and they should listen carefully to the patient's hopes, concerns and expectations. The conversation should include all the relevant medical facts about the patient's condition and prognosis. It should also include, as appropriate, specific topics such as advance directives, artificial nutrition, end of life preferences, code status and specific life events (such as a daughter's wedding) that are of particular importance to the patient. The surgeon and patient should then work together to formulate realistic goals of care.

The goals of care are not limited merely to treating the patient's organic disease. Rather, the treatment plan can be directed toward more overarching goals that include relieving suffering, improving quality of life and helping patients to achieve specific and unique life goals. Prior to the twentieth century, physicians had few tools with which they could effectively treat disease and so the identification and management of these more overarching goals of care played a large role in the physician's work. As modern medicine developed, the technical mastery of a growing arsenal of therapeutic approaches demanded increased focus from physicians. As a result, the over-arching goals of care were sometimes lost in the details of treating the disease. Indeed, it is perhaps increasingly challenging for surgeons today to balance the "big picture" with the meticulous attention to detail demanded by modern surgical therapy. The concept and discipline of palliative care has emerged to address this challenge.

Palliative care aims to alleviate suffering (when possible) and to improve the quality of life for those affected by serious illness. It is not limited to end of life care. The scope of palliative medicine is broad: a patient need not have a terminal illness to receive palliative care and those considered to be affected by a serious illness include not only the patient but also the patient's family. Suffering is also broadly construed: it is not limited to physical pain. As Eric Cassell has argued, a patient can suffer not only physically but also psychologically, socially and spiritually. Patients may experience non-physical suffering when they have concerns and fears about things such as the loss of independence, being a burden to their loved ones and facing mortality. In addition, patients are often anxious about the goals of care. By establishing realistic goals of care, the surgeon can often alleviate a great deal of the anxiety and suffering that patients experience.

Palliative medicine employs an interdisciplinary approach to improve the quality of life for patients and their loved ones by: (1) optimizing doctor/patient communication; (2) assessing and treating the patient's symptoms; (3) offering psychological, spiritual and bereavement support; and (4) assisting in advanced care planning and the coordination of care. In recognition of the increasingly specialized skills needed for effective palliative care, palliative medicine was recognized as a specialty by the American Board of Medical Specialties in 2006. Palliative medicine physicians can be an important resource in negotiating goals of care and formulating treatment plans. However, the surgical oncologist continues to play an essential role in discerning the goals of care and developing appropriate treatment plans. Indeed, surgical oncologists continue to lead in the development of palliative medicine.

When formulating the goals of care and making plans to treat the patient's disease and his or her suffering, surgeons are encouraged to pursue curative and palliative therapies simultaneously. They can address palliative issues on their own or in consultation with a palliative medicine team. The aim is to have a comprehensive plan for care of the whole patient, not only physically but also psychologically, spiritually and socially. When an appropriate plan has been formulated, the surgeon should strive to have an ongoing dialogue with the patient about how best to implement it, or how to modify it when

necessary. For example, during the course of therapy, the patient's commitment to the plan of care may falter. He or she may even wish to give up on the surgical recovery or chemotherapy. On some occasions, such despair may be a realistic assessment of the clinical facts and further aggressive treatment might not be in the patient's best interest. On other occasions, however, the clinical facts may not warrant such despair and the surgeon may have the responsibility to encourage, persuade and even cajole the patient to hold the course. Determining the correct path to take between these two extremes requires the practical wisdom acquired over time from the experience of caring for many such patients.

Palliative care is not dependent on the patient's disease or prognosis. Indeed, any patient who suffers from a serious illness stands to benefit from palliative care. When curing a patient's disease is no longer realistic, however, palliative therapies become the primary form of care, often in the form of hospice. Hospice is dedicated to providing end-of-life care to patients and their families and it specializes in relieving the suffering specific to dying patients. **Table 3-1** shows a comparison between palliative care and hospice. Any patient with a life expectancy of six months or less qualifies for hospice care under Medicare. Medicare's hospice benefit does not expire, however, if the patient lives longer than six months: a patient remains eligible for hospice indefinitely as long as his or her life expectancy is less than six months.

Informed Consent and Advance Directives

After discussing at some length the patient's hopes and fears for treatment of his rectal cancer, the patient and surgeon agree that the best option will be neoadjuvant chemoradiation followed by low anterior resection (LAR). Their discussion includes a focused, but thorough, review of the risks and benefits of the procedure including how intraoperative findings might modify the operative plan regarding the choice of procedure [LAR vs abdominoperineal resection (APR)] and the need for a diverting ileostomy. Although this discussion meets all the necessary criteria for "informed consent", the surgeon elects to wait until a time closer to the planned operation to complete the paperwork that will formalize the patient's consent to treatment. However, before concluding the interview, the surgeon asks one more critical question: "I expect that this plan of treatment will go well and you will recover rapidly from your surgery, but as we discussed, we may encounter real problems during and after the operation. In the unfortunate event that you get so sick that you can't speak for yourself, who should I talk to regarding decisions about your treatment?"

TABLE 3-1	Palliative care and hospice compared	
	Palliative care	**Hospice (Medicare benefit)**
Eligibility	• May be initiated by physician referral at the time of diagnosis of any serious illness regardless of prognosis • No renewal criteria because of lack of prognosis requirement • All illnesses, ages	• Patient is eligible for Medicare Part A • Patient certified (two physicians) to have probable survival of six months or less if disease, untreated, pursues its natural course • Patient (surrogate if patient not competent) must sign form electing hospice benefit • Eligibility may be renewed as long as patient continues to meet admission criteria • All terminal illnesses • Medicare benefit does not require. Do not Resuscitate (DNR) for eligibility • Medicare benefit does not require primary care-giver in the home • Hospice care must be provided by a Medicare-certified hospice program
Venues of service	• Hospitals including Veteran's Administration hospitals • Health care clinics • Assisted living facilities • Nursing homes • Home	• Majority cared for at home • Hospitals including Veteran's Administration hospitals • Assisted living facilities • Nursing homes
Treatments	• Palliative and disease-directed therapies such as chemotherapy and dialysis	• Palliative only • Some hospice programs will authorize continued dialysis, total parenteral nutrition, tube feedings and chemotherapy
Insurance	• Some treatments and medications covered by Medicare, Medicaid and private insurers	• More defined and comprehensive than palliative care reimbursement. • Medicare covers all expenses related to hospice care: medications, procedures, consultant's fees, durable medical equipment, nursing home visits, bereavement services up to one year after the date of death • Medicaid benefit similar to Medicare in almost all states • Most insurance plans have a hospice benefit
Team composition	• Interdisciplinary, including physicians, nurse practitioners, physician assistants, social workers, bereavement counselors, psychologists, chaplains, nurses, complementary medicine practitioners • Composition flexible depending on clinical setting	• Interdisciplinary • Medicare requires physician, nurse, social worker and a volunteer as core team members • Patient may retain primary physician or be followed by hospice medical director

Reproduced with permission from Brunicardi R, et al, Schwartz's Principles of Surgery, 9th edition, McGraw Hill, New York, 2009. All rights reserved.

Since the mid-1970s, the concept of informed consent has been promoted as the preferred way to protect a patient's autonomy when he or she needs medical intervention. Informed consent consists of five components. First, the patient must have the *capacity* to understand and evaluate possible treatment options. A patient's capacity is not a static entity: it can fluctuate depending on his or her health status and medications. It can even fluctuate with the time of day. Second, the surgeon must *disclose* to the patient the risks and benefits of the various treatment options, including no treatment. Third, the patient must demonstrate an *understanding* of the treatment options.

A complete understanding is not necessary and in many cases may not even be possible, but a patient's consent is not considered "informed" until he or she recognizes at least some of the possible consequences of his or her decision. Fourth, the decision should be *voluntary* without coercion or undue influence. In presenting and discussing the various treatment options, neither the surgeon nor the family members are required to be neutral. They can advocate for a certain course, but they should be sensitive to the ways that their advocacy might unduly limit the voluntariness of the patient's choice. It should be noted, moreover, that many patients, especially those with cancer, often feel that the realities of their disease compel them to act in certain ways. Finally, the patient gives *authorization* for a particular medical intervention to be performed.

Obtaining informed consent is not simply a matter of getting the patient's signature. Indeed, a patient does not give his or her informed consent simply by signing a form. The ethical and legal adequacy of consent depends more on the evidence of a substantial conversation than on the presence or absence of a physical signature. Generally speaking, the minimum legal requirement is that the surgeon and patient discuss the risks and benefits of the proposed procedure and any alternatives to it, including no treatment. From an ethical perspective, obtaining informed consent often requires discussing much more than the minimum legal requirements. A wide range of issues may need to be covered, as appropriate; some of these are listed in **Table 3-2**. After this conversation has occurred, the patient's signature on the form documents the content of the conversation between physician and patient. Obtaining informed consent is a skill that is mastered only with practice, just like suturing. And just like suturing, residents can improve their skills in this area by working with experienced clinicians and seeking their constructive feedback.

Whenever possible, surgeons should solicit their patient's informed consent. However, not all patients have the capacity to make an informed decision (e.g. the

TABLE 3-2	Elements of informed consent
Disclosure	Explicitly explain the process of consent and the patient's role in it.
	What are the indications that have led your doctor to the opinion that an operation is necessary?*
	What, if any, alternative treatments are available for your condition?*
	What will be the likely result if you don't have the operation?*
	What are the basic procedures involved in the operation?*
	What are the risks?* (Explain all common risks with probabilities ranging from 1-5%. Also explain any serious risks with a probability greater than or equal to 1 in 1000)
	How is the operation expected to improve your health or quality of life?*
	Is hospitalization necessary and, if so, how long can you expect to be hospitalized?*
	What can you expect during your recovery period?*
	When can you expect to resume normal activities?*
	Are there likely to be residual effects from the operation?*
	What are the qualifications, experience and personal success rate of the surgeon?
	What are the non-conventional treatment options?
	How long will the procedure take?
	Who will participate or assist with the operation?
	Make a clear recommendation, acknowledging the limits of knowledge and opinion.
Understanding	Explicitly ask the patient to explain their understanding of the diagnosis and treatment.
	Consider asking the patient to repeat the risks and benefits in their own words.
	Explore the potential impact of the surgery on the patient's own life.
	In the treatment of this disease, what is most important to you?
	Invite questions and clarification
Authorization	Explicitly ask for consent.
	Explicitly state that refusal is permissible and no offense will be taken.

*From the American College of Surgeons (American College of Surgery. Giving your informed consent. http://www.facs.org/public_info/operation/consent.html. Accessed January 23, 2008).

patient's capacity might be compromised by delirium, coma or deep sedation). In these instances, somebody besides the patient must make the decisions. An advance health care directive (also known as an advance directive) is one way for a person to give instructions about how medical decisions should be made if he or she incapable of making them for himself or herself. In 1990, the United States Congress passed the Patient Self Determination Act, which mandates that hospitals receiving Medicare funding must inform all admitted patients about their rights under state law regarding advance directives.

The strongest form of an advance directive is a durable power of attorney (POA), also known as a health care proxy. The patient (or principal) designates another person (or agent) to make medical decisions if he or she becomes incapacitated. The agent's power is "durable" because he or she is authorized to make decisions while the principal is incapacitated [A standard POA (i.e. non-durable) becomes ineffective if the principal becomes incapacitated]. Living wills are another form of advance directive. In a living will, the patient gives written instructions about medical interventions that should be provided or withheld in specific circumstances. For example, a person may declare that a ventilator should be withheld if he or she has a terminal illness.

Living wills and durable POAs are both formal advance directives. Informal advance directives exist when the patient verbally expresses his or her wishes to family or friends but does not put those wishes in writing. For example, a man with a terminal illness may tell his family that he doesn't want his life to be extended by any procedure that requires intubation. In instances like this, the patient has an informal advance directive and the family should communicate the patient's instructions to the physicians.

When the patient does not have an advance directive, a surrogate must be found or appointed to make decisions for the patient if and when he or she is incapacitated. A court-appointed guardian for a patient can give directives that supersede all other directives except those stemming from a formal advance directive. When the patient has no guardian, most states have laws specifying a hierarchy of decision makers. For example, a common hierarchy is as follows: spouse, adult children, siblings, other family members, friend and finally the patient's physician (in the absence of other decision-makers). Surgeons should familiarize themselves with the applicable laws for the state(s) in which they practice. The American Bar Association's Commission on Law and Aging publishes a document on its website entitled "Surrogate Consent in the Absence of an Advance Directive", which provides a comparison chart of the laws for each state. (http://www.abanet.org/aging/legislativeupdates/home.shtml).

The strength of a living will is that it expresses the patient's own judgment. However, the instructions of a living will are often difficult to interpret because it is not always clear that the existing clinical context is the kind of context in which the patient would have wanted his or her instructions to be followed regarding mechanical ventilation, defibrillation, vasoactive medications, etc. Because durable POAs identify a specific decision-maker, they are often more useful in guiding clinical decisions because the POA is able to apply what they know about the patient's values to the specific clinical scenario. At least one study, however, has found that patients and their POAs, when presented with a hypothetical scenario, often make different decisions regarding medical interventions. The limitations of living wills and POAs reinforce the importance of frequent and explicit discussions between families, patients and clinicians throughout the course of treatment to clarify patients' wishes in the event that they are incapacitated.

Surgeons treating cancer patients should strongly encourage their patients to have frequent, open and detailed discussions with their family members early in the course of their illnesses about end-of-life issues. In addition, patients should be encouraged to assign a person to be their durable POA, as this is the strongest form of an advance directive. Studies have shown that patients often feel uncomfortable raising the issue of advance directives with their physician and they frequently want the physician to initiate the discussion. Surgeons should thus do this soon after they begin caring for a patient. In addition, patients should be asked to bring with them to the hospital any advance directives they already have. A copy of any advance directives should be put in the patient's chart. In many ways, identification of an advanced directive or surrogate should be a part of any preoperative checklist—like DVT prophylaxis or perioperative antibiotics. Surgeons of all kinds, especially those caring for cancer patients, are encouraged to make this a part of the routine History and Physical and all pre-operative workups.

Spirituality in Patient Care

The patient tells the surgeon that because his wife is institutionalized with advanced dementia, he wants his younger son (a medical doctor) to be his surrogate decision-maker. However, the patient has not formalized this with a POA. Given the impending surgery, the patient agrees to make his younger son his POA and to draw up a living will.

Over the course of the neoadjuvant chemoradiation, the surgeon continues to see the patient in clinic, but as the date of surgery approaches, the surgeon notices that the patient is increasingly distressed about the risks of surgery. He is not depressed, but he seems very uneasy about facing mortality. The surgeon finds a seat in the exam room and says, "It's OK to be scared about surgery and about your disease. The possibility of death is frightening. I'm wondering what resources you have for coping with all of this. Many patients find some support from their spiritual community. Do you consider yourself a religious or spiritual person?"

Nearly 90% of Americans describe themselves as either "religious" or "spiritual but not religious." For simplicity's sake, this section will use the terms "spiritual" and "spirituality" to refer to both of these categories. Broadly speaking, spirituality can be defined as the values and beliefs that give purpose and meaning to a person's life. A person's spirituality might be grounded in traditional religious beliefs, nature, art, interpersonal relationships, etc. Numerous studies suggest that spirituality is important to most patients, particularly in the context of severe illness and death. Furthermore, studies have found that many patients wish to have their spiritual needs addressed in the context of their medical care. Surgeons and other physicians, however, are often reluctant to ask patients about spirituality. One reason is that they themselves are often much less spiritual than their patients. For example, one study found that surgeons are only half as likely as their patients to be religious. A second reason is that physicians often feel unqualified to address a patient's spiritual needs.

One method to broach the topic of a patient's spirituality is to include questions about spirituality when taking the social history. Patients are frequently reluctant to volunteer information about their spiritual beliefs, but they will often respond when asked. The surgeon should listen carefully and respectfully and should not pry if the patient declines to answer. **Table 3-3** outlines the FICA, one of several tools that have been developed for taking a spiritual history. The detail of the spiritual history can be adapted to the clinical context. For example, it may not be necessary to obtain a spiritual history from a patient being treated for basal cell carcinoma because the prognosis is usually so favorable. On the other hand, a thoughtful and detailed inquiry into spirituality may be essential for a patient who has just been diagnosed with stage IV lung cancer.

After taking a patient's spiritual history, the surgeon must exercise good judgment in order to determine how best to address a patient's spiritual needs. One approach is to refer the patient to the pastoral care services that are offered in the hospital. Surgeons should familiarize themselves with the many pastoral services that are offered in most hospitals. They can refer a religious patient to an appropriate minister, while offering music therapy to a patient whose spirituality is grounded in music. Another way to be attentive to patients' spirituality is simply to listen to their spiritual concerns. Patients might be angry at God because they are ill and they might not feel comfortable expressing this anger within their religious communities. Simply listening respectfully without trying to offer an answer may be all that is necessary (and is often greatly appreciated by the patient). In other circumstances, it may be appropriate for the surgeon to engage the patient's spiritual questions directly, but again, this requires the surgeon to discern the appropriate boundaries for the discussion.

Medical Errors

After being asked about his spirituality, the patient admits that he is very upset about the possibility of dying. He asks that the hospital chaplain visit him everyday while he is recovering from his surgery. The surgeon makes an appropriate referral.

The surgery proceeds as planned. However, during a difficult dissection of the rectum, the surgeon injures the left ureter. The surgeon is able to repair the injury without delay, but as they are closing the fascia, the chief resident asks the surgeon if he plans to tell the patient and family about the ureter.

TABLE 3-3	Taking a spiritual history	
F	Faith and Belief	"Do you consider yourself spiritual or religious?" or "Do you have spiritual beliefs that help you cope with stress?" If the patient responds "No", the physician might ask, "What gives your life meaning?" Sometimes patients respond with answers such as family, career, or nature.
I	Importance	"What importance does your faith or belief have in our life? Have your beliefs influenced how you take care of yourself in this illness? What role do your beliefs play in regaining your health?"
C	Community	"Are you part of a spiritual or religious community? Is this of support to you and how? Is there a group of people you really love or who are important to you?" Communities such as churches, temples and mosques, or a group of like-minded friends can serve as strong support systems for some patients.
A	Address in care	"How would you like me, your health care provider, to address these issues in your health care?"

Reproduced with permission from Puchalski C. Spiritual assessment tool. Journal of Palliative Medicine 2000;3(1):131. Mary Ann Liebert, Inc, publishers. All rights reserved.

In 1999, a landmark report on medical errors by the Institute of Medicine (IOM) estimated that between 44,000 and 98,000 people die each year in the United States as the result of medical errors. More Americans die from medical errors than from motor vehicle accidents (43,458) and breast cancer (42,297). Approximately 60% of these errors are the result of a failure at the systems level, with the remainder attributable to the failure of an individual. It is estimated that three to four percent of all hospital patients suffer some form of harm as the result of error.

While the IOM report describes all types of medical errors, smaller studies have looked more specifically at surgical errors. It was found that surgical errors contribute to a significant proportion of the adverse events that patients suffer (An adverse event has been defined as an unintended result of medical therapy that causes increased morbidity and mortality, or a prolonged hospital stay). One study found that 66% of all adverse events were due to surgical procedures and 59% of these adverse events were preventable. Another study found that 39% of surgical patients had complications, 18% of which were due to error. It is thought that these numbers may be underestimates because of the difficulty in attributing an adverse event to error as opposed to other causes.

Part of the challenge of accurately measuring errors is that the definition of the term itself is controversial. The IOM report defines medical error as the failure to complete the correct action as intended (a failure of execution) or as a failure to choose the correct plan (a failure of planning). A second approach defines it as a failure to follow the standards of practice that results in a negative outcome. A third approach maintains that a medical error is a potentially harmful act or omission that would be judged wrong by a knowledgeable observer. Excluded from these definitions are foreseeable complications of a correct course of action, or the failure of a disease to respond to an appropriate treatment.

While scholarly inquiry continues to clarify the definition of medical error, other recent work examines the obligations that physicians have to disclose an error once it has occurred. The AMA Code of Medical Ethics maintains that physicians are obligated to be open and honest with their patients. They must give full disclosure to patients when a medical error has occurred and they must not let potential legal liability affect their truthfulness. As it turns out, this approach may be prudent independent of its ethical soundness. Recent studies have shown that patients are less likely to sue when their erring physicians give them a full disclosure and an apology. Patients' anger is often due to a failure of their physicians to be forthcoming about their errors and not due to the errors themselves. In other words, a failure of communication sends the patient to the malpractice attorney more often than a failure of surgical skill.

When an error occurs, the surgical or medical team should first come to an agreement about what happened. They should then decide whom should be informed about the error. Sometimes it is appropriate to report the error only to the institution and not to the patient. For example, if the wrong drug is delivered to the ICU but is never given to a patient, this error need be reported only to the staff members in charge of drug delivery within the institution. Similarly, if a surgical incision is erroneously made 2 millimeters to the left of the intended location and this will in no way affect the patient's recovery, this need not be disclosed. A full disclosure must be made when a patient suffers injury as the result of error.

Merely disclosing a harmful error is not enough. The way in which the disclosure is performed is essential. The attending surgeon should meet with the patient (and his or her family and/or representatives). A quiet room should be used if at all possible and the disclosure should never be rushed. If at all possible, the surgeon should sit down—a simple action that independently improves patient perceptions of the time and quality of the interaction. When the disclosure has been made, the surgeon should stop talking and allow the patient time to process the information and to react. Space and time for silence are essential. The surgeon should then respond to the patient's questions and concerns with forthright transparency and empathy. The content of the disclosure should include: (1) a description of the error, including when and how it occurred and the harms it caused; (2) actions initiated to mitigate the harm of the error and to prevent similar errors in the future; (3) an apology; and (4) a description of the next steps in the care of the patient. Disclosing these components in an empathetic manner is not easy. It is a skill that takes time to learn. Residents should observe experienced clinicians making such disclosures so that they too can become proficient.

Aggressive Care

Responding to the resident, the surgeon says, "Why don't you come with me when I talk with the family? I'll show you how I'm going to tell them about the ureter."

Happily, the patient has an uneventful postoperative course. During a routine follow-up appointment several months later, however, he reports that he noticed some blood in his stool during the past week. He also reports a 10 pound weight loss. A work-up reveals that the patient's cancer has recurred and has metastasized throughout his body.

The patient tries the standard chemotherapy protocols, but none of them is able to halt the advance of his cancer and he is finding the side effects oppressive.

He seeks out his surgeon for advice about how to proceed. Based on their previous discussions about the goals of care and on the patient's current peace with his rapidly approaching death, the surgeon and the patient agree to pursue hospice care.

Two days later, the surgeon gets a call from one of his colleagues who is also following the case. The colleague accuses the surgeon of "giving up on his patient" and demands that he refer him for an experimental chemotherapy protocol.

Several recent studies have examined whether cancer patients receive overly aggressive care when they are terminally ill. Measures of aggressive care included the overuse of chemotherapy (i.e. whether a patient received chemotherapy within the last two weeks of life), unwarranted surgical intervention and the underuse of hospice service (as determined by a patient not being enrolled in hospice or only being enrolled within the last three days of life). While further work needs to be done on this topic, initial findings suggest that aggressive care is becoming more common and that it is associated with worse patient quality of life.

Many reasons have been offered as to why patients receive aggressive care. One is that physicians are sometimes reluctant to discuss end of life issues because they fear that doing so will destroy hope in their patients. Contrary to this perception, however, at least one study has shown that end-of-life discussions do not destroy hope and do not cause psychological harm to patients. Another reason stems from patients' desire to "do everything". If patients do not accurately understand their prognosis or the likely success of the proposed intervention, they may assume that doing "something" is better than doing "nothing". Indeed, much of the previous discussion about goals of care can be directed to recognizing that the decision to stop aggressive treatment of the cancer need not imply that the physician and patient have decided to do "nothing". Rather the goals of care should be refocused to "do" symptom management and quality of life.

Patients often seek the care of a surgical oncologist precisely because he or she is aggressive in the treatment of cancer. In many ways, it is the surgical oncologist's job to hate the cancer even more than the patient hates the cancer. It is the surgical oncologist's work to help patients discern how far and how long to fight the disease. In the best of hands, the surgical oncologist becomes a coach, encouraging, pushing and inspiring patients to go further than they ever thought possible. But just as a running coach must realize that only a few people want to run a four minute mile (and even fewer people actually have the capacity to do so), the surgical oncologist must be constantly attentive to the goals and capacities of each individual patient. To do otherwise can result in cruelty to vulnerable patients.

Medical Futility

Responding to his colleague's concern for the patient's best interest, the surgeon explains the clear communication he had shared with the patient over the previous months regarding the patient's goals for care. In the end, the surgeon is able to reassure his colleague that hospice is the wisest choice of action for the patient.

Unfortunately, the patient's older son is very upset when he learns about the plan to pursue home hospice care. He feels that "more" should be done. Two weeks later, when the patient develops an obstruction secondary to carcinomatosis, the older son convinces the younger son that they should rush their father to the emergency room. The surgeon is called to the bedside where he finds the patient to be acidotic, tachycardic and hypotensive with free air on X-ray. In desperation, both sons demand that the surgeon operate.

The concept of medical futility became a topic of debate within medical ethics in the late 1980s. Initially the term was used by families who disagreed with the standard of care at the time and wished to withdraw life support from their loved ones. More recently, it has been increasingly used by surgeons and other physicians who contend that inappropriate medical interventions are being requested by the families of patients with terminal conditions.

One reason the topic of medical futility is contentious is that there is no widely accepted definition of the term itself. Generally speaking, it refers to medical interventions that will not significantly benefit the patient. *Quantitative futility* refers to situations in which the odds are very low that an intervention will benefit the patient. Some consider the threshold for futility to be when the odds that the patient will benefit are less than one percent, while others consider it to be when the intervention is "highly unlikely" to benefit the patient. *Qualitative futility* refers to situations in which an intervention will likely produce only an insignificant benefit to a patient. For example, aggressive treatment of congestive heart failure in a patient dying of pancreatic cancer may produce a benefit, but the benefit is likely to be insignificant because the patient is still going to die from the cancer.

When applied to a particular case, a patient's expectations also play a role in determining how medical futility should be defined. For example, suppose two women are both dying of metastatic breast cancer. One of them may decide that CPR is medically futile because it will in no way change her long term outcome: she will eventually die from cancer whether or not the CPR is performed. So she makes it clear to her physicians that she does not want CPR. The second patient, however, is waiting for some of her out-of-town family members to come visit her. She wants to live until she sees them. So she does not consider CPR futile, at least until her family members arrive.

Open and frank discussions between patients and their surgeons regarding the goals of care are thus essential in order to address effectively the concept of medical futility. The specific goals of care significantly shape what may or may not be futile in a particular case and they should be discussed early in the doctor-patient relationship. As noted above, patients should be encouraged to complete an advance directive to guide decisions in the event that they are unable to speak for themselves.

Ethical Aspects of Research and Innovation

The surgeon explains to the brothers that their father had made his wishes very clear regarding the goals of care and in fact, he had documented those wishes in his living will. The surgeon further explains that given the advanced cancer and the obvious bowel perforation, no surgical intervention could possibly benefit their father. As such, the patient is moved to a quiet room where the palliative care team manages his symptoms in the last hours until he dies.

Several weeks later, the two sons stop by the surgeon's office to thank him for taking care of their father. The surgeon shares with them that, in the course of repairing their father's injured ureter, he figured out a new and potentially better way to repair ureteral injuries. He tells them that he plans to propose a study of the new technique to the Institutional Review Board at the hospital.

Federally funded scientific research involving human subjects is regulated by the Code of Federal Regulations, Title 45, Part 46 (commonly referred to as 45 CFR 46). Ethical principles that inform 45 CFR 46 were expressed by a committee of ethicists in the 1979 Belmont Report. Surgeons can familiarize themselves with these principles for human subject research (and receive up to 7.5 hours of CME credit) via the booklet *Protecting Study Volunteers in Research*.

The currently accepted gold standard for scientific research is the double-blinded randomized controlled trial (RCT). Surgical research faces several ethical challenges in trying to meet this standard. For example, a truly "blinded" study of a surgical procedure requires that some of the subjects undergo a sham surgery in which they receive anesthesia and at least some surgical incisions but not the potentially therapeutic portion of the procedure. Because sham surgeries themselves carry some risks,

scholars have debated under what conditions, if any, they are ethically justifiable. Other challenges involved in conducting surgical research include: (1) establishing whether clinical equipoise exists between two alternative therapies (e.g. is there a legitimate need for a randomized trial of resection versus chemoradiation in the setting of pancreatic cancer?) and (2) the challenges of obtaining voluntary informed consent in the context of critical illness and among vulnerable populations such as children, the elderly and the incapacitated.

Surgical oncology involves constant innovation, but that innovation often transpires outside the narrowly defined context of "research" as defined by 45 CFR 46. Some of these innovations are pre-planned and some are spontaneously devised during a case. Some are part of formal research protocols, but many times a spontaneous innovation occurs because of unforeseen complications in a case. The surgeon will improvise and find an alternative course which eventually proves to be superior to the standard technique. The newly devised technique might then become the new standard.

Because surgical innovation is, in many ways, qualitatively different from medical innovation, the Society of University Surgeons (SUS) has employed the terms *variation*, *innovation* and *research* in order to clarify the ethical ambiguities that surround surgical innovation. A *variation* is a minor change to a procedure that does not pose an increased risk to the patient. An *innovation* is a new procedure that may pose an increased risk and the outcome of which has not been studied. *Research* involves systematic inquiry that seeks generalizable knowledge. The SUS recommends the creation of institutional Surgical Innovations Committees (SIC) that would review proposed innovations. **Table 3-4** summarizes the SUS proposals regarding variations, innovations and research. **Table 3-5** lists the SUS guidelines regarding when an innovation should require formal review.

For surgeons whose institutions do not have a SIC, one possible approach to pursuing an innovation is as follows: First, follow any institutional guidelines already in place. Second, see if it has been done before: search the literature and query the surgical innovations registry that is maintained by the American College of Surgeons (http://web.facs.org/innovations/innovationsdefault.htm). This registry enables surgeons to share information and avoid duplication of negative results. Third, discuss the innovation with colleagues and seek their critical feedback. Fourth, ask the department chairperson to form an *ad hoc* committee that will formally review the innovation. This approach, like the SIC, enables surgical innovation to proceed via a middle path between no regulation and the formal IRB review process, the lengthiness of which can sometimes be a barrier to valuable innovation.

TABLE 3-4	Ethics of surgical innovation		
Term	**Definition**	**Example**	**Proposed ethical status**
Variation	Minor variation of a surgical procedure that is unlikely to pose and increased risk to the patient.	A surgeon performs an appendectomy via a periumbilical incision.	Normal informed consent required. Information about the variant need not be disclosed.
Innovation	A new or modified surgical procedure that differs from standard practice, the outcomes of which have not been studied and which may pose and increased risk to the patient.	A surgeon employs a natural orifice transluminal endoscopic surgery (NOTES) in order to remove a patient's appendix.	(1) Informed consent that includes a full disclosure of the innovation. (2) Formal review by a surgical innovations committee (SIC).
Research	Systematic investigation designed to contribute to generalizable knowledge.	A surgeon decides to perform appendectomies via both NOTES and periumbilical incisions and then compare patient outcomes.	(1) Informed consent (2) IRB approval

TABLE 3-5	Surgical innovations requiring formal review
If the innovation is planned*, AND :	
The surgeon seeks to confirm a hunch or theory about the innovation;	
OR:	
The innovation differs significantly from currently accepted local practice;	
OR:	
Outcomes of the innovation have not been previously described;	
OR:	
The innovation entails potential risks for complications;	
OR:	
Specific or additional patient consent appears appropriate,	
Then: a) The described review by a local surgical innovations committee is required, plus b) submission to the national innovations registry is required and c) additional informed consent is required of the patient specific to the nature of the proposed innovation.	

*If an innovation occurred unplanned, it should be regarded as performed on an individual as-needed basis for the benefit of that particular patient, unless it meets any of the other five criteria. In such instances, postoperatively, the patient or patient's surrogate should be informed of the innovative nature of the procedure. If it does not meet any of the criteria, the innovation falls under acceptable modifications of surgical technique. (Reproduced with permission from Biffl, W, et al. Responsible Development and Application of Surgical Innovations: A Position Statement of the Society of University Surgeons. Journal of the American College of Surgeons. 206(6): 1204-1209. Elsevier publishers. All rights reserved. Original adapted from: Reitsma AM, Moreno JD. Ethics guidelines for innovative surgery: Recommendations for national policy. A position statement from the Committee on the Development of National Policy Recommendations for Innovative Surgery. In: Reitsma AM, Moreno JD (Eds). Ethical guidelines for innovative surgery. Hagerstown, MD: University Publishing Group, Inc: 2006)

Summary

- Ethics are important because every clinical decision, no matter how mundane, is invested with moral content.
- Good surgeons must have *practical wisdom* to discern the best course of action in each clinical situation.
- Early and frequent discussions about the goals of care with patients and their families should inform clinical decision making and can often mitigate difficulties posed by questions of futility and overly-aggressive treatment.
- Palliative care is an interdisciplinary effort that aims to relieve suffering and improve quality of life for patients and their families in the context of serious illness. It should not be confused with non-curative treatment of the dying.
- Cancer affects the whole patient, physically, psychologically, socially and spiritually. The FICA is one way to explore how a patient's spirituality may be relevant to their cancer care.
- Encourage all patients to have some form of advance directive.
- Medical and surgical errors are not uncommon and a full and honest disclosure should be made when an error causes harm to a patient.
- Familiarity with current guidelines regarding surgical innovations can streamline innovation while also protecting patients and surgeons.

Landmark Papers

1. Bosk C. Forgive and Remember (2nd edn). Chicago: University of Chicago Press; 2003 (1979).
2. Cassell EJ. The Nature of Suffering and the Goals of Medicine. N Engl J Med 1982; 306:639-45.
3. Committee on the Quality of Health Care in America. To Err is Human: Building a Safer Health System United States: National Academies Press, 2000.
4. Engelhardt HT, Jr. The Foundations of Bioethics (2nd edn). New York: Oxford University Press, 1996.
5. McCullough LB, Jones JW, Brody BA (Eds). Surgical Ethics. New York: Oxford University Press, 1998.
6. McGrath MH, Risucci DA, Schwab A (Eds). Ethical Issues in Clinical Surgery. Chicago, IL: American College of Surgeons, 2007.
7. National Commission for the Protection of Human Subjects of Biomedical and Behavioral Research. The Belmont Report: Ethical Principles and Guidelines for the Protection of Human Subjects of Research. Washington, DC: US Government Printing Office, 1979.

Fundamentals and Basics of Cancer

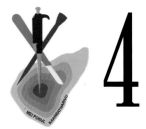

4

Molecular and Cellular Biology of Cancer

Tara J Loux, Pawel Kalinski

Introduction

As described in detail by Dr Robert Weinberg (see Landmark Papers), cancerous cells all display several hallmarks which are necessary and sufficient for tumor formation and can constitute the targets for therapeutic intervention. The following hallmarks of cancer represent the key seven aspects of aberrant cellular behavior **(Figure 4-1)**:
- potential for replication without limit
- self-sufficiency of growth signals
- insensitivity to anti-growth signals
- evasion of apoptosis
- genomic instability
- ability to manipulate angiogenesis
- ability to invade surrounding tissues and metastasize distantly.

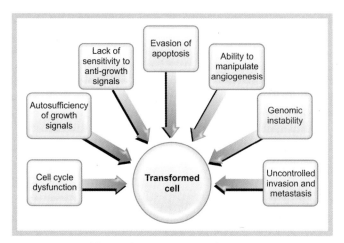

Figure 4-1: Hallmarks of cancer

Some of the key aspects of cancerous transformation take place at the genetic level, i.e. direct mutations of the genome allowing one of the seven hallmarks above to be accomplished. In general, these are separated into gain of function mutations (activation of protooncogenes), requiring a change in only one allele and loss of function mutations (silencing of tumor suppressor genes), requiring a change in both alleles. In accordance with the

seven hallmarks, carcinogenesis is generally thought to require a series of genetic alterations in both categories which accumulate in an affected cell over time.

However, recent investigations show that focusing solely on mutation events in the cancer cell may foster a narrow viewpoint of carcinogenesis. Emphasis is now being placed on study of the entire tumor microenvironment, which has been shown to comprise surrounding endothelial cells needed to feed the arising tumor, circulating and extravasating members of the immune system (dendritic cells, granulocytes, monocytes, macrophages and many types of lymphocytes), able not only to control tumor growth, but also in some cases boost tumor survival, as well as stromal cells, including fibroblasts and myoepithelial cells that provide key growth factors and support. Thus, the arising tumor's changing pattern of interactions within its microenvironment is just as important a factor in its growth and development as the mutations found within its genome.

The molecular biology associated with each hallmark is often complex and overlapping and thus, can be difficult to separate completely between one hallmark and another. For instance, regulation of the cell cycle is dependent both on growth factors and anti-growth factors, many of which interact with neighboring cells and extracellular matrix components via various adhesion molecules. Factors regulating the cell cycle and involved in the repair of DNA damage call direct the cell to or from apoptosis. Angiogenesis allows delivery of growth signals and transport and extravasation of circulating cells to support the tumor microenvironment.

This chapter will address these seven hallmarks as separate entities, in an attempt to tame this complex and only partially understood topic. We will begin each segment by outlining the normal biology associated with each hallmark. This will be followed by description of the abnormal phenomena related to each hallmark which create unique tumor-specific targets for chemotherapy and result in neoantigenicity of cancer cells. Finally, each segment will culminate by briefly noting therapeutic modalities associated with utilization of each particular

TABLE 4-1	Commonly used anti-neoplastic agents and their molecular mechanisms		
Family	**Members**	**Mechanism of action**	**Related to hallmark**
Nucleoside inhibitor	Methotrexate	Interfere with DNA synthesis	Cell cycle
Nucleoside analogues	6-mercaptopurine, 6-thioguanine, 5-fluorouracil	Interfere with DNA synthesis	Cell cycle
	Gemcitabine	Inhibits ribonucleotide reductase	Cell cycle
Alkylating agents	Busulfan, streptozocin, chlorambucil, melphalan cyclophosphamide	Crosslink DNA	Cell cycle
Platins	Cisplatin, carboplatin, oxaliplatin	Crosslink DNA	Cell cycle
Antibiotics	Actinomycin D	Intercalates between DNA strands	Cell cycle
	Bleomycin	Causes double strand DNA breaks	
Rubicins	Daunorubicin, doxirubicin Etoposide	Inhibit DNA topoisomerase Inhibit DNA topoisomerase	Cell cycle Cell cycle
Vinca alkaloids	Vincristine, vinblastine	Inhibit microtubule function	Cell cycle
Taxols	Paclitaxel, docetaxel	Inhibit microtubule function	Cell cycle
Interleukins	IL-2	Immunomodulation	Growth factors
Interleukin monoclonal antibodies	IL-6 mAB	Blockade of growth stimulation	Growth factors
Myelostimulants	Hematopoietins, IL-3, IL-11	Treatment of myelosuppression	Growth factors
EGF receptor family monoclonal antibodies	Cetuximab (Erbitux), trastuzumab (Herceptin)	Bind various members of EGF receptor family	Growth factors
Tyrosine kinase inhibitors	Erlotinib	Inhibit signaling of EGF receptor	Growth factors
	Imatinib (Gleevec)	Inhibit signaling of PDGF receptor, c-kit and Bcr-Abl	
Cyclooxygenase inhibitors	Non-steroidal anti-inflammatory agents	Inhibit prostaglandin formation, decrease VEGF expression	Growth factors/ Angiogenesis
Interferons	Interferon-alpha	Direct tumor cell toxicity, induction of apoptosis, decreased replication of tumor-causing viruses	Anti-growth factors/ Apoptosis
TNF family	TNF	Direct tumor cell toxicity, induction of tumor cell apoptosis	Anti-growth factors/ Apoptosis
VEGF monoclonal antibodies	Bevacizumab (Avastin)	Inhibition of new nutrient vessel formation	Angiogenesis

neoantigenic phenotype to accomplish cancer cell killing while sparing normal cells. **Table 4-1** summarizes pertinent molecular mechanisms of the most common current anti-neoplastic agents.

Replication and its Limitations

The cell replication cycle is composed of several discrete stages characterized by specific regulatory and effector proteins. G1 is the initial growth phase. It is followed by S phase, during which the cell's genome is duplicated. G2 is a secondary growth phase, in which the genome is assessed for accuracy and integrity prior to M phase, in which the cell divides into two daughter cells. Both of these daughter cells now find themselves back in G1 phase after division, completing the cycle. Exit of the cell cycle is possible and occurs via reversible quiescence (also described as G0) or irreversible terminal differentiation, which involves the acquisition of specialized functions ensuring inability to further replicate.

Disinhibition of the cell cycle, leading to limitless replicative potential, can occur via one of two major mechanisms: (1) bypass of cellular regulatory checkpoints for repair of DNA damage and mitotic spindle integrity, or (2) dysregulation of senescence, a mechanism by which cells cease dividing after a finite number of divisions.

Abnormalities in both these areas generally are necessary for neoplastic transformation of the cell.

Regulatory Checkpoints

Various proteins have been noted as vital for progression of the cell cycle. *Cyclins* form complexes with specific *cyclin-dependent kinases* (cdks), which are then activated by phosphorylation and act as gene transcription factors, allowing transcription of appropriate genes needed for progression of the cell cycle **(Figure 4-2)**.

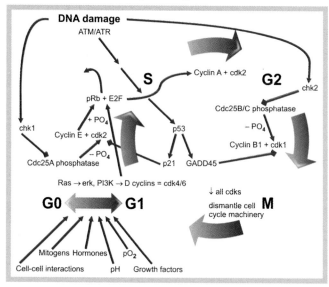

Figure 4-2: Cell cycle

There are 15 identified cyclins, which are transcribed only at the appropriate point in the cell cycle and 9 identified cdks which are ubiquitously available in the cell throughout the cycle. Cyclin activating kinases and Cdc25 phosphatases are responsible for the phosphorylation status of the cyclin/cdk complex. Cdks are further regulated through various inhibitors, including the INK4 family (p15, 16, 17 and 19) which target cdk4 and cdk6, the Cip/Kip family (p21, 27 and 57) which targets cdk 1 and cdk 2 and the pRb protein family (Rb, p107 and p130) which specifically target cdk2 in complex with cyclins E and A.

Cells are continuously sampling the extracellular environment, receiving signals from mitogens, hormones, growth factors, contact with other cells and metabolic conditions such as hypoxia or acidosis. Re-entry into the cell cycle from G0 requires growth factor receptor coupling mediated by Ras, which then activate several protein kinase cascades including erk (extracellular-signaling related kinase) and PI3K (phosphoinositide 3 kinase). These cascades result in transcription of G1-related genes, including D cyclins, which complex with cdk4 and cdk6, in addition to activating proteins necessary to assemble mRNA translation machinery in the cytosol. The cyclin

D/cdk4,6 complex stimulates the cell to continue proliferating or to leave G0 and begin proliferating. During mid to late G1, levels of cyclin E begin to rise, which complexes with cdk2. This is known as the cellular *restriction point*. Once passing this point, an event tightly regulated by the retinoblastoma protein (pRb), the cell is dedicated to continue progression through one cell cycle.

Cyclin D/cdk4,6 and cyclin E/cdk2 complexes phosphorylate pRb, which while hypophosphorylated is bound to the E2F transcription factor. E2F influences transcription of genes necessary for progression to S phase. As pRb is phosphorylated, it frees E2F which then translocates to the nucleus and acts on the genome. Subsequently, levels of cyclin A begin to rise and this cyclin complexes with cdk2, along with the E cyclins to drive the cell from S phase into G2. G2 transitions into M phase via dephosphorylation of cyclinB1/cdk1 complexes by Cdc25 B/C. Once mitosis is complete, daughter cells re-enter G1. Accumulation of cells in G1 leads to down-regulation of cdks and dismantling of cell cycle machinery.

Cells entertain several checkpoints in this progression in order to sense and correct DNA prior to its transmission to daughter cells. Progression can be halted mid-G1, mid-S and mid-G2 phases in DNA damage is sensed. The main sensors of DNA damage are two DNA-bound atypical protein kinases called ATM and ATR. Once damage is sensed, this information is transmitted to downstream regulators, which activate p53. p53 activates transcription of p21 which inhibits cdk2 to halt G1 and GADD45 which inhibits cdk1 to halt G2. The chk1 and chk2 effector protein kinases can also sense DNA damage and on doing so, degrade Cdc25A and Cdc25C, resulting in inability to dephosphorylate cdk2 and cdk1 respectively. This then causes buildup of inactive cyclin/cdk complexes in the cytosol and halts G1 and G2 respectively until DNA damage is repaired. Further, as a last checkpoint in M phase, mitotic spindle integrity is ensured through an activation cascade that is induced only once proper and appropriate attachment of sister chromatids to the spindle kinetochore has occurred.

Senescence

Cellular senescence is an irreversible state of quiescence that occurs after a certain number of replicative events. It can be induced by shortening of telomeres, severe DNA damage, oxidative stress or oncogene expression and is promoted by the INK4/ARF family of proteins. Telomeres are 6 base pair repeats at the ends of chromosomes that prevent end-to-end chromosomal fusion. Each time DNA is replicated, approximately 50 base pairs are lost from the end of the chromosome, causing telomeric shortening and threatening the ability to protect the chromosome ends. Once telomere dysfunction or shortening is sensed by a normal cell, it will be routed toward senescence or apoptosis. Several telomere-binding proteins (TRF1 and 2, Pot1) regulate telomere length and protect telomeres from activating DNA repair mechanisms.

Telomerase is a multiunit enzyme complex which adds telomere segments to the ends of chromosomes. It is highly expressed in embryonic and stem cell populations which require the ability for continuous growth and division, but repressed in adult cells as a defense against unfettered growth.

Transformations Related to Cell Cycle and Replicative Potential

Carcinogenic transformations related to the cell cycle machinery include mutations in the pRb family, which lead to dysregulated activation of cyclin/cdk complexes, downregulation of cdk inhibitors such as p21 and p16 and mutations in p53 or chk2, which promote tumor cell immortalization via bypassage of checkpoints. **Table 4-2** outlines various congenital mutations associated with cancer-causing syndromes and can be used as a reference throughout the chapter. Transformations related to cellular replicative potential include mutations in INK4a and INK4b which lead to increase phosphorylation of pRb and therefore increase the activity of E2F and mutations in ARF, which inhibits the MDM2-regulated degradation of p53, causing destabilization of the p53 system.

Additionally, the telomerase enzyme may play a paradoxical role in carcinogenesis. Initially, during early stages of neoplastic growth, lack of telomerase activity and telomere attrition may strongly promote chromosomal rearrangement via repeated breakage-fusion-bridge cycles. Breakage points may cause misreplication or chromosomal fusion. Decreased telomerase activity allows for multiple deleterious mutations to accumulate, precipitating a cellular crisis where the majority of cells experience programmed death secondary to genetic instability. In a small number of remaining cells, telomerase may subsequently become re-activated and release of its repression encourages future cancer cell immortalization through reconstitution of the telomere complement.

Therapeutic Opportunities Related to Cell Cycle and Replicative Potential

Many of the initial chemotherapeutic modalities targeted cells at weak points in their cell cycle. However, this makes them relatively non-specific for tumor cells and can allow them to target any rapidly dividing cell line. Methotrexate inhibits the enzyme dihydrofolate reductase, an enzyme necessary for purine synthesis, leading to depletion of nucleotide precursors. 6-mercaptopurine, 6-thioguanidine and 5-fluorouracil are all nucleoside analogues which interfere with DNA synthesis in some manner.

Gemcitabine inhibits ribonucleotide reductase, causing abrupt termination of DNA chains. Alkylating agents and the platin family cross link DNA, limiting the ability to replicate. Actinomycin D intercalates between DNA strands, also forming a barrier to replication. The rubicin family and etoposide inhibit DNA topoisomerase. Bleomycin directly cleaves DNA causing double strand breaks. The vinca alkaloids and paclitaxel inhibit microtubule function, leading to inability to arm the mitotic spindle and culminate mitosis.

In addition to creating tumor-specific targets for chemotherapy, the aberrant expression of some of the key components of replicative cycle makes it possible to design vaccines against any cells overexpressing such factors.

Tumorigenic Growth Factors and Downstream Signaling

As previously mentioned, growth signals are important determinants of cell cycle initiation and progression. Several sub-categories of growth factors have been identified: cytokines (including interleukins, colony-stimulating factors, interferons and tumor necrosis factors), platelet-derived growth factor (PDGF), epidermal growth factor (EGF) family, scatter factor protein family, vascular endothelial growth factor (VEGF) family, chemokines, neuropeptides and prostanoids. Many of these families have similar or overlapping functions, indicating the evolutionary sensitivity of these factors in promoting survival. These growth factors signal through a number of different downstream signaling pathways, including Janus kinase/signal transducer and activator of transcription (JAK/STAT), G protein-coupled signaling, Ras adaptor protein utilizing mitogen-activated protein kinase (MAP kinase), PI3 kinase and Src adaptor protein utilizing Myc transcription factor, pathways. Carcinogenic transformations can occur not only in the secretion or reception of growth signals, but also in their downstream signaling pathways. A summary of growth factors pertinent to tumorigenesis is provided in **Table 4-3.**

Factors with Predominantly Tumor-supporting Functions

Hematopoietins: Colony-stimulating factors (CSFs) include G(granulocyte)-CSF, M(macrophage)-CSF, GM(granulocyte/macrophage)-CSF, stem cell factor (SCF), erythropoietin and thrombopoietin, which stimulates megakaryocyte production of platelets.

Interleukins are cytokines secreted mainly by cells of hematopoietic lineage, with differential effects on proliferation and activity of other hematopoietic effectors. **Table 4-4** provides a limited overview of the major characteristics of interleukins.

TABLE 4-2 Congenital and familial syndromes associated with known genetic mutations

Gene mutated	Defect in	Associated syndrome	Associated conditions
pRb	Control of cell cycle	Retinoblastoma	Retinoblastoma (bilateral), soft tissue and osteosarcomas
p53, chk2, ARF	Decreased ability for apoptosis	Li Fraumeni	Breast cancer, brain cancers, bone and soft tissue sarcomas, adrenocortical carcinoma, leukemia
INK4a, INK4b	Activation of pRb, inhibition of tumor suppression	Familial melanoma, familial pancreatic carcinoma	Melanoma, pancreatic cancer
Met	Response to growth factor	Hereditary papillary renal carcinoma (HPRC)	Multiple bilateral renal papillary cancers
VHL	Decreased sensitivity to tissue oxygen levels, increase in VEGF secretion	Von Hippel Lindau	Hemangioblastomas, renal clear cell carcinoma, pancreatic islet cell tumors, pheochromocytoma, CNS angiomas
MLH1, MSH2, MSH6, PNS2	Mismatch repair genes	Lynch syndrome (hereditary non-polyposis colon cancer or HNPCC)	Colon (especially cecal/ ascending), ovarian, uterine including cervix, gastric and renal cancers
XPA, B, C, D, E, F & G	Nucleotide excision repair	Xeroderma pigmentosum	Hypersensitivity to sunlight, neurologic defects, skin cancers
CSA, CSB	Nucleotide excision repair	Cockayne syndrome	Hypersensitivity to sunlight, growth and mental retardation, NO increased incidence of cancer
ATM	Double strand breakage repair	Ataxia telangiectasia (AT)	T cell defects, cerebellar degeneration, predisposition to epithelial and lymphoid cancers
MRE11	Double strand breakage repair	AT-like disorder	Similar to AT
Nbs1	Cell cycle checkpoints	Nijmegen breakage syndrome	Humoral/T cell defects, radiosensitivity, lymphoma, rhabdomyosarcoma, neuroblastoma
BRCA1, BRCA2	Homologous recombination	Familial breast and ovarian cancer syndromes	Breast cancer, ovarian cancer
RECQL4	DNA helicase	Rothmund-Thompson syndrome	Hypersensitivity to sunlight, osteogenic sarcomas, squamous cell carcinomas
BLM	DNA helicase	Bloom syndrome	Immunodeficiency, leukemia/ lymphoma, breast and intestinal cancers
WRN	DNA helicase	Werner syndrome	Premature aging, with age-associated diseases and malignancies, soft tissue sarcoma, melanoma, thyroid cancer
MEN1	Telomerase suppression, suppression of transcription factors and downstream signaling	MEN I	Parathyroid hyperplasia (100%), pituitary adenoma, endocrine pancreatic tumors, bronchial and thymic carcinoid
RET	Membrane tyrosine kinase signaling constitutively activated	MEN IIa, MEN IIb, familiary medullary thyroid cancer (MTC)	IIa: MTC (100%), parathyroid hyperplasia, pheochromocytoma IIb: MTC (100%), pheochromocytoma, mucosal neuromas, Marfanoid habitus, megacolon
APC	Adhesion, nuclear transcription factor signaling	Familial adenosis polyposis (FAP)	Colon cancer, duodenal/ periampullary carcinoma, hepatoblastoma, desmoids tumors

TABLE 4-3	Growth factors families, their main members and receptors and their roles in tumorigenesis		
Family	**Members**	**Receptors**	**Role in tumorigenesis**
Hematopoietins/ Interleukins	G-CSF, M-CSF, GM-CSF, SCF, erythropoietin, thrombopoietin, interleukins 1-33 (see **Table 4-2**)	Various individual receptors	Tumors express receptors for growth-promoting factors or usurp downstream signaling pathways
PDGF	A,B,C and D isoforms	PDGFR α/β subunits	Tumors overexpress PDGF isoforms or experience automatic stimulation of receptors
EGF	EGF, TGF-α, HB-EGF, amphiregulin, epiregulin, beta-cellulin	ErbB1-4	Constitutively activated receptors, increased secretion of ligands
Scatter factors	HGF, MSP, semaphorins	Met, Ron, plexins	Receptor overexpression or constitutive activation
VEGF	VEGF-A, B, C & D, PlGF	VEGFR-1, VEGFR-2	Overexpression of VEGF isoforms, loss of VHL activity
Chemokines	CCL family, CXCL family, CX3CL1 (fractalkine), XCL1 (lymphotactin)	CCR family, CXCR family, CX3CR1, XCR family	Tumors overexpress both chemokines and receptors, which may aid in homing of metastatic cells
Neuropeptides	Thrombin, bombesin, calcitonin, bradykinin, substance P, endothelin, neurotensin, serotonin, gastrin, CCK	Various individual receptors	Tumors overexpress various neuropeptides which enrich microenvironment and stimulate growth.
TGF-β	TGF-β, activin, inhibin, BMPs, GDFs, MIF	TβR-I, TβR-II	Overexpression promotes growth and differentiation of tumors of mesenchymal origin. Epithelial tumors may contain mutations which inactivate the receptor
Eicosanoids	Prostaglandins (especially PGE2), leukotrienes	EP 1-4	Tumor overexpression of PGE2 leads to immunosuppression, changes in vascular tone and tumor cell proliferation

The receptors for many hematopoietins, including erythropoietin, G-CSF, GM-CSF and IL-11 are found on multiple different lineages of solid and hematologic malignancies. Tumor cells may usurp the downstream signaling pathways of these receptors for their own growth and proliferation.

PDGF: Platelet-derived growth factor is a major element in the growth, survival and migration of mesenchymal cell types and has been shown important in the biology of cancer. It is stored in the alpha granules of platelets, but also secreted by many other cell types. It regulates interstitial fluid pressure, stimulates regeneration of connective tissue during wound healing and supports angiogenesis via stimulation of pericytes. The A,B,C and D isoforms of PDGF come together in homo- or hetero-dimers which join the α and β subunits of the PDGF receptor with differing specificities, leading to divergent downstream signals and thus different effects on growth and chemotaxis.

PDGF is overexpressed by many tumor types, including sarcomas and glioblastomas. Some of these tumors do not express PDGF receptors themselves, indicating that PDGF may be secreted as a paracrine factor influencing cells in the tumor microenvironment. Retroviruses express an oncogene called *v-sis* which shares significant homology with the PDGF B chain and aids in transformation via autocrine stimulation of the cell by a PDGF-like factor. The E5 oncoprotein of bovine papillomavirus is able to crosslink and homodimerize the PDGFR β-chain, causing stimulation of the receptor. Overexpression of PDGF is also noted in other proliferative diseases such as atherosclerosis and fibroses.

EGF family: Members of the epidermal growth factor (EGF) family include EGF, transforming growth factor-alpha (TGF-α), heparin binding EGF-like growth factor (HB-EGF), amphiregulin, epiregulin and beta-cellulin. EGF is secreted from mucosal cells into their respective secretions (e.g. saliva, urine, tears, breast milk, seminal

TABLE 4-4	Major known interleukins, along with the main cell of their effect and the resulting function	
Interleukin	**Major target cells**	**Function**
IL-1	T cells, macrophages, dendritic cells	Activation, support for the production of tumor-enhancing factors
IL-2	CD8+ T cells, NK cells	Proliferation, activation, predominant antitumor effects; possible tumor-enhancing activity
IL-3	All hematopoietic cells	Multi-lineage stimulator of proliferation
IL-4	B cells, Th cells, macrophages	Clonal expansion of antigen-specific B cell, activation of Th2 response, macrophage activation
IL-5	Eosinophils	Proliferation/IgA differentiation
IL-6	B cells	Differentiation into antibody secreting plasma cell, promotes expansion and survival of hematologic tumor cells
IL-7	Pre-B and pre-T cells; memory T cells	Growth and expansion; promotes survival of memory T cells
IL-8	Neutrophils, basophils, T cells	Chemoattractant for immune cells
IL-9	Mast cells	Activation
IL-10	Th1 cells, DCs, macrophages	Inhibits activation and cytokine release; promotes tumor resistance to immune elimination
IL-11	All hematopoietic cells	Multi-lineage stimulator of proliferation
IL-12	NK cells, CTLs, Th1 cells	Activation of antitumor effector functions, indirect antiangiogenic and antitumor effects mediated by reduced blood supply and immune effects
IL-13	B cells, macrophages, Th1 cells	Proliferation of B cells, inhibition of cytokine production from macrophages and Th1 cells
IL-15	CD8+ T cells, NK cells	Proliferation, activation, enhanced survival
IL-16	CD4+ T cells, monocytes, eosinophils	Chemoattractant
IL-17	Fibroblasts/epithelial cell/neutrophils	Cytokine production and secretion, activation
IL-18	CD8+ and CD4+ T cells, NK cells	Interferon-gamma secretion
IL-23	CD8+ and CD4+ T cells, NK cells	Promotes the production of IL-17, proinflammatory effects; may promote or suppress growth of different tumors
IL-27	CD8+ and CD4+ T cells, NK cells	Promotes the production of IFNγ; may promote or suppress growth of different tumors
IL-33	Similar to IL-1	Similar to IL-1

fluid), with a primary function of maintaining the integrity of the mucous membrane. All family members are membrane-bound glycosylated proteins that are enzymatically shed for secretion purposes. They are potent stimulators of proliferation and migration. They signal via the EGF receptor family, which consists of erbB1 (EGFR), erbB2 (Her-2/neu), erbB3 (Her-3) and erbB4 (Her-4). These tyrosine kinase receptors form heterodimers and transphosphorylate when activated by ligand. erbB2 has no natural ligand, but is the preferred heterodimerization partner of the other three receptors; thus it functions mainly as a co-receptor. Downstream signaling is via MAP kinases such as Erk1, Erk2, Erk5, Jun and stress-activated p38 kinase.

A constitutively activated EGF receptor is over-expressed in many tumor types, including lung and head/neck cancers (erbB1) and breast, gastric, ovarian, lung and oral cancers (erbB2). Tumors with activation of the Ras oncogene, especially pancreatic cancer, secrete supernormal quantities of EGF receptor ligands that act in an autocrine fashion. HB-EGF expression is enhanced in hepatocellular, pancreatic, gastric and breast cancers.

Scatter factor protein family: Members of this family include hepatocyte growth factor (HGF) and macrophage-stimulating protein (MSP). Scatter factors promote invasive growth, which under normal conditions, signifies orderly growth of epithelial tubules into the surrounding cell stroma. They additionally promote terminal differentiation and polarization of epithelial and endothelial cells, guide axonal movement in proliferating neuronal tissue, stimulate red blood cell precursors to leave the bone marrow and join the peripheral circulation and recruit osteoclasts to participate in bone remodeling. The HGF receptor is the Met protooncogene tyrosine kinase, while the MSP receptor is the Ron protooncogene tyrosine kinase.

Semaphorins are proteins involved in emitting repulsion signals, whose receptors, the plexins share significant homology with the scatter protein family receptors. Plexins mediate repulsion signals in almost all tissues, resulting in dissociation of packed cells, a process similar to scatter. These two families appear to share overlapping functions.

Patients with germ-line missense mutations of Met (the receptor for HGF) form multiple bilateral papillary renal cancers. Similar spontaneous mutations are found in patients affected by sporadic renal carcinoma or juvenile hepatocellular carcinoma. Met mutations have been shown to confer transformational and apoptosis-evading capabilities, but only in the presence of the HGF ligand. Met overexpression is also found in human tumors, including colorectal carcinoma and sarcoma. Semaphorins are overexpressed in invasive and metastasizing tumors, in which they can sustain motility, invasion and cell survival.

VEGF family: Members of this family include VEGF-A, B, C and D and placental growth factor (PlGF). VEGF-A is a highly specific and potent mitogen of vascular endothelial cells. It stimulates endothelial cell (EC) division, induces EC migration, enhances EC survival by up-regulating anti-apoptotic mediators and mobilizes EC progenitors from the bone marrow to sites of angiogenesis. In addition, it strongly promotes vascular permeability. VEGF-B is important in the recruitment and mobilization of hematopoietic stem cells and EC progenitors from the bone marrow. VEGF-C is a major regulator of lymphangiogenesis. VEGF-D can induce both vascular angiogenesis and lymphangiogenesis and likely plays a role in repair of vasculature after injury.

Under normoxic conditions, the von Hippel-Lindau (VHL) protein regulates levels of the hypoxia-inducible transcription factor (HIF)-1α by targeting it for ubiquitin-mediated degradation. Hypoxia stabilizes levels of HIF-1α, allowing it to translocate to the nucleus, heterodimerize with HIF-1β, bind to hypoxia response elements in the genome and enhance transcription of the downstream genes. VEGF is one of the major genome elements that contains a hypoxia response element in its promoter sequence.

Receptors are VEGFR-1 and VEGFR-2. VEGFR-2 mediates the majority of proangiogenic signaling, via upregulation of phospholipase C-γ and activation of the protein kinase C cascade. VEGFR-1 has little signaling capability but 10-fold higher binding affinity and occurs in a soluble form which may negatively regulate physiologic angiogenesis.

VEGF-A is overexpressed by most human and animal cancer. Oncogenes and non-functional tumor suppressor genes induce upregulation of its expression. VEGF-D is also overexpressed in a range of human tumors including melanoma, glioma, breast and lung carcinomas. Loss of activity of VHL leads to highly vascularized tumors such as renal cell carcinoma, pheochromocytoma and orbital hemangioblastomas. Further discussion of angiogenesis is detailed below.

Chemokines: Chemokines are small peptides with potent chemoattractant ability for monocytes and neutrophils that are secreted by nearly every cell type. They may also serve functions in regulation of adhesion, degranulation, hematopoiesis and genesis of lymphoid organs. They are classified and named according to disulfide bonding between paired cysteine residues. These bonds form between cysteines 1 and 3 and cysteines 2 and 4. Nomenclature depends on the number of intervening amino acids between the first and second cysteine residues. α chemokine ligands have one intervening amino acid between C1 and C2 and thus are named CXCL. β chemokines have no intervening amino acid and are named CCL. γ chemokines have only one cysteine pair and are named XCL. The only known member of this sub-family is lymphotactin (XCL1). δ chemokines have three intervening amino acids and are named CX3CL. The only known member of this sub-family is fractalkine (CX3CL1).

Chemokine receptors are sub-family specific (CXCR, CCR, XCR or CX3CR) and belong to the seven-trans-membrane domain G-protein coupled receptor family. The biologic effects of chemokines are in general pro-inflammatory, although they may also serve homing, homeostatic and developmental functions as well.

Chemokines and their receptors have variously been shown to be overexpressed on non-small cell lung carcinoma, Kaposi sarcoma, breast cancer, glioblastoma, ovarian cancer, melanoma and many other cancers. Certain chemokines have been loosely linked with improved survival in cancer patients, mostly due to leukocyte recruitment and infiltration in the tumor. These include CCL2 in pancreatic cancer, CCL5 and CCL22 in non-small cell lung cancer and CCL4, CCL5, CXCL9 and CXCL10 in renal cell carcinoma.

Expression of most chemokines, however, is linked with poorer prognosis. CXCL12/CXCR4 is a chemokine and receptor pair that has been identified as a homing mechanism directing metastatic breast cancer cells toward bone, lung and liver. CCR7, whose ligand CCL21 is found in the lymph nodes, is expressed by many cancers and high expression has been found to correlate highly with lymph nodal metastasis. CCR5 (also known as RANTES) expression in non-small cell lung cancer has been found to correlate with an increased risk for invasion and death. In addition to their role in metastatic homing, chemokines may be produced by tumors to control leukocyte infiltration, support angiogenesis and promote their own growth and survival.

Neuropeptides: There is a gamut of peptides responsible for signaling throughout the central, peripheral and enteric nervous systems which, along with their receptors, are expressed by a variety of solid tumors and can serve as mitogens for poorly differentiated cancer cells. Some of these include thrombin, bombesin, calcitonin, brady-kinin, substance P, endothelin, neurotensin, serotonin, gastrin and cholecystokinin. Various neuropeptides are overexpressed in breast, lung, prostate and colorectal cancer, in addition to a variety of other solid tumors.

Transforming growth factor-beta: Transforming growth factor-beta (TGF-β) is a superfamily of over 100 related proteins including TGF-β, activin, inhibin, bone morpho-genetic proteins (BMPs), growth and differentiation factors (GDFs) and Mullerian inhibitory factor (MIF). These family members generally favor inhibition of normal cells (especially those of epithelial lineage), by keeping pRb in a hypophosphorylated state, arresting cells in late G1 and preventing progression into S phase.

Paradoxically, TGF-β promotes growth and differen-tiation of mesenchymal cells as well as collagen produc-tion and deposition and is especially active and important during wound healing. It initially acts as a potent chemoattractant for inflammatory cells, but later in the wound healing process has more immunosuppressive activity. It is not a classic pro- or anti-oncogenic cytokine, as its role seems to change according to cell type and microenvironment as well as timing of inflammatory response.

Receptors are TβRI and TβRII, transmembrane serine/threonine kinases which form a hetero-tetramer in response to TGF-β ligation. Intracellular downstream effectors are the SMAD protein family.

TGF-β overexpression or inactivation is found in several different types of cancers, emphasizing its complex role in regulation of cell proliferation and differentiation. TβR mutations conferring an inactive receptor are found in a majority of colorectal, hepatocellular, biliary tract and gastric cancers. Mutations in SMAD4 intracellular signaling molecule are very common in pancreatic cancer.

Eicosanoids: Eicosanoids comprise the prostaglandins, leukotrienes and other related compounds. They are fatty acid-derived chemicals though to act mainly in paracrine or autocrine fashion on nearby smooth muscle cells to effect contraction or relaxation, depending on the situation. Prostaglandin E2 (PGE2) affects vascular tone, platelet aggregation and inflammatory responses, among other duties. PGE2 signals through 4 different receptors, EP1, EP2, EP3 and EP4, which carry out diverse effects based on their differential expression in different tissues.

Prostanoids, particularly PGE2, have been shown to be overproduced in colorectal cancer and multiple other tumor types and have been implicated in directly promoting tumor cell proliferation. In addition, a potent immunosuppressive activity of PGE2, mediated by inhibition of the proinflammatory and cytotoxic functions of CD4+ and CD8+ T cells, NK cells and antigen-presenting cells such as macrophages and dendritic cells, has been shown to contribute to tumor-induced immune dysfunction.

Transformations Related to Growth-promoting Factors

In addition to the above-mentioned transformations related to growth factors themselves, downstream signaling components of cytokines and growth factors may also be transformed in tumors. For instance, the JAK/STAT pathway is constitutively activated in many different leukemias and lymphomas. Downstream components of the PDGF receptor may be abnormally active in chronic myelomonocytic leukemia. c-Kit, a cellular protein tyrosine kinase, is constitutively activated in many gastrointestinal stromal tumors.

Therapeutic Interference with Growth-promoting Factors

The main role of the hematopoietin family in cancer therapy is to reconstitute the bone marrow population after bone marrow cytotoxic chemotherapies. Due to the wide expression of hematopoietin receptors on various tumors, administration of hematopoietic growth factors may be detrimental to the cancer patient in stimulating proliferation of malignant cells. However, some hematopoietins are being studied in an adjunctive role to conventional chemotherapies by thrusting the cancer cell into a vulnerable state of proliferation at which time the chemotherapy may be more effective.

Various interleukins have been used either in recombinant form or in blockade via antibody as therapies for specific cancer entities. IL-1 is produced by various types of leukemia and IL-1 receptor blockade is currently being tested in trials. IL-1 may also inhibit proliferation in certain solid tumors. Multiple myeloma depends on IL-6 for survival and IL-6 antibodies have been shown to be very effective in combination with conventional chemotherapies for this entity, as well as post-transplant lymphoproliferative disease. IL-2 treatment is used in renal cell cancer and metastatic melanoma. IL-3 and IL-11 may show promise in treating myelosuppression related to conventional chemotherapies which obliterate rapidly dividing cells, including hematopoietic cell lines.

The EGF receptor family is a significant target of biological therapies for breast and colorectal cancers. The monoclonal antibody cetuximab *(Erbitux)* binds the erbB1/EGFR and has been used successfully in treating colorectal cancer and squamous cell carcinomas of the head and neck. The monoclonal antibody trastuzumab *(Herceptin)* antagonistically binds the erbB2/Her2/neu receptor and is used commonly in Her2/neu positive breast cancers. Multiple other monoclonal antibodies and small molecule inhibitors have been tested against different components of EGF receptors and their downstream receptor tyrosine kinase signaling pathways. Erlotinib is a small molecule tyrosine kinase inhibitor of the EGFR which has shown to induce substantial and durable responses in a small minority of patients with non-small cell lung cancer.

Antagonization of certain chemokines and/or their receptors may prove to be beneficial in a prophylactic manner to prevent metastases from early stage disease. Others whose expression has been linked to an improved prognosis might be beneficial when given supplementally by mobilizing certain immune system effectors against tumor cells. There is some promising animal model research in this area, however to date no treatment studies have been done with therapeutic chemokines or chemokine- and chemokine receptor-blocking agents in human cancers.

Imatinib *(Gleevec)* is a tyrosine kinase inhibitor initially noted to block ATP binding and use of the PDGFR kinase domain. Subsequently, it was found to also inhibit the Philadelphia chromosome gene product (Bcr-Abl receptor tyrosine kianse) and the c-kit protein tyrosine kinase, which is overexpressed in many gastrointestinal stromal tumors (GISTs). It is used to treat chronic myelogenous leukemia and unresectable or metastatic GISTs or as adjuvant therapy after surgical resection.

Although PGE2-inhibiting factors, particularly selective or non-selective inhibitors of cyclooxygenases 1 and 2, have been extensively applied in the prevention and treatment of multiple types of cancer, as yet clear benefit for their use has only been convincingly demonstrated in the case of colorectal cancer.

In addition, growth factors may function as adjuvants in tumor-antigen vaccines. Cytokine-tumor antigen fusion proteins, for example those involving GM-CSF, represent a novel twist on this approach as they facilitate uptake of tumor antigen by antigen-presenting cells via the normal process of cytokine ligand-receptor internalization.

Endogenous Inhibitors of Cancerous Growth

Factors with Predominantly Tumor-inhibitory Functions

Interferons: Interferons (IFNs) confer non-specific resistance to a broad range of viral infections, affect cell proliferation and modulate immune responses. Type I interferons (alpha, beta, tau and omega) have anti-tumor, immunomodulatory, antiparasitic and antiproliferative properties. Type I interferon receptors are formed by the interaction of two proteins, IFNAR-1 and IFNAR-2, which signal via JAK/STAT and PI3K pathways. Interferon regulatory factors (IRFs) regulate interferon expression at many levels. IRF-3 and IRF-7 are DNA-binding proteins that regulate transcription of IFN-α. Regulation of cell growth has been shown to depend in part on the ratio of IRF-1 and IRF-2 and any change that interferes with the balance of these two factors can result in significant alteration in cell proliferation.

Type II interferon (gamma) is produced mainly by activated T cells, natural killer (NK) cells and NK-T cells. It has innate antiviral and antitumor activities, but plays a much larger role in the maturation and function of both innate and adaptive immune systems. It acts as the major activator of macrophages, promotes the growth of Th1 cells while inhibiting Th2 development, enhances NK cytotoxic activity, promotes the switch to IgG2a production by B cells and enhances antigen presentation by activating dendritic cells and inducing expression of both class I and class II MHC molecules on the surfaces of target cells. IFN-gamma has been shown to inhibit growth and induce apoptosis of a number of cells, including tumor cells. The receptor is composed of two proteins, IFNGR-1 and IFNGR-2, which signal mainly via the JAK/STAT pathway.

Tumor necrosis factor family: Tumor necrosis factors (TNFs) consist of TNF-α and TNF-β, both of which have essentially identical functions. The former is produced primarily by macrophages and the latter, also known as lymphotoxin, is produced by lymphocytes. These cytokines are the central mediators of LPS-induced shock. TNF is primarily an effector molecule of the innate immune system, produced in copious quantities in response to microbial "signature" molecules called pathogen-associated molecular pattern molecules, or PAMPs, that herald infection of the host. TNF-related apoptosis-inducing ligand (TRAIL) signals through receptors of the TNF family and has been found to induce apoptosis mainly in transformed and cancer cells.

TNF synthesis is activated by LPS via the toll-like receptor 4 (TLR4) with recruitment of the MyD88 adaptor protein. It is synthesized as a membrane-bound homo-trimeric protein, which is released from the membrane through the action of the matrix metalloproteinase TACE (TNF-alpha converting enzyme). TNF's biological effects include activation of neutrophils, induction of coagulant effects on vascular endothelium, especially in tumor vasculature, enhancement of cellular microbicidal activity, including improving the efficacy of radical oxygen species (ROS) production, stimulation of proteolytic enzyme synthesis and induction of apoptosis in sensitive tumor cells. It provides defense against viruses, gram-positive bacteria, mycobacteria and protozoa, as well as transformed "self" cells.

There are two types of TNF receptors: Type I receptors (p55) have a "death domain" which permits heterotypic interaction with signaling molecules such as Fas-associated death domain (FADD), TNF receptor-associated death domain (TRADD) and receptor-interacting protein (RIP), which have similar domains and can initiate cellular apoptosis. Type II receptors (p75) lack a death domain, are engaged by TNF receptor-associated factor (TRAF) family of signaling molecules and use the NF-κB downstream signaling pathway. Gene knockout investigations have established that the majority of TNF toxicity, including its tumoricidal effect, is mediated through the p55 receptor complex.

Transformations Related to Loss of Anti-growth Signals

It goes without saying that many cancers will have become insensitive to anti-growth signals as those mentioned above. Genes encoding interferon-regulatory factors have been found to be dysregulated in the cells of patients with Li-Fraumeni syndrome, resulting in an increased ability of the cells to spontaneously immortalize. In some human cancer cell lines, downregulation of the STAT1 pathways confers resistance to interferon-alpha. Also, Bcr-Abl transformation of hematopoietic cell lines has been shown to suppress IFN-activated signaling pathways.

Chronic TNF production is thought to mediate the catabolic cancer cachexia syndrome of anorexia and weight loss. Tumors which evade apoptosis can have mutations anywhere in the death-receptor mediated pathway triggered by the TNFs.

Therapeutic use of Anti-growth Factors

Interferon-alpha has been extensively used in the treatment of hematologic malignancies, metastatic renal cell cancer and melanomas which have become metastatic, or those whose morphology and staging portend a high risk of locoregional recurrence or systemic metastasis. In addition, treatment of hepatitis B or C with interferon-α has been shown to reduce risk of hepatocellular cancer (HCC) by 50% in all those treated. When treated patients are broken down into groups based on response to

interferon treatment, the majority of risk improvement occurs in the group with a complete response to treatment, implying that viral suppression, leading to decreased hepatocellular turnover and slower progression to cirrhosis confer a significant benefit in terms of HCC risk.

Isolated limb perfusion with TNF has found some success to treat localized tumors, such as locally advanced melanomas without visible metastasis. However, outside of loco-regional use, TNF carries too much toxicity to be employed in the systemic anti-tumor armamentarium.

Aberrations of Cell Death in Cancer

Cell death can occur in one of two major ways—apoptosis and necrosis. Necrosis is pathologic cell death associated with severe injury that rapidly overwhelms cellular survival mechanisms. Histologically, it is characterized by vacuolization of the endoplasmic reticulum, cell swelling, membrane disruption and spillage of intracellular contents into the extracellular matrix. Necrotic cell death is invariably accompanied by a strong inflammatory response.

Apoptosis is the classically understood programmed cell death necessary for removal of irreversibly stressed, dying, excess, mutant or harmful cells for the protection of the organism. It can either be physiologic or pathologic in nature. Histologically, apoptosis is characterized by cell shrinkage, nuclear fragmentation, chromatin fragmentation and cytoplasmic blebbing. These blebs are recognized by macrophages and neighboring cells to be ingested and degraded. Apoptosis is thought to incite minimal, if any, inflammatory response. Cancer cells develop mechanisms allowing them to evade apoptotic cell death despite their mutant status.

Pathways of Initiation of Apoptosis

There are four known pathways for initiation of apoptosis. Integral to all these pathways are the activation of caspases. The caspases are a family of enzymes which degrade key elements in the cell once the programmed cell death pathway has been chosen. They have affectionately been referred to as the "cellular demolition squad". Initiator caspases (caspases 2, 8, 9 and 10) convert procaspases into an active form. Executioner caspases (caspases 3, 6, 7 and 14) target certain integral proteins for cleavage. These include DNA repair proteins such as polyadenosine diphosphate ribose polymerase (PARP), anti-apoptotic proteins such as Bcl-2, DNA-dependent protein kinases such as AKT-1, structural proteins such as lamins and actin, cell cycle progression factors such as pRb, PKC and MDM2 and DNA-fragmentation factor (DFF), which mediates the internucleosomal cleavage of DNA.

The *extrinsic pathway* of apoptosis is initiated via ligation of death receptors Fas (also known as APO or CD95), tumor necrosis factor receptor 1 (TNFR1), DR3 (alternatively known as TRAMP), tumor necrosis factor-related apoptosis-inducing ligand-receptor 1 (TRAIL-R1, alternatively known as DR4), TRAIL-R2 (alternatively known as DR5) and DR6. These receptors carry intracellular death domains which associate with Fas-associated death domain (FADD), TNF-receptor-associated death domain (TRADD) and pro-caspase 8, resulting in autocatalytic cleavage of the pro-enzyme to its active form.

The *intrinsic (mitochondrial) pathway* of apoptosis is initiated by ultraviolet radiation, growth factor starvation and hypoxia, in addition to other cellular metabolic stresses. It is mediated via the Bcl-2 family of molecules. This family is a conglomerate of related balancing factors, some of which are pro-apoptotic, others of which are anti-apoptotic. The ratio between pro- and anti-apoptotic members of the family present in a cell can tip the balance of power toward or away from apoptosis. The family is separated into three main groups: *triggers* (Bid, Bik, Bmf, Puma, Noxa, Bad and Bim) which are pro-apoptotic factors acting upstream of the killer proteins, *arbitrators* (Bcl-2, Bcl-XL, Bcl-W, Mcl-1 and A1) which are anti-apoptotic factor and *killers* (Bax and Bak). Bcl-2 binds to pRb and keeps it in a hypophosphorylated state, which stabilizes its binding of the E2F transcription factors, holding the cell cycle in check at late G1. Downstream from the trigger proteins, Bax (located in the cytosol) oligomerizes with Bak (located in the inner mitochondrial membrane), directly affecting permeability of the mitochondrial membrane and allowing leakage of cytochrome c. Upon its release, cytochrome c binds APAF-1 in the cytosol and pro-caspase 9 is recruited to form the apoptosome complex, which begins the intracellular caspase cascade.

The *cell-mediated pathway* is initiated via interaction of cytotoxic lymphocytes with MHC class I molecules. Lymphocytes subsequently induce perforin-mediated pore formation on the cell surface and inject granzymes into the cell, which initiate the caspase cascade. A more recently discovered pathway, called the *integrin-mediated pathway*, is mediated by cell surface interaction and communication molecules. Integrins, when unligated or antagonized, can stimulate caspase 8 activity independent of death-receptor activation.

Apoptosis is highly regulated by an important complement of cellular surveillance proteins, which include the p53 family of molecules. p53 is activated by any sort of perceived cellular stress. Activated p53 halts the cell cycle and, if injury is found to be irreversible, initiates programmed cell death. Under normal circumstances, p53 is maintained inactive via ubiquitin-mediated degradation. When activated, however, it becomes a transcription factor for genes involved in apoptosis and cell cycle arrest, such as the cdk inhibitors and Bcl-2 family members.

Akt, a downstream protein in the PI3K pathway, is an anti-apoptotic factor that regulates p53 expression via phosphorylation of MDM2, which can then translocate to the nucleus and degrade p53. It also phosphorylates IκB kinase, which degrades IκB and allows NFκB to translocate to the nucleus and activate gene transcription for cellular survival mechanisms. Akt may also phosphorylate some of the trigger proteins of the Bcl-2 family, leading to their sequestration and inability to activate the killer protein subset.

Transformations Related to Dysregulation of Cell Death

p53 is ubiquitously non-functional or mutated in all human tumors. Many tumor cells express Fas ligand (FasL), which can initiate apoptosis in cytotoxic T cells responding to tumorigenesis. Tumors can also express decoy receptors which lack an intracellular death domain, resulting in inability to initiate apoptosis via the death receptor pathway. Loss of caspase 8 or integrins has been associated with a metastatic phenotype. Various isoforms of Akt are found in gastric, ovarian and pancreatic cancers. Elevated NFκB has been implicated in many solid tumors, including gastric and breast cancers, promoting cell survival mechanisms. In metastatic melanoma, APAF-1 can be silenced, leaving the cell unable to assemble the apoptosome.

Therapeutic Opportunities Related to Programmed Cell Death

Many of the chemotherapeutic agents aforementioned (and those mentioned following) are thought to work by causing irreparable DNA damage and inducing apoptosis in susceptible tumor cells via one pathway or another. The fundamental basis of radiotherapy is a similar induction of cell "suicide" via apoptosis engendered through damage of tumor DNA.

Small-molecule drugs that occupy the ATP-binding pocket of the catalytic domain of Akt may represent an approach to restoration of apoptosis sensitivity in cancers. As discussed above, TNFα is a powerful inducer of tumor cell apoptosis. It is used as an antitumor factor upon local intratumoral administration.

Gene Stability and DNA Repair Mechanisms

DNA damage can be produced by many naturally occurring and manmade entities. Mutations can be spontaneous alterations in the chemical structure. They can be a by-product of infidelity of the DNA replication machinery in base-pairing. They can be due to reactive oxygen species (ROS), UV radiation from sunlight, ionizing radiation (usually in the form of gamma radiation), exogenous natural chemicals such as ozone or radon, or exogenous manmade chemicals ingested or absorbed following exposure from use in manufacturing or agriculture. UV radiation tends to cause formation of pyrimidine dimmers, while gamma radiation causes DNA double strand breaks.

Classes of DNA damage include point mutations, frame shift mutations such as translocations, amplifications or deletions, microsatellite instability involving amplification of simple repeating sequences which can cause defects in DNA mismatch repair and whole chromosome loss or gain.

Mechanisms of DNA Repair

To repair DNA damage, the cell employs several mechanisms. Enzymatic photoreactivation involves DNA lyases in combination with energy from the visible light spectrum which restores pyrimidine dimers to their natural state. Transferase enzymes can perform dealkylation of purines in a suicide mechanism resulting in deactivation of the enzyme. Repair of double strand breaks can be performed directly by DNA ligase. Homologous recombination is a method by which an identical sister chromatid or homologous chromosome is used as a template sequence to reconstruct damaged DNA.

Base excision repair involves excision of damaged or inappropriate bases by DNA glycosylases. These empty apurinic or apyrimidinic (AP) spaces are then recognized by specific AP endonucleases which create a larger gap in the sugar-phosphate backbone. DNA polymerases then can fill in the gap using the opposite DNA strand as a template and DNA ligases seal the new bases in place.

Mismatch excision repair utilizes much of the same machinery as base excision repair, however mismatch recognition proteins, e.g. MutH, MutL and MutS, recognize the newly formed DNA strand based on transient hypomethylation of GATC sequences on the new strand, as compared with normal methylation of the parent template strand.

Nucleotide excision repair involves excision of oligonucleotide strands of bulky damage of multiple bases, which requires recognition of the damage by the *repairosome*. This entity consists of DNA helicase for unwinding of the affected DNA segment and formation of an *excision repair bubble*, as well as specific endonucleases which identify the injured strand and excise an approximately 30 base pair sequence around the damaged segment. In this case, strand specificity to distinguish the newly replicated strand from the template requires the products of the CSA and CSB genes.

Transformations Related to Dysfunction of DNA Repair Mechanisms

Defects in a variety of mismatch repair genes create Lynch syndrome, a syndrome of familial colon, ovarian, uterine, gastric and renal cancers. Many other familial diseases with increased malignancy rates involve defects in other pathways for repair of DNA damage (Table 4-1).

Therapeutic Opportunities Related to DNA Repair Mechanisms

Tumors with defects in DNA repair mechanisms, which cause favorable oncogenic phenotypes, may also be more susceptible to chemotherapy which confers overwhelming DNA damage. This, of course, is modulated by the tumor's sensitivity to apoptotic mechanisms still present in the tumor cell. If DNA repair mechanisms could be manipulated in a tumor-selective fashion, it might be possible to enhance chemotherapy-associated DNA damage in tumor, leading to lethal accumulation of mutations. O6-benzylguanine is a DNA-repair inhibiting compound but it has not yet been studied with respect to anti-tumor pharmacology. However, any non-selective inhibitor of DNA repair would likely display high toxicity.

In particular, hematopoietic cells are essentially defenseless against inhibition of DNA repair. Given this susceptibility, current areas of research include viral transfection with DNA repair genes including MGMT or selective chemotherapy. Cells derived prior to therapy would be reinjected before, during or after treatment with DNA repair inhibitors or other chemotherapies with significant bone marrow toxicity. Treatment of the bone marrow cells in this way would provide an advantage over tumor cells by providing selective resistance to DNA damaging chemotherapy.

Angiogenesis

There are several sequential steps involved in the formation of new blood vessel networks in and around tumors. Tumors secrete various proangiogenic factors and enzymes involved in extracellular matrix (ECM) degradation. This is followed by breakdown of the venule wall basement membrane. Migration of endothelial cells into the extracellular matrix results in a new capillary sprout. The endothelial cells divide and proliferate and endothelial progenitor cells are recruited from the bone marrow. Once proliferation has achieved a substantial mass of new endothelial cells, a lumen develops. The basement membrane re-forms around the new capillary loops. Pericytes are then recruited to form a vascular support network.

This sequence of events is quite similar to that which occurs during wound healing and in embryonic development, however tumor vascular networks are often very abnormal in comparison, exhibiting dilated and tortuous vessels and often lacking basement membrane or pericyte support.

Pro- and Anti-angiogenic Factors

Angiogenic factors: Factors which promote angiogenesis are split into two groups: primary or direct factors, whose receptors are found specifically on endothelial cells and secondary or indirect factors, which essentially enhance or upregulate production of the primary factors. Primary factors include the VEGF family and their receptors, the angiopoietins and their receptors and the Notch receptor family and its ligands. IL-6, IL-8, PDGF, G-CSF, acidic and basic fibroblast growth factors (FGFs), TGF-α, TGF-β, steroid sex hormones and EGF receptor ligands have all been found to be secondary, stimulatory factors.

The VEGF family has been described in greater detail previously in this chapter. The angiopoietins are especially important for the later stages of vessel maturation and stabilization. Ang-1 promotes endothelial cell survival and pericyte coverage, while Ang-2 has the opposite effect. Their receptor is tie-2, a tyrosine kinase receptor. Ligands of the Notch receptor family include the delta-like ligands (DLLs) and the Jaggeds. Vascular endothelial cells express notch 1 and notch 4 receptors, as well as DLL4 and Jagged 1. Notch receptors have an intracellular domain which, when stimulated by ligand, is cleaved and translocates directly to the nucleus to act as a transcription co-factor. In embryonic development, this system is required for angiogenesis, however in tumors, it appears to negatively regulate angiogenesis in a paradoxical fashion.

Endogenous inhibitors of angiogenesis: Cytokines such as platelet factor 4, interferons alpha and beta and thrombospondin-1 have been shown to endogenously inhibit angiogenesis. Angiostatin, endostatin and vasostatin are cleaved fragments of the clotting cascade or extracellular matrix proteins (plasminogen, type XVII collagen and calreticulin, respectively) which inhibit angiogenesis. Vasohibin is a paracrine hormone secreted by endothelial cells as a negative feedback mechanism on stimulation with proangiogenic factors such as VEGF.

Transformations Related to Angiogenesis

As previously noted, most invasive tumors overexpress VEGF and/or its receptors. The abnormal vasculature in and around tumors may promote for invasive behavior due to increased vascular permeability.

Therapeutic Opportunities Related to Angiogenesis

Avastin (bevacizumab) is a monoclonal antibody to VEGF, which is given in combination with conventional chemotherapies in the treatment of breast, colorectal and renal cell cancers. Several other VEGF antibodies, receptor inhibitors or soluble receptors are currently being investigated for anti-tumor potential. In addition, cyclo-oxygenase 2 (COX2) inhibitors decrease expression of VEGF and may be important partners in anti-tumor therapy and prevention of primary neoplasia, although their use is still currently being studied.

Invasion and Metastasis

In order to spread from their primary tissue of origin, cancer cells must achieve a number of useful characteristics. First of all, they must exhibit motility. Cell-cell dissociation and loss of adhesion molecules are the first steps in this process, which then allows migration through the tissues, via cytoskeletal reshaping and ECM digestion. Scatter factors (described above) are instrumental in this first step. Cells then migrate utilizing chemotactic gradients such as pH and oxygen tension that polarize them toward blood vessels. The tumor microenvironment may promote or retard invasive behavior by its complement of growth factors, degradative enzymes, cytokines and motility factors, as well as the components of its ECM.

Cellular Adhesion Molecules

Cellular adhesion molecules (CAMs) are molecules containing intracytoplasmic, transmembrane and extracellular domains, whose main functions are anchoring the cell and communicating extracellular information to and from the cell cycle machinery. They can be divided into four groups: integrins, immuno-globulin (Ig)-like CAMs, cadherins and selectins. *Integrins* form heterodimers between α and β subunits, generally attach to ECM components such as fibronectin and lamellin and serve important functions in cell-cell and cell-ECM signaling (including providing an alternative pathway for apoptosis as noted above). *Ig-CAMs* are expressed mainly on nervous tissues (NCAM) and in the vasculature (VCAM and ICAM) and are important for pairing with integrins of leukocytes needed for adhesion and emigration of leukocytes through vessel walls. *Cadherins* (N/neural, P/platelet and E/endothelial varieties) form homologous zippers by binding to an opposite cadherin in a calcium dependent fashion. Their cytoplasmic domains are anchored to the cytoskeleton by catenins. They localize in adherence junctions forming adhesion belts which connect with the actin-containing cytoskeleton and play important roles in morphogenesis and histogenesis. *Selectins* mediate the early, weaker adhesion of flowing leukocytes to the endothelium (also known as rolling) as a precursor to the Ig-CAM-mediated firmer adhesion and emigration. They bind to the carbohydrate ligand sialyl Lewis X (affectionately referred to as "sticky sugar"). L-selectin is expressed on the leukocytes, P-selectin on the platelets and E-selectin on the endothelium.

ECM degradation is performed by four families of enzymes: matrix metalloproteinases (MMPs, which include interstitial collagenases, stromelysins and gelatinases), adamalysin-related membrane proteinases, bone morphogenetic protein type 1 (BMP1) metallo-proteinases and tissue serine proteases such as tissue plasminogen activator (tPA), urokinase, thrombin and plasmin. The major substrates of these enzymes are 13 types of collagens, proteoglycans, laminins, fibronectins and vitronectins. Separate ECM compartments contain different complements of these matrix materials; for instance, collagens I and III are found mainly in the stroma, whereas the basement membrane includes mostly collagens IV and V.

Once cancer cells have reached the vasculature, they must be able to intravasate into surrounding blood or lymph vessels, requiring an ability to degrade the basement membrane of the vessel. Intravasation may be enhanced by the abnormal peri-tumoral vasculature which tends to have increased permeability and may even lack a basement membrane in some areas. MMP-2 and MMP-9 (also known as gelatinases A and B) are type IV collagenases involved in breakdown of the basement membrane and can be secreted by tumor cells.

Once they have entered the vasculature, cancer cells must survive in the circulation against significant physical stressors. They encounter the shear forces inherent in blood flow and mechanical arrest in small diameter vessels. In the hepatic sinusoids, mechanical impaction by tumor cells activates the hepatocytes to secrete nitric oxide, which can cause apoptosis of the arrested tumor cells. They must evade the immune system's surveillance cells which are capable of killing them, either directly via the perforin-granzyme pathway or indirectly through engaging them with TNF-related molecules such as FasL (CD95L) or TRAIL. Endothelial cells also protect against wandering tumor cells through expression of DARC, one of the Duffy blood group glycoproteins. DARC interacts with KAI1, a metastasis suppressor gene expressed on many tumor cells which, when ligated, causes them to enter senescence.

Arrest of the cancer cell can be caused by cancer cell-endothelial cell interactions via surface adhesion molecules, or can be due to a tumor cell or thrombus simply getting physically lodged in a capillary bed through which it is too big to travel. If cancer cells do survive impaction in a distant organ's capillary bed, they must then extravasate, or at least physically disrupt the capillary through intravascular growth in order to enter the parenchyma. Some tumor cells express selectins,

allowing them to extravasate in a manner similar to leukocytes. Many also overexpress VEGF, which can result in increased vascular permeability and loosening of endothelial cell junctions, aiding tumor cell egress through capillary walls.

Finally, a tumor cell must adapt to growth in its new microenvironment to sustain itself. Organ tropism describes the phenomenon by which certain tumors appear predictably in certain organs when metastasizing. For some tumors, this predictability may have to do with the first capillary bed or the next closest organ that the tumor cell encounters upon invasion. For instance, ovarian cancers frequently spread directly onto the peritoneum and liver capsule and breast cancers will often spread into the chest wall. Colon cancer often metastasizes to the liver and ovarian cancer and sarcomas to the lung (the first capillary beds encountered).

However, this is overly simplistic when noting that breast cancer also often spreads to the liver or ovaries, lung cancer to the adrenals and bone in the form of osteoclastic lesions and prostate cancer to the bone in the form of osteoblastic lesions. Clearly there must be other mechanisms by which tumor cells select their bed of metastatic spread (or vice versa). Circulating leukocytes and stem cells are known to use chemokines mechanisms to home in on specific organs. Chemokines may additionally play a large role in organ tropism of metastatic tumor cells.

Cancer-related Disturbance of Cell Adhesion, Interaction and Invasiveness

While well-differentiated tumors tend to retain E-cadherin expression, poorly differentiated tumors with greater invasive potential have often lost this CAM. E-cadherin can be down-regulated in a number of manners, including decreased transcription (by growth factors or transcriptional repressors like SNAIL, SLUG and TWIST), phosphorylation resulting in degradation and hypermethylation of encoding DNA, resulting in epigenetic silencing. The end result remains decreasing cell-cell contact inhibition. Cancer cells also tend to alter the integrins that they express, switching to those that promote survival and migration, through mechanisms such as recruitment of matrix metalloproteinases to the leading edge of cancer spread.

Therapeutic Opportunities Related to Cell Adhesion, Interaction and Invasion

The possibility to treat cancer using small molecule inhibitors of matrix metalloproteinases (particularly MMP9) involved in cancer cell invasiveness and anti-integrin antibodies is a subject of current preclinical studies and multiple clinical trials. Although there is no currently established therapy based on the paradigm of the inhibition of cell adhesiveness or cell motility, recent mouse studies demonstrated the promise of such approaches in limiting the metastatic spread of cancer as well as survival of tumor cells.

Conclusion

The normal human cell counts on multiple overlapping and multi-step protective mechanisms to impede malignant transformation. Because of the complementary and interdependent nature of many of these biological pathways, more than one transformation is needed to turn a normal cell into a malignant one. After multiple deleterious genomic changes occur, normal cells can acquire the phenotypic characteristics needed for malignant growth, as noted in the seven segments above. Though the biology is quite complex and still not entirely understood, recent research has come a long way in understanding the many genetic and biologic alterations affecting cancerous cells and this knowledge base informs future therapeutic possibilities. As our knowledge of the cellular and molecular biology of cancer continues to grow, new therapies with increased efficacy and decreased toxicity can be developed to treat the complex system of dysfunction at work in the cancer cell.

Landmark Papers

1. Hanahan D, Weinberg RA. The hallmarks of cancer. Cell 2000;100: 57-70.
2. Kanduc D, et al. Cell death: apoptosis vs necrosis. Int J Oncol 2002;21: 165-70.
3. Hirohashi S, Kanai Y. Cell adhesion system and human cancer morphogenesis. Cancer Sci 2003;94: 575-81.
4. Yang L, Moses HL. Transforming growth factor beta: tumor suppressor or promoter? Are Host Immune Cells the Answer? Cancer Res 2008;68: 9107-11.
5. Zhao RC, Zhu YS, Shi Y. New hope for cancer treatment: exploring the distinction between normal adult stem cells and cancer stem cells. Pharmacol Ther 2008;119: 74-82.
6. Eichhorn ME, et al. Angiogenesis in cancer: molecular mechanisms, clinical impact. Langenbecks Arch Surg 2007;392: 371-9.
7. Hunter KW, et al. Mechanisms of metastasis. Breast Cancer Res 2008;10 Suppl 1: S2.
8. Budzowska M, Kanaar R. Mechanisms of dealing with DNA-damage induced replication problems. Cell Biochem Biophys 2009;53: 17-31.

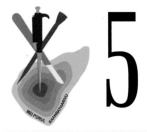

5

Methods of Investigation of Cancer

Jan Franko, Pragatheeshwar Thirunavukarasu

This chapter focuses on health care driven cancer research by clinicians. Aspects of translational, clinical and population research are discussed. Laboratory research is an important component of surgical oncology investigation, however, it is not a subject of this chapter.

The key elements of fruitful and beneficial clinical research are as follows:

- Established research question
- Assembled and motivated team
- Development of protocol
- Implementation and continued re-evaluation of protocol
- Data analysis and description
- Critical discussion of outcomes
- Selection of publication methods
- Subsequent and follow-up research.

Formulating a Research Question

Formulating a good research question is first and a crucial part in research design. Obscurity and ambiguity should be avoided while formulating the theme question. In essence, the central question of the research design should be made explicitly clear.

A good research question originates from a deep understanding of problem and available knowledge. Literature research helps to establish and shape a good question. Good literature research also avoids researching irrelevant questions. Oftentimes, a good question comes from a mentor. The research questions should be:

- *Interesting:* Once you have your research question you can imagine possible outcomes of your study. A simple test is to ask, *"Who cares?"* or *"So what?"* If no difference in is made by these simple tests, it is likely that the research question is not interesting and relevant.
- *Feasible*: There should be enough resources to actually conduct study. Many studies fail because of low number of subjects and/or events. Similarly, a long follow-up of poorly selected end-point may preclude successful study completion. Technical expertise may not be available for studied subject. Prohibitive and

unforeseen costs can stop any project. Too many end-points and research questions within a single study usually result in no meaningful outcome.

- *Novel*: Studies of well-established facts are likely to fail to produce valuable outcomes. However, research that invalidates theories based on prior research may be valuable. Novel inquiries, the answering of which furthers understanding and leads to more inquiries that may further potentiate better understanding are the most welcome in the field of research.
- *Ethical*: If the study has ethical limitations (e.g. unjustified risk or privacy loss), it will not be approved by the IRB (Institutional Review Board) and should not be attempted. Difficult ethical dilemmas should be discussed with institutional ethicist and the IRB. A minimum education in ethics is advisable for all researchers. The NIH provides one of these programs online (http://phrp.nihtraining.com/index.php).
- *Relevant*: Relevant research outcomes, whether positive or negative, have an important impact on our understanding, diagnosis, treatment and decision making in cancer care. Irrelevant questions are not only a waste of time but also resources. Questions with uncertain relevance require additional literature research and discussion to establish their worthiness to study. Many irrelevant questions may, however, become highly relevant with time and new scientific developments. For example, ability of modern chemotherapy to downsize liver colorectal cancer metastases opened a substantial research field on survival benefit in previously unresectable patients and on associated hepatotoxicity. Without development of modern chemotherapy, there would be no reason to consider inoperable patients for further surgical research.

Primary and Secondary Research Questions

Primary research question is related to a *primary end-point*. It is the most important outcome measure. Additionally, statistical considerations are typically tied to the primary end-point, for example, calculation of study power and sample size are related to primary-end point.

Nevertheless, valuable information can be obtained for secondary questions. They typically lack determination of statistical power, but may elucidate some questions and be a basis for future theories. *Secondary end-points* cannot therefore provide level I evidence, but frequently are an important source of clinical information. For example, the primary end-point of CONKO-1 trial in pancreatic cancer was disease-free survival. One of the secondary questions answered in that trial was that efficacy of gemcitabine is present for both completely resected and incompletely resected pancreatic cancer patients.

Assembling and Motivating Research Team

All current cancer research is done by a team and not by a single individual. Even "simple" retrospective research by students, residents and/or fellows usually involves a faculty member. Selection of appropriate team members with expertise and acceptable interpersonal relationships can make or fail research. This becomes even more prominent while designing larger studies, especially large international prospective randomized studies. At absolute minimum, the team involves cancer researcher and/or clinician plus a statistician. Retrospective studies frequently involve honest brokers, basic scientists and supportive staff. Prospective study teams additionally involve ethicists, regulatory and administrative personnel, data and safety monitoring personnel and interviewers.

Motivation of team members is of a great importance. Although major studies typically employ salaried personnel, much basic and retrospective research is done because of personal interest of team members. Early determination of authorship and development of presentation plan help appropriate motivation.

Development of Protocol

Study plan is described in a *research protocol*. This document covers all aspects of the study which includes:
- Background, rationale and objective
- Methods
- Study subjects and population, together with inclusion and exclusion criteria
- Preplanned analysis, calculation of statistical power and risk thresholds
- Expected method of reporting
- Timeline
- Budget and financial considerations
- Personnel aspects
- Ethical considerations

Well-written protocol is a great referral for future problems with the study as well as a base for writing scientific reports. Time spent in developing a protocol allows for anticipation of many problems and helps solving unanticipated problems. Implementation and continued re-evaluation of protocol is a natural process during all studies. Good initial planning is, however, essential to avoid major changes, which may invalidate all completed parts of research. Research protocol evolves from a single sentence (*research question*) to *study outline* (key elements of the study), *study protocol* (expansion of outline) and *operations manual* (specific instructions and details of each research component).

Data Description and Analysis

Data Management

Data management is seemingly unimportant until one or more of the following problems occur:
- data loss because of insufficient back up
- unrecognized data loss and mismatch while repeatedly updating master data file
- problem with analysis because data type does not fit statistical package.

Additionally, data management and safety are of concern because of possible personal information loss. IRBs require adequate security measures for paper, electronic and other data storage systems. Most researchers use a Windows based platform. Although back up can be automated, researcher has to assume a significant role in data safety and perform periodic back ups. Macintosh based systems can easily be set-up for periodic back up procedure.

Power, Sample Size and Effect Size

Selection of study type, appropriate data format and planned procedures for analysis should be done before data collection. Exhaustive description of statistical procedures is outside of this chapter scope. There are numerous statistical guides in medical literature. Excellent series were published in the *British Medical Journal* (Greenhalgh 1997a; Greenhalgh 1997b; Vickers and Altman 2001). Please refer to section "Statistical software and Internet resources" (below) for links to online statistical resources.

Study power $(1-\beta)$, *type II error* (β), *type I error* (α), *sample size* and *effect size* are related measures of effectiveness of study to reach or refute hypothesis. Too small study with too small effect size cannot be expected to answer a clinical question—it can happen only by a chance—a process we attempt to avoid in science. Prospective studies without appropriate power are to be considered unethical, because they expose subjects to unjustified risk (no chance to detect the truth) and waste resources. Statistical power of the study (ability to detect difference if one truly exists) is increased when more subjects are involved, difference between study groups is large, variability of subjects within groups small and observation period is long. Type I error (α) is usually set to 0.05 (5%) or less. It describes

TABLE 5-1	Factors affecting power and sample size	
Factors		**Power**
↓ Significance level (higher α)		↑
↑ Group difference (effect size)		↑
↑ Number of events (~ follow up time)		↑
↑ Standard deviation within groups		↓
↑ Sample size		↑
Factors		**Sample size**
↑ Standard deviation within groups		↑
↑ Group difference (effect size)		↓
↑ Significance level (lower α)		↓
↑ Number of events (~ follow up time)		↓
↑ Power (1 - β)		↓

the chance that the results of the study are achieved by pure chance and therefore do not represent the truth. Type II error is by convention 0.2 or 0.1, but can achieve any value between 0 and 1. It describes probability that we fail to detect the difference, which actually truly exists. Therefore (1-β) expression relates to power to find the difference if one exists. For more information, see **Table 5-1**. The longer the observation in survival studies, the higher power is achieved. Power in survival studies is actually related to number of events, which is obviously a function of time **(Figure 5-1)**. Easy way to estimate power and sample size for various studies is by a freely available program *Power Sample Size* (see below).

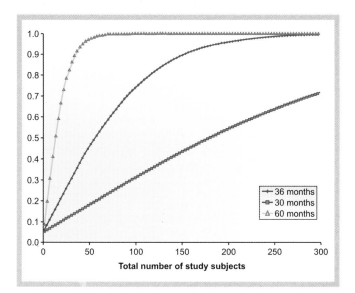

Figure 5-1: Relationship of a required number of study subjects and study power. Assumes median survival 24 months in control group. Effect size is expressed as a median survival in experimental group 1 (30 months median survival, red line), group 2 (36 months median survival, blue line) and group 3 (60 months median survival, yellow line)

Statistical Software and Internet Resources

A statistical software is essential to perform adequate analysis. Microsoft Excel provides basic functions, which can be extended by add-ons. There are several available spreadsheets with automated functions for easy calculation of basic statistics and sample size (http://www.epibiostat.ucsf.edu/dcr). Specialized statistical software can be open source (i.e. free) or commercially available. Open source projects include both simple products like OpenStat (http://www.statpages.org/miller/openstat/), or for high-end statistics platform like R-project (requires substantial experience, http://www.r-project.org/). Power and sample size calculation can be easily performed using an excellent Windows-based program *PowerSampleSize* made freely available by William Dupont and Walton Plummer (http://biostat.mc.vanderbilt.edu/twiki/bin/view/Main/PowerSampleSize). There are many available commercial software products with perhaps some are used more commonly. The author has experience with several comprehensive packages, including STATISTICA (www.statsoft.com), SPSS (easy to use, www.spss.com), SAS (complex high-end product, www.sas.com) and STATA (stands somewhere between SPSS and SAS in robustness and complexity, www.stata.com). There are many great resources on the Internet, including web-based textbooks (http://www.statsoft.com/textbook/stathome.html, http://www.statpages.org). UCLA provides easy-to-use website with guides for major statistical packages (http://www.ats.ucla.edu/stat).

Whatever software used, there are two following steps to perform before actual pre-planned analysis:
- Always summarize data before you perform other analyses;
- Always plot data.

After these steps one looks for outliers and identifies their explanation. Inputting errors may constitute 15-20% of all errors in large datasets. Before rejecting any observation as an outlier, specific tests for outliers have to be employed. It is not acceptable to reject data as outliers after performing planned analysis, especially if removing outlier changes the outcome of analysis. Such outliers that heavily influence outcome are called *influential points*. In some cases, *analysis of missing data* can be performed. Additionally, there are methods to "predict" missing data, such as *imputation*.

Cancer Epidemiology

Occurrence of cancer is described in epidemiological terms. *Incidence* refers to a number of *new* cases and *prevalence* refers to all active cases. Useful terms are defined in **Table 5-2.** Two items have to be clearly declared when using epidemiological terms: the *population* and *time period*

TABLE 5-2	Mathematical expressions of epidemiological terms	
Term	**Definition**	**Description**
Incidence	$\dfrac{\text{\# new cases}}{\text{\# population at risk}}$	Number of newly diagnosed cases during a specific time period.
Prevalence	$\dfrac{\text{\# cases alive}}{\text{\# population at risk}}$	Number of cases of a disease that are present in a particular population at a given time.
Mortality rate	$\dfrac{\text{\# cancer deaths}}{\text{\# population at risk}}$	Number of deaths due to cancer in a particular population at a given time.
Case fatality rate	$\dfrac{\text{\# disease death}}{\text{\# population with disease}}$	Ratio of number of deaths due to disease to number of cases diagnosed with the particular disease.
Proportional mortality ratio	$\dfrac{\text{\# disease deaths}}{\text{\# total deaths}}$	Ratio of deaths due to a particular disease to total number of deaths in a given population.
Odds ratio	$\dfrac{\text{\# Exposure odds cases}}{\text{\# Exposure odds controls}}$	The ratio of the odds of an event occurring in one group to the odds of it occurring in another group.
Relative risk	$\dfrac{\text{Incidence exposed}}{\text{Incidence unexposed}}$	Relative risk is a ratio of probability of the event occurring (incidence) in the exposed group versus a non-exposed group.
Attributable risk (ATR)	incidence exposed – incidence unexposed	The difference in the incidence of a disease between exposed and non-exposed groups.
Relative risk reduction (RRR)	RRR = (ER control - ER experimental)/ ER control ER = Event Rate	Percent reduction in risk in the experimental group as compared with the control group.
Absolute risk reduction (ARR)	ARR= ER control - ER experimental	The difference between the control group's event rate and the experimental group's event rate.
Number needed to treat (NNT)	NNT=1/ARR	Number of patients that would need to be treated over the time course of the study to prevent one bad outcome.

in question. Substantial differences may exist among different populations in different time periods. For example, incidence of melanoma in some Australian regions is as high as 50 new cases per 100,000 inhabitants per year since late 1980s. Swedish population at the same time has approximately only 15 new cases. A rising trend in melanoma was documented in Sweden (10 to 30-fold increase since 1960s till 1990s) and many other countries, including the USA. Some other cancers have decreasing trends, notably gastric cancer and lung cancer in men (but not in women). Incidence, prevalence and mortality can have discordant trends, as evidenced for breast cancer. Although the incidence of breast cancer never declined, mortality after year 2000 declined, presumably due to withdrawal of hormonal replacement therapy, improved diagnostics and treatment.

Much of epidemiological data needs to be *adjusted* (*standardized*) for influential factors before any reasonable comparison is made. Age-adjustment is most common type of data adjustment. Consider a theoretical example of pancreatic cancer incidence in coastal city with a large retirement community compared to a nearby college town. Since pancreatic cancer is more common in elders,

unadjusted incidence rates will clearly point to an unknown "risk factor" in our costal city, because more elderly people live there. Standardization calculates incidence rates across age strata (e.g. by age decades: incidence for 20+ year old, 30+ year old, etc.). Age stratum-specific rate is then applied to a population of entire geographic area. Adjustment is a critical necessity when comparing data across populations and institutions. Substantial differences exist among populations presenting to major tertiary centers versus community hospitals. For example, to adjust for initial patient differences, multiple preoperative factors are analyzed in the *National Surgical Quality Improvement Project*. This risk-adjustment was initially developed in Veteran Affairs hospitals (Daley, Forbes, et al 1997) and then successfully implemented outside of the VA system to report risk-adjusted quality outcomes.

Number needed to treat (NNT) is the number of patients that would need to be treated over the time course of the study to prevent one bad outcome. Similarly, one can express *number needed to harm* in toxicology studies and adverse reaction studies. Both patients and physicians are more likely to favor a particular therapy if it is expressed in terms of *relative risk reduction* (usually large number), as opposed to *number needed to treat*. Number needed to treat is however preferred because it takes in account *absolute risk reduction* (usually small number).

Epidemiologic data and diagnostic tests are related through contingency tables. The basic contingency table is 2 × 2 table. Common definitions of measures of diagnostic tests are presented in **Tables 5-3 and 5-4**.

The most important measures of test performance are sensitivity and specificity. Predictive values are dependent on particular population, but sensitivity and specificity of the test remains stable. The specific cut-off values for a diagnostic test are established by a test developer from what is called *Receiver Operator Curves* (ROC).

A *likelihood ratio* (LR) is the proportion of sick people with a given test result divided by the proportion of well people who have the same test result. Ideally, positive (= abnormal) test results are more common in sick people than well people (high LR+) and negative (= normal) test results are more common in well people than sick (low LR -). Likelihood ratios relate pre- and post test probability of disease and therefore should greatly impact clinical judgment. Likelihood ratio of 1 is completely unhelpful: there is no influence of a test on post-test probability of disease. LR >10 helps to rule in the diagnosis and LR < 0.1 helps to rule out the diagnosis.

TABLE 5-3	2 x 2 Contingency table for diagnostic test performance.		
		Disease status (M)	
		M+	M-
Test results	Positive	'a' True positives	'b' False positives
	Negative	'c' False positives	'd' True negatives

More complex tables involving indeterminate test results can be constructed (e.g. 3 x 2)

Cross-sectional Studies

Cross-sectional studies provide a 'snapshot' characteristic for any given malignancy. These studies have purely descriptive character. Therefore they provide a reflection of association but do not study cause-effect relationship. Generalizations from cross-sectional studies may be significantly misleading unless appropriate sampling is used. If a cross-sectional study of gastric cancer selects its sample from San Francisco area (high percentage of Asian immigrants) generalization on national level will lead to overestimate of gastric cancer incidence and related characteristics. One of the well-known cross-sectional studies is the National Health and Nutrition Examination

TABLE 5-4	Measures of performance of the diagnostic test	
Measure of performance	**Expression**	**Question addressed**
True-positive rate (*sensitivity*)	$\dfrac{a}{a+c}$	How good is this test at picking up people with this disease?
False-negative rate	$\dfrac{c}{c+a}$	How likely is this test to fail to identify people with disease
True-negative rate (*specificity*)	$\dfrac{d}{b+d}$	How good is this test at correctly excluding people without the disease?
False-positive rate	$\dfrac{b}{b+d}$	How likely is this test to wrongly identify people without disease as sick?
Positive predictive value	$\dfrac{a}{a+b}$	If a person tests positive, what is the probability that he/she actually has the condition?
Negative predictive value	$\dfrac{d}{c+d}$	If a person tests negative, what is the probability that he/she actually does not have the condition?
Accuracy	$\dfrac{a+d}{a+b+c+d}$	What is the overall precision of the test?
Likelihood ratio positive	$= (a/a+c)/(b/b+d)$	How much more likely is a positive test found in someone with the disease than in someone without it?
Likelihood ratio negative	$(c/a+c)/(d/b+d)$	How much more likely is a negative test found in someone with the disease than in someone without it?

Survey (NHANES, www.cdc.gov/nchs/nhanes.htm). This study has collected broad U.S. nutrition and health information. Estimates of weight (including pediatric), blood pressure, infectious disease (e.g. HIV, HCV, STD, HPV) and thyroid and liver function tests were established. Pediatric growth charts were created using data from this study and removal of lead from gasoline and paint products was legislated after data collection from this study as well.

Case-control Studies

Case-control studies represent an important research tool. They are especially suited for study of rare events, such as: cancer, development of malignant bowel obstruction in colorectal cancer patients, prevalence of extrapancreatic cancers in patients with pancreatic intraductal papillary mucinous neoplasms, development of lung metastases from follicular cell thyroid cancer or ventricular tachycardia among patients receiving adriamycin. Risk is expressed as *odds ratio*. Study population generally consists of two groups: (1) *cases*, group with 'disease', for example, bowel obstruction from colorectal cancer and (2) *controls*, group with similar characteristics, but without 'disease', for example, patients with colorectal cancer but no bowel obstruction. Selection of control group is usually challenging and actually more important than case-group. *Selection bias* and *recall bias* are common and may result in false findings.

Ability to study rare events is the main strength of this study design. They are also very useful in generating hypotheses, because they can readily identify many potential risk factors. On the other hand, there is little information about population characteristics and susceptibility to bias is very high. A good way to minimize bias is to perform matching. *Matching* procedure selects case and control with similar characteristics in selected features. This ensures that cases and controls are comparable with respect to matched factors. Typical matching variables include gender, age, disease stage, etc. Matching can greatly improve comparability of study groups. Unfortunately, matching can be done on known risk factors only. Unknown risk factors can be equally distributed in randomized studies only. *Frequency matching* ensures that both case and control group are matched, but no individual case-control pair is matched. *Systematic matching* ensures that specific case-control cases are matched to selected variables (e.g. age, gender and cancer stage). Latter technique requires specific statistical methods for analysis, whereas frequency matching can be analyzed using common methods.

Modifications of case-control study are (1) studies with two or more control groups, (2) *case-cohort studies* and (3) *case-crossover studies*. Each of these study types can be 'nested' within other larger study, which can reduce costs

further. Nested design is used when (1) certain laboratory measurements are expensive, or (2) certain laboratory measurements are not available or known when samples are collected. Typically, (1) a dataset of a large cohort study performed for other reason is available and (2) entire cohort study has banked specimen of interest. Investigators then identify cases and controls and only then perform expensive testing on samples stored from the past.

How to Detect Causality

Association of factors may or may not represent *causality*, or *cause-effect* relationship. It is known that majority of pancreatic cancers carry *KRAS* mutation. It remains unproven, however, whether *KRAS* mutation is a cause or effect of pancreatic cancer. Additionally, *spurious association* due to *random error* is common, unless study α is set low (type I error).

Confounding is present when a third factor associates with both cause and effect. Typical confounder in early melanoma studies was sunscreen exposure. In fact, many early melanoma studies from 1960s pointed sunscreen exposure as a risk factor for melanoma, rather than sunburn. Causality is favored if results are *consistent* with prior experience, association is *strong*, *dose-response* association is seen, appropriate *temporal relationship* exists (cause precedes effect) and relationship is *biologically plausible*.

Causal effect can be underestimated due to confounders. There are many strategies used to deal with confounders, including propensity scoring, stratification, adjustments and /or matching.

Prospective Trials

Prospective trials are experimental studies evaluating active therapy for cancer. Therefore their character is experimental, rather than observational. A subset of these studies, *phase III prospective trials*, have *randomized* and often *blinded* character. Phase III studies represent highest available experimental evidence available to date.

Testing of a new candidate drug in humans goes through a series of rigorous experimental studies. Pharmacokinetic studies on healthy volunteers are done prior to phase I studies and are sometimes referred to as phase 0 trials. The initial dose for phase 0 and phase I trial is determined from animal studies and is usually at 10% of LD_{10}. As one can expect, there are many drug going into phase I trials, but only a few reach phase III and even fewer reach clinical practice.

A *phase I trial* is typically a nonrandomized experimental study with a single experimental group. Such a study evaluates safety and efficacy of a new treatment, with emphasis on safety. Safety of each drug/approach is tested first in a phase I trial. For example, neurotoxicity of oxaliplatin was published with early phase I trial among patients with various advanced cancers. The primary endpoint of typical phase I trial is a *phase II recommended dose* (P2RD: optimal dose, which will be tested in phase II study). Some drugs, like gemcitabine, have gone directly into phase II studies.

Phase II studies again test safety and efficacy, but scientific emphasis is on efficacy. A typical phase II study is larger than phase I. By design it may be either a randomized trial of two groups, or a single experimental group, comparing efficacy to historical controls. It may be combined with the first phase to form phase I/II study. Phase II study is sometimes split into two segments: IIA further refines issues of dosing; IIB is purely designed to investigate the efficacy. Clinical efficacy can be measured in various ways: (1) radiological response, for example, RECIST criteria **(Table 5-5)**; (2) biochemical response, for example, drop in PSA in prostate cancer; (3) overall or progression-free survival; (4) quality of life and other ways. Favorable response rates and progression-free survival were observed for both oxaliplatin for metastatic colorectal cancer and gemcitabine for pancreatic cancer in phase II studies.

Phase III trials form a backbone of our understanding and clinical knowledge. The number of patients is typically 400 and more, sometime up to tens of thousands. These are *prospective randomized* studies, many times *single blinded* (evaluating clinicians are blinded) or *double-blinded* (both patient and clinicians blinded). It is nearly impossible to create a surgical trial with blinded patients, although it has been done before. A famous study in orthopedic surgery randomized patients to arthroscopic washout and cartilage debridement versus placebo operation without any intervention (Moseley, O'Malley et al 2002). The patients had spinal anesthesia; therefore length of shame operation was made appropriate. In fact, TV monitors played back an unrelated tape of some other arthroscopic operation creating a perfect illusion to patients. Arthroscopic surgery was found of no value in knee osteoarthritis is this blinded study.

Although it would be difficult to create such a trial in surgical oncology, several examples document ethically sound trials with substantially different surgical approach between study arms; for example, wide local excision versus amputation for extremity sarcoma or NSABP trial of mastectomy versus lumpectomy for breast cancer. These trials established current standard of care, but at the time of their inception and presentation they were revolutionary.

Randomization is the only protection against bias. Loss of randomization invalidates entire trial. The purpose of randomization is to evenly distribute all risk factors among the experimental group, keeping in mind that many disease risk factors are not fully known or understood even today. There are several statistical methods to deal with confounders and group imbalances. There is, however, no better method than randomization to establish groups comparable at baseline. It is the only method, which evenly distributes even unknown prognostic and predictive factors. In this respect, one has to acknowledge, that there may be patients who are unwilling to randomize and therefore they will not enter trial. These subjects may be bearers of traits important for disease and/or treatment. Therefore characterization and reporting of *screened* versus *enrolled* patients is important.

Worse, subjects who are unwilling to get randomized and are not blinded, may *withdraw consent* and further participation. This violates *intention-to-treat* analysis and if there are many subjects withdrawing, the trial may fail. Intention-to-treat and randomization are two cornerstones of proper phase III trial conduct and reporting. Reporting *per treatment* (treatment actually received, rather than assigned) may generate interesting hypotheses and be clinically useful. There is, however, little if any scientific value to such reporting. *Modified intention-to-treat analysis* is sometimes presented. In such an analysis some randomized patients are removed post-randomization from analysis. Acceptable reasons to perform post-randomization removal from the study include inappropriate entry to randomization and some others.

Measures of Outcome and Endpoints

Each study investigates its objective by specific outcome measures. Outcome measures are defined and measurable factors. There has to be a reliable and accurate tool to perform such measurements. Outcome measures of prospective studies are classically called endpoints.

Outcome measures can be simple factors as weight, concentration of tumor marker, or length of survival from randomization. There are more complex endpoints in some trials: for example "clinical benefit", defined as a combination of weight, pain and performance status, was studies in advanced symptomatic pancreatic cancer by Burris et al. That landmark study led to approval of gemcitabine for treatment of advanced pancreatic cancer. Similar quality of life measures are increasingly common.

Radiologic response of tumors has been long considered an important surrogate for drug effectiveness. After modification of several schemes most commonly used are Response Evaluation Criteria in Solid Tumors (RECIST, http://ctep.cancer.gov/protocolDevelopment/docs/quickrcst.doc) (see **Table 5-5**). There are, however, many problems with these criteria. For example, GIST tumors and many CNS tumors do not shrink despite favorable response and associated clinical benefit. Many other factors are being investigated, among them CT density, metabolism on PET scan, etc.

TABLE 5-5		Response evaluation criteria in solid tumors (RECIST). All radiologic lesions are classified as either *target* or *non-target*. There are specific requirements for target lesion (e.g. a minimum 10 mm diameter on CT)
Complete response	CR	Disappearance of all target lesions
Partial response	PR	30% Decrease in the sum of the longest diameter of target lesions
Stable disease	SD	Small changes that do not meet other categories
Progressive disease	PD	20% Increase in the sum of the longest diameter of target lesions

Overall survival is a relatively easy measurable endpoint, typically calculated from randomization or study inception till death from any cause. Overall survival will remain the most important indicator of treatment effectiveness together with quality of life. Because it may take many years to establish reasonable overall survival difference or equality, other measures obtained over shorter period were developed. *Disease-free survival* is the length of time during which a patient survives with no sign of a specific disease. It has been accepted as a reasonable endpoint of trials for metastatic colorectal cancer, therefore it serves as a *surrogate endpoint*. Pancreatic cancer usually leads quickly to demise of patients and therefore a need for surrogate endpoint is less needed. One has to remember that a surrogate endpoint is an approximation to other clinical variable. For example, overall survival of mastectomy versus lumpectomy was not significantly different after five years of observation in NSABP study, whereas disease-free survival was. This changed with longer follow-up reports.

Progression-free survival (PFS) is a term used to describe the length of time from randomization to first documentation of objective tumor progression, or to death due to any cause, whichever occurs first.

Time to progression (TTP, *time to recurrence*) is defined as the time from randomization/observation to the first documented disease recurrence. For subjects who had not recurred at the time of analysis, TTR is censored at their last date of evaluation.

Duration of response (DR) is defined as the time from the first documentation of objective tumor response (complete response [CR] or partial response [PR]) that is subsequently confirmed to the first documentation of objective tumor progression or death due to any cause. DR can be calculated for the subgroup of patients with objective response only.

Objective response rate (ORR) is defined as the percent of patients with confirmed complete response or

confirmed partial response according to the RECIST, relative to the total analysis population. Confirmed responses are those that persist on repeat imaging study ≥ 4 weeks after initial documentation of response. Designation of best response of SD requires the criteria to be met at least 6 weeks after randomization/study start.

Traditional and Alternative Clinical Trial Design

Phase I trials are traditionally designed according to modified Fibonacci schema **(Figure 5-2)**.

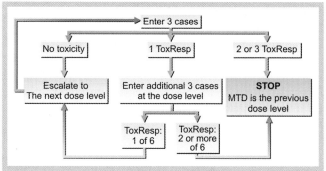

Figure 5-2: Modified Fibonacci schema. ToxResp = toxic response is any Grade III or higher toxicity as defined by Common Terminology Criteria for Adverse Events (CTCAE). MTD = maximum tolerated dose.

The starting dose is usually defined based on preclinical studies on at minimum 2 subhuman species, where LD_{10} is defined (lethal dose for 10% of experimental animals). Phase I starting dose is usually one-tenth of LD_{10} of the most sensitive animal species.

To standardize toxicity reporting the National Cancer Institute implemented *Common Terminology Criteria for Adverse Events* (CTCAE) with the most recent version (3rd edn) published in 2006 (http://ctep.cancer.gov/protocolDevelopment/electronic_applications/ctc.htm#ctc_v30).

Fibonacci scheme eliminates high-risk of toxicities, but requires many patients to be treated at relatively ineffective doses. Those patients are unlikely to derive significant benefit. With many drugs available and needed to be tested, there is not enough patients to enter phase I trials. More importantly, this schema may be ethically outdated because of a large number of undertreated individuals. Therefore several alternative designs were proposed, although there is no consensus how to approach this ethical and resource dilemma. Pharmacologically guided trials define drug area under curve from preclinical studies and modify enrollment schema. Stochastic predictive model is used to determine relationship of *dose-limiting toxicity* in *continuous reassessment*. Accelerated Phase I design receives a lot of attention because it uses (1) a single patient at initial and early doses and (2) large increment in next dose level until grade II toxicity is observed. It then reverts into traditional Fibonacci schema. Therefore fewer patients are exposed to lower and ineffective drug treatment. Some also recommended to initiate phase I trials with higher initial dose, especially with drugs where favorable toxic-to-therapeutic ratio is expected. This may be particularly true for biological agents.

Similar ethical and resource dilemmas are faced in phase III trial design. The appropriate research question is the most important initial consideration for phase III trials. These studies consume large financial and personnel resources. To justify utilization of large financial and personnel resources and patients sacrifice, a true clinical *equipoise* has to exist. If a knowledgeable researcher cannot make rational decision on treatment (even for self or a close family member), than the equipoise (dilemma) probably exists. For example, mastectomy was the traditional treatment of breast cancer based on 19th century case observations formulated by Halsted. Although many practitioners and patients alike refused to follow up traditional "standard of care", it was not until NSABP trials when equality of mastectomy and lumpectomy plus radiation was established. Treatment is also expected to bring a *substantial* benefit. For example, in 2005, FDA approved the use of erlotinib for treatment of advanced pancreatic cancer based on a study, which demonstrated statistically significant survival benefit ($p = 0.038$). Not often it is known that the length of this benefit was approximately 13 days longer survival (5.9 versus 6.4 months). On the other hand, there is very limited information on how to treat pancreatic cancer patients who fail their first line chemotherapy (5-FU or gemcitabine).

Phase III trials require a certain number of subjects to be enrolled. Some of the most successful trials enrolled ten thousand and more patients. For example, Physician Health Study I asked all AMA-registered male physicians ($n = 261,248$) to respond and finally enrolled 33,223 male physicians to address, whether aspirin does or does not protect against coronary events and 44% reduction of myocardial infarction was found. Oncology trials cannot involve so many patients and surgical trials usually involve much less.

There is a reverse relationship between study population size (and events and length of observation) and effect size. The smaller effect size, the more events are necessary to document significant difference (i.e. more enrolled patients and longer follow-up to produce a higher number of events). Because surgical oncology trials cannot practically involve thousands patients, alternative or adaptive trial designs are need to be considered. In classical trials the probability of randomization into control or experimental treatment is 0.5 (50% to one or the other arm). In adaptive trials the probability of randomization to one of two treatments is skewed away from 0.5 according to results obtained on so far enrolled patients. This way randomization preferentially occurs in a fashion favoring early determination of statistical significance or absence of it.

Statistical Analysis of Survival Endpoints

Survival is an important endpoint. More broadly, it is considered *time-to-event analysis*. Time-to-event studies, especially in life sciences and health care, are frequently challenged with incomplete data. Therefore it remains unknown whether the event did not happen because not enough time was allowed, or simply because the particular subject is less prone to the event. Events, which did not occur yet, are called *censored* (censored from observation). If our cancer study does have a complete follow-up and most events occur at the very end of observation period, we call it right censoring. Robust methods dealing with incomplete of data and time-to-event analysis include Kaplan-Meier survival estimator, Cox proportional hazard model and some others.

Time-to-event analysis centers on survival and hazard functions. *Survival function* describes a probability to survive till particular time. *Hazard function* defines the instantaneous failure rate, given that one has survived up to particular time. There are two general methods to estimate survival function: (1) Kaplan-Meier method and (2) Nelson-Aalen estimator.

Kaplan-Meier estimated survival function is a step function with jumps at observed event times. The size of these jumps depends on the number of events observed at each event time and on the pattern of prior censored observations. Two main assumptions are important for proper application of Kaplan-Meier estimates: (1) independence between the survival times and (2) that the censoring is independent of the event of interest. This means in practice that each patient's disease course is independent of other patients. *Nelson-Aalen estimator* is also a non-parametric estimator of the cumulative hazard function based on a sample that is subject to right censoring. The estimated cumulative hazard rate based on the Nelson-Aalen estimator has better small-sample-size performance than the estimator based on the Kaplan-Meier estimator.

Comparison between groups is made using most commonly *log-rank test* without giving any weight to any observations. *Breslow's test* (generalized Wilcoxon test) gives more weight to the earlier failure times when more subjects are at risk. Therefore this test is more powerful with data from a lognormal survival distribution, but may have low power if there is heavy early censoring (early drop offs = too many subjects with no event and short observation time). *Tarone-Ware* method also favors earlier time events, but not so much as Breslow test. The test is less susceptible to the censoring patterns. Given its intermediate weighting scheme, it is designed to have good power across a wide range of survival functions, although it is not the most powerful of the three tests in a particular situation. The *Peto-Peto-Prentice test* uses a special weight function and is not susceptible to differences in censoring patterns among groups.

The *stratified log-rank* test compares survival in groups while at the same time correcting for the effects of other factors that are related to survival and are differently distributed in the groups (stratified variable). For example, compare survival between *Her-2/neu* positive and negative breast cancer within strata (estrogen receptor status) and combine information to one test.

When investigating influence of *predictive factors* (here termed as *covariates*) on survival, *Cox proportional hazard model* is often used. Advantage is that the baseline survival function does not have to be known. This method compares experimental group(s) against this baseline function and determines whether risk of event is higher or lower.

A coefficient (expressed as coefficient β or as *hazard ratio*—HR) for each predictor variable indicates the direction and degree of flexing that the predictor has on the survival curve. A coefficient of zero ($\beta = 0$, HR=1) means that a variable has no effect on the curve, that is, it is not a predictor at all. A positive coefficient ($\beta > 0$, or HR > 1) indicates that larger values of the variable are associated with greater risk (mortality).

Sometimes so-called *parametric hazard models* (e.g. exponential or Weibull) are preferred. Typically a correct functional form of hazards is known and proportional hazard assumption is violated. Otherwise, Cox model is a safe choice. Each Cox model should include checking the *proportional hazards assumption*. Some of more common methods include *log-log survival plot*, plot of *Schoenfeld residuals versus time* and *Grambsch and Therneau's* method. If proportional hazard assumption is violated, either parametric model can be fitted, or *stratified Cox model* can be constructed. The *stratified Cox model* is a modification of the Cox proportional hazards model that allows for controlling by "stratification" of a predictor that does not satisfy the proportional hazard assumption. Predictors that are assumed to satisfy the proportional hazard assumption are included in the model, whereas the predictors being stratified are not included.

Calculation and fitting of Cox proportional hazard model is a long and iterative process best done in conjunction with a statistician. In my experience, statisticians alone usually fit unreasonable models (no biological or clinical meaning), whereas doctors alone usually fit wrong models (do not represent truth, but what they intend to find).

Using Existing Database for Research

Research on existing databases can quickly and inexpensively address important questions. There are generally three types of existing database research: (1) secondary data analysis, (2) nested studies and (3) meta-analysis.

Secondary data analysis exploits existing database(s) to investigate questions, for which the database was not specifically initiated. These data typically originate from tumor registries, Department of Veterans Affairs databases, San Francisco Mammography Registry, or various insurance carrier registries. Some databases can be joined to make available clinical and financial data (e.g. tumor registry and Medicare data). National Cancer Data Base (http://www.facs.org/cancer/ncdb/index.html) collects approximately 80% incident cancer in the USA since 1985 and is a data source for many studies. Similarly, the SEER database (Surveillance, Epidemiology and End-Results Project, seer.cancer.gov) has a publicly available dataset. Many of these datasets have incomplete data and suffer from early non-informative censoring. Linking against National Death Index (http://www.cdc.gov/nchs/ndi.htm), which lists all United States deaths since 1978, may overcome this problem. Closed databases from large prospective projects usually do not suffer from non-informative censoring due to superior data collection. For example, validations of OncotypeDX genetic signature for prediction of breast cancer outcomes was performed on dataset from NASBP (http://foundation.nsabp.org/default.asp) breast study. There are several methods and specialized software for linking of unrelated databases. Linking of clinical outcome database (e.g. NCBD or SEER) to financial data available from Medicare or other insurance carriers can be used in *cost effectiveness analysis*.

Nested studies perform research on a subset of patients initially researched in a large prospective study. Selection of patients originates from primary research database. Banks of stored serum, tissue banks, repositories of pathology departments, etc. represents a great opportunity for secondary or nested studies.

A *meta-analysis* combines the results of several studies that address a set of related research hypotheses. This is normally done by identification of a common measure of effect size and complex regression methods. Systematic review performs analysis of published results, whereas true meta-analysis is a true statistical analysis of raw data pooled from many prior studies. Therefore each meta-analysis requires access to entire dataset from each original study. Nevertheless, if done correctly, enormous statistical power can be generated. Examples are publications assessing utility of intraperitoneal chemotherapy for ovarian carcinomatosis or resectable gastric cancer.

Selection of Publication Methods

Appropriate forum for publishing surgical oncology results is as important as the study itself. Spectrum ranges from publication in Journal of Clinical Oncology, where the audience is almost entire oncology community to Annals of Surgical Oncology, as a specialized surgical oncology journal with a high impact factor. Experimental laboratory, translational and clinical research can be published in many journals. Conferences range from broad topic annual meeting of the Society of Surgical Oncology (www.surgonc.org) to more specialized ones such as meetings of Society for Surgery of Alimentary Tract (http://www.ssat.com), American Hepatopancreaticobiliary Association (http://www.ahpba.org). Some very specialized meetings have only 50-60 active participants from the US and Europe (e.g. International Symposium on Regional Cancer Therapies, http://www.regionaltherapies.com/).

A great list of instructions for authors is maintained by University of Toledo medical library (http://mulford.meduohio.edu/instr/). One can find links to thousands of medical journals in one place, plus links to ASSERT (A Standard for the Scientific and Ethical Review of Trials), CONSORT (Consolidated Standards of Reporting Trials) and COPE (Committee on Publication Ethics) statements.

Landmark Papers

1. Daley J, Forbes MG, et al. Validating risk-adjusted surgical outcomes: site visit assessment of process and structure. National VA Surgical Risk Study. J Am Coll Surg 1997;185(4): 341-51.
2. Emanuel EJ, Wendler D, et al. What makes clinical research ethical? JAMA 2000;283(20): 2701-11.
3. Greenhalgh T. How to read a paper. Statistics for the non-statistician. I: Different types of data need different statistical tests. BMJ 1997;315(7104): 364-6.
4. Greenhalgh T. How to read a paper. Statistics for the non-statistician. II: "Significant" relations and their pitfalls. BMJ 1997;315(7105): 422-5
5. Hulley S, Cummings S et al. Designing Clinical Research: An Epidemiologic Approach. Philadelphia, Lippincott Williams & Wilkins, 2006.
6. O'Quigley J, Pepe M et al. Continual reassessment method: a practical design for phase 1 clinical trials in cancer. Biometrics 1990;46(1): 33-48
7. Rosenberger WF, Seshaiyer P. Adaptive survival trials. J Biopharm Stat 1997;7(4): 617-24.
8. Simon R, Freidlin B et al. Accelerated titration designs for phase I clinical trials in oncology. J Natl Cancer Inst 1997; 89(15): 1138-47.
9. Therasse P, Arbuck SG, et al. New guidelines to evaluate the response to treatment in solid tumors. European Organization for Research and Treatment of Cancer, National Cancer Institute of the United States, National Cancer Institute of Canada. J Natl Cancer Inst 2000;92(3): 205-16.
10. Vickers AJ, Altman DG. Statistics notes: Analysing controlled trials with baseline and follow up measurements. BMJ 2001; 323(7321): 1123-4.
11. Wassmer G. Planning and analyzing adaptive group sequential survival trials. Biom J 2006; 48(4): 714-29.
12. Collins JM, Grieshaber CK, et al. Pharmacologically guided phase I clinical trials based upon preclinical drug development. J Natl Cancer Inst 1990; 82(16): 1321-6.
13. Vickers AJ, Altman DG. Statistics notes: Analysing controlled trials with baseline and follow up measurements. BMJ 2001; 323(7321): 1123-4.
14. Wassmer G. Planning and analyzing adaptive group sequential survival trials. Biom J 2006; 48(4): 714-29.

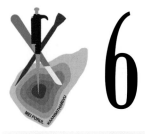

6

Principles of Pathology

Leo A Neimeier, Jon M Davison

Introduction

Surgical pathology is the art and science of establishing a diagnosis through the evaluation of human tissue samples. In America this multispecialty discipline evolved from the clinical practice and scientific inquiry of several ground-breaking surgeons and physicians who practiced in the late 1800s and early 1900s. Early pioneers in the application of the science of pathology to the diagnosis and treatment of human neoplasia came to recognize the paramount importance of accurately characterizing a neoplasm at the microscopic level prior to definitive surgical intervention. Consequently, the need developed for experienced clinicians to evaluate intraoperative frozen sections and diagnostic biopsies in addition to surgical resections. This necessity, coupled with recognition of the importance of having all forms of laboratory testing managed by trained physicians, were forces which helped surgical pathology evolve into a separate clinical specialty.

Early on, the practice of surgical pathology was influenced by innovations in microscope design, development of histologic techniques and the use of the intraoperative frozen section. Technological innovation and changing understanding of biology of disease require today's surgical pathologist to employ and integrate a wider array of adjunctive techniques to the classification of human neoplasia: electron microscopy; immuno-fluorescence and immunohistochemistry; as well as molecular techniques. None of these technological advancements has supplanted the need for the fundamental skills of the surgical pathologist: astute clinical observation, careful gross inspection and histological pattern recognition. It is well beyond the scope of this chapter to provide an introduction to the pathologic classification of human neoplastic disease. Rather, this chapter will introduce the general approach surgical pathologists use in order to arrive at a diagnosis. It will also attempt to introduce some of the ancillary testing methods which are increasingly germane to this process. It is hoped that carefully chosen examples will illustrate these general principles.

Communicating with the Surgical Pathology Laboratory

On a given day, a pathology laboratory may manage thousands of patient samples and an individual surgical pathologist may see cases from dozens of different patients. In order to ensure patient safety, to maximize the benefit of a diagnostic or therapeutic intervention and to ensure that all important clinical questions are addressed in the pathology report, all surgical specimens should be properly labeled and accompanied by relevant clinical information. Improper labeling of specimens and insufficient communication of clinical history are major causes of delay in diagnosis and diagnostic error in surgical pathology. We discuss below some of the most important information which must accompany a specimen submitted for analysis to the pathology lab.

Patient Identification

A surgical specimen must be identified with the patient's date of birth, hospital identification number (medical record number) and full name. An improperly labeled specimen cannot be accepted by the pathology laboratory. Specimen mislabeling may profoundly impair patient safety, by causing unnecessary delays in diagnosis, inappropriate or unnecessary surgical procedures or unnecessary exposure to chemotherapeutic drugs among other serious consequences. Specimen labeling should take place in the operating room at the time of the procedure to reduce the risk of errors.

Identification of the Patient's Physicians

The identity of physicians responsible for the patient's care should accompany all pathology specimens. These are the clinicians to whom final pathology reports will be sent, critical values and preliminary results will be communicated and questions about the patient will be directed. Including this information can avoid unnecessary delays in reporting results.

Pertinent Medical History and Directed Clinical Questions

Pathologists with access to a patient's medical record will review this information as a routine part of the process of evaluating a tissue specimen. This underscores the need for timely entry of operative reports and clinical history into the medical record. However, some aspects of the patient's medical history should be highlighted on the pathology requisition form to ensure that they are not overlooked:

- Prior pathologic diagnoses relevant to the current procedure
- Prior malignancy or treatment for malignancy of any type
- History of immunosuppression, organ transplant
- Other systemic medical conditions which may cause pathology
- Familial or genetic syndromes
- Specific clinical questions which need to be addressed in the pathology report.

Review of Previous Pathology

Relevant surgical pathology specimens should be reviewed by the treating institution's pathologists prior to definitive surgical or medical treatment. There are several reasons for this: (1) to confirm the nature of the neoplasm which is being treated (benign versus malignant, primary tumor versus metastasis, tumor type, etc.); (2) confirm the location of the tumor; (3) to allow local pathologists the opportunity to examine the morphologic features of a tumor prior to evaluating frozen sections, thereby reducing the chance of error made at the time of frozen section; (4) reduce the need for confirmatory diagnostic procedures at the local institution; (5) allow comparison of new tumors (possible metastases or local recurrences) to previously resected primary tumors. The value of outside pathology review was affirmed in a study performed at a large academic institution wherein the authors documented that 1.4% of diagnoses had a major change after review, resulting a significant modification of the patient's management or prognosis.

Care of the Surgical Specimen Prior to Pathologic Evaluation

Surgical resection specimens should be transported to the pathology laboratory as soon as possible so they may be assessed and processed. Standard formalin fixation preserves tissues for routine morphologic evaluation, special histochemical stains and immunohistochemistry and permits accurate diagnosis in the vast majority of cases. Fresh tissue is needed in cases requiring microbiologic cultures, enzyme histochemistry (detection of enzyme activity), immunofluorescence, flow cytometry, electron microscopy, conventional cytogenetics and high quality nucleic acid extraction. If the diagnosis of a tumor has not been established, intraoperative consultation with a surgical pathologist may be required to optimize the allocation of tissue for different diagnostic tests. This is particularly true when the differential diagnosis includes lymphoma. A pathologist may need to perform a rapid histological assessment ("frozen section") if a preoperative diagnosis is not known and if there is a question about whether adequate, viable and diagnostic tissue has been procured.

Specimen Orientation by Surgeon

Determining the anatomic extent of a neoplasm and its relationship to surgical margins is a fundamental concern of oncologic surgical pathology. In order to accurately describe the relationship of a tumor to specific anatomic structures and margins of resection, the correct anatomical orientation of the specimen needs to be apparent. The orientation of the majority of surgical specimens can be deduced from the gross anatomy of the specimen itself. Surgeons can facilitate the identification of important anatomic or surgical landmarks by judicious use of sutures, surgical clips or other indicators for specimens that would otherwise be difficult or impossible to orient (e.g. breast lumpectomy, wide skin excisions, partial neck dissection).

In order to orient a mass in three dimensions, three non-opposing surfaces must be identified either anatomically or by the use of sutures or clips. **Figure 6-1** illustrates how a breast lumpectomy is oriented in the surgical pathology laboratory and subsequently inked in order to assess margins microscopically and report the relationship of the tumor to margins.

Intraoperative Surgical Pathology Consultation

Formal consultation with a surgical pathologist during an operative procedure requires the pathologist to be familiar with the patient's prior medical and surgical history, clinical or operative findings, laboratory and radiographic data. This information can be essential to an accurate intraoperative diagnosis, particularly if the pathologist is evaluating a biopsy specimen. Ideally, the consulting pathologist should have the opportunity to review relevant outside pathology, especially diagnostic biopsies and prior resections of malignancy if recurrence or metastasis is in the differential diagnosis. All intraoperative consultations require the pathologist to perform a thorough gross assessment of the submitted specimen. This is even true for biopsy specimens which occasionally cannot (or should not) be entirely submitted for frozen section. The biopsy is evaluated grossly to determine which tissue should be evaluated intraoperatively. On resection specimens, the

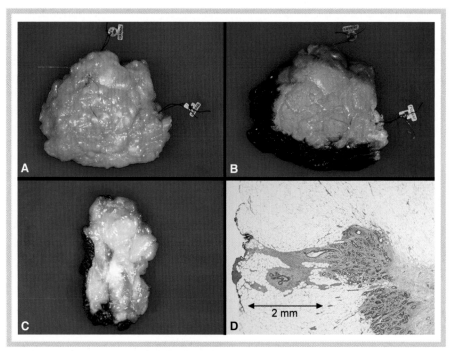

Figure 6-1: Gross and histologic evaluation of a breast lumpectomy specimen. (A) Breast lumpectomy specimen oriented by the surgeon with a short suture designating the cranial margin (top of picture) and longer suture designating the lateral margin (right side of picture). A localizing needle identifies the anterior surface. (B) Same lumpectomy specimen with differentially inked peripheral margins. As you can appreciate, the pathologist arbitrarily decides based on the shape of the resection where one margin begins and another ends. (C) Complete cross-section of a lumpectomy demonstrating the relationship of the grossly visible, white, fibrous tumor to the inked margins. (D) Histologic examination of a breast carcinoma in relationship to the inked margin

pathologist makes a decision about which margins should be evaluated microscopically and whether microscopic evaluation of the resected lesion is required. The clinical judgment of the surgeon is given appropriate weight in these situations as pathologists recognize the value of the surgeon's intraoperative assessment of the lesion and their clinical judgment regarding the adequacy of the therapeutic procedure.

There are two indications for the utilization of an intraoperative frozen section:
1. The diagnosis rendered will guide an intraoperative therapeutic decision.
2. To confirm that adequate tissue has been obtained when the purpose of the surgical procedure is to obtain a biopsy for diagnosis.

The technique can play an invaluable role in answering focused clinical questions such as:
1. Has diagnostic tissue been procured?
2. Is this a neoplasm? If so, is it benign or malignant? Many times it is possible to broadly subclassify a lesion (carcinoma, sarcoma, lymphoma, melanoma, etc.) when necessary to determine the therapeutic approach.
3. Is this a high grade or a low grade tumor?
4. Are the surgical margins free of tumor?

5. Should tissue be obtained for special studies (e.g. flow cytometry, cytogenetics, etc.)?
6. Is there metastatic disease present?
7. Are there microorganisms whose identification would allow therapy to begin immediately (e.g. fungal organisms)? Does tissue need to be submitted for microbiological cultures?

Attempts to answer subtler questions can be successful, but risks of error increase due to the limitations of the procedure. Freezing tissue distorts histologic features which may be critical to an accurate diagnosis. In most cases, limited sampling of a lesion is required (introducing the possibility of sampling error). Lastly, inherent properties of certain types of tissue may preclude quality frozen sections (e.g. ossified or fatty tissue).

A frozen section is inappropriate and potentially harmful to the patient:
1. When the results will not influence the operative procedure.
2. When subjecting tissue to freezing and thawing introduces artifacts which preclude a definitive diagnosis on permanent sections (e.g. when an entire lesion or biopsy is submitted for frozen section and additional diagnostic tissue is not available).

This can usually be avoided by discussing the necessity of intraoperative frozen section with the pathologist and agreeing on strategies for obtaining tissue for routine processing and ancillary testing prior to terminating a diagnostic surgical procedure.

The Surgical Pathology Report

The final pathology report for a surgical specimen incorporates many elements, including a final diagnosis, a gross description, a microscopic description and results of ancillary testing as well as other data.

Final Diagnosis

This section of the pathology report is, generally speaking, the most likely portion of the report to be read by a non-pathologist. It should contain a succinct statement of the final diagnosis which includes the following basic components: (1) classification of the tumor; (2) grading and staging information; (3) assessment of surgical margins; (4) assessment of any pathologic features, which are of known prognostic significance (e.g. vascular invasion and perineural invasion); (5) documentation of other important pathologic findings.

Tumor Classification

Tumors are classified on the basis of the line of differentiation of the cells which comprise the tumor: epithelial (carcinomas, neuroendocrine tumors, etc.); mesenchymal (sarcoma, etc.); hematolymphoid tumors (lymphoma, etc); melanocytic (melanoma, etc.); glial (astrocytoma, oligodendroglioma, etc.); and so on. Tumors are then rather extensively subclassified based on anatomic, morphologic, clinical, radiographic, immunophenotypic (i.e. antigen expression) and molecular characteristics. The World Health Organization and Armed Forces Institute of Pathology are two organizations which promote standardization of nomenclature and criteria for pathologic classification of tumors. One of the ways in which this is accomplished is through the publication of widely used series of atlases. Current morphology-based tumor classification systems allow patients to be stratified into appropriate treatment groups, facilitate development of new treatment modalities for defined patient groups, help to determine prognosis, define associations with risk factors and even predict molecular changes which are involved in the pathogenesis of the tumor.

Tumor Grading

Histologic grade is an assessment of the degree to which a tumor recapitulates the architectural and cytologic features of normal tissues. Grading criteria are tumor specific. Morphologic features which are evaluated in determining tumor grade may include: presence of architectural features of normal tissue, degree of cellularity, cell size, nuclear size and shape, mitotic activity, tumor necrosis, etc. For example, a well-differentiated squamous cell carcinoma retains many of the histologic characteristics of normal squamous epithelium (e.g. keratin formation, formation of desmosomes, etc.). A poorly differentiated, malignant tumor may require immunohistochemical stains to accurately classify it as epithelial, mesenchymal, hematopoietic, etc. Tumors are usually graded on a three to four grade scale: well-differentiated, moderately differentiated, poorly differentiated, undifferentiated. Generally speaking, more poorly differentiated tumors exhibit more aggressive clinical behavior. However, the extent to which tumor grade is predictive of biological behavior is relative to the type of tumor. For some tumors, tumor grade is an important and independent prognostic factor (e.g. many sarcomas, adenocarcinoma of the prostate); for other tumors, all grades of tumor behave rather similarly (e.g. pancreatic adenocarcinoma).

Pathologic Staging

Pathologic staging is a description of the anatomic extent of a tumor as determined by an evaluation of a surgical resection specimen. The most widely used system for staging epithelial tumors and melanoma is the TNM staging system which classifies the primary tumor on the basis of its size and extent of local invasion (T), the presence, size, number and location of regional lymph node metastases (N) and the presence and location of distant metastases (M). Different TNM combinations with similar survival rates are grouped into broader stage groupings Stage 0 through Stage IV. These stage groupings should have survival rates distinct from one another for a given anatomic site and tumor type.

Other histopathologic features can be of prognostic significance:

1. Lymphatic invasion (presence of tumor cells within lymphatic spaces) may be predictive of lymph node metastases.
2. Venous invasion (tumor cells within lumen of a vein) may reflect an increased risk of distant or hematogenous metastases.
3. Perineural invasion may reflect the tendency of a tumor to invade insidiously beyond the palpable or grossly visible tumor mass along nerves and thus correlate with an increased risk of local recurrence.
4. Extranodal invasion (tumor metastatic to a lymph node which invades the surrounding peri-nodal soft tissue from within the lymph node) can be an adverse prognostic factor.

Once again, the relative prognostic importance of these findings is dependent upon the tumor type and anatomic site.

Assessment of Surgical Margins

To the pathologist, a surgical margin is a tissue plane which has been created by the surgical procedure. In most resection specimens, these margins are anatomically obvious (bronchovascular margins in a pneumonectomy; ureteral margins in a nephrectomy, etc.). Surgical margins are assessed by the pathologist to determine the likelihood of localized residual disease after a resection has been performed. In cases where it would be possible to perform a wider resection, it is desirable to assess margins intraoperatively. This is a primary indication for intraoperative consultation with a surgical pathologist and the performance of frozen sections. Occasionally, tumor will be present in the lumen of a vessel or lymphatic space at a margin some distance from the main tumor mass. Technically, such a margin is involved by tumor, but additional surgery is unlikely to benefit the patient. This should be communicated clearly by the pathologist at the time of intraoperative consultation or in the final pathology report to facilitate decisions on the prudent use of additional surgery.

Techniques for the Assessment of Surgical Margins

There are multiple techniques a pathologist may employ to assess a surgical margin and each has its advantages and disadvantages. An *en face* or "shave" margin is obtained by shaving the edges of specimen parallel to the plane of resection and microscopically evaluating whether or not there is invasive or *in situ* tumor present in the shaved tissue. The advantage of this technique is that it allows the pathologist to evaluate a more extensive surface area. The disadvantage is that it does not allow a precise measurement of the distance of a tumor to the margin itself—any tumor present in the shave is considered a positive margin, even if the shaved tissue is 2 millimeters thick. In actuality, the true margin may be microscopically free of tumor, but because the tumor was within 2 millimeters, it is regarded as positive. Conversely, when the shaved tissue is free of tumor, one does not know how close the tumor approached the margin (technically, the tumor is greater than 2 millimeters from the margin).

Sections can be cut perpendicular to the surgical margin, toward the tumor **(Figure 6-1C)**. This technique is essential in cases where it is necessary to have an accurate estimate of the microscopic distance of an invasive or *in situ* tumor to the margin of resection. For the pathologist, it allows one to view the tumor as well as the surrounding tissue and adjacent margin. This can be an invaluable frame of reference when interpreting a difficult specimen. There are drawbacks to the use of perpendicular sections to assess a surgical margin: (1) perpendicular sections are an incomplete representation of the margin due to the thickness of the tissue sections; (2) it may require many more tissue blocks to completely evaluate a margin. This fact often precludes the evaluation of a large surface area in this way at the time of an intraoperative consultation. If the specimen is carefully evaluated to determine exactly where to obtain the representative sections, perpendicular margins will allow an accurate assessment of the margin.

Some surgeons prefer to submit a resection specimen (e.g. a breast lumpectomy) and separate portions of tissue which represent margins of interest. Pathologists regard these separately submitted portions of tissue as representative of the true surgical margin.

Gross Description

All biopsies and surgical specimens require a gross description which is included in the pathology report. Part of the function of this description is to maintain a "chain of custody", ensuring that each specimen can be linked back to a particular patient. Therefore, this portion of the report documents the condition of the specimen when it was received in the laboratory and the way it was labeled (i.e. with the patient's name and any other designations). The gross examination of the specimen is an essential component of accurate diagnosis and staging because only a small fraction of a large resection specimen will be submitted for histologic examination. The pathologist dissects the specimen to evaluate the size and local extent of the resected tumor and its relationship to surrounding anatomic structures and surgical margins. Serial cross sections allow the pathologist to evaluate tumor color, consistency, degree of circumscription/extent of invasion, presence of necrosis, presence of vascular invasion, serosal or capsular invasion, background pathology which may have predisposed to the formation of a tumor, etc. Ink is utilized to identify surgical margins in histologic sections **(Figure 6-1)**. The pathologist also carefully examines the specimen for evidence of metastasis involving regional lymph nodes. In routine cases, representative tissues are submitted for histologic evaluation in order to confirm the stage of the tumor as assessed grossly, to microscopically classify and grade the tumor and to look for microscopic evidence of metastatic disease.

Microscopic Description and Ancillary Tests

The initial histologic evaluation of a tumor specimen involves the examination of sections of formalin-fixed, paraffin embedded tissue which have been stained with hematoxylin and eosin (H&E). In most cases, it is possible to classify and stage a resected tumor utilizing this traditional methodology. There are a variety of scenarios which may require the use of ancillary tests: more refined tumor classification, staging, determining prognosis, evaluating a tumor for sensitivity to targeted therapy. I will first discuss the different tests and then provide illustrative examples of common uses for these tests.

Immunohistochemistry (Table 6-1)

Immunohistochemistry (IHC) is a method of analyzing the expression of protein antigens in cells and tissues. The method involves incubating tissues with antibodies, allowing these antibodies to bind to antigens they specifically recognize. After the antibodies have bound, the presence of bound antibody can be detected using one of several sensitive techniques. These techniques result in the deposition of a pigmented chromogen on the tissue in areas where antibodies have bound. The chromogens can be visualized with the conventional light microscope **(Figure 6-2)**. Some common scenarios in which immunohistochemistry has applications:

1. Benign or malignant: For example, in breast lesions, the use of cell markers (p63, smooth muscle myosin heavy chain, calponin, etc.) to identify myoepithelial cells that can help to distinguish between invasive carcinoma and carcinoma *in situ* or completely benign lesions such as sclerosing adenosis.

2. Tumor classification: **Figure 6-2** illustrates the use of immunohistochemistry to classify a soft tissue tumor.

3. Differentiating primary tumor from a metastasis: A solitary lung tumor in a patient with a history of colorectal adenocarcinoma may be a new primary or metastatic disease. Morphologic features may be diagnostic, but immunohistochemistry can provide additional evidence supporting one interpretation over the other. Colorectal adenocarcinoma almost always expresses the intermediate filament protein cytokeratin 20 and the transcription factor CDX2. Yet it does not typically express the transcription factor TTF-1 or the intermediate filament protein cytokeratin 7. Primary lung adenocarcinoma most frequently has the opposite protein expression pattern.

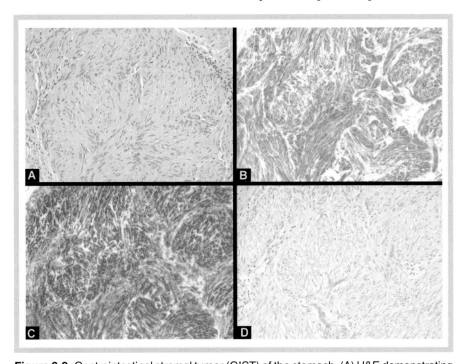

Figure 6-2: Gastrointestinal stromal tumor (GIST) of the stomach. (A) H&E demonstrating a tumor comprised of spindle-shaped cells with abundant eosinophilic cytoplasm. The histologic differential diagnosis includes GIST, leiomyoma and schwannoma among other entities. (B) Immunohistochemistry detects expression of the C-KIT protein in the tumor cells (brown pigment). A blue counterstain is also used in order to visualize the cells which do not express the C-KIT antigen. (C) Immunohistochemistry also detects expression of CD34. Expression of C-KIT and CD34 is typical of GIST and not characteristic of leiomyoma or schwannoma. (D) Further support for the diagnosis of GIST is the lack of expression of antigens that characterize tumors in the differential diagnosis: S100 protein (expressed in schwannoma), smooth muscle actin and desmin (expressed in smooth muscle tumors) are all negative. Negative staining for S100 is depicted

TABLE 6-1	Typical immunohistochemical markers used in the differential diagnosis of tumors. Table presents typical immunohistochemical markers used to identify common (mostly epithelial) neoplasms in the head/neck, thoracic cavity, gastrointestinal tract and genitourinary tract. Immunohistochemical markers are always interpreted in the context of a specific clinical and pathologic differential diagnosis. Few markers are truly specific to a given neoplasm. In this table, + means most frequently positive; +/- means approximately 50% are positive; − means most frequently negative

Tissue/tumor	Typical immunohistochemical markers
Epithelial markers	Cytokeratin (CK), EMA, CEA, Ber-EP4, MOC-31
Squamous markers	CK5/6, p63
Lymphoid marker	CD45/LCA
B-cell markers	CD20, CD79a
Plasma cell markers	kappa/lambda light chain, CD138, CD38
T-cell markers	CD3, CD2, CD5, CD7, CD4, CD8
Myeloid markers	Myeloperoxidase , lysozyme
Melanocytic neoplasm (e.g. malignant melanoma)	S100 +, Melan-A +, HMB45 +, MITF +
Nerve sheath tumors (e.g. schwannoma, malignant peripheral nerve sheath tumor)	S100 +
Smooth muscle tumors (e.g. leiomyoma, leiomyosarcoma)	Smooth muscle actin +, desmin +, HHF-35 +
Vascular tumors (e.g. angiosarcoma)	CD34 +, CD31 +
GI stromal tumors (GIST)	C-KIT +, DOG1 +, CD34 +
Neuroendocrine tumor (e.g. carcinoid, small cell carcinoma)	CK +, synaptophysin +, chromogranin +, CD56 +
Breast carcinoma, ductal	CK7+, CK20-, ER +, PR +, GCDFP +/-, mammaglobin +/-
Breast carcinoma, lobular	CK7+, CK20-, ER +, PR +, GCDFP +/-, mammaglobin +/-, loss of E-cadherin
Urinary bladder (transitional cell) carcinoma	CK7 +, CK20 + , thrombomodulin +, uroplakin III +
Prostate adenocarcinoma	CK7 -, CK20 -, PSA +, racemase/P504S +, prostein/P501S + androgen receptor +
Renal cell carcinoma	CK7 -, CK20 -, EMA +, RCC +, CD10 +
Endometrioid carcinoma	CK7 +, CK20 -, ER +
Serous carcinoma	CK7 +, CK20 -, WT-1 +, ER +, p53+
Endocervical adenocarcinoma	CK7 +, CK20-, p16+
Dysgerminoma/classic seminoma	PLAP +, C-KIT(CD117) +, OCT4 +
Embryonal carcinoma	PLAP +, CK +, CD30 +, OCT4 +
Choriocarcinoma	PLAP +, CK +, hCG +
Yolk sac tumor	PLAP +/-, CK +, AFP +/-
Sex cord stromal tumors	Inhibin +, calretinin +, Melan-A +
Lung adenocarcinoma	CK7 +, CK20 -, TTF1 +, surfactant +
Mesothelioma	CK7 +, CK20 -, CK5/6 +, calretinin +, WT-1+, D2-40 +, Ber-EP4 -, CEA -, MOC31 -
Esophageal/gastric/small bowel adenocarcinoma	CK7 +, CK20 +/-, CDX2 +/-, villin +/-
Colon adenocarcinoma	CK7 -, CK20 +, CDX2 +, villin +
Pancreaticobiliary adenocarcinoma	CK7 +, CK20 +/-, CA 19-9 +, loss of SMAD4
Hepatocellular carcinoma	CK7 -, CK20 -, HepPar1 +, pCEA + (cannalicular), CD10+ (cannalicular), glipican 3 +, AFP+/-
Thyroid carcinoma	CK7 +, CK20 -, TTF-1 +, Thyroglobulin +
Thyroid medullary carcinoma	CK +, calcitonin +, TTF1 +, synaptophysin +, chromogranin +, thyroglobulin -
Pheochromocytoma	CK-, chromogranin +, S100 positive (sustentacular pattern)
Adrenal cortical carcinoma	CK 7 -, CK 20 -, Inhibin +, Melan-A +, calretinin +
Thymic carcinoma	CK +, CD5 +/-

4. Predicting response to therapy: For example, breast tumors which express estrogen receptor are more responsive to anti-estrogen treatment regimens and have a favorable prognosis relative to tumors which do not express estrogen receptor.

Cytogenetics and Molecular Cytogenetics

Cytogenetic analysis involves growing tumor cells in short-term culture, arresting cells in metaphase (so that chromosomes are maximally elongated) and evaluating changes in number and structure of the chromosomal complement of individual tumor cells. Fresh tumor tissue with viable tumor cells is required for successful cytogenetic analysis. Chromosomal analysis plays a significant role in the diagnosis of mesenchymal and hematolymphoid tumors and also plays a more limited role in the diagnosis of solid tumors of other lineages. An example would be the diagnosis of a "round blue cell" tumor. The differential diagnosis is broad, including diverse entities such as Ewing's sarcoma, rhabdomyosarcoma, lymphoma, neuroendocrine carcinoma and melanoma. Clinical presentation, morphology, immunohistochemistry and cytogenetics will all play a role in the diagnosis of such a tumor. Ewing's sarcoma is characterized by recurrent chromosomal translocations involving the EWS gene on chromosome 22. Positive identification of a chromosomal rearrangement involving this region of chromosome 22 would be diagnostic of Ewing's sarcoma. Molecular cytogenetic techniques such as fluorescence in situ hybridization (FISH) or array-based techniques may substitute for traditional cytogenetic analysis to evaluate structural and/or copy number changes in chromosomes. For example, FISH is routinely used to detect genomic amplification of the *ERBB2* (*HER2*) gene in breast cancer specimens as a means of identifying cancers which may respond to therapy with agents that target this molecular pathway. FISH and array-based techniques can be utilized with a wider range of specimens (e.g. paraffin embedded tumor or archival frozen tumor tissue) and are playing an increasing role in the diagnosis of human cancers **(Figure 6-3)**.

Diagnostic Molecular Pathology

Diagnostic molecular pathology as applied to cancer diagnosis and treatment is a rapidly evolving field. It is a discipline which is founded principally on the characterization of nucleic acid (DNA and RNA) changes which occur in tumor cells (e.g. oncogenic mutations in DNA sequence, changes in gene expression at the mRNA level, etc.). These changes have been described during several decades worth of research into the molecular genetics of tumors. Many different techniques are utilized to detect these changes. The most commonly used

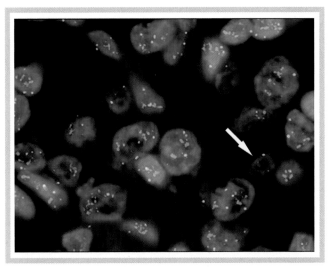

Figure 6-3: Fluorescence in situ hybridization (FISH) detecting amplification of the *ERBB2 (HER2)* gene in paraffin embedded breast carcinoma tissue. All nuclei are counterstained with blue fluorescent dye, allowing them to be visualized. The majority of nuclei are tumor cell nuclei. A red fluorescently tagged DNA probe uniquely hybridizes to the ERBB2 region of chromosome 17. Two signals are seen in the normal stromal cell nucleus (arrow), but numerous signals are present in tumor cell nuclei, indicating amplification of this gene. By comparison, a green fluorescently tagged DNA probe which uniquely hybridizes to the chromosome 17 centromere is present in two to three copies per cell (green signals). This indicates that it is not the entire chromosome which is present in multiple copies, but amplification of the *ERBB2* genomic region. Breast carcinomas with amplification of ERBB2 are more likely to respond to targeted systemic chemotherapies. ERBB2 status may also predict response to other forms of systemic chemotherapy

techniques involve polymerase chain reaction (PCR) to amplify nucleic acid sequences of interest and allow their detection and analysis. Some nucleic acid changes occur only in tumor cells. The presence of such changes can be diagnostic of a tumor. For example, clonal immunoglobulin or T-cell receptor gene rearrangements in the diagnosis of lymphoma. Other nucleic acid changes are associated with response to therapy. Patients with metastatic colorectal adenocarcinoma treated with inhibitors of epidermal growth factor receptor (EGFR) signaling do not respond if the tumor harbors an oncogenic mutation in the gene encoding K-ras. It is becoming a standard practice to analyze a tumor for an oncogenic K-ras mutation prior to initiating this type of therapy **(Figure 6-4)**. Because most assays which fall under this general rubric require the use of nucleic acid, care must be taken when submitting specimens to ensure that they are submitted to the pathology laboratory in a timely fashion to prevent RNA (and to a lesser extent DNA) degradation.

Another major role for molecular genetics in the care of cancer patients is in the identification of patients with

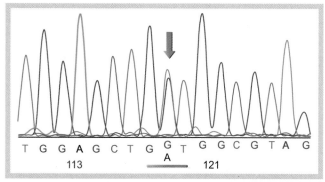

T G G A G C T G G T G G C G T A G
113   A   121

Figure 6-4: Electropherogram depicting the DNA sequence of exon 1 of the gene encoding the K-ras oncoprotein from a colorectal adenocarcinoma metastatic to the liver. Because the tumor retains at least one normal copy of the gene encoding K-ras, the normal DNA sequence at codon 12 (GGT, two black peaks followed by a red peak, underlined) is observed. However, there is an abnormal green peak in codon 12 (arrow), signifying that one copy of the gene encoding K-ras has the codon 12 sequence GAT (black peak, green peak, red peak), a point mutation encoding aspartic acid in place of glycine. The glycine to aspartic acid mutation is a common oncogenic mutation in the K-ras protein. Patient's whose colorectal adenocarcinomas harbor oncogenic K-ras mutations do not respond to therapy with cetuximab, an inhibitor of the epidermal growth factor receptor

hereditary cancer predisposition syndromes. Patient age, tumor morphology, family history, pattern and number of primary tumors all play a role in determining whether or not a patient may have a hereditary cancer predisposition syndrome. For example, patients with numerous adenomatous polyps in the colon should be evaluated for germline mutations in the APC or MYH genes after appropriate genetic counseling is offered. Identification of a germline mutation involves analyzing DNA extracted from normal tissue (usually peripheral blood).

Cytopathology

Cytopathology is concerned with the examination of individual cells and cell clusters which have been spread onto the surface of a glass slide and stained. Cytology specimens can be obtained from body fluids (e.g. cerebrospinal fluid, nipple discharge, ascites, urine), from scraping a mucosal surface (e.g. cervical smear, bile duct brushings) or obtained by needle aspiration (e.g. needle aspiration of a pancreatic, thyroid or pulmonary mass). The major advantage to the clinician and patient is that diagnostic material can usually be obtained through a relatively non-invasive procedure. Moreover, sample adequacy can quickly be assessed on site if a cytopathologist is present when the material is obtained, thus increasing the probability of a definitive diagnosis for a

given procedure. If sufficient material is obtained, cytology specimens can be prepared in order to permit immunohistochemical staining to aid in diagnosis.

Since cytology specimens are composed of disaggregated cells and small clusters of cells, diagnostic certainty can be limited by the absence of tissue architecture. Tissue architecture can be crucial to a definitive diagnosis of malignancy. In such cases, needle core or mucosal biopsy or staged surgical procedure with or without intraoperative frozen section may be required to establish a diagnosis. Thyroid lesions provide a useful example to illustrate this. Fine-needle aspiration of a thyroid lesion can accurately discriminate between benign and malignant lesions with a very high degree of sensitivity and specificity. However, it is not possible to discriminate between an encapsulated well-differentiated follicular carcinoma and a cellular, benign follicular lesion on the basis of fine-needle aspiration. The diagnosis of follicular carcinoma, in this case, requires identification of the architectural features of capsular invasion or vascular invasion. These features can only be identified in tissue sections.

Summary

The clinical role of the surgical pathologist is that of a consultant. From the initial evaluation of a cytology specimen or biopsy to evaluation of intraoperative frozen sections and final characterization and pathologic staging of a resected neoplasm, the pathologist aids the surgical oncologist, medical oncologist and radiation oncologist among others in making optimal management decisions. Pathologists have always made use of available technology to gain insight into the nature of a pathologic process and provide the most useful information to guide patient care decisions. The light microscope, formalin, paraffin, hematoxylin and eosin are the tried and true technological mainstays of the practice of surgical pathology. This will likely remain so for the foreseeable future given the depth of insight, speed and relative low cost associated with these traditional methods. Increasingly, however, pathologists are asked to bring a wider and wider array of technology to bear on the classification of human neoplasia as targeted therapies become more commonplace and insights into the biology of human neoplasia are translated into novel therapies.

Landmark Papers

1. Fechner RE. The Birth and Evolution of American Surgical Pathology, in Guiding the Surgeon's Hand: The History of American Surgical Pathology. Rosai J (Eds). American Registry of Pathology: Washington, DC 1997;7-21.
2. Rosai J. Some Considerations on the Origin, Evolution and Outlook of American Surgical Pathology, in Guiding the

Surgeon's Hand: The History of American Surgical Pathology, J. Rosai (Ed). American Registry of Pathology: Washington, DC 1997;1-6.

3. Nakhleh RE, Gephardt G, Zarbo RJ. Necessity of clinical information in surgical pathology. Arch Pathol Lab Med 1999;123(7): 615-9.

4. Nakhleh RE, Zarbo RJ. Surgical pathology specimen identification and accessioning: A College of American Pathologists Q-Probes Study of 1,004, 115 cases from 417 institutions. Arch Pathol Lab Med 1996;120(3): 227-33.

5. Wagar EA, et al. Specimen labeling errors: a Q-probes analysis of 147 clinical laboratories. Arch Pathol Lab Med 2008; 132(10): 1617-22.

6. Makary MA, et al. Surgical specimen identification errors: a new measure of quality in surgical care. Surgery 2007;141(4): 450-5.

7. Kronz JD, Westra WH, Epstein JI. Mandatory second opinion surgical pathology at a large referral hospital. Cancer 1999;86(11): 2426-35.

8. Ackerman LV, Rosai J. The pathology of tumors, part three: frozen section, gross and microscopic examination, ancillary studies. CA Cancer J Clin 1971;21(5): 270-81.

9. WHO Classification of Tumours, Kleihues P, Sobin LH (Eds). 2000-2009, Lyon: IARC Press.

10. AFIP Atlas of Tumor Pathology, 4th Series. Silverberg SG, Sobin LH (Eds). 2004-2009, Washington, DC: American Registry of Pathology.

11. AJCC Cancer Staging Manual (6th edn). Greene FL, et al (Eds). New York: Springer-Verlag, 2002.

12. Dabbs DJ (Eds). Diagnostic Immunohistochemistry (2nd edn). Churchill-Livingstone: Philadelphia, PA, 2006.

13. Lerwill MF. Current practical applications of diagnostic immunohistochemistry in breast pathology. Am J Surg Pathol 2004;28(8): 1076-91.

14. Barbareschi M, et al. CDX-2 homeobox gene expression is a reliable marker of colorectal adenocarcinoma metastases to the lungs. Am J Surg Pathol 2003;27(2): 141-9.

15. Gown AM. Current issues in ER and HER2 testing by IHC in breast cancer. Mod Pathol 2008; 21(Suppl 2): S8-S15.

16. Payne SJ, et al. Predictive markers in breast cancer—the present. Histopathology 2008;52(1): 82-90.

17. Keen-Kim D, Nooraie F, Rao PN. Cytogenetic biomarkers for human cancer. Front Biosci 2008;13: 5928-49.

18. Leonard DGB (Eds). Molecular Pathology in Clinical Practice. Springer: New York, 2007.

19. Karapetis CS, et al. K-ras mutations and benefit from cetuximab in advanced colorectal cancer. N Engl J Med 2008;359(17): 1757-65.

20. Ogilvie JB, Piatigorsky EJ, Clark OH. Current status of fine needle aspiration for thyroid nodules. Adv Surg 2006;40: 223-38.

21. Baloch ZW, LiVolsi VA. Fine-needle aspiration of the thyroid: today and tomorrow. Best Pract Res Clin Endocrinol Metab 2008;22(6): 929-39.

7

Diagnostic Imaging in Cancer

Gregory Vorona, Frances Austin, Kurian Puthenpurayil

Introduction

Today many imaging options are available following more than a century of technological development and clinical studies to refine these techniques. We have entered an era where several modalities are capable of whole body imaging and of small tumor detection long before patients are symptomatic. As radiology continues to expand its role in the management of cancer patients, a basic understanding of a variety of diagnostic examinations and interventional procedures greatly facilitates effective utilization of diagnostic imaging.

Overview of Imaging by Modality

X-ray Examinations

Still the backbone of radiology, the X-ray was discovered in the late 1800s. Although not the first scientist to produce X-rays in the laboratory, Wilhelm Roentgen is considered the father of radiology for first clearly demonstrating the diagnostic potential of X-rays for which he won the Nobel Prize in Physics in 1901. X-rays produced for radiographs, fluoroscopic procedures, mammograms, and CTs are all generated in a similar fashion. A voltage across an X-ray tube propels a current of electrons from the cathode to the anode where they lose energy by interacting with nuclei within the tungsten anode. Some of the energy they lose is given off as X-rays via bremsstrahlung ("braking") reactions, wherein the negatively charged electrons are decelerated by passing in close proximity to the positively charged nucleus. The maximum penetrating energy (expressed in kilovolts, kV) is equal to the voltage applied across the tube, and the intensity of X-rays (expressed in milliamperes, mA) is proportional to the current. The X-ray beam spectrum is narrowed by a filter before transmission through the subject to expose an image receptor. Contrast agents such as barium and iodine are high atomic number materials which absorb diagnostic energy X-rays to add information to the image. Mammography, fluoroscopy, and CT all utilize the same basic principles, but differ in the type of image receptor and in the energy and current (kV and mA) of X-rays.

X-ray detectors traditionally have been screen/film systems, but now most modern projection radiography utilizes either computed radiography (CR) or digital radiography (DR). These are both distinctively different than computed tomography (CT), which will be discussed later. Although the details of these two systems extend beyond the scope of this chapter, both involve techniques whereby the detector absorption pattern is translated directly into digital images for storage/viewing on computers. The typical imaging matrix for a digital chest X-ray is 2,500 pixels × 2,000 pixels with a normal field of view of 43 cm × 35 cm. In other words, 43 cm in "real life" is divided into 2,500 pixels (and 35 cm into 2,000 pixels) on the display monitor. Spatial resolution is defined as field of view (FOV) divided by matrix size, and in this instance, this calculation results in a hypothetical resolution of 0.17 mm (43 cm/2,500 pixels). Additionally, with CR and DR systems, there is a generous dynamic range that permits the viewer to manually modify the image contrast in order to optimize viewing conditions.

Mammography

In 1931, Stafford Warren described his technique for imaging the architecture of the breast. Twenty years later, Raul Leborgne would be recognized for developing early mammography. His use of a compression pad and cone produced better images of mammary pathology.

As the X-ray attenuation differences between normal and cancerous breast tissues are minimal, imaging the breast requires specifically designed X-ray equipment. Mammography is a modified form of projection radiography, in which (in addition to other differences) the traditional tungsten target is replaced with a molybdenum or rhodium target and a lower tube voltage is used. This results in a lower average energy of the emitted X-rays which makes them less penetrating, and enhances detection of low contrast masses. The detection of microcalcifications is also improved. As with standard

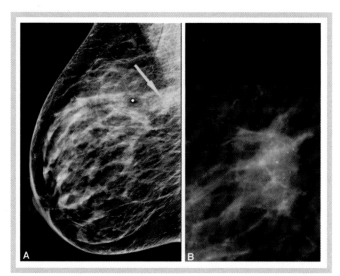

Figures 7-1A and B: A-46-year old female presented with a palpable right breast mass (arrow). A metal marker was placed the area where the patient felt "a lump", and an underlying soft tissue mass was seen on the MLO (mediolateral oblique) view (A) A spot compression XCCL view of the right breast mass demonstrated spiculation and small, pleomorphic calcifications (B) These findings were highly suggestive of malignancy. The patient was found to have invasive ductal carcinoma on biopsy

projection radiography, mammographic screen/film systems are being replaced with full field digital detector systems. These images typically have a matrix size of 3,000 × 4,000 pixels, and have an average pixel size of 0.08 mm. Optimal mammography requires the use of breast compression, which further enhances low-contrast detection and improves image resolution by decreasing patient movement and exposure times **(Figure 7-1)**.

Many exciting tools are currently in varying stages of development to improve the diagnostic sensitivity and accuracy of mammography. Some contemporary mammographic digital systems utilize computer aided diagnosis (CAD) software and while these systems have sensitivities as high as 90% for detecting breast cancer, current software has a high false-positive rate (up to 1-2 false positives per image). Digital tomosynthesis systems, in which multiple projection images of the breasts are obtained at different angles in order to create tomographic maps, are expected to further enhance early breast cancer detection. Although not yet FDA approved, digital tomosynthesis systems have been used in clinical practice in Europe since 2008. Designated portable positron emission tomography (PET) mammographic units are also currently being assessed for clinical utility.

CT

The commercial success of the Beatles contributed to the development of CT by providing capital to the British company, Electric and Musical Industries, Ltd (EMI), which developed the first commercial CT scanner in the early 1970s under the direction of Sir Godfrey Hounsfield. Sir Hounsfield and Allan MacLeod Cormack shared the 1979 Nobel Prize in Medicine for their independent roles in the development of CT.

Both axial and helical CT function by rotating an X-ray tube and a bank of detectors around the patient to form a density map which is converted into an image. Density is quantified using an arbitrary scale named for Sir Hounsfield. Water is assigned a Hounsfield density of 0, air a density of negative 1000, and bone a density of roughly 800-1000.

CT scanners are categorized by the number of rows of detectors (4, 16, 64, 128, 256, 320, etc.) that are available to obtain information at a given moment, which impacts how quickly an image can be acquired. CT images usually have 512 pixels by 512 pixels display matrix. This results in a pixel size of 0.5 mm for a typical head scan (25 cm FOV), and of 0.8 mm for a normal body scan (40 cm FOV). Although the resolution of CT is vastly inferior compared with projection radiography, CT is superior in detecting very small differences in density between adjacent structures. Each pixel normally represents 12 bits, or 4,096 shades of gray.

In addition to resolution, it is also very important to consider the slice thickness in which a study is viewed. Although an individual detector element in a traditional 64 slice CT unit may have a longitudinal (aligned with the long axis of the patient) thickness of 0.6 mm, multiple "slices" are typically fused on the workstation to view the study in 3-5 mm axial "cuts". Thinner acquisitions allow for clearer reformatted images in multiple planes. Many CT examinations are tailored specifically to best address the clinical question by altering slice thickness, by varying type and timing of contrast administration, and by performing various volumetric and/or multi-planar reconstructed images.

The use of oral and/or IV contrast agents in CT depends on the particular circumstances. Generally, oral contrast is used for all abdominal CTs except for renal stone CT protocols, CT angiograms and some specific CT protocols which use water or a water density oral contrast agent such as CT urography, pancreatic mass CT protocols and CT enterography. There is very little difference between water-soluble, iodine based oral contrast agents and barium oral contrast agents from an imaging point of view. Water soluble iodinated contrast agents are typically preferred if there is suspicion of a bowel perforation as they are more readily absorbed from the peritoneal cavity, but they are associated with increased risk of pneumonitis if accidentally aspirated. IV contrast is desirable in virtually all staging or restaging CT examinations. An initial CT scan of the liver without contrast is also obtained in evaluation of breast cancer and colorectal cancer.

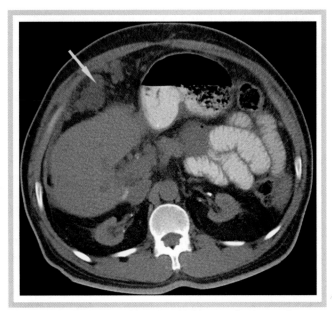

Figure 7-2: A 58-year-old male with history of colorectal cancer presented with chronic renal failure and a small bowel obstruction (notice the atrophic kidneys and the dilated small bowel loops). Multiple nodular soft tissue densities were seen throughout the mesentery (arrow), keeping with "omental caking" and peritoneal carcinomatosis. Only PO contrast was administered. (*Courtesy* Dr. Matthew Hartman, West Penn Allegheny Health System)

The increasing use of CT in a variety of applications has focused increasing attention on its risks. IV contrast can be nephrotoxic, particularly in patients with underlying renal dysfunction. Iodinated contrast agents should be avoided in patients with a glomerular filtration rate of less than 30cc/minute, and less nephrotoxic agents and/or decreased dye load should be considered in patients with milder renal dysfunction. Level I evidence supports aggressive hydration to prevent nephrotoxicity, while some patients may further benefit from the use of N-acetylcysteine (Mucomyst). Allergic-like reactions to IV dye are common. Premedication with steroids (typically 50 mg doses of oral Prednisone given 13 hours, 7 hours, and 1 hour before IV dye administration) and diphenhydramine (50 mg orally one hour before IV dye) can reduce the risk and severity of allergic reactions.

CT is now one of the largest sources of medical radiation exposure in the United States, and its use has been increasing at a rate of 10% per year over the past decade. Although there are many ways to measure radiation exposure for a specific radiographic study, the most clinically useful unit is the Effective Dose. The Effective Dose, measured in Sieverts (Sv), is calculated by assessing the dose distribution and relative radio-sensitivity of the irradiated organs in order to estimate the risk of radiation-induced stochastic (oncogenesis and hereditary) effects. According to the FDA, a single CT of the abdomen is approximately 8 mSv. By comparison, a typical plain film of the chest has an effective dose of about 0.02 mSv. The International Commission of Radiological Protection (ICRP) in their most recent 2008 risk estimate (Publication 103) places the nominal cancer detriment at 5.5% per Sv exposure. In other words, a standard single phase CT of the abdomen would result in approximately 8 mSv of exposure, and impart a slightly greater than 1/2500 risk of developing cancer from the study to the average patient. This dose would be increased if the pelvis was included. Risks of exposure are believed to be cumulative over the patient's lifetime. In comparison, the average individual is exposed to annual background radiation of 3 mSv, mostly from environmental radon.

PET and PET/CT

The first commercial combined PET/CT scanner was introduced in 2001. In a very short time, PET/CT has become the imaging examination of choice for an increasing variety of malignancies. Positron emission tomography utilizes a radioisotope that decays by positron emission, usually Fluorine-18. In most clinical PET/CT examinations, F-18 is bound to glucose to form 6-F-18 fluorodeoxyglucose which is taken up by cells and phosphorylated. This traps the radioisotope within cells and highlights metabolically active cells preferentially utilizing glucose. Most cancers primarily use glucose for metabolism. In addition, there is typically high activity in the brain and spinal cord, and variable, but often elevated uptake in cardiac and bowel wall and variable uptake in skeletal muscle, liver, spleen, salivary glands, and marrow. F-18 FDG is also excreted in urine, highlighting the kidneys, collecting systems, and urinary bladder.

Combining the functional imaging of PET with the anatomic information of CT allows greater specificity for most imaging findings than allowed by PET alone. CT is also used to correct for attenuation of radioactivity by the body. Clinical indications for F-18 FDG PET/CT approved by Medicare now include diagnosis, staging, and restaging of breast cancer, lymphoma, melanoma, colorectal cancer, lung cancer, esophageal cancer, head and neck cancer, and restaging of thyroid cancer. PET/CT has clearly demonstrated its usefulness in evaluation of many additional malignancies including, but not limited to, pancreatic cancer, ovarian cancer, cervical cancer, urothelial cancer, and adrenal cancer. In addition, PET is particularly useful in evaluation of cancer of unknown primary and in evaluation of pulmonary nodules greater than 8 mm in diameter.

Protocols vary by institution, but when a PET/CT is ordered with a diagnostic CT, oral and intravenous contrasts are often utilized to improve the accuracy of the CT portion of the PET/CT examination. A number of trials across a variety of imaging indications have indicated that

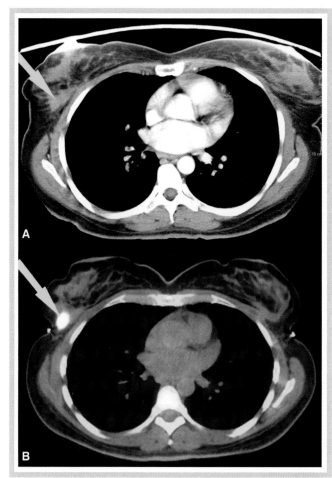

Figures 7-3A and B: Enhanced CT (A) and non-enhanced PET/CT (B) of the previously described 46-year-old woman with invasive ductal carcinoma of the right breast. An enhancing, minimally calcified deep-seated soft tissue density in the right breast measured 3.3 x 2.0 cm and correlated with the patient's known breast cancer (arrow). A hypermetabolic focus correlating with the soft tissue mass was present in the deep soft tissues of the right breast (arrow). The SUV (standard uptake value) was 7.9. In general, a SUV >2.5 is considered suspicious for malignancy

combined PET/CT has higher accuracy than PET alone, and most imaging departments are transitioning to combined PET/CT scanners. Effective doses in PET imaging are about 10 mSv, and the radiation from the CT component can range from an approximate additional 5 mSv (for attenuation correction images) to 15 mSv (a full diagnostic CT).

Nuclear Medicine

Nuclear medicine involves imaging a radiopharmaceutical that is introduced into the body. A radiopharmaceutical is a radionuclide that emits radiation (usually gamma rays) that is typically combined with a molecule that allows disproportionate uptake in a tissue of interest.

Therefore, unlike other fields of radiology, nuclear medicine is focused on evaluating function rather than anatomy. The most commonly used radionuclide in clinical practice is Technetium 99m, which has the characteristics of (a) being easily combined with a number of carrier molecules and (b) produced relatively easily through a Molybdenum-99 based generator system. Radionuclides can also be produced from cyclotrons (i.e. I-123, F-18) and nuclear reactors (I-131), although these usually have to be shipped to the hospital daily.

Images in nuclear medicine can be acquired either through planar scintillation cameras or by single photon emission computed tomography (SPECT) units. The most important salient difference between the two types of imaging is that the scintillation camera is stationary in the former, and that it rotates around the patient at certain defined intervals in the latter. Planar imaging produces single images (AP, oblique, etc.), while SPECT utilizes reconstruction algorithms that permit viewing in multiple planes (similar to CT). SPECT images can also be fused with CT data (i.e. Ind-111 octreotide SPECT/CT to image metastatic carcinoid tumor). In general, the resolution of images in nuclear medicine is variable, and usually they are inferior compared with other modalities. Typical imaging matrixes are 64 × 64 pixels or 128 × 128 pixels, although whole body images can be up to 256 × 1024 pixels.

Apart from PET, the examination most commonly utilized in surgical oncology is the bone scan. Technetium 99m is a metastable isomer which decays by gamma emission and emits a 140 keV gamma ray. When bound to a diphosphonate (Tc-99m methylene diphosphonate), the isotope accumulates within bone with increased avidity in areas of more rapid bone turnover such as bony metastases. Bone scan has lower sensitivity in lytic metastases. Virtually any metastasis can be primarily lytic, but classically, metastases from urothelial carcinoma or multiple myeloma can be missed on bone scans. Typically, lytic-predominant metastases are high grade malignancies, and will be avid on PET imaging.

Radioactive iodine plays an important role in staging and restaging of thyroid carcinoma. Sensitivity of iodine imaging is lower in poorly differentiated thyroid carcinoma, and again, PET is often strongly positive in these patients. I-123 is always utilized for imaging, while I-131 can be used for both imaging and treatment (metastatic thyroid cancer, Grave's Disease, etc.).

Sentinel node imaging for breast carcinoma and melanoma usually involves intradermal injection of Technetium 99m Sulfur Colloid injected either periareolar or at the site of tumor or tumor resection. The nodes which first take up the radiotracer are the nodes which would first be exposed to tumor spread via the lymphatic system. For melanoma, lymphoscintigraphy permits the surgeon to avoid unnecessary nodal basin resection if the sentinel

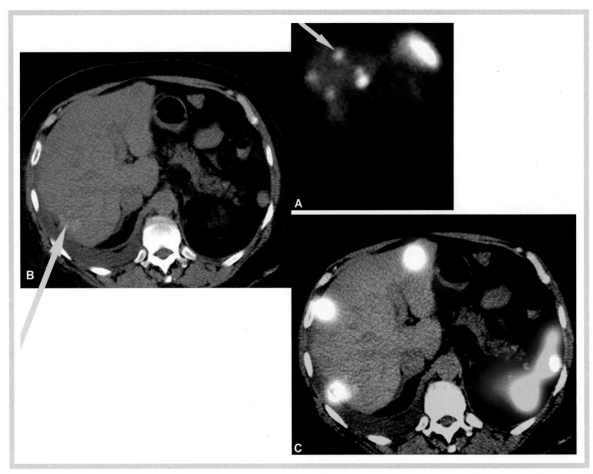

Figures 7-4A to C: A 70-year-old male with a history of small bowel carcinoid presented with abdominal pain and elevated liver enzymes. AP planar Indium-111 Octreotide scan imaged at 24 hours after injection (A) demonstrated multiple areas of abnormal uptake within the liver (arrow). The patient had a CT scan performed prior to the nuclear medicine study without IV contrast due to a history of renal failure, and some non-specific calcifications were seen in the posterior right hepatic lobe (arrow) (B). When the SPECT images were fused with the CT study (C), the locations of the patient's carcinoid metastasis within the liver were much easier to identify

node is negative as "skip" metastases are rare (<2%). For breast cancer, lymphoscintigraphy using an Intraoperative gamma probe has greater than 90% accuracy for detecting sentinel nodes, and a histopathologically negative node has a very high negative predictive value for metastatic axillary involvement.

Radionuclides can also be combined with monoclonal antibodies for both diagnostic and therapeutic indications. Complexes exist for imaging metastatic colorectal, lung, prostate and ovarian cancer. Y-90 Ibritumomab tiuxetan (Y-90 Zevalin) is a murine IgG1 kappa monoclonal antibody that targets the CD20 receptor on lymphocytes, and this agent has showed significant success in the treatment of refractory non-Hodgkin's lymphoma.

Magnetic Resonance Imaging

Nuclear Magnetic Resonance (NMR) is a complex method of imaging that utilizes magnetism and radio waves. Its long history began in 1882 with the discovery of the Rotating Magnetic Field by Nikola Tesla, for whom the Tesla unit was named. In 1946, Felix Bloch and Edward Purcell, worked independently, observed atomic spectra via NMR; a one dimensional image was created. It was not until 1971 that Damadian claimed that NMR could be used to diagnose cancer through measurements of relaxation times, called T1. He had observed that tumor samples *in vitro* had significantly greater relaxation time than normal tissue. He patented NMR technology in 1972, claiming NMR would be used to scan the human body for cancer, with no knowledge of how a 2D image would be generated.

In 1973, Lauterbur demonstrated that he could localize two test tubes in water, thereby creating the first 2D image from NMR. His paper was initially rejected by *Nature* because they believed that NMR was not a sufficiently significant development. Mansfield, in 1977, was credited with analyzing the mathematical signals from MRI

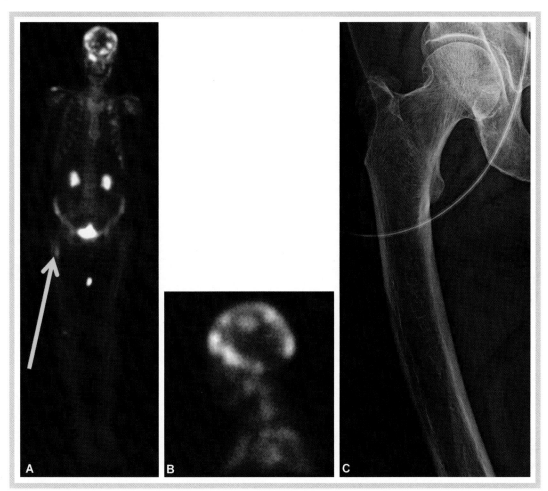

Figures 7-5A to C: A 82-year-old female treated 8 years prior with radiation and chemotherapy for breast cancer. AP full body Tc-99m MDP bone scan (A) demonstrated multiple foci of increased uptake within the calvarium, thorax, and the right femur (arrow). Lateral skull view (B) showed the extent of calvarial involvement. Plain film of the right femur obtained at that time (C) did not demonstrate any evidence for metastasis. The site within the femur seen on the bone scan was biopsied, and was found to be metastatic lobular breast carcinoma

making it possible to generate a useful image. He was also credited with discovering how rapid images could be achieved by developing the MRI protocol for echo- planar imaging. The first MRI scanner was built by Damadian and on July 3, 1977 it took close to 5 hours to generate one image of a human lung. A year later he imaged a patient with cancer. Lauterbur and Mansfield received the 2003 Nobel Prize for their contributions to MRI. Damadian demanded to be recognized for his contributions, taking out full-page ads in the Washington Post, the New York Times, and the LA Times.

The most complex imaging modality, a MRI generates images by placing the patient in a strong magnetic field. Within the patient, spinning protons (hydrogen nuclei) induce their own magnetic fields, and a disproportionate number will align with the machine's strong field (or B0 field). Radiofrequency waves (or the B1 field) are applied which alter the axis of spinning protons and cause a

shifting of their net magnetic field. As the protons realign their spins with the main magnetic field (B0) when the B1 field is "turned off", energy is released in the form of radio waves. These waves are detected by the current that they induce in RF receiver coils. Through a complex reconstruction method an image is generated. Closer specifically-designed RF coils (head coils, knee coils, etc.) produce higher signal, and superior image quality in certain indications, compared with the body coil within the magnet. In general, MR provides spatial resolution approximately equivalent to CT, with pixel sizes of 0.5 mm to 1.0 mm. Typical image matrixes range in size from 128 × 128 pixels to 1024 × 512 pixels.

Protons in different environments (i.e. tissues) realign their spins with the main magnetic field (B0) at different speeds, allowing for differentiation on an image. Imaging in MR is fundamentally based on the T1 and T2 relaxation times. T1 signal represents how quickly the spinning

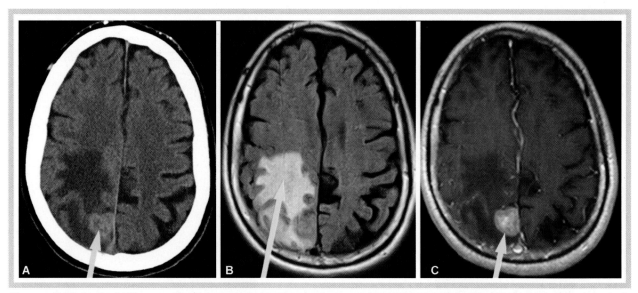

Figures 7-6A to C: A 74-year-old man presented to the emergency room with acute left-sided hemiplegia. The hospital's stroke protocol was initiated, and the patient had an immediate head CT (A). A hyperdense right parietal parafalcine mass was seen (arrow) with surrounding vasogenic edema. Subsequent MRI better demonstrated the surrounding edema on the T2 weighted FLAIR (fluid attenuated inversion recovery) sequence (arrow) (B), as well as an enhancing mass (arrow) on the T1 post-contrast sequences (C). The mass was removed and found to be metastatic melanoma. The patient reported having had a melanoma removed 20 years prior from his arm.

protons realign with the unit's main magnetic field (B0). Tissues with short T1 times (i.e. fat) realign quickly, and appear bright on T1 weighted images. Conversely, tissues which retain their altered magnetic alignment are known to have long T2 times (i.e. CSF, water), and appear bright on T2 weighted images. T1 weighted images are generally superior in providing anatomic detail, while T2 weighted images are generally better in demonstrating pathology (as damaged tissue is usually edematous). Contrast enhanced images are almost always T1 weighted. There are, of course, numerous variations and exceptions to these general principles. For example, fat is bright in a very common sequence known as a T2 fast-spine-echo (FSE) used to image the abdomen, requiring a process known as "fat saturation" to remove the signal from fat. Different institutions have varying protocols for different MRI indications, and the reader is encouraged to discuss any uncertainties with the radiologist.

It is important to realize that the magnetic field used in most clinical MR is generated by a strong current running through a superconducting coil which is always on (even when the machine appears to be off). The strong magnetic field will interact with ferromagnetic objects such as stethoscopes, steel oxygen cylinders, most stretchers, hairpins, or electronics containing iron. Ferromagnetic objects are drawn to the center of the coil and can injure a patient within the coil. At least one death has occurred in this manner. Because of the potential for the strong magnetic field to induce currents within a circuit, anyone with a pacemaker should not enter the MRI room at any time. Patients should also be prescreened for any metal objects that they may have within their bodies. This can range from metal shards in the orbits (if the patient has a history of working with metal), to certain older cerebral aneurysm clips. In the case of an emergency, an MRI magnet can be "quenched", in which the liquid cryogens used to cool the superconducting magnet are exposed to the atmosphere and boil off rapidly. This will result in rapid deactivation of the MRI unit, but with considerable damage to the machine. There is also the theoretical risk of suffocation if the room is improperly vented. Even if the patient has non-ferromagnetic metal within their body that is within the field of imaging, the RF pulses (B1) can cause the metal to heat, resulting in burns to the patient. Finally, there is a concern for Nephrogenic Systemic Fibrosis (NSF) in patients with renal failure who receive IV gadolinium contrast. The FDA recommends avoiding gadolinium in patients with an estimated GFR <30 ml/min and recommends checking serum creatinine and estimated GFR before giving IV gadolinium or IV iodinated contrast.

MRI is perhaps best utilized in oncology for specific purposes such as the characterization of adrenal, ovarian, renal or liver masses, the evaluation of local extent of disease of endometrial cancer or prostate cancer and the evaluation of bony metastatic disease, especially in the spine. MRI with contrast has the highest sensitivity for intracranial metastases. MRI has sensitivity equal to or higher than CT in the evaluation of liver metastases, particularly in the setting of a fatty infiltrated liver.

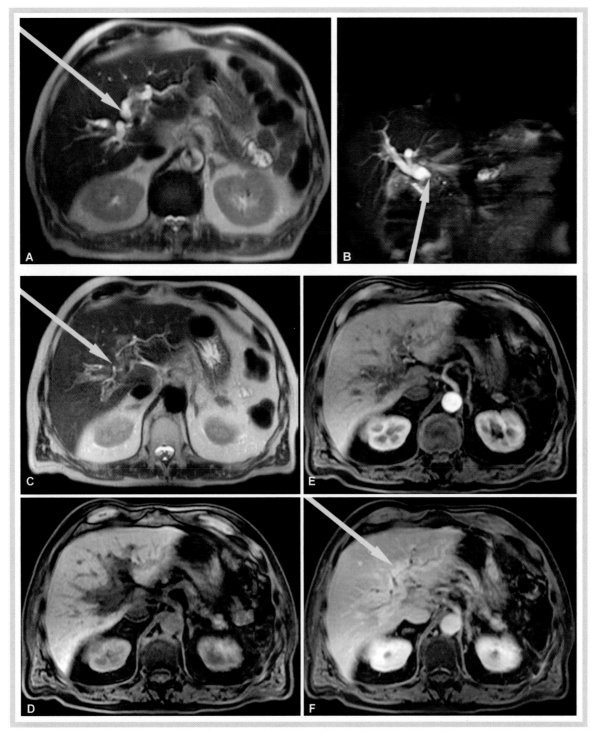

Figures 7-7A to F: A 74-year-old male presented with jaundice. Initial MRI of the abdomen (A,B) demonstrated marked intrahepatic biliary tract and proximal common bile duct dilation (arrow, A) , ending in an abrupt termination (arrow, coronal view, B). Both of these images were from T2 weighted sequences.

Subsequent enhanced MRI of the abdomen (C,D,E,F) performed 6 months later. The patient had an interval ERCP with biliary stent placement (notice the decompressed intrahepatic biliary ducts, marked, C, on this T2 weighted sequence). Timed interval T1 enhanced images (D = before contrast, E = arterial phase, F = "delayed phase" 5 minutes after the initial contrast injection) demonstrated characteristic delayed enhancement of an infiltrating central cholangiocarcinoma (arrow, F).

Ultrasound

Underwater sonar predated the use of medical ultrasound by over thirty years, and the first medical ultrasound machines were introduced in the 1940s. Ultrasound examinations play a role in virtually all facets of modern medicine and are second only to radiographs in the number of imaging studies performed each year in the United States. Ultrasound images are generated from a probe with many individual transducer elements. Each element has an individual piezoelectric crystal which is able to convert electrical energy into ultrasonic energy and vice-versa. When exposed to an electric voltage, a crystal will resonate at a particular frequency depending upon its thickness, and this produces a sound wave. This sound wave travels through the patient's tissues, and when it encounters a tissue interface, some of the sound wave will be reflected back towards the probe. If during the "echo listening period" the crystal element detects this reflected sound wave, the crystal will generate an electric signal, and the location of the object can be estimated on an image. The image is produced using (a) the length of time it takes the echo to return to the transducer and (b) the amplitude of the returning echo.

Although the typical matrix of a displayed ultrasound image is 512 × 512 pixels, the actual resolution of the acquired image can vary considerably. The axial resolution, which separates two objects along the direction of the beam, is limited by the transducer frequency. Higher frequency transducers provide superior axial resolution, but as higher frequency sound waves are attenuated more easily, this is at the cost of decreased potential imaging depth. For a 2 MHz probe the axial resolution is about 1 mm, and for a 4 MHz probe it is about 0.5 mm. Higher frequency probes are used when the object being imaged is close to the ultrasound probe (i.e. transvaginal ultrasound, thyroid imaging, etc.), and lower frequency probes are used when deeper imaging is necessary (i.e. gallbladder). Ultrasound is generally considered to be safe at the intensity levels used in diagnostic imaging, although there are theoretical risks of tissue heating and cavitation (the creation and collapse of microscopic bubbles in the tissue).

Ultrasound is widely utilized as imaging guidance for a variety of biopsy or fine needle aspiration particularly involving the thyroid, breast, liver, or superficial nodes. It is also useful intraoperatively when assessing for liver metastasis undetected by other imaging modalities. However, the quality of a diagnostic ultrasound is highly dependent on the skill of the sonographer. This limitation, in addition to its limitations in tissue penetration, has made ultrasound less successful as a screening modality and less successful in staging/restaging of cancer. There has been recent interest in developing microbubble contrast agents and techniques for ultrasound imaging that could potentially increase its sensitivity for cancer detection.

Interventional Radiology

The role of interventional radiology in oncology has expanded from venous access and biopsy procedures to direct treatment as intra-arterial chemotherapy and percutaneous ablation procedures have grown in acceptance.

Radiofrequency ablation has demonstrated effectiveness in treating a variety tumors of the liver, kidney, lung, adrenal gland and bone. Radiofrequency probe insertion may utilize ultrasound, CT, or even MR guidance. Radiofrequency ablation (RFA) can be done percutaneously, laparoscopically, or during open surgery, and is very effective for tumors 3 cm or less in size. RFA has a role in larger tumors as well, but recurrence rates typically increase with increasing tumor size. A variety of alternative ablation procedures such as cryoablation, microwave ablation and ethanol vary in availability by institution.

Intra-arterial chemotherapy and embolization can significantly improve lifespan as palliative treatment of non-operable hepatocellular carcinoma or hepatic metastatic disease, especially hypervascular hepatic metastases such as neuroendocrine carcinoma or melanoma. Transarterial delivery of Yttrium-90 microspheres has also proved effective for localized radiotherapy of hepatic neoplasm.

Assessment of Imaging Modalities for the Detection of Malignancy

With the multitude of different imaging modalities and techniques currently available, it is important to have an objective means to assess diagnostic performance for a given indication. Without this, the clinician lacks the reference for what tests to order. Unfortunately, there is no single measurement that does this both successfully and comprehensively. Rather, multiple different methods have been developed to assess the varying aspects of diagnostic performance, which are reviewed briefly below:

True positive: A positive test result in a person with the disease.

True negative: A negative test result in a person without the disease.

False positive: A positive test result in a person without the disease.

False negative: A negative test result in a person with the disease.

Sensitivity: Percentage of positive tests in a group of patients with the disease, or,
Sensitivity = True Positives / (True Positives + False Negatives).

Specificity: Percentage of negative tests in a group of patients without the disease, or,
Specificity = True Negatives / (True Negatives + False Positives).

Positive Predictive Value: Percentage chance that a person with a positive test has the disease, or,
Positive Predictive Value = True Positives / (True Positives + False Positives).

Negative Predictive Value: Percentage chance that a person with a negative test is disease free, or,
Negative Predictive Value = True Negatives / (True Negatives + False Negatives).

A high sensitivity is desirable in a screening test. In other words, a screening test (i.e. mammography) should detect the majority of patients with a given disease. Alternatively, a high specificity is desirable for a confirmatory test (i.e. ultrasound-guided biopsy of a breast lesion). A test with a high specificity should accurately describe the majority of normal patients as being disease-free.

Imaging tests are often analyzed using the **receiver operating characteristic** (ROC) curve in which sensitivity is plotted on the Y-axis vs. the false positive fraction (1 – specificity) on the X-axis. Typically, as the sensitivity of a test is increased (i.e. Lowering the threshold value to obtain a positive test), the specificity of a test decreases due to a larger number of false positives. Examinations can be mathematically optimized by finding the threshold for a positive test which maximizes the area under the ROC curve. A random test such as a coin flip to detect the presence of disease would appear as a straight, diagonal line bisecting the graph with an area under the curve of 0.5. A perfect test with 100% specificity and 100% sensitivity has a point at the upper left corner of the graph and has a theoretical area under the curve of 1.0 (**Figure 7-8**). The receiver operator curve is considered a good scientific way of comparing two imaging modalities. One logistic difficulty of ROC analysis knows the actual clinical truth that is necessary to compute sensitivity and specificity.

A phenomenon at the intersection of diagnostic radiology and oncology, stage migration, is an important factor in the evaluation of cancer treatment. **Stage migration** occurs when patients in a clinical trial are staged with the newest and best imaging modalities. Often, highly sensitive modalities such at PET/CT detect disease which would not have been detected in the past. For example, the detection of a solitary extra-nodal metastasis

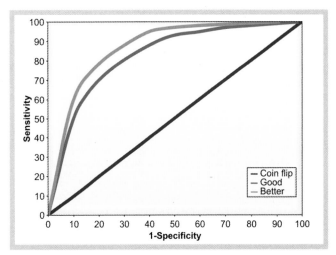

Figure 7-8: Receiver-operating characteristic curve

could upstage a breast cancer patient from stage III to stage IV. In the past, this patient would remain stage III. The hypothetical patient would be expected to have a mortality risk higher than the average stage III patient, but lower than the average stage IV patient with more extensive metastatic disease. By moving the patient from stage III to stage IV based on more sensitive imaging, the overall mortality of both stage III and stage IV patients improves. On a larger scale, this phenomenon can make a new treatment strategy appear more effective when compared to prior mortality data obtained when less sensitive imaging techniques were used for staging.

Examples of Imaging Utilization with Specific Cancers

Colorectal Carcinoma

Colorectal carcinoma is the second leading cause of cancer death in the United States, with a yearly incidence of 61.2 men and 44.8 women per 100,000 people. There were an estimated 147,000 new cases of colorectal carcinoma diagnosed in 2009, and approximately 50,000 deaths from colorectal carcinoma in the US in 2009. Innovation continues in diagnostic imaging with the hopes of detecting colorectal cancer earlier, providing more accurate staging, and improving restaging of treated patients.

Non-radiological screening programs targeted at detecting colorectal cancer in the population have focused primarily on fecal occult blood testing (FOBT) and colonoscopy. Traditional FOBT is, at best, approximately 33 to 50% sensitive for detecting cancer. Most advanced adenomas (>10 mm diameter or villous histological features) are usually not detected by means of FOBT. Conversely, colonoscopy is >90% sensitive for detecting lesions >10 mm in diameter and case-control studies have demonstrated an approximate 50-75% reduction in the incidence of colorectal cancer and a 30% reduction in mortality from the routine use of colonoscopy as a screening tool. However, few randomized, controlled trials are available to confirm this reduced incidence or mortality. Colonoscopy also has a high initial cost, requires bowel preparation, necessitates special expertise and is invasive (with 3-5 "serious" adverse events per 1000 examinations).

CT colonography represents another developing screening study for colorectal carcinoma. It is most appropriate for the average-risk patient in which the chance of having a large lesion necessitating colonoscopy is low, or for asymptomatic patients for whom screening with colonoscopy is unnecessarily risky (bleeding diathesis, risk for sedation, etc.). The sensitivity for polyp detection is similar to that of colonoscopy (90% for polyps >= 10 mm, 78% for polyps > 6 mm), and this sensitivity is likely to further improve as more advanced CT units are developed. CT colonography involves bowel preparation similar to traditional colonoscopy, although some imaging protocols permit the digital subtraction of stool and require minimum patient preparation. The colon is insufflated with air or carbon dioxide, and the patient is imaged via traditional CT. Two and three dimensional images are viewed on the workstation, and computer assisted detection (CAD) software can be used to increase cancer detection. The estimated radiation dose is similar to a regular body CT, and has been reported to be about 5-10 mSv. There is a smaller risk of serious adverse events compared with colonoscopy (1% vs. 3-5%), but approximately 15-25% of patients would be referred for colonoscopy if a 6 mm polyp size criteria was used. Although the American Cancer Society (ACS) recommended CT colonography as a preferred screening test in its 2008 guidelines, the Centers for Medicare and Medicaid Services (CMS) have recently ruled to deny routine coverage for Medicare recipients.

For colorectal cancer, the prognosis and choice of therapy are determined by the stage of the tumor at the time of diagnosis. Therefore, it is imperative that imaging adequately assess for the depth of invasion into the colonic wall, spread into pericolonic tissues and distant metastasis. Early studies with CT had a sensitivity of approximately 60% for determining local invasion compared with the TMN classification. The current sensitivity of CT is likely significantly higher due to contemporary multi-detector technology and improved spatial resolution. High resolution multi-planar MRI with surface coils compares favorably with CT in assessing for local extension of disease. CT and MRI can also be utilized to assess for regional and distant lymph node metastases by evaluating lymph node size, with MRI demonstrating superior sensitivity after the administration of ultra-small particles of iron oxide (which can detect metastatic disease in lymph nodes 3 to 4 mm in size). However, increasing evidence suggests that PET/CT should be used as the first test to assess metastatic disease and lymph node involvement in patients with intermediate to high pre-test probability of metastatic disease.

Staging of rectal cancer provides additional radiographic challenges. Specifically, the depth of mural involvement by the tumor and the distance from the tumor to the mesorectal resection plane need to be accurately characterized to guide treatment. Endorectal ultrasound is an established modality for evaluating the integrity of the rectal wall layers and has 65-95% accuracy in assessing for transmural/perirectal extension. However, it is unable to characterize lymph nodes out of range of the transducer and it cannot penetrate completely through bulky tumors, making it less useful for staging advanced rectal cancer. MRI has many advantages over ultrasound: it images the entire pelvis, it allows for clear delineation of the mesorectal fascia, it has the ability to differentiate malignant tissue from the muscularis propria, and it can detect extramural vascular invasion. Conversely, CT demonstrates a staging accuracy of approximately 50-75%.

As approximately 50% of patients will develop liver metastases over the course of their disease, early detection of liver metastases can help select patients who may significantly benefit from more aggressive surgical approaches. Computed tomography is the most widely used technique, and with studies utilizing helical CT and thin slice thicknesses (5 mm or less), the sensitivity for detecting liver metastases is believed to be between 70-90%. PET imaging has a very high sensitivity (>90%) for the overall detection of liver metastases, but this sensitivity drops when considering lesion-by-lesion sensitivity. Emerging evidence also suggests that PET may have a very low detection rate for small (<1 cm) liver metastases. PET imaging alone is not sufficient for visualization of the number and location of liver metastases before liver surgery, and should be combined with a full diagnostic CT study (PET/CT including IV contrast). In superparamagnetic iron oxide (SPIO) – enhanced MRI imaging of the liver, normal Kupffer cells take up the administered iron oxide and appear dark on T2 weighted imaging. As colorectal liver metastases have no SPIO uptake, and are typically bright on T2-weighted sequences, the metastasis-to-liver contrast is significantly improved. The sensitivity for detecting liver metastasis utilizing this technique is between 70-98%, higher than for routine gadolinium enhanced MRI. Intraoperative ultrasound is routinely used to assess for liver metastasis not detected by other imaging modalities, with a reported sensitivity of 80-98% compared with pathological examination.

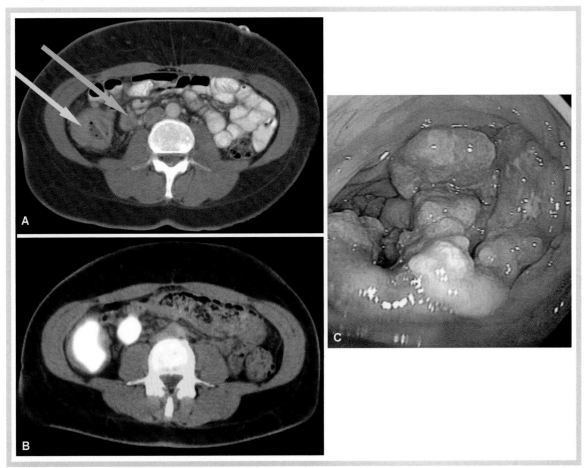

Figures 7-9A to C: A 46-year-old female with an incidentally detected colon cancer (the same unlucky patient with the right breast invasive ductal carcinoma previously illustrated). Enhanced axial CT (A) demonstrated abnormal cecal mural thickening (arrow, yellow), as well as an enlarged mesenteric lymph node (arrow, green). These areas correlated with increased FDG uptake on PET/CT (B). The patient's cecal mass was confirmed at colonscopy (C)

Breast Cancer

Breast cancer is the second most common cause of cancer death among US women. Over 200,000 cases are diagnosed each year and women have a 1 in 8 lifetime risk of developing the disease. Screening for breast cancer has been recommended for many decades in women older than 40 in the United States. There has been recent controversy regarding screening between ages forty and fifty, but screening after age fifty remains the gold standard, generally complemented by clinical and self breast exams.

The clinical breast exam is performed on only two thirds of US women over 40. Sensitivity of clinical breast exam is low, between 40% and 70%. Indeed, the US. Preventive Services Task Force (USPSTF) in their recent 2009 report assessed that "the current evidence is insufficient to assess the additional benefits and harms of clinical breast examination beyond screening mammo-graphy in woman 40 years or older". Canadian physicians have increased the rate of breast cancer detection based on their physical exams, traditionally believed to result from a more through systematic clinical exam. Less than one-third of US women regularly perform self breast exams. The USPSTF actually recommends against clinicians teaching women how to perform breast self-examinations over concern of the resulting unnecessary anxiety, imaging studies, and biopsies. The sensitivity of the breast self exam is believed to range 10-40%, and is age-dependant.

Screening mammography has been shown to statistically reduce breast cancer mortality in women ages 50 to 69 years. In general, breast cancers detected by mammography are smaller and have more favorable histological and biological features compared to tumors first found by clinical exam. The benefit of screening women in their 40s is reduced by the relatively low incidence of breast cancer in this age group, by the presence of dense breast tissue which confounds interpretation of the study and by the increased incidence of rapidly growing tumors in these patients. Recent studies suggest that, in women 39 to 49 years of age, approximately 1900 women need to be screened by mammography to prevent one breast cancer death. For women 50 to 59 years of age, approximately 1300 would need to be screened to prevent one death. For women 60 to 69, approximately 400 would require screening. On the other hand, there may be little benefit to screening women with multiple co-morbidities and or with a life expectancy of less than 5 years. The sensitivity of mammography is above 75% and the specificity above 90% across all ages and breast types.

Full-field digital mammography and Computer Aided Detection (CAD) programs use ionizing radiation like standard mammography. The image is captured digitally enabling the radiologist to manipulate the image on the computer or print and view the image. Currently this technology is more expensive. Computer Aided Detection (CAD) programs recognize potential pathologic patterns in breast images consistent with cancer and mark them for the radiologist to look at. They have increased radiologist recall rate and breast cancer detection, but larger studies are needed to prove its clinical benefit. Currently Medicare and Medicaid will allow additional billing for this technology.

Magnetic resonance imaging is currently not approved as a general screening modality in the US. It may prove helpful in women who are at increased risk of developing breast cancer at a younger age, such as women who are known carriers of *BRCA1* or *BRCA2*. It can be recommended for woman with dense breasts and for patients with implants. MR is also useful to assess for multifocal disease and for recurrence. MRI has an increased sensitivity but decreased specificity in comparison to mammography in women, potentially resulting in unnecessary further exams and biopsies. MRI screening will probably not be available in the immediate future to the general population due to its high cost and low specificity compared to mammography.

Ultrasound is problematic for screening the general population because it requires a well trained operator and data indicates a high false positive rate. Ultrasound screening is best utilized in selected populations such as younger women in whom radiation exposure is a greater concern, women with dense breast tissue and women with high risk factors for breast cancer. Ultrasound has an extremely important role in the characterization of breast masses and cysts.

If a patient has a concerning lesson on a screening exam, a biopsy is often necessary. Biopsies can be performed via ultrasound, X-ray, CT, or MRI guided techniques. The

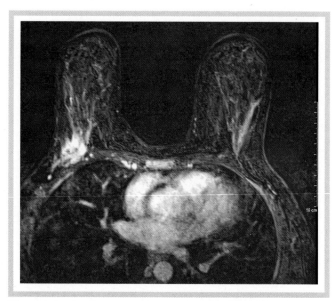

Figure 7-10: T1 post-contrast subtracted axial image demonstrated an enhancing right breast mass invading the underlying pectoralis muscle in a patient with invasive ductal carcinoma

lesion or the margins of a lesion can also be clearly defined by wires placed in or around the lesion to facilitate surgical removal.

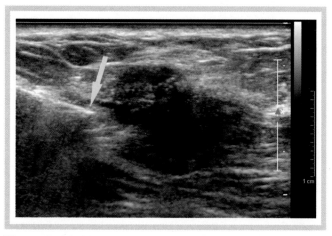

Figure 7-11: Ultrasound guided biopsy of an irregular, hypoechoic breast mass using a 14 gauge core biopsy needle. A metallic localization clip was also placed. Pathology was returned as invasive ductal carcinoma (The needle tip is marked with arrow)

Primary staging and follow up may require a multimodality approach including mammography, X-ray, ultrasound, MRI, CT, or PET scans. In particular, PET/CT has proven very useful for staging patients with advanced disease, and restaging recurrent disease. PET is superior in detecting distant metastases in the chest, liver, and bone compared with conventional modalities.

As mentioned previously, PET and technetium bone scan play complementary roles in detecting bony metastasis; the former is better at detecting lytic lesions, and the latter at detecting sclerotic metastasis. Some research also suggests that PET can be utilized to asses for treatment response, as "responding" tumor will demonstrate decreased metabolic activity on interval PET scanning. It should be noted, however, that certain well-differentiated and slow-growing tumors (i.e. lobular carcinoma and DCIS) have been known to occasionally demonstrate false-negative PET findings.

A significant number of women diagnosed with breast cancer are at risk of tumor recurrence. Follow-up examinations are necessary after primary treatment for breast cancer. Early detect of recurrence is of paramount importance for ideal treatment. Follow-up programs based on a regular physical exam with an oncologist and yearly mammograms should be utilized. Additional imaging should be based on the patient's symptoms, with consideration given to MRI and PET/CT.

Pancreatic Cancer

Pancreatic adenocarcinoma is the fourth leading cause of cancer-related death in the United States. It is an aggressive and almost universally fatal malignancy, with only approximately 3% of diagnosed patients surviving for five years. As complete surgical removal is the only therapy with curative intent, it is imperative to properly stage patients in order to identify the 10-20% of patients that are potentially resectable.

Computed tomography is the primary method for diagnosing pancreatic adenocarcinoma. Most pancreatic protocols for CT involve imaging slightly after the arterial phase in order to maximize contrast between tumor and the normal pancreatic parenchyma, and imaging during the portal-venous phase to assess for regional and distant metastasis. CT angiography is also sometimes utilized in order to better ascertain potential vascular involvement by tumor. CT has been shown to have a very high sensitivity for detecting larger pancreatic lesions, approaching 100% for tumors >1.5 cm in size. However, this sensitivity drops for smaller tumors, with one recent study showing a 67% sensitivity for tumors <1.5 cm.

CT is also very commonly used to stage pancreatic adenocarcinoma. Signs of unresectability on CT include involvement of adjacent major vascular structures, extension of tumor beyond the margins of the pancreas, tumor invasion of adjacent organs, liver metastases, and carcinomatosis. Although CT has been shown to have >90% sensitivity and specificity in detecting vascular invasion, it is however less successful for accurately detecting nodal metastases. If a 10 mm short-axis cutoff is used to diagnose pathologic lymphadenopathy (which

is common practice), one recent study suggested 14% sensitivity for detecting lymph node invasive due to early micrometastases. The sensitivity increased to 77% when a 5 mm cutoff was used. CT performs well for detecting hepatic metastases >= 1 cm, with decreased sensitivity for smaller lesions. Peritoneal carcinomatosis can be difficult to diagnose by any imaging modality in its early stages, but its presence can be suggested on CT when ascites is present.

Other imaging modalities that are useful in the treatment of pancreatic adenocarcinoma include magnetic resonance imaging and PET. The former offers superior imaging of fluid-filled structures (such as the pancreatic and biliary ducts), and can sometimes detect small hepatic metastases not seen on CT. It has been shown to be slightly less sensitive than CT (approximately 85% vs. 90%) for the detection of pancreatic adenocarcinoma, with about equivalent accuracy in predicting resectability. MRI also offers the advantage of improved visualization of tumor in the setting of pancreatic inflammation compared with CT, and can be used in patients with poor renal function. The research to substantiate the routine use of PET/CT for pancreatic adenocarcinoma diagnosis and staging is ongoing, with studies suggesting a >95% sensitivity for the detection of cancer.

Up to 20% of patients undergoing routine cross-sectional radiological examination may have incidental pancreatic cystic lesions, with the majority of these representing pseudocysts. Correlation with the patient's medical history is important, as prior pancreatitis can strongly suggest this diagnosis. However, 10-15% of these lesions statistically will represent primary cystic masses of the pancreas. It is imperative to properly categorize these lesions, which many times appear radiographically similar, as they have the potential for malignancy that ranges from negligible (serous cystadenoma) to approximately 90% (main branch intraductal papillary mucinous neoplasm, IPMN). Although endoscopic ultrasound (EUS) and endoscopic retrograde cholangiopancreatography (ERCP) play increasing roles in the diagnoses of these lesions, our discussion will focus on the cross-sectional imaging performed by the radiology department. Specifically protocoled pancreatic MRI with contrast is preferable to enhanced CT for the characterization of cystic pancreatic masses as MR has higher sensitivity for contrast enhancement and MR better evaluates for mural nodularity and for communication with the pancreatic duct.

Serous cystic neoplasms are pancreatic tumors with minimal malignant potential, although there are case reports of malignant transformation. They are most frequently cystadenomas, and comprise about 25% of primary cystic masses of the pancreas. Demographically they present most commonly in middle-aged and older

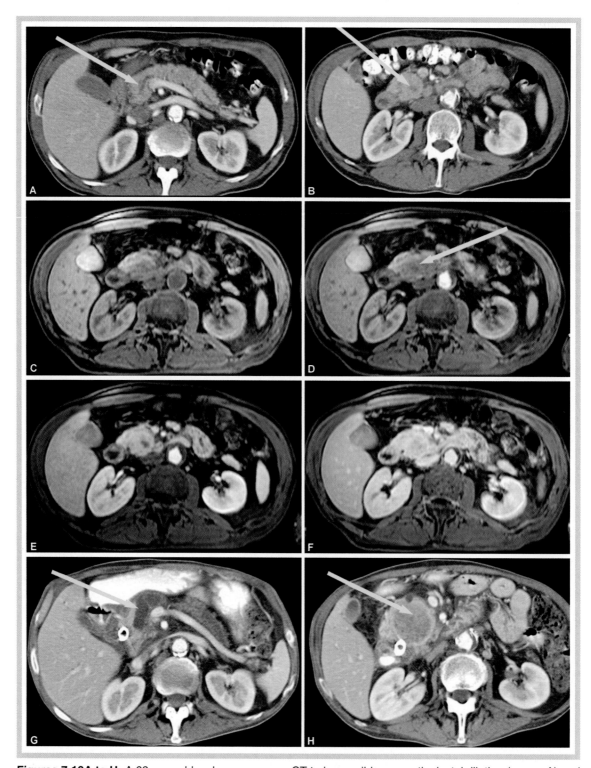

Figures 7-12A to H: A 63-year-old male was seen on CT to have mild pancreatic ductal dilation (arrow, A) and a subcentimeter focus within the pancreatic uncinate process (marked B). Findings were concerning for a small mass. Subsequent enhanced MRI of the abdomen (C, D, E, and F). Timed interval T1 enhanced images (C = before contrast, D = arterial phase, E = portal-venous phase, and F = delayed phase 5 minutes after the initial contrast injection) more clearly demonstrated a 3 cm tumor in the pancreatic head, best seen on arterial phase imaging as a hypovascular mass (arrow, D). Repeat CT in 4 months demonstrated significant interval increase in pancreatic ductal dilation (arrow, G) and pancreatic parenchymal atrophy. The pancreatic head mass (pancreatic adenocarcinoma) was also much larger (arrow, H). A biliary stent had been placed since the prior study

women, and are found equally distributed throughout the organ. They can either appear as a well-circumscribed mass of innumerable small cysts, or in a unilocular form. Serous cystadenomas often have a characteristic central stellate scar with associated calcification.

Mucinous cystic neoplasms comprise approximately half of the discovered primary cystic pancreatic neoplasms. All are low-grade mucinous cystadenocarcinomas. These traditionally occur in middle-aged females, and approximately a quarter are found to be malignant. Most tumors occur in the pancreatic body or tail. They appear on imaging as multiloculated cysts with thin, enhancing septa. These tumors do not communicate with the ductal system, and may be associated with peripheral calcifications.

Intraductal papillary mucinous neoplasms (IPMN) arise from the epithelium lining the pancreatic ducts, with histology that ranges from hyperplasia to adenocarcinoma. They are predominately found in elderly males, and may present clinically as pancreatitis. IPMN's comprise approximately 25% of the primary cystic pancreatic neoplasms, and are divided into "main branch" and "side branch" variants. The former has a malignancy potential of 60-90%, and the latter of 5-45%. On imaging, tumors that arise from the main pancreatic duct can produce marked ductal dilation and secondary atrophy of the pancreatic parenchyma. Conversely, side-branch IPMN's usually produce a multicystic mass, with a majority occurring within the head and uncinate process.

Solid pseudopapillary tumors of the pancreas (SPN) are rare tumors that occur predominately in younger women. They are distributed evenly throughout the pancreas. On imaging they are well-circumscribed tumors, may be predominately solid, and have uniformly enhancing soft tissue components. Although they have a low malignant potential, SPN's are typically removed as they have imaging characteristics overlapping with neuroendocrine tumors and mucinous cystadenocarcinomas.

The last category of pancreatic tumors we will discuss are the pancreatic neuroendocrine tumors. Functioning tumors produce clinical syndromes due to the hormones that they secrete, and usually present when the tumors are small. They vary in malignant potential from 10% (insulinoma), to 60% (gastrinoma), to 80% (glucagonoma). Approximately 80% of non-functioning islet cell tumors are malignant, and usually present when they are large. Small (<4 cm) tumors tend to be homogenous on imaging, with intense enhancement during the arterial phase. Larger tumors are usually more heterogeneous. Staging should include imaging of the liver to assess for metastases. Approximately 20% of islet cell tumors can have cystic components, and therefore have overlapping imaging characteristics with the previous described

pancreatic cystic tumors. Indium-111 DTPA Octreotide scans are sometimes helpful in assessing for extend of disease, particularly for gastrinoma and carcinoid.

Landmark Papers

1. Baron Richard L, et al. Hepatocellular carcinoma: Evaluation with biphasic, contrast-enhanced, helical CT. Radiology 1996;199(2): 505.
2. Beyer, Thomas, et al. A combined PET/CT scanner for clinical oncology. The Journal of Nuclear Medicine 2000; 41(8): 1369.
3. Brenner, David, et al. Estimated risks of radiation-induced fetal cancer from pediatric CT. American Journal of Roentgenology 2001; 176 (2): 289.
4. Bushberg J. The essential physics of Medical Imaging (2nd edn) Lippincott Williams & Wilkins: Philadelphia, 2002.
5. Elmore JG, et al. Screening for Breast Cancer. JAMA 2003; 293(10); 1245-56.
6. Hollett Michael D, et al. Dual-phase helical CT of the liver: Value of the arterial phase scans in the detection of small (< 1.5 cm) malignant hepatic neoplasms. American Journal of Roentgenology 1995;164(4): 879.
7. Huda W. Review of Radiologic Physics. Lippincott Williams: Baltimore, 2010.
8. Hutchins G, Draganov P. Diagnostic Evaluation of Pancreatic Cystic Malignancies. Surg Clin N America 2010;90: 399-410.
9. Kalb B, Sarmiento J, et al. MR Imaging of Cystic Lesions of the Pancreas. Radiographics 2009;29: 1749-65.
10. Kinney T. Evidence-Based Imaging of Pancreatic Malignancies. Surg Clin N America 2010;90: 235-49.
11. Korobkin Melvyn, et al. Delayed enhanced CT for differentiation of benign from malignant adrenal masses. Radiology 1996;200(3): 737.
12. Lasser EC, et al. Pretreatment with corticosteroids to alleviate reactions to contrast material. New England Journal of Medicine 1987;317(14): 845.
13. Lieberman DA. Screening for Colorectal Cancer. The New England Journal of Medicine 2009;361:1179-87.
14. Lu David SK, et al. Local staging of pancreatic cancer: Criteria for Unresectability of major vessels as revealed by pancreatic-phase, thin-section, helical CT. American Journal of Roentgenology 1997;168(6): 1439.
15. McWhirter E, et al. Baseline radiological staging in primary breast cancer: impact of educational interventions on adherence to published guidelines. Journal of Evaluation in Clinical Practice 2007;13: 647-50.
16. Nystrom Lennarth, et al. Long-term effects of mammography screening: Updated overview of the Swedish randomized trials. Lancet 2002;359(9310): 909.
17. Pickhardt PJ. Noninvasive radiologic imaging of the large intestine; a valuable complement to optical colonoscopy. Current Opinion in Gastroenterology 2009;25:61-68.
18. Rappeport ED, et al. Liver metastases from Colorectal Cancer: imaging with super-paramagnetic iron oxide (SPIO)-enhanced MR imaging, computed tomography and positron emission tomography Abdominal Imaging 2007; 32:624-634.

19. Rockey DC. Computed Tomographic Colonography: Current perspective and Future Directions. Gastroenterology 2009;137: 7-17.

20. Rossi S, et al. Percutaneous treatment of small hepatic tumors by an expandable RF needle electrode. American Journal of Roentgenology 1998;170(4): 1015.

21. Russell EJ, et al. Multiple cerebral metastases: Detestability with Gd-DTPA-enhanced MR imaging. Radiology 1987; 165(3): 609.

22. Schmidt GP, et al. Whole Body MRI and PET-CT in Oncology: Top Mgn Reson Imaging 2007;18(3): 193-202.

23. Som P, et al. A fluorinated glucose analog, 2-fluoro-2-deoxy-D-glucose (F-18): Nontoxic tracer for rapid tumor detection. Journal of Nuclear Medicine 1980;21(7): 670.

24. Soto JA. Imaging of Colorectal Carcinoma. Cancer treatment and research 2008;143: 255-280.

25. US Preventive Services Task Force. Screening for Breast Cancer: U.S. Preventive Services Task Force Recommendation Statement. Ann Intern Med 2009; 151 (10): 716-26. W-236.

26. Wahl RL, et al. Metabolic monitoring of breast cancer chemohormonotherapy using positron emission tomography: Initial evaluation. Journal of Clinical Oncology 1993;11: 2101.

27. Webb R, Brant W, Major N. Fundamentals of Body CT (3rd edn). Saunders Elsevier 2006;253-8.

28. Weinmann, Hanns-Joachim, et al. Characteristics of Gadolinium-DTPA complex: A potential NMR contrast agent. American Journal of Roentgenology 1984;142(3): 619.

29. Ziessman HA, et al. Nuclear Medicine (3rd edn). Elsevier Mosby: Philadelphia, 2006

30. The History of Magnetic Resonance Imaging, The University of Manchester http://www.isbe.man.ac.uk/ personal /dellard/dje/history_mri/history%20of% 20mri.htm

Level of Evidence Table

What is the best imaging test for...	Best choice	Level of evidence	Disadvantages	Comments	Alternatives	References
Staging or restaging of lymphoma	PET/CT	Level 1	Cost. Ionizing radiation. PET may show low uptake (false negative) in MALT or low grade follicular lymphoma	Most sensitive and specific modality. PET evaluation of metabolic activity improves specificity for tumor viability after treatment	CT	Tatsumi M, et al. Direct comparison of FDG PET and CT findings in patients with lymphoma: Initial experience. Radiology 2005;237: 1038. / Buchman I, et al. 2-(Fluorine-18) Fluoro-2-Deoxy-D-Glucose positron emission tomography in the detection and staging of malignant lymphoma. A Bicenter Trial. Cancer 2001;91(5): 889.
Evaluation of intracranial metastases	MRI with and without contrast	Level 1	Cost, contraindicated in patients with pacemaker	Most sensitive and specific modality for intracranial metastases	Head CT with and without contrast. PET may be more useful in evaluation of viability of treated intracranial lesions	Schellinger PD, et al. Diagnostic accuracy of MRI compared to CCT in patients with brain metastases. Journal of Neuro-Oncology 1999;44: 275-81.
Evaluation of spinal metastases	MRI with and without contrast	Level 1	Cost, pacemaker contraindication. Relatively long imaging times especially if imaging of entire spine is performed	High sensitivity and excellent anatomic characterization	Bone scan and PET have excellent sensitivity, and specificity is improved by adding CT. CT myelography may be a useful alternative to MRI when evaluating for cord compression	Algra PR, et al. Detection of vertebral metastases: Comparison between MR imaging and bone scintigraphy. Radiographics 1991;11(2): 219.
Evaluation of hepatic masses	MRI with and without contrast	Level 1	Cost, pacemaker contraindication	Accuracy varies by type of malignancy and technique	PET/CT has higher sensitivity for specific metastases such as colorectal cancer. CT with and without contrast (with arterial phase imaging for hypervascular tumors) also has excellent sensitivity and specificity	Stark DD, et al. Hepatic metastases: randomized, controlled comparison of detection with MR imaging and CT. Radiology 1987;165: 399. / Bipat S, et al. Colorectal liver metastases: CT, MR imaging, and PET for diagnosis—meta-analysis. Radiology 2005;327-123.
Evaluation of pulmonary metastases	PET/CT	Level 4	Cost. Ionizing radiation	Highly sensitive and specific	CT alone is less specific, but often is preferred due to lower cost and wide availability. Few studies comparing PET/CT to CT alone	Strobel K, et al. High-risk melanoma: Accuracy of FDG PET/CT with added CT morphologic information for detection of metastases. Radiology 2007;244: 566. / Schulthess GK, et al. Integrated PET/CT: Current applications and future directions. Radiology 2006;238: 405.

Contd...

Contd...

What is the best imaging test for...	Best choice	Level of evidence	Disadvantages	Comments	Alternatives	References
Evaluation of bony metastases	PET/CT	Level 1	Cost. Ionizing radiation	Allows for evaluation of visceral metastases	Bone Scan offers lower cost and high sensitivity, particularly with sclerotic metastases	Shie P, et al. Meta-analysis: comparison of F-18 FDG-positron emission tomography and bone scintigraphy in the detection of bone metastases in patients with breast cancer. Clinical Nuclear Medicine 2008; 33 (2): 97. Gallowitsch HJ, et al. F-18 fluoro-deoxyglucose positron-emission tomography in the diagnosis of tumor recurrence and metastases in the follow up of patients with breast carcinoma: A comparison to conventional imaging. Investigative Radiology 2003; 38(5):250.
Characterization of adrenal masses	CT with and without contrast	Level 3	Ionizing radiation. IV contrast often necessary.	Widely available	MRI has comparable specificity and requires no contrast. PET has limited specificity, as adrenal adenomas are occasionally FDG avid	Peña C, et al. Characterization of indeterminate (lipid-poor) adrenal masses: Use of washout characteristics at contrast-enhanced CT. Radiology 2000; 217:897.
Screening of breast cancer in women over age 40	Mammography	Level 1	Ionizing radiation	Widely available	MRI has high sensitivity and specificity, but is limited in evaluation of microcalcifications ultrasound	Nystrom L, et al. Long term effects of mammography screening: updated overview of the Swedish randomized trials. Lancet 2002; 359 (9320):909.
Screening of breast cancer in women under age 40 (where indicated)	MRI	Level 4	Cost. Requires Gadilinium injection. Limited availability	Particularly useful in women with dense breast tissue	Mammography and ultrasound	Hall F. The rise and impending decline of screening mammography. Radiology 2008; 247:597.
Restaging of metastatic breast cancer	PET/CT	Level 1	Cost. Ionizing radiation	Highest sensitivity and specificity for Stage IV disease	CT and bone scan are likely adequate for stage II and stage III disease	Rosen E, et al. FDG PET, PET/CT, and breast cancer imaging. Radiographics 2007; 27:215.
Initial evaluation of symptomatic or palpable thyroid nodule/mass	Ultrasound	Level 4	Imaging quality depends on skill of sonographer. High sensitivity, but poor specificity	No radiation. Inexpensive. Ultrasound guidance often used for biopsy	CT	Won-Jin M, et al. Benign and malignant thyroid nodules: Ultrasound differentiation—Multicenter retrospective study. Radiology 2008; 247:762

Contd...

Contd...

What is the best imaging test for...	Best choice	Level of evidence	Disadvantages	Comments	Alternatives	References
Staging/ Restaging of metastatic thryoid cancer	PET/CT	Level 4	Cost. Ionizing Radiation	Best utilized in patients with elevated thyroglobulin levels and negative Radioiodine scans	Radioiodine whole body imaging. Ultrasound for recurrence in the neck.	Palmedo H, et al. Integraded PET/CT in differentiated thyroid cancer: diagnostic accuracy and impact on patient management. Journal of Nuclear Medicine 2006; 47:4616.
Evaluation of parathyroid adenoma	Dual phase Technicium Sestimibi scan	Level 4	Limited anatomic information. Limited specificity	Best used in patients with elevated parathyroid hormone	CT and/or ultrasound are useful adjuncts for anatomic information	De Feo ML, et al. Parathyroid glands: Combination of 99mTc MIBI scintigraphy and ultrasound for demonstration of parathyroid glands and nodules. Radiology 2000; 214:393.
Hepatocellular cancer screening	MRI with and without contrast or triphasic CT	Level 1	Cost. Pacemaker contraindication. Requires IV gadolinium	Widely available	Triphasic CT has very comparable sensitivity and specificity	Willatt J, et al. MR imaging of hepatocellular carcinoma in the cirrhotic liver: Challenges and controversies. Radiology 2008; 247:311.
Hepatocellular carcinoma Staging and restaging	MRI with and without contrast or triphasic CT, particularly if chest imaging is also desired	Level 1	Ionizing radiation. Requires IV contrast	Widely available	MRI is excellent for liver imaging, but limited for whole body imaging for lung and bony metastases	Willatt J, et al. MR imaging of hepatocellular carcinoma in the cirrhotic liver: Challenges and controversies. Radiology 2008; 247:311.
Gallbladder carcinoma	CT	Level 4	Ionizing radiation. Requires IV contrast	Widely available	MRI also useful in assessment of local extent of disease	Kalra N, et al. MDCT in the staging of gallbladder carcinoma. American Journal of Roentgenology 2006; 186:758.
Evaluation of resectability of pancreatic adenocarcinoma	Pancreatic mass protocol CT	Level 1	Ionizing radiation. Requires IV contrast	Highest spatial resolution for depiction of vascular encasement. Water may be used as oral contrast	MRI depicts the pancreatic duct well, but is limited in evaluation of vascular involvement with tumor	Nishiharu T, et al. Local extension of pancreatic carcinoma: assessment with thin-section helical CT versus with breath-hold fast MR imaging—ROC analysis. Radiology 1999; 212:445. Kalra MK, et al. State-of-the-art imaging of pancreatic neoplasms. British Journal of Radiology 2003; 79:857.
Restaging pancreatic carcinoma after resection or therapy	CT with contrast	Level 4	Ionizing radiation. Requires IV contrast	Widely available	PET or PET/CT most useful for problem solving for indeterminate findings at CT.	Tamm E, et al. Diagnosis, staging, and surveillance of pancreatic cancer. American Journal of Roentgenology 2003;180:1311.

Contd...

Contd...

What is the best imaging test for....	Best choice	Level of evidence	Disadvantages	Comments	Alternatives	References
Pancreatic islet cell tumors/ Neuroendocrine tumor	Triphasic CT	Level 2	Ionizing radiation. Requires IV contrast	Widely available. Water often used as an oral contrast agent in this setting	MRI has comparable accuracy in evaluation of the pancreatic mass and in evaluation of hepatic metastases, but is less useful in whole body imaging	Ichikawa T, et al. Islet cell tumor of the pancreas: Biphasic CT versus MR imaging in tumor detection. Radiology 2000; 216:163.
Characterization of pancreatic cystic masses	MRI without and with contrast	Level 2	Cost. Pacemaker contraindication. Requires Gadolinium contrast	CT and MRI have comparable sensitivity, and both have limited specificity. MR best depicts relation to pancreatic duct	CT PET can be very useful in differentiating metabolically active malignancies from benign pancreatic cystic masses	Visser BC, et al. Characterization of cystic pancreatic masses: Relative accuracy of CT and MRI. American Journal of Roentgenology 2007;189 (3):648.
Evaluation of local extent of esophageal cancer	Endoscopic Ultrasound	Level 4	Invasive. Cost.	Potential for biopsy at same procedure	Barium esophagram useful in depicting extent of luminal involvement and may aid operative planning	Rice TW, et al. Role of clinically determined depth of tumor invasion in the treatment of esophageal carcinoma. The Journal of Thoracic and Cardiovascular Surgery 2003;125:1091.
Staging or restaging esophageal cancer	PET/CT	Level 1	Ionizing radiation. Requires IV contrast	Best single examination to evaluate for local recurrence and metastatic disease after surgery	CT with contrast. Endoscopic Ultrasound often used to assess response of primary mass	Westerterp M. et al. Esophageal cancer: CT, endoscopic US, and FDG PET for assessment of response to neoadjuvant therapy—Systemic review. Radiology 2005; 236:841.
Staging or restaging of gastric cancer	CT with contrast	Level 3	Ionizing radiation. Requires IV contrast	Multiplanar and additional specialized reformatted images improve evaluation of local disease	PET/CT may play a role in surveillance, particularly if the primary is known to be FDG avid	Kim H.J, et al. Gastric cancer staging at multi-detector CT gastrography. Comparison of transverse and volumetric CT scanning. Radiology 2005; 236: 879. Lim J S, et al. CT and PET in stomach cancer: prospective staging and monitoring of response to therapy. Radiographics 2006; 26:143.
Evaluation of small bowel adenocarcinoma	CT enterography	Level 5	Ionizing radiation. Requires IV contrast	CT enterography uses low density luminal contrast agent and IV contrast to better evaluate the small bowel wall	CT enteroclysis. PET/CT also useful, but can be limited in evaluation of bowel due to variable physiologic bowel uptake of FDG	Paulsen S, et al. CT enterography as a diagnostic tool in evaluating small bowel disorders: Review of clinical experience with over 700 cases. Radiographics 2008; 26:641.
Staging or Restaging of metastatic colorectal cancer	PET/CT	Level 1	Cost. Ionizing radiation	PET/CT has excellent sensitivity and specificity for colorectal carcinoma	CT without and with contrast has slightly lower sensitivity and specificity	Soyko J, et al. Staging pathways in recurrent colorectal carcinoma: Is contrast-enhanced 18F-FDG PET/CT the diagnostic tool of choice? Journal of Nuclear Medicine 2008; 49(3):354.

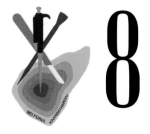

8

Vascular Access and Infusion Pumps

Theodore H Yuo, Rabih A Chaer

Overview

The surgical oncology patient often requires vascular access for the ongoing administration of chemotherapy and parenteral nutrition. Many of the agents used are vesicants and can result in local tissue damage if extravasation were to occur, as well as phlebitis and venous thrombosis if infused in smaller veins. Administration therefore requires central venous access in order to avoid such complications and provide large bore access. In addition, many chemotherapeutic regimens require periodic treatment and as such, long-term central venous access is often necessary. The purpose of this chapter is to review the current indications and techniques of vascular access for the surgical oncology patient.

Venous Access

Techniques

Central venous access is based on the Seldinger technique, named after the Swedish radiologist Sven-Ivar Seldinger who first described the eponymous technique in the 1950s, in which a needle accesses a vascular channel, a wire is advanced through the needle, the needle is removed, a catheter is advanced over the wire into the vascular channel and the wire is removed. As with all invasive procedures, informed consent should be routinely obtained, unless an emergent situation exists. Coagulopathy should be corrected, including an INR of less than 1.5 and a platelet count of at least 50,000 per microliter. Finally, Trendelenburg position, ultrasound guidance, continuous monitoring of cardiac rhythm, sterile technique and appropriate analgesia, with local anesthetic (e.g. lidocaine) are essential, as well.

Subclavian Venous Access

The specific technique to obtain subclavian access is described in a number of publications. In general, the first step is to identify the mid-point of the clavicle. Although ultrasound guidance can be useful, visualization of the subclavian vein is limited and familiarity with anatomic landmarks is essential **(Figures 8-1 and 8-2)**.

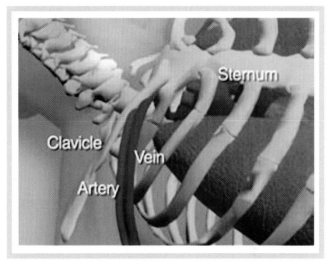

Figure 8-1: Important anatomy for subclavian vein access (see footnote)

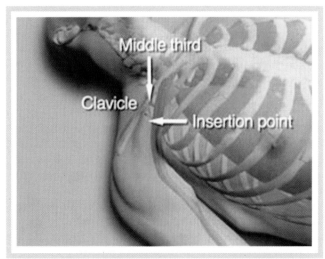

Figure 8-2: Localization of anatomic landmarks for subclavian vein access (see footnote).

Reprinted with permission from Braner et al. Videos in clinical medicine: central venous catheterization—subclavian vein. *New England Journal of Medicine* 2007 Dec 13;357(24):e26. Copyright © 2007 *Massachusetts Medical Society. All rights reserved.*

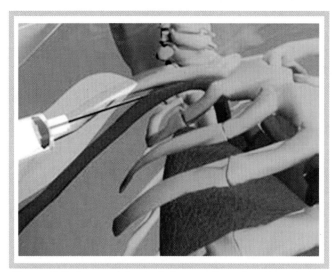

Figure 8-3: Appropriate angle for needle and syringe during subclavian vein access (see footnote on page 95)

An insertion point approximately 2 cm caudad and 2 cm lateral to the mid-point of the clavicle is chosen. The site should be free of significant skin lesions, cellulitis or other infectious process. Local anesthesia should be infiltrated into the area with special attention to the periosteum of the clavicle. Starting 2 cm lateral to the bend of the clavicle and approximately 2 cm caudal, the catheterization needle is inserted through the skin at a 30-degree angle and aimed toward the sternal notch. A finger of the nondominant hand placed in the sternal notch can help to identify the landmark. Once the needle is under the skin, the needle and the syringe are lowered in order to run parallel to and posterior to the clavicle **(Figure 8-3)**.

Some practitioners advocate hitting the clavicle with the needle and then walking the needle posteriorly (down) the clavicle in order to dive deep to the clavicle and access the subclavian vein without potentially causing a pneumothorax. Access to the vein typically occurs just beneath the clavicle, but it may occur at a depth of several centimeters under the skin, depending on the patient's body habitus. Once venous access has been obtained, the needle is carefully stabilized and the syringe removed. The J-tipped end of the guidewire is inserted into the needle. The wire should thread easily and without resistance until well beyond the end of the needle. If ectopic cardiac beats appear on a cardiac monitor, the wire should be pulled back until the ectopic beats disappear. The needle is then removed, leaving the wire in place. Maintaining control of the wire is essential, as the wire can be lost into the circulation and can lodge in the heart or pulmonary vasculature. A small, 2-mm incision should be made in the skin at the insertion point to facilitate dilator passage. The dilator is advanced over the wire into and through the skin and then a few millimeters into the vessel. Note that the dilators are stiff and overdilating risks puncturing the back

wall of the vessel. Once the tract is dilated, the dilator is removed and hemostasis is achieved with manual compression. After ensuring that the side ports are clamped to avoid air emboli, the line is quickly advanced over the guidewire, maintaining control of the wire before passing the catheter into the skin. Excessive skin contact with the catheter is to be avoided in order to minimize the risk of infection. The insertion length can be estimated by tracing the course of the catheter externally and is typically longer for left sided access. The guidewire is then removed and blood return from all ports is ensured. Ports are then flushed and appropriate caps placed, before securing the catheter in place using suture. A sterile dressing should be applied before removing the drapes. A post-procedure chest X-ray is essential to ensure proper placement and for the evaluation for possible pneumothorax.

The catheter tip should lie at the cavoatrial junction, as placement of the catheter tip high in the SVC can result in a higher incidence of thrombosis and may not adequately flush because of apposition to the caval wall. In addition, since wire insertion is not routinely guided by fluoroscopy, the catheter can inadvertently be placed into the internal jugular vein.

Internal Jugular (IJ) Venous Access

The most commonly used technique is the anterior approach in which the internal jugular vein is punctured where it passes just deep to the supraclavicular triangle. This triangle is defined by the sternal and clavicular heads of the sternocleidomastoid muscle. The needle should be aimed toward the ipsilateral nipple with an angle of 30-45 degrees from the sagittal (horizontal) plane. Of note, the carotid artery is just medial to the internal jugular vein and must be avoided when cannulating the IJ.

The catheter tip should lie in the cavoatrial junction, as described above. A post-procedure chest X-ray to confirm position and exclude pneumothorax is essential.

Use of ultrasound guidance is recommended, given the results of randomized controlled trials that demonstrate fewer complications, failures and time required for insertion. Its use avoids inadvertent arterial puncture, ensures patency of the target vein and allows prompt and easy access. Ultrasound guidance utilizes high frequency sound waves to produce a two dimensional image. To obtain IJ access, a cross sectional transverse image of the vessels allows visualization of the target vessel and structures to be avoided, especially the common carotid artery **(Figure 8-4)**.

The artery can be distinguished from the vein by several characteristics:
1. The carotid artery is medial to the internal jugular vein.
2. The carotid artery in general is smaller, with a thicker wall.
3. The carotid artery is pulsatile.
4. The carotid artery is non-compressible **(Figure 8-5)**.

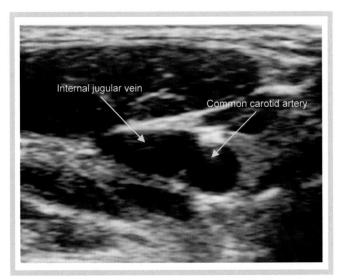

Figure 8-4: Ultrasound image of the internal jugular vein and common carotid artery during internal jugular vein access

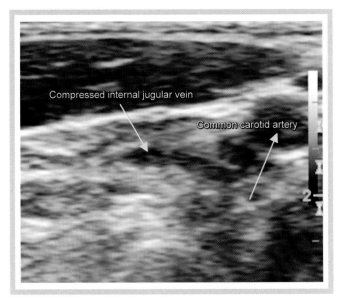

Figure 8-5: Compressed internal jugular vein and non-compressible common carotid artery

After advancing the needle through the skin, the wall of the internal jugular will become deformed as the needle impinges on it. As the needle punctures the vessel, the wall will spring back to its original position and dark blood return should be obtained.

For questionable situations, a subclavian or jugular line can be connected to a pressure transducer to exclude arterial access, or a blood gas can be checked for the same purpose.

Femoral Venous Access

The femoral vein is easily accessed and is ideal for emergent situations that require prompt large bore venous access. To identify the anatomic landmarks, the femoral artery is palpated just inferior to the inguinal ligament and the vein is assumed to be immediately medial to it. In some cases, the vein is tortuous and lies deep to the artery. In these cases, ultrasound guidance can be valuable to better identify the anatomy. After access is obtained, the catheter is placed as described above using the Seldinger technique.

Because of its location, though, the femoral vein is less desirable than the internal jugular or subclavian vein for placement of medium or long-term central venous access, due to increased risk of infection and difficulty with ambulation.

Peripherally Inserted Central Catheters (PICCs)

PICCs are non-tunneled, central catheters inserted through a peripheral vein of the arm. The insertion of PICCs can be performed at the bedside with the use of ultrasound guidance. In many hospitals, specialized teams of nurses can perform bedside placement but patients with limited venous access may require placement in the angiography suite. Multiple insertion sites are possible at the arm and include the brachial, basilic or cephalic vein and may be associated with fewer infectious complications. The superficial veins, however, should be preserved in patients needing permanent access for hemodialysis. PICCs lines are suitable for outpatient use as the United States Food and Drug Administration (FDA) has approved their use for up to 12 months. The principal disadvantage to the use of PICCs is their low-flow rates due to their smaller caliber and long length.

Acute Complications

Cannulation of a central vein carries substantial risk that should be discussed with the patient or decision-maker prior to performing the procedure. In addition, management of possible complications and avoidance techniques should be reviewed.

Pneumothorax: Although this may be more common with subclavian access, it can certainly occur with jugular access. An upright chest X-ray should be obtained after venous cannulation in order to exclude the possibility of pneumothorax and to check for placement. If a pneumothorax results, the patient should be placed on high-flow oxygen to facilitate air resorption and monitored carefully for respiratory insufficiency and the development of tension pneumothorax. Small (less than 30%), asymptomatic pneumothoraces can be observed with supplemental oxygen and serial chest X-rays. Larger, symptomatic pneumothoraces should prompt thoracentesis or chest tube placement. This complication can be avoided by minimizing the number of needle passes.

Air embolism: A potentially fatal air bolus can be drawn into the patient's circulation if the venous pressure becomes significantly lower than the atmospheric pressure. The patient should immediately be placed in left lateral decubitus position and an urgent consult to cardiothoracic surgery should be obtained for possible aspiration. To avoid this complication, the patient should be in the Trendelenburg position in order to increase the venous pressure and deep inspiratory movements should be avoided.

Arrhythmias: The guidewire and the catheter should not be advanced too far to avoid irritation of the myocardium. Observing the cardiac rhythm on a monitor during catheter insertion can be helpful, as can a post-procedure chest X-ray.

Carotid artery puncture/cannulation: The use of ultrasound is essential and can facilitate puncture of the correct lumen. In addition, pressure transduction can be helpful as can determining the blood's oxygen pressure. Finally, a post-procedure chest X-ray can help determine if the catheter is in the correct system. If the carotid artery is punctured, the needle should be removed and gentle, non-occlusive pressure applied for hemostasis. If the carotid is cannulated, an urgent vascular surgery consult should be obtained, as leaving the catheter in place risks stroke and may require operative exploration for safe removal.

Subclavian artery puncture/cannulation: This is a relatively unusual complication, as the subclavian artery lies posterior to the vein, but the same principles for the IJ/carotid system described above apply here, as well, in that a needle puncture can be managed by prompt removal of the needle and direct pressure. Cannulation requires urgent vascular surgery consultation for safe removal, as the local anatomy can make obtaining adequate control of the artery difficult without operative exploration.

Femoral artery puncture/cannulation: The femoral artery is frequently punctured during venous catheterization and can be recognized by the presence of bright red, pulsatile blood. The needle or catheter should be removed and pressure applied directly over the arterial puncture site until hemostasis is obtained. Cannulation is managed through removal of the catheter and placement of direct pressure over the puncture site until hemostasis is obtained.

Retroperitoneal hematoma: This complication of femoral venous cannulation can be recognized by the presence of hypotension, precipitous anemia, lower abdominal or flank pain or neurological changes in the lower extremity from nerve compression. Management is initially conservative and involves blood transfusion, reversing anticoagulation and manual compression. Operative evacuation and arterial repair is indicated if neurologic changes exist or ongoing bleeding is evident.

Chylothorax: Unique to the left IJ approach, disruption of the thoracic duct is a distinct complication that can be avoided by minimizing the number of punctures performed, using ultrasound guidance and preferentially accessing the right internal jugular vein.

Venous thrombosis: Acute thrombosis is a rare complication, but when it occurs, it is usually treated with removal of the catheter and anticoagulation. Lytic therapy should be considered for acute DVT of the iliofemoral system for functional patients with a life expectancy of at least one year and no contraindications for lysis. Thrombolysis will not only provide symptomatic relief but will also minimize the development of post- thrombotic sequelae. The role of lysis in upper extremity DVT management has not yet been as clearly defined, much less its role in the hypercoaguable milieu of the oncology patient. The issue has been studied with multiple case series and small prospective cohort studies, providing evidence that selected patients with acute upper extremity DVT can benefit from clot lysis. However, large, well controlled randomized trials have not yet been performed and as a result, current guidelines do not recommend either systemic or local lysis, unless appropriate expertise and resources are available and only for patients with primary (i.e. spontaneous) upper extremity DVT. The restriction to primary DVTs essentially excludes patients with secondary causes for their DVT, like cancer or central venous catheters. However, given the paucity of data, it is our practice to offer upper extremity DVT lysis to carefully selected, severely symptomatic patients without contraindications to anti-coagulation.

Long-term Complications

Venous thrombosis: The mere presence of a central venous catheter (CVC) predisposes cancer patients to DVT, which can lead to pulmonary embolism, loss of catheter function, catheter related bloodstream infections, swelling and post-thrombotic syndrome of the affected extremity. Interestingly, subclavian catheterization carries the lowest risk of subsequent DVT, with one-fourth the risk of internal jugular catheterization and approximately one-tenth the risk of a femoral line.

In an attempt to prevent DVT, low-dose warfarin at 1 milligram per day has been studied. Results have been mixed, with an increased risk of bleeding complications. As a result, current consensus recommendations do not recommend the use of warfarin as prophylaxis against upper extremity DVT in cancer patients with central catheters. Similarly, prophylactic low molecular weight heparin (LMWH) has been studied, with mixed results. As with warfarin, consensus recommendations do not support routine use of LMWH as prophylaxis against DVT in cancer patients with central catheters. However, when these patients are hospitalized for either medical or surgical care, they should be treated with routine thrombo-prophylaxis that is appropriate for the type of surgery.

Catheter associated DVT is initially managed with anticoagulant therapy. Since most cancer patients with extremity DVT associated with a CVC still require central venous access and require anticoagulation, retaining the catheter is often the best choice. Mandatory indications for removal of the catheter in the setting of thrombus include: infected thrombus, malpositioning of the tip and irreversible occlusion of the lumen.

Finally, the use of long-term anticoagulation has a large role in the management of catheter-associated DVT. The 2008 guidelines of the American College of Chest Physicians suggest at least 3 months of therapy, even if the CVC has been removed. In lieu of coumadin, LMWH is an alternative but should be used with caution in patients with renal failure.

Infection: Catheter related bloodstream infections (CRBSI) in the cancer patient are frequent due to the underlying immunosuppression that cancer patients suffer. Prevention starts with insertion of the catheter, where meticulous attention to sterile technique including use of a cap, mask, sterile gown, sterile gloves and large sterile drape substantially reduces the incidence of CRBSI compared with standard precautions (e.g. sterile gloves and small drapes).

Once infection is suspected, though, careful thought regarding the next steps in management is warranted, as immediate catheter removal runs the risk of unnecessary waste and the need for an operation if a port is involved.

For non-tunneled catheters, once CRBSI is suspected, removal of the catheter is usually required along with commencement of antibiotic therapy. If necessary, a temporary replacement catheter at a different location can also be placed. Tunneled catheters present a larger problem, as replacement of the catheter usually requires the resources of an operating room, so catheter removal should only be undertaken if the catheter is not salvageable. Indications for removal include complicated infections like tunnel infection, port abscess, septic thrombosis, endocarditis or osteomyelitis. Infections with *Candida* species also require catheter removal. Infection with *Staphylococcus aureus* and Gram-negative bacilli can be treated with antibiotic lock therapies, though the catheter should still be removed if the patient continues to clinically deteriorate.

In neutropenic patients, antibiotic lock therapies have achieved some success in preventing CRBSI. This technique involves filling the lumen of the catheter with an antibiotic solution, usually vancomycin and leaving the solution to dwell in the lumen. The principal risk of this technique is the development of vancomycin resistant enterococcus (VRE) and as such is not routinely recommended.

Ointments placed at the insertion site of catheters to prevent CRBSI have had mixed success. One study showed that povidone-iodine ointment applied at the insertion site of hemodialysis catheters reduced the incidence of exit-site infections, catheter-tip colonization and CRBSI compared with no ointment at the insertion site. However, use of other antibiotic ointments has been associated with the development of antibiotic resistance and the colonization of catheters by fungal species without clear evidence of reduced rates of CRBSI. As a result, with the exception of dialysis catheters, CDC guidelines explicitly state that topical antibiotic ointments and creams should not be used on catheter insertion sites.

Scrupulous care of catheter exit sites is essential to avoid infectious complications. Either sterile gauze or sterile, transparent, semipermeable dressings should cover the catheter site at all times. Prompt replacement of damp, loosened or visibly soiled catheter site dressings and at least weekly dressing changes are also important adjuncts to keeping infectious complications low.

Tunneled Catheters

Tunneled catheters are designed for long-term repeated use and are more resistant to infection. Their use, however, should be avoided in the setting of systemic infection.

Choice of Number of Lumens

Various systemic chemotherapeutic agents and regimens will require different access techniques, with the use of double or triple lumen catheters being essential if the agents are not compatible with one another. One common scenario is a patient simultaneously receiving a chemo-therapy infusion, maintenance intravenous fluids and an additional medication (e.g. antiemetic therapy). Although convenient for administration, the presence of multiple lumens increases the risk of line infection. One meta-analysis suggested that for every 20 single-lumen catheters inserted, one CRBSI will be avoided that would have occurred had multi-lumen catheters been used.

Indwelling Ports

Totally implanted ports consist of a reservoir connected to a central venous catheter. The reservoir is placed sub-cutaneously and is accessed using a Huber needle. Of some interest, the principal limitation to flow is not the catheter diameter, but rather the diameter of the Huber needle.

Among the advantages of ports over catheters are the lower reported rates of CRBSI. However, most ports have only one lumen, which makes them best suited for long-term intermittent chemotherapy, especially in patients with solid tumors. Ports allow for improved quality of life and enable bathing and swimming. However, they are more expensive to purchase, insert and remove and they leave larger scars. In general, implanted ports are more suitable for children and long-term use (more than 2 to 3 months) with less-frequent need for access, especially in patients receiving intermittent bolus chemotherapy for solid tumors.

Coated Catheters

Catheters coated with antimicrobials have recently become available and may prove to be valuable in terms of preventing catheter-associated infections. In addition, coating with antithrombotic substances may prevent thrombosis. However, there are some controversial reports on the potential of adverse reactions due to silver- and antiseptic-coated catheters.

Cuffed Catheters

Catheters with a cuff that lies subcutaneously have been shown to prevent colonization, presumably by providing a mechanical barrier to microbial migration from the skin into the bloodstream on the catheter. Use of these catheters is associated with lower rates of CRBSI, as compared to uncuffed catheters. Ionic silver has also been used in subcutaneous cuffs attached to central venous catheters and was associated with lower CRBSI rates. The theory is that the ionic silver provides antimicrobial activity while the cuff provides a mechanical barrier to the migration of microorganisms along the external surface of the catheter.

Venous Access for Nutrition

Parenteral nutrition often requires high osmolality fluids, with solutions containing greater than 10% glucose or 5% amino acids. As a result, central venous access is essential to avoid causing peripheral vein damage and sclerosis. Peripheral parenteral nutrition can be given through a short peripheral cannula or through a midline catheter when the osmolarity of the nutrient solutions, which may contain lipids, does not exceed 800 mOsm/Liter.

Hepatic Arterial Infusion for Colorectal Cancer

This is a brief description of the technical considerations surrounding hepatic arterial infusion pumps. Detailed information about the indications for this technique can be found in the chapter on Surgical Management of Metastases.

Overview

Colorectal cancer often metastasizes to the liver, with up to 60% of patients being affected. Prognosis is uniformly poor without treatment, with median survival of 6 months

and almost no survival at 5 years. For carefully selected patients with isolated liver metastases, surgical resection can provide hope for a cure. This group, however, represents less than 20% of patients. In these patients, hepatic arterial infusion pumps could be appropriate adjuncts.

The rationale for HAI is based on several observations:

1. Tumor from gastrointestinal malignancies spreads hematogenously via the portal circulation, which makes the liver the first site of metastasis in the majority of patients.
2. Once hepatic metastases grow above 2-3 mm in size, they derive their blood supply from the hepatic artery, while normal hepatocytes are perfused by the portal circulation. As a result, infusion of chemotherapy via the hepatic artery can achieve toxic levels in tumor cells with relative sparing of normal hepatic parenchyma.
3. The liver acts as a filter, extracting the chemotherapeutic agent from the hepatic arterial circulation. As a result, high local concentrations of the drug can be achieved with less systemic toxicity.

Patient Selection

Candidates for regional therapy with HAI must only have metastases localized to the liver and be medically suitable for the surgical procedure. Extensive hepatic metastases (>70% replacement with tumor), moderate or severe hepatic insufficiency and poor performance status are relative contraindications, as perioperative morbidity and mortality in those situations are high. In addition, patients with portal vein thrombosis are at risk for significant hepatic ischemia and HAI should be considered a treatment of last resort. Preoperative evaluation should include a computerized tomography (CT) scan of the chest, abdomen and pelvis to rule out extrahepatic disease, as well as a recent colonoscopy for patients with metachronous disease. CT angiography to define the hepatic arterial anatomy is also required in order to ensure that the patient does not have anatomic variants that would preclude perfusion of the entire liver. The goal is to have complete and specific perfusion of the liver with minimal impact to the rest of the systemic circulation.

Pump Placement

At laparotomy, portal lymph nodes are biopsied to rule out extrahepatic disease. The catheter is inserted into the gastroduodenal artery and distal vessels that supply the stomach, duodenum and pancreas are ligated to avoid perfusing these organs with the chemotherapeutic agent. In addition, cholecystectomy is an important adjunct, in order to avoid chemically induced cholecystitis from subsequent chemotherapy. Finally, the pump **(Figure 8-6)** is placed in the subcutaneous tissues and the catheter in the gastroduodenal artery is connected.

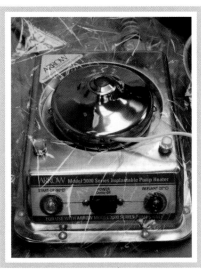

Figure 8-6: Intra-arterial infusion pump being heated before implantation

Key Complications

Early complications, though rare, include hepatic artery thrombosis, pump pocket hematoma, wound infection, hypoperfusion of the liver and extrahepatic perfusion. Late complications are more common and include catheter thrombosis or displacement, infection of the pump pocket, hepatic artery thrombosis, pump failure and gastric or duodenal ulceration.

Conclusions

Vascular access is essential and at times challenging in the surgical oncology patient to maintain chemotherapeutic and nutritional therapy. Although jugular access is preferred, other access sites can be successfully used. Sterile technique, line care and adjunctive endovascular interventions are key elements of catheter maintenance and contribute to prolonged access longevity.

Level of Evidence Table		
Recommendation	**Best level of evidence**	**References**
Use ultrasound guidance when placing internal jugular catheters in order to reduce the risk of failed catheterization and complications.	1a	Hind D, Calvert N, McWilliams R, et al. Ultrasonic locating devices for central venous cannulation: meta-analysis. BMJ 2003; 327:361.
In cancer patients with central venous catheters (CVC), whose only indication for DVT prophylaxis is the presence of the CVC, use of low-dose warfarin or therapeutic doses of low-molecular weight heparin (LMWH) for deep venous thrombosis (DVT) prophylaxis is ineffective, is potentially associated with serious bleeding complications and should be avoided.	1a	Geerts WH, Bergqvist D, Pineo GF, Heit JA, Samama CM, Lassen MR, Colwell CW; American College of Chest Physicians. Prevention of venous thromboembolism: American College of Chest Physicians Evidence-Based Clinical Practice Guidelines (8th edn). Chest 2008; 133(6 Suppl):381S-453S.
A CVC with associated DVT should be retained as long as it is functional and there is an ongoing need for it. Therapeutic anti-coagulation should be started if the patient can tolerate it.	1a	Kearon C, Kahn SR, Agnelli G, Goldhaber S, Raskob GE, Comerota AJ. American college of Chest Physicians. Antithrombotic therapy for venous thromboembolic disease: American College of Chest Physicians Evidence-Based Clinical Practice Guidelines (8th edn). Chest 2008;133(6 Suppl):454S-545S. Kovacs MJ, Kahn SR, Rodger M, Erson DR, Reou R, Mangel JE, Morrow B, Clement AM, Wells PS. A pilot study of central venous catheter survival in cancer patients using low-molecular-weight heparin (dalteparin) and warfarin without catheter removal for the treatment of upper extremity deep vein thrombosis (The Catheter Study). J Thromb Haemost 2007; 5(8):1650-3.
Subclavian catheterization carries a lower risk of subsequent DVT as compared to internal jugular and femoral catheterization.	4	McGee DC, Gould MK. Preventing complications of central venous catheterization. N Engl J Med 2003;348(12):1123-33.

Contd...

Contd...

Recommendation	Best level of evidence	References
Acute upper and lower extremity DVT should be treated with therapeutic doses of LMWH, unfractionated heparin or fondiparinux, regardless of whether or not the catheter is removed.	3a	Kearon C, Kahn SR, Agnelli G, Goldhaber S, Raskob GE, Comerota AJ. American College of Chest Physicians. Antithrombotic therapy for venous thromboembolic disease: American College of Chest Physicians Evidence-Based Clinical Practice Guidelines (8th edn). Chest 2008;133(6 Suppl):454S-545S.
Lytic therapy should be considered for acute DVT of the iliofemoral system for functional patients with a life expectancy of at least one year and no contraindications for lysis.	3a	Kearon C, Kahn SR, Agnelli G, Goldhaber S, Raskob GE, Comerota AJ. American College of Chest Physicians. Antithrombotic therapy for venous thromboembolic disease: American College of Chest Physicians Evidence-Based Clinical Practice Guidelines (8th edn). Chest 2008;133(6 Suppl):454S-545S.
Long-term anticoagulation for DVT should be continued for at least 3 months, even after a catheter has been removed.	3a	Kearon C, Kahn SR, Agnelli G, Goldhaber S, Raskob GE, Comerota AJ. American College of Chest Physicians. Antithrombotic therapy for venous thromboembolic disease: American College of Chest Physicians Evidence-Based Clinical Practice Guidelines (8th edn). Chest 2008;133(6 Suppl):454S-545S.
Mandatory indications for removal of a CVC in the setting of thrombus include: infected thrombus, malpositioning of the tip and irreversible occlusion of the lumen.	3a	Gallieni M, Pittiruti M, Biffi R. Vascular access in oncology patients. CA Cancer J Clin 2008;58(6):323-46.
The incidence of CRBSI can be reduced with the use of cap, mask, sterile gown, sterile gloves and large sterile drape as compared with standard precautions (e.g. sterile gloves and small drapes).	1a	O'Grady NP, Alexander M, Dellinger EP, et al. Guidelines for the prevention of intravascular catheter-related infections. Centers for disease control and prevention. MMWR Recomm Rep 2002;51(RR-10):1–29.
Patients with non-tunneled CVCs that demonstrate erythema or purulence overlying the catheter exit site, or clinical signs of sepsis should be treated with catheter removal and the tip should be cultured.	2a	Mermel LA, Farr BM, Sherertz RJ, et al. Guidelines for the management of intravascular catheter-related infections. Clin Infect Dis 2001;32:1249–72.
For salvage of a tunneled CVC in patients with uncomplicated infections, antibiotic lock therapy can be used for 2 weeks with standard systemic therapy for treatment of catheter-related bacteremia due to Staphylococcus aureus, coagulase-negative staphylococci and gram-negative bacilli for suspected intraluminal infection in the absence of tunnel or pocket infection.	3a	Mermel LA, Farr BM, Sherertz RJ, et al. Guidelines for the management of intravascular catheter-related infections. Clin Infect Dis 2001;32:1249–72.
Patients with tunneled CVCs that have complicated infections (e.g. tunnel infection, port abscess, septic thrombosis, endocarditis, or osteomyelitis) should be treated with catheter removal and administration of 4-6 weeks of antibiotics (6-8 weeks in the case of osteomyelitis).	2a	Mermel LA, Farr BM, Sherertz RJ, et al. Guidelines for the management of intravascular catheter-related infections. Clin Infect Dis 2001;32:1249–72.
The presence of multiple lumens increases the risk of line infection and single lumen central catheters should be considered where clinically feasible.	1a	Zürcher M, Tramèr M, Walder B. Colonization and bloodstream infection with single- versus multilumen central venous catheters: a quantitative systematic review. Anesth Analg 2004;99:177–82.

Landmark Papers

1. Geerts WH, Bergqvist D, Pineo GF, Heit JA, Samama CM, Lassen MR, Colwell CW. American College of Chest Physicians. Prevention of venous thromboembolism: American College of Chest Physicians Evidence-Based Clinical Practice Guidelines (8th edn). Chest 2008;133(6 Suppl):381S-453S.
2. Hind D, Calvert N, McWilliams R, et al. Ultrasonic locating devices for central venous cannulation: meta-analysis. BMJ 2003; 327:361.
3. Kearon C, Kahn SR, Agnelli G, Goldhaber S, Raskob GE, Comerota AJ. American College of Chest Physicians. Prevention of venous thromboembolism: American College of Chest Physicians Evidence-Based Clinical Practice Guidelines (8th edn). Chest 2008; 133(6 Suppl):454S-545S.
4. O'Grady NP, Alexander M, Dellinger EP, et al. Guidelines for the prevention of intravascular catheter-related infections. Centers for disease control and prevention. MMWR Recomm Rep 2002;51(RR-10):1–29.

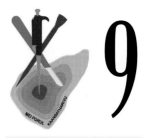

9

Endovascular Applications in Surgical Oncology

Donald T Baril, Rabih A Chaer

Introduction

Endovascular procedures provide minimally invasive diagnostic and therapeutic interventions for the management of a number of different malignancies and malignancy-related processes. Although the primary means of cancer treatment remain surgery and chemoradiation therapy, endovascular applications have increasingly complemented the traditional treatment of the cancer patient. These procedures can be performed on an outpatient basis with minimal anesthesia, which, in turn, provides a less expensive and less invasive option for select patients with cancer.

Endovascular applications within the field of surgical oncology are intended to assist in diagnosis and help in planning for further treatment, providing a method of definitive treatment and furthermore, treating complications arising from malignancies or their treatment.

Diagnostic Applications of Endovascular Techniques

Endovascular Biopsies

Although less commonly utilized than computed tomography (CT) or ultrasound-guided biopsy, endovascular biopsy offers similar less invasive means of tissue diagnosis. The most common utilization of this technique is transjugular liver biopsy which is associated with less risk of post-biopsy bleeding compared to conventional transcutaneous biopsy. Prior to performing this procedure, the anatomic relationship between the IVC and hepatic veins should be evaluated with CT imaging. Patency of the hepatic artery and vein, portal vein and IVC may also be assessed prior to biopsy with Doppler ultrasonography. The procedure is performed under local anesthesia in the supine position with continuous hemodynamic and cardiac monitoring. The right or left internal jugular vein is accessed using the Seldinger technique and a 9-French sheath and 5-French catheter are inserted. Under fluoroscopic control, the catheter is advanced into the IVC and into the hepatic vein which

corresponds with the lobe of interest using a 0.035-in wire. Hepatic venography is performed to evaluate patency of the hepatic vein outflow at the junction of the IVC and hepatic vein prior to introducing the biopsy device cannula. In cases of acute angulation between the IVC and the hepatic vein, a stiff 0.035-in wire may be used to introduce the biopsy device cannula. After removal of the wire, a 14-gauge stainless steel automated biopsy device loaded with an 18-gauge Quick-Core biopsy needle is advanced through the cannula and the biopsy is performed. A venogram is then acquired through the cannula in the hepatic vein to identify intrahepatic or subcapsular collections of contrast medium or intraperitoneal leaks. Manual jugular compression of the puncture site is maintained for 5-10 minutes following removal of the cannula and sheath. The complication rate of transjugular liver biopsy is reported to be 0-8% and is primarily related to hepatic hemorrhage.

Applications of this technique have also been described for biopsies of primary vena caval tumors, as well as intrcardiac tumors.

Preoperative Evaluation of Tumor Arterial Supply

Although CT and magnetic resonance (MR) angiographies provide excellent imaging for preoperative tumor evaluation, conventional contrast angiography remains the gold-standard to evaluate arterial supply. These diagnostic studies may be performed using percutaneous access of the femoral or brachial arteries and insertion of a 5-French sheath. Subsequently, 4- or 5-French catheters or even smaller microcatheters may then be directed into the vessel of interest to best delineate the contribution of a particular artery to a given tumor. Such studies can typically be performed with a relatively small amount of contrast compared to CT angiography and will provide more detailed anatomy of the arterial tree. In addition to delineating anatomy, the angiographic appearance of a tumor may aid in its diagnosis. In particular, pancreatic neuroendocrine tumors have distinct angiographic findings: insulinomas are seen as well-defined, round or oval vascular blushes that are of increased vascularity when compared with the surrounding normal pancreatic parenchyma; gastrinomas tend to be less intensely vascular than insulinomas and may only be identified on superselective studies, especially when involving peripancreatic lymph nodes or duodenum.

Angiography also provides information with regards to tumor vessel involvement, which may determine the course of therapy. Findings on angiography indicative of tumor involvement include filling defects, vessel wall irregularities and vessel occlusion. However, with improvements in other modalities, it appears that CTA and MRA may be more sensitive and specific in determining tumor vessel involvement. Furthermore, for pancreatic tumors, endoscopic ultrasound also appears to be more sensitive in determining vascular involvement when compared to conventional angiography.

Venous Sampling

The technique of percutaneous venous sampling is most useful in assisting in the diagnosis of benign adrenal disorders and of select pancreatic tumors. In particular, pancreatic neuroendocrine tumors may fail to be identified on multiple imaging modalities despite clinical suspicion only to be identified using venous sampling.

The localization of both insulinomas and gastrinomas rely on the arterial stimulation using calcium. A hyperosmolar concentration of calcium in the vessels supplying the tumor will cause degranulation of cells within the neoplasm and release of insulin or gastrin into the portal venous system, resulting in a detectable rise in insulin or gastrin in venous samples obtained from the hepatic veins. Calcium gluconate is selectively administered into the vessels supplying the pancreas, which will cause a temporary several-fold increase in molar concentration of calcium within the injected vessels. The splenic, gastroduodenal, superior mesenteric and proper hepatic arteries are those vessels most commonly studied during this technique; an appropriate rise in the level of insulin or gastrin in the hepatic vein (sampled through a second catheter introduced via a femoral venous approach) will localize the insulinoma or the gastrinoma to the pancreatic body/tail, anterosuperior portion of the pancreatic head and posteroinferior portion of the pancreatic head, respectively.

Specifically, for insulinomas, after the diagnostic angiogram, a venous catheter is introduced into the right or the middle hepatic vein close to their point of drainage into the inferior vena cava; 1 ml of 10% calcium gluconate is diluted with normal saline to a volume of 4 ml and is injected into each of the vessels supplying the pancreas sequentially. The rate of injection varies depending on the size of the vessel catheterized and the flow within it as judged by the preliminary injection of a small amount of contrast medium. It is vital that the calcium does not spill into adjacent branches and potentially localize the insulinoma to an incorrect site. Venous samples are obtained from the hepatic vein catheter before and 30, 60, 90, 120 and 180 seconds after the calcium injection. A twofold or greater rise in insulin above baseline is considered a diagnostic elevation. The injection of calcium into subsequent vessels should be performed no sooner than two minutes after the final venous sample to allow any rise in insulin concentration that may have occurred after the previous injection to return to baseline levels. If a tumor blush has been demonstrated angiographically, then the vessel supplying this area is usually studied last. Based on the results of the selective angiogram performed immediately prior to the venous sampling, further injections may be made into other vessels supplying an area of angiographic abnormality.

The technique of arterial stimulation venous sampling is identical to that used for insulinomas. Originally, secretin was used as the secretogogue, but equal results using the same dose of calcium gluconate as that used for the localization of insulinomas have been demonstrated. When injected into the vessel supplying a gastrinoma, both secretin and calcium gluconate will produce a significant rise in gastrin concentration in the hepatic vein of at least 25% at 20 seconds or 50% at 30 seconds after administration. It should be noted that a similar rise does not occur when the injection is made into a vessel supplying normal territory. Although there has been some concern that H2-antagonists and proton pump inhibitors increase fasting gastrin levels and may interfere with the results of arterial stimulation venous sampling, discontinuation of these dose not seem necessary for localization of gastrinomas despite the higher basal levels of gastrin. Furthermore, the risks of gastrointestinal bleeding and perforation outweigh the need to discontinue these medications prior to attempts at tumor localization.

Although relatively rare, complications associated with these procedures may directly be related to the angiography itself including access issues (hematomas, pseudoaneurysms, dissections), contrast-related issues (allergic reactions, contrast-induced nephropathy) or related to the induction of tumor activity (hypoglycemia).

Therapeutic Applications of Endovascular Techniques

Transcatheter Embolization

Transcatheter embolization allows the selective delivery of small caliber materials (both solid and liquid) to end organ arteries for a number of different applications, including achieving hemostasis, inducing ischemia and delivering chemotherapeutic agents. Initial access may be achieved either through the femoral or brachial arteries using a 5-French sheath. Selective angiography is obtained by accessing individual aortic branches and then through wire and catheter techniques, subsequent superselective angiography may then be performed utilizing micro-catheters (whose distal tips may measure as small as 1.7 French) and 0.014" guidewires.

Hemostasis

Gastrointestinal bleeding or intra-abdominal bleeding not uncommonly complicates patients with malignancies. Although bleeding may stop spontaneously, many patients will go on to require endoscopic control. When cannot be controlled or isolated using endoscopic techniques, endovascular techniques allow for localization and potential treatment of gastrointestinal bleeding prior to subjecting patients to open, often blind surgical resections. Furthermore, the conventional treatment for bleeding from solid organs has been surgical. Unfortunately, many of these patients may have advance tumors and may not medically tolerate such operations performed under emergent conditions with the associated hemodynamic instability from ongoing hemorrhage. The endovascular approach is therefore attractive and offers a minimally invasive alternative to an emergent open operation.

Transcatheter infusion of vasopressin has been the traditional first line endovascular approach to controlling hemorrhage from the gastrointestinal tract. Vasopressin causes generalized vasoconstriction through a direct action upon vessel walls, especially the arterioles, capillaries and venules. Infusion of vasopressin leads to a rapid reduction in local blood flow which returns to normal several hours following termination of the infusion. Vasopressin use has been shown to be efficacious for patients with hemorrhagic gastritis, those with poor collateral supply (following intestinal surgery) and those with anastomotic ulcers. Additionally, vasopressin has been demonstrated to be useful both in upper and lower gastrointestinal bleeds.

The majority of patients will respond to a vasopressin infusion of 0.2 units/minute. Angiography is performed 30 minutes following the initiation of the infusion and the rate is increased to 0.4 units/minute if the bleeding persists. If the bleeding is controlled, the infusion is continued in an intensive care setting for 24-36 hours and then tapered over 24 hours. Patients who are not responding to an infusion rate of 0.4 pressor units/minute are unlikely to respond to higher doses and will likely require operative intervention.

Transcatheter embolization uses either temporary or permanent agents to occlude end arteries which are the source of hemorrhage. Patients who may benefit from embolization include patients who have failed a vasopressin infusion, patients with high rate bleeds which are clearly visible on angiography, patients with pyloro-

duodenal bleeding, patients with hemobilia or hemorrhage into pancreatic pseudocysts and patients with underlying coagulopathy.

A number of different temporary and permanent agents are available for transcatheter embolization control of hemorrhage. Gelfoam (Upjohn, Kalamazoo MI) is a long-acting, biodegradable sponge that causes hemostasis upon contact when injected into a vessel. Gelfoam comes as a powder or as small blocks which may be cut to the desired size. Polyvinyl alcohol is a permanent embolic agent that is available as small microspheres or sheets. Permanent occlusion is achieved through mechanical impaction. In addition to polyvinyl alcohol, there are a number of mechanical blocking agents such as steel coils, platinum microcoils, balloons and silk thread. Permanent agents are best used when bleeding occurs from a lesion which is not expected to heal spontaneously such as a tumor, aneurysm or arteriovenous communication.

Initial angiography is used to confirm the bleeding site and to identify anomalous or variant vascular anatomy, particularly relevant in patients who have undergone prior surgical resection **(Figure 9-1)**. An end-hole catheter should be inserted into the selected artery in order to avoid reflux of embolic materials into undesired vessels. Embolic materials may then be injected into the selected artery utilizing saline or pushed into place using a guidewire. Repeat angiography is subsequently performed to confirm hemostasis. Some of these agents may take several minutes to induce complete thrombosis so care should be taken not to immediately declare an embolization unsuccessful

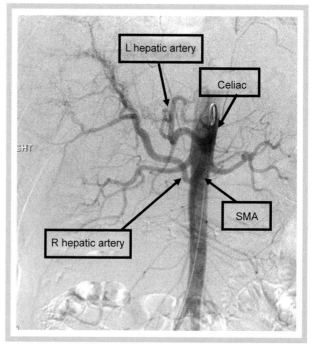

Figure 9-1: Aortogram demonstrating anomalous anatomy: right hepatic artery arising from superior mesenteric artery

if there is persistent bleeding on initial post-embolization angiography.

As with other endovascular techniques, access-related complications may arise. Specific to the use of vasopressin, patients may suffer cardiac arrhythmias and coronary vasoconstriction as there is some degree of systemic circulation despite selective catheter administration of the drug. For patients undergoing embolization, bowel or organ infarction is the most serious complication. Although the gastrointestinal tract has a rich collateral blood supply, care should be taken in patients who have undergone prior bowel resections, elderly patients, patients with underlying peripheral vascular disease and patients with colonic bleeds. Furthermore, although superselective, catheterization decreases the risk of bowel infarction it certainly does not eliminate it.

Preoperative Use of Transcatheter Embolization

Transcatheter embolization may be used preoperatively to either decrease blood supply to a given tumor and allow for a safer surgical resection or, in the case of hepatic tumors, to induce compensatory hypertrophy of the remaining organ.

Splenic malignancies are the most common tumors to undergo preoperative embolization to decrease the risk of intraopertive blood loss. Additionally, with the majority of splenectomies now being performed laparoscopically, preoperative embolization induces splenic shrinkage and may decrease the complexity of the operation. Patients who have Hodgkin's lymphoma, non-Hodgkin's lymphoma, chronic B-cell lymphocytic leukemia and hairy cell leukemia may all benefit from splenectomy. Of these patients, those with marked splenomegaly will benefit from preoperative embolization. This can be accomplished using the same techniques described earlier in the chapter whereby catheter selection of the distal splenic artery is performed and embolization with any of the available agents is carried out. Of note, acute tumor lysis syndrome has been described following preoperative splenic embolization and awareness should exist of this complication, particularly in the setting of massive splenomegaly from tumor. In addition to splenic malignancies, preoperative embolization has been used for carotid body tumors, pulmonary tumors, musculoskeletal tumors, gynecologic and urologic tumors.

Unlike these tumors, preoperative portal vein embolization (PVE) prior to major liver resection is performed to induce hypertrophy as postoperative mortality is most strongly associated with the degree of hepatic reserve. PVE has been shown to reduce the risk of postoperative liver failure after major hepatectomy and increases the number of patients who are candidates for resection. PVE redirects portal flow to the intended future liver remnant (FLR) to initiate hypertrophy of the nonembolized segments.

Preprocedure determination of the future liver remnant is vital to successful portal PVE and subsequent surgical resection. CT is used to measure the disease free liver remnant size which is then compared to the total liver volume (based on an individual patient's body surface area). A ratio of these two values then provides information of anticipated liver remnant and operative outcome based on prior studies. CT images should be obtained immediately before PVE and approximately 3-4 weeks after PVE to assess the degree of liver remnant hypertrophy.

There are three standard approaches to performing PVE: the transhepatic contralateral (portal access via the functional liver remnant), transhepatic ipsilateral (portal access via the liver to be resected) and intraoperative transileocolic venous approaches. These approaches are selected on the basis of operator preference, type of resection planned, extent of embolization and type of embolic agent used.

The transhepatic contralateral approach is the most commonly used technique. A branch of the left portal system is accessed and a 6-French balloon occlusion catheter is advanced through an introducer into branches of the right portal tree for embolization. The major advantage of this approach is that catheterization of the desired right PV branches is more direct via the left system than via the right system, making the procedure technically easier. However, the disadvantage of this technique is the risk of injury to the FLR parenchyma and the left PV. In particular, migration of embolic material with use of the contralateral approach may compromise the FLR and may make the planned resection more difficult.

The transhepatic ipsilateral approach differs in that a peripheral PV branch in the liver to be resected is accessed and a 6-French sheath is advanced through it. Standard angiographic catheters are used for combined particulate and coil embolization. The major advantage of the ipsilateral approach is that the anticipated liver remnant is not instrumented. However, catheterization of the right PV branches may be more difficult because of severe angulations between right portal branches and the technique usually requires the use of reverse-curved catheters. Another potential disadvantage of this approach is that some embolic material could be displaced on catheter removal, leading to nontarget embolization.

The transileocolic venous approach is performed during laparotomy by direct cannulation of the ileocolic vein and advancement of a balloon catheter into the PV for subsequent embolization. This approach is preferred when a percutaneous approach is not feasible, or when additional treatment is needed during the same surgical exploration. Disadvantages of this method are the need for general anesthesia and laparotomy, with their inherent risks.

The ideal embolic agent should cause permanent embolization of the portal vein with minimal risk of recanalization. Additionally, it should easily be administered and not cause an inflammatory reaction. With this as the background, many embolic materials have been used for PVE without significant differences in degrees or rates of hypertrophy. These include fibrin glue, gelatin sponge and thrombin, cyanoacrylate and lipiodol, polyvinyl alcohol, absolute alcohol, microspheres and microcoils. Polyvinyl alcohol is safe, easy to use and produces minimal inflammation and creates durable portal vein occlusion when used in combination with metal coils. Polyvinyl alcohol, microspheres, or gelfoam provide occlusion to small outflow vessels in the tumor bearing segments, while the metal coils provide large vessels inflow occlusion. This accounts for more permanent occlusion associated with the combination of coils and PVA. Cyanoacrylate produces reliable portal vein occlusion, which persists for four weeks after PVE, whereas gelfoam and thrombin may produce only transient PVE with recanalization of the vessels reported. As with alcohol, a marked inflammatory reaction can be seen with cyanoacrylate, making the subsequent surgical procedure more difficult.

Complications with PVE occur in 9-13% of cases and include subcapsular hematoma, hemoperitoneum, hemobilia, pseudoaneurysm, arteriovenous fistula, arterioportal shunts, PV thrombosis, transient liver failure, pneumothorax and sepsis. The majority of technical complications occur in the punctured lobe, which has led many to recommend that the transhepatic ipsilateral approach be utilized first.

Transcatheter Therapies for Hepatic Tumors

Despite advances in intraoperative and perioperative care of patients with hepatic tumors, surgical resection remains an option only for a minority of patients. Transcatheter arterial approaches to these tumors provide an alternative therapy to deliver either "bland" or chemotherapeutic agents directly to tumors and induce ischemia and/or cytotoxicity. These therapies are based on the principle that liver tumors derive the majority of their blood supply from the arterial circulation. Selective delivery of cytotoxic or ischemia-inducing materials into selective branches of the hepatic artery allow for preferential necrosis of tumors while sparing the remaining normal liver parenchyma. Furthermore, such directed therapy allows for increased drug concentrations at the target tissue while reducing the systemic toxicity of the particular agents.

A variety of techniques are used to perform transarterial chemoembolization with the greatest discrepancy revolving around the number and type of agents used, the selectivity of catheter positioning and the type of embolic material used. In general, the technique involves standard arterial access using the Seldinger technique via either the femoral or the brachial artery. A catheter is advanced in the aorta and selective celiac trunk and superior mesenteric arteriography is performed with late-phase imaging of the portal venous anatomy. This serves to determine the arterial supply to the tumor, detect variations in hepatic arterial supply, identify the arteries that should be avoided during treatment delivery and determine the patency of the portal vein or the presence of hepatopetal flow through collaterals to the liver in cases of portal vein thrombosis. Once the arterial anatomy is defined, a catheter is advanced superselectively into the right or left hepatic artery, depending on which lobe contains the greatest tumor volume **(Figures 9-2 and 9-3)**. A 4-French hydrophilic Cobra catheter (Cook Medical, Bloomington, IN) used with a hydrophilic guidewire is often used. Catheter size should be selected to allow for rapid injection of the viscous chemoembolic emulsion while still allowing flow. Smaller vessels and branches which cannot be accessed with a standard angiographic catheter can be catheterized with a variety of microcatheters **(Figure 9-4)**. There are particular catheters that are different from standard microcatheters in that they have a slightly larger inner lumen and shorter overall length, which makes the injection of viscous chemoembolic emulsions easier. These include the Cragg wire (Boston Scientific, Natick, MA), the Turbo Tracker Infusion Catheter (Boston Scientific) and the Renegade Hi-Flo (Boston Scientific) microcatheters. When the catheter is

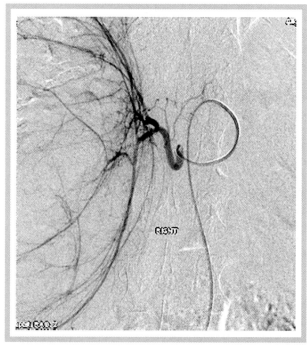

Figure 9-2: Right hepatic artery angiogram showing distortion of the normal branches by a large hepatocellular carcinoma

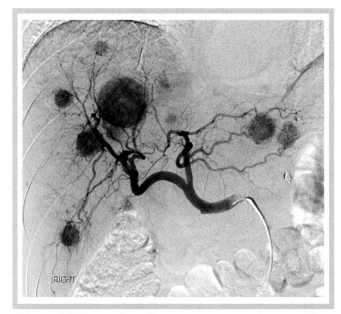

Figure 9-3: Proper hepatic artery angiogram demonstrating multiple tumors in both the right and left hepatic lobes

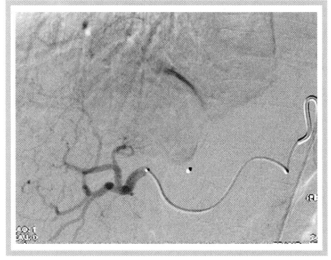

Figure 9-4: Microcatheter placed selectively within the right hepatic artery

positioned, it is important to perform an arteriogram to confirm the anatomy before injecting any chemotherapy as this superselective injection may reveal findings not depicted in the celiac or superior mesenteric artery injection. The end point of the procedure is visualization of the complete blockage of the tumor-feeding branch. It is essential to check for extrahepatic collateral arterial supply to the tumor; in particular, the right inferior phrenic artery is the most common collateral pathway and should be evaluated.

Post-procedure, patients should be treated with vigorous hydration, antiemetic therapy and optional antibiotics. After three to four weeks the patient returns

for a second procedure directed at the other segment or lobe of the liver. Depending on the arterial anatomy, two to four procedures are required to treat the entire liver. Thereafter, response is assessed by repeated imaging studies and tumor markers.

Worldwide, the most commonly used chemotherapeutic agent is doxorubicin. In the United States, the preferred treatment is a combination of cisplatin, doxorubicin and mitomycin. Lipiodol (iodized oil), an oily contrast medium which persists more selectively in tumor nodules for a few weeks up to some months when injected into the hepatic artery, is nearly always used because of its properties as a drug carrier and tumor-seeking agent.

Embolization to induce ischemia is also typically used at the end of these procedures since it reduces blood supply to the tumor, thereby increasing contact time of the chemotherapeutic agents with the tumor. A variety of agents are used including Gelfoam particles, polyvinyl alcohol, starch microspheres and metallic coils. Gelfoam is the most commonly used agent which only occludes the artery temporarily with recanalization taking place within two weeks. Polyvinyl alcohol particles can cause a permanent or semi-permanent arterial occlusion and achieve more distal obstruction because of their smaller size (50-250 μm in diameter). Embospheres, trisacryl gelatine microspheres (100-700 μm), offer the advantage of being able to penetrate deeper and to embolize smaller and more peripheral vessels.

Complications of transarterial chemoembolization include access related complications as well as the well-described post-embolization syndrome. This syndrome, which complicates up to 10% of all procedures, consists of right upper quadrant pain, nausea, vomiting and fever along with a mild elevation in liver enzymes. Treatment is supportive and the syndrome is self-limiting with full recovery in 7-10 days. Other reported complications include cholecystitis, pancreatitis, gastric erosions and renal dysfunction. Although very rare, the most devastating complication of transarterial chemoembolization is liver failure, which may occur in patients with compromised liver function.

In addition to the standard approaches to chemoembolization, two more recent modifications of the technique have been utilized. The first of these is to load polyvinyl alcohol based microspheres with doxorubicin to increase the amount of drug which can selectively be delivered to a tumor. In select studies, these drug-eluting beads have demonstrated a more pronounced initial tumor response when compared to the conventional techniques. Furthermore, drug-eluting beads loaded with irinotecan are being investigated for the treatment of patients with colorectal cancer metastases to the liver. The second modification to conventional chemoembolization has been the targeted delivery of radioisotopes to hepatic tumors. Such isotopes, including iodine 131 and yttrium 90, have been compounded with lipiodol and microspheres for the treatment of both primary and metastatic liver tumors. Although randomized data is lacking, these modalities offer promise of an additional means of managing patients with advanced liver tumors.

Isolated Limb Infusion

Isolated limb perfusion for the treatment of extremity sarcomas and melanomas provides the opportunity to salvage limbs that might otherwise require amputation because of a locally advanced or recurrent tumor. The technique was originally described in 1958 by Creech and involves open cannulation of the femoral vessels and subsequent connection to an extracorporeal bypass circuit, requiring a cardiopulmonary bypass machine operated by a suitably trained perfusionist. The circulating blood is mechanically oxygenated and warmed. A large catheter size is needed, varying up to 14 French for the arterial access and from 14 to 16 French for venous access. An alternative type of regional chemotherapy treatment, isolated limb infusion, was described by Thompson in 1998. This technique involves percutaneous access of an artery and vein using high flow catheters, along with use of a pneumatic tourniquet proximally to isolate the extremity. Isolated limb infusion differs from isolated limb perfusion in that it circulates blood in the isolated extremity at a much slower rate and for a shorter time period than isolated limb perfusion.

To perform this procedure, either antegrade access in the affected leg or contralateral 'up-and-over' cross-over access to the affected side may be achieved with 5 French or 6 French sheaths. Combinations of ipsilateral or contralateral access may be used for the arterial and venous catheters. Special considerations should be made in oncology patients. In particular, patients with melanoma may have had prior groin dissection or lymphadenectomy making arterial or venous access difficult or not feasible. Once access has been achieved, sidehole catheters should then be positioned in the popliteal artery and vein. Additionally, these sheaths are connected to continuous heparinized saline infusions (1000 units/1 L saline at 25 ml/hr).

Following appropriate positioning of the catheters, the limb is elevated and drained of venous blood. A pneumatic tourniquet is inflated proximally enabling effective isolation of the limb vasculature from the systemic circulation. Integrity of the limb tourniquet is critical to avoiding whole-body toxicity from the high-concentration locally infused chemotherapy. The limb is warmed using a heating blanket as hyperthermia improves cytotoxic efficacy. The cytotoxic agent, added to prewarmed heparinized saline, is hand injected into the arterial catheter and withdrawn from the venous catheter. Cyclical

reinjection and withdrawal is carried out over approximately 30 min. The infusate is then washed out with saline and the venous effluent is discarded. The isolating tourniquet is deflated and the catheters are removed.

Several studies have demonstrated equal efficacy of isolated limb infusion to isolated limb perfusion for the treatment of melanoma and sarcoma. Furthermore, isolated limb infusion avoids the larger sheath sizes and the full anticoagulation that are necessary for isolated limb perfusion. Isolated limb infusion, although less invasive, still carries the potential risks related to access including dissection, thromboembolism, contrast allergy and hemorrhage, as well as toxicity from the infusion agent. Additionally, the actual limb toxicity is related to total cytotoxic dose, duration and limb temperature and is similar to isolated limb perfusion. This may manifest as erythema, edema, myositis or, in severe cases, compartment syndrome. Although still relatively novel, this modality offers an additional, less invasive treatment option for select patients with extremity melanomas and sarcomas.

IVC Filter Placement

Cancer patients are hypercoagulable and are commonly affected by venous thromboembolism. This has a negative impact on survival since the probability of death within six months after an initial thromboembolic event may be twice as compared to cancer patients with no venous thromboembolism. A large percentage of patients with malignancy may have contraindications to anticoagulation as definitive treatment of deep vein thromboses (DVT). For such patients, inferior vena cava (IVC) filters have proven to be a viable alternative to anticoagulation therapy for the prevention of life-threatening pulmonary emboli (PE). In addition to patients with known DVT, prophylactic retrievable filters may be used in patients with malignancies at the time of surgery, when they are at most risk for thromboembolic events and may not safely be treated with pharmacologic prophylaxis.

There are a number of permanent and retrievable filters available for percutaneous use though either a femoral or jugular vein approach using local anesthesia with or without light sedation. Standard Seldinger technique is used for venous access and an initial venogram is performed to identify the renal veins. Although standard technique is to place the filter infrarenally, suprarenal filter placement has been proven to be safe when necessitated by extension of thrombus above the renal veins or in cases of renal vein thrombosis. Following initial venography, the filter is then deployed via an introducing sheath, which range in size from 6 French to 12 French depending on the filter. Completion venography is then performed to confirm the position of the filter **(Figure 9-5)**.

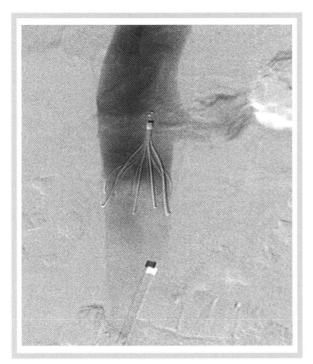

Figure 9-5: Venogram following IVC filter insertion

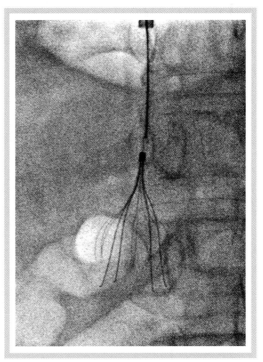

Figure 9-6: Snare around proximal hook of IVC filter prior to removal via a jugular approach

IVC filter retrieval is performed percutaneously as well under local anesthesia with or without light sedation. Depending on the filter used, this can be achieved via the jugular or femoral approach. Following venous access, an IVC venogram is performed to detect clot in the IVC and filter, which might preclude removal. Following venography, a sheath is placed into the IVC and subsequently a snare is used to capture the filter **(Figure 9-6)**. The filter is then collapsed and resheathed and removed. Postretrieval IVC venography is then obtained to inspect for complications, specifically IVC injury or thrombosis.

Complications are rare following IVC filter insertion and include insertion site injury, filter migration, filter erosion through the IVC wall and adjacent organs and IVC thrombosis.

Conclusion

The management of patients with cancer has become more complex and continues to evolve as more challenging patients are considered for aggressive therapies. The use of less invasive techniques is therefore attractive for diagnostic and therapeutic purposes. In particular, endovascular techniques have enabled patients to safely and effectively be treated for a variety of malignancies using minimally invasive procedures as adjunctive or primary therapeutic modalities. As endovascular technologies for the cancer patient continue to be refined, it is likely that a multimodality approach including the use of endovascular techniques will be applied to an increasing number of patients with cancer.

Summary

- Endovascular liver biopsy offers a less invasive means of tissue diagnosis, with less risk of post-biopsy bleeding compared to conventional transcutaneous biopsy.
- Arteriography remains the gold-standard in determining tumor arterial supply.
- Endovascular venous sampling appears to be the most sensitive modality to identify and localize select pancreatic neuroendocrine tumors.
- Transcatheter embolization allows for percutaneous selective delivery of small caliber materials to end organ arteries for a number of different applications, including achieving hemostasis, inducing ischemia and delivering chemotherapeutic agents.
- Isolated limb infusion offers a less invasive and equally efficacious alternative to isolated limb perfusion for the treatment of select extremity melanomas and sarcomas.
- IVC filters are a viable alternative to anticoagulation therapy for the prevention of life-threatening pulmonary emboli in patients with contraindications to anticoagulation.

Landmark Papers

1. Abulkhir A, Limongelli P, Healey AJ, Damrah O, Tait P, Jackson J, et al. Preoperative portal vein embolization for major liver resection: a meta-analysis. Ann Surg 2008; 247(1):49-57.

2. Awad SS, Colletti L, Mulholland M, Knol J, Rothman ED, Scheiman J, Eckhauser FE. Multimodality staging optimizes resectability in patients with pancreatic and ampullary cancer. Am Surg 1997;63(7):634-8.

3. Doppman JL, Chang R, Fraker DL, Norton JA, Alexander HR, Miller DL, et al. Localization of insulinomas to regions of the pancreas by intra-arterial stimulation with calcium. Ann Intern Med 1995;123(4):269-73

4. Kinoshita H, Sakai K, Hirohashi K, Igawa S, Yamasaki O, Kubo S. Preoperative portal vein embolization for hepatocellular carcinoma.World J Surg 1986;10(5): 803-8.

5. Llovet JM, Real MI, Montaña X, Planas R, Coll S, Aponte J, Ayuso C, Sala M, Muchart J, Solà R, Rodés J, Bruix J. Barcelona liver cancer group. Arterial embolisation or chemoembolisation versus symptomatic treatment in patients with unresectable hepatocellular carcinoma: a randomised controlled trial. Lancet 2002;359(9319): 1734-9.

6. Moncrieff MD, Kroon HM, Kam PC, Stalley PD, Scolyer RA, Thompson JF. Isolated limb infusion for advanced soft tissue sarcoma of the extremity. Ann Surg Oncol 2008; 15(10): 2749-56.

7. Thompson JF, Kam PC, Waugh RC, Harman CR. Isolated limb infusion with cytotoxic agents: a simple alternative to isolated limb perfusion. Semin Surg Oncol 1998; 14(3):238-47.

8. Wallace MJ, Jean JL, Gupta S, Eapen GA, Johnson MM, Ahrar K, et al. Use of inferior vena caval filters and survival in patients with malignancy. Cancer 2004;101(8): 1902-7.

9. Yamada R, Sato M, Kawabata M, Nakatsuka H, Nakamura K, Takashima S. Hepatic artery embolization in 120 patients with unresectable hepatoma. Radiology 1983;148(2):397-401.

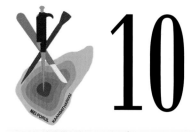

10

Nutrition in Surgical Oncology

Deepa Magge*, Fateh Entabi*, Juan Ochoa

Introduction

This chapter summarizes the importance of a thorough nutritional evaluation and the development of a logical nutritional intervention strategy in the care of the oncologic patient undergoing surgical intervention. Clinical data demonstrate that nutritional status is an essential independent predictor of outcome. Yet, despite, realizing the importance of nutrition, a careful plan for nutrition intervention is often not instituted during patient care.

In this chapter we will use the term "nutritional intervention" to describe any changes we make in the patient's nutritional intake. Similar to any intervention we do in medicine: nutritional interventions have their own risks and may certainly be harmful. Thus, every surgeon should know the principles of nutritional intervention and be able to formulate a plan to provide the patient with optimum nutrition that is individualized and is part of the overall medical care plan. To do that, physicians need to carefully evaluate the patient's nutritional state in order to present a treatment plan, evaluate risk of complications and determine the best forms of nutritional intervention. Learning about nutrition intervention is a worthwhile effort for the physician that will result in significant benefits if carefully delivered or increase risks if poorly done. Nutritional intervention is not intuitive and this chapter will point to practical aspects of the nutritional care of the oncologic patient and hopefully will be able to guide the physician toward providing better care of the patients.

In the 1940s, in the midst of the World War II, classic forms of nutritional deficiencies were extremely common (Marasmus, Kwashiorkor). These were easily defined and identified. The agricultural revolution after the war, along with better understanding of the nutritional needs, gave widespread access to multiple food products with high caloric values and low-cost. As a result, physicians are now challenged with a different set of nutrition pathologies, better called "*Dysnutrition*", which become

particularly important when other illnesses, such as cancer, are diagnosed. A pathologic nutritional state with a significant deficiency is observed in up to 30% of the patients at a given moment in our hospitals. The presence of widespread obesity makes the diagnoses of nutritional deficiencies even more difficult. The surgeon therefore, must remain vigilant regarding the nutritional state of the patient.

Although most clinicians currently realize the crucial role nutrition plays in the outcomes of their patients, it took a significant amount of effort in the twenteeth century to understand how dramatically malnutrition affects outcomes. In fact, malnutrition remains the single most important independent predictor of postoperative morbidity and mortality in any given surgical disease. The critical role of the surgeon was clearly recognized in 1955, as Williams and Zollinger published in the American Journal of Clinical Nutrition: "Since the surgeon understands time effects of poor nutrition, the correction of either deficits or excesses should not be delegated completely to other personnel".

Starvation and Malnutrition

According to Dorland, malnutrition is defined as poor nourishment resulting from an inadequate or improper diet or from some defect in metabolism that prevents the body from using its food properly. Starvation refers to the physiologic responses that occur in response to inadequate food intake. In other words, starvation is a genetically coded physiologic response to protect the organism in the face of inadequate nutritional supply that aims to preserve organ function. When the nutritional deficit reaches a certain point, the physiologic mechanisms fail to keep up with the deficit. At this point, malnutrition ensues and is accompanied by significant pathology and organ dysfunction **(Figure 10-1)**. How long a starved patient can compensate before malnutrition ensues depends on many factors including the acuity of illness,

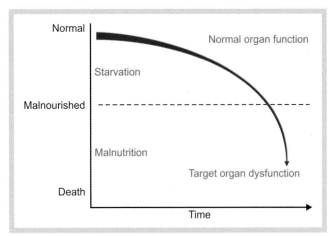

Figure 10-1: Progression to malnutrition

nutrition demands imposed for recovery and the overall nutritional state prior to the onset of starvation.

Malnutrition is very common in hospitalized patients and is observed in up to 50% of the patients hospitalized for two weeks or more. The association between a higher likelihood of postoperative morbidity and mortality and nutritional depletion was first pointed out by Studley in 1936: Chronic peptic ulcer patients undergoing gastrectomy had a 3.5% mortality rate if they had less than 20% preoperative weight loss, but a 33% mortality rate if they had lost more than 20%.

Malnutrition negatively affects the function of all organs and systems and renders the patient prone to multiple increased complications. Wound healing is negatively affected with decreased collagen deposition and increased surgical wound breakdown. Mainous, et al showed that malnutrition leads to immune system dysfunction by impairing complement activation and production, bacterial opsonization and the function of neutrophils, macrophages and lymphocytes. One series of underfed patients found subnormal skin reactions to Candida and low levels of antibodies to various phytomitogens, suggesting that both humoral and cell mediated immunity are affected. Haydock, et al also demonstrated slower rates of wound healing.

Activities of daily living are also negatively affected by malnutrition. This includes the capacity to get out of bed (mobility) and to maintain adequate pulmonary toilet, which becomes very important after surgery. This renders the patient increasingly susceptible to the development of atelectasis and pneumonia. Also, the development of decubitus ulcers, a devastating postoperative complication, is almost always associated with malnutrition. Early recognition of the presence of severe malnutrition is essential in surgical risk stratification and in planning nutritional intervention strategies that improve outcome.

Nutritional Requirements

Nutritional requirements in patients are divided into macronutrients and micronutrients. Macronutrients include carbohydrates, lipids and proteins. In adults of stable weight, energy requirements should balance energy expenditures. Carbohydrates are the principal source of energy in a normal diet, meeting 40-55% of energy requirements in the western diet. Carbohydrates are the principal energy substrate for the brain. Carbohydrate intake reduces ketone body production, facilitates storage of triglycerides in fat tissue and helps to preserve body protein by reducing the need for gluconeogenesis from amino acids. The metabolic and long-term health effects of carbohydrates depend on their glycemic index rather than their biochemical structure. Intake of food with a moderate to high glycemic index can provide immediate energy and spares glycogen stores. When glycogen stores are exhausted, muscle has to rely entirely on fatty acids for fuel.

Lipids are ingested as triglycerides, phospholipids or sterols. Triglycerides are composed of fatty acids and glycerol. Lipids are an important source of energy and carriers of fat-soluble vitamins A, D, E and K. Fatty acids are substrates for fat formation in subcutaneous adipose tissue, which is the major energy reserve during fasting. Fatty acids are also precursors for synthesis of eicosanoids that modulate immune function and contribute to the feeling of satiety after eating by slowing gastric emptying. The minimal fat allowance to ensure adequate absorption of fat-soluble vitamins is thought to be between 10% and 15% of energy intake. Fat consumption should not exceed 30-35% of total energy intake.

Proteins are involved in tissue synthesis and are the primary constituents of hair, skin, nails, tendons, bones, ligaments, major organs and muscle. Their building blocks are amino acids, which are also the precursors of neurotransmitters. Amino acids, which also form the major part of antibodies, enzymes, transporters of ions and substrates in blood, are acid-base buffers and act as initiators of muscle contraction. The recommended minimum daily protein intake is 0.8-1.0 g/kg for healthy adults. Amino acids are classified as non-essential, conditionally essential and essential. Conditionally essential amino acids, such as glutamine and arginine, may become essential in certain pathological situations. Excessive protein and amino acid intake lead to formation of undesirable quantities of urea and other compounds that may exceed the capacity of the liver and kidney to clear them.

Micronutrients include trace elements and vitamins, which are required in the diet in very small amounts. The fact that only a small intake is necessary is in contrast to their critical importance in both health and disease.

Micronutrients can be used as cofactors in metabolism, as coenzymes in metabolism, as control factors, as structural components and as antioxidants. Examples of important micronutrients include zinc, which serves as a cofactor for many enzymes and selenium, which is required within the enzyme glutathione peroxidase. Riboflavin and niacin are required to play active roles within the electron transport chain. Vitamins E and A serve as antioxidants to prevent bodily harm created by oxidative reactions, thus, both macronutrients as well as micronutrients are critical in human function.

Nutrition and the Systemic Inflammatory Response Syndrome

The impact of the systemic inflammatory response syndrome (SIRS) caused by sepsis/trauma on metabolism can be divided into three phases according to Cuthbertson's work on trauma patients in the middle of the past century.

The first phase "Ebb" lasts around 12-24 hours and is characterized by a decrease in all metabolic activities, hyperglycemia secondary to the hepatic glycogen breakdown and hypoperfusion. It represents the initial response to injury. These adaptive changes reflect activation of the sympathetic nervous system and the pituitary-adrenal axis, resulting in a rapid rise in the plasma concentrations of epinephrine and norepinephrine, adrenocorticotropic hormone, growth hormone, cortisol and other corticosteroids.

The second "flow" phase, which lasts for the remainder of the acute illness, is marked by hyper-catabolism and is primarily mediated by catecholamines. This phase is accompanied by a negative nitrogen balance. This negative balance is universal and cannot be reversed by any modality of nutrition support. The only way to alter this negative balance is to alter the cause of the inflammatory response. The catabolic response is universal after surgery and is also present in infection as well as in advanced cancer.

The third or "anabolic" phase, which begins with the onset of recovery from the acute illness, is characterized by normalization of vital signs, improved appetite and diuresis. During that phase the body starts acquiring a positive nitrogen balance again.

The duration and severity of these phases varies based on the nature of the insult and its management.

The Myth of Hyperalimentation

Intuitively, investigators, nutritionists and clinicians in the 1970s pursued the goal of providing high-calorie nutrition support or "hyperalimentation". This was based on the observation that metabolic requirements were increased in surgical patients and that this increase appeared to be proportional to the degree of stress. Based on this notion, formulas were created to provide large amounts of nutrients to meet the increased metabolic demands. Unfortunately, a positive nitrogen balance, regardless of the amount of nutrients provided, is frequently not achieved until the systemic inflammatory response is controlled. In addition, this strategy easily leads to overfeeding, which is associated with increased complications including prolonged ventilator dependence and liver damage. The emphasis has therefore shifted to controlling SIRS (e.g. antibiotics, surgery, etc.) as a primary target. Once the inflammatory catabolic response is controlled, nutrition intervention can produce the desired results of reversing negative nitrogen balance. This can be achieved with the provision of moderate amounts of nutrients in the order of 20-25 kcals/kg/day.

Malnutrition in Patients with Cancer

The word cachexia comes from the Greek words "kakos" meaning "bad things", and "hexus" meaning "state of being". Cachexia is a general weight loss and wasting occurring in the course of a chronic disease or emotional disturbance. It occurs in association with chronic infection, AIDS, heart failure, rheumatoid arthritis and chronic obstructive pulmonary disease. Although body composition changes are not identical in all of these disease states, the term cachexia is used in all of these settings. Cachexia in cancer is a result of the patients' inflammatory state and significant similarities can be seen in patients with severe infections or patients in the post-surgical setting. Anorexia is common among cancer patients. However, it is critical to realize that the profound weight loss suffered by patients with cachexia cannot entirely be attributed to poor caloric intake. In contrast to simple starvation, which is characterized by a caloric deficiency that can be reversed with appropriate feeding, the weight loss of cachexia cannot adequately be treated with aggressive feeding.

Weight loss is the most obvious manifestation of cancer cachexia and is a marker for both progression of the syndrome and prognosis. In a multi-institutional, retrospective review of 3047 clinical protocol cancer patients from the Eastern Cooperative Oncology Group, weight loss of more than five percent of premorbid weight prior to the initiation of chemotherapy was predictive of early mortality. Weight loss was a risk factor to poorer outcome and it was independent of the disease stage, tumor histology and patient performance status. There was also a trend toward lower response rates with the use of chemotherapy among weight-losing patients, but this trend reached statistical significance only among patients with breast cancer. Cachexia may be a direct cause of death in approximately one percent according to an autopsy study of 486 cancer patients.

Nutritional Assessment in the Surgical Patient

Nutritional screening addresses four issues: recent weight loss, recent food intake, current body mass index and disease severity. A good detailed clinical assessment including a detailed history and physical exam is clearly the most important tool. A more detailed assessment should be performed if initial screening indicates a patient is at risk for malnutrition. The detailed assessment may include a thorough history and physical, height and weight to calculate the BMI (kg/m^2), functional assessment (mental and physical), as well as anthropometry to measure the anatomical changes associated with change in nutritional status, midarm circumference and triceps skin-fold thickness. Functional tests including hand dynamometry to measure voluntary handgrip strength, direct muscle stimulation, respiratory function via peak flow and FEV1 and immune function have also been shown to correlate with the presence of malnutrition.

Body composition can be measured using bioelectrical impedance spectroscopy. This is based on measuring the conducting properties of different tissues. Tissues containing large amounts of water and electrolytes (e.g. muscle) are good conductors while fat, air and bone are poor conductors. Bioelectrical impedance is a useful tool to estimate the proportion of muscle to fat and determine nutritional status. Acute inflammatory status, including that induced by surgery, can alter the proportion of water and electrolytes in tissues, thereby significantly altering bioelectrical impedance. Thus, in these individuals, bioelectrical impedance is less useful for estimating nutritional status.

Biochemical parameters can also be used to diagnose malnutrition. Some of the tests found to be useful include urinary excretion of creatinine (which reflects muscle mass), serum protein evaluation including prealbumin, transferrin and most importantly albumin. In particular, albumin levels measured prior to surgery are most useful at diagnosing malnutrition.

Like other tests, the accuracy of albumin and other biochemical parameters is lost once the patient undergoes surgical intervention or becomes critically ill. The patient's inflammatory state and measurements, including CRP and sedimentation rate, have been shown to be important in assessing a patient's nutritional status. If markers of inflammation are elevated, assessment of a patient's nutritional status is more difficult because albumin and prealbumin levels may be inaccurately low.

The National Veteran's Administration (VA) Surgical Risk Study of 54,215 patients followed prospectively showed that mortality increased steadily from approximately 1% to 29% as albumin declined from values greater than 4.6 gm/dl to values less than 2.1 gm/dl. Also, albumin level was evaluated against 61 other preoperative risk variables, including other lab tests and comorbidities. Compared to other parameters, albumin was found to be the best predictor of surgical outcome. Serum albumin level also detected risk in a subset of patients who scored low on other risk factors and whose risk might not clinically be apparent. It was also estimated that measuring albumin as a way to target nutritional support could reduce costs by $116 to $215 per VA surgical patient through reduction of complications and shorter hospital stays.

Out of the many parameters to evaluate nutritional status and its clinical consequences, serum albumin levels provide an excellent marker for the preoperative evaluation. For the surgical patient, it is easily obtainable, objective and is backed by strong evidence. It is only valuable preoperatively. Once a patient enters an acute phase response, albumin loses its specificity.

Nutritional Interventions

So far, we have demonstrated that malnutrition negatively affects outcome. The next question to answer is whether nutritional intervention benefits the patient. It is now clear that well focused, carefully tailored nutritional interventions can be very beneficial. Poor nutritional interventions on the other hand can produce significant increases in morbidity and mortality. Nutritional intervention follows the same rules as any other medical intervention with beneficial, unproven and negative effects associated with it.

It is inevitable that a clinician will be faced with the decision of providing a nutritional intervention plan. Thus, "doing nothing" is in and of itself a plan, albeit most likely, a poor one. In oncologic patients it is best to define a nutritional intervention strategy prior to any surgical or chemotherapeutic intervention. For example, one might plan for preoperative TPN in the severely malnourished patient prior to surgery. The surgeon should try to answer several questions:

1. Nutritional status: What is the patient's current nutritional status and the expected impact of the planned surgery on his nutrition?
2. Timing: Should the nutritional intervention be started prior to surgery?
3. Operative consideration: Can oral intake be started in the postoperative period, and how soon?
4. Gut function and ability to eat: Can the gastrointestinal tract be used? Should oral intake or enteral feeding be used?
5. Need for TPN: Does the patient need TPN?
6. Need for macro and micronutrients: What types should be given?

Preoperative Nutrition

Fortunately, most oncologic patients do not present as emergencies. Therefore, there tends to be enough time (7-14 days) for carefully targeted nutritional interventions. These interventions, if done well, can greatly benefit patient outcomes.

The first goal is to characterize the patient's nutritional state. Measuring albumin, history of recent weight loss and BMI are essential when meeting a possible surgical candidate. If severely malnourished, preoperative nutritional intervention becomes essential. In the severely malnourished patient that cannot eat or will not eat, a short course of total parenteral nutrition (TPN) (seven days preoperative and three days postoperative) is associated with significant improvement in outcome. In the VA TPN cooperative study, the use of TPN in the above mentioned fashion decreased complication rates from 45% in the control group to 6% in the experimental group. Interestingly, the use of preoperative TPN in well-nourished patients significantly increased postoperative complications.

In patients with significant malnutrition but adequate oral intake, the use of preoperative and postoperative immunonutrition (given as a supplement) could be beneficial as demonstrated by a randomized controlled study by Marco Braga. In this study, a dietary supplement enriched with arginine, RNA and ω3 fatty acids was given to cancer patients for seven days preoperatively and continued postoperatively, resulting in significantly decreased infectious complications.

Postoperative Nutrition

Typically, the postoperative period is characterized by a certain period of nil per os (NPO) status especially after major abdominal surgeries. From this starting point, nutritional intervention includes: (1) Keeping patients NPO; (2) Providing patients with enteral nutrition; (3) Instituting total parenteral nutrition; and (4) Providing oral supplements.

The first option involves keeping patients NPO for limited to extended periods of time. This is based on the idea that a postoperative ileus prevents successful oral intake. In addition, it is suggested that food could threaten the integrity of an intestinal anastamosis. Postoperatively, patients frequently receive an nasogastric (NG) tube, particularly after abdominal surgery. Removal of the NG tube is determined on clinical grounds when resolution of the ileus is evident by the presence of peristaltic bowel sound, a decrease in the volume of NG output, the passage of flatus and the presence of bowel movements. Traditionally, oral intake is advanced gradually and is often started with clear liquids and advanced slowly to a regular diet.

There are a growing list of concerns that challenge the validity and safety of this traditional approach. Postoperative ileus tends to be short lived or non-existent particularly in the small bowel and does not preclude oral intake. Ileus is exacerbated by the use of narcotics as the only mode of analgesia and excessive amounts of intravenous (IV) fluids. Ileus also appears to be prolonged in patients that are kept NPO suggesting that careful oral intake postoperatively is actually therapeutic and may promote resolution of the ileus. There is also no clear evidence that the presence of clinical markers of peristalsis, are predictive of successful resolution of ileus or the success of oral intake. Finally, a growing amount of evidence both in human clinical trials and animal studies suggest that intestinal anastamoses are not placed at risk by early postoperative enteral or oral intake; on the contrary it appears that they are actually protected. Furthermore, prolonged periods of maintaining the patients' NPO or keeping them on clear fluids may cause significant morbidity including prolonged starvation, significant fluid and electrolyte imbalances and complications arising from the NG tube itself.

Challenges to maintaining the patients' NPO have prompted the European Society of Parenteral and Enteral Nutrition (ESPEN) and other entities and individuals to explore alternatives. A concerted effort to resume early oral intake requires the careful coordination of a team to be successful. The prevention of excessive amounts of perioperative intravenous crystalloids and the provision of multimodality analgesic therapy with the addition of nonsteroidal anti-inflammatory drugs (NSAIDs) are paramount to the success of early oral intake. These interventions decrease the incidence of nausea and vomiting and may decrease intestinal edema. In addition extensive education of the patient, their families and other personnel is important. Early oral intake does not mean liberal and uncontrolled food ingestion. Rather, small quantities of food containing balanced amounts of macronutrient are encouraged and tested. The presence of nausea and/or vomiting prompts clinicians to keep the patients NPO for short amounts of time with prompt resumption of feeding. Early oral intake has resulted in significant benefits including decreased infection rates and decreased mortality with shorter lengths of stay, cost and an obvious improvement in patient satisfaction.

In patients that are unable to take adequate amounts of nutrients by mouth, the use of enteral nutrition via a feeding tube, a gastrostomy or a jejunostomy should be considered. As with oral intake, early enteral nutrition is associated with significant benefits, which are evident in the critically ill surgical patient. Enteral nutrition is indicated even in patients without obvious under-nutrition, if it is anticipated that the patient will be unable to eat for more than seven days perioperatively. In these situations, nutritional support should be initiated without delay. Delay of surgery for preoperative enteral nutrition is also recommended for patients at severe nutritional risk, defined as: weight loss > 10-15% within six months, BMI < 18.5 kg/m², subjective global assessment Grade C, serum albumin < 3 gm/dl. Altogether, it is strongly recommended not to wait until severe under-nutrition has developed, but to start enteral nutrition therapy early, as soon as a nutritional risk becomes apparent. Whenever feasible, the enteral route should be used except in the presence of intestinal obstructions or ileus, severe shock, or intestinal ischemia.

Inadequate oral intake for more than 14 days is associated with a higher mortality. Thus, patients with severe nutritional risk benefit from 10 to 14 days of nutritional support prior to major surgery even if surgery has to be delayed. Also, patients who do not meet their energy needs from normal food should be encouraged to take oral nutritional supplements during the preoperative period.

Tube feeding should be applied in patients in whom early oral nutrition cannot be initiated. Special regard should be given to those undergoing major head, neck or gastrointestinal surgery for cancer, with severe trauma, with obvious undernutrition at the time of surgery and in whom oral intake will be inadequate (< 60%) for more than 10 days. Patients undergoing major head, neck or abdominal cancer surgeries often exhibit nutritional depletion before surgery and run a higher risk of developing septic complications postoperatively. Additionally, oral intake is often delayed postoperatively due to swelling, obstruction or impaired gastric emptying. It is also delayed in order to prevent straining the anastamosis, making it difficult to meet nutritional requirements. Nutritional support reduces morbidity with an increasing protective effect of enteral nutrition and immune-modulating formulae.

Once the diagnosis of malnutrition is established, the question of what is the best intervention comes next. While it seems intuitive that feeding malnourished patients perioperatively should improve outcomes, there are risks specific to each route of nutritional support. These risks plus the added cost must be balanced with the potential benefit.

The literature is rich with a plethora of studies to evaluate the risks and benefits of the different nutritional interventions. However, it is quite difficult to interpret the data, as the majority of trials are small and not randomized. The wide variety of the inclusion criteria and the severity of malnutrition in the different studies must be considered. In the next section we will explore all the possible interventions and the data behind them.

Different Options for Nutritional Interventions

Perioperative Enteral Feeding (For All Operations)

A meta-analysis evaluated a total of 44 randomized controlled trials of enteral nutrition (EN) in the perioperative period. Trials were grouped into three comparisons: EN versus no nutritional treatment, EN versus parenteral nutrition and volitional nutritional supplements (oral supplemental feeding) versus no artificial nutrition. EN was associated with decreased risk of infectious complications when compared to no nutritional intervention or total parenteral nutrition (TPN).

Perioperative Enteral Feeding (In GI Malignancies)

Perioperative enteral feeding may confer benefit in the severely malnourished patients with GI malignancy. A systematic review of available RCT demonstrated fewer complications when postoperative feeding was accomplished by the enteral rather than parenteral route. Bozzetti, et al randomly assigned 317 malnourished patients to either postoperative enteral or parenteral nutritional support, starting the morning after surgery and continuing until oral intake was adequate. Although the incidence of adverse effects related to feeding was greater in the enteral group (35 versus 14%), the incidence of postoperative complications was significantly less in this group (34 versus 49%), as was the length of hospital stay (15 versus 13.4 days).

As with oral intake, pre- and postoperative enteral intake requires the careful orchestration of a team approach and can produce complications if poorly implemented. In most patients early EN fails to meet caloric goals during the first week. Indeed, attempts at overly aggressive EN may be deleterious as was reported in a small study of 30 patients undergoing a Whipple procedure for pancreatic cancer. In these patients EN was associated with prolongation of gastric ileus and the need for prolonged NG decompression.

Parenteral Feeding

Interpreting the data regarding the use of parenteral feeding is quite challenging. Like any other medical intervention TPN produces dramatic benefits when used adequately but can significantly increase complications when poorly used. TPN is not a substitute for oral or enteral intake and should only be used when adequate attempts at using the patients' gastrointestinal tract have failed.

Overfeeding can easily occur with TPN and may explain the results of studies showing that TPN increases sepsis.

The Veterans Affairs Total Parenteral Nutrition Cooperative Study Group remains the most important large scale randomized control study to address perioperative TPN in surgical patients. The trial published in 1991 (NEJM) was designed to test the hypothesis that perioperative TPN decreased the incidence of serious complications after major abdominal or thoracic surgical procedures in malnourished patients. It included 395 malnourished patients (99% of them were male) who required laparotomy or noncardiac thoracotomy. They were randomly assigned to receive either TPN for 7-15 days before surgery and three days afterward (the TPN group) or no perioperative TPN (the control group). The patients were monitored for complications for 90 days after surgery. This study demonstrated similar rates of major complications during the first 30 days after surgery between the two groups (TPN group, 25.5%; control group, 24.6%), as well as the overall 90-day mortality rates (13.4% and 10.5%, respectively). There were more infectious complications in the TPN group than in the controls (14.1 vs 6.4%; P = 0.01; relative risk, 2.20; 95% confidence interval [1.19-4.05]), but slightly more noninfectious complications in the control group (16.7 vs 22.2%; P = 0.20; relative risk, 0.75; 95% confidence interval, [0.50-1.13]). The increased rate of infections was confined to patients categorized as either borderline or mildly malnourished and these patients had no demonstrable benefit from TPN. In contrast, severely malnourished patients who received TPN had fewer noninfectious complications than controls (5 vs 43%; P = 0.03; relative risk, 0.12; 95% confidence interval, [0.02-0.91]), with no concomitant increase in infectious complications. *In summary, the trial demonstrated that the use of preoperative TPN should be limited to patients who are severely malnourished unless there are other specific indications.*

Perioperative Parenteral Feeding (All Operations)

The largest meta-analysis included 41 trials of parenteral nutrition, provided before and/or after surgery. Parenteral nutrition had no effect on postoperative mortality; there was no significant effect on postoperative complication rates, although trends for all evaluated outcomes favored TPN over no nutrition. In these trials however, there was significant variability in the indication for starting TPN. Enteral therapy was purported as superior to parenteral nutrition when tolerated, while TPN is associated with less procedure-related complications than EN (peg/gastric tube placement) and is beneficial in the treatment of malnutrition.

Perioperative Parenteral Feeding (GI Malignancies)

Patients with hepatocellular carcinoma undergoing partial hepatectomy were randomly assigned to 14 days of preoperative cyclical TPN or placebo. Both groups included patients with only mild malnutrition, as indicated by

the fact that fewer than 20% of patients in either group had sustained a >10% weight loss and the median serum albumin was greater than 4.0 gm/dL in both groups. There was no difference in mortality when compared to controls, but supplemental TPN was associated with less postoperative morbidity (34 vs 54%), better liver function, less ascites and a reduction in the need for diuretics.

Similar results were noted in a trial of 90 patients who were undergoing resection for gastric or colorectal tumors and who had lost >10% of their usual body weight. Compared to control patients, those who were randomly assigned to perioperative TPN for ten preoperative and nine postoperative days had fewer postoperative complications (37 vs 57%), including noninfectious complications (12 vs 34%).

Data from studies of postoperative TPN alone are less favorable. One study of patients undergoing pancreatic resection for malignancy found that those who received postoperative TPN had higher rates of major complications including fistulae, abscesses, peritonitis and anastamotic breakdown (45 vs 23%). The rate of infectious complication was also higher in the TPN group, predominantly due to intra-abdominal abscesses that were thought to be secondary to increased bacterial translocation from lack of enteral feeding. One systematic review found that preoperative parenteral nutrition (13 randomized trials) decreased postoperative complications by 10%, while postoperative TPN alone (8 randomized trials) resulted in a 10% increase in complication rates. These findings were not confirmed by a subsequent meta-analysis. Another meta-analysis (26 randomized trials, although three were not in surgical patients) found that parenteral nutrition decreased hospital complications in studies where lipid-free solutions were used and for patients who were malnourished (not consistently defined). These findings were also not confirmed by another study, which found greater benefit for TPN in trials where lipids were used and in trials evaluating well-nourished patients.

Nutritional Intervention in Specific Cancers

Nonsurgical Cancer Treatment

PN causes net harm to cancer patients undergoing chemotherapy or radiation therapy. There was no apparent positive or negative effect from the enteral provision of nutrients (either through a tube or by volitional consumption).

Esophageal Cancer

The role of nutritional support in patients with localized esophageal cancer treated with concurrent chemotherapy and RT followed by surgery is unclear. Many of these patients present in a nutritionally depleted state from progressive dysphagia and some degree of malnutrition is present in up to 80% of patients at presentation. Although some reports suggest that nutritional support can improve the higher mortality associated with preoperative nutritional depletion in patients undergoing esophagectomy, randomized trials have failed to demonstrate either improved tolerance to therapy or a survival benefit. Like other patients, adequate nutritional evaluation prior to surgical intervention will allow the design of the best form of nutritional intervention for a given individual.

Advanced Cancer

Severe malnutrition and cancer cachexia is a cause of increased anxiety and is particularly distressing for the families of the patients that suffer from it. Many nutritional intervention strategies in the treatment of cancer cachexia have been attempted with most of these trials failing to improve measurable outcomes. It may be of benefit for families and patients to understand that starvation at the end of life may not increase the suffering of the patients. Indeed studies in palliative care suggest that the ketosis associated with starvation diminishes the sensation of hunger and decreases anxiety. In general, despite the subjective perception of benefit, TPN should be avoided at the end of life, as it appears to increase complications including infections, hyperglycemia and may cause unnecessary hospitalizations.

Summary

Malnutrition is a prevalent condition with important implications for the patient undergoing surgery. The consultant asked to evaluate a malnourished patient for possible intervention should first assess the patient's nutritional status by performing a history and physical examination. Judicious use of a small number of laboratory tests aimed at assessing protein and vitamin stores may be helpful. Data regarding outcomes of nutritional interventions in the perioperative period are extensive and difficult to compare, given the broad range of surgical settings and interventions. However, the following general recommendations can be made:

- Early use of the gut is most beneficial, if possible. Among patients who have had general anesthesia, resumption

of oral intake is usually possible within 24 hours and no supplemental nutrition is required during this time.

- Given the lack of clear benefit and documented risks, patients who are not malnourished or who have only mild to moderate malnutrition should not have surgery deferred for TPN or enteral feeds and should not have routine postoperative TPN. Earlier intervention may be appropriate in patients who are malnourished at baseline, or who have a complicated postoperative course.

- Patients with severe malnutrition derive clear benefit from preoperative nutritional intervention. As in all patients the presence of adequate oral intake or the availability of an enteral route should be used, if possible. In severely malnourished patients preoperative use of TPN is clearly beneficial when the gastrointestinal tract cannot successfully be used.

- The use of dietary supplements containing arginine and ω3 fatty acids have been shown in over 30 different surgical trials to decrease infection rates, shorten length of stay and cost in patients undergoing high-risk surgical interventions and is independent of their nutritional status. These should be used for short amounts of time (five days preoperatively and 5-10 days postoperatively) as they are costly and their beneficial effect has only been observed in the perioperative period.

- Nutritional support is not efficacious for patients undergoing chemotherapy or RT for advanced disease unless prolonged periods of GI toxicity are expected. There is little if any justification for the use of nutritional support in patients with advanced cancer or those who are terminally ill. Reasonable justification can be found for administering adjunctive nutritional therapy to malnourished cancer patients who are undergoing major visceral surgery, for prophylaxis during hematopoietic cell transplantation and during therapy for head and neck cancer.

- The role of nutritional support in patients with localized esophageal cancer who are treated with concurrent chemotherapy and RT followed by surgery is unclear and should be decided on a case-by-case basis. Further clinical trials are necessary to corroborate the results of earlier trials and to identify other subgroups of cancer patients who might derive similar benefits from nutritional interventions.

Landmark Papers

1. Bozzetti F, Braga M, Gianotti L, Gavazzi C. Postoperative enteral versus parenteral nutrition in malnourished patients with gastrointestinal cancer: a randomised multicentre trial. Lancet 2001; 358:1487.

2. Bozzetti F, Gavazzi C, Miceli R, et al. Perioperative total parenteral nutrition in malnourished, gastrointestinal cancer patients: a randomized, clinical trial. JPEN J Parenter Enteral Nutr 2000; 24:7.

3. Braga M, Gianotti L, Radaelli G, Vignali A. Perioperative immunonutrition in patients undergoing cancer surgery: results of a randomized double-blind phase 3 trial. Arch Surg 1999; 134:428.

4. Brennan MF, Pisters PW, Posner M, et al. A prospective randomized trial of total parenteral nutrition after major pancreatic resection for malignancy. Ann Surg 1994; 220:436.

5. Detsky AS, Baker JP, O'Rourke K, Goel V. Perioperative parenteral nutrition: a meta-analysis. Ann Intern Med 1987; 107:195.

6. Dewys, WD, Begg C, Lavin PT, et al. Prognostic effect of weight loss prior to chemotherapy in cancer patients. Eastern Cooperative Oncology Group. Am J Med 1980; 69:491.

7. Fan ST, Lo M, Lai EC, et al. Perioperative nutritional support in patients undergoing hepatectomy for hepatocellular carcinoma. N Engl J Med 1994; 331:1547.

8. Heslin MJ, Latkany L, Leung D, Brooks AD. A prospective, randomized trial of early enteral feeding after resection of upper gastrointestinal malignancy. Ann Surg 1997; 226:567.

9. Kortez RL, et al. Does enteral nutrition affect clinical outcome? A systematic review of the randomized trials. Am J Gastroenterol 2007;102:412.

10. Kudsk KA, et al. Preoperative albumin and surgical site identify surgical risk for major postoperative complications. JPEN 2003;27(1):1-9.

11. Percentage of weight loss: a basic indicator of surgical risk in patients with chronic peptic ulcer. 1936. Studley HO Nutr Hosp 2001;16(4):141-3; discussion 140-1

12. Ravasco P, Monteiro-Grillo I, MArques Vidal P, Camilo ME. Impact of nutrition on outcome: a prospective randomized controlled trial in patients with head and neck cancer undergoing radiotherapy. Head Neck 2005; 27:659.

13. Sandstrom R, et al. The effect of postoperative intravenous feeding (TPN) on outcome following major surgery evaluated in a randomized study. Ann Surg 1993; 217(2): 185-95.

14. Schloerb PR, Skikne BS. Oral and parenteral glutamine in bone marrow transplantation: a randomized, double-blind study. JPEN J Parenter Enteral Nutr 1999; 23:117.

15. The Veterans Affairs Total Parenteral Nurition Cooperative Study Group, Perioperative Total Parenteral Nutrition in Surgical Patients. The New England Journal of Medicine 1991;325(8):525-32.

Level of Evidence Table			
Recommendation	**Grade**	**Best level of evidence**	**References**
Enteral nutrition within 24 hrs of surgery including gastrointestinal procedures should be considered generally safe with potential reductions in complications and length of stay.	A	1a	1, 2
Enteral versus parenteral is the nutritional support route of choice when possible and if needed.	A	1a	3-5
Preoperative albumin level should be routinely used to help stratify perioperative risk.	B	1b	6
The consideration of pre- and/or postoperative nutritional support by any route should be limited primarily to severely malnourished surgical patients. Benefits for well-nourished surgical oncology patients are less clear.	B	1a	7-10
Permissive underfeeding is associated with better outcomes in critically ill patients.	C	3	11

References

1. Andersen HK, Lewis SJ, Thomas S. Early enteral nutrition within 24 h of colorectal surgery versus later commencement of feeding for postoperative complications. Cochrane Database Syst Rev 2006;4:CD004080.
2. Lewis SJ, Andersen HK, Thomas S. Early enteral nutrition within 24 h of intestinal surgery versus later commencement of feeding: a systematic review and meta-analysis. J Gastrointest Surg 2009;13(3):569-75.
3. Braga M, Gianotti L, Gentilini O, Parisi V, Salis C, Di Carlo V. Early postoperative enteral nutrition improves gut oxygenation and reduces costs compared with total parenteral nutrition. Crit Care Med 2001;29(2):242-8.
4. Marik PE, Zaloga GP. Meta-analysis of parenteral nutrition versus enteral nutrition in patients with acute pancreatitis. BMJ 2004;328(7453):1407.
5. Koretz RL, Avenell A, Lipman TO, Braunschweig CL, Milne AC. Does enteral nutrition affect clinical outcome? A systematic review of the randomized trials. Am J Gastroenterol 2007;102(2):412-429; quiz 468.
6. Gibbs J, Cull W, Henderson W, Daley J, Hur K, Khuri SF. Preoperative serum albumin level as a predictor of operative mortality and morbidity: results from the National VA Surgical Risk Study. Arch Surg 1999; 134(1): 36-42.
7. Goonetilleke KS, Siriwardena AK. Systematic review of peri-operative nutritional supplementation in patients undergoing pancreaticoduodenectomy. JOP 2006;7(1):5-13.
8. Gianotti L, Braga M, Biffi R, Bozzetti F, Mariani L. Perioperative Intravenous Glutamine Supplemetation in Major Abdominal Surgery for Cancer: A Randomized Multicenter Trial. Ann Surg 2009.
9. Wu MH, Lin MT, Chen WJ. Effect of perioperative parenteral nutritional support for gastric cancer patients undergoing gastrectomy. Hepatogastroenterology 2008;55(82-83):799-802.
10. Perioperative total parenteral nutrition in surgical patients. The Veterans Affairs Total Parenteral Nutrition Cooperative Study Group. N Engl J Med 1991;325(8):525-32.
11. Caba D, Ochoa JB. Gastrointestinal Endoscopy Clinics of North America 2007;17(4):703-10.

11

Pain and Palliative Care in Surgical Oncology

Julie W Childers, Linda King, Robert Arnold

Patients with cancer often experience significant physical and psychological symptoms from the time of diagnosis through the final stages of their disease. Palliative treatments can and should coexist with medical care that seeks to cure disease or extend life. In order to provide the best care to cancer patients, surgical oncologists need to know about the range of symptoms their patients may experience, and how to effectively treat them. A majority of patients with cancer experience pain and other bothersome physical symptoms including nausea, shortness of breath, depression and fatigue.

Palliative medicine is an approach to patients with cancer and other life-limiting illnesses that attempts to maximize quality of life and relieve suffering. Palliative medicine addresses psychological, spiritual as well as physical suffering. Surgeons who treat cancer patients must have the basic skills needed to effectively treat their patients' symptoms. Since many surgical treatments for cancer, such as debulking to decrease tumor burden or surgical management of malignant small bowel obstruction, are palliative in nature, the surgeon's efforts to improve quality of life and control symptoms are paramount.

The importance of palliative medicine in surgery is highlighted because of adoption by the American Board of Surgery (ABS) of a set of principles guiding care at the end of life, which include the management of pain and other symptoms, as well as providing access to palliative and hospice care. In addition, the ABS was one of the nine boards who joined together to support a palliative medicine subspecialty. These palliative medicine specialists are available to help surgeons handle more complex situations much like cardiologists help with complex cardiac problems.

This chapter addresses the management of symptoms often encountered in cancer patients, including pain, nausea, dyspnea, fatigue, depression, anorexia/cachexia, etc. In addition, we review guidelines for referral to a palliative care specialist and hospice.

PAIN

Approximately 75% of cancer patients experience significant pain. However, by following some general principles, up to 90% of this pain can be successfully treated. The first step in treating a patient with pain is to assess the pain accurately and identify a mechanism (or mechanisms) to guide management.

Assessment of Pain

Pain is subjective. Similar stimuli result in different levels, durations and qualities of pain in different individuals. Observation of patient behavior and vital signs cannot substitute for patient report, as physiologic and behavioral adaptations affect how patients express pain. Research has shown that when clinicians do not ask patients to rate their pain, they are more likely to underestimate and undertreat pain. Accordingly, pain should be assessed using a standardized scale on every encounter. A numerical rating scale, where 0 is no pain and 10 is the worst pain imaginable, is commonly used. For children and patients with limitations to communicate, a visual scale using facial expressions may be more suitable **(Figure 11-1)**. In addition, other dimensions of pain should be assessed: location, quality of pain, diurnal variation, provoking and relieving factors, previous treatments and their effect and the impact of the pain on the patient's mood and functioning.

Clinicians should assess and document pain at each encounter with the patient. Pain related to cancer is dynamic and requires close monitoring and frequent adjustments to the treatment plan. A focused physical examination with appropriate imaging and laboratory studies can determine the etiology of pain and guide treatment.

Pain Mechanisms

Understanding the etiology of pain can guide decisions about pain treatment. Clinically, pain is described as nociceptive, due to inflammation or local tissue injury;

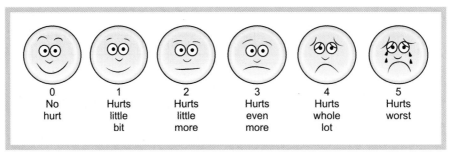

Figure 11-1: Wong-Baker FACES pain rating scale (*Courtesy:* Hockenberry MJ, Wilson D: *Wong's Essentials of Pediatric Nursing* (8th edn), St. Louis, Mosby, 2009. Used with permission. Copyright Mosby

visceral, due to injury to a hollow organ; or neuropathic, due to nerve damage. In the first two cases, the pain is caused by abnormal tissue signaling to normal nerves; in the third case, the nerves are damaged. *Nociceptive (somatic) pain* is a result of activation of nociceptors in the cutaneous or deep tissues. In cancer, this pain can be due to bone or soft tissue metastases, incisional or postsurgical pain, as well as inflammation or spasm. This type of pain is usually well-localized and may be sharp, dull, or aching in quality. *Visceral pain* results from infiltration, compression or distention of deep thoracic or abdominal structures. This can occur in patients with liver metastases that stretch the hepatic capsule, as well as pancreatic cancer. Visceral pain is often described as "dull" or "squeezing", and sometimes is referred to a different cutaneous site. *Neuropathic pain* is a result of damage to the central or peripheral nervous system and is often described as sharp, lancinating or as "tingling" or "numb". Some examples of neuropathic pain in cancer are lumbar or sacral plexopathy from locally advanced gynecologic, rectal and prostate cancers and peripheral neuropathy from chemotherapy or other medications. Frequently, pain in cancer is due to a combination of etiologies and differentiation between types of pain can be difficult.

Management of Pain

Most cancer pain will require treatment with both pharmacologic and nonpharmacologic modalities. Medications to treat cancer pain include opioids, nonsteroidal anti-inflammatory drugs (NSAIDs) and adjuvant medications such as steroids, antidepressants and anticonvulsant medications. Effective pharmacologic pain management includes using adequate starting doses and titrating doses regularly, dispelling patient misconceptions about pain management and anticipating and promptly treating any side effects.

Nonpharmacologic modalities to treat cancer pain include physical measures such as heat, transcutaneous electrical nerve stimulation (TENS) as well as psycholo-gical strategies such as distraction and relaxation. A multidisciplinary team, including chaplaincy, social work and sometimes psychologists and trained counselors, can best address factors that increase perception of pain. Interventional modalities, such as nerve blocks and implantable drug delivery systems, are also useful in treating cancer pain. In fact, some data show that interventional modalities may offer better pain control, less toxicity and even prolonged survival when used earlier in cancer pain treatment.

Pharmacologic Management of Cancer Pain

Opioids

Opioids are potent analgesics frequently required in cancer-associated pain. Opioids act by binding to μ and κ receptors in the central and peripheral nervous system. Opioids are available in both short-acting formulations with a peak-onset of 30-60 minutes and duration of action of 3-4 hours and long-acting formulations which have a slower-onset but a longer duration of action (12-72 hours). Short-acting opioids are used to control acute pain such as pain related to surgery or in patients just starting on opioid therapy.

Patients with chronic or persistent pain are most typically prescribed a long-acting opioid on a scheduled basis with a short-acting opioid ordered as needed as a rescue or breakthrough medication to manage episodes of acute or incident pain. Breakthrough doses of short-acting opioids are usually 5-20% of the total 24-hour dose of the long-acting preparation and should be used every 2-4 hours as needed.

Opioid requirements vary greatly between patients. Careful titration is necessary to achieve adequate pain relief. Opioid doses can be titrated as often as every 24 hours when the pain is moderate and more frequently when the pain is severe. When titrating opioids, if pain continues to be moderate, the dose should be increased by 20-50%, while for severe pain the dose should be increased by 50-100%.

Choice of Opioid Agent

Short-acting opioids: In most patients who are opioid-naïve, there is little indication to choose one initial oral opioid over another. Mixed preparations, such as *codeine/acetaminophen* (Tylenol #3 and Tylenol #4), *oxycodone/acetaminophen* (Percocet and Roxicet) and *hydrocodone/acetaminophen* (Vicodin and Lorcet), are often chosen as initial agents for acute pain. However, the overall daily dose of these medications is limited by the maximum dose of acetaminophen that can safely be given (four grams per day). Generally, patients with persistent pain requiring regular doses of opioids must be changed to an alternative opioid regimen. Morphine, oxycodone, hydromorphone and oxymorphone (a newer agent) are all available in various oral formulations and strengths, allowing easy titration to achieve rapid pain control. Another potent ultrashort acting opioid, fentanyl, is available in an oral transmucosal form on a stick (the "fentanyl lollipop" or Actiq) or as a buccal lozenge (Fentora). A portion of the fentanyl diffuses across the oral mucosa and avoids first-pass metabolism, making oral transmucosal formulations useful in patients with poor GI absorption. Analgesic effect occurs in five minutes and continues for 2.5-5 hours. The lowest available dose of these transmucosal forms of fentanyl is quite potent; therefore, *these should not be used in opioid-naïve patients and should only be prescribed by clinicians experienced in their use.*

Meperidine (Demerol), an opioid sometimes used for hospitalized patients, has toxic metabolites that build up with repeated dosing and is not recommended for chronic cancer pain or ongoing dosing. *Propoxyphene* (Darvon and Darvocet) should also be avoided, particularly in the elderly, because of neurologic side effects and relatively ineffective analgesia.

Long-acting opioids: When a patient's pain has been stabilized with short-acting opioids and is expected to continue for weeks to months, clinicians should prescribe long-acting opioids to decrease pill burden and provide more even analgesia. Long-acting opioids include sustained-release oral formulations of oxycodone, morphine and oxymorphone as well as transdermal preparations of fentanyl. *Oxycodone* (Oxycontin) and morphine (MS Contin and SR Oramorph) are available in formulations that provide analgesia for 8-12 hours and are dosed on a scheduled basis 2-3 times per day. *Morphine* is also available in 24-hour formulations usually dosed once or twice daily (Kadian and Avinza). These long-acting oral opioids cannot be crushed or chewed, though Kadian and Avinza capsules can carefully be opened and administered to patients with large bore feeding tubes or mixed with sauces for patients who cannot swallow pills. *Fentanyl* is available in a transdermal patch form for ongoing treatment of stable, chronic pain. Doses of 12, 25, 50, 75 and 100 mcg/hr are available. These doses have been shown to be equivalent to hourly IV fentanyl doses (e.g. a patient on a 25 mcg/hr drip can be converted to a 25 mcg patch). The manufacturer provides a table converting fentanyl patches to oral morphine equivalent. A rule of thumb is that the fentanyl patch dose in mcg/hour can be doubled to convert to a 24-hour morphine equivalent. Patients who have been using opioids in the range of 30-75 mg of oral morphine a day should start with a 25 mcg patch. Relatively opioid-naïve patients and those, such as elderly patients, who may be sensitive to opioid side effects should start with a 12 mcg patch. In patients who require higher doses than 100 mcg/hr, multiple patches can be used at once. Patches are replaced and rotated to a different site every 72 hours. When first applied, the fentanyl patch takes effect after 12-16 hours and titration to an effective dose may take several days. Short-acting opioids must be used during this period to achieve effective analgesia.

Methadone, though often associated with its use in addiction, is also available for use as a second-line agent in chronic pain. However, due to its highly variable half-life and multiple interactions with drugs metabolized by the cytochrome p450 system, consultation with a palliative care or pain specialist is advised when prescribing methadone.

Opioid Conversions

Frequently, whether due to inadequate effect, intolerance of side effects or concern about renal toxicity, clinicians need to change patients from one opioid to another. An equianalgesic table is used to determine appropriate doses when switching between different opioids and different routes of administration. The first step is to convert the total 24-hour use of all opioid used by a patient to the equivalent amount of oral morphine and then to convert this dose into the new opioid regimen. Fifty to seventy-five percent of the previous analgesic dose should be prescribed when starting the new agent, due to incomplete cross-tolerance. Prescribers then should adjust the dose regularly. Dose adjustments can be made based on the severity of the patient's pain and response to the new opioid. **Table 11-1** depicts equivalencies of commonly used opioids.

Use of Patient-Controlled Analgesia

Hospitalized patients with acute pain or postoperative pain may benefit from the use of patient-controlled analgesia, or PCA. Studies of PCA use in postoperative pain show that patients achieve better analgesia with an overall lower dose of opioids compared with patients managed without a PCA. With a PCA, the patient self-delivers a fixed dose

TABLE 11-1	Opioid equivalencies	
Opioid	**Parenteral**	**Oral**
Morphine	10	30
Fentanyl	0.1	not available
Hydromorphone	1.5	7.5
Oxycodone	not available	20-30
Oxymorphone	1	10
Codeine	130	300
Hydrocodone	not available	25-30

of an intravenous opioid at a fixed interval by pressing a button. Patients using a PCA must be alert and cognitively intact, as well as physically able to press a button for pain relief. For patients in acute pain, an intravenous bolus dose can be given prior to initiating the PCA. This loading dose is usually in the range of 2-4 mg IV morphine or 0.4-0.8 mg of hydromorphone in opioid-naïve patients, repeated every 15 minutes until the patient is comfortable. The PCA dose is a lower dose that the patient will receive when she presses the button and is allowed every 8-15 minutes. In patients who have been on chronic opioids, allow an hourly maximum PCA dose which is three to five times the previous average hourly opioid dose.

Opioid Choice in Renal and Hepatic Failure

Morphine, as well as codeine, which is metabolized to morphine, should be avoided in renal failure and dialysis patients due to risk of accumulation of toxic metabolites. Fentanyl, which is not renally cleared, may be the safest drug, although there is little data. Liver failure decreases the clearance of most opioids, increasing the risk of side effects and toxicities. Morphine and fentanyl may be the least risky opioids to use in hepatic failure. In either renal or hepatic impairment, one should start with a low dose and slowly titrate the dose upward.

Opioid Dependence

Patients are often reluctant to take opioids because of fear of addiction. This fear arises from the popular image of opioids as drugs of abuse and a misunderstanding of the nature of addiction and physical dependence. All patients who are taking opioids regularly in doses greater than approximately 30 mg of morphine a day will become physically dependent upon their medication and will suffer withdrawal if it is abruptly stopped. Tolerance, the need for increasing amount of a substance to achieve the same analgesic effect, may develop in any patient taking opioids and should be treated by increasing the dose of the current opioid, switching to a different opioid or adding an adjuvant medication to the current regimen.

Addiction is a pattern of escalating use and craving that persists despite substantial harm. For cancer patients, substantial research has shown that the risk of developing a substance abuse disorder is very low. Clinicians should explain the difference between addiction and physical dependence to patients who are concerned that they will become addicts. The analogy of a diabetic who is dependent on insulin, or a patient with congestive heart failure who requires diuretics might be useful.

Patients with histories of substance abuse also develop cancer and severe pain. In general, they should be treated by the principles discussed in this chapter. Physicians should discuss the history of addiction openly with the patient but that background should not preclude the use of opioids. Simple precautions such as establishing a single provider for opioid prescriptions and periodic screening with urine drug tests may be appropriate. It can also be helpful to involve additional individuals such as sponsors or addiction counselors to monitor safe use of opioids.

Management of Opioid Side Effects

Constipation is the only opioid side effect that does not wear off with time. All patients on opioids should proactively be prescribed a laxative such as senna. The dose of laxative can be titrated until the patient experiences a bowel movement every day or every other day. If the patient does not have a bowel movement in a 48-hr period, a stronger laxative such as bisacodyl, milk of magnesia or lactulose should be added. Sometimes it is worthwhile to use laxatives with different mechanisms of action. For example, senna and dulcolax are both stimulants of peristalsis, but lactulose works by an osmotic mechanism and may be added when bowel stimulants have been maximized. If constipation continues, a clinician should perform a rectal examination to rule out impaction. If there is no impaction, it is appropriate to add another agent or administer an enema.

Nausea and vomiting symptoms, if they occur at all, usually are present for only the first three days to one week of opioid therapy. Patients with a history of nausea with a specific opioid should be treated with a different opioid and receive scheduled antiemetics such as metoclopromide or haloperidol for the first three to five days of opioid treatment. Serotonergic agents such as ondansetron, which are more expensive, can also be used.

Sedation may be the most troublesome during the first two to five days of opioid use. Often, patients sleep more when effective pain relief is provided if they have been tense and sleepless for some time with uncontrolled pain. However, if somnolence is troublesome to the patient, consider decreasing the opioid dose and adding a coanalgesic such as a nonsteroidal anti-inflammatory drug (NSAID). Rotating to a different opioid may also be effective. Finally, some patients will need a psychostimulant to help them tolerate the opioid and maintain an acceptable level of alertness. In some cases, decreased alertness will be difficult to avoid with the doses of opioid needed to achieve adequate pain relief. In those situations, physicians should discuss with the patient and family the relative value they place on wakefulness versus adequate pain control.

Confusion, hallucinations and cognitive impairment are opioid side effects that can be difficult to distinguish from progression of disease and the metabolic abnormalities that come with serious illness. If the opioid therapy is suspected, the opioid can be rotated to a different one at the lowest dosage possible. In some cases, confusion may not be able to be reversed. Low-dose haloperidol (0.5 mg IV or PO tid) can be started to alleviate confusion if it is distressing to the patient or family.

Non-opioid Analgesics

Non-opioid analgesics include acetaminophen and nonsteroidal anti-inflammatory drugs (NSAIDs).

Acetaminophen has central analgesic effects rather than inhibiting peripheral inflammation. Its main advantage is lack of toxicity and its safety even in long-term use. The dose ceiling of four grams per day before hepatic toxicity occurs limits its use alone and in combination with opioids. It is rarely indicated for use alone in cancer pain, but often can be useful with other agents.

NSAIDs are common first line agents in nonmalignant pain and can be useful in cancer pain as well, usually in combination with an opioid, particularly for treating bony metastases. They relieve pain by multiple mechanisms, including inhibiting the cyclo-oxygenase (COX) enzyme peripherally and reducing the production of prostaglandins, as well as by central analgesic mechanisms. There is no evidence that any one NSAID is more efficacious than another, though individuals may respond more to one NSAID than another. If a patient does not respond to an NSAID within one class, a better response might be obtained from one from a different chemical class. For example, ibuprofen and naproxen are proprionic acids; sulindac and etodolac are indolacetic acid and might be tried if ibuprofen and naproxen fail to provide relief. Side effects, including GI upset, platelet inhibition and potential renal toxicity, are common and may limit long-term use in susceptible patients.

Adjuvant Analgesics

Adjuvant analgesics are drugs with other indications that have been found to be effective for treatment for specific types of pain. In cancer patients, adjuvant analgesics are most typically used for treatment of neuropathic pain, bone pain or pain related to inflammation. Antiepileptic agents, tricyclic antidepressants and corticosteroids are the adjuvants that are most commonly used for cancer pain. Adjuvant medications generally are not sufficient therapy for acute and severe pain, as significant time is required to titrate to an appropriate dose.

Adjuvant Agents for Neuropathic Pain

Neuropathic pain is a frequent complication of cancer. A variety of cancers can cause the sharp, lancinating pain that is characteristic of neuropathy: for example, pancreatic cancer frequently causes celiac plexopathy; locally advanced gynecologic, rectal and prostate cancers can cause lumbosacral and sacral plexopathies and lung and breast cancer can cause brachial plexopathy. Other neuropathies, such as postmastectomy pain, postsurgical neuralgia and chemotherapy-related peripheral neuropathy, are iatrogenic.

Neuropathic pain is challenging to treat. Clinicians must individualize pharmacologic regimens and implement them in a stepwise fashion with frequent adjustments of medications. First-line recommendations include antiepileptics such as gabapentin and pregabalin; tricyclic antidepressants (TCAs) and serotonin-norepinephrine reuptake inhibitors (SNRIs) and topical lidocaine. Choice of a particular agent depends on cost, convenience, side effects and coexisting symptoms.

Gabapentin (Neurontin), a gamma-aminobutyric acid (GABA) analogue, originally developed as an anticonvulsant, is the best-studied medication for neuropathic pain. It is typically dosed three times a day, with a starting dose of 300 mg at night and slow titration (every three days to one week) to a maximum of 3600 mg daily. A trial of two weeks at an effective dose should be completed before concluding that the drug is not effective. Sedation is the main side effect. Dosage should be decreased in renal failure. *Pregabalin* (Lyrica) is a newer GABA analogue which was approved in 2004 for the treatment of diabetic neuropathy and postherpetic neuralgia. Pregabalin has similar side effects and cautions as gabapentin but may have added benefit in patients with anxiety disorders.

TCAs are a less costly alternative to GABA analogues but can have more side effects. Common side effects of TCAs include dry mouth, orthostatic hypotension, sedation and urinary retention. *Nortriptyline* (Pamelor) and *desipramine* (Norpramin) are the preferred TCAs for neuropathic pain, as they have fewer anticholinergic side effects than amitriptyline (Elavil); however, all TCAs should be used with caution in patients with heart disease, particularly arrhythmias. Starting doses are 25 mg at bedtime and can be increased by 25 mg every three to seven days as tolerated to a maximum of 150 mg/day. As with other medications for neuropathic pain, a trial of several weeks is required to see an effect.

Duloxetine (Cymbalta) and *venlafaxine* (Effexor) are selective serotonin-norepinephrine reuptake inhibitors

(SNRIs) that have been shown to be effective in some types of neuropathic pain. Both work as antidepressants and anxiolytics, but have also been shown to have independent analgesic effects. Duloxetine has few side effects. Nausea is the most frequent patient complaint, but this can be mitigated by starting at a dose of 30 mg daily and increasing to 60 mg after one week. Venlafaxine is used for neuropathic pain in doses of 150-225 mg/day and is available in both short-acting (dosed twice daily) and long-acting (dosed once daily) formulations. Venlafaxine can cause very mild elevations in blood pressure. Patients who are stopping venlafaxine should be tapered to avoid a discontinuation syndrome.

Five percent lidocaine patches are useful in patients with localized neuropathic pain, especially those with postherpetic neuralgia. Up to three patches at once can be applied, but there should be a patch-free period of twelve hours daily. The lack of systemic effects makes topical lidocaine advantageous in the elderly and those with concerns about sedation.

Corticosteroids for Pain Caused by Inflammation and Edema

Corticosteroids are useful for pain from bony metastases and from tumor compression. Patients with large tumor burden compressing structures such as the trachea or the superior vena cava, as well as those with brain metastases, may experience relief with corticosteroid-induced decrease in peritumoral edema. Steroids can also help with decreasing pain from distention of the hepatic capsule. Dexamethasone at 8-12 mg/day is useful for pain, while higher doses are used to treat brain metastases or spinal cord compression.

Interventional Modalities

Though systemic analgesics have proven efficacy for cancer pain, two to ten percent of patients with advanced cancer still experience severe pain despite maximal treatment with opioids and adjuvant analgesics. Patients who have pain that is uncontrolled with systemic analgesics and those who experience intolerable side effects from analgesics are candidates for spinal analgesia and other interventional approaches to pain management. In addition, patients with pain localized to a specific nerve distribution may benefit from blockade of a peripheral nerve. Most of these procedures are performed by anesthesiologists or other physicians who have completed training in interventional pain management.

Administration of opioids or non-opioid medications directly into the epidural or subarachnoid space through an implantable pump or a tunneled epidural catheter delivers analgesics directly to receptors in the dorsal horns of the spinal cord. Concentrations of opioids attained in the cerebrospinal fluid are much higher than in the systemic circulation and greater analgesia can be obtained with doses that are small fractions of what are required for oral or intravenous administration. As a result, systemic side effects such as sedation and nausea are limited. Adverse effects from spinal analgesia can include common opioid side effects and device-related complications, including infection and fibrosis. There is some data suggesting that the use of intrathecal analgesics is both clinically superior and less expensive than using oral opioids for patients who continue to have pain despite large doses of oral pain medications.

Another modality which interventionalists may provide is spinal cord stimulation, which involves implantation of an electrical stimulator directly into the epidural space at the spinal cord level corresponding to the level of pain. Generally, patients who are considered for implantation of a device to deliver medications or stimulation of the spinal cord should have a fairly good performance status and a prognosis of at least months and be able to perform activities of daily living.

Nerve blocks use local anesthetics, steroids, chemical neurolytic agents or thermal neurolysis to produce small lesions in nociceptive pathways and interrupt the transmission of pain signals. An initial block can be used as a diagnostic technique to determine if there is potential for a more long-lasting one. Types of blocks performed in cancer patients include hypogastric plexus blocks for pelvic or rectal pain such as that caused by metastatic colon cancer or cervical cancer. Celiac plexus blockade is used for abdominal pain caused by cancers of the stomach, pancreas or gallbladder and can be done either as a transcutaneous procedure or at the time of surgery or via endoscopic ultrasound. Consultation with an interventional pain specialist can help identify patients who would most benefit from these interventions.

Non-pharmacologic Modalities

Non-pharmacologic treatments are useful adjuncts to pharmacologic and interventional methods of treating pain and can be effective opioid-sparing agents in patients who have difficulty tolerating or are reluctant to take analgesics. Though there are few randomized trials, some methods which have shown benefit are relaxation techniques, transcutaneous electrical nerve stimulation (TENS) and acupuncture. *Relaxation and distraction techniques* taught by a psychologist can ease breakthrough and procedural pain. *TENS* is a noninvasive intervention in which a device electrically stimulates the skin over a painful area and reduces the perception of pain. Units may initially be set-up and titrated to effect by a physical therapist and are then available for home use by prescription. *Acupuncture,* a 3,000-year-old therapy that is part of Traditional Chinese Medicine, involves needle stimulation of predetermined points. This technique has been shown to release serotonin and endogenous opioids, which may explain its effect on pain. It is traditionally given in a series of treatments by licensed practitioners and may not be covered by health insurance plans. Acupuncture is generally safe, even for patients who are moderately thrombocytopenic or anticoagulated.

Cancer Pain Syndromes

1. Bone pain is often present in patients with bony metastases, though not all bone metastases are painful. Common sites of bone metastases include vertebrae, long bones, pelvis, skull and ribs. Patients typically present with persistent, localized pain that is often worsened by weight-bearing or movement. Diagnosis can be confirmed by imaging including plain films and/or bone scan, though CT scans have the most sensitivity and specificity in identifying bone metastases.

Monthly bisphosphonates are the standard of care for metastatic skeletal disease and may relieve pain as well as prevent fractures. Treatment of bone pain often requires use of multiple modalities; for example, medical treatments such as opioids in addition to NSAIDs or corticosteroids are useful. Bone pain is also an indication for radiation therapy; single dose radiation therapy can often definitively treat pain from an isolated bone metastasis. When multifocal bone metastases occur and pain is not controlled with analgesics, radioisotopes such as samarium-153 and strontium-89 can provide effective palliation. Surgical intervention is sometimes necessary to prevent impending fracture or neurological injury from spinal cord or nerve root compression.

2. Abdominal pain in pancreatic cancer and other upper abdominal malignancies may be caused by pain fibers that travel with the sympathetic afferents, through the celiac plexus. A neurolytic celiac plexus block is frequently used to manage pancreatic cancer pain. Limited evidence from randomized controlled trials suggests that patients who undergo the procedure require fewer opioids post-procedure, especially for patients with cancer in the head rather than the tail of the pancreas. Possible side effects from the procedure include diarrhea and hypotension. Neurolytic celiac plexus block has been shown to alleviate pain for up to seven years, but its use is usually limited to patients with a prognosis of less than one year due to risk of a post-neurolysis pain syndrome.

3. Malignant bowel obstruction, common in patients with gynecologic and colon cancer, often is treated surgically. However, when the patient's condition or goals of care prohibits surgical intervention, medical treatments are available. These include anticholinergic agents such as *hyoscyamine* (0.125 mg PO or SL every four hours as needed) which help to relieve spasmodic and colicky pain

due to bowel wall distention. When the patient cannot take oral medication sublingual hyoscyamine, transdermal scopolamine or parenteral glycopyrrolate can be used. Octreotide, a somatostatin analogue which can be administered via intravenous infusion, subcutaneous injections or intramuscular depot injection, markedly reduces upper GI secretions and is very effective in controlling nausea and vomiting associated with small bowel obstructions, though its cost is often prohibitive. In addition, corticosteroids can sometimes provide relief by shrinking bowel wall edema. If symptoms are intractable, gastric decompression may be required via nasogastric tube, though the discomfort of the nasogastric tube should be weighed against the bowel obstruction symptoms. Placement of a venting gastrostomy tube is a longer-term solution to relieve pain with inoperable bowel obstruction.

NON-PAIN SYMPTOMS

Nausea and Vomiting

Rates of nausea and vomiting in cancer patients ranged from 4 to 44% in one review. Nausea is a debilitating symptom that can interfere with a patient's nutritional status as well as quality of life. The first step in treating nausea in a cancer patient is a history and physical examination to identify a cause, or combination of causes. Common etiologies of nausea in cancer patients include chemotherapy, constipation, bowel obstruction, GI tract infiltration of tumor, brain metastases, metabolic abnormalities such as hypercalcemia, and dysmotility caused by opioids or medications with anticholinergic properties.

Understanding the cause and mechanism of nausea guides the choice of treatments. Whenever possible, treat the underlying cause of the nausea. For nausea caused by bowel obstruction, surgical treatment or placement of a nasogastric tube may provide relief. Aggressive management of constipation and correction of metabolic abnormalities will often alleviate nausea. Chemotherapy-induced nausea is mediated primarily by 5HT3 receptors; first-line antiemetics include 5HT3 antagonists such as *ondansetron* (Zofran) and *granisetron* (Kytril). *Mirtazipine* (Remeron) also binds to 5HT3 receptors and is a less expensive choice for nausea control and can also benefit depression. Opioid-induced nausea is caused by several factors, including direct chemical stimulation, gastroparesis and constipation. Dopamine antagonists such as *haloperidol* and *prochlorperazine* are useful in treating nausea due to these causes. Haloperidol is the strongest dopamine antagonist available and can be very effective in treating nausea in much lower doses than that used for psychosis: a common starting dose is 0.5 mg IV or PO q 6 hrs around the clock, with additional PRN doses.

Metoclopramide also has antidopaminergic activities as well as improving motility and can be useful in chemically-mediated nausea as well as that caused by partial bowel or gastric outlet obstruction.

Antihistamines such as cyclizine, meclizine and promethazine can be useful in motion-induced nausea, as well as in nausea caused by increased intracranial pressure. Cyclizine is the least sedating of the antihistamines.

Nonpharmacologic treatments can be useful adjuncts to antiemetics. Instruct patients in simple behavioral measures such as taking in small, frequent meals and avoiding foods with strong odors. Some patients find techniques such as relaxation and imagery helpful. In addition, some studies have shown that *acupuncture* can be an effective antiemetic.

Mild intermittent or infrequent nausea can be treated with use of an antiemetic on an as-needed basis. For severe or persistent nausea, patients should receive antiemetics on a scheduled basis with an additional PRN agent available. When nausea is not controlled with one medication on a scheduled basis, a second drug with a different mechanism of action can be added.

Dyspnea

Dyspnea, or shortness of breath, is discomfort in breathing. Twenty-one to seventy-eight percent of cancer patients experience dyspnea with a wide variety of underlying etiologies. Whenever feasible, treatment of the underlying cause of shortness of breath, such as pneumonia, pleural effusion, congestive heart failure or pulmonary embolism, provides the most effective relief. However, dyspnea is not always due to a specific cardiac or pulmonary etiology; it is a poorly understood symptom with a complex pathophysiology that is also influenced by psychological and social factors.

Sometimes dyspnea responds to correction of hypoxia. Opioids are effective in treating the sensation of dyspnea across a wide range of illnesses. No opioid has any advantage over another, despite the common practice of choosing morphine for dyspnea. If the patient is already taking opioids for pain, the one that he or she is using should simply be titrated to effect. If the patient is opioid-naïve, use small doses of opioids such as 2.5-5 mg of oxycodone every four hours or 0.2 mg of IV hydromorphone every three hours. The dose can be increased and the interval decreased for uncontrolled dyspnea. Unfortunately, aerosolized opioids are not effective in relieving dyspnea.

In addition to opioids, nonpharmacologic methods for treating dyspnea include positioning the patient in a more upright position and reducing the need for exertion. Providing air circulation with a fan or open windows, using a dehumidifier or air conditioner and avoiding strong odors, including perfume and smoke, can also help relieve shortness of breath. Clinicians may address anxiety by encouraging social support, teaching relaxation and using anxiolytics when necessary. Evidence from trials with COPD patients suggests that acupuncture as well as breathing retraining may relieve dyspnea.

Delirium

Delirium is common in hospitalized patients, particularly in patients nearing the end of life and is often distressing for patients and families. Delirium is characterized by its acute onset, fluctuating course and altered mental status. It is important to note that patients who are somnolent or unresponsive may in fact be in a hypoactive delirium. A validated bedside test for delirium in intubated patients is the Confusion Assessment Method, or CAM-ICU. In this population, it is 93% sensitive and 89% specific. In non-ICU patients, standardized methods of assessing delirium such as the CAM are available. **Table 11-2** summarizes the CAM-ICU.

Delirium may be reversible if clinicians identify and treat the underlying cause. Drugs, especially benzodia-

TABLE 11-2	Confusion assessment method (CAM) ICU for the diagnosis of delirium	
	Feature	**Assessment**
1.	Acute onset and fluctuating course AND	Ask family or friends of the patient, nursing staff, other clinicians
2.	Inattention: patient is easily distracted	Abnormal digit span: Inability to repeat a series of five digits (Start with reading aloud a string of two random digits and then increase). Vigilance A: Read a list of 10 letters with 4 As. Ask patient to tap or squeeze your hand when an A is read.
	PLUS	
3.	Disorganized thinking: > 2 errors	Ask: 1) Can a rock float? 2) Are there fish in the sea? 3) Is one pound more than two pounds? 4) Do you use a hammer to pound a nail? Tell patient "Hold up this many fingers" using two fingers and then repeat with the other hand with a different number of fingers
	OR	
4.	Altered level of consciousness	Hyper-alert, drowsy, stuporous, or unarousable.

zepines, opioids and those with anticholinergic properties such as diphenhydramine, are the most common causes of delirium in the hospital setting. Metabolic derangements such as hypo- or hypercalcemia, as well as infections, drug or alcohol withdrawal and CNS pathology, are also culprits. Delirium is usually multifactorial, however and often persists despite addressing the etiology, especially in elderly patients and those nearer the end of life.

The first steps in treating delirium are nonpharmacologic interventions. Staff and family should frequently reorient the patient to time and place. The presence of familiar people at the bedside can also be helpful. Restraints, IVs and catheters can all exacerbate delirium; these should be removed when possible. A regular sleep cycle should be encouraged by reducing stimulation, including interventions such as blood draws, at night.

Pharmacologic treatment should be administered to patients to whom delirium is distressing, or for whom delirium is impeding their recovery. Antipsychotics are given not only to agitated patients, but also to hypoactively delirious patients, with the goal of restoring patients to their baseline. The most common and well-studied pharmacologic intervention in delirium is *haloperidol,* which can be administered PO, SL, SC or IV. A frequent starting dose is 0.5 mg IV q 6-8 hrs around the clock, with 0.5 mg every four hours as needed for agitation. The clinician should reassess the patient frequently and titrate the dose until effective with a usual maximum of 3.5 mg per 24 hours. Haloperidol is generally safe in these doses, with a small risk of dystonic reactions and prolonged QTc interval. Newer antipsychotics such as *risperidone* (Risperdal) and *olanzapine* (Zyprexa) can also be used with fewer extrapyramidal effects and less risk of QT prolongation. Risperidone is usually started at 0.25 mg orally at night and can be titrated to 0.5 mg twice daily. Olanzapine is useful for patients who need more sedation and is given at doses of 2.5-5 mg orally once daily. The latter agents are not available intravenously which may limit their use in some patients.

Fatigue

Cancer-related fatigue is often the most severe and troubling symptom to patients. It is usually due to a combination of factors, which may include medications, treatments such as radiation and chemotherapy, deconditioning, metabolic abnormalities and the disease itself. In some cases it may be possible to treat the underlying cause: blood transfusions can be provided for symptomatic anemia and physical therapy can improve muscle strength.

Medications also have some effectiveness in treating cancer-related fatigue. Some patients benefit from psychostimulants such as *methylphenidate* (Ritalin), which

should be initially dosed as 5 mg in the morning and 5 mg in the early afternoon. Providers should be aware that higher doses and long-term use brings risks, including sleeplessness and possible cardiac effects. Short-term use of *steroids,* such as a daily 4 mg dose of dexamethasone, can also enhance both energy and appetite. The effect of steroids is likely to wane if used for over a month. Some recent evidence also shows that *modafinil* (Provigil), a non-amphetamine-based stimulant, can improve severe cancer-related fatigue.

Education and support to mitigate the effect of fatigue on the patient's quality of life is also essential. Health professionals may be able to provide information about support services to help with daily activities such as self-care and cleaning. Clinicians should encourage patients to observe their own patterns of energy and develop realistic expectations about the amount which they can accomplish in a day. At the same time, light exercise can improve well-being and energy in patients with cancer, even those with advanced disease.

Anorexia and Cachexia

In advanced cancer, anorexia and cachexia are often the inevitable results of a metabolic, endocrine and cytokine-mediated cascade of events and are a poor prognostic factor. Patients sometimes benefit from treatment of reversible causes such as depression, uncontrolled pain, xerostomia, gastrointestinal dysfunction and oral candidiasis.

Unfortunately, no medication for cancer cachexia has been shown to change a patient's prognosis. Some medications may increase appetite and/or weight and thus improve quality of life. *Megestrol acetate* (Megace), a synthetic progesterone, has been studied as an appetite stimulant in cancer. Evidence shows that it is effective in promoting weight gain in 15% of patients with cancer and it is well-tolerated. However, the weight that is gained is primarily adipose rather than muscle. Megestrol acetate also increases the risk of thromboembolism, which is a significant concern in cancer patients. It is often prescribed as an elixir and begun at 400 mg/day, with titration to a maximum dose of 800 mg/day.

Dronabinol (Marinol) is a cannabinoid that has been shown to be effective in improving appetite in AIDS patients, but the evidence in cancer patients is weaker. It also has antiemetic effects. Side effects of dronabinol include effects on mental status, including somnolence, confusion and perceptual disturbance. A number of other drugs—ranging from growth hormone to androgenic steroids—are actively under investigation for cachexia.

Artificial nutrition, which may provide benefit in some patients, is addressed in more detail in another chapter. However, advanced cancer patients who are no longer candidates for life-prolonging treatments often have cancer cachexia that is difficult to treat and does not resolve with artificial nutrition. Families, who associate the sharing of food with love, often strongly encourage or even force food on the patient. In these situations, clinicians may wish to encourage friends and family to identify other means of expressing care such as sharing stories, listening to music together or giving gentle massages.

Depression

Depression is treatable, even in patients who are terminally ill and is not an inevitable consequence of a cancer diagnosis. Guidelines recommend screening for depression in all patients with cancer, as studies have shown that advanced cancer is a risk factor for psychosocial distress. Screening is particularly recommended for patients with newly advanced disease, who are starting on chemotherapy and those who express a desire for hastened death. However, because decreased appetite, sleep disturbance and loss of energy are common in cancer patients, screening should focus on psychological and cognitive symptoms such as worthlessness, hopelessness and guilt.

Screening for depression can be accomplished with a very short test such as the two questions: "Have you been feeling either depressed or hopeless most of the time over the last two weeks?" and "Have you found little brings you pleasure or joy over the past two weeks?"

One step in treating depression is to address uncontrolled pain, which is a risk factor for depression. Supportive counseling, whether provided by a psychologist, social worker, psychiatrist or hospice nurse, can help the patient to identify fears about the dying process, concerns about effects on family members and to develop ways to find meaning and hope within his or her life limitations.

Choice of pharmacologic treatment of depression in patients with advanced disease depends on prognosis. SSRIs and SNRIs are effective but often take up to four weeks to produce an effect. These drugs are best used for patients with a life expectancy of at least several months or more. For patients with a prognosis of less than one to three months, depression may be relieved by initiation of a psychostimulant, such as methylphenidate. Methylphenidate can be dosed once to twice daily, with a starting dose of 2.5-5.0 mg and a maximum daily dose of 40 mg for depression.

Suicidality is more common in patients with medical illness especially as their disease progresses; clinicians should be comfortable assessing patients for suicidal risk.

Hospice

When patients are no longer receiving curative treatments, ongoing palliative care may be provided through a hospice program. Hospice represents one component of palliative care. Hospice care is administered by community-based organizations that provide care to patients in their homes, in freestanding hospice facilities, or in hospitals or nursing homes. Patients who enroll in hospice are certified by a physician to have a prognosis of less than six months if their disease runs its typical course and are no longer receiving treatments directed at curing their disease. The referring physician continues to direct the patient's care and provides all orders for medications and other treatments.

Most U.S. hospice patients receive hospice care through the Medicare Hospice Benefit but many commercial insurance companies and medical assistance plans also include a hospice benefit. The hospice benefit generally covers medication related to the terminal illness, nursing and home health aide services, durable medical equipment, medical supplies, physical and occupational therapy and five days of respite care. Visits to the referring physician continue to be covered under the patient's Medicare Part B component or under their commercial insurance. Hospice patients can also utilize the services of a hospice team physician, which may include home visits.

Table 11-3 outlines where hospice care takes place and common issues with each setting.

More than 95% of patients in hospice continue to receive care at home and the hospice provides support in the form of visiting nurses, home health aides, social work

TABLE 11-3	Locations of hospice care
Home	• Family members must be available to provide most of the care • Hospice team members visit intermittently • Telephone support and nursing visits available for acute issues 24/7 • Medications related to disease and medical equipment are provided by hospice benefit
Long-term care facility	• Medicare hospice benefit does not cover room and board charges of the facility • Hospice care provided to residents *in addition* to usual care provided by the facility • Individual hospice organizations must establish a contract with the facility
Hospice inpatient unit	• Dedicated hospice unit • Freestanding or as part of a hospital or long term care facility • Patients admitted for symptom control or sometimes when actively dying • Length of stay and admission policies vary by facility
Hospital	• For symptom control or actively dying patients • Length of stay limitations dependent on facility • Hospice organization must have a contract with the facility

and chaplaincy and volunteers. Many hospice agencies have a palliative home care component which provides similar services to patients who are still receiving active treatments including radiation, chemotherapy or surgical interventions.

Patients may revoke the hospice benefit at any time if their decision to forgo curative therapy changes. Hospice also provides ongoing bereavement support to family for thirteen months after a patient's death.

Palliative Care Specialists

Palliative medicine physicians are increasingly available to provide consultation for cancer patients. Specialists in palliative medicine work with surgeons and oncologists to provide palliative care to patients in both inpatient and outpatient settings, including patients who are receiving potentially curative treatments and those who are near the end of life. Surgeons may request palliative medicine assistance with pain and non-pain symptom assessment and providing psychological support. In addition, when appropriate, the palliative care team is available to assist with difficult decisions such as continued use or withdrawal of treatments such as feeding tubes, dialysis

or ventilators and with planning for the most appropriate care setting and caregivers to meet patient goals for end-of-life care. Palliative care physicians generally work as part of an interdisciplinary team, involving social work, chaplaincy and nursing providers.

Patients may have negative associations with palliative care and hospice, thinking that their physicians are "giving up" by referring them to these services. As with any consult, the referring surgeon should discuss the consultation and its reason with the patient or family before the consultant appears. Often this conversation is best begun by asking the patient about goals, asking about hopes for symptom control and where he or she would like to be (often home). To broach the topic of a palliative care consultation, the surgeon may find phrases such as "To best meet some of the goals we've been discussing, I'd like to ask the palliative care team to see you" helpful. Emphasis is on the positive aspects of what palliative care or hospice can provide, such as aggressive symptom control and improving quality of life, rather than on accepting death and dying or "withdrawing care". It is helpful to mention that you will discuss the palliative care recommendations with the patient and continue seeing him or her.

Level of Evidence Table			
Recommendation	**Best level of evidence**	**Grade of recommendation**	**Literature**
Evaluate pain with a comprehensive pain assessment, including location, quality, time course, physical examination and diagnostic studies.	5	A	National Comprehensive Cancer Network. Practice Guidelines in Oncology 2008;1.
Use opioids alone or in combination with non-opioids for patients with pain despite maximal non-opioid therapy, for more severe pain at onset and for patients who cannot tolerate non-opioids or for whom the risks outweigh the benefits.	2a	B	Marinangeli F, et al. Use of strong opioids in advanced cancer pain: a randomized trial. J Pain Symp Management 2004;27(5): 409-16.
In a patient with difficult-to-treat side effects from an opioid medication, consider rotating to a different opioid.	2a	C	Quigley C. Opioid switching to improve pain relief and drug tolerability. Cochrane Database of Systematic Reviews 2004;3: CD004847. DOI: 10.1002/14651858.CD004847.
Treat delirium first by looking for reversible causes and then with low-dose antipsychotics and nonpharmacologic methods such as re-orientation and elimination of restraints.	5	A	National Comprehensive Cancer Center. Practice Guidelines in Oncology 2008;1.
Low-dose antipsychotics agents such as haloperidol (< 3.5 mg/day), risperidone and olanzapine are equally effective in treating delirium, with few adverse effects	1a	A	Lonergan E, Britton AM, Luxenberg J. Antipsychotics for delirium. Cochrane Database of Systematic Reviews 2007;2: CD005594. DOI: 10.1002/14651858.CD005594.pub2.
In patients with serious illness at the end of life, clinicians should use therapies of proven effectiveness to manage dyspnea,	1b	A	Jennings AL, Davies AN, Higgins JPT, Broadley KE, Anzures-Cabrera J. Opioids for the palliation of breathlessness in terminal illness. Cochrane

Contd...

Contd...

Recommendation	Best Level of evidence	Grade of recommendation	Literature
which include opioids in patients with unrelieved dyspnea and oxygen for short-term relief of hypoxemia.			Database of Systematic Reviews 2001;3.CD002066. Evidence-based interventions to improve the palliative care of pain, dyspnea and depression at the end of life: a clinical practice guideline from the American College of Physicians.
Predict, recognize and treat side effects of opioid therapy such as constipation, sedation and nausea.	5	A	Management of opioid side effects in cancer-related and chronic noncancer pain: a systematic review. The Journal of Pain 4(5): 231-56.
Consider treating neuropathic pain with SNRIs, anticonvulsants and topical analgesics for neuropathic pain	1a	A	Wiffen PJ, McQuay HJ, Edwards JE, Moore RA. Gabapentin for acute and chronic pain. Cochrane Pain, Palliative and Supportive Care Group Cochrane Database of Systematic Reviews 2005;3. Dworkin RH, et al. Pharmacologic management of neuropathic pain: evidence-based recommendations. Pain 2007;132:237-51.
5HT3 antagonists are beneficial in chemotherapy-related nausea and vomiting; haloperidol is likely to be effective for other causes of nausea.	2a	C	Jantunen IT, Kataja VV, Muhonen TT. An overview of randomised studies comparing 5-HT3 receptor antagonists to conventional anti-emetics in the prophylaxis of acute chemotherapy-induced vomiting. Eur J Cancer 1997;33:66–74. Critchley P, Plach N, Grantham M, et al. Efficacy of haloperidol in the treatment of nausea and vomiting in the palliative patient: a systematic review. J Pain Symptom Manage 2001;22:631-4.
Consider use of psychostimulants for cancer-related fatigue.	1a	A	Minton O, Stone P, Richardson A, et al. Drug therapy for the management of cancer related fatigue. Cochrane Database Syst Rev 2008;1: CD006704.

Landmark Papers

1. American Board of Surgery. Statement of principles of palliative care. Bulletin of the American College of Surgeons 2005;90(8).
2. Back AL, Arnold RM, Tulsky JA. Mastering communication with seriously ill patients: Balancing honesty with empathy and hope. Cambridge University Press, 2009.
3. Block SD. Assessing and managing depression in the terminally ill patient. ACP-ASIM End-of-Life Care Consensus Panel. American College of Physicians - American Society of Internal Medicine. Annals of Internal Medicine 2000;132(3):209-18.
4. Casarett D, Inouye SK. Diagnosis and management of delirium near the end of life. Ann Int Med 2001; 135 (1): 32-40.
5. Chang VT, Janjan N, Jain S, et al. Update in cancer pain syndromes. J Palliat Med 2006;9(6):1414-34.
6. Dworkin RH, O'Connor AB, Backonja M, et al. Pharmacologic management of neuropathic pain: evidence-based recommendations. Pain 2007;132:237-51.
7. Marinangeli F, Ciccozzi A, Leonardis M, et al. Use of strong opioids in advanced cancer pain: a randomized trial. J Pain Symptom Management 2004; 27(5):409-16.
8. Mercadante A, Fulfaro F. Management of painful bone metastases. Curr Opin Oncol 2007; 19:308-14.
9. Mercadante S, Casuccio A, Mangione S. Medical treatment for inoperable malignant bowel obstruction: a qualitative systematic review. J Pain Symptom Manage 2007;33(2):217-23.
10. Morrison RS, Meier DE. Palliative care. N Engl J Med 2004;350:2582.
11. Principles of analgesic use in the treatment of acute pain and cancer pain (5th edn). Glenview IL: American Pain Society, 2003.
12. Schofield P, Carey M, Love A, et al. 'Would you like to talk about your future treatment options'? Discussing the transition from curative cancer treatment to palliative care. Palliative Medicine 2006;20(4):397-406.
13. Smith TJ, Coyne PJ, Staats PS, et al. An implantable drug delivery system (IDDS) for refractory cancer pain provides sustained pain control, less drug-related toxicity and possibly better survival compared with comprehensive medical management (CMM). Ann Oncol 2005;16(5):825-33.
14. The SUPPORT Principal Investigators. A controlled trial to improve care for seriously ill hospitalized patients. The study to understand prognoses and preferences for outcomes and risks of treatment (SUPPORT). JAMA 1995; 274:1591-8.
15. Thomas JR, von Gunten CF. Clinical management of dyspnea. Lancet Oncol 2002;3(4):223-8.
16. Wood GJ, Shega JW, Lynch B, et al. Management of intractable nausea and vomiting in patients at the end of life "I was feeling nauseous all of the time . . . nothing was working". JAMA 2007;298(10):1196-207.

Principles and Philosophy of Cancer Therapy

12

Principles of Surgical Therapy

Jason A Breaux, Steven A Ahrendt

Introduction

The effectiveness of surgical extirpation in the treatment of cancer has been recognized since ancient times. The most well preserved early writings on the subject are by the Roman physician Galen who observed that some breast cancers could be cured by complete surgical removal of the tumor. Later, the Scottish surgeon John Hunter (1728-1793) described methods of patient selection and techniques of cancer surgery including wide excision for margins and lymphadenectomy for superficial cancers. The introduction of anesthesia and aseptic technique in the late 19th century paved the way for a rapid growth in surgical oncology, as more extensive resections to remove tumor became feasible.

The concept of radical operations to completely remove tumors en bloc with a margin of normal tissue, along with the lymphatic drainage, was developed during this period straddling the turn of the 20th century. The classic example is the Johns Hopkins surgeon William S Halsted and his development of the radical mastectomy. Other examples of oncologic surgery milestones during this time period include Billroth's development of partial gastrectomy and total laryngectomy and Miles' abdominoperineal resection (APR). Halsted and most others during this period believed that cancer cells spread outside the primary tumor in a linear, stepwise fashion via the lymphatic drainage basin of the involved organ and then on to distant sites. Therefore, the aim of these procedures was to remove the tumor and the appropriate anatomical lymphatic basin, which theoretically should result in a cure. Local control rates for solid tumors with these new techniques approached 90%, a tremendous improvement from previous less-radical procedures. However, their results in terms of improving overall survival were much less impressive and most patients went on to die from distant disease. Furthermore, these procedures were morbid, often producing significant disability and disfigurement. Alternative theories during this period by surgeons such as Paget, Matas and others that the hematogenous route of metastasis may be

significant were prophetic but largely discounted at the time due to a lack of understanding of cell biology and mechanisms of cancer metastasis.

More recently advancements in the understanding of tumor biology, the diagnosis of tumors at an earlier stage and the development of effective adjuvant therapies have resulted in a general trend toward less radical operations for cancer. Cancer, even at early stages, is being thought of and approached as a systemic disease warranting a systemic approach for effective treatment. Surgical therapy today is one component, albeit oftentimes the most important, in the multidisciplinary approach to treatment of solid tumors. A prime example of this trend is the evolution of the surgical treatment of breast cancer. There has been a progression from radical to modified-radical to segmental mastectomy and from extensive axillary node dissection to sentinel lymph node biopsy. A better understanding of the biology and behavior of breast tumors combined with developments in the fields of radiation oncology and medical oncology have made this less-radical approach not only feasible, but also *more* effective than previous more morbid procedures with regard to overall survival. Other examples include sphincter-sparing operations for rectal cancer largely replacing abdominoperineal resection and limb-sparing surgery for sarcoma. This trend parallels an increased understanding of tumor biology, increasingly efficacious adjuvant therapy and has been validated through randomized, prospective trials such as those pioneered by the NSABP and others. Further, as the choices of when and how to apply adjuvant therapies becomes more complex, the role of surgery in the accurate staging of malignancy has become essential.

Despite the trend toward less radical surgery for cancer, the role of surgical therapy remains paramount in the treatment of most localized solid tumors. The importance of sound surgical therapy remains vital as widespread screening for common malignancies produces trends toward diagnosis at early stages, when surgery is most effective and can be curative as a primary modality.

Today, very few solid tumors can be cured with non-surgical therapies and adequate resection is the most essential part of most treatment algorithms. In fact, for most solid tumors, the single most important favorable prognostic indicator of recurrence-free survival is a *margin-negative surgical resection* of the primary tumor. In addition, some malignancies such as melanoma, hepatocellular carcinoma and pancreatic adenocarcinoma currently lack broadly effective adjuvant therapies. In these patients complete surgical extirpation offers the only chance at long-term survival. Finally, the role of surgery in the treatment of patients with metastatic cancer has expanded with recent advancements in surgical technique and systemic chemotherapy. The best example of this is the modern treatment of colorectal liver metastasis. Once a virtual death sentence, advancements in surgical technique and adjuvant chemotherapy have resulted in 5-year-survival rates of over 50% after complete resection of hepatic metastases in several recent series from large cancer centers.

The importance of surgical treatment, therefore, has not diminished but rather changed with improved understanding of tumor biology and with the development of effective adjuvant therapies. Likewise, the indications for surgery in cancer have expanded to meet the needs of increasingly complex treatment algorithms to not only include removal of the tumor, but also play a crucial role in the diagnosis, staging, prevention and palliation of cancer. The most recent advancement has been the incorporation of minimally invasive surgical techniques widely applied in surgery for benign disease, to surgical oncology. While this process is still very much in evolution, it stands to reason that this represents the future of both oncologic surgery and surgical therapy in general.

Indications and Rationale for Surgical Intervention in Cancer (Table 12-1)

Diagnosis

A tissue sample for histopathologic examination is the most critical part of diagnosis of solid tumors. A specific anatomic site can produce a variety of tumors each with completely different biologic behavior and patterns of spread. An accurate diagnosis is therefore essential for planning the operative approach and making decisions about adjuvant therapy. An example that highlights importance of this is in the stomach where both gastrointestinal stromal tumor (GIST) and gastric adenocarcinoma may occur. Though both present as solid tumors of the stomach, the operative therapy and adjuvant treatments are completely different making an accurate diagnosis essential. Also, recent advances in immunohistochemistry and tumor genetics make an adequate

TABLE 12-1	Indications for surgical therapy in cancer
Indication	**Examples**
Diagnosis	Excisional biopsy suspicious skin lesion Excisional biopsy suspicious lymph node(s) Incisional biopsy soft tissue tumor Laparoscopic core-needle biopsy of liver or other lesion
Staging	Sentinel lymph node biopsy Lymphadenectomy during resection of solid tumor Supraclavicular lymph node biopsy to confirm distant (stage IV) disease
Definitive therapy	Wide excision of early-stage melanoma Colectomy for early-stage colon cancer Mastectomy for DCIS or early-stage breast cancer
Multimodal therapy	Wide local excision and sentinel lymph node biopsy for breast cancer Colectomy for node-positive or locally advanced colon cancer Sphincter-sparing low anterior resection for rectal cancer Liver resection for colorectal liver metastasis
Cytoreduction	Debulking procedure for ovarian cancer Debulking procedure with heated intraperitoneal chemotherapy (HIPEC) for carcinomatosis Liver resection for metastatic neuroendocrine tumor
Palliation	Gastrojejunostomy and/or biliary bypass for advanced pancreatic cancer Bowel resection/bypass for malignant obstruction with metastatic disease "Toilet" mastectomy for locally advanced and metastatic breast cancer
Prophylaxis	Bilateral Mastectomy in BRCA1 & 2, or strong family history, LCIS Total proctocolectomy for FAP or Ulcerative colitis Thyroidectomy in MEN2 syndrome

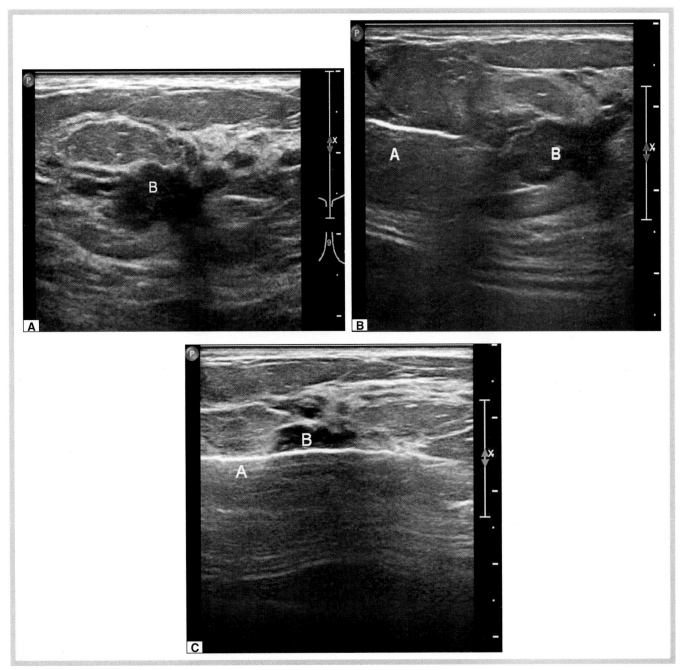

Figures 12-1A to C: Ultrasound images during real-time image-guided biopsy of suspicious breast mass. The first image shows the suspicious lesion (B). The subsequent images show the needle (A) approaching the mass and then after firing, confirming placement within the lesion

tissue sample ever more important. Information gained with these techniques may influence decisions on timing of therapeutic modalities, the use of specific biologic therapies and/or referral for genetic counseling. Parallel advances in radiographic and endoscopic methods for obtaining biopsies have complemented the surgeon's role in diagnosis. Percutaneous, image-guided biopsies utilizing mammography, ultrasound and CT technology

are now commonly used when appropriate to obtain tissue via fine-needle or core-needle biopsy **(Figures 12-1A to C)**.

Similarly, technologic advancements in endoscopy especially endoscopic ultrasound have allowed for diagnostic tissue sampling using these techniques as well. However, in some circumstances the lesion is in an anatomic position that is not amenable to these methods due to fear of tumor dissemination or potential injury to adjacent structures and a surgical biopsy may be indicated. In other cases, such as suspected lymphoma where flow cytometry is needed for an accurate diagnosis, a larger tissue sample is required and the surgeon is called on to obtain adequate tissue. Therefore, the surgical oncologist needs to understand the various methods available and their limitations, for obtaining an accurate diagnosis of a solid tumor. Also important when considering surgical or other forms of biopsy is whether the results will change the management. If resection will be indicated regardless of biopsy results, then the surgeon should forgo other attempts at diagnosis and proceed with an oncologic resection as the ultimate "biopsy". For many lesions, the biopsy results will change the operative strategy, the decision to use preoperative chemotherapy/radiation, or both. Biopsy should then be undertaken in the most efficient manner available prior to formulating a final treatment plan. As always, a thoughtful approach is required to produce the best results while minimizing patient risk.

Staging

As options for surgical and adjuvant therapies for cancer become more numerous and complex, so do decisions about when and how to use them. The most important information about a tumor with regard to treatment options and prognosis is the stage of disease. While clinical staging is important for initial treatment planning, accurate final pathologic staging on a resected tumor utilizing the combined UICC/AJCC staging criteria is essential for complete prognostic evaluation and multimodal treatment planning. Under or over staging of disease may result in inappropriate treatment with significant consequences for the patient. The UICC/AJCC staging systems for solid tumors utilize specific information that often can only be gathered at operation such as number of positive lymph nodes, depth of tumor penetration/invasion and involvement of surrounding structures or distant sites **(Table 12-2)**.

Therefore, the surgeon must keenly be aware of what is needed to accurately stage a given tumor and plan the operation accordingly or else this critical information may be lost. For example, some tumors have a propensity to spread to regional lymph nodes and others do not. The surgeon must understand this biology and know when an elective lymphadenectomy or sentinel lymph node biopsy is indicated and when it is not. Melanoma and breast cancer studies have demonstrated that a sentinel lymph node biopsy may be used for initial sampling of the lymphatic basin and if negative a more extensive lymphadenectomy can be avoided. This is in contrast to

gastric and colon cancers, which also have a propensity to locoregional lymphatic spread, where sentinel lymph node biopsy has not proven useful and an adequate lymphadenectomy at the time of resection is critical for accurate staging. Further, the surgeon must be aware of likely sites of distant metastasis for a given tumor type and examine these sites at operation for staging purposes as preoperative clinical staging can be inaccurate.

Finally, surgeons are sometimes called upon to obtain biopsies to confirm disseminated disease. These should be approached in the least invasive way possible, while still obtaining adequate tissue for diagnosis. The most accessible location of suspected distant disease should be sought out and used for the biopsy, such as a superficial lymph node (supraclavicular node in breast or gastro-intestinal tumors). Minimally invasive approaches should be used liberally such as endoscopic or laparoscopic techniques to obtain deeper tissue samples. Quality of life issues and minimal morbidity are especially important to consider in these patients in whom survival may be limited to months if metastatic disease is confirmed.

Definitive Therapy

Despite advances in systemic chemotherapy and radiation therapy, surgical resection is the only curative therapeutic modality for some common malignancies. Surgery alone can be curative for thin/node-negative melanomas, early-stage breast cancer when mastectomy is utilized and early-stage colon cancer and low grade/early-stage sarcomas. In diseases such as colon cancer, routine screening practices have resulted in detection of early stage cancers amenable to primary surgical resection with high rates of cure and no need for adjuvant therapies. Other malignancies such as pancreatic cancer, hepatocellular carcinoma and cholangiocarcinoma have only marginally effective adjuvant therapies. In these cases, the only long-term survivors are those who have had a complete resection, warranting an aggressive surgical approach despite the poor overall survival. However, surgical therapy used alone has limitations, especially in patients with more advanced stage malignancies who are assumed to have systemic disease at the time of diagnosis. Specifically, surgery can only address locoregional disease and while it may be curative in cases where disease is limited, it cannot address distant microscopic metastases, which will ultimately lead to the patient's demise. Further, the ability to predict the presence of these microscopic, occult metastases are currently extremely limited and can only be estimated based on stage. This fact along with the development of effective adjuvant therapies to treat microscopic disease, including radiation and systemic chemotherapy, has resulted in a multidisciplinary approach to most solid tumors.

TABLE 12-2	UICC/AJCC staging systems
Primary Tumor (T)	**Description**
Tx	Cannot be assessed
T0	No evidence of tumor
Tis	Carcinoma in situ
T1	Tumor invades submucosa
T2	Tumor invades muscularis propria
T3	Tumor invades through muscularis propria into subserosa or nonpertinonealized pericolic tissue
T4	Tumor directly invades surrounding organs or structures and/or perforates visceral peritoneum
Regional Lymph Nodes (N)	**Description**
Nx	Cannot be assessed
N0	No regional lymph node metastasis
N1	Metastasis in 1- 3 regional lymph nodes
N2	Metastasis in 4 or more regional lymph nodes
Distant Metastasis (M)	**Description**
Mx	Cannot be assessed
M0	No distant metastasis
M1	Distant metastasis

Stage	T	N	M	Estimated 5-year survival
0	Tis	N0	M0	> 95%
I	T1/T2	N0	M0	93%
IIA	T3	N0	M0	85%
IIB	T4	N0	M0	83%
IIIA	T1/T2	N1	M0	72%
IIIB	T3/T4	N1	M0	64%
IIIC	Any T	N2	M0	44%
IV	Any T	Any N	M1	8%

Multimodal Therapy

In the modern era of cancer treatment, surgical therapy is most commonly employed as a part of a multimodal approach applied to each individual patient. In this approach, en bloc surgical extirpation of the tumor (and its regional lymphatic basin, when appropriate) is viewed as the primary destruction of the bulk of disease and the principal modality for local control of the tumor. This step is the most critical part of most multimodal treatment algorithms. Radiation and chemotherapy are thus utilized to deal with occult microscopic disease, improving local control rates and preventing distal metastasis, respectively. Though surgery is the most vital aspect of treatment in most cases, rare exceptions include anal canal squamous cell cancer as well as certain head and neck cancers in which primary chemoradiation are often curative. Surgery for these tumors is generally reserved as a second- or third-line therapy.

In addition to the primary role that surgical therapy plays in multimodal therapy, significant progress has been made in developing effective adjuvant therapies, such that they have become essential to the successful treatment of many solid tumors. Radiation, chemotherapy, biological and hormonal therapies act to treat microscopic/systemic disease and prevent or delay recurrence. Their addition to the multimodal treatment algorithm results in increased survival for many surgically resected tumors (**Table 12-3**).

Furthermore, the addition of these therapies has allowed for a definite trend toward less radical/morbid surgical procedures, as seen in the current treatment of breast and low rectal cancers. However, the absolute benefit of these therapies in some cases may be minimal and therefore must be weighed against the risks of therapy to the patient and the impact on patient quality of life. Further, in the modern era of multimodal cancer therapy

TABLE 12-3	Benefits of multimodal therapy. Examples of the use of multimodal therapy and its benefit in select solid tumors, compared to resection alone.	
Tumor	**Modality**	**Benefit**
Breast	Chemotherapy	Doxorubicin/Cyclophosphamide plus Taxane in node-positive and/or tumor > 1 cm results in up to 10% increased survival (absolute benefit) depending on other risk factors
	Radiation	Addition of radiation after lumpectomy reduces local recurrence from 39-10%
	Hormonal therapy	Tamoxifen therapy postoperatively for 5 years associated with 47% decreased risk of recurrence and 26% decreased risk of death
	Biologic therapy	The addition of the monoclonal antibody trastuzumab (Herceptin) to standard chemotherapy results in 12% improvement in disease-free survival
Colon	Chemotherapy	5-FU/Leucovorin based regimens associated with 30% improvement in survival in node-positive patients
Rectal	Radiation	Addition of radiation to total mesorectal excision decreased local recurrence by 5-15%
	Chemoradiation	5-FU based therapy combined with radiation decreased local recurrence by 18% and increased survival by 14%
Gastric	Chemotherapy	5-FU, epirubicin, cisplatin given both pre- and postoperatively improved survival by 13%
	Chemoradiation	5-FU/leukovorin and radiation increased survival by 9% (3 year) and decreased local recurrence rate by 10%
Thyroid	Radiation	Radioactive iodine (^{131}I) ablation postoperatively associated with 50% reduction in recurrence and disease-specific mortality in well-differentiated cancer
	Hormonal therapy	Suppression of TSH with replacement thyroid hormone shown to decrease recurrence and disease-specific mortality in retrospective studies

important decisions must be made about when to administer adjuvant therapy in relation to surgical therapy.

Traditional approaches to multimodal therapy for solid tumors included surgical resection followed by postoperative adjuvant radiation, chemotherapy, or both. The goal of postoperative adjuvant therapy is to destroy microscopic tumor cells left behind after resection and/or cells that have escaped the primary site. The aim of radiation therapy in most cases is to control microscopic tumor deposits left in the original tumor bed and enhance local control of disease. Likewise, systemic therapy eradicates microscopic tumor cells that have escaped the primary tumor site and could result in distant metastatic disease. In some cases chemotherapy can act to sensitize the tumor to radiation, as with 5-FU and radiation used for rectal cancer, improving local control rates over each modality alone. Theoretical advantages to postoperative therapy include no delay in definitive surgical resection. Also, complete pathologic staging is available after resection to guide treatment and may spare a patient who may have been over-staged clinically. Limitations to this approach include administering radiation to a surgically altered field where oxygen tension levels may be decreased, thereby lowering efficacy. Also, organs

susceptible to toxicity (i.e. small intestine) may have shifted to occupy the space where the tumor resided. Others shortfalls include the inability to monitor response to therapy and a delay in treating systemic disease if complications occur postoperatively.

A variation in this algorithm is the administration of the adjuvant therapies preoperatively, classically known as neoadjuvant therapy. Theoretically, this approach offers several advantages **(Table 12-4)**.

Firstly, neoadjuvant therapy treats systemic disease without delay. This is an important consideration, especially in locally advanced tumors, given that distant disease is by far the most deadly form of treatment failure. Also, many major resections have the potential for morbidity that may significantly delay or even preclude subsequent adjuvant therapy, a consequence avoided with neoadjuvant therapy. Secondly, preoperative therapy permits an opportunity to monitor response to therapy of an *in situ* tumor; so that changes in the regimen can be made or surgical resection can be undertaken in non-responders. Contrast this with postoperative therapy where there is almost no way to know if first-line therapy is effective. Similarly, patients who progress rapidly during therapy, indicating aggressive tumor biology can be spared unnecessary surgery. Thirdly an advantage is

TABLE 12-4	Preoperative/Neoadjuvant vs Postoperative/Adjuvant therapy. Theoretical advantages and disadvantages to preoperative vs postoperative adjuvant therapy as part of the multimodal approach to treatment of solid tumors	
Type of therapy	**Advantages**	**Disadvantages**
Postoperative/ Adjuvant therapy	• Complete pathologic staging • No delay in surgical therapy • Avoid adverse tissue-healing effects of therapy	• Delay in treatment of systemic disease • Delayed or omitted adjuvant therapy due to postoperative complications • Treatment delivered to surgically-altered tissues may be less efficacious
Preoperative/ Neoadjuvant therapy	• No delay in treating systemic disease • Ability to monitor in-situ tumor response to therapy • Selects out aggressive tumors and avoids unnecessary surgery • Diminished radiation toxicity to surrounding structures • Improved efficacy of therapy in non-surgically altered field • Gain prognostic information based on response to therapy • Downsized tumor allows for less radical surgery • Convert tumor from unresectable into resectable	• Overtreatment of clinically overstaged patients • Potential tissue-healing complications from therapy • Loss of initial pathologic staging information

that when administering preoperative radiation the tumor can act as a spacer, keeping organs susceptible to radiation injury out of the radiation field. Further, radiation is also theoretically more efficacious in a well-oxygenated, non-operated field. Fourthly, preoperative therapy can offer important prognostic information, as complete responders generally have improved long-term survival compared to incomplete responders. Finally, preoperative therapy can potentially shrink the primary tumor mass to decrease the extent of surgical therapy or, in rare cases, convert an unresectable lesion into a resectable one. A very common application of this approach is seen with locally advanced breast cancer, where many women can be spared the need for total mastectomy after reduction in tumor size resulting from preoperative chemotherapy. Another standard use today for preoperative chemoradiation is in locally advanced rectal cancer, an approach, which can often yield all of the advantages, listed above, not the least of which is the high likelihood of conversion from an APR to a sphincter-sparing surgical resection.

Regardless of the sequence used, the surgical oncologist plays a central role in this multidisciplinary approach. The surgeon must not only be able to skillfully complete the surgical arm of treatment, but also thoughtfully coordinate multimodal therapy. He or she must be astutely aware of the indications for adjuvant therapy and options available for a given situation. The decision to apply adjuvant therapies and whether to apply them pre- or post-operatively depends on both tumor-specific and patient-related factors. Communication between the surgeon, radiation oncologist and medical oncologist should be free-flowing and the surgeon should be keenly aware of

the issues important to the medical specialists and vice versa. The best results seem to come from treatment planning during multidisciplinary discussions or tumor boards involving all specialties, conducted *prior* to initiating therapy. Overall, advancements in multimodal therapy have resulted in improved survival, decreased local recurrence rates and less radical surgical procedures for many solid tumors.

Cytoreduction

Traditional oncologic principles limited surgical therapy to the treatment of locoregional disease and patients with diffusely metastatic disease were only offered palliative treatments or supportive care. Ovarian and many gastrointestinal tumors have a predilection toward tumor rupture and dissemination throughout the peritoneal cavity. In recent years, some have suggested that diffuse metastatic disease isolated to the peritoneum represents an extension of locoregional disease and locoregional therapies including surgery could be applied. Approaches utilizing cytoreductive surgery combined with intra-cavitary and/or systemic chemotherapy have been subsequently developed to address this. An example of an instance in which this treatment is now standard is in the management of ovarian cancer with peritoneal meta-stases utilizing cytoreductive surgery. In these patients, optimal surgical tumor debulking wherein complete cytoreduction is achieved with no macroscopic residual disease, followed by systemic therapy can result in significant long-term survival. Further, survival rates have been shown to be directly proportional to the extent of cytoreduction achieved at surgery suggesting that the surgical debulking plays a central role in treatment efficacy.

These concepts have now been applied to many gastrointestinal tumors with peritoneal dissemination, a disease state with a previously dismal prognosis with standard chemotherapy regimens. Several centers are now performing cytoreductive surgery on these patients, with the goal of reduction of residual disease to nodules approximately < 3 mm in size. As an adjunct to debulking, hyperthermic intraperitoneal chemotherapy (HIPEC) is utilized to maximize destruction of residual disease and prevent or delay recurrence. Intraperitoneal chemotherapy has been shown to maintain a high concentration gradient between peritoneal and plasma drug levels, as well as providing high levels of intratumoral drug concentration up to a depth of approximately 2.5-3 mm. Hyperthermia also has direct toxic effects on cancer cells, as well as an indirect synergistic effect with certain chemotherapeutic agents, increasing their penetration and toxicity. Promising recent work is focused on the efficacy of these techniques for mesothelioma, colon, gastric and other cancers with peritoneal dissemination. A recent prospective, randomized trial and several retrospective studies have shown improved (and some long-term) survival in colon cancer patients with peritoneal carcinomatosis treated with cytoreductive surgery and combined systemic/intraperitoneal chemotherapy versus patients treated with conventional systemic chemotherapy. As with ovarian cancer the most important prognostic indicator in these studies is whether a complete cytoreduction is achieved. In fact, patients with an incomplete cytoreduction often have dismal outcomes equivalent to non-surgical treatments. Further, while studies from high-volume centers demonstrate low perioperative mortality, these extensive procedures have a high major morbidity rate. These issues make patient selection crucial to a positive outcome. Cytoreductive surgery with HIPEC should therefore not be offered to patients with evidence of extraperitoneal disease, poor functional status and / or clinical evidence that the extent of disease precludes complete cytoreduction.

Another indication for the use of cytoreductive surgery is in the case of indolent tumors that may cause significant symptomatology or take years to cause death. A common example is patients with indolent low-grade mucinous neoplasms of the appendix or ovaries with extensive peritoneal dissemination (e.g. pseudomyxoma peritonei). These patients clearly benefit from multiple debulking procedures sometimes years apart (usually with addition of HIPEC). Cytoreduction in these cases dramatically improves symptoms and overall survival with treatment failure occurring only after debulking becomes no longer feasible. A more controversial, but well described

application of debulking surgery is in metastatic neuroendocrine tumors. These have a tendency to present with bilobar liver metastasis and generally demonstrate otherwise indolent tumor biology. Even complete resection of gross disease in these patients could be viewed as debulking, as recurrence and ultimate death from disease after many years is generally the rule after resection. However, numerous retrospective reviews have demonstrated a substantial survival benefit with resection of all or most (>90% is general recommendation) gross disease. Another important aspect of this disease are the debilitating syndromes associated with these tumors (e.g. severe hypoglycemia in insulinoma and diarrhea/flushing in carcinoid syndrome) especially when metastases to the liver occur. In these extremely symptomatic patients, resection of all or most of gross disease results in significant improvement or interval resolution of these symptoms for the majority of patients, an important quality of life issue considering the indolent nature of these tumors and poor response to systemic therapy. Given the low chance for cure with resection, some have advocated utilizing minimally invasive and ablative techniques to approach these lesions. However, formal comparisons of the efficacy of these modalities versus traditional surgical debulking in these tumors have not been made.

Metastatic Disease

The development of distant metastases from solid tumors classically portended a dismal prognosis precluding surgical intervention and curative therapies were generally unavailable. However, astute clinicians noted that some tumors tended to metastasize to specific sites, with progression in this single site ultimately leading to death. This lead to the idea that metastases could be resected with intent to cure. This was coupled with the fact that increasingly effective adjuvant therapies caused some tumors to behave more indolently, perhaps opening the door for resection before further metastases developed and potentially addressing the issue of residual micrometastases. Building on these concepts, pioneering efforts by surgeons and further advancements in systemic therapies have made long-term survival in many patients with metastatic disease a realistic possibility.

A prime example is the success of surgical resection of hepatic and pulmonary metastases from colorectal carcinoma. This was made possible by the development of safe hepatic resection techniques, new interventional radiology technologies and effective systemic therapies. As these therapies have improved, now even patients with multiple bilobar hepatic metastases may be candidates for resection and / or ablation. Long-term survival in appropriately selected patients approaches 50% as reported and confirmed by recent studies in high-volume centers. Successful metastasectomy followed by long-term survival has been observed in other solid tumor types including sarcoma, melanoma, breast, neuroendocrine and renal cell cancers. Additionally, case series have demonstrated that other sites of metastasis can successfully be treated with resection, including metastases to adrenal, distant soft tissue/lymphatic and isolated visceral locations. Despite these advancements in the surgical treatment of some types of metastatic disease, thoughtful patient selection for this type of therapy remains critical. Patient and tumor-related factors are considered when resection of metastases is indicated **(Table 12-5)**. Patients must be able to tolerate major surgery and preoperative evaluation of comorbidities and functional status are critical. Comorbidities related to the target organ must be focused on, such as underlying pulmonary disease when considering lung resection, or liver disease when considering hepatic resection. Patients with metastatic disease from tumors with aggressive biology and a tendency toward early widespread dissemination such as pancreatic, bile duct and esophageal cancers are generally not considered for surgery. If resection is to be considered, the status of the primary tumor is important. While most lesions present metachronously, synchronous presentations also occur and can be resected concurrently in cases where the two resections will be straightforward; however this decision is rather subjective, requiring mature surgical judgement and may be influenced by intraoperative findings. A short interval between resection of the primary tumor and the development of multiple metastases may also suggest aggressive tumor biology, warranting a trial of adjuvant therapy and restaging before considering resection.

TABLE 12-5	Issues to consider when evaluating a patient with metastatic disease for possible surgical therapy.

- Patient comorbidities, functional status
- Tumor biology
- Status of primary tumor
- Adequate and current preoperative staging
- Anticipated complexity of resection in synchronous primary and metastatic lesions
- Disease-free interval for metachronous tumors
- Ability to completely treat all evident disease
- Ability to leave adequate remnant of target organ

There are two major tumor-related criteria that must be met when considering surgical therapy of metastatic disease: First, that all clinically evident disease can safely be resected or ablated with negative margins and second, that the remnant target organ after resection is sufficient enough for adequate function **(Table 12-5)**. For example, volumetric measurements are sometimes performed on the future liver remnant before extended resections with a goal of at least a 20-25% remnant volume postresection to ensure adequate hepatic function. Also, a current and accurate staging work-up must be completed prior to proceeding with resection to confirm that disease is limited to the organ to be resected. For instance, in colorectal liver metastasis, full-body PET/CT scans are used liberally to search for extrahepatic disease, a finding that precludes resection when present. High-quality preoperative imaging is also critical to evaluating extent of disease within the organ involved and confirming that adequate resection with preservation of function is possible.

Surgery for Palliation

Performing a major surgical procedure on a cancer patient with disseminated disease and a limited life expectancy is controversial and requires mature surgical judgement. The prospect of a terminally ill patient spending much of their remaining lifespan recovering from major surgery, or dealing with complications is highly undesirable. Alternatively, proper patient selection can lead to a surgical intervention that produces an improved quality of life for a person with limited time. This has lead to controversy over when palliative surgery is indicated. Traditionally, palliative surgery was recommended for patients experiencing complications related to their tumor including most commonly obstruction and/or bleeding. Major operations to resect or bypass the area may lead to temporary relief but some studies suggest a high recurrence rate of symptoms and high surgical morbidity in this patient population. Therefore, the surgeon must weigh the potential benefit of operative intervention against the patients estimated life expectancy, medical comorbidities, current performance status and personal wishes and also must reach a consensus with other members of the multidisciplinary team before proceeding.

When symptoms arise in a patient with disseminated disease, tumor biology and extent of disease, available nonoperative therapies, and estimated life expectancy all need to be considered. In certain metastatic cancers with effective systemic therapies and a more indolent course such as breast cancer, resection of a locally advanced and symptomatic primary tumor will result in improved quality of life for the patient. Similarly, obstructed colorectal cancer patients with disseminated disease often benefit symptomatically from resection or diversion in all but the most terminal cases. Palliative procedures in these patients can allow for delivery of systemic therapy with sometimes significant responses and prolonged survival. On the other hand, when small bowel, gastric outlet or biliary obstruction occurs in patients with metastatic disease from aggressive neoplasms like gastric or pancreatic cancer, the decision to intervene operatively is more complex. Small bowel obstruction may be due to surgical adhesions, just as in non-cancer patients and easily remedied with conservative management and operation if necessary. If malignant obstruction is confirmed the approach is more controversial, as some case series have noted a very poor prognosis in these patients. A recent Cochrane Database review examined the available literature on surgical intervention for malignant small bowel obstruction and noted highly variable symptom relief, re-obstruction rates and morbidity. The authors concluded that a "best evidence" approach cannot currently be formulated and treatment remains empiric. Similar controversies exist in the literature with regards to gastric outlet and biliary obstruction. However, if unresectable or disseminated disease is discovered during an attempted curative procedure, most would advocate biliary and/or intestinal diversion to palliated current or anticipated obstruction, as these carry generally low morbidity. A common example is when operating for pancreatic cancer and operative findings preclude resection. Most surgical oncologist in this setting will perform both gastric and biliary bypass for palliation. Biliary bypass may be omitted if endoscopic stenting has already been successful, but should be included if not, because even today endoscopic stenting is sometimes unsuccessful.

Fortunately, advancements in endoscopic and interventional radiologic procedures have offered effective non-operative palliation of symptoms. Endoscopic placement of gastrostomy (PEG) and jejunostomy feeding tubes have offered palliation to patients with end-stage disease and obstruction, with minimal discomfort and morbidity. Long metal biliary stents offer excellent palliation for biliary obstruction in advanced disease. Enteric stents have some success, especially in esophageal cancer. Their role in obstructive colon and rectal lesions is evolving and shows promise. Stents for gastric outlet and small intestinal obstruction have thus far been less effective and surgical intervention should strongly be considered in appropriate patients. Laparoscopic techniques for gastric bypass, biliary bypass and even small bowel obstruction have developed rapidly over the past decade and should be utilized whenever possible, depending on the clinical situation and surgeon skill level. Overall, the risks and benefits of surgery in these situations must carefully be weighed, realistic discussions with the patient and family must be had and the decision to operate must highly be individualized. Minimally invasive techniques that limit morbidity should be utilized in these situations whenever available to maximize quality of life in these unfortunate patients.

Preoperative Assessment

History and Physical Examination

The preoperative assessment begins with a thorough history and physical examination. History taking should generally focus on two fronts. First, an assessment should be made of severity and duration of tumor-related symptoms including pain, neurological symptoms, obstructive symptoms and/or other subjective findings to suggest extent of disease based on the anatomic location of the tumor. Symptoms suggestive of metastatic disease should be sought including pain outside of the anatomic location of the primary, neurological symptoms, fever, night sweats and profound weight loss. Prior cancer history as well as family history should be elicited. Patterns of inheritance for hereditary cancer syndromes should be carefully sought out and genetic counseling offered when appropriate. All details regarding previous or ongoing treatment for the current disease must be gathered.

Second, the surgeon should inquire about history and symptoms of significant comorbidities which could influence operative risk and might require preoperative intervention to optimize patient status for surgery. The presence of disorders such as coronary artery disease, pulmonary disease, diabetes mellitus, renal insufficiency and congestive heart failure may have a significant impact on operative planning. Severity and stability of disease as well as efficacy of current treatment should be evaluated. Additionally, a history of bleeding disorders or hypercoagulable states should be noted. Symptoms suggestive of malnutrition should be recorded such as degree of weight loss and ability to tolerate oral intake. Overall functional status should be evaluated both to assess severity of comorbid conditions as well as predict the patient's postoperative needs. A thorough social history including tobacco and alcohol use, as well as extent of the patient's support network, aids in risk assessment and postoperative planning. Careful review of a patient's current medications is essential for appropriate cessation of anticoagulation and antiplatelet medications and to ensure inclusion of important cardiovascular agents such as beta-blockers in the perioperative treatment plan. A review of systems is important to identify symptoms and risk factors for undiagnosed comorbidities.

Physical examination should be complete and yet focused on obtaining information about extent of disease and patient comorbidities for operative planning. This begins with simple observation of the patient. If the patient enters the office in a wheelchair, requires significant assistance onto the examination table or appears obviously cachectic or jaundiced this may indicate advanced disease and/or high operative risk. Examination of the head and neck can reveal subtle findings of jaundice or lymphadenopathy. Careful examination of the heart, lungs and extremities may reveal significant findings related to known or unknown comorbidities. Abdominal examination should focus on identifying palpable masses, hepatosplenomegaly, previous scars and signs of portal hypertension.

Evaluation of the primary tumor, if palpable, includes assessment of size, firmness, fixation and relationship to surrounding structures. Any involvement or changes in the overlying skin should be noted. Previous surgical biopsy sites should be identified and their locations documented. All major superficial lymphatic basins should be surveyed with focus on the anatomically appropriate basin for the given primary tumor. If abnormal lymph nodes are identified, their number, size and any evidence of fixation or matted nodes should be noted.

Laboratory Studies

Routine laboratory studies to assess hematologic parameters, electrolytes, renal function and nutritional status are appropriate for any patient undergoing major surgical procedures. With regard to operations for cancer, information regarding extent of disease may be obtained from specific lab studies. For example, in patients with hepatobiliary malignancies focus on the hepatic profile including degree of jaundice and hepatic dysfunction may influence preoperative care. Tumor markers may offer some insight into extent of disease in certain tumors and pre- and postoperative levels may be useful in gauging response to therapy and identifying recurrences.

Imaging Studies

Preoperative imaging studies have become essential for the accurate staging and evaluation of solid tumors prior to resection. Imaging now identifies the majority of unresectable tumors preoperatively, preventing many patients from undergoing nontherapeutic exploratory procedures **(Figure 12-2)**.

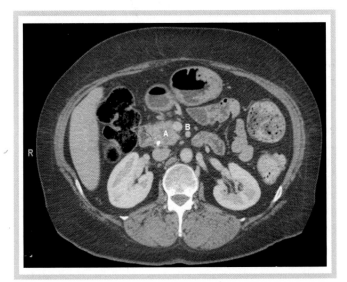

Figure 12-2: Preoperative imaging showing resectable pancreatic head mass (A) with clear fat planes circumferentially around superior mesenteric artery (B)

In general, the surgical oncologist should be aware of which imaging modalities most accurately stage the tumor being evaluated. For high-risk neoplasms, the likely locations of metastatic disease for a given tumor should be investigated with appropriate imaging. The surgeon, in addition to reviewing radiologists' reports, should always review images personally. Extent of disease and relationships to critical anatomic structures should be noted and can greatly influence preoperative therapies and operative approach. Knowledge of individual case specifics and surgical anatomy can sometimes result in discordance between the surgeon's impression and the imaging report. These issues should be clarified preoperatively through clear and open lines of communication between surgeon and radiologist. Most importantly, careful review of high-quality imaging should provide a road map for the surgeon in planning operative strategy.

Operative Risk Assessment and Management

In addition to adequate treatment of the tumor, a central principle of surgical therapy for cancer is the minimization of postoperative complications. The majority of patient-related operative mortality results from cardiac and pulmonary events postoperatively. A systematic approach to preoperative risk assessment in these areas is therefore warranted. Also important is an objective assessment of the patient's preoperative level of function so that an accurate prediction of the patient's postoperative needs and functional outcome can be made. Nutritional status also plays a key role in surgical outcomes and the evaluation and treatment of preoperative malnutrition is covered in a separate chapter. Finally, thromboembolic events and surgical site infections have been identified as common preventable causes of postoperative morbidity and appropriate prophylactic measures based on evidence-based guidelines is essential.

The potential for cardiac events after major surgery and the often-lethal nature of these events has sometimes led to unnecessary preoperative cardiology consults for "clearance" prior to surgery. In reality, true clearance cannot be obtained and all that can be realistically measured is a patient's overall risk for a cardiac event. This is further complicated by the controversy whether preoperative cardiac interventions influence mortality in patients undergoing non-vascular major surgical procedures. These and other issues have prompted the American College of Cardiology (ACC) and American Heart Association (AHA) to jointly publish evidence-based guidelines on preoperative cardiac risk assessment and intervention. This assessment begins with the surgeon during his initial evaluation of the patient and may involve cardiologists when appropriate. This includes thorough history taking combined with physical exam findings to identify active cardiac conditions, clinical risk factors for cardiac events and assess functional capacity.

The ACC/AHA recommendations for patients over age 50 with known cardiac disease or clinical risk factors have been published in literature. Active cardiac conditions requiring further evaluation and treatment preoperatively include unstable coronary syndromes (unstable angina, recent myocardial infarction within 30 days), decompensated heart failure, significant arrhythmia (*not* including *rate-controlled* atrial fibrillation) and severe valvular disease. Clinical risk factors in the most recent guidelines are limited to history of ischemic heart disease, history of compensated heart failure, cerebrovascular disease, diabetes mellitus and renal insufficiency. Surgical oncologic procedures are classified as intermediate risk (intrathoracic, intraperitoneal, head, neck and prostate) or low risk (superficial and breast). The key cutoff for functional capacity is defined as the ability to perform four or more metabolic equivalents (METs), which is the energy required to climb a flight of stairs or perform light house work, without symptoms. Patients undergoing low or intermediate risk surgery who are able to perform four METs can be excluded from preoperative testing, even in the presence of clinical risk factors. Patients with clinical risk factors and lower or unknown functional capacity are candidates for noninvasive testing such as stress testing and echocardiography if the management will be changed based on results **(Figure 12-1)**. Interventions for coronary artery revascularization are recommended based on standard indications, but the risk of cardiac events must carefully be weighed against the risk of delay in surgery.

Another issue that has emerged in recent years is the widespread use of percutaneous coronary revascularization and specifically, intraluminal stents. These require extended periods of uninterrupted therapy with potent antiplatelet agents such as clopidogrel (Plavix®) and can create a dilemma for a patient who needs major surgery, as these agents drastically increases the risk for bleeding. On the other hand, cessation of antiplatelet agents can lead to stent occlusion and infarction, especially with newer drug-eluding stents. The ACC/AHA has recognized these issues and has the following recommendations. Patients undergoing solely angioplasty can undergo operation with aspirin alone after two weeks. Those with bare-metal stents should delay major operation and continue clopidogrel for 4-6 weeks before cessation for surgery with aspirin alone. Those with drug-eluting stents are recommended to delay elective surgery for one year. This final group creates the biggest dilemma for the cancer surgeon and current recommendations state that "urgent" surgery can be performed after cessation of clopidogrel, but with maintenance on aspirin therapy during the perioperative period. Patients with drug-eluting stents should be counseled on their risk for stent occlusion and infarction and antiplatelet therapy should be resumed as soon as safely possible postoperatively. Furthermore, if percutaneous intervention is recommended preoperatively there should be communication between the surgeon and the cardiologist to formulate an appropriate treatment plan. This may include withholding the use of drug-eluding or bare metal stents depending on the urgency of operative intervention. Finally, according to the current guidelines beta-blockers should be continued perioperatively in patients already receiving them and should be considered in patients not receiving them who have more than one clinical risk factor undergoing intermediate risk surgery.

Pulmonary complications after major operation can prolong hospital stay significantly and contribute to postoperative mortality; therefore identification of high-risk patients is important. Generally, younger patients with well-controlled asthma are not at increased risk. High-risk patients as identified by the National Veterans Administration Surgical Improvement Program include those age > 60 years, history of chronic obstructive pulmonary disease (COPD), serum albumin < 3 gm/dl, BUN > 30 mg/dl and those undergoing upper-abdominal or thoracic procedures. Routine use of preoperative pulmonary function tests (PFTs) has not been shown to be effective in stratifying risk in non-thoracic surgery. Patients with multiple risk factors, or those with significant functional impairment from COPD, should have preoperative pulmonary consultation for risk assessment and optimization. Smokers should be encouraged to quit preoperatively, although the maximum benefit is not seen for approximately two months. Pulmonary infections should aggressively be treated and resolved prior to any operative intervention. Some studies suggest that the use of epidural pain catheters or regional nerve blocks postoperatively reduce the risk of pulmonary complications in high-risk patients. Postoperative care includes early ambulation, aggressive pain control, continuation of bronchodilators, inhaled steroids and incentive spirometry.

Pulmonary embolism and its antecedent deep venous thrombosis have been identified as largely preventable causes of postoperative morbidity and mortality. This is especially relevant to the surgical oncologist as malignancy increases the risk of thromboembolic events. The routine use of prophylactic measures including graduated compression stockings (GCS), intermittent pneumatic compression devices (IPC) and pharmacologic prophylaxis can greatly reduce this risk. Inconsistent and non-standardized use of these adjuncts has led to the development of evidence-based guidelines, the most extensive of which are those published by the American College of Chest Physicians (ACCP), most recently updated in 2008.

The recommendations include the following: low-risk patients undergoing minor procedures (same-day breast, thyroid, skin/soft-tissue) need no specific prophylaxis other than early and frequent ambulation. Cancer patients undergoing major operations should receive pharmacologic prophylaxis with low-dose unfractionated heparin (LDUH) three times daily, low molecular weight heparin (LMWH) or fondaparinux, as these have been shown to be more effective than mechanical prophylaxis. Cancer patients with multiple risk factors should receive both mechanical (GSC and IPC) and pharmacologic prophylaxis, as the two augment each other. The therapy should be initiated 1-2 hours before induction of anesthesia and continued during the postoperative hospital course. Early and frequent ambulation should also be strongly encouraged even when other prophylactic measures are utilized. The highest-risk patients should be considered for prolonged therapy after discharge for up to one month postoperatively. The risk of major bleeding complications in patients receiving pharmacologic prophylaxis has been shown to be equivalent to placebo. Minor bleeding episodes (wound hematoma) are slightly increased (2%).

Another cause of postoperative morbidity is surgical site infection, the second most common nosocomial infection and urinary tract infection being the first. While complete prevention of surgical site infections is not currently feasible, multiple entities including the Center for Disease Control have weighed the evidence and published guidelines on practices that will significantly reduce the incidence of this postoperative complication. Patient-related factors such as poorly controlled diabetes, smoking and poor nutritional status should be addressed preoperatively. Much of the focus around prophylaxis has centered on antimicrobial agents given in the perioperative period. Current recommendations for antimicrobial prophylaxis include the use of a first or second generation cephalosporin, depending on the expected flora involved, with second generation agents used when the gastrointestinal, biliary or urinary tract will be entered. Broad-spectrum penicillins have been advocated for higher risk procedures. In beta-lactam allergic patients, clindamycin or a combination of a fluoroquinolone and metronidazole is used. Antimicrobial agents should be administered so that at the time of incision, peak plasma concentration has been reached. The current recommendations are 60 minutes prior to incision for all but the fluoroquinolones, which require 120 minutes. Antibiotics should be redosed appropriately based on their serum and tissue half-lives throughout the procedure and discontinued within 24 hours. In cases that require hair removal, electric clippers rather than a razor should be used. Standard iodine or chlorhexidine based aseptic skin preparation solutions should be used. Surgical technique including gentle tissue handling, meticulous hemostasis and minimization of contamination are essential. In colon surgery the use of both mechanical bowel preparation and oral antibiotics preoperatively are standard, though recent studies have called their usefulness over appropriate single-dose preoperative parenteral antibiotics into question.

Operative Approach

Surgical Principles: Diagnosis and Staging

The basic surgical tenets for the management of cancer vary based on the indication for surgery. The goal during procedures for diagnosis is adequate tissue sampling to confirm the diagnosis and gather biologic information about the tumor to guide therapy. The least invasive way to obtain a diagnosis of malignancy is via fine-needle aspiration (FNA). This can be done in the office setting, with no anesthesia required. Ultrasound guidance is preferred to confirm needle placement within the lesion **(Figure 12-1)**, but not necessary. A 22-25-gauge needle is attached to a 10 cc syringe and the lesion is immobilized with the non-dominant hand. The needle is inserted into the lesion and suction applied to the plunger. Several passes through the lesion in slightly different planes are made, introducing cells into the needle. Suction is released prior to removal of the needle from the tissue, the needle is detached from the syringe that is then filled with air and reattached to the needle. The sample is placed on a glass slide for smear preparation by a pathology technician, who should be available at the time of the procedure. Alternatively, commercially available solutions are utilized to transport the sample to the cytopathology lab for preparation. FNA has the advantages of a very high positive predictive value for identification of malignancy. It is limited by a relatively low negative predictive value and an inability to distinguish invasive from *in situ* disease due to lack of cellular architecture in the specimen. It is most useful in the evaluation of neck masses, thyroid nodules, suspicious lymph nodes and breast lesions. It is also being utilized extensively during endoscopic ultrasound (EUS) to confirm malignancy and sample suspicious lymph nodes for staging purposes.

The most commonly utilized technique for obtaining tissue for diagnosis is core-needle biopsy. Manual core needle devices have largely been supplanted by automatic spring-loaded or vacuum assisted needles in the 11-14-gauge range that obtain a cylindrical sample of tissue. The major advantages over FNA are the greater volume of tissue obtained and maintenance of cellular structure allowing for a more accurate histopathologic assessment including identification of invasion and grade of disease. Core needle biopsies can be obtained on palpable lesions in similar fashion as FNA. Several core biopsies should be obtained to minimize sampling error. Core tissue samples should be placed in formalin for routine histopathology, or sent fresh for flow cytometry if there is a suspicion of lymphoma. Image guidance utilizing ultrasound **(Figure 12-1)**, mammography, computed tomography, endoscopic ultrasound and most recently magnetic resonance imaging allows for tissue sampling in most anatomic locations.

Occasionally these techniques are inadequate or unfeasible and operative biopsy is required for diagnosis. Excisional biopsy is utilized for small (< 2 cm) lesions and superficial lymph nodes. Suspicious skin lesions should be excised down to the subcutaneous tissue, as depth of the lesion is critical in the staging of melanoma. Shave biopsies should strictly be avoided in suspicious lesions for this reason. Incisional biopsy is used for larger lesions, which includes punch biopsy of suspicious skin lesions. Thoughtful placement and orientation of incisions for biopsy is *critical*, with *future definitive surgical procedures* always kept in mind. Also, potential contamination of otherwise unaffected tissue planes with tumor cells should be considered and avoided. In general, incisions on the extremities should be longitudinally oriented to allow for future wider excision, if necessary. On the trunk and face, incisions can be made parallel to the skin's natural lines of tension for cosmetic outcomes. For excisional biopsy of lymph nodes, incisions should be made along the line of a potential future lymph node dissection incision. Drawing the full incision with a marking pen and placing the biopsy incision on this line is helpful. Incisions on the breast should be amenable to resection during potential future mastectomy. The surgical technique should involve as little dissection, flap formation and disruption of natural tissue planes around the tumor as possible, as the entire operative field will be contaminated and require resection at definitive surgery. Meticulous hemostasis should be ensured as hematoma formation may disrupt tissue planes and make any subsequent wide excision much more difficult. Large hematomas may also contribute to local tumor cell dissemination and increase local recurrence rates. Failure to follow these simple principles universally results in a much larger tissue defect when definitive resection is undertaken. This leads to otherwise unnecessary plastic surgical procedures/tissue transfers for closure, poorer cosmetic outcomes and compromises oncologic outcome.

Accurate staging of solid tumors is also a critical consideration during surgery for malignancy. Different types of solid tumors have unique qualities of invasion and patterns of locoregional spread. Much tumors spread via lymphatics, and lymphatic sampling at operation is critical to proper staging. Therefore, an understanding of the lymphatic drainage patterns of different tumor locations is essential. Still other tumors such as sarcomas

and gastrointestinal stromal tumors rarely involve lymph nodes and a nodal dissection is unnecessary if gross disease is not present. The surgical oncologists must keenly be aware of these tumor qualities in order to obtain adequate staging information during surgery. This information usually must be gathered at the initial resection or else be lost, leading to difficulty in planning adjuvant therapy, as well as physician and patient angst. A prime example is in melanoma where the depth of the lesion is critical for staging and therefore with inadequate depth of excision or biopsy (e.g. shave technique) staging the disease will be impossible. Other examples include gastrointestinal malignancies such as colon and gastric cancer, where inadequate lymphadenectomy can result in staging inaccuracies and omission of needed postoperative adjuvant therapies or over-treatment of patients with incompletely staged early stage tumors. In fact, AJCC staging for these malignancies now include a minimal number of nodes to be removed and examined and the surgical oncologist must work in concert with the pathologist to achieve these staging goals.

Sentinel lymph node biopsy (SLNB) has emerged as a minimally invasive way to stage breast cancer and melanoma, which generally follow a stepwise pattern of metastasis to regional nodes. Elective lymph node dissections accurately stage these cancers, but carry a significant morbidity rate (i.e. lymphedema, nerve injury, etc.) and are not necessary for patients that ultimately are found to be node-negative. SLNB is based on the concept that cancer cells shed from the primary tumor into lymphatics will appear in the first node(s) in the chain of regional nodes that drain that anatomic site. This node(s) is thus referred to as the sentinel node(s). This concept led to the development of techniques to identify this node for removal, with the idea that the status of this node (positive or negative for metastasis), would accurately predict the status of the nodal basin. The smaller number of nodes sampled using SLNB can be more closely scrutinized by the pathologist, leading to more accurate staging of disease. Currently, the most common method used for SLNB involves peritumoral or intradermal injection of 1 mCi of Tc99 technetium sulfur colloid, anytime from 20 minutes to 4 hours preoperatively. This is done in conjunction with lymphoscintigraphy in head/neck and truncal melanomas to identify lymphatic drainage patterns, which may vary in these locations. This is followed by subcutaneous injection of 3-5 ml of isosulfan or methylene blue dye peritumorally in the minutes after induction of anesthesia in the operating room. The hand held gamma probe and visual identification of blue-stained lymphatics are then used to identify the sentinel node(s). Using this combined technique the accuracy of SLNB exceeds 95% in breast cancer and melanoma cases. Also, there is no apparent increase in locoregional nodal recurrence or cancer-related death when SLNB is utilized versus traditional elective nodal dissections. Further there is a definite decrease in the incidence of major morbidity including lymphedema and ipsilateral extremity symptoms, which can have a dramatic impact on patient quality of life after therapy. Sentinel lymph nodes removed are sent for preliminary frozen section or touch-prep analysis and, if positive, a completion lymph node dissection is performed. Other malignancies such as gastric adenocarcinoma and colon cancer have a more varied pattern of metastasis and require a more extensive lymphadenectomy both for locoregional control and adequate staging. SLNB has not proven to be a useful tool as of yet in these and other tumors, but its role is currently under investigation

Surgical Principles: Definitive and Multimodal Therapy

Definitive and multimodal surgical approaches to cancer treatment revolve around a central common goal, complete extirpation of the primary tumor. Many basic tenets of sound oncologic surgery that were recognized decades ago still apply today **(Table 12-6)**. These include the goals of *en bloc* tumor resection with a margin of normal tissue and adequate lymphadenectomy for both local control and accurate staging. Historically, tumors were given wide berth during resection with large margins and much normal tissue resected, which improved local control dramatically but with significant impacts on form and function. Examples of the use of this radical approach to resection included the radical mastectomy and, at one time a > 50% amputation rate for extremity sarcomas. Over time, the trend has been toward less radical surgery and more effective adjuvant therapies. This is based on better understanding of tumor biology; comparative randomized controlled trials and the development of more effective adjuvant therapies. For example, breast conservation is now routinely practiced due to improved understanding of the disease including patterns of recurrence and more effective adjuvant therapy in the form of radiation, with little impact on local recurrence rates and no impact on long-term survival compared to more radical approaches, based on randomized controlled studies. Similarly, the amputation rate for extremity sarcoma has dropped to < 5% with better understanding of the local behavior of the disease and the use of radiation to improve local control. Close margins are sometimes acceptable in areas near vital structures (essential neurovascular bundles), especially when adjuvant therapies can be used and proven to be effective. However, despite this trend of decreasing radicalness of surgery, the importance of adequate resection cannot be overstated, as many solid tumors' prognosis directly correlates with the ability to achieve negative surgical margins. Complete excision, therefore, remains the most basic core tenant, just as Halsted and others recognized 100 years ago. Advancements in the understanding of tumor behavior and development of multimodal approaches have only refined this idea.

Other tenets that should be part of the surgical oncologist's mindset involve other strategies for prevention of locoregional recurrence of disease. For most tumors, previous operative biopsy sites should be included *en bloc* in the resection. Needle tracts from percutaneous biopsies can be excluded from this principle, as studies have shown extremely low incidence of recurrence within these tracts. Gentle handling of the tumor mass to prevent rupture and dissemination are essential, especially in cystic, mucinous or locally advanced tumors that have already penetrated natural anatomic barriers such as serosa. Numerous studies have demonstrated higher recurrence rates and lower survival for many tumor types when intraoperative tumor violation has been documented. These include increased risks for the development of carcinomatosis in colon cancer, GISTs, ovarian tumors and hepatocellular carcinoma. This very ominous and often deadly consequence may be prevented with sound surgical oncologic technique. Isolation of vascular pedicles and the bowel lumen in gastrointestinal tumors before tumor manipulation, the so called "no-touch" technique, has not been definitively proven to decrease recurrence or spread of disease, but this is controversial and some studies have shown lower recurrence and improved survival with this technique. However, despite this debate, the basic tenets of careful tumor handling and adequate mesenteric resection for bowel lesions are critical for adequate control of disease.

TABLE 12-6	Core principles of oncologic surgery. Basic tenets of surgical therapy for solid tumors

- Complete tumor excision with circumferential margin of normal tissue
- Adequate lymphadenectomy
- Obtain accurate staging information
- Excise sites of previous biopsy or excision *en bloc*
- Gentle tumor and tissue handling to prevent rupture/dissemination
- Use natural tissue planes and anatomic boundaries to advantage
- *En bloc* resection of involved structures, always assume adhesions to be malignant
- Properly orient and prepare specimen for pathologic evaluation
- Check margins with pathologist
- Preserve function
- Consider available adjuvant therapies and their effectiveness
- Consider effects of neoadjuvant therapy on tissue healing

Planes of dissection around the tumor should generally follow natural tissue planes, except when involved with tumor. Dissection should not be continued through areas where planes become fused or involved with tumor. Adhesions or attachments to surrounding structures should be assumed to be malignant and no attempt should be made to detach the tumor from these structures. Distinguishing between malignant and benign adhesions or inflammation intraoperatively is impossible and should not be attempted. Furthermore, numerous studies have shown that while up to half of these adhesions may be benign, dividing adhesions in attempts to detach the tumor leads to much higher recurrence rates and lower survival. In these cases, *en bloc* resection of the tumor and its attachments, including a section or all of an involved structure is the preferred technique. This may require complex vascular or other reconstructions, which should be anticipated by the surgeon based on preoperative imaging. For instance, in locally advanced sigmoid colon cancers it may be necessary to resect portions of the bladder or small bowel *en bloc* along with the tumor. Pancreatic cancers may require *en bloc* resection of the portal or superior mesenteric vein with reconstruction. Rarely, structures of vital importance with tumor abutment may be left in place with plans to treat residual microscopic disease with adjuvant therapy, as in extremity sarcoma with major neurovascular involvement in which limb preservation is desired. However, it must be emphasized that radiation and/or chemotherapy cannot substitute for complete surgical resection as adequate treatment for most solid tumors and gross disease or clearly involved structures should generally not be left behind. Anatomic borders such as fascia and peritoneal boundaries can be included in areas of close margins, as many solid neoplasms will respect these anatomic constraints. For example, when a major nerve is abutted by tumor, removal of the perineurium *en bloc* may allow for both tumor clearance and preservation of function. The surgical oncologist must therefore have a three-dimensional and cross-sectional understanding of the anatomy related to the area of resection and use this to both avoid inadvertent injury of vital structures while maintaining an adequate surgical margin.

The extent of the surgical margin at the time of resection is often based on several factors. Tumor biology and patterns of spread are the most important factors to consider when planning the resection margin. For example, tumors such as gastric adenocarcinomas which spread in an infiltrating and diffuse manner, mandate a wide (5-6 cm) margin of normal tissue relative to the tumor, in addition to *en bloc* lymphadenectomy. This requires a major or sometimes complete gastric resection and reconstruction. Gastrointestinal stromal tumors (GISTs) of the stomach, on the other hand, are usually

well localized and confined to the apparent tumor margins. Consequently, GISTs of the stomach can effectively be managed with a simple wedge resection with 1-2 cm margin, as a more extensive gastric resection would be unnecessary to clear the disease and could lead to needless morbidity. Therefore, a clear understanding of a tumor's biology and characteristics are essential for the surgical oncologist in order to plan adequate resection margins, with the minimal required long-term morbidity. Also important in planning margin width is the availability of effective adjuvant therapies. Along with a better understanding of tumor biology, improved adjuvant therapy has contributed to less radical and yet more effective surgery. A prime example is the surgical management of rectal cancer. Careful study has shown that rectal tumors spread in radial fashion and the previous fears of submucosal distal spread were unfounded. Therefore, surgical management now includes a focus on total mesorectal excision to maximize radial margin clearance, with less emphasis on distal margin. This, along with effective adjuvant therapies, has led to less radical surgery (much fewer abdominoperineal resections) with a better functional and oncologic outcome.

In the modern era of multimodal cancer therapy and with the use of preoperative chemotherapy and radiation therapies the surgeon must consider the effects of these treatments on wound healing. Most standard chemotherapeutic agents cause bone marrow suppression with subsequent decreases in cell counts including hemoglobin, lymphocytes and platelets. The resultant anemia, immunosuppression and thrombocytopenia can all have detrimental effects on surgical outcomes. Therefore, when preoperative therapy has been administered the patient must be given time to recover from these effects, generally requiring about four weeks, before proceeding with surgery. Newer biologic agents such as bevacizumab (Avastin) that act on EGF receptors also have a significant effect on wound healing which requires 6-8 weeks for resolution. Another issue is the effect of prolonged therapy on the target organ. This issue is highlighted in patients being considered for resection of hepatic metastases where prolonged preoperative chemotherapy can cause hepatic steatosis. These patients require larger remnant hepatic volume and this must be part of the operative strategy. When planning neoadjuvant therapy followed by resection, these issues should be coordinated with the medical oncologist. Radiation therapy also has a long-lasting effect on wound healing due to radiation-induced fibrosis in the treatment area. This requires a thoughtful approach because surgical wounds created in radiated fields heal very poorly. Plastic surgical procedures involving transferring non-radiated tissue to the wound for closure should be applied liberally here. Also, when dealing with anastomoses in radiated fields such as in low rectal tumors, non-radiated bowel should be used for anastomosis and proximal diversion should strongly be considered.

Surgical Principles: Cytoreduction and Metastatic Disease

Surgical therapy for locoregionally disseminated or metastatic disease seems to be counter to the core tenets of oncologic surgery, in that it is assumed that small amounts of macroscopic and/or microscopic disease will be left behind. While some controversy certainly still exists, the role of this type of surgery has been established for many tumor types and metastatic sites. However, despite the seemingly unconventional nature of this approach, the goals of cytoreductive surgery are similar to surgery to completely remove a tumor in that cytoreductive surgery centers on a strategy of maximal resection of gross disease. This allows for adjuvant therapy, whether systemic or regional in nature, to have the best chance at eliminating remaining disease. When intraperitoneal chemotherapy will be used, experimental data confirms that drug penetration is confined to a depth of less than 3 mm. This highlights the importance of complete surgical debulking when using this modality. This concept is validated by current evidence in disseminated ovarian and other peritoneal-based tumors, which correlates long-term survival with extent of surgical cytoreduction. In fact, patients with incomplete cytoreduction often have similar outcomes to historical controls. This emphasizes the importance of aggressive and meticulous surgical cytoreduction in these patients and strongly discourages reliance on adjuvant therapy to do the work of clearing gross disease.

Surgery for metastatic lesions follows the same principles as those applied to primary tumors. Complete extirpation with negative margins continues to be the goal. During the course of these operations the initial focus should be to define the extent of disease and confirm that there is no evidence of disease outside the target organ. This may require the use of adjunctive methods of evaluation, such as the use of intraoperative ultrasound in liver surgery or frozen section analysis of distant lymph nodes suspicious for disease. These measures help to confirm that surgical therapy is indicated and will clear all evident disease. For example, intraoperative ultrasound in liver surgery has been shown to change the initial operative strategy in up to 30% of cases, so surgeons engaging in this endeavor should be facile with its use. Preservation of function is also an important consideration during surgery for metastatic disease, especially when performing hepatic and pulmonary metastasectomy. Wedge resections of metastases are used when anatomically feasible and have been shown to be as effective as anatomic resection when negative margins are achieved, with less impact on overall function. Alternative forms of surgical therapy such as radiofrequency ablation should be utilized when necessary to preserve function. However, there are limitations to their use and efficacy, therefore margin-negative resection is preferable even when larger anatomic resections are required.

Minimally Invasive Surgical Oncology: Present and Future

The rapid development of minimally invasive surgery over the past decade has led to the adoption of these techniques for a wide range of indications. This has sometimes been based on good evidence and sometimes been driven by patient request and industry forces. The integration of these approaches into the surgical treatment for cancer has been more guarded, largely due to fears that one would sacrifice oncologic principles for the sake of smaller incisions and shorter postoperative recovery. However, as the technology advanced and minimally invasive skills of surgeons increased, many have adopted minimally invasive approaches to many solid tumors. The evolution of laparoscopic colectomy for colon cancer is the prime example. Initially criticized due to fears of unsound oncologic surgery and laparoscopic port site recurrence, pioneers in this field continued to pursue it and these fears ultimately were proven to be unfounded. A multicenter randomized controlled trial (COST trial) confirmed the benefits of this approach to colon cancer and showed no difference in oncologic outcome. As the skills of surgeons have increased in this area, minimally invasive approaches have also been applied and refined to treat many other solid tumors, including gastric, pulmonary, pancreatic and liver lesions. The use of robotic-assisted surgery has widened the indications for these approaches in some instances and this technology is still being developed. Endoscopic techniques for treating superficial rectal, esophageal and gastric tumors are also being developed, in addition to non-surgical palliation of advanced lesions. The full range of indications and applications for these techniques are discussed in detail in other chapters. Overall, while many of these techniques are currently only being applied at tertiary centers and in the setting of clinical trials, others have become commonplace and this certainly seems to represent a significant part of the future of surgical therapy for cancer.

13

Principles of Chemotherapy

Benedito A Carneiro, Nathan Bahary

Introduction

The observation that soldiers exposed to mustard gas during the World War I developed lymphoid atrophy and myelosuppression spurred the modern era of systematic investigations to identify chemical agents with antitumor activity. Clinical trials showing significant responses of lymphoma to nitrogen mustards increased the interest in these compounds leading to the discovery of their mechanism of action as DNA alkylating agents, which in turn became the first class of chemotherapy drugs. Shortly thereafter, antifolates were discovered to induce remission of childhood acute lymphoblastic leukemia (ALL) by inhibiting the synthesis of nucleotides. During the 1950s and 1960s, the first cure of a solid tumor (choriocarcinoma) by chemotherapy and the demonstration that combination of chemotherapy agents could overcome drug resistance and lead to long-lasting remissions of lymphoma and ALL brought additional enthusiasm to the field. In 1974, surgical resection of osteosarcoma followed by single agent methotrexate was shown to decrease recurrence rates, creating the concept of adjuvant chemotherapy and simultaneously highlighting the importance of multi-modality therapy. Utilizing *in vivo* and *in vitro* experimental models, taxanes, camptothecins and Vinca alkaloids were discovered during the next 40-50 years using various preclinical antiproliferative-screening platforms. Almost all the drugs developed through this screening approach exert their anticancer effects by blocking DNA synthesis, causing DNA damage, or disrupting mitosis.

Anticancer drug development was revolutionized in the early 1990s when advances in molecular cancer biology and genetics started to reveal numerous dysregulated signaling pathways in cancer cells. Most of these aberrant pathways were involved in cell proliferation, invasion or cell death mechanisms and immediately became potential therapeutic targets **(Figure 13-1)**. The early observation that *HER2* gene overexpression in breast carcinomas correlate with decreased patient survival and time to progression was the basis for the development of

trastuzumab, a monoclonal antibody (mAb) against the growth factor receptor HER2 that inhibits its internalization and downstream signaling. Trastuzumab (Herceptin®) was the first targeted anticancer agent approved by the FDA for the treatment of breast carcinoma in 1998, and it represented the proof of concept that mAbs against cell surface growth factor receptors could successfully be incorporated into cancer therapy.

The refinement of bioinformatics, molecular computer modeling and high throughput screening of chemical libraries was also critical for the rapid development of drugs directed at these abnormal molecular signals. Imatinib mesylate (Gleevec®) was the successful prototype of small-molecule tyrosine kinase inhibitors (TKI), another class of targeted therapies had a significant impact on the management of chronic myelogenous leukemia (CML) and gastrointestinal stromal tumor (GIST) and helped shift anticancer drug discovery from serendipitous identification of antiproliferative compounds to development of drugs specific against molecular defects contributing to carcinogenesis. Imatinib was developed as an inhibitor of the BCR-ABL constitutively active tyrosine kinase resulting from the chromosome translocation 9:22, a pivotal event in the pathogenesis of CML. Imatinib also inhibits KIT and platelet-derived growth factor receptor-β (PDGFR-β) tyrosine kinases, which are involved in the progression of GIST. This drug was approved for treatment of CML and GIST in 2001 and 2002, respectively.

The delineation of the epidermal growth factor pathway and the role of receptor tyrosine kinases in signal transduction provided the framework for several new therapeutic interventions. Epidermal growth factor receptors (EGFR/HER1, HER2, HER3, HER4) are overexpressed in numerous epithelial tumors and regulate cell proliferation and survival. The subsequent approval of the anti-EGFR/HER1 antibodies cetuximab (Erbitux®) and panitumumab (Vectibix®) for the treatment of advanced colorectal cancer further validated the EGFR family members as important targets for anticancer drugs. The demonstration that mutations in the ATP-binding pocket of EGFR blocked its tyrosine kinase acitivity and

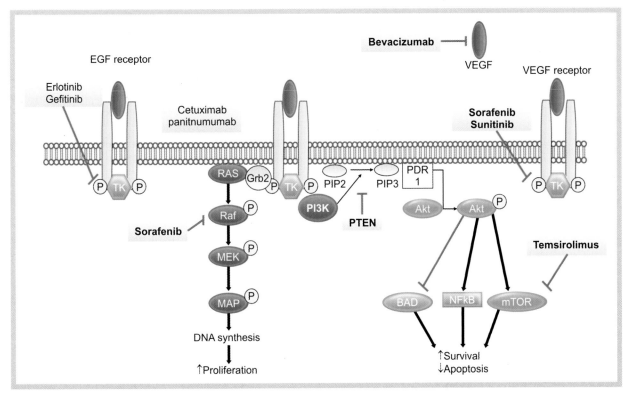

Figure 13-1: Signaling pathways involved in tumor growth. Cell signaling pathways can be inhibited by monoclonal antibodies (mAbs;cetuximab and panitumumab) against growth factors or their receptors. Tyrosine kinase inhibitors (TKIs; erlotinib and gefitinib) also block multiple cancer cell signaling pathways involved in carcinogenesis and cell proliferation. Tumor angiogenesis and growth can be inhibited by bevacizumab, a monoclonal antibody against the vascular growth factor A (VEGFA), or by TKIs of VEGF receptor such as sorafenib or sunitinib. Sorafenib also inhibits the serine/threonine kinase Raf. Temsirolimus inhibits the mammalian target of rapamycin (mTOR) kinase. PI3K, phosphoinositide 3-kinase; Akt, protein kinase B; PTEN, phosphatase and tension homolog; BAD, Bcl-2 antagonist of cell death; NF-kB, nuclear factor kB; PIP2, phosphatidylinositol 4,5-trisphosphate; PIP3, phosphatidylinositol 3,4,5-trisphosphate;Raf, Raf serine/threonine kinase; MEK, mitogen-activated protein kinases; MAP, mitogen-activated protein kinase; Grb2, SH2 and SH3 domain-containing adaptor protein

downstream signaling supported the development of TKIs such as gefitinib and erlotinib that were later approved for treatment of non-small cell lung cancer and pancreatic cancer respectively.

Judah Folkman's insights into the central role that angiogenesis, the creation of new vasculature, plays in sustaining tumor proliferation and metastasis guided the development of several anti-angiogenesis drugs. The anti-vascular endothelial growth factor A (VEGFA) antibody bevacizumab (Avastin®) was the first approved drug in this category. Bevacizumab in combination with chemo-therapy prolongs survival in advanced colorectal and non-small cell lung cancers and improves progression-free survival in metastatic breast cancer. Small molecule inhibitors (e.g. sunitinib and sorafenib) that block VEGF receptor tyrosine kinases have subsequently been appro-ved for the treatment of advanced renal cell carcinoma based in part on their anti-angiogenesis activity. These

successes with EGFR and VEGF-based therapies promo-ted the development of numerous other drugs and technologies capable of modulating networks underlying the malignant phenotype.

This historical transition of cancer therapy from con-ventional cytotoxic agents to targeted agents represents one of the major therapeutic advances of the last century, but several challenges remain. Improved biomarkers are needed to identify the patients likely to benefit from these therapies; otherwise, we will continue to treat numerous patients empirically to benefit only a few with unacceptable cost and toxicities. Basic principles of drug resistance driven by mutations on drug target also apply to the targeted agents. Although small-molecule TKIs and mAbs can be less toxic than cytotoxics, clinicians need to be aware of important side effects associated with these drugs. Lastly, many of these targeted agents are cytostatic and do not cause dramatic reduction in the size of tumors, which affects conventional outcome measures and benefits seen during clinical trials. Disease stabilization and improvement of progression-free survival without significant response rates may become a more frequent finding with targeted agents. Taken together, the benefits and challenges of this new generation of drugs have important implications for the care of cancer patients.

Combination Chemotherapy

The early enthusiasm brought by significant clinical responses to single chemotherapy agents was counterbalanced by the short duration of these responses attributed to the rapid growth of clones of cancer cells resistant to chemotherapy. Guided by the mechanisms of drug resistance and kinetics of cancer growth, Dr Frei and his colleagues showed for the first time that a combination of drugs could result in durable remission of childhood ALL overcoming the development of resistance. This approach also led to cures in Hodgkin's and diffuse large B-cell lymphomas and was further supported by mathematical models showing that the most effective way to circumvent spontaneous drug resistance mutations in cancer cells is to use multiple chemotherapy agents over a short period of time. The concepts of dose intensity and dose density were also formulated during this time when cytotoxicity was shown to correlate with dose of chemotherapy and tumor volume. These ideas led to the log-kill hypothesis which states that the percentage of cells killed by a certain drug is constant and independent of tumor volume; therefore, smaller tumors have a higher chance of cure with chemotherapy. This hypothesis formulated the concept of adjuvant chemotherapy; chemotherapy given after the surgical removal of tumors to eradicate residual microscopic disease. Drugs used in combination should have activity as single agents, different mechanisms of action to enable synergistic or additive effects, and distinct toxicity profiles to allow the use of maximum individual doses. It is also important to combine drugs that elicit distinct resistance mechanisms.

Drug Resistance

Resistance to cytotoxic agents is a major challenge inherent to chemotherapy. Most known resistance mechanisms relate to genetic abnormalities preventing the execution of programmed cell death (apoptosis), positioning of cell in the cell cycle, defects in drug transport or delivery, or modification of drug targets. Cytotoxic agents causing DNA damage or impairing DNA repair trigger apoptosis that is tightly regulated by a complex interplay between death receptors, anti- and pro-apoptotic Bcl-2 family of proteins and caspases. Cancer cells have developed a wide range of sophisticated mechanisms to block apoptosis

including overexpression of anti-apoptotic Bcl-2 protein, which, in fact, has been investigated as a therapeutic target. Agents that interfere with DNA synthesis (e.g. antimetabolites) or mitosis (e.g. taxanes and vinca alkaloids) are most active on cells undergoing DNA synthesis (e.g. S and G2 phases of cell cycle), whereas drugs that cause DNA damage (e.g. alkylating agents, anthracyclines and platinum agents) are toxic to cells in all stages of the cell cycle including the resting G1 and G0 phases. Mechanism of resistance related to cell cycle kinetics is the physiologic basis for prolonging infusion of chemotherapy agents to capture cells in susceptible cell cycle stages.

Biochemical or genetic alterations of drug transporters and targets resulting in resistance can be present constitutively or develop during therapy. The most common disturbance in drug transport is the overexpression of cell surface P-glycoprotein that lead to efflux of drugs such as taxanes, vinca alkaloids and anthracyclines. Overexpression of *MDR1* gene encoding P-glycoprotein in renal and colon cancers is responsible in part for their resistance to these agents. Ongoing research is exploring the use of P-glycoprotein inhibitors as a strategy to overcome resistance. Malignant cells can also develop mutations on cell surface drug transporters blocking drug access to the intracellular targets, or have mutations or alterations in the expression of targets resulting in significant sensitivity or resistance to treatments. For instance, increased expression of dihydrofolate reductase (DHFR) and thymidylate synthase (TS) leads to resistance to methotrexate and 5-fluorouracil, respectively.

Treatment Modalities

Chemotherapy when used alone can be curative in only a small number of malignancies (e.g. Hodgkin's disease, Non-Hodgkin's lymphoma, germ cell tumors, choriocarcinoma, ALL, Burkitt's lymphoma, Wilms' tumor and embryonal rhabdomyosarcoma) but combinations of chemotherapy with surgery, radiation therapy and /or hormonal agents increase the cure rates of several malignancies. Neoadjuvant or adjuvant chemotherapy is frequently combined with surgery to increase cure rates and prevent recurrences. Neoadjuvant chemotherapy refers to chemotherapy given prior to definitive surgical treatment of tumors, whereas adjuvant chemotherapy refers to chemotherapy administered after complete surgical resection of tumors designed to treat micrometastases. Neoadjuvant or induction chemotherapy reduces the tumor burden facilitating less morbid surgery than might otherwise be required, and it can make surgery a feasible therapeutic option when tumors are initially felt to be unresectable. In addition, this approach treats micrometastatic disease present at the time of diagnosis and provides information regarding tumor sensitivity to the drugs utilized that can guide future therapy. Some chemotherapy agents are also used concomitantly with radiation therapy given their tissue radiosensitization properties and potential to improve local control. Lastly, chemotherapy is frequently used alone in the treatment of advanced or metastatic disease where other modalities have no beneficial role.

Neoadjuvant chemotherapy has a well-established role in the management of locally advanced breast cancer. Many patients are able to avoid a radical mastectomy with this modality and those achieving complete pathological responses have higher rates of both disease-free and overall survival. For instance, four cycles of preoperative chemotherapy with doxorubicin, cyclophosphamide and docetaxel in patients with locally advanced breast cancer led to a complete pathological response rate of 26%, and a 71% five-year disease-free survival rate. This paradigm has also been applied successfully to the treatment of larynx, esophageal, gastric, osteosarcomas, bladder, and anal cancers. Higher rates of larynx and anal canal preservation are obtained with combined neoadjuvant chemotherapy and radiation compared to first-line surgery. A phase III trial comparing induction chemotherapy with cisplatin and 5-fluorouracil followed by radiation therapy to upfront laryngectomy and postoperative radiation in patients with advanced laryngeal carcinoma showed significant improved rates of larynx preservation (64%) and complete clinical response (31%) among patients receiving induction chemotherapy. Patients with locally advanced anal squamous cell carcinoma treated with induction chemotherapy followed by concomitant radiation with 5-FU and mitomycin achieved an impressive 82% complete response rate and 68% four-year survival rate. The benefit of perioperative chemotherapy in locally advanced gastric cancer was demonstrated in the MAGIC trial that randomized approximately 500 patients to either surgery alone or perioperative chemotherapy (three cycles of preoperative and three cycles of postoperative epirubicin, cisplatin and 5-FU). The group receiving perioperative chemotherapy had significantly higher five-year (36% vs 23%) and progression-free survival rates.

Adjuvant chemotherapy was first shown to be beneficial in the treatment of osteosarcoma, yet its application in breast cancer treatment consolidated its use in clinical practice. Adjuvant chemotherapy in lymph node positive breast cancer reduces annual breast cancer death rate by approximately 30% based on recent meta-analyses and have contributed substantially to the increased cure rates from this disease since the seminal trials led by Drs Bernard Fisher and Gianni Bonadonna. Genomic profiling of early stage, lymph node negative tumors have been able to identify those patients with the highest risk of recurrence for which adjuvant chemotherapy should also be considered. The benefit of adjuvant chemotherapy was further validated in the treatment of stage III (lymph node positive) colorectal cancer where it decreases the 5-year overall survival (OS) by approximately 20-40%; more recently, it has shown to improve the outcome of patients with resectable non-small cell lung, gastric and pancreatic cancers as well. Cisplatin-based adjuvant chemotherapy for early stage non-small cell lung cancer results in an absolute increment of 5.4% in 5-year-overall survival (HR .89; P = .005). For gastric cancer, perioperative chemotherapy improves OS by 17-20% and it is accepted as the standard of care in many European countries, whereas in the United States adjuvant chemoradiation has widely been adopted based on the results of the intergroup trial 0116 that showed a significant improvement in median survival from 27 to 36 months with 5-FU/leucovorin-based regimen combined with radiation therapy. The role of adjuvant chemotherapy for resected pancreatic adenocarcinoma was demonstrated in the CONKO-001 trial in which six months of gemcitabine increased 5-year survival from 9% to 21% and disease-free survival from 13.4 to 6.9 months compared to placebo.

In the setting of incurable metastatic disease, chemotherapy is a well-established palliative measure to treat cancer-related symptoms, complications, improve quality of life and , in many cases, prolong survival. These benefits are achieved through reduction of tumor burden, improvement of clinical symptoms and reduction in tumor growth rate. The major challenge with palliative chemotherapy, however, is to weigh acute and chronic toxicities against expected benefits. The benefits of palliative chemotherapy are quite apparent in diseases such as breast and colorectal cancers in which treatment prolongs survival significantly, whereas in other diseases such as non-small cell lung, gastric, pancreatic and renal cell cancers the benefits are less robust requiring careful selection of patients according to performance status and comorbidities. Nonetheless, the treatment of metastatic colorectal and breast cancers provides a good example of the progress and benefit of palliative chemotherapy. The median survival of patients with metastatic colorectal cancer has improved from six months with best supportive of care to greater than two years with 5-fluorouracil-based chemotherapy regimens (e.g. 5-FU, leucovorin plus irinotecan or oxaliplatin; FOLFOX and FOLFIRI chemotherapy regimens) combined with molecular targeted agents.

Although only 23% patients with metastatic breast cancer survive beyond five years, chemotherapy for metastatic disease can preserve the quality of life for prolonged periods of time and achieve median survival of approximately 24 months. The incorporation of targeted therapies such as trastuzumab and bevacizumab into chemotherapy regimens for metastatic breast and colorectal cancers, respectively, changed the natural history of these diseases and proved the potential of these new drugs to prolong survival without significant side effects. This paradigm has been expanded to non-small cell lung cancer where the combination of carboplatin, paclitaxel plus bevacizumab increased modestly median survival in selected patients with metastatic disease and it is been actively explored in many other malignancies.

Chemotherapy can also be combined with radiation therapy for more effective local treatment of tumors. Drugs with radiation sensitization properties that result in synergistic activity against malignant tumors include cisplatin, carboplatin, 5-fluorouracil, gemcitabine and paclitaxel. This strategy is particularly important when superior local control of disease can influence overall survival (e.g. locally advanced head and neck cancers), or result in organ preservation (e.g. larynx, anal and rectal carcinomas). Concurrent chemoradiation is also standard of care in locally advanced lung cancer and esophageal carcinomas. An important limitation of this approach is the additive toxicity of both modalities. Patients receiving chemoradiation for head and neck cancers, for instance, can develop severe mucositis requiring prophylactic gastrostomy tubes for nutritional support. In this regard, molecularly targeted agents have shown to enhance radiation effects without significant toxicity to normal tissues. The combination of cetuximab (anti-EGFR monoclonal antibody) with radiation therapy for locally advanced head and neck cancers improved local control and overall survival without significant additional toxicity. These results provided the proof of principle that anti-EGFR agents can be effective and well-tolerated radiosensitizers.

The role of immunotherapy has been investigated alone or in combination with cytotoxic agents based on the potential enhancement of antitumor effects through activation of immune system. One year of high dose interferon alpha as adjuvant treatment of high-risk (stages IIB, IIC and III) melanoma, has been shown to consistently increase relapse-free survival by 20-30% and some studies suggested a survival benefit particularly among patients with lymph node positive disease (stage III). These results led to the approval by FDA of interferon alpha as the standard adjuvant regimen for high-risk melanoma. Newer generations of immunotherapy drugs such as the monoclonal antibodies against cytotoxic T-lymphocyte-associated antigen 4 (anti-CTLA4) that can reverse tumor-induced immunosuppression and activate T-lymphocytes have shown promising results in metastatic melanoma and are undergoing clinical evaluation in other diseases such as colon, prostate and pancreatic cancers.

Standard Chemotherapy Drug Classes

Alkylating Agents and Related Drugs

The main groups of alkylating agents used as anticancer drugs include the nitrosoureas (e.g. carmustine [BCNU], lomustine [CCNU], semustine [methyl-CCNU]), nitrogen mustards, ethyleneimines (cyclophosphamide, ifosfamide, chlorambucil, melphalan) and alkylsulfonates (e.g. busulfan) **(Table 13-1)**. Platinum derivatives (e.g. cisplatin,

TABLE 13-1	Standard chemotherapy drugs

Alkylating agents
  Nitrosoureas (carmustine, lomustine and semustine)
  Nitrogen mustards
  Cyclophosphamide, ifosfamide, chlorambucil and melphalan
  Busulfan
  Platinum derivatives: cisplatin, carboplatin and oxaliplatin
  Dacarbazine and Temozolomide

Antimetabolites
  Purine inhibitors
      Fludarabine, cladribine, 6-mercaptopurine and 6-thioguanine
  Pyrimidine inhibitors
      5-fluorouracil, capecitabine, cytarabine and gemcitabine
  Folic acid antagonists
      Methotrexate and pemetrexed

Natural products
  Vinca alkaloids
      Vinblastine, vincristine and vinorelbine
  Taxanes
      Paclitaxel, docetaxel and albumin-bound paclitaxel
  Camptothecins
      Topotecan and irinotecan
  Anthracycline antibiotics
      Doxorubicin, epirubicin, daunorubicin, idarubicin and mitoxantrone
  Epipodophyllotoxins
      Etoposide (VP-16) and teniposide

Hormonal agents
  SERM
      Tamoxifen and raloxifene
  SERD
      Fulvestrant
  Aromatase inhibitors
      Formestane and Exemestane
      Anastrozole, letrozole and aminoglutethimide
  LHRH agonists
      Leuprolide and goserelin
  Androgen receptor antagonists
      Flutamide, bicalutamide and nilutamide

Miscellaneous
  Dactinomycin D, bleomycin and mitomycin
  Thalidomide and lenalidomide

Abbreviations: SERM: selective estrogen-receptor modulator; SERD: selective estrogen-receptor downregulator; LHRH: luteinizing hormone-releasing hormone

TABLE 13-2	Major adverse effects of chemotherapy drugs	
Drug classes	**Drugs**	**Major adverse effects**
Anti-EGFR	Erlotinib, gefitinib, cetuximab, and panitumumab	Papulopustular rash, dry skin, abnormal scalp and eyelashes hair growth, nail changes and periungual inflammation
Anti-VEGF	Bevacizumab	Hypertension, proteinuria, hemorrhage, arterial thrombosis, GI perforation, impaired wound healing and RPLS
Multikinase inhibitors	Sorafenib and sunitinib	Hypertension, fatigue, hand-foot syndrome, rash/desquamation and lymphopenia
Alkylating agents	Cyclophosphamide and ifosfamide	Myelosuppression, N/V, hemorrhagic cystitis, CNS toxicity and secondary leukemias
Platinum derivatives	Cisplatin, carboplatin and oxaliplatin	Nephrotoxicity, peripheral neuropathy[1], N/V and myelosuppression
Antimetabolites	5-FU, capecitabine, MTX, Ara-C, gemcitabine and pemetrexed	GI toxicity, myelosuppression, hand-foot syndrome[2], flu-like symptoms[3], pulmonary toxicity[4] and rash[5]
Vinca alkaloids	Vinblastine, vincristine and vinorelbine	Myelosuppression and peripheral neuropathy
Taxanes	Paclitaxel, docetaxel and albumin-bound paclitaxel	Myelosuppression, hypersensitivity reaction[6], peripheral neuropathy, arthralgias and fluid retention[7]
Camptothecins	Topotecan and irinotecan	Myelosuppression and diarrhea
Anthracyclines	Doxorubicin, epirubicin, daunorubicin, idarubicin and mitoxantrone	Myelosuppression, mucositis, cardiotoxicity, myelodysplastic syndromes and secondary leukemias
Epipodophyllotoxins	Etoposide (VP-16) and teniposide	Secondary leukemias
Miscellaneous agents	Bleomycin	Pulmonary toxicity and skin toxicities
	Mitomycin	Myelosuppression, mucositis, dermatitis, pulmonary fibrosis, HUS and nephrotoxicity
	Thalidomide and lenalidomide	Fatigue, peripheral neuropathy, myelosuppression and thrombosis[8]
	Bortezomib	Thrombocytopenia, fatigue, peripheral neuropathy and diarrhea
Estrogen-receptor modulators (SERMs)	Tamoxifen and raloxifene	Endometrial cancer[9], thrombosis, vaginal discharge, hot flushes and cataract
Aromatase inhibitors	Anastrozole and letrozole	Myalgias, arthralgia and osteoporotic fractures
LHRH agonists	Leuprolide and goserelin	Fatigue, hot flushes, erectile dysfunction, weight gain, muscle atrophy, osteoporosis and hyperlipidemia

Abbreviations: 5-FU: 5-fluorouracil; Ara-C: cytarabine; MTX: methotrexate; 6-MP: 6-mercaptopurine; HUS: hemolytic uremic syndrome; LHRH: luteinizing hormone-releasing hormone; GI: gastrointestinal; RPLS: reversible posterior leukoencephalopathy; CNS: central nervous system; N/V: nausea and vomiting

1. Oxaliplatin-induced neurotoxicity can present shortly after the intravenous infusion with paresthesias triggered or potentiated by cold exposure including difficulty swallowing; these symptoms develop in 85-95% of patients and resolve within days. However, 10-20% of patients treated with oxaliplatin develop chronic sensory neuropathy that can result in permanent disability. While carboplatin induces mild sensorimotor neurotoxicity in 25% of patients, cisplatin administration can result in severe chronic sensory neuropathy in >50% of patients receiving > 500 mg/m^2 cumulative doses. Nephrotoxicity and ototoxicity are important adverse effects associated mostly with cisplatin.
2. Hand-foot syndrome is associated with oral 5-FU prodrug capecitabine and prolonged infusional 5-FU.
3. Flu-like symptoms, fever, HUS and pulmonary toxicity can be associated with gemcitabine.
4. Pulmonary toxicity can be associated with methotrexate
5. Pemetrexed can cause severe myelosuppression and a significant erythematous rash requiring the use of dexamethasone to prevent these adverse effects.
6. Hypersensitivity reactions occur in 8-45% of patients receiving paclitaxel and it is likely caused by the excipient Cremophor EL (polyoxyethylated castor oil). These reactions are very rare with docetaxel or albumin-bound paclitaxel preparations that do not contain Cremophor EL.
7. Fluid retention syndrome is specifically associated with docetaxel and can be prevented by dexamethasone.
8. Both thalidomide and lenalidomide are associated with thrombotic events including deep vein thrombosis and pulmonary embolism particularly when combined with dexamethasone for treatment of multiple myeloma. Antithrombotic prophylaxis with aspirin, low-molecular weight heparin or warfarin should be given to all patients treated with these drugs. Sedative effects and neurotoxicity are negligible with lenalidomide compared to thalidomide but both are associated with myelosuppression.
9. Incidence of endometrial cancer is lower with raloxifene compared to tamoxifen (seven years cumulative incidence 14.7 per 1000 patients for tamoxifen vs 8.1 per 1000 for raloxifene). Thromboembolic events and cataracts also occur less frequently with raloxifene, but there are no differences in the incidence of strokes and osteoporotic fractures.

carboplatin and oxaliplatin), procarbazine, dacarbazine and temozolomide are grouped as alkylating agents because alkylation is part of their mechanism of action. These agents transfer an alkyl group to several cellular components including DNA bases guanine, resulting in interstrand DNA crosslinks that ultimately induce cell death. Major toxicities common to this class are bone marrow suppression, nausea, vomiting, mucositis, alopecia and increased risk of secondary leukemias **(Table 13-2)**. This subtype of leukemias is frequently associated with chromosomes 5 and 7 deletions and most cases occur 4-5 years after treatment. These agents are used in a variety of diseases from chronic leukemias, Non-Hodgkin's lymphoma, sarcomas, bone marrow transplantation regimens to numerous epithelial cancers and have specific side effects with significant clinical implications.

Cyclophosphamide and its analog ifosfamide are associated with potentially life-threatening hemorrhagic cystitis caused by the metabolite acrolein. This cystitis is preventable by coadministration of mesna (2-mecapto-ethanesulfonate) and intravenous hydration. Ifosfamide in high doses can also be nephrotoxic and cause central nervous system adverse events such as seizures, mental status changes, coma or cerebellar ataxia. Busulfan can cause adrenal insufficiency, pulmonary fibrosis and skin pigmentation. Procarbazine has been associated with central nervous system depression. Cisplatin side effects include nephrotoxicity requiring aggressive hydration, peripheral sensory neuropathy and ototoxicity. Carboplatin has less nephrotoxicity and neurotoxicity but is more myelosuppressive. Oxaliplatin—a third generation platinum—causes acute and chronic peripheral sensory neuropathy, myelosuppression, diarrhea and mild renal toxicity. Neurotoxicity related to oxalipatin presents with cold sensitivity and dysesthesias on hands and feet; it can result in major debilitation and premature interruption of therapy.

Some alkylating agents are available orally (e.g. cyclophosphamide, temozolomide, busulfan, melphalan and chlorambucil) and carry similar toxicity profile compared to intravenous administration.

Antimetabolites

The drugs in this class inhibit critical enzymes involved on nucleotide and nucleic acid synthesis thereby blocking DNA and RNA production. The antimetabolites can be subgrouped as purine (e.g. fludarabine, cladribine, 6-mercaptopurine [6-MP] and 6-thioguanine [6-TG]), pyrimidine (e.g. 5-fluorouracil, capecitabine, cytarabine [ara-C] and gemcitabine) and folic acid antagonists (e.g. methotrexate and pemetrexed).

Fludarabine and cladribine are purine analogs activated intracellularly to triphosphate forms that are incorporated into DNA resulting in inhibition of DNA polymerases, DNA repair and synthesis machineries. Fludarabine has a central role on the treatment of chronic lymphocytic leukemia with some activity in non-Hodgkin's lymphoma, whereas cladribine is important for the treatment of hairy cell leukemia. Both drugs are associated with important immunosuppression given their cytotoxicity against CD4 and CD8 lymphocytes. 6-mercaptopurine and 6-thioguanine are oral agents used in childhood and adult leukemia and both inhibit *de novo* purine nucleotide synthesis.

The preferential utilization of uracil for DNA synthesis by rat hepatomas provided the rationale to the development of 5-fluorouracil by Heidelberger and his colleagues in 1956 and represented one of the earliest examples of targeted drug development. Fluoropyrimidines (5-FU, capecitabine and 5-F-deoxyuridine [5-FUdR]) are prodrugs that require activation to nucleotide metabolites to exert their cytotoxic effects. 5-FU is converted to three main metabolites: 5-fluoro-2′-deoxyuridine-5′-monophosphate (FdUMP), 5-fluorouridine-5′-triphosphate (FUTP) and 5-fluorodeoxyuridine-5′-triphosphate (FdUTP). FdUMP binds to thymidylate synthase (TS) in combination with 5-10 methylenetetrahydrofolic acid blocking the synthesis of thymidine triphosphate, a deoxynucleotide required for DNA synthesis. This appears to be the main mechanism of anticancer activity of 5-FU and its modulation alters the sensitivity to 5-FU. The administration of folic acid as 5-formyl-tetrahydrofolate (leucovorin) concomitant with 5-FU increases the stability and formation of the FdUMP, TS and folate complex, thereby enhancing 5-FU effects in colorectal cancer. On the other hand, increased expression of TS creates resistance to 5-FU. The cytotoxicity of 5-FU also results from the incorporation of FUTP into RNA and FdUTP into DNA that disrupt mRNA processing and DNA synthesis, respectively.

Gastrointestinal toxicity (e.g. mucositis and diarrhea) and bone marrow suppression are the major limiting toxicities of 5-FU. Deficiency of the enzyme dihydropyrimidine dehydrogenase (DPD) responsible for 5-FU inactivation potentiates these side effects and should be excluded prior to additional doses of 5-FU when applicable. Capecitabine is an oral 5-FU prodrug activated in the liver, plasma and tumor cells with similar spectrum of anticancer activity as 5-FU. In addition to 5-FU described adverse events, capecitabine also may cause hand and foot syndrome characterized by palmar and plantar erythema, dysesthesia, tenderness and desquamation in approximately 50% of patients. 5-FUdR is a fluoropyrimidine used mostly for treatment of hepatic metastases from colon cancer through hepatic artery infusion, which allows the local delivery of high doses without significant systemic toxicity. This modality, however, can result in cholestasis, elevation of transaminases and biliary sclerosis. Fluoropyrimidines can rarely lead to coronary artery vasospasm and ultimately angina and myocardium infarction.

The deoxycytidine analogs cytarabine and gemcitabine play an important role on the treatment of acute leukemia and several solid tumors, respectively. These drugs are converted intracellularly to their respective triphosphate nucleotide forms followed by incorporation into RNA and DNA. Cytarabine is also a potent inhibitor of DNA polymerase involved in DNA synthesis and repair and leads to programmed cell death. Its clinical use is restricted to hematologic malignancies since it lacks activity in solid tumors. Important side effects of cytarabine include myelosuppression, mucositis, conjunctivitis, noncardiogenic pulmonary edema, dermatitis and elevation of transaminases.

Gemcitabine is widely used in the management of pancreatic, breast, ovarian, bladder and lung cancers. The major toxicity of gemcitabine is myelosuppression, particularly when given as a prolonged intravenous infusion. The drug undergoes deamination in the plasma with rapid clearance, which varies significantly among patients. Elderly patients can have a slower clearance and should be monitored for severe myelosuppression. In addition, specific polymorphisms of the cytidine deaminase gene decrease its clearance and toxic levels of gemcitabine metabolites can be achieved. Other side effects include fever, flu-like symptoms, pulmonary toxicity, hemolysis and hemolytic-uremic syndrome.

5-azacytidine and decitabine are also cytidine analogs that induce cellular differentiation approved for the treatment of myelodysplasia. Once incorporated into the DNA, these drugs inhibit cytidine methylation leading to expression of genes silenced by epigenetic modifications. They have also cytotoxic activity through inhibition of DNA synthesis and induction of apoptosis. In general, they are well tolerated with myelosuppression being the major side effect.

Folic acid antagonists are best represented by methotrexate and pemetrexed. The development of methotrexate was driven by the understanding of the role of folic acid as a crucial enzymatic cofactor and carbon group donor during the synthesis of thymidylate and purines. Methotrexate is a potent inhibitor of the enzyme dihydrofolate reductase (DHFR) and causes depletion of tetrahydrofolate cofactors with significant impairment of DNA synthesis. Methotrexate also forms intracellular polyglutamates that inhibit other enzymes involved with purine synthesis (i.e. thymidylate synthase) and prolong the action of methotrexate. This drug is very active in tissues with high cell turnover such as bone marrow and intestinal epithelium, hence its associated myelosuppression and marked mucositis. In addition, methotrexate administration can cause pneumonitis, hepatic fibrosis and cirrhosis. It does not undergo metabolism and is excreted mostly through the kidneys requiring dose adjustment and close monitoring of serum levels when given to patients with renal insufficiency. For these same reasons, nephrotoxic drugs should be avoided during treatment with methotrexate including non-steroidal anti-inflammatory drugs. Methotrexate can accumulate in peritoneal, pericardium or pleural effusions resulting in prolonged elevated serum levels. Leucovorin is usually given concomitant with high-dose methotrexate to replenish intracellular folate levels and to prevent excessive toxicity to normal tissues. Hemodialysis is not effective for management of toxic serum levels of methotrexate, however the enzyme carboxypeptidase G can be used to rapidly decrease methotrexate plasma levels by cleaving the drug. Methotrexate has a well-established and central role in the treatment of childhood ALL, CNS lymphoma, osteosarcoma, choriocarcinoma and breast carcinoma among others.

Pemetrexed has a very similar mechanism of action compared with methotrexate but it is a more potent inhibitor of thymidylate synthase. Its side effect profile is comparable to methotrexate but it can cause a distinct erythematous rash in approximately 20-40% of patients. Prophylactic administration of dexamethasone is recommended to reduce the rash, as well as vitamin B_{12} and folic acid starting one week prior to treatment to prevent severe myelosuppression. Pemetrexed is approved for treatment of mesothelioma and non-small cell lung cancer. Interestingly, pemetrexed in combination with cisplatin was more active in adenocarcinoma and large-cell carcinoma histologic subtypes of lung cancer compared with squamous cell histology. This difference may possibly relate to the higher expression of thymidylate synthase in squamous cell carcinomas compared to adenocarcinomas but additional investigations are ongoing.

Natural Products

Vinca Alkaloids

Vinca alkaloids—vinblastine, vincristine, vinorelbine— inhibit the formation of microtubules by binding to β-tubulin and preventing its polymerization with α-tubulin. Consequently, cells do not build a functional mitotic spindle during methaphase resulting in cell death. Vinblastine and vincristine are used to treat Hodgkin's and Non-Hodgkin lymphomas, acute lymphocytic leukemia, sarcomas and testicular cancers. Vinorelbine has significant activity in non-small cell lung and breast cancers. These drugs are metabolized through cytochrome P450 (CYP3A4) and their side effect profile is most notable for peripheral neuropathy and myelosuppression. Vinblastine causes more myelosuppression and less peripheral neurotoxicity compared to vincristine. Vinorelbine limiting side effect is myelosuppression but can also cause mild peripheral neuropathy. Other side effects observed with these agents include elevation of transaminases, syndrome of inappropriate secretion of antidiuretic hormone, autonomic dysfunction and ileus.

Taxanes

The taxanes—paclitaxel, docetaxel and albumin-bound paclitaxel (Abraxane®)—are used in a variety of solid tumors including breast, ovarian, head and neck, lung and bladder cancers. They bind to β-tubulin in a distinct site used by vinca alkaloids and promote stabilization and formation of microtubules that lead to mitosis arrest and apoptosis. Given their metabolism through the P450 system, they have a number of relevant drug interactions with other anticancer agents (e.g. doxorubicin, cisplatin and gemcitabine) and CYP3A4 inducing anti-epileptics (e.g. phenytoin and phenobarbital). The major toxicity with these agents is neutropenia and patients usually require growth factor support during therapy. Hypersensitivity reactions during infusion occur in approximately 5% of patients and it is likely related to the solvent cremaphor. Abraxane does not require this solvent and it is not associated with such reactions. Paclitaxel can also cause peripheral neuropathy, myalgia, arthralgia and bradycardia. Fluid retention syndrome is specifically associated with docetaxel after several cycles of therapy and it can be prevented by dexamethasone.

Camptothecins

Topotecan and irinotecan are potent inhibitors of topoisomerase I with clinical activity in small cell lung carcinoma, colorectal and ovarian cancers. These drugs form complexes with DNA and topoisomerase I leading to single-strand DNA breaks that contribute to the formation of lethal double-strand DNA breaks. Topotecan is used in the treatment of ovarian and small cell lung cancers and its major toxicity is myelosuppression. Dose adjustment is necessary in patients with renal dysfunction given its predominant renal excretion.

Irinotecan is a prodrug converted to its active metabolite SN-38 in the liver with marked activity in colorectal cancer by itself or when combined with 5-FU and leucovorin. SN-38 is inactivated by diphosphate-glucuronosyltransferase (UGT) which is deficient in individuals with Gilbert's syndrome that carry the UGT1A1*28 polymorphism. Serum levels of irinotecan increase significantly in these patients, at times resulting in life-threatening diarrhea and/or myelosuppression. Baseline hyperbilirubinemia and family history of Gilbert's syndrome warrant further testing to exclude this polymorphism. In addition to its myelosuppressive effects, irinotecan causes significant diarrhea in approximately 30-40% of patients. An acute diarrhea

attributed to a cholinergic reaction develops within 24 hours of drug administration and it can be treated with atropine. Another form of diarrhea occurs 2-4 days later and can be more severe and result in significant morbidity. Patients should be monitored closely and treated with aggressive regimens of loperamide and intravenous hydration.

Anthracycline Antibiotics

The anthracycline antibiotics can both intercalate with DNA and/or inhibit topoisomerase II. The enzyme topoisomerase II catalyzes the relaxation of supercoiled DNA through the creation of transient DNA double-strand breaks to allow strand passage and it subsequently reseals the DNA break. This enzyme is crucially important in DNA replication, transcription and repair and chromosome segregation. The anthracyclines include doxorubicin, epirubicin, daunorubicin, idarubicin and mitoxantrone. Doxorubicin and epirubicin have been used mostly in breast cancer, sarcomas and lymphomas, whereas daunorubicin and epirubicin are important for the treatment of acute myelogenous leukemia (AML). Mitoxantrone is used in hormone-refractory prostate cancer and relapsed AML. Side effects common to this class include myelosuppression, mucositis, alopecia, cardiotoxicity and increased risk of myelodysplastic syndromes and secondary AML.

The cardiotoxicity caused by free-radicals generated by the anthracyclines is related to the cumulative dose administered and it manifests acutely with EKG changes and arrhythmias, or chronically with congestive heart failure. The incidence of symptomatic cardiomyopathy with total cumulative dose of doxorubicin below 450 mg/m^2 ranges from 1% to 10% and it increases to greater than 20% with doses above 550 mg/m^2. Monitoring of cardiac function with echocardiogram or MUGA scan is required for patients receiving these drugs and doses need to be reduced in the presence of hepatic dysfunction in light of their hepatic metabolism. Other chemotherapy drugs (e.g. paclitaxel and trastuzumab) and chest irradiation can potentiate the risk of cardiotoxicity. Liposomal formulations of doxorubicin and daunorubicin may have less cardiotoxicity and are approved for treatment of platinum-refractory ovarian cancer and Kaposi's sarcoma, respectively.

Epipodophyllotoxins

The derivatives of mayapple plant product podophyllotoxin—etoposide and teniposide—are also inhibitors of topoisomerase II. Etoposide (VP-16) is active in testicular tumors and small cell lung cancer. Its side effect profile is notable for myelosuppression. Teniposide (VM-26) is used in childhood acute lymphoblastic leukemia and causes myelosuppression and mucositis as its main side effects. This class of drug is associated with increased risk of secondary AML that can present 1-3 years after treatment and involve balanced translocations in the long arm of chromosomes 11 (11q23) and 21(21q22).

Hormonal Agents

Hormonal agents play a significant role in the treatment of breast, prostate and endometrial cancers. Up to 70% of breast cancer cells overexpress estrogen receptors (ERs) and those respond to estrogen proliferative effects through transcription of genes involved in cellular proliferation, differentiation and survival. The pharmacological manipulation of estrogen levels or its receptor activity has had a profound impact on the management of ER-positive breast cancer. A somewhat similar paradigm applies to endometrial cancers expressing ER and progesterone receptors, although the clinical impact of hormonal therapy is less than in breast cancer. The pivotal role of androgens in prostate carcinogenesis and progression is well documented and lowering of androgen levels and/or blocking androgen-dependent cell signaling represents a major component of prostate cancer treatment. This section will focus on the main hormonal strategies used in breast and prostate cancers.

Hormonal Therapy in Breast Cancer

The antiestrogen drugs utilized in the treatment of breast cancer include selective estrogen-receptor modulators (SERMs), selective estrogen-receptor downregulators (SERDs) and aromatase inhibitors (AIs). SERMs bind to estrogen receptors and have estrogenic or anti-estrogenic effects depending on the target organ. Complex signaling pathways connecting estrogen receptor activation and gene transcription in part explain these distinct effects. Tamoxifen—the first agent developed in this class—was introduced in late 1970s for the treatment of metastatic breast cancer. Given its efficacy and favorable side effect profile, its application has expanded to prevention and therapy of early ER-positive breast cancer. Tamoxifen is indicated for:
- primary prevention of breast cancer in individuals at high risk for invasive carcinoma.
- risk reduction of invasive cancer in patients with ductal carcinoma *in situ* (DCIS) treated surgically.
- adjuvant treatment of early stage ER-positive invasive breast cancer.
- palliative treatment of metastatic disease in both pre- and postmenopausal women.

The pivotal National Surgical Adjuvant Breast and Bowel Project (NSABP) P-1 trial demonstrated the role of tamoxifen as an effective strategy to prevent invasive breast carcinoma in high-risk women (i.e. 60 years of age or older, 35-59 years of age with five year predicted risk for breast cancer >1.66% according to Gail model, or history of lobular carcinoma *in situ*). Patients were randomized to receive tamoxifen 20 mg daily or placebo for five years. The incidence of invasive breast cancer was reduced by 49% in the tamoxifen group. Tamoxifen use was however, associated with an increased incidence of early stage endometrial cancer, higher rates of stroke, pulmonary embolism and deep vein thrombosis, as well as cataract, vasomotor symptoms and vaginal discharge. Conversely, tamoxifen reduced the incidence of fractures by 21%, which is consistent with its estrogenic effects improving bone mineral density. These results were corroborated by other clinical trials and led to the approval of this drug for primary prevention of breast cancer.

Raloxifene, a second generation SERMs with distinct tissue specificity compared to tamoxifen, was found to reduce incidence of breast cancer during early trials evaluating its potential to treat osteoporosis. The effects of tamoxifen and raloxifene in preventing breast cancer were directly compared in the NSABP STAR trial involving nearly 20,000 postmenopausal women at increased risk for breast cancer. The results showed that both raloxifene and tamoxifen reduced invasive breast cancer to similar extent, but fewer cases of endometrial cancer were seen in the raloxifene arm. The incidence of thromboembolic events and cataracts were lower with raloxifene and there were no differences in regard to strokes and osteoporotic fractures. Both drugs are currently approved for breast cancer prevention. Raloxifene is favored in postmenopausal patients and tamoxifen continues to be the standard option for premenopausal women until safety data on raloxifene becomes available in this population.

In the adjuvant setting, five years of tamoxifen reduces breast cancer mortality by approximately 30%. The benefits of tamoxifen in overall survival and recurrence rates are irrespective of age, lymph node status and remain significant 15 years later. Tamoxifen is also the therapy of choice for hormonal treatment of metastatic breast cancer in premenopausal women. Tamoxifen is metabolized through the cytochrome P450 system and specific polymorphisms of the gene *CYP2D6* lead to lower serum levels of the active metabolite endoxifen. This observation is relevant because commonly used selective serotonin reuptake inhibitors can suppress the CYP2D6 activity. Toremifene is a tamoxifen analogue with significantly less estrogenic activity, but in clinic trials, this reduced estrogenic activity did not translate into consistent improvement of side effects. However, similar overall efficacy and toxicity led to the approval of this agent as an alternative to tamoxifen in front-line treatment of metastatic breast cancer.

The only approved selective estrogen-receptor down-regulator (SERD) for treatment of breast cancer is fulvestrant. This drug has the advantage of blocking and inducing degradation of estrogen receptors without the agonist activity of tamoxifen. Fulvestrant is given as a monthly 250 mg intramuscular injection and has comparable efficacy to tamoxifen in the first-line treatment of metastatic breast cancer. It is also active in tamoxifen-resistant breast cancer with similar efficacy to the aromatase inhibitor anastrazole in the second-line setting. Oral SERD EM-800 is also active in tamoxifen-refractory breast cancer but it is not available in the United States.

While the ovaries produce most of the estrogen during the premenopausal state, after menopause the primary sources of estrogen are from peripheral conversion of adrenal androgens by aromatase enzyme present in fat, muscle and liver. For this reason, aromatase inhibitors have emerged as important therapeutic tools in the management of postmenopausal breast cancer patients as they demonstrate higher efficacy in this setting and are better tolerated than tamoxifen.

The two groups of aromatase inhibitors (AIs) in clinical use are the type 1 steroidal inhibitors (e.g. formestane, exemestane) and the type 2 nonsteroidal inhibitors (e.g. aminoglutethimide, anastrozole and letrozole) with only partial cross-resistance between both groups. Steroidal inhibitors bind irreversibly to aromatase causing permanent inactivation, whereas the nonsteroidal AIs are reversible inhibitors. The two type 1 inhibitors exemestane and formestane are not widely utilized. Exemestane is used in second-line treatment only, whereas formestane has a better side effect profile compared to aminoglutethimide but it is not available in the United States. The first generation type 2 inhibitor aminoglutethimide is associated with multiple side effects and has been replaced by more specific and better-tolerated AIs. The newer type 2 inhibitors anastrozole and letrozole are approved for first- and second-line treatment of metastatic breast cancer. Anastrozole is also indicated for adjuvant treatment of postmenopausal patients with early stage disease based on results of a phase III trial comparing anastrozole to tamoxifen. In this trial, anastrozole was associated with longer disease-free survival, time to recurrence and significant reduction in the incidence of contralateral breast cancer compared to tamoxifen. Patients receiving anastrozole had less ischemic cerebrovascular events, deep vein thrombosis, hot flashes, vaginal bleeding and discharge and endometrial cancer. Anastrozole was associated with significantly higher rates of myalgias, arthralgias and osteoporotic fractures compared to tamoxifen. These side effects are also common to letrozole and exemestane. Anastrozole and exemestane are metabolized through the liver, whereas letrozole is excreted through the kidneys.

In summary, the SERMs tamoxifen and raloxifene are approved options for breast cancer prevention. Tamoxifen is also indicated for adjuvant treatment of ER-positive premenopausal breast cancer patients, whereas the options for adjuvant treatment for postmenopausal patients include tamoxifen and AIs (e.g. letrozole and anastrozole). Tamoxifen or AIs are appropriate choices for first-line treatment of postmenopausal women with advanced breast cancer taking into consideration the distinct side effect profiles, although there is data showing greater efficacy of AIs in this setting. Premenopausal patients with advanced disease should receive tamoxifen as the first-line treatment and ovarian ablation as a second-line therapy. Ovarian ablation using luteinizing hormone-releasing hormone (LHRH) agonists was evaluated alone or in combination with tamoxifen in premenopausal women with metastatic breast cancer. This combination results in higher response rates and progression-free survival with a small overall survival benefit. These marginal benefits have guided some clinicians to adopt this combined strategy. LHRH agonists can also be and used after tamoxifen failure in the second-line setting.

Alternative hormonal strategies for patients with progression of metastatic breast cancer after tamoxifen, AIs and SERDs include progestins, estrogens or androgens. Progesterone derivatives megestrol acetate and medroxyprogesterone reduce serum estrogen levels through unclear mechanisms and can lead to reasonable control of disease at the cost of increased risk of thromboembolic events, fluid retention and weight gain. Heavily pretreated patients with other hormonal strategies can potentially respond to high dose estrogens and androgens but their use has extremely been limited because of untoward side effects.

Hormonal Therapy in Prostate Cancer

Androgens mediate the physiological development and growth of the prostate and are implicated in carcinogenesis. Androgen suppression plays an important role in the treatment of metastatic disease and in the adjuvant treatment of localized disease. Androgen deprivation is the standard first-line treatment option for metastatic prostate cancer. Approximately 80-90% of the patients with metastatic disease obtain significant relief of symptoms, but, unfortunately, a significant percentage will develop resistance to hormonal therapy within two years at which point the palliative therapeutic options are second-line hormonal therapy or chemotherapy. Hormonal therapy has also been shown to improve survival of patients with localized prostate cancer with lymph node positive treated primarily with surgery or radiation therapy and these findings established the role of adjuvant hormonal therapy.

Androgen ablation can be achieved surgically through bilateral orchiectomy or medically with LHRH agonists (e.g. leuprolide and goserelin) and androgen receptor antagonists, adrenal androgen synthesis inhibitors and estrogens. The efficacy of LHRH agonists is similar to surgical castration and has become the preferred treatment option. Leuprolide and goserelin can be administered monthly or every 3-4 months as depot preparations. LHRH agonists have been combined with androgen receptor inhibitors to block the action of androgens produced by the adrenal glands achieving complete androgen ablation, although the benefits of this combined strategy awaits definitive prove. The antiandrogens available in the United States are flutamide, bicalutamide and nilutamide. Once patients develop progression of disease with these antiandrogen modalities, other agents with benefit of less magnitude include ketozonazole and hydrocortisone that block extragonadal androgen synthesis and diethylstilbestrol. The use of estrogens, however, has been limited by its cardiovascular complications.

Despite its benefits, hormonal therapy for prostate cancer has a significant negative impact on quality of life. Side effects of hormonal therapy include fatigue, hot flushes, loss of libido, erectile dysfunction, weight gain, gynecomastia, muscle atrophy and decreased bone mineral density. Patients also develop hyperlipidemia and insulin resistance, which coupled with weight gain and decreased exercise tolerance might contribute to the higher incidence of diabetes and cardiovascular disease seen in patients treated chronically with androgen suppression. Hence, cardiovascular risk mitigation is critical to the optimal use of antiandrogen therapy; for example, screening for diabetes and regular physical activity should be encouraged to this patient population. Vitamin D and calcium supplementation are recommended for prevention of osteoporosis and regular monitoring of bone mineral density is beneficial as well. Biphosphonate therapy is a reasonable approach once patient develops osteoporosis or presents with osteoporotic bone fracture.

Miscellaneous Agents

Dactinomycin or actinomycin D was the first antibiotic with anticancer activity discovered. This agent binds to DNA and blocks transcription by RNA polymerase. Side effects include myelosuppression, oral mucositis and skin desquamation and cause severe skin necrosis, if extravasation occurs. It is mostly used in Wilms' tumor and rhabdomyosarcoma.

Bleomycin is another antibiotic that causes oxidation of nucleotides resulting in single- and double-strand DNA breaks. It is excreted mostly through the kidneys requiring dose adjustment in patients with renal insufficiency. Significant pulmonary injury develops in 5-10% of patients treated with bleomycin and manifests from mild dyspnea with dry cough to irreversible and lethal pulmonary fibrosis. Risk factors for pulmonary injury are total doses exceeding 500 mg/m^2, underlying pulmonary disease, age > 70 years old, radiation therapy and exposure to high concentrations of inspired oxygen. Unfortunately, there is no proven effective therapy. Steroids have been used based on uncontrolled studies. Skin toxicity manifestations include hyperpigmentation, erythema and ulcerations. In spite of these serious adverse effects, bleomycin continues to be used in testicular cancer, lymphomas and squamous carcinoma of cervix and vulva given its high effectiveness.

Mitomycin, an antibiotic with DNA alkylating effects, has clinical use limited to the treatment of squamous cell carcinoma of the anal canal where it is given in combination with 5-FU and radiation. It is a potent radiosensitizer associated with significant side effects such as myelosuppression, mucositis, dermatitis, pulmonary fibrosis, renal toxicity and hemolytic uremic syndrome.

Thalidomide was first approved as a sedative and antiemetic agent used during pregnancy in 1950s but it was withdrawn from the market because of teratogenicity. Significant clinical activity in erythema nodosum leprosum (ENL) identified in late 1960s renewed the interest in thalidomide and fostered further investigation that eventually resulted in the discovery of its activity in multiple myeloma, myelodysplastic syndrome (MDS), as well as in various non-malignant conditions. Thalidomide and its derivative lenalidomide were respectively approved for the treatment of newly diagnosed and refractory multiple myeloma in 2006. Lenalidomide has also shown significant activity in patients with MDS, particularly those with chromosome 5q31.1 deletion. Thalidomide inhibits cytokines (e.g. TNF-α, IL1-β and IL-6) production, block nuclear factor kB (NF-kB) and activate T-cells. In addition to these immunomodulatory activities, thalidomide inhibits VEGF and beta fibroblast growth factors (FGFs) synthesis in tumor and bone marrow stromal cells and suppresses endothelial cell proliferation resulting in significant antiangiogenesis effects. Furthermore, antiproliferative activity in malignant cells have been demonstrated as well as proapoptotic effects by enhancing death receptor signaling, increasing expression of caspase-8 and inhibiting anti-apoptosis Bcl-2 family members. The exact mechanism of action responsible for thalidomide's clinical activity in multiple myeloma and MDS has not been clearly defined but appears to derive from a combination of immunomodulatory action, anti-inflammatory effects in the bone marrow microenvironment and antiangiogenesis. The limiting side effects of thalidomide and lenalidomide are fatigue, sedation, peripheral neuropathy, myelosuppression and increased risk of thrombosis including deep vein thrombosis and pulmonary embolism requiring prophylactic anticoagulation. The use of more potent and less toxic thalidomide analogs such as lenalidomide in other hematologic and solid organ malignancies is being investigated.

A better understanding of the mechanisms of intracellular protein degradation by proteasomes has led to the successful development of proteasome inhibitors as anticancer agents. Bortezomib, a dipeptide boronic acid analog, is a first-in-class agent currently approved for treatment of multiple myeloma and refractory mantle cell lymphoma. It blocks the 26S proteasome complex that plays an important role in the degradation of misfolded or damaged proteins and regulation of cell survival, cell cycle progression, several transcription factors and mediators of apoptosis. The therapeutic effects of bortezomib in multiple myeloma appears to be closely related to its inhibitory action on NF-kB pathway through decreased degradation and stabilization of IκB, which prevents the nuclear translocation of NF-κB and downstream transcription of genes involved in cell growth, angiogenesis, antiapoptosis mechanisms and production of cytokines. Bortezomib also regulates other cell signaling pathways (e.g. c-jun kinase and 3-kinase/Akt pathways, heat shock proteins expression and DNA repair machinery) that contribute to its action beyond NF-κB inhibition. The most common adverse effects associated with bortezomib are peripheral neuropathy, fatigue, diarrhea and thrombocytopenia.

Molecularly Targeted Agents

Advances in the understanding of the molecular and biochemical mechanisms involved in carcinogenesis and tumor growth have led to development of drugs targeting specific molecular pathways. These molecularly targeted therapies are currently used in several cancers either alone or combined with cytotoxic agents. In some cancers where a single signaling pathway is primarily responsible for tumor pathogenesis, these new therapies (such as the use of imatinib in GIST and CML) have revolutionized the outcome of the disease. However, multiple interconnected signaling networks requiring therapeutic strategies beyond single target inhibition drive most tumor growth and development. Indeed, to date most of the benefits from these agents have been achieved through combination with standard chemotherapy drugs. Among these complex signaling networks—EGFR, VEGF, RAS and PI3K-Akt-mTOR—pathways are the best characterized and explored therapeutically **(Figure 13-2)**. Drugs affecting specific components of each pathway are either approved for clinical use or are in advanced stages of clinical development.

Tyrosine Kinase Pathways as Targets for Anticancer Drugs

Protein tyrosine kinases are enzymes capable of transferring phosphates from ATP to a variety of protein residues.

Tyrosine kinases can be found as transmembrane receptors (receptor tyrosine kinases or RTKs) or as intracellular proteins located in the cytoplasm, nucleous or in the juxtamembrane region. RTKs have an extracellular ligand binding domain, a transmembrane segment, a juxtamembrane sequence, a carboxy-terminal domain and a tyrosine kinase domain that undergoes autophosphorylation after ligand binding resulting in receptor activation. Examples of groups of RTKs include ErbB family (EGFR/ErbB1, ErbB2 or HER2/neu, ErbB3 or HER3 and ErbB4 or HER4), platelet derived growth factor receptor (PDGF), vascular endothelial growth factor receptors (VEGFR1/Flt-1 and VEGFR2/Flk-1) and insulin growth factor receptors. An example of an intracellular kinase is cytoplasmically localized ABL kinase, which in CML is usually constitutively activated by autophosphorylation of its kinase domain through BCR mediated dimerization.

Several abnormalities in the function of tyrosine kinases have been implicated in carcinogenesis. The major mechanisms of tyrosine kinase dysregulation are: (1) overexpression of RTKs or their ligand (e.g. HER-2/neu and PDGF); (2) constitutive activation of TKs by mutations of extracellular or tyrosine kinase domains of RTKs, fusion of cytoplasmic TKs with partner proteins (e.g. BCR-ABL); (3) loss of factors that attenuate TK activity such as tyrosine phosphatases and inhibitory proteins.

Ras small GTP-binding proteins are central components of the multiple RTKs signaling. The family of these membrane-bound molecules consists of ten members including H-, N- and K-RAS. These molecules cycle between a GDP-bound inactive form and a GTP-bound active state; this switch is mediated by guanine nucleotide exchange factors recruited to the juxtamembrane region after activation of RTKs and GTPase activating proteins that induce GTP hydrolysis. The oncogene *RAS* is mutated in ~ 15% of all malignancies and most of these mutations result in a constitutively active molecule by decreasing the GTP-hydrolysis that leads to downstream signaling independently of upstream ligand-binding and activation of RTKs. This mechanism is believed to underlie the resistance of KRAS mutant colorectal tumors to EGFR blockade. The major effector downstream of *RAS* is the serine/threonine kinase RAF that is found in three isoforms (A-Raf, B-Raf and C-Raf). Raf kinases phosphorylate the kinase MEK, which in turn activates mitogen-activated protein kinases (MAPKs) 1 and 2 (also known as ERK) that translocate to the nucleus resulting in the phosphorylation of several transcription factors effecting DNA synthesis and proliferation. This pathway has been validated as a target for cancer therapy though the development of small-molecule MEK inhibitors (e.g. AZD6244 and PD 0325901) that have favorable toxicity profile and encouraging efficacy based on early clinical trials in solid tumors. In addition, sorafenib, an oral multi-

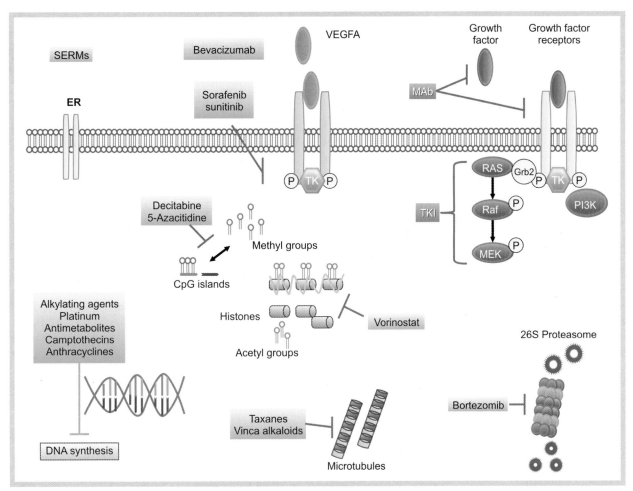

Figure 13-2: Molecular targets of anticancer agents. The small-molecule tyrosine kinase inhibitors (TKI) inhibit epidermal growth factor (EGF) receptors though competition with the ATP binding to the intracellular kinase domain of the receptor. Monoclonal antibodies (MAb) against EGF receptors extracellular domain also inhibit this pathway. Sorafenib inhibits multiple targets including the serine/threonine kinase Raf and the vascular endothelial growth factor (VEGF) receptor tyrosine kinase. Sunitinib also targets several receptor tyrosine kinases including VEGFR. Bevacizumab is a monoclonal antibody against the VEGF with potent anti-angiogenic properties. Intracellular degradation of proteins can be inhibited by 26S proteasome complex inhibitor bortezomib. Taxanes and Vinca alkaloids interfere with formation and stabilization of microtubules resulting in mitosis arrest and cell death. Alkylating agents, platinum derivatives, antimetabolites, camptothecins and anthracyclines cause DNA damage and inhibit DNA synthesis and repair machineries through distinctive mechanisms. Epigenetic changes regulate gene expression in numerous tumors and can be modulated by blocking the methylation of CpG islands in gene promoter regions with decitabine or 5-azacitidine, or through histone deacetylation inhibitors such as Vorinostat. Estrogen receptor modulators (SERMs; tamoxifen and raloxifene) inhibit the growth signaling associated with estrogen. PI3K, phosphoinositide 3-kinase; MEK, mitogen-activated protein kinases; Grb2, SH2 and SH3 domain-containing adaptor protein

kinase inhibitor approved for clinical use in advanced renal cell carcinoma and unresectable hepatocellular carcinoma, was initially developed as a potent inhibitor of RAF kinases but later found to also block VEGFR, PDGFR, c-KIT and FLT3 kinases.

Another critical pathway downstream of multiple growth factor receptors involves the phosphatidylinositol 3-kinase (PI3K), Akt and mTOR kinases that play an important role in cell survival. PI3K phosphorylates the inositol group of the phospholipid $PI(4,5)P_2$ at the plasma membrane generating $PI(3,4,5)P_3$ which activates Akt that in turn stimulate cell survival through activation of mTOR protein kinase and inhibition of proapoptotic Bcl-2 proteins BAD and other protein involved in the control of cell cycle (e.g. GSK-3 tyrosine kinase). The phosphatase PTEN converts $PI(3,4,5)P_3$ to $PI(4,5)P_2$ functioning as a negative regulator of PI3K. Mutations of the PI3K pathway have been implicated in numerous malignancies and include activating mutations of PI3K gene (e.g. PI3KCA) or deletion of PTEN suppressor function. The mTOR inhibitor temsirolimus is currently approved for the treatment of renal cell carcinoma. Several PI3K inhibitors are in clinical development with promising anticancer activity.

The Therapeutic Role of Antiangiogenesis Strategies

Early demonstration of the importance of angiogenesis to sustain tumor growth and metastatic potential led extensive research that resulted in the discovery of endogenous factors that promote and inhibit formation of blood vessels in physiologic and pathologic conditions. The factors that promote vasculogenesis include vascular endothelial growth factor A (VEGFA), basic fibroblast growth factor (bFGF), angiopoietins (ANG 1 and 2) and platelet-derived growth factor (PDGF); thrombospondin, endostatin and tumstatin inhibit the formation of blood vessels. The identification of VEGFA along with evidence showing the critical role of VEGFA in tumor angiogenesis and growth converged in the discovery of bevacizumab, a monoclonal antibody targeting VEGFA, which has been the most successful anti-angiogenesis therapeutic strategy. Bevacizumab was approved in 2004 for the treatment of metastatic colorectal cancer based on improvement of survival of patients with metastatic colorectal cancer that received chemotherapy and bevacizumab compared to those treated with chemotherapy alone; subsequent studies also showed a significant survival benefit in advanced non-small cell lung and progression-free survival in breast cancer. This drug prevents VEGFA from binding to tyrosine kinase receptors (e.g. VEGFR 1 or Flt-1 and VEGFR-2/Flk-1) in endothelial cells where it activates downstream PI3K, Src and protein kinase C pathways modulating proliferation, cellular migration and vessel permeability.

Other agents in clinical use also exert their anticancer effects partially through inhibition of angiogenesis. The receptor tyrosine kinase inhibitors sorafenib and sunitinib approved for treatment of renal cell cancer block VEGFA and PDGF receptors, the EGFR small-molecule inhibitor erlotinib reduces the expression of VEGF and newer drugs that block both VEGF and EGFR tyrosine kinase receptors are under development. Moreover, drugs classified as immunomodulators, including thalidomide and interferon-α, also exhibit anti-angiogenic activity.

Modulation of Epigenetic Changes in Cancer Treatment

The molecular control of gene expression or silencing through epigenetic changes has been explored as a target for cancer therapy. The two major mechanisms of epigenetic gene expression regulation include the methylation of CpG islands in gene promoter regions and the enzymatic deacetylation of histones. Both pathways

lead to aberrant silencing of multiple genes including tumor suppressor genes with important role in carcinogenesis. Distinct from mutations in the DNA sequence, gene silencing by hypermethylation of promoter regions or by histone deacetylation can be reversed biochemically and targeted for cancer treatment or prevention. Agents such as 5-azacitidine and 5-aza-2′-deoxycytidine (decitabine) inhibit DNA methyltransferases responsible for methylation of cytosine residues in CpG islands. These drugs reactivate the expression of genes such as the cyclin-dependent kinase inhibitor p15, translating into significant responses in myelodysplastic syndromes for which these drugs were approved. The transfer of acetyl groups to histone lysine residues contributes to the switch between an open chromatin favoring gene transcription and a closed or condensed chromatin that precludes gene expression. Acetylation of histones leads to gene expression by relaxing the chromatin and deacetylation by histone deacetylase (HDAC) attenuates gene expression. HDAC inhibitors such as vorinostat enhance the expression of several genes and ultimately lead to G0 and G1 cell cycle arrest and apoptosis. Vorinostat is approved for the treatment of cutaneous T-cell lymphoma and other drugs in the same class are undergoing clinical evaluation in other hematologic malignancies and mesothelioma.

Side Effects of Targeted Agents: New Challenges

The specificity of newer biological agents carries the hope of mitigating normal tissue toxicity. Nevertheless, they are associated with side effects not usually observed with standard chemotherapy. These unique adverse events and their management are discussed below.

Epidermal Growth Factor Receptor (EGFR)-related Rash

Both classes of EGFR inhibitors—monoclonal antibodies (mAbs) against EGFR extracellular domain [cetuximab and panitumumab] and small-molecule tyrosine kinase inhibitors (TKIs) that block the ATP binding to the intracellular kinase receptor domain [erlotinib and gefitinib]—have been associated with a papulopustular rash. This rash occurs in vast majority of patients and frequently involves the face, upper back and chest. EGFR important role in keratinocytes maturation, migration and survival along with a proinflammatory response triggered by EGFR inhibition are postulated as the mechanisms for EGFR inhibitors-related rash and other skin toxicities. The rash is dose-related causing significant physical and psychological distress and, in severe cases, leads to treatment interruption. Rash usually occurs during the first three weeks of therapy and its intensity correlates with higher response rates and improved treatment outcomes in colorectal, head and neck, pancreatic and non-small cell lung cancers. Exposure to sunlight aggravates the rash, which might explain its higher incidence in fair-skinned patients and its location in sun-exposed areas. Other toxicities associated with EGFR blockade include skin exfoliation, skin fissure, dry skin, abnormal scalp and eyelashes hair growth and nail changes with periungual inflammation. The management recommendations are mostly based on retrospectively analyses given the limited number of controlled prospective trials addressing this toxicity.

Topical steroids (e.g. hydrocortisone 2.5% or alclometsone dipropionate cream 0.05%) or topical clindamycin 1% gel are recommended for mild rash (grade 1). For moderate to severe rash (grade 2 or 3), oral antibiotics minocycline or doxycycline (100-200 mg/day for 4-6 weeks) are added to the topical regimen. A short course of oral steroids should be considered in absence of improvement. Clinical suspicion for secondary bacterial and viral infections warrants further evaluation with cultures and treatment with appropriate antimicrobials. Oral antibiotics have been used in patients with marked xerotic skin who have a higher risk of infections such as impetigo caused by *Staphylococcus aureus*. Patients with severe rash, neutropenia and history of colonization by Methicillin-resistant *Staphylococcus aureus* (MRSA) require close monitoring given disruption of skin barrier and risk of bacteremia. Topical immunomodulators (e.g. tacrolimus and pimecrolimus) have been used for short period in refractory cases, but its indication should be discussed in consultation with dermatology. Maintenance therapy with minocycline or doxycycline (50-100 mg/day) can be considered in cases of rash recurrence.

Dry skin frequently associated with rash is managed with emollients in combination with antihistamines (e.g. diphenhydramine and hydroxyzine). Sunscreens containing zinc oxide or titanium oxide have been suggested for rash prophylaxis but confirmatory studies are pending. Prophylaxis with minocycline upon initiation of treatment with cetuximab reduced the severity of the rash during the first month of therapy but it did not show any benefit eight weeks later. Topical retinoids or benzoyl peroxide commonly used for acne should be avoided given lack of proven benefit in this setting and, in fact, they can cause irritation and worsening of symptoms.

Side Effects Related to Vascular Endothelial Growth Factor (VEGF) Inhibition

Anti-angiogenic agents including mAbs against VEGF (e.g. bevacizumab) and VEGF receptor TKIs (e.g. sorafenib and sunitinib) have a favorable safety profile and do not appear to potentiate chemotherapy toxicities. The most common toxicities of these agents include hypertension, asymptomatic proteinuria, hemorrhage, arterial thrombosis, gastrointestinal perforation, impaired wound healing and reversible posterior leukoencephalopathy (RPLS). These adverse effects were somewhat unexpected given the notion that VEGF had a limited role in adult vascular physiology, but multiple studies have challenged this paradigm by demonstrating the importance of VEGF to vascular homeostasis in normal adult organs.

New onset of hypertension was observed in up to 34% patients treated with bevacizumab in colorectal cancer trials and in 15-28% of the patients receiving sunitinib or sorafenib. In most cases, the hypertension is mild, manageable with standard antihypertensive medications and does not lead to interruption of therapy. Nevertheless, it can require multidrug therapy in 10-15% of the cases. The hypertension resolves after treatment. One proposed mechanism for the hypertension is decreased production of nitric oxide by endothelial cells resulting in peripheral arteriolar vasoconstriction.

Approximately 20% of patients treated with bevacizumab can also develop dose-dependent and asymptomatic proteinuria that usually resolves after stopping bevacizumab without major or lasting impact on renal function. Rare cases of significant proteinuria (e.g. $\geq$ 2 gm/24 hr) and nephrotic syndrome have been reported with bevacizumab and are indications to discontinuation of the drug. The proteinuria seems to result from blockade of VEGF signaling in endothelial cells and podocytes that plays an important role in maintaining the glomerular filtration barrier.

Bevacizumab has also been associated with mild and self-limited mucocutaneous bleeding (e.g. epistaxis and gingival and vaginal bleeding) and rarely with fatal pulmonary hemorrhage in lung cancer trials. Serious hemorrhage was documented in 3-9% of patients with colorectal and non-small cell lung cancer receiving bevacizumab. As squamous cell lung cancers have a significantly higher risk of bleeding, they should not be treated with bevacizumab. Patients with CNS metastases have been excluded from trials with antiangiogenic drugs, therefore limited information is available regarding risk of CNS hemorrhage. However, studies using bevacizumab in glioblastomas have not shown a significant risk of intracranial bleeding. Patients receiving anticoagulation can be cautiously treated with these agents.

Arterial thrombotic events such as myocardial infarction, angina, stroke, transient ischemic attack and subarachnoid hemorrhage are additional possible serious adverse effects of bevacizumab particularly in patients older than 65 years with significant history of cardiovascular disease or thrombosis. The incidence of arterial thromboembolic events among patients receiving bevacizumab with chemotherapy for lung, colorectal and breast cancers is approximately 4% with 0.8% mortality rate.

Several mechanisms are proposed to explain both bleeding and arterial thrombotic events. The bleeding tendency may result from blocking the key role of VEGF in endothelial cell proliferation and maintenance of vascular architecture. Disruption of endothelial cell lining can also lead to exposure of procoagulants such as phospholipids and subendothelial collagen that combined with anti-VEGF suppression of nitric oxide production greatly enhances the risk of thrombosis.

Another important challenge with bevacizumab is the rare but life-threatening occurrence of gastrointestinal perforation observed in approximately 1.5% of patients with colorectal carcinoma receiving bevacizumab and chemotherapy. The risk factors for GI perforation include acute diverticulitis, bowel obstruction, abdominal carcinomatosis, history of abdominal radiation and tumor at the site perforation. These patients warrant close monitoring for new onset of abdominal pain and intestinal obstruction during treatment. Regression of intestinal villi capillaries observed with VEGF inhibition in experimental animals could contribute to the pathogenesis of gastrointestinal perforation.

Reversible posterior leukoencephalopathy—neurological syndrome of headache, mental status changes, seizures, visual changes, hypertension and occipital-parietal cerebral edema—has been observed in patients treated with bevacizumab, sunitinib and sorefenib. This entity is associated with hypertensive encephalopathy and results from endothelial dysfunction leading to disruption of blood-brain barrier and cerebral edema. It also happens with cytotoxic drugs and immunosuppressive agents. Brain magnetic resonance imaging can show areas of enhancement as well as nonenhancing leukoencephalopathy changes. Discontinuation of drug and control of hypertension are imperative for treatment of his rare condition.

Wound healing can be impaired in patients receiving bevacizumab and an interval of 4-6 weeks between discontinuation of therapy and surgery is recommended given its prolonged half-life. Lastly, reduction of left ventricular ejection fraction was observed in patients receiving sunitinib and sorafenib with coronary ischemia occurring in 3% of patients with renal cell carcinoma treated with sorafenib.

Despite these rare and potentially life-threatening side effects, the anti-angiogenic drugs alone or in combination with chemotherapy are in general better tolerated than cytotoxic agents and have certainly improved progression-free and overall survival in multiple malignancies.

Predicting Response to Targeted Agents

Molecular predictors of response or resistance to targeted agents identified during clinical drug development are building the foundations for individualized therapies in cancer and some have already reached the clinical practice. Genetic exploration of the fact that females, Asians, non-smokers with adenocarcinoma of the lung obtain greater benefit from EGFR TKIs (e.g. erlotinib and gefitinib) compared to the general population led to the discovery of somatic mutations in the EGFR kinase domain that can predict both sensitivity (L858R point mutation in exon 21 and exon 19 deletion) and resistance (T790M mutations) to these agents. Non-small cell lung cancer tumors carrying activating EGFR mutations seem to depend significantly on the EGFR pathway for their growth explaining their sensitivity to TKIs. Other mutations such as T790M, seem to alter the binding kinetics of reversible EGFR TKIs and decrease their effectiveness. These findings further advanced the attempts to match the tumor genetics profile with therapeutic options. Indeed, the current use of anti-EGFR mAbs in advanced colorectal cancer is guided by the mutational analysis of components of the EGFR cascade such as KRAS and BRAF. Clinical studies in metastatic colorectal cancer have shown consistently that only patients without KRAS mutations benefit from cetuximab and panitumumab anti-EGFR mAbs. BRAF mutations also seem to predict resistance to these drugs but require further validation. KRAS mutational analysis is currently used in clinical practice to exclude approximately 40% of patients with advanced colorectal cancer that carry KRAS mutations and should not be exposed to these drugs.

Another example of molecular predictors can be seen in the treatment of GIST with imatinib. The majority of GISTs have activating mutations of the transmembrane tyrosine kinase KIT that drive tumor growth. KIT mutations are commonly located in the exons 11 (approximately 66% of cases) and 9 (15.4% of the cases) and rarely involve exons 13 and 17. GISTs harboring activating exon 11 mutations have higher clinical responses to imatinib compared to those with exon 9 mutations or no detectable mutations on KIT (67%, 40% and 39%, respectively).

Novel gene and protein profiling of tumors have provided a significant amount of information regarding prognosis through a more accurate classification of heterogeneous diseases such as non-small cell lung cancer. Gene signatures able to predict benefit from chemotherapy regimens have been validated in breast cancer and will likely be expanded to other cancers. The establishment of these molecular predictors of response to anticancer drugs will not only protect patients from inactive drugs and their side effects but also decrease the exposure of cancer cells to ineffective agents that can foster resistance to other drugs.

Conclusions

The last 60 years since the discovery of the first chemotherapy drugs witnessed a major evolution on treatment of cancer and drug development strategies that have translated into improved prognosis of numerous malignancies. The shift in anticancer drug discovery from serendipitous identification of antiproliferative compounds to development of drugs specific to molecular defects contributing to carcinogenesis, resulted in targeted agents already incorporated into clinical practice and hundreds of new compounds are undergoing clinical testing.

The enormous enthusiasm brought by these new drugs has been tempered by the relative lack of efficacy when these drugs are used alone showing the need to inhibit several pathways simultaneously in the complex molecular network that drives tumor growth. Adverse effects not seen previously with cytotoxic agents also represent a new challenge with these drugs. Nevertheless, significant advances in disease control and survival have been achieved through the addition of molecularly targeted agents to standard chemotherapy regimens in several malignancies. For instance, the median survival of patients with metastatic colorectal cancer more than doubled over the past decade (21-24 mo vs 10-12 mo) as a result of a number of factors including the efficacy of new cytotoxics (e.g. irinotecan and oxaliplatin), innovative administration of 5-FU and the addition of bevacizumab and cetuximab.

The availability of more effective supportive drugs such as anti-emetics and bone marrow growth factors over the past two decades has also contributed to improve patients' quality of life and the delivery of chemotherapy drugs. Furthermore, the foundations of personalized therapies in oncology built through the identification of molecular biomarkers able to identify the patients likely to benefit from novel therapies has evolved significantly in the last decade with numerous examples of molecular predictors used in clinical practice (e.g. KRAS mutational analysis to predict effectiveness of EGFR-based therapies in colorectal cancer; EGFR tyrosine kinase mutations that predict both resistance and sensitivity to EGFR therapies in lung cancer; gene signatures that indicate the likelihood of benefit from chemotherapy in early stage breast cancer). The combination of rapidly growing knowledge of the molecular underpinnings of carcinogenesis with the emergence of novel drugs will continue to contribute to the reduction of global cancer burden.

Landmark Papers

1. Druker BJ, Talpaz M, Resta DJ, et al. Efficacy and safety of a specific inhibitor of the BCR-ABL tyrosine kinase in chronic myeloid leukemia. N Engl J Med 2001;344:1031-7.
2. Fisher B, Costantino JP, Wickerham DL, et al. Tamoxifen for prevention of breast cancer: report of the National Surgical Adjuvant Breast and Bowel Project P-1 Study. J Natl Cancer Inst 1998;90:1371-88.
3. Folkman J. Tumor angiogenesis: therapeutic implications. N Engl J Med 1971;285:1182-6.
4. Fry DW, Kraker AJ, McMichael A, et al. A specific inhibitor of the epidermal growth factor receptor tyrosine kinase. Science 1994;265:1093-5.
5. Howell A, Cuzick J, Baum M, et al. Results of the ATAC (Arimidex, Tamoxifen, Alone or in Combination) trial after completion of 5 years' adjuvant treatment for breast cancer. Lancet 2005;365:60-2.
6. Hurwitz H, Fehrenbacher L, Novotny W, et al. Bevacizumab plus irinotecan, fluorouracil and leucovorin for metastatic colorectal cancer. N Engl J Med 2004;350:2335-42.
7. Leung DW, Cachianes G, Kuang WJ, Goeddel DV, Ferrara N. Vascular endothelial growth factor is a secreted angiogenic mitogen. Science 1989;246:1306-9.
8. Lynch TJ, Bell DW, Sordella R, et al. Activating mutations in the epidermal growth factor receptor underlying responsiveness of non-small-cell lung cancer to gefitinib. N Engl J Med 2004;350:2129-39.
9. Miller K, Wang M, Gralow J, et al. Paclitaxel plus bevacizumab versus paclitaxel alone for metastatic breast cancer. N Engl J Med 2007;357:2666-76.
10. Oettle H, Post S, Neuhaus P, et al. Adjuvant chemotherapy with gemcitabine vs observation in patients undergoing curative-intent resection of pancreatic cancer: a randomized controlled trial. JAMA 2007;297:267-77.
11. Paez JG, Janne PA, Lee JC, et al. EGFR mutations in lung cancer: correlation with clinical response to gefitinib therapy. Science 2004;304:1497-500.
12. Paik S, Tang G, Shak S, et al. Gene expression and benefit of chemotherapy in women with node-negative, estrogen receptor-positive breast cancer. J Clin Oncol 2006;24:3726-34.
13. Sandler A, Gray R, Perry MC, et al. Paclitaxel-carboplatin alone or with bevacizumab for non-small-cell lung cancer. N Engl J Med 2006;355:2542-50.
14. Slamon DJ, Clark GM, Wong SG, Levin WJ, Ullrich A, McGuire WL. Human breast cancer: correlation of relapse and survival with amplification of the HER-2/neu oncogene. Science 1987;235:177-82.
15. Slamon DJ, Leyland-Jones B, Shak S, et al. Use of chemotherapy plus a monoclonal antibody against HER2 for metastatic breast cancer that overexpresses HER2. N Engl J Med 2001;344:783-92.

14

Principles of Radiotherapy

Joel S Greenberger

Introduction

In the modern era, the principles of clinical radiation oncology/radiation therapy include a wide expanse of new topics which extend beyond those originally defined by the pioneers of the field. In clinical radiotherapy, the dose/time/fractionation principles have been modified to include consideration of dose rate, transit volumes, dose/volume histograms and X-ray drug interactions. There is also concern for quality of the radiation beam, concerns for "field within a field" radiation boost techniques and the molecular biology of radiation repair. In radiation therapy physics, the principles of high linear energy transfer (LET) beams have now been extended to include concerns for secondary photon-generated high LET particle scatter in patients receiving intensity modulated radiotherapy (IMRT) using high energy photons but now with moving multileaf collimators that require longer beam-on time and more neutron scatter from photons hitting the primary collimator jaws and multileaf collimator secondary jaws. Finally, radiation biology has witnessed an explosion of new ideas including insight into an understanding of the molecular mechanisms of irradiation damage, the capacity to generate targeted small molecule radiation protectors and radiation sensitizers for specific tissues or tumors and the concept of the "cancer stem cell" which adds a new dimension to the basic four Rs of radiation biology (see inset). Furthermore, normal tissue stem cells involvement in tissue repair presents a new opportunity.

Four "Rs" of Radiation Biology
Reoxygenation
Redistribution
Repopulation
Repair

The availability of new potent chemotherapeutic agents and biological response modifiers that are used in combined modality protocols with irradiation promises a high degree of radiocontrollability of tumors in a variety of anatomic locations. However, these new targeted agents pose a challenge for radiation oncologists who now must be more concerned about the primary goal of radiation oncology, namely improving the therapeutic ratio. This chapter will address contemporary concerns about the radiation oncologist's approaching to care of the cancer patient, new concerns in the team approach (surgeon/medical oncologist/radiation oncologist) and new strategies which must apply to ensure safe, effective and high quality of care.

Therapeutic Ratio

Henry S Kaplan, MD, member of the National Academy of Sciences, past Chairman of the Department of Radiation Oncology at Stanford University School of Medicine and pioneer in the treatment of Hodgkin's Disease, was also a phenomenal teacher. When visiting the Harvard Joint Center for Radiation Therapy in 1970s and lecturing the then residents he said:

"When one is required to aim a beam, one is obligated to have a higher level of intellectual curiosity".

For physicians learning the principles of radiation oncology in 1970s, the then available 3-dimensional treatment planning tools presented 2-dimensional printouts of radiation isodose curves. There was the availability of an atlas of human anatomy, opportunity to view 3-D CT scans and opportunities for intraoperative observation of anatomy at the time of surgical radioseed and radiation brachytherapy source placement. These tools provided some guide in planning external beam radiotherapy of cancer relative to normal tissue anatomy. The ability to go to the operating room and participate with the surgeon in the identification of treatment volumes at risk for tumor local recurrence was then not easily replaced by scans or X-rays.

Current residents in radiation oncology training programs have available additional tools to complement their armamentarium in radiation therapy treatment planning, including algorhythms to plot dose/volume histograms (the percentage of an organ, for example lung, that receives 70% of the prescribed tumor dose, the percent that receives 30% of the tumor dose, etc.). Elaborate computer-based work stations in which anatomic representations of normal anatomy and tumor volume can be rotated in 3-dimensions and perhaps most importantly the availability of sophisticated radiation oncology delivery devices that can tailor dose within millimeters to irregularly shaped tumor volumes. These devices include IMRT, beams, image guided radiotherapy (IGRT) devices such as cone beam CT (which attaches to the linear accelerator for daily field checks) and sophisticated small volume/high fraction delivery devices including CyberKnife, Trilogy and Synergy Systems.

In the modern era, it is even more critical to heed Dr Kaplan's admonition. The standard of care in Radiation Oncology and our quality assurance programs demand attention to a higher level of detail. The radiation oncologist must ask: What am I targeting? Why? What is the expected toxicity? The concept of the therapeutic ratio has not changed since 1970s. Simply stated, the principle means that if radiation dose escalation to a tumor target is to be achieved by increasing the fraction size (daily dose), total volume of tissue treated, or total cumulative dose delivered in an attempt to control or prevent the regrowth of cancer in that particular target volume, then one must also account for the expected added damage to normal tissue. Another concern which has not changed is the awareness of acute and chronic radiation side effects, most of which are exacerbated by the addition of new systemic chemotherapeutic agents and biological response modifiers to combined modality regimens.

The therapeutic ratio (damage to tumor/normal tissue) is dependent upon not only ionizing radiation but also other agents in the cancer treatment program.

The process of decision making for lung cancer patients serves as an excellent model for all anatomic sites. For example, the use of Carboplatinum and Taxol chemotherapeutic agents in the management of patients with locally advanced non-small cell lung cancer presents concerns for acute radiotherapy complications including esophagitis and pneumonitis. Radiotherapy treatment planning for each patient also must account for past surgery, degree of postoperative recovery and comorbid medical conditions such as emphysema. Treatment planning requires not only attention to detail for radiation therapy but also the heightened degree of "intellectual curiosity" as to outcome of the total program as cited above.

For example, in treating a patient with Stage IIIB non-small cell lung cancer of the left lung, involving multiple visible hilar nodes on CT, PET-CT, or other image scans, the radiation oncologist must decide whether or not to include all sites of these positive nodes as well as the area of gross disease in the primary tumor volume, one must also plan for conedown/reduced field radiotherapy volume to any residual disease seen on a second PET/CT scan carried out after the primary treatment course is completed. If Carboplatinum and Taxol, Etopicide, Navelbine or other effective chemotherapy drugs are to be included in the regimen and if surgery is not contemplated, a seven and a half week course of radiotherapy or even longer course may be planned. The volume of the primary treatment field will determine the incidence and severity of esophagitis which is observed in over a third of patients requiring a treatment break, or possibly hospital admission for treatment of dehydration, severe nutritional deficit and severe dysphagia.

Lung inhomogeneity correction dose calculations in treatment planning, use of multifield conformal techniques and the availability of IMRT and respiratory gating can decrease the normal tissue volume treated in many patients and may reduce the percent of normal tissue receiving a significant portion of the dose fraction by dose volume histogram calculation. However, adding Carboplatinum and Taxol may act against this careful planning and increase the toxicity to levels expected before such planning. Sophisticated planning techniques are now routine and expected in modern radiotherapy approaches to such a patient. However, "intellectual curiosity" that must accompany the treatment planning has not changed. Radiation oncologists are asking the same questions with regard to combined modality treatment of lung and other thoracic cancers, compared to those questions asked in 1970s regarding the toxicity of the then new drug Adriamycin.

The radiation oncologist must always plan treatments considering the following issues: Should all suspected gross disease detected in diagnostic scanning be included in the primary tumor volume? Should sites of suspected microscopic disease based on known natural history of a particular cancer be included in the primary treatment volume? What is a safe dose and fraction size required to achieve local control of gross disease? Is a reduced field/conedown/boost therapy course safe to deliver to this patient?

There may be selected stage IIIA and IIIB NSCLCA patients who may benefit from surgical excision after the initial course of radiotherapy. The radiation oncologist must ask: What would be the expected improvement in the quality of life for patients completing a reduced field 7½ week radiotherapy compared to those receiving instead the initial field radiotherapy 5½ weeks and surgical excision?

Whenever a new biological response modifier, or new chemotherapy drug becomes available, to add to protocols for management of non-small cell lung cancer as well as any other forms of cancer, these questions must again be asked and answers reviewed in detail. The answers may be very different.

Normal Tissue Tolerance and Modern Principles of Radiotherapy

Modern radiotherapy treatment planning techniques and sophisticated treatment delivery devices are now routinely used to optimize radiotherapeutic approaches for the cancer patient. Modern PET/CT scan fusion techniques, MRI scans and novel techniques for imaging hypoxic regions within visibly gross cancer, as well as microscopic invisible areas through scanning for tumor antigen positive regions, present new challenges to the treatment planning strategy **(Figure 14-1)**. Surgical staging has improved dramatically and minimally invasive techniques for sampling nodal stations and modern molecular biologic histopathology techniques (including the use of polymerase chain reaction for detection of tumor gene transcripts in microscopic nodal disease), allow a higher degree of certainty in tumor positive and tumor negative areas compared to that available forty years ago. However, patients in the modern era experience the same toxicity of normal tissue damage from radiotherapy as did patients treated with a plan based upon less reliable diagnostic evaluation. Acute radiation side effects can clearly be reduced by decreasing the total treatment volume. This strategy becomes more difficult, as sophisticated preoperative diagnostic staging techniques add more options to the decision process. Radiotherapy fraction size reduction also decreases acute side effects.

However, basic radiobiology has not changed and fraction sizes below 1.8 Gy per day may not be effective in producing local control without increasing the overall number of fractions and treatment duration time, which reintroduces the same concern for increased toxicity.

Further improvements in therapeutic ratio have been attempted by investigators seeking to tip the balance of the ratio in favor of normal tissue by either increasing relative sensitivity of tumor cells or increasing the relative radioresistance of normal tissues.

Tumor Radiosensitizers

Attempts to increase the therapeutic ratio by sensitizing tumors have been the most attractive approach in clinical radiotherapy trials over the past 30 years. Administration of radiosensitizers requires bioavailability of the drug to tumor cells, thus, a conundrum rapidly emerges. If large tumors have hypoxic or hypovascular areas, how will the intravenously administered sensitizer get to the tumor **(Figure 14-1)?** Fractionated radiotherapy and multiple administrations of tumor radiosensitizers led to the discovery that the vascular supply to hypoxic areas does shift and does change during a multiweek radiotherapy fractionated course. Thus, delivery of radiosensitizers to tumors may not be clinically feasible. Many clinical trials of tumor radiosensitizations have included those with BUdR, p53 (given to p53 deficient lung cancer), EGFR receptor modulators for squamous tumors and others. While some optimistic results have been obtained from these trials, actual clinical alterations of therapeutic ratio leading to improved outcome have been difficult to conclude. Normal tissue toxicity of radiotherapy has remained a persistent problem. One possible interpretation of these studies is that the potential success of tumor radiosensitization motivated some investigators to increase overall radiotherapy dose, thus increasing normal tissue toxicity as described above.

Normal tissue radioprotectors are another approach to improving the therapeutic ratio. These have included a wide variety of agents administered either systemically or locally into specific organs. Systemic administration of WR2721 (Amifostine) has led to increased uptake in the salivary glands and associated radioprotection. Protection of other normal tissues selectively compared to tumor has been more difficult to demonstrate. Organ specific radioprotection by administration of manganese superoxide dismutase-plasmid liposomes has been successful in experimental model systems with respect to protection of the lung, esophagus, oral cavity, bladder and intestine and new evidence suggests protection from not only the acute but also chronic side effects of total body irradiation in mice.

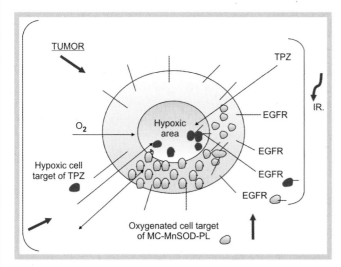

Figure 14-1: Tumor biology as related to definitive or perioperative radiation therapy. Diagram of poorly vascularized hypoxic areas in tumor, expression of epidermal growth factor receptor (EGFR) and strategies to radiosensitize tumor cells by plasmid mini circle-manganese superoxide dismutase (mc-MnSOD)(20) and Tirapazamine (TPZ) administration. These combinations may improve the radiocontrollability of human tumors without increasing normal tissue toxicity

Selective Tumor vs Normal Tissue Radiobiologic Effects

The ideal method by which to improve the therapeutic ratio would be one in which administration of the specific agent or agents would simultaneously protect normal tissue of sensitized tumors. The pioneering work of Larry Oberley and his colleagues first suggested that differences in the redox balance within tumor cells might provide a way to exploit such selective normal tissue protection/tumor radiosensitization. Oberley, St. Clair, Spitz and their colleagues demonstrated that squamous cell tumors, both human and experimental animal showed a decreased availability of manganese superoxide dismutase. One possible explanation was the shift to anaerobic metabolism of hypoxic and anoxic areas within tumor cells, obviating the need for cells to produce significant numbers of mitochondria and mitochondrial associated respiratory chain enzymes. Less production of free radicals from oxygen metabolism led to decreased requirement for a free radical neutralizing enzyme, such as manganese superoxide dismutase (MnSOD), which is mitochondrial localized. This logic led Oberley and his colleagues to investigate whether the adaptation of tumor cells to anaerobic metabolism could be used against them by reintroducing MnSOD through transgene administration. They reasoned that tumor cells having down regulated MnSOD might also have down regulated products used for neutralization of the MnSOD product, namely Hydrogen Peroxide. If this were the case, then tumor cells would demonstrate Hydrogen Peroxide toxicity and the introduction of MnSOD might actually produce a beneficial tumorcidal effect. These hypotheses were in fact proven correct. In other studies, MnSOD-PL transgene therapy showed a similar paradoxical increase in tumor local control with simultaneous normal tissue protection in both lung cancer and oral cavity cancer models.

Benefits of Minimally Invasive Surgery in Radiotherapy Patients

Normal tissue toxicity from radiotherapy is exacerbated by the toxicity of chemotherapeutic agents and also by the cytokine and trauma of the healing from surgery. In the example of lung cancer patients, replacement of standard thoracotomy with minimally invasive surgical approaches to segmentectomy, lobectomy, bilobectomy and minimally invasive techniques for surgical staging, including mediastinoscopy and microscopic staging using endobronchial ultrasound greatly reduced the normal tissue damage experienced by the patient, who is coming to start a plan of radiotherapy or chemoradiotherapy. Thus, initiation of a radiotherapy program was greatly improved in the patient experiencing a healing process

from a minimally invasive surgical approach compared to a large surgical field approach.

Preoperative radiotherapy followed by minimally invasive surgical techniques for lung cancer resection, or minimally invasive esophagectomy, in the case of preoperative radiotherapy for esophagus cancer, also produces significantly less toxicity and decreases acute radiotherapy side effects.

Benefits of Continuous Low Dose Infusion Chemotherapy in Radiotherapy Patients

The four Rs of radiotherapy include repopulation and redistribution of cells in the cell cycle. The timing of cell entry into chemotherapy sensitive phases of the cell cycle may not coincide with the time of the delivery of the 1 – 2 minute radiotherapy fraction. This logic led to the use of brachytherapy techniques in which radioisotope seed or brachytherapy sources were implanted into patients for continuous low dose rate irradiation. This principle still applies in patients receiving radioiodine or Gadolinium seed implantation for treatment of prostate cancer and radioiodine brachytherapy mesh techniques are still used in some lung cancer patients, who have a positive resection margin in the chest wall. For those patients receiving fractionated radiotherapy, usually one fraction per day, the addition of continuous infusion chemotherapy adds a new dimension to tumor control. Continuous infusion of 5-FU has proven a valuable addition to the combined modality protocol for patients with esophagus cancer and colorectal cancer. It is likely that the continuous infusion of other biological response modifiers and new chemotherapeutic agents will be added to protocols for radiotherapy patients and will provide further benefit with reduction of toxicity.

Radiotherapy in Cancer Care of the Future

Clinical radiotherapy is now linked very closely to diagnostic radiologic scanning techniques both for treatment planning and for monitoring accuracy of treatment delivery. It is likely that these radiologic scanning techniques will incorporate further new improvements in molecular biologic imaging. Imaging for hypoxic areas in tumors will allow the possibility for dose intensity modulation to areas of hypoxia giving relatively higher doses to these areas within the tumor. Since these areas may shift day to day, real time daily imaging of hypoxic areas may allow beam modulation techniques to focus on these sites. Treatment of microscopic deposits of cancer with multiple microbeams of irradiation can avoid normal tissue damage. As molecular imaging techniques become more sophisticated and the resolution of positive areas compared to negative areas appears feasible, the use of frameless stereotactic radiosurgery techniques can be applied to treat multiple metastatic lesions in the abdomen, chest and multiple sites. These techniques have already been applied successfully by utilized Gamma Knife for treatment of multiple brain metastases, now adding the techniques of CyberKnife, Trilogy and Synergy (Stereotactic Radiosurgery). The use of CyberKnife for treatment of multiple individual metastatic lesions in the liver, lung, head and neck region and multiple spinal metastases is also a common option for radiation oncologists. Adaptation of this kind of technique to external beam radiotherapy in which IMRT-like modulation of the beam can occur in real time linked to areas of positive scanning that day and change day to day will undoubtedly facilitate more normal tissue sparing and better targeted tumor therapy.

The area of normal tissue radioprotectors and tumor radiosensitizers has just begun to come of age. Understanding the molecular mechanism of tumor cell physiology at the single cell and 3-dimensional tumor level including changes in vascularity will allow design of new small molecule agents that can target tumor in normal tissue simultaneously and produce different effects. The different effects should include protection of normal tissue, adding sensitization to the tumor and the final benefit of preventing transformation at a later date of normal cells in the irradiated volume to secondary cancers.

Studies of the late effects of radiotherapy in cancer survivors continues to provide evidence of radiotherapeutic induction of new malignancies. Examples include a detection of breast cancer in patients cured of Hodgkin's disease and a detection of lung cancer in breast cancer patients cured of their breast cancer. The radiation induction of soft tissue sarcomas in previously high dose treated areas has been known for decades. Modulation of radiotherapy techniques to minimize normal tissue malignant transformation as well as acute toxicity will be a persistent goal for the future.

Conclusions

Modern radiation oncology demands attention to classic principles of cancer patient management. The availability of new techniques in radiotherapy treatment planning and precise dose delivery tools has posed a tempting argument that higher doses can be delivered to larger volumes of tissues while maintaining a safe outcome for the patient. Adding toxic chemotherapeutic drugs and biological response modifiers to the modern radiotherapy approach further poses a challenge to stay within acceptable levels of normal tissue toxicity. More than ever, the radiation oncologist must collaborate closely with surgeon, medical oncologist and all physicians caring for the cancer patient to ensure that a safe therapeutic dose is delivered with minimal toxicity.

Landmark Papers

1. Vistad, Ingvild, Cvancarova, Milada, Fossa, Dorothea S, Kristensen, Gunnar B. Postradiotherapy morbidity in long-term survivors after locally advanced cervical cancer: how well do physicians' assessments agree with those of their patients? Int J Radiation Oncology Biol Phys 2008; 71(5):1335-42.

2. Azria, David, Rosenstein, Barry S, Ozsahin, Mahmut. Radiation-induced side effects with or without systemic therapies: Prime time for prediction of individual radiosensitivity. Int J Radiation Oncology Biol Phys 2008; 71(5):1293-4.

3. Suzuki, Osamu, Yoshioka, Yasuo, Isohashi, Fumiaki, et al. Effect of high-dose-rate ^{192}Ir source activity on late rectal bleeding after intracavitary radiation therapy for uterine cervix cancer. Int J Radiation Oncology Biol Phys 2008;71(5):1329-34.

4. Hall Eric J, Phil D. Intensity-modulated radiation therapy, protons and the risk of second cancers. Int J Radiation Oncology Biol Phys 2006;65(1):1-7.

5. Schultheiss, Timothy E. The radiation dose-response of the human spinal cord. Int J Radiation Oncology Biol Phys 2008; 71(5):1455-9.

6. Bakkenist CJ, Kastan MB. DNA damage activates ATM through intermolecular autophosphorylation and dimmer dissociation. Nature 2003;421:499-504.

7. Hill Richard P. Identifying cancer stem cells in solid tumors: Case not proven. Cancer Res 2006;66(4):1891-6.

8. Epperly MW, Gretton JE, Bernarding M, Nie S, Rasul B, Greenberger JS. Mitochondrial localization of copper/zinc superoxide dismutase (Cu/ZnSOD) confers radioprotective functions in vitro and in vivo. Radiation Research 2003;160:568-78.

9. Kaplan HS. The radical radiotherapy of regionally localized Hodgkin's disease. Radiology 1962;78:553-61.

10. Hall EJ. In Radiobiology for the Radiologist (4th edn). Philadelphia, PA, JB Lippincott, Inc., 1999.

11. Chute JP, et al. Transplantation of vascular endothelial cells mediates the hematopoietic recovery and survival of lethally irradiated mice. Blood 2007;109:2365-72.

12. Greenberger JS, Epperly MW. Radioprotective antioxidant gene therapy: potential mechanisms of action. Gene Ther Mol Biol 2004;8:31-44.

13. Oberley LW, Oberley TD. Free radicals, cancer and aging. In Johnson JE, Walford R, Harmon D, Miquel J (Eds): Free Radicals, Aging and Degenerative Diseases. R Liss, Inc., 1986;325-81.

14. Zhong W, Oberley LW, Oberley TD, St Clair DK. Suppression of the malignant phenotype of human glioma cells by overexpression of manganese superoxide dismutase. Oncogene 1997;14:481-90.

15. Spitz DR, et al. Oxygen toxicity in control and H_2O_2-resistant Chinese hamster fibroblasts. Archiv Biochem Biophys 1990;279:249-60.

16. Nair CKK, Parida DK, Nomura T. Radioprotectors in radiotherapy. J Radiat Res 2001;42:21-37.

17. Hahn SM, et al. Identification of nitroxide radioprotectors. Radiation Research 1992;132:87-93.

18. Basu Swati K, Schwartz Cindy, Fisher Susan G, Hudson Melissa M, Tarbell Nancy, Muhs Ann, et al. Unilateral and bilateral breast cancer in women surviving pediatric Hodgkin's disease. Int J Radiation Oncology Biol Phys 2008;72(1):34-46.

19. Epperly Michael W, Smith Tracy, Wang Hong, Schlesselman James, Franicola Darcy, Greenberger Joel S. Modulation of total body irradiation induced life shortening by systemic intravenous MnSOD-plasmid liposome gene therapy. Rad Res (in press).

20. Zhang Xichen, Epperly Michael W, Kay Mark A, Chen Zhi-Ying, Smith Tracy, Franicola Darcy, et al. Radioprotection in vitro and in vivo by minicircle plasmid carrying the human manganese superoxide dismutase transgene. Human Gene Therapy 2008;19:820-6.

21. Evans JW, et al. Homologous recombination is the principal pathway for the repair of DNA damage induced by Tirapazamine in mammalian cells. Cancer Res 2008;68:257-65.

15

Principles of Biologic Therapy

Antonio Romo de Vivar Chavez, Michael E de Vera, Michael T Lotze

Introduction

Biologic therapy represents a relatively new treatment strategy that involves the use of agents that modify the tumor-host interaction and elicit tumor regression. Rather than targeting intracellular pathways, this type of therapy primarily targets the cell surface expression of stress factors or novel tumor peptides expressed in major histocompatability molecules. As such, biologic therapy promotes and restores a host antitumor response as well as diminishes tumor immune escape mechanisms. Examples of biologic agents include recombinant cytokines such as Interleukin (IL)-2, interferon γ, as well as cytotoxic cells and viral therapy. Initially aimed to modify immune response to tumor, hence also called immunotherapy current biologic therapy involves strategies that seek to modify cell death mechanisms, cell metabolism and the tumor microenvironment. Recent evidence suggests a link between the immune response, the redox state of tumor cells, pH regulation and cell death mechanisms. The individual sites of action of immuno-therapy or biologic therapy are illustrated in **Figure 15-1**.

Inflammation and Immune Responses in the Origin, Progression and Treatment of Cancer

Rudolf Virchow suggested in 1863 that the origin of cancer was at sites of chronic inflammation. He observed that irritants and inflammation enhanced cellular proliferation. Today, we know that cancer is not only a hyperpro-liferative disorder but also that cell proliferation alone does not cause cancer, rather, the development of malignant cells is tightly related to a disorder or lack of cell death. Growing evidence suggests that the setting in which cell proliferation takes place plays a crucial role in the development of cancer. DNA damaging agents coupled with an environment rich in inflammatory cells, activated epithelial and stromal cells, cytokines and growth factors, certainly potentiate neoplastic risk. These proneoplastic factors come together in the setting of chronic tissue damage.

The host's efforts to repair damage and fight infection are now known to be mediated by "alarm signals" derived from tissues, also known as damage associated molecular pattern (DAMP) molecules. These molecules, although crucial for tissue repair during wound healing, may contribute to tumor growth, progression and invasiveness and even disrupt the cell mediated host antitumor immune response. Furthermore, a chronic inflammatory state by itself can induce or promote neoplastic transformation. Production of free radicals such as reactive oxygen intermediates hydroxyl radicals (OH.-) and superoxide (O2.-) and /or reactive nitrogen intermediates such as nitric oxide (NO.) and peroxinitrite (ONOO.), initially described as antimicrobial molecules, may have a "double-agent" role in the development of cancer by leading to oxidative damage and nitration of DNA bases, promoting DNA mutations.

As the tumor progresses over time, due to "Darwinian" selection, emerging tumor cells become capable of maintaining this pro-survival/pro-proliferative environment independent of a wound like stroma. Regulating and manipulating this complex tumor-host interaction is the basis for biologic therapy. The principles of some of the current approaches in biologic cancer therapy will be discussed in this chapter.

Brief History of Biologic Therapy

Immunotherapy or biologic therapy is a relatively new approach in cancer therapy. Biological therapy has been used in medicine for more than 200 years, dating back to the development of vaccines. Edward Jenner utilized fluid from cattle infected with cowpox to inject humans and reported benefits and further studies led him to develop the smallpox vaccine. Jenner's smallpox immunization studies also provided early experimental support for the concept of immune memory. A century later, immune modifiers were used to treat cancer patients by a German physician, Busch and then by a New York surgeon, William Coley. Coley observed spontaneous tumor regression following bacterial, fungal, viral and protozoal infections.

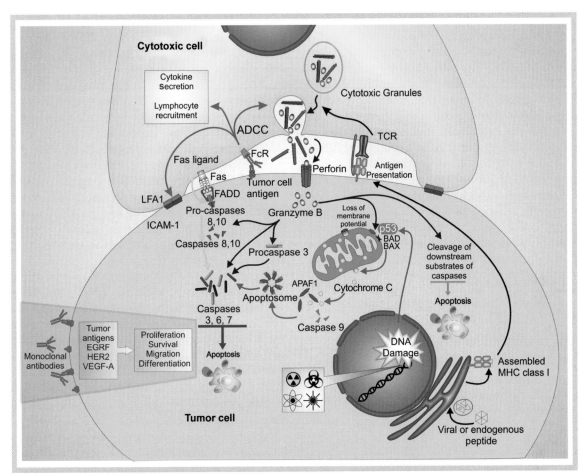

Figure 15-1: Diagram of the cell illustrating sites of action of available and emerging therapies. Overexpressed molecules on the tumor cell surface (box), also called tumor-associated antigens (TAAs), can be receptors that transduce critical signal pathways such as cell proliferation, survival, differentiation and migration. Epidermal growth factor receptor (EGFR) is an overexpressed receptor present in tumors and is the target of Cetuximab, matuzumab and panitumumab. HER2 is a glycoprotein involved in signal transduction pathways leading to cell growth and differentiation, overexpressed in invasive breast cancer, trastuzumab and pertuzumab target HER2 and block signal transduction. Antibodies making use of the Fc portion of the molecule induce antibody-dependent cell-mediated cytotoxicity (ADCC) (green arrows) or complement-dependent cytotoxicity (CDC) (not shown). ADCC contributes to the anti-tumor effects of trastuzumab. FcR bearing effector cells play a predominant role in the *in vivo* anti-tumor effects of Rituximab. During ADCC, three components are required: the antigen bearing cancer cell, an Fc receptor (FcR) bearing effector cell and the antibody that will mediate the formation of an immunological synapse between these two cells stabilized by LFA1 to ICAM. Effector cells when activated also release cytokines and chemokines, such as interferon(IFN)-γ, that also have antitumor effects, inhibiting cell proliferation and angiogenesis, promoting autophagy and upregulating the expression of MHC molecules leading to better tumor antigen presentation (black arrows). NK cells express a Fas-receptor ligands (FasL) on the cell surface that interacts with Fas on the tumor cell to activate the so called extrinsic apoptotic pathway (yellow arrows). Two apoptosis signaling pathways are illustrated. The intrinsic pathway (red arrows), initiated by caspase 9, is dependent on mitochondrial signals. This pathway involves p53-mediated activation and cytochrome C release from mitochondria. The extrinsic pathway (yellow arrows) involves activation of caspase 8 and represents a p53-independent apoptosis. Fas-FasL interaction activates its associated intracellular death domain and subsequently activates caspase 8 which in turn activates downstream caspases 3, 6 and 7 or effector caspases which are the start of the common pathway of apoptosis (Purple arrow). Cytotoxic cells (mainly NK cells) have also alternative mechanisms for killing their targets, which primarily involve the perforin-mediated trafficking of a family of proteases, the granzymes. CTL/NK cells deliver these proteins by mobilization of secretory granules into the immunological synapse. The recognition of a target cell triggers a rearrangement of microtubules polarized towards the immunological synapse and directs granules towards the plasma membrane followed by delivery of the granule contents into the synaptic space. Perforin embeds in the target cell plasma membrane forming a pore through which granzymes can pass directly into the cytosol. Granzyme B interacts with apoptotic processes at several levels (blue arrows), it directly cleaves and activates caspase-3, -6, -7, -8 -9 and -10 and indirectly activates caspase-2, -6 and -9 through caspase-3 cleavage; triggers mitochondrial permeabilization and release of cytochrome C followed by the formation of the apoptosome and activation of the downstream caspases; cleaves downstream substrates of caspases (orange arrow), disrupting structural proteins and DNA with alteration of the mitotic potential of tumor cells

This inspired Coley to work in the development of cancer immunotherapy and developed a killed bacterial vaccine for cancer in the late 1800s. Indeed the immune system can discriminate between healthy cells and cancerous cells. In the early 1900s, Nobel Prize winner Paul Ehrlich described "side chain" molecules carried on the surfaces of the cells. Ehrlich believed that antibodies could bind these molecules and suggested the possibility of creating antibodies to deliver drugs or toxins to tumor cells, a concept he called the "magic bullet". Decades later Georges Köhler, César Milstein and Niels Kaj Jerne shared the 1984 Nobel Prize for the discovery of monoclonal antibodies. In 1980s, the FDA approved the use of interferon for the treatment of hairy-cell leukemia, chronic myelogenous leukemia and Kaposi's sarcoma. In 1992, recombinant IL-2 received FDA approval for the treatment of metastatic kidney cancer and several years later for melanoma.

Immunotherapy

Approaches to Immunotherapy

Immunotherapy can be either active or passive. The active approach elicits a host generated immune response in the patient to target malignant cells. The passive approach involves administration of immune molecules or effector cells that have direct effects on the tumor.

Passive Immunotherapy (Antibodies, T-cells and NK-cells)

Antibodies can be targeted toward overexpressed molecules on the tumor cell surface, also called tumor-associated antigens (TAAs), against specific soluble molecules, or work through signaling mechanisms. Overexpressed antigens can be receptors that transduce very critical signal pathways such as cell proliferation, survival, differentiation, migration, etc. Epidermal growth factor receptor (EGFR) is one example of an overexpressed receptor and is present in up to 50% of all cancers and in up to 80% of metastatic colon cancer. Cetuximab, matuzumab and panitumumab are all monoclonal antibodies directed against this receptor. HER2, a glycoprotein involved in signal transduction pathways leading to cell growth and differentiation, is overexpressed primarily due to gene amplification in 25-30% of invasive breast cancer and is correlated with poor survival and drug resistance. The natural ligand for HER2 has not been identified but trastuzumab and pertuzumab target this glycoprotein and inhibit signal transduction.

VEGF stimulates proliferation and migration and inhibits apoptosis of endothelial cells. It also increases vascular permeability and vasodilatation. Bevacizumab is a monoclonal antibody directed against VEGF-A. Used as an antiangiogenic agent, it has improved response duration and survival rates in colorectal cancer patients receiving the drug as part of a chemotherapy regimen as compared with standard chemotherapy alone. Survival benefits in patients with non-small cell lung cancer and breast cancer are also seen.

Another group of antibodies now approved for cancer treatment work in a more physiological way by making use of the Fc portion of the molecule to induce antibody-dependent cell-mediated cytotoxicity (ADCC) or complement-dependent cytotoxicity (CDC). Trastuzumab is a monoclonal antibody specific for HER2 and is thought to act by multiple mechanisms to exert its antitumor effects. *In vitro* studies have shown that trastuzumab kills HER2 positive but not HER2 negative cancer cells through ADCC. *In vivo* studies suggest that ADCC contributes to the antitumor effects of trastuzumab. Rituximab is a monoclonal antibody against CD20, which is widely expressed on B-cells from early stages of differentiation and lost in mature antibody-producing plasma cells. Rituximab is used in the treatment of B cell non-Hodgkin's lymphoma, B-cell leukemias and some autoimmune disorders. Although the exact mode of action of rituximab is unclear, FcR bearing effector cells play a predominant role in the *in vivo* antitumor effects of this agent, non-ADCC mechanisms have also been identified.

During ADCC, antibodies direct the effector limb of the innate immune response to kill cancer cells expressing a specific antigen. Three components are required for the process of cell mediated cytolysis: the antigen bearing cancer cell, an Fc receptor (FcR) bearing effector cell and the antibody that will mediate the formation of an immunological synapse between these two cells stabilized by LFA1 to ICAM **(see Figure 15-1)**. The binding of the FcR to the Fc portion of the antibody activates the cytotoxic cell. NK or other effector cells when activated not only induce tumor cell death but also release cytokines and chemokines, such as interferon(IFN)-γ, that also have antitumor effects, inhibiting cell proliferation and angiogenesis, promoting autophagy and upregulating the expression of MHC molecules leading to better tumor antigen presentation. As illustrated in **Figure 15-1**, NK cells release cytotoxic granules containing perforin and granzymes that induce tumor cell death in both caspase-dependent and caspase-independent pathways. NK cells also express a Fas-receptor ligand (FasL) on the cell surface that interacts with Fas on the tumor cell to activate the so called extrinsic apoptotic pathway. Furthermore, antigen stimulated cytotoxic T lymphocytes (CTLs) and activated NK cells produce a variety of cytokines. This cytokine-dependent cell cytotoxicity (CDCC) activates local macrophages and lymphocytes mainly through TNF and IFN-γ secretion and promotes a TH1 response, further stimulating differentiated CTLs. Multiple chemokines also released during the immune reaction help recruit additional lymphocytes. NK cells also produce GM-CSF,

IL-5, IL-10 and IL-13 which provide them immune regulatory capabilities.

During malignant transformation, tumor cells down regulate expression of MHC class I molecules either by somatic mutation or selection, sometimes resulting in the complete loss of the antigen presenting machinery and leading to ineffective host CTL effector functions. NK cells, on the other hand, are part of the innate immune system and execute their function by either eliminating cells in which MHC class I molecules are down regulated on the cell surface or stressed cells expressing NKG2D ligands. Several mechanisms for the loss of the antigen presenting capability important for CTL recognition and effector responses resulting in tumor "escape" mechanisms have been identified. The loss of HLA expression by itself, however, is insufficient to confer NK cell activation and cytotoxicity against tumor cells and several mechanisms may be at play. NK cells may not efficiently reach the target cell within the tumor, or an NK activating receptor (such as NKG2D) may be down regulated or not inducible. CTL and NK cells also likely play other functional roles by the release of interferons, thereby promoting enhanced autophagic flux in some threatened epithelial cells.

Other approaches to passive immunotherapy include the use of tumor-specific effector cells. This cellular immunotherapy requires the presence of specific antigens expressed on the surface of tumor cells (TAAs) that effector cells can target selectively, minimizing toxicity to the normal host tissue. The presence of specific antigens in tumor cells and the lack of control of the tumor by the immune system suggest that antigen recognition by itself is not sufficient to achieve an appropriate immune response against cancer cells. Tumor cells, even in the presence of MHC class I, may lack costimulatory signals, rendering T cells to a state of anergy in which they not only fail to activate, but are also unresponsive to subsequent stimuli, particularly when the T cells gain access to secondary lymphoid sites. Furthermore, the presence of regulatory T (T_{reg}) cells and other lymphocytes may interefere with tumor cell cytotoxicity. Therefore, cell therapy approaches often apply effector cells that have been manipulated either by cytokine activation, genetic manipulation and/or *in vitro* expansion.

Adoptive Cellular Therapy

Adoptive cellular therapy (ACT) most frequently consists of using the patient's own T lymphocytes that have been stimulated and expanded *ex vivo* and reinfused into the patient. The use of autologous tumor infiltrating leuko-cytes (TIL) has shown to be effective ACT in patients with metastatic melanoma. Application of TIL plus high dose IL-2 showed an overall response rate of 36% in 86 patients. Response rates positively correlate with several factors including the ability of T cells to traffic to tumor deposits,

the proliferative potential of TIL and the ability to lyse autologous tumor cells *in vitro*; telomere length also correlates with responsiveness which is also tightly related with the TIL proliferative potential. Use of high dose IL-2 and preparative application of nonmyeloablative chemo-therapy and radiation therapy appear to also be critical for TIL effectiveness.

In vitro cultured lymphokine activated killer (LAK) cells have also been shown to induce regression of small pulmonary metastases and prolong survival in preclinical studies. Clinical studies have shown complete tumor responses in patients with advanced cancer receiving adoptive immunotherapy; however, there have been no significant outcome differences in patients receiving LAK cells plus IL-2 compared with IL-2 alone.

T_{reg} cells are found reciprocally with effector cells within the immune system and have the ability to suppress effector T-cell functions. T_{regs} act to inhibit autoimmune responses but also may suppress tumor-specific T-cell responses. There is an increase in T_{reg} cells in cancer patients both at the tumor site and within the circulation. Not surprisingly, strategies that deplete T_{regs} have been used and shown to improve responses to therapy. ACT objective responses benefit from prior lymphodepletion due to the abolition of T_{reg} cells and probably the depletion of normal lymphocytes competing for regulatory cytokines.

Active Immunotherapy (Vaccination, DCs, etc.)

Tumor-specific immunity is initiated critically and then regulated by antigen presenting cells. Dendritic cells (DCs) play a critical role in the development of primary immunity as well as tolerance. DCs are professional antigen presenting cells capable of fully activating naïve T cells. Its dual role depends on the type of DC. Immature DCs are localized at sites of antigen capture in the tissues and express costimulatory signals weakly; the lack of costimulatory signals renders the T-cell anergic, promoting tolerance. In contrast mature DCs are located at sites of high T-cell traffic within secondary lymphoid sites and their costimulatory signals and inflammatory cytokine expression is unregulated, making them potent stimulators of effector T-cells. Several trials have been carried out by administering single or multiple peptides from tumor-associated antigens designed to couple T cells with MHC class I or II molecules.

To be effective, vaccination with antigens requires intact mechanisms of antigen presentation, recognition and the appropriate costimulation of effector cells. Vaccination strategies using single tumor antigens, although potentially targeting an immune response to specific cancer cells, are likely to be unsuccessful due to immune escape mechanisms that lead to tumor establish-ment in the first place.

Cancer patients often have quantitative and functional deficiencies in DCs associated with tumor immune tolerance. Within the tumor microenvironment, DC maturation is inhibited by tumor secreted molecules such as VGEF, TGFβ and IL-10, thus promoting tolerance. In patients with multiple myeloma, factors from within the bone marrow inhibit DC maturation and function, mediated in part by local release of IL-6 and TGFβ. One approach to overcome immune escape mechanisms is the use of autologous DCs that are pulsed *in vitro* with single antigens or tumor cell lysates and reinfused into the patient. DCs are the most powerful antigen-presenting cells and can present tumor antigens to CD8+ and CD4+ T cells as well as activate NK cells and regulate antibody mediated immunity. This approach has resulted in objective clinical responses in a small number of patients in individual clinical trials. Although tumor specific immunity can be induced, a correlation with significant and durable clinical responses has rarely been achieved. Clinical trials use various methods for DC isolation, maturation, stimulation and loading for DC vaccination and a standard protocol has not been established. DC immunotherapy, however, has proven to be very safe and to induce tumor-specific immune responses. The development of treatment related toxicity and the incidence of autoimmunity is rare when compared with other types of immunotherapy. Future efforts may focus on combining DC vaccination with other therapies to enhance clinical efficacy.

Modern Immunotherapy

Enhancing Non-necrotic Cell Death

Effector cells within the immune system target cell death mechanisms to eliminate infected or malignant cells. Biologic therapy strategies involving these pathways have been developed. Tumor cells often present with defects or resistance in one or more components of the programmed cell death pathways. The apoptosis pathway has been studied extensively, particularly in cancer research in the last two decades. Two major apoptosis signaling pathways are recognized. The intrinsic pathway, initiated by caspase 9, is dependent on mitochondrial signals and is also the major target of chemotherapy or irradiation-induced cell death (see Figure 15-1). This pathway involves p53-mediated activation and cytochrome C release from mitochondria. The extrinsic pathway, by contrast, is initiated through death receptors on the cell surface, which include various members of the extended tumor necrosis factor (TNF) receptor superfamily. This pathway involves activation of caspase 8 and represents an alternative target that can induce p53-independent apoptosis in cancer cells that are resistant or have a defective intrinsic pathway of apoptosis. The extrinsic pathway can be initiated by cytotoxic cells through the expression of Fas or other members of the TNF receptor family expressed on the surface of target cells. Fas ligand (FasL) and TRAIL receptors play a role in driving these apoptosis pathways. They can activate the extrinsic apoptotic pathway which interestingly is defective in some tumor cells. These so-called death receptors and their intracellular or death domains are necessary for the transmission of apoptotic signals via the caspase cascade. As illustrated in **Figure 15-1**, Fas-FasL interaction activates its associated intracellular death domain and subsequently activates caspase 8. This initiates the extrinsic apoptosis pathway that activates downstream caspases 3, 6 and 7. In some tumors this pathway is impaired. Some melanomas overexpress FLICE inhibitory protein (FLIP), a caspase 8 inhibitor, making the tumor cells resistant to death domain-mediated apoptosis. Down regulation of Fas has been also found in some tumor cells including non-Hodgkin's lymphoma, multiple myeloma and melanoma as well as mutations detected in some mediators of the downstream pathways, although this remains an area checkered with controversy given the lack of assuredness of detection systems. TRAIL-induced apoptosis defect has also been found in tumor cells, either by down regulation of the TRAIL receptor (TRAIL-1) or by up-regulating "decoy" receptors such as TRAIL-DR3 and TRAIL-DR4.

Cytotoxic cells have also evolved alternative mechanisms for directly killing their targets and NK cells appear to rely predominantly in these mechanisms which primarily involve the perforin-mediated trafficking of a family of proteases, the granzymes. CTL/NK cells deliver these proteins by mobilization of secretory granules into the immunological synapse. This is the so-called perforin/granzyme pathway or "granule-dependent" killing. The recognition of a target cell triggers a rearrangement of microtubules polarized toward the immunological synapse and directs granules toward the plasma membrane followed by delivery of the granule contents into the synaptic space. Perforin, a pore forming protein, embeds in the target cell plasma membrane, presumably forming a pore through which granzymes can pass directly into the cytosol.

Granzymes are a family of serine proteases stored in CTL and NK cell granules. The human repertoire of granzymes include A, B, H, K and M with granzymes A and B being the most abundant and most extensively studied. Interestingly, granzyme B interacts with apoptotic processes at several levels, providing alternative means to activate cell death mechanisms. For example, it directly cleaves and activates caspase-3, -6, -7, -8 -9 and -10 and indirectly activates caspase-2, -6 and -9 through caspase-3 cleavage. Granzyme B also triggers mitochondrial permeabilization in a caspase independent manner involving release of cytochrome C followed by the formation of the apoptosome and activation of the downstream caspases cascade independently of p53. However, even in the absence of caspase activity, granzyme B effects on the mitochondria eventually leads to a decrease in ATP production. Furthermore, granzyme B cleaves downstream substrates of caspases, disrupting both structural proteins and DNA with consequent alteration of the mitotic potential of tumor cells.

Cytotoxic T cells are sensitive to cytokines such as IL-2 and IFN-γ, regulating their functional activity. Unlike CTL, NK cells have innate killing capacity that does not require exposure to previous stimuli, although recent information suggests that NK cells can expand and contract over shorter time periods with essentially a short-term memory phenotype. Both CTL and NK cells demonstrate significant increases in killing capacity when stimulated by cytokines and proinflammatory signals, becoming so-called lymphokine activated killer (LAK) cells.

Regulation of Suppressor Cells

CD4+ regulatory T cells are generated naturally during the development of the immune system in the thymus along with CD4+ T helper cells and CD8+ T cells. These cells enter the bloodstream and regulate effector T cells that escape thymic selection and thereby maintain peripheral tolerance against self-antigens and limit autoimmunity. T_{regs} express high levels of the alpha chain of IL-2 (CD25) critical for their maintenance, function and survival. T_{regs} do not produce IL-2 and, therefore, depend on IL-2 produced by other cells. The naturally occurring T_{regs} also express the more specific cell surface marker Foxp3. However, naïve T cells that are primed in the periphery under suboptimal conditions for effector T cell induction such as in a non-inflammatory microenvironment or inadequate TCR activation can also render a suppressive phenotype to the T cell. These cells are called adaptive T_{regs}.

The presence of T_{regs} within the tumor greatly affects the host immune response and the clinical outcome. These cells include natural T_{regs} (e.g. CD4+ CD25+ and Foxp3+) and tumor induced adaptive T_{regs} especially within epithelial sites. Depletion of local CD4+ T cells or blocking IL-10 *in vivo* results in increased effector function of CD8+ effector T cells and eradication of tumor in preclinical studies. Antibodies against CD25 enhance proliferation of effector T cells and increase production of IFN-γ. However, CD8+ T cells can also become adaptive T_{regs} in the tumor microenvironment and facilitate tumor escape. T_{regs} play an important role in controlling cancer immunity. Depletion of CD25+ T cells by monoclonal antibodies results in delay of tumor growth or even regression of already established tumors in murine models. Removal of T_{regs} before immunotherapy improves

antitumor efficacy in adoptive T cell therapy.

Cyclophosphamide is an alkylating agent with cytotoxic effects that can reduce the number and function of CD4+CD25 + T_{regs}. Cyclophosphamide treatment enhances apoptosis and decreases proliferation of T_{regs}. Expression of GITR and Foxp3 is down-regulated following administration, which decreases the suppressor function of T_{regs}. Selective elimination of CD4+CD25^{high} T_{regs} can also be achieved by administration of ONTAK, a recombinant IL-2 diphtheria toxin conjugate. This agent is thought to decrease protein synthesis due to delivery of the diphtheria toxin to cells with expression of high affinity IL-2 receptors (e.g. CD25). Treatment of patients with metastatic renal cell carcinoma showed a significant increase in the number of tumor-specific T cells following vaccination with RNA transfected DCs compared with vaccine alone. In ovarian cancer patients, a single dose of this IL-2/toxin decreased the number of circulating T_{regs}. The remaining T_{regs} showed diminished suppressor effects on effector T cells to a substantial degree. The IL-2/toxin, however, failed to eliminate T_{regs} in patients with metastatic melanoma.

Antibodies targeting the cytotoxic T lymphocyte antigen (CTLA)-4 have shown promising results in the treatment of patients with melanoma. CTLA-4 is one of two surface molecules, along with cell surface CD28, that counterbalances T cell inhibition and activation, respectively. The CTLA-4-CD28 axis has been an area of great interest in cancer immunotherapy. CTLA-4 effectively induces T-cell anergy and inhibits secretion of IL-2. CD28, in contrast, is a costimulator of T cell proliferation and IL-2 production. Ipilimumab and tremelimumab are under investigation in melanoma as a monotherapy, with vaccination, or in combination with chemotherapy with dacarbazine or IL-2 with overall response rates ranging from 13% to 17% and 22%, respectively. Ongoing phase I/II clinical trials for ONTAK and phase II/III for ipilimumab as well as other T_{regs} suppressor drugs are being evaluated as a potential role to improve current immunotherapy strategies.

Tumor Evasion of Immunity

Treatment Strategies

Increase antigen presentation: The interferons
Interferons were discovered in 1957 and described by Lindemann and Isaacs as secreted proteins that "interfered" with the ability of a virus to infect cells. There are two types of interferons characterized in humans (type I and type II), both of which can induce a state in which viral replication is impaired.

Type I interferons include IFN-α, IFN-β and IFN-ω. The genes for α interferons are redundant. At least 14 separate genes encode structurally distinct forms of these molecules. However, the receptor for type I interferons, termed IFNα/β, is the same and their actions are similar although their potencies do differ. This receptor is composed of two subunits—IFNAR1 and IFNAR2. Both IFNα and IFNβ increase the cytolytic activity of NK cells. INFNAR1 knockout mice have normal lymphoid development but are extremely susceptible to infections. Lymphokine-activated killer (LAK) cell activity is also increased with exposure to these agents. The antiviral action of type I interferons is one of its major effects. These molecules act on all cells to inhibit viral replication as well as cellular proliferation. The major mechanisms involve the inhibition of protein translation, upregulation of MHC class I and downregulation of MHC class II in addition to the promotion of autophagy. The type II interferon family has only one member, interferon-γ. IFN-γ is a major activator of macrophages, increasing their cytolytic potential by increasing production of ROS and RNS including hydrogen peroxide, nitric oxide and indoleamine dioxigenase. It upregulates MHC class II expression and acts on CD4+ T cells to promote Th1 differentiation while inhibiting Th2 cells. IFN-γ promotes maturation of CD8+ T cytotoxic cells and augments cytolytic function of NK cells.

Figure 15-2 illustrates the signaling pathway for type I and type II interferons. In addition to their effects on immune responses, interferons have non-immunologic, direct effects on tumor cells. Type I interferons inhibit

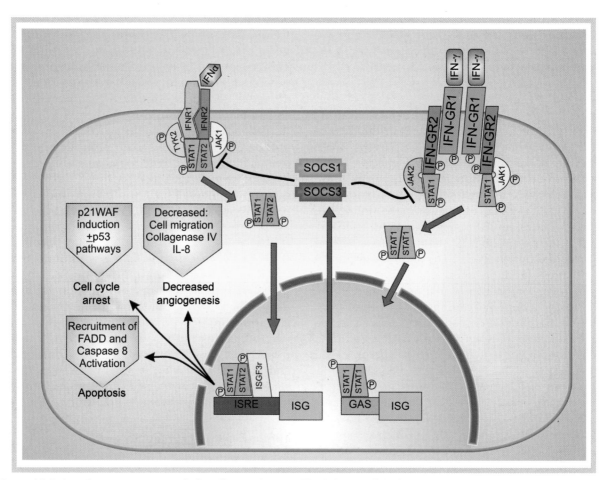

Figure 15-2: Interferon receptor and signaling pathways. The left side of the figure shows receptor for type I interferons (e.g. α); the right side shows the receptor for type II interferons (e.g. γ). The binding of IFNs to the receptors initiate phosphorilation of the cytoplasmic domains and subsequently of cytoplasmic proteins which results in nuclear translocation and binding to interferon-stimulated response elements (ISRE) and γ-activating sequences (GAS) which leads to regulation of interferon-stimulated genes (ISG). The potent interferon signaling is regulated by a negative feedback that inhibit interferon-stimulated signal transduction using the suppressor of cytokine signaling SOCS1 and SOCS3.

p21waf is a cycling-dependent kinase inhibitor that functions as a mediator of p53 activity controlling cell growth arrest; p21waf can also be induced by p53-independent pathways which result in growth arrest or differentiation. Type I interferons inhibit endothelial cell migration and inhibit the synthesis of basic fibroblast growth factor (bFGF), IL-8 and type IV collagenase, all of which have proangiogenic functions. Interferons can cause cell death receptor FADD and activation of caspase 8. The expression of apoptosis effector molecules, the caspases, increases with interferon treatment.

endothelial cell migration and inhibit the synthesis of basic fibroblast growth factor (bFGF), IL-8 and type IV collagenase, all of which have proangiogenic functions. The clinical significance of these effects has been shown in the therapy of infantile hemangiomas, hemangioblastomas and giant cell tumors of the mandible. IFNα is FDA approved for the treatment of AIDS-related Kaposi's sarcoma, a virally induced endothelial tumor as well as hepatitis B and C. In tumor cells, interferons can induce proapoptotic proteins and cause cell cycle arrest as a direct effect or indirectly in combination with other therapies. INFα induces p21waf in lymphoma cell lines. p21waf is a cyclin-dependent kinase inhibitor that functions as a mediator of p53 activity controlling cell growth arrest; p21waf can also be induced by several p53-independent pathways which result in growth arrest or differentiation. Furthermore, interferon can cause cell death in chronic myelogenous leukemia and myeloma cells through recruitment of the cell death receptor FADD and activation of caspase 8 **(Figure 15-1)**. Basal cell carcinoma, melanoma and cholangiocarcinoma can be sensitized to Fas ligand mediated apoptosis through application of type I interferons, in part through TRAIL-mediated mechanisms. The expression of apoptosis effector molecules, the caspases, increases with interferons in the treatment of patients with breast cancer, colon cancer and melanoma.

As with many cytokines, one limitation of the use of interferons is its broad range of side effects. Much of the side effects related with interferons are schedule and dose dependent and highly variable between individuals. The most common side effects are constitutional but individual organ toxicities can also be observed such as confusion, liver toxicity and strangely hairy eyebrows. Pharmacologic modification of interferons to increase its short half life and reduce the peak plasma concentrations has been evaluated to increase its therapeutic index.

Damage Associated Molecular Pattern Molecules (DAMPs)

The host has the ability to detect tissue damage and to induce immune responses. These responses restore local homeostasis, protect the host from further damage and initiate wound healing. How does the immune system communicate with the damaged site, or how do damaged tissues call in immune cells even in the absence of infection? This communication requires an interaction of so-called "danger" signals from infecting agents or from damaged tissues, so called Pathogen or Damage Associated Molecular Pattern molecules (PAMPs or DAMPs respectively) with their cognate receptors. DAMPs are molecules with specific locations and specific roles within cells that usually lack leader secretory sequences. These molecules can be secreted in a typical way by myeloid and lymphoid cells as well as from parenchymal (e.g. hepatocytes) and epithelial cells especially during stress or during autophagy and subsequent cell death.

Solid tumors grow at a faster rate than normal tissue and eventually reach a point where blood vessels can't proliferate as fast and a characteristic necrotic center starts to develop. This limited blood supply may change the microenvironment to one of hypoxia and chronic inflammation that promotes angiogenesis, stromagenesis and epithelial proliferation. These changes modify systemic and local immune responses, creating a "wound healing" microenvironment that is an ideal setting for tumor progression, growth and metastasis. All of these changes are believed to be orchestrated by the release of DAMPs from stressed cells within the tumor microenvironment.

Individual DAMPs are often overexpressed in tumor cells when compared to normal epithelium. High Mobility Group Box 1 (HMGB1), a nuclear DNA binding protein recently characterized as an extracellular factor involved in the response to infection, injury and inflammation, is probably the best characterized DAMP. DAMP molecules, including HMGB1, are leaderless secretory proteins (LSPs) that can be released by stressed cells particularly during nonapoptotic death. Cancer cells may have defective apoptotic pathways and are prone to undergo autophagy and subsequently necrotic cell death which increases the release of DAMPs, further increasing cell stress, inhibiting apoptosis and perpetuating the state of inflammation within the tumor microenvironment.

Interestingly, the release of DAMPs is also related to individual apoptotic pathways. HMGB1 is released following melanoma cell death induced by cytolytic lymphoid cells. However, HMGB1 is not released following intracellular delivery of granzyme B via adenoviral infection. CTLs and NK cells kill tumor cells not only by the perforin/granzyme pathway but also by ligation of death receptors in the extrinsic apoptotic pathway. HMGB1 release is thus caused not only by necrotic cell death but may also be released following caspase-dependent apoptosis of tumor but not normal cells. Anticancer treatment favoring caspase independent apoptosis may create a less tumorigenic microenvironment.

Other molecules have been identified as DAMPs as well including the S100 family of molecules, purinergic metabolites including ATP, adenosine monophosphate and uric acid and heat shock proteins. These molecules are usually located within the cytosol and when released into the extracellular space, can activate immune responses. Several receptors that bind these molecules have been identified and include the toll like receptor (TLR)-2, TLR-4, TLR-9, CD24/Siglec 10 and the Receptor for Advanced Glycation Endproducts (RAGE). Signaling through these receptors promotes inflammatory cell recruitment, wound healing responses with associated stromagenesis, angiogenesis, epithelial proliferation and modulation of the immune response. Pronounced expression of HMGB1 and RAGE is associated with increased cancer progression and metastatic potential. Similarly, S100 proteins are overexpressed in various tumors including breast, pancreas, lung and colorectal cancer. The spontaneous tumor regression of metastatic lesions observed in a small percentage of patients with metastatic renal cell carcinoma may be due to a reduction of DAMPs released from the primary tumor following nephrectomy.

HMGB1 release and cell death.
The circumstances under which cell death ensues following chemotherapy, hormonal therapy, radiation therapy or naturally and whether it induces an immune response has been subject of intense research. Many have thought that such death was immunologically silent or

tolerogenic. Whether or not apoptotic/necrotic cells are immunogenic or tolerogenic is a crucial question, the answer to which is not well understood.

Apoptosis and necrosis/necroptosis are two different pathways of cell death. Apoptosis or 'programmed cell death' is thought to confer tolerance and the latter to stimulate a vigorous inflammatory response. In contrast autophagy or 'programmed cell survival' can carry the cell through stressful periods and represent a means of cellular survival, particularly following chemotherapy **(Figure 15-3)**.

Most chemotherapeutic agents do not kill cells by inducing apoptosis, but rather necrosis. Not all agents have the capacity to induce immunogenic cell death. Tumor cells treated with oxaliplatin or anthracyclins were far more immunogenic than other agents when implanted in immunocompetent mice. Radiation treatment shows a similar response behavior indicating that the efficacy of these treatments depends on the active contribution of the host immune system.

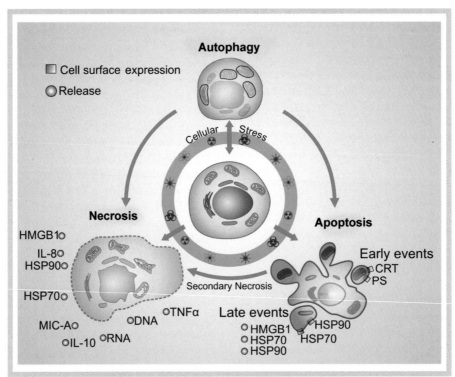

Figure 15-3: Cell death and cell survival. The cell response to stress can be classified in necrotic cell death, apoptotic cell death and autophagic cell survival. These responses are mostly classified based in morphological features but have also specific immunological profiles. Autophagy is characterized by formation of autophagosome vesicles in response to stress and can lead to cell adaptation and survival. Apoptosis usually shows nuclear fragmentation and cell blebbing. At later stages of apoptotic cells can acquire characteristics of necrotic cell death; this is called secondary necrosis and is characterized by swelling and cell membrane rupture. This different forms of cell death and survival have characteristic immunogenic profiles as well and are dictated by of damage associated molecular patterns (DAMPs) that are secreted (blue circles) or expressed on the cell surface (green squares).

Autophagy involves the sequestration of cellular material into double or multi-membrane autophagosomes with subsequent degradation of its contents upon fusion with lysosomes. Autophagy represents a major turnover mechanism to eliminate damaged or supernumerary organelles, intracellular pathogens, aggregate-prone proteins and excess portions of cytoplasm. By promoting catabolic reactions, autophagy generates metabolic substrates to meet the energy needs of the cell during periods of stress. However resources are limited by the amount of intracellular substrate and when the cell is depleted of critical organelles and proteins it can lead to a caspase independent form of cell death **(Figure 15-3)**. Autophagic flux can be induced by p53 and p53-dependent genes, however, in the absence of p53, autophagy can be induced by transcription independent mechanisms.

During autophagy cells usually fail to manifest signs of apoptosis (e.g. chromatin condensation) suggesting that enhanced autophagic flux can correlate with inhibition of apoptotic cell death.

HMGB1 is released when cells undergo necrotic cell death. However both apoptotic and autophagic cells can release HMGB1 under specific circumstances. HMGB1 is released from the nucleus of dying cancer cells to the cytoplasm and subsequently to the extracellular space in necrotic cells or late apoptotic stages, later it represents a crucial step in the activation of antigen presenting cells. TLR-4 binding of HMGB1 inhibits the phagosome-lysosome fusion, therefore preventing the degradation of tumor antigens in APCs. Blocking TLR-4 or HMGB1 abolishes the capacity of dying tumor cells to elicit an anticancer immune response *in vitro* and *in vivo*.

Enhanced autophagic flux can regulate the amount of cell death, but evidence suggests that the amount of HMGB1 released from dying cells is also dependent on autophagy. Increasing autophagy in dying cells selectively release HMGB1 without causing lysis of the cell membrane and necrosis.

Interleukin Therapy

IL-2

IL-2 was first described in 1976 and recognized as a T cell growth factor, it was one of the first cytokines to be studied in detail. IL-2 is produced mainly by activated T cells and in an autocrine fashion is required for and induces the progression of T cells from the G1 to the S phase of the cell cycle. IL-2 also determines the magnitude of T-cell and Natural Killer (NK) cell responses, augmenting cytolytic activity and inducing IFN-γ secretion. IL-2 is required for expansion of CD8+ memory T cells during viral infections and as a growth factor induces class switching in B-cells. Observations in mice with targeted

IL-2 and IL-2 receptor deletions suggest that IL-2 has a role in preventing autoimmune disease and other lymphoproliferative diseases.

IL-2 structure and IL-2 receptor

IL-2 was initially termed T-cell growth factor. It is a 15 kd polypeptide made up of 153 amino acids including a signal sequence 20 amino acids long that is cleaved during secretion. Two cysteine residues at positions 58 and 105 form a disulfide bridge and a third residue at position 125 is not essential for biological activity. IL-2 binds to specific surface receptors to execute its biological effects. The expression of this receptor as well as the expression of IL-2 itself is induced by signaling through the T cell antigen receptor. The IL-2 receptor consist of 3 subunits: α, β and γ chains. The α subunit has a large extracellular domain which binds to IL-2 with low affinity and its short intracellular domain has no known biological activity nor is necessary for IL-2 signaling. The β subunit also has a large extracellular domain as well as a large intracellular domain that is essential for signaling. The γ subunit is a 64 kd protein that physically associates with the β chain and it has paired cysteines at two sites within the extracellular domain and a perimembrane WSXWS motif. This is probably related with binding to several molecules including HMGB1 which could facilitate cytokine/receptor interactions **(Figure 15-4)**. All three chains are upregulated after antigenic stimulation. Resting NK cells express β chain constitutively and when exposed to IL-2 or IL-12, α and γ chain expression is induced. IL-2R signaling is primarily mediated through the activation of JAK1 and JAK3 kinases that physically associate with the cytoplasmic domain of receptor subunits, with subsequent phosphorylation and activation of the signal transduction and activators of transcription (STAT). IL-2 also induces the recruitment and subsequent tyrosine phosphorylation of the adaptor protein Shc to the β chain resulting in the downstream activation of p21^{ras} and subsequently protein kinases erk-1 and erk-2 **(Table 15-1)**.

Downstream effects

In addition to its proliferative effects, IL-2 can induce the synthesis of a number of secondary cytokines including IL-1, TNF, IFN-γ, IL-6 and lymphotoxin. These other cytokines may also contribute to the efficacy and side effects of IL-2 therapy and are found to decrease after IL-2 treatment is terminated.

Proliferation of T cells

One of the most important effects of IL-2 treatment in the setting of anticancer immunotherapy is the enhancement of the cytolytic activity of antigen-specific cytotoxic T lymphocytes and NK cells. This effect was characterized almost three decades ago; however, the exact mechanism for this enhancement is not completely understood.

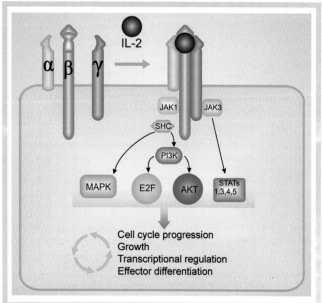

Figure 15-4: The high affinity interleukin-2 (IL-2) receptor and signaling pathways. The IL-2 receptor has 3 subunits: the α chain also known as CD25; the β chain also known as CD122 and the γ chain also known as CD132. The three subunits are not assembled in the absence of IL-2. Upon binding of IL-2 to the α chain, the β and γ chains associate to form a stable heterotrimer leading to initiation of signal transduction. The cytoplasmic domains of the β and γ chains contain several tyrosines that, when phosphorilated, represent activation sites for downstream kinases that affect cell cycle progression, growth and differentiation

TABLE 15-1	Mechanisms of tumor escape and IL-2 antitumor mechanisms. Which of these mechanisms are responsible for IL-2 response in patients with RCC is still unclear and more studies are needed to answer this question. A better understanding of the IL-2 biology is necessary to develop treatment strategies with higher response rates, improve patient selection and minimize side effects

Tumor escape mechanism	IL-2 mechanism
Down-regulation of HLA	Increase HLA independent cytotoxicity
Decreased or defective blood vessels:	Promotes adhesion and migration (LAF-1)
– Low effector T cell access	Increases iNKT cells
– Down-regulation of NK receptors (e.g. NKG2D)	– increases IFN gamma
	– activates NK, DCs, CD4+, CD8+ T cells
Immunosuppressive tumor microenvironment	Increases NK cells
Overexpression of transporter proteins for	Activation and proliferation of T cells, IFN gamma production
chemotherapeutics (e.g. MDR1Pgp)	Promotes p53 independent apoptosis
Death Receptor Defects	
Complete loss of caspases pathways or activity	Death receptor independent cytotoxicity (perforin/granzyme)
T cell anergy:	Granzyme mediated mitosis disruption
– low costimulatory T cell signals (e.g. B7)	Prevent and reverses T cell anergy
– increase anergy costimulatory signals (e.g. B7H1)	
Defective iNKT cell numbers and/or function	Increases cytolytic activity
	– increases cytotoxic granule components (Perforin/Granzyme)
Increased T regulatory cells	Decreases regulatory T cells
Acidic microenvironment	Better treatment response in CAIX overexpression tumors
– HIF	
– CAIX	
Overexpression of DAPM receptors (e.g. RAGE)	
Release of DAMPs during necrotic death	
– Release of HMGB1	
Reduced microenvironment	
Overexpression of DAMPs (e.g. HMGB1)	
Altered metabolism	
– Aerobic glycolytic pathways	
– Lactic acidosis	

Enhancement of the cytolytic activity of T cells and NK. Is thought to be to some extent due to the increased expression of genes encoding for the granule cytotoxic components of the cytotoxic cells (the perforin/granzyme pathway), as well as adhesion molecules like LAF-1 thus facilitating leukocyte adhesion and migration to tumor site.

Increased HLA restricted cytotoxic activity of CTLs. The effect of IL-2 treatment is not only restricted to the enhancement of antigen specific or HLA restricted killing of cytotoxic cells. Peripheral blood lymphocytes exposed only to IL-2 showed an increased capacity for killing tumor cell lines and freshly isolated tumor cells *in vitro*. This HLA unrestricted killing is carried out by cells termed lymphokine-activated killer (LAK) cells. LAK cells where initially used along with IL-2 in the initial trials using IL-2 to treat cancer patients. Further studies using high dose IL-2 with or without LAK cells failed to show a significant benefit of LAK cells observed in preclinical studies to justify their continued use.

Toxicity
The greatest limitation for IL-2 treatment has been the wide range of side effects that high dose IL-2 causes not only precluding treatment for a great number of patients that do not fulfill the pretreatment characteristics but also, not infrequently, selected patients have to stop the proposed treatment due to serious or uncontrollable effects. However, over the years, physician experience and the use of routine antibiotic prophylaxis and extensive cardiac screening has lead to a significantly diminished profile of side effects in current treatment as compared with early reports. Common side effects include fever, chills lethargy, diarrhea, nausea, anemia thrombocytopenia, eosinophilia, diffuse erythroderma, hepatic dysfunction and confusion. More serious side effects include myocarditis in around 5% of the patients.

Capillary leak syndrome: A number of serious side effects of high dose IL-2 administration are associated with the "capillary leak syndrome" which leads to fluid retention, hypotention, prerenal azotemia and more serious conditions such as adult respiratory distress syndrome and myocardial infarction. Interestingly, this effects, similar to a generalized delayed type hypersensitivity reaction (DTH), may be an important aspect of IL-2's efficacy. Patients on high dose IL-2 treatment present a higher risk of developing infections especially with gram positive bacteria. This is probably due to a chemotactic defect in neutrophils observed in these patients. Prophylactic antibiotics and intravenous fluids may be required. Acetaminophen and NSAIDs are now routinely used both prophylactic and as needed basis for the management of side effects.

Interleukin 12
Interleukin 12 was discovered in 1989 and first described as a lymphocyte maturation factor and a cytotoxic T cell maturation factor. IL-12 plays an important role in the development of a Th1 type of immune response and the production of IFN-γ. In preclinical studies IL-12 can inhibit tumor growth and metastasis in mouse models.

Activation of immunity by IL-12
IL-12 is crucial for driving CD4+ T cells toward a Th1 phenotype. APCs activate the T cell receptor and produce IL-12 upon antigen presentation. This promotes CD4+ T cell proliferation, IFN-γ and IL-1 production and upregulation of the IL-12 receptor β2 (IL-12Rβ2) which is the main regulator of IL-12 responsiveness. Coexpression of IL-12Rβ2 and IL-12Rβ1, normally expressed in resting lymphocytes, synergistically increases the affinity of both receptors to IL-12. CD4+ Th1 cells then induce antigen specific proliferation of CD8+ cells and development of cytotoxic T lymphocytes. IL-12 also induces NK cell proliferation and IFN-γ production, B-cell IgG production and activation of neutrophils. IFN-γ in turn induces the upregulation of MHC molecules and activates macrophages and NK cells; furthermore IFN-γ induces IL-12 production by APC forming a positive feedback loop between APCs and T cells. In addition of TRC activation by APCs, ligation of CD2 and CD 28 on T-cells also augments the response to IL-12.

Cell mediated IL-12 antitumor effects
The antitumor effects of IL-12 have been attributed at least in part to cytotoxic CD8+ T cells. Tumors from both mouse models and humans have shown CD8+ T cells infiltrating the tumor after treatment with hrIL-12. Furthermore depletion of CD8+ T cells in mouse experiments resulted in the lost of antitumor effects of IL-12 whereas NK and CD4+ T cell depletion had little to no effect in that setting.

A subpopulation of CD8 negative T cells denominated Vα14 NKT cells may also play a role in IL-12 mediated tumor effects. Selective depletion of these cells in murine tumor models without manipulation of CD8+ or NK cells resulted in loss of IL-12 mediated tumor rejection. The role of NK and CD4+ cells in IL-12 tumor immunity is not clear. Mice studies indicate that neither NK nor CD4+ T-cells play an essential role in IL-12 treated tumor models with otherwise normal immune systems. However, in the absence of T and NKT cells, NK cells can effectively mediate antitumor response following IL-12 stimulation. Similarly, CD4+ T cells enhance antitumor effects of IL-12 in CD8+ depleted mice.

IL-12 binds neutrophils and causes a CA++ dependent activation and increases production of reactive oxygen species. In a murine mammary tumor model, mice were treated with IL-12 and showed neutrophilic infiltration and showed neutrophil depletion decreased the effect of IL-12 on survival.

IFN-γ and IL-12 antitumor effects

IL-12 treatment has both direct and indirect effects in IFN-γ production. This cytokine is central to the IL-12 response. IFN-γ plays a role as an activator of immune effector cells, induction of cytokines and chemokines including IL-12 and has direct effects in tumor cells. The mechanism of IFN-γ has been discussed earlier in this chapter; not surprisingly, neutralization of IFN-γ abolishes the antitumor effects of IL-12. It also has antiangiogenic effects through the increased production of IP-10, Mig and I-TAC, collectively called CXC3 chemokines. CXC3 receptors are found on intraepithelial lymphocytes, macrophages, dendritic cells and endothelial cells. CXC3 chemokines facilitate T-cell migration and inhibit angiogenesis. Despite significant antitumor activity of IL-12 documented in preclinical studies, clinical trials have shown minimal efficacy. Several clinical trials have been done investigating effects of IL-12 in patients with advanced solid tumors and hematologic malignancies, either as a monotherapy or in combination with other therapies. With few exceptions efficacy was minimal, with objective responses rating ranging between 0% and 11%. More effective application of this cytokine and recently identified IL-12 family members (e.g. IL-23 and IL-27), should be investigated as possible therapeutic agents in cancer patients.

Viral Therapy

The possibility of using viruses to treat cancer has been studied for many years. Anecdotal cases of cancer regression in patients with concurrent viral infections lead to the first clinical trials in which cancer patients were infected with bodily fluids containing animal or human viruses. Although responses were obtained in a number of patients, the morbidity related to infection of normal tissue was unacceptable. The limited technology and ethical implications placed this area of research on standby for a number of decades. In the 1950s, the idea was revisited with the advent of tissue culture techniques and the ability to grow viruses in specific cultures and tissues, again, with the limitation of the absence of means to improve efficacy of infection by manipulating virus properties.

Today we know that cancer cells represent a better environment for viral replication than non-transformed cells. Defects in antigen presenting machinery and other means used by the tumor cell to escape the immune system recognition may help the virus to replicate and been unnoticed by the immune system and ultimately cause cell lysis. Recognition of infected cells in non-transformed cells results in viral eradication by the immune system. This results in a specific lysis of tumor cells infected with viruses, or oncolytic virotherapy (OV). While very promising in theory, an oncolytic virus needs to have specific characteristics to efficiently eradicate tumors while sparing normal cells. These characteristics include a tropism to cancer cells and low infectivity to normal tissues as well as means to visualize viral distribution and quantity. A need for tools to modify virus characteristics becomes crucial, three basic modifications are the goal for a good oncolytic virus: improve targeting, shielding the virus and arming with specific biomolecules. Targeting increases cancer specificity and increases the therapeutic index. Shielding may be capsular modifications that protects the virus from immediate immune system recognition and elimination. The addition of biomolecules including expression of molecules that improve tumor killing such as prodrug proteases and activators of cell death pathways have also been considered and applied.

Retargeting oncolytic viruses

Current knowledge in cancer biology, virology and genetic engineering has allowed great advances in the targeting of oncolytic viruses and development of viruses. Targeting specific molecules in the tumor not only improves tumor tropism but can also activate cell death pathways and elicit host antitumor immune responses to further eliminate tumor cells. The selectivity of the tumor is crucial for a successful approach in OV. One strategy is to select a virus with a natural tropism for a given tissue. One example is the use of HSV to treat glioblastoma: the strategy here becomes to modify the virus so it does not harm normal neurons while maintaining its oncolytic efficacy. One alternative is to reprogram a virus with only partial tropism to target cells; this strategy benefits from a natural low toxicity. This last strategy requires modifying the virus to a tumor-specific characteristic.

Viral replication relies on the use of host proteases. For example, enveloped viruses, such as influenza or HIV-1, require protease cleavage of viral glycoproteins for successful internalization following receptor recognition. Therefore, tumor-specific proteases or proteases highly expressed in tumor cells can be exploited for tumor targeting. Matrix metalloproteinases (MMPs), for example, are endopeptidases that are overexpressed in almost every human cancer. Structural changes in fusion proteins of measles virus and Sendai virus changed these proteins from a phenotype of susceptibility to ubiquitous proteases to becoming uniquely susceptible to MMP. Mice infected with modified measles virus which retained full oncolytic activity in MMP positive subcutaneous tumor did not infect and kill the mice compared to wild type measles virus infection.

Other determinants of viral tropism include the cell surface receptors that the virus binds to prior to internalization. Individual tumor markers on the cell surface can be targeted by modifying both enveloped and naked oncologic virus to bind. This approach is challenging and often the combination of individual ligands with some viruses is incompatible. In addition entry of a virus into a cell sometimes depends on multiple cell surface receptors and multiple ligands expressed on the surface of the virus. Successful retargeting virus requires inactivation of the virus natural entry mechanism. For example, the measles virus requires a CD150 and CD46 molecules for infection. Specific residues in the measles virus hemagglutinin that were required for either CD150 or CD46 dependent cell entry were mutated in a recombinant virus by reverse genetics. After tropism inactivation, targeting to receptor proteins in cancer cells is the next step. Here a specificity domain of the epidermal growth factor (EGF) or insulin-like growth factor (IGF)1 which bind to the extracellular domain of the viral hemagglutinin. Replication capabilities are observed in previous non-susceptible cells expressing EGF and IGF1 receptors.

For a successful viral infection and subsequent replication a virus needs to gain control of the translational machinery of their host cells. For this to happen the infected cell must have a phenotype that favors such interaction. This adds an additional layer of viral tropism and even in the case the virus is internalized, failure to interface properly with the translational machinery may result in an abortive infection and greatly restrict viral replication. Furthermore, the virus must seize control of the cell's translational control to their own benefit. To our advantage this specificity can be exploited to interfere with the oncolytic virus's ability to properly regulate translation in a specific kind of cancer cell.

Targeting can also be accomplished by deactivating certain viral capabilities. Adenoviruses normally inhibits p53 in the host cell using a protein encoded in the E1B region of the viral genome. p53 inactivation allows the virus to replicate without the cell initiating the intrinsic apoptotic pathway. Targeted deletion of 827 Bp in the E1B region will impair this mechanism and cause normal cells infected with the virus to undergo apoptosis and tumor cells with defective p53 pathways to allow viral replication. This retargeting strategy, described by Berk more than 20 years ago although theoretically interesting, its selectivity for cells without p53 function was unfortunately a rather oversimplification of the biology. Alternative mechanisms in both the tumor cell and the virus lead to a comparable replication efficacy between this mutated virus (ONYX-015) and wild type adenovirus. A similar approach targeting the A1 region of the adenoviral genome targets the virus to cells with defective RB pathway and has shown promising results in animal models.

Shielding

One challenge to oncolytic biotherapy is overcoming the immune response to the virus in immunocompetent cancer patients. Strategies are needed for the oncolytic virus and the host immune system to coexist or even act synergistically. Pre-existing antibodies can rapidly neutralize the incoming viruses following injection. Even in the absence of performed antibodies, the initial treatment can induce the formation of neutralizing antibodies that will affect subsequent injections. This is important when designing protocols for oncolytic virotherapy and takes advantage of stages of immuno-suppression. For example, patients with multiple myeloma have low levels of antibodies and could have better rates of infection in tumor cells. Alternatively, chemotherapeutics such as cyclophosphamide has immunosuppressive side effects that can increase oncolysis when used in combination therapy. In the case of immunocompetent patients other approaches can be used. Changing the capsid, and therefore the serotype of the virus, can allow evasion from neutralizing antibodies. Mice that are treated with Ad2 serotypes vector for the first time developed neutralizing antibodies against Ad2. In the second round Ad5 could be used with little reduction in transduction. This approach requires using multiple different serotypes for each subsequent injection. Alternatively chemical coating with polymers such as polyethylene glycol or other hydrophilic polymers can be cross-linked to viruses to shield them from neutralizing antibodies. Although this modification can significantly reduce virus infection *in vitro*, it's been suggested that shielding can in some cases enhance tumor infection by reducing virus uptake by normal tissue.

Cell-viral biotherapy is another mechanism by which the virus can reach the tumor without being neutralized or recognized by the immune system. One example is the combination of immune effector cell population with oncolytic virus. Cytokine activated killer (CIK) cells pre-infected with vaccinia virus in preclinical studies allowed the virus to remain hidden until the cell interacted with the tumor. The CIK cells remained capable to traffic and to infiltrate the tumor, effectively before releasing the virus.

Arming oncolytic viruses

The efficiency of oncolytic viruses can be enhanced by arming or supplementing the virus with genes that confer additional biologic effects. These genes, when transcribed, can have a biologic effect within the cell, within the tumor microenvironment, systemically or act in combination with other forms of cancer therapy.

Prodrug convertases.

These proteins cleave nontoxic non-bioactive substances into drugs that can have anticancer effects either locally or systemically. Ganciclovir is a nucleoside analog that inhibits DNA elongation when phosphorylated by cellular kinases. Therefore, the use of HSV armed with thymidine kinase adds susceptibility to the infected cell to ganciclovir. Furthermore, ganciclovir only affects cells that are dividing. Cancer cells infected with this virus are more susceptible than infected normal cells.

Apoptosis inducers

Oncolytic virus can be armed with molecules capable of inducing apoptosis in tumor cells. In theory promising, this strategy can induce early apoptosis in the infected cell and decrease viral replication and further infection of more tumor cells. Therefore, an approach could be made in which apoptosis is induced in late stages of viral replication. In this scenario, apoptosis improves virus yield and release from infected cells. Adenovirus armed to express TRAIL are more oncolytic than parental viruses in tumor cells lines *in vitro* and in animal tumor models. p53 armed virus increases apoptosis in *in vitro* assays but sadly show no increased antitumor activity *in vivo*.

Antisense Therapy

Current cancer therapy is associated with substantial secondary effects and narrow therapeutic indices. Biologic therapy approaches are not an exception. Continuous research efforts identifying strategies to increase efficacy without increasing, or potentially decreasing toxicity, are being sought. One of the best ways to achieve this goal, conceptually at least, is by targeting mRNA containing the sequence to be translated by the ribosome into a specific protein. If this protein is responsible for the growth, invasiveness, viability of the tumor cell, then knocking down its expression may lead to tumor cell death or will render the cell susceptible to other types of cancer therapy.

The mRNA sequence is defined as "sense" a complementary, antiparallel sequence is "antisense". All that is required is the sequence of the mRNA and an antisense piece of DNA or siRNA can chemically be synthetyzed. Binding the antisense oligonucleotide to its target mRNA forms an mRNA-DNA hybrid that will inhibit translation of that mRNA into protein. This strategy offers an extremely high specificity for the targeted molecules.

The antisense based therapy in theory makes sense, however translation into clinical practice has been difficult to achieve for a number of reasons. DNA oligonucleotides have phosphodiester bounds and are rapidly digested in human plasma, mostly by exonuclease activity. Oligonucleotides cannot pass through lipid bilayers. Some forms of oligonucleotides bind to heparin binding proteins, both within the plasma and to cell surface proteins, thus affecting their bioavailability and potentially causing toxicity and/or non-antisense effects.

The role of phosphorothioates

Phosphorothioates are a class of oligonucleotide in which an oxygen atom is replaced with sulfur in a non-bridging position at each phosphorous (changing the P-ester to a P-thioate bound). Because sulfur and oxygen are isoelectric, the charge is maintained and so is the aqueous solubility of the nucleotide. Phosphorothioates are much more resistant to nucleases (though not nuclease-proof). mRNA binding to complementary phosphorothioates is relatively stable with a lower melting temperature than mRNA-phosphodiester oligonucleotide complexes. Another chemical property of phosphorothioates is a high affinity to bind heparin-binding proteins such as FGF, PDGF, HMGB1 and VEGF. This binding can render the protein inactive and cause dose dependent toxicity. Binding to factors IX and VIII is associated with coagulopathy. This interaction, however, can also affect the tumor environment and account for the non-antisense effects commonly observed both *in vitro* and *in vivo*.

Targeting Bcl-2 mRNA: G3139

Cytotoxic chemotherapy induced apoptosis can be prevented in tumor cells by expression of Bcl-2 or other antiapoptotic proteins. The Bcl-2 family of proteins consist of 25 pro- and antiapoptotic molecules that maintain a balance between new cells and senescent cells. The Bcl-2 protein is overexpressed in most types of cancer including chronic lymphocytic leukemia lymphomas, colon, breast and prostate cancer. Overexpression of this protein is related to chemoresistant tumor cells to a wide variety of agents including, cisplatin, topoisomerase II inhibitors, alkylating agents, antimetabolites and radiation.

G3139 (Oblimersen) is an 18-mer phosphorothioate antisense oligonucleotide designed to bind to the first six codons of the human bcl-2 mRNA. Oblimersen is the first agent targeting Bcl-2 that entered clinical trials and has been tested in combination with other anticancer chemotherapeutic agents in CLL, AML, multiple myeloma, small cell lung cancer, non-Hodgkin's lymphoma and melanoma with promising initial results.

Conclusion

Adult, but not childhood, tumors arise in the setting of chronic inflammation driven by the metabolic disturbances in the tumor and its microenvironment. Thus the tumor and inflammatory cells are intimate associates during the Darwinian evolution of the tumor occurring over several years. Biologic therapy, by definition, focuses on the tumor from the cell membrane out, something we have termed 'epicrine' to contrast it with the notion of 'epigenetic' events occurring within the tumor cell which modify it as well as the host's behavior. As such, antibodies targeting the cell surface molecules including interferon, TGFβ and TNF family member receptors; the rich inflammatory cells recruited to the tumor microenvironment including macrophages, T cells, dendritic cells and on occasion full tertiary lymphoid sites embedded within the tumor, can all be considered suitable areas for investigation and therapeutic development. Modern biologic therapies greatest successes have been in the application of cytokines, antibodies and soon, we believe, with the application of T, NK and dendritic cell therapies.

Landmark Papers

1. Atkins MB, et al. High-dose recombinant interleukin 2 therapy for patients with metastatic melanoma: analysis of 270 patients treated between 1985 and 1993. J Clin Oncol 1999:17(7):2105-16.
2. Balkwill F, Mantovani A. Inflammation and cancer: back to Virchow? Lancet 2001;357(9255): 539-45.
3. Brassard DL, Grace MJ, Bordens RW. Interferon-alpha as an immunotherapeutic protein. J Leukoc Biol 2002;71(4): 565-81.
4. Green DR, et al. Immunogenic and tolerogenic cell death. Nat Rev Immunol 2009;9(5): 353-63.
5. Guo ZS, Thorne SH, Bartlett DL. Oncolytic virotherapy: molecular targets in tumor-selective replication and carrier cell-mediated delivery of oncolytic viruses. Biochim Biophys Acta 2008;1785(2): 217-31.
6. Hurwitz H, et al. Bevacizumab plus irinotecan, fluorouracil and leucovorin for metastatic colorectal cancer. N Engl J Med 2004;350(23): 2335-42.
7. Kepp O, et al. Immunogenic cell death modalities and their impact on cancer treatment. Apoptosis 2009;14(4): 364-75.
8. Lotze MT, et al. The grateful dead: damage-associated molecular pattern molecules and reduction/oxidation regulate immunity. Immunol Rev 2007;220: 60-81.
9. O'Brien S, et al. Randomized phase III trial of fludarabine plus cyclophosphamide with or without oblimersen sodium (Bcl-2 antisense) in patients with relapsed or refractory chronic lymphocytic leukemia. J Clin Oncol 2007; 25(9): 1114-20.
10. Rosenberg SA, et al. Adoptive cell transfer: a clinical path to effective cancer immunotherapy. Nat Rev Cancer 2008; 8(4): 299-308.
11. Rosenberg SA, Yang JC, Restifo NP. Cancer immunotherapy: moving beyond current vaccines. Nat Med 2004; 10(9): 909-15.
12. Smith I, et al. 2-year follow-up of trastuzumab after adjuvant chemotherapy in HER2-positive breast cancer: a randomised controlled trial. Lancet 2007;369(9555): 29-36.
13. Tanaka H, et al. Depletion of CD4+ CD25+ regulatory cells augments the generation of specific immune T cells in tumor-draining lymph nodes. J Immunother 2002;25(3): 207-17.
14. Vander Heiden MG, Cantley LC, Thompson CB. Understanding the Warburg effect: the metabolic requirements of cell proliferation. Science 2009;324(5930): 1029-33.

Section 4

Superficial Tissues

16

Nonmelanoma Skin Cancer

A Serhat Gur, Bulent Unal, Atilla Soran, Howard Edington

Nonmelanoma skin cancer (NMSC) is the most commonly diagnosed malignancy in the United States, accounting for 33% to 50% of all the newly diagnosed cancers each year. More than one million new cases are diagnosed in the United States and three million in the world every year. The incidence of NMSC is difficult to determine, however, as many cases are not reported because the cancer is not typically followed in tumor registries. The incidence of NMSC is thought to be increasing. A primary care physician can expect to diagnose 6-7 cases of basal cell cancer, 1-2 cases of squamous cell cancer and approximately 1 case of melanoma every year, according to population-based studies. Of patients with squamous cell carcinoma, 30% will develop an additional squamous cell carcinoma after five years and over 50% will develop an additional nonmelanoma skin cancer. More than one-third of patients with basal cell carcinoma will develop an additional basal cell carcinoma after five years.

Basal cell carcinoma (BCC, 75%) and squamous cell carcinoma (SCC, 20%) account for the vast majority of NMSC (> 95%). Because of their slow growth and negligible risk for metastasis, the mortality associated with these cancers is low. It is for this reason they attract relatively little attention from the medical and lay communities; however, they cause considerable functional and cosmetic deformity. The cost of treatment is significant and resulting in an annual cost to Medicare alone of $500 million. 'Stage and histological grade are the most important parameters to effect the treatment options and survival in patients with NMSC **(Table 16-1)**.

Risk Factors in Skin Carcinogenesis

The low and high risk with clinicopathologic correlation are shown in **Tables 16-2 and 16-3**. The pathophysiology of NMSC is multifactorial. Relevant causes or associations can be considered in terms of environmental and intrinsic factors. Intrinsic risk factors may include skin type, immune competence and genetically predisposing syndromes. In contradistinction to a number of other malignancies, the importance of environmental influences is established. Relevant environmental exposures include ionizing radiation and a variety of chemical agents.

Host Factors

Phenotype

A significant constitutional risk factor for all skin cancers seems to be skin type and specifically how the skin responds to sun exposure. The incidence of NMSC is much lower in non-whites than in Caucasians. The Fitzpatrick skin type classification is widely used to classify individuals according to their skin reaction to sun exposure **(Table 16-4)**.

A number of genetic disorders exist that are characterized by an increased incidence of NMSC.

Xeroderma Pigmentosum

This is a rare autosomal recessive disorder (prevalence 1/250,000) characterized by a defect in the normal detection and repair mechanism of the UV-induced DNA damage. Patients have increased photosensitivity, exaggerated sunburn response and prolonged erythema with early onset actinic changes **(Figure 16-1)**. A marked

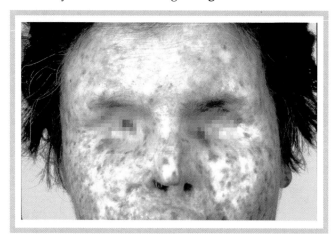

Figure 16-1: Patient with xeroderma pigmentosum. In addition to cutaneous malignancies, ocular neoplasms are common

TABLE 16-1	Staging classification of NMSC*

Primary Tumor (T)

TX	Primary tumor cannot be assessed
T0	No evidence of primary tumor
Tis	Carcinoma in situ
T1	Tumor ≤ 2 cm
T2	Tumor 2.1-5 cm
T3	Tumor > 5 cm
T4	Tumor invades deep extradermal structures (e.g. cartilage, skeletal muscle or bone)

Regional Lymph Nodes (N)

NX	Regional Lymph Nodes cannot be assessed
N0	No regional lymph node metastasis
N3	Regional lymph node metastasis

Distant Metastasis (M)

MX	Distant metastasis cannot be assessed
M0	No distant metastasis
M1	Distant metastases

Stage

0	=	Tis, N0, M0
I	=	T1, N0, M0
II	=	T2-3, N0, M0
III	=	T4, N0, M or Any T, N1, M0
IV	=	Any T, any N, M1

Histologic Grade (G)

GX	=	Grade cannot be assessed
G1	=	Well differentiated
G2	=	Moderately differentiated
G3	=	Poorly differentiated
G4	=	Undifferentiated

Abbreviations: T = tumor; N = nodal; M = metastasis; G = grade.

Used with the permission of the American Joint Committee on Cancer (AJCC), Chicago, Illinois. The original source for this material is the AJCC Cancer Staging Manual, Sixth Edition (2002) published by Springer-Verlag, New York

TABLE 16-2	High-risk factors for basal cell carcinoma and squamous cell carcinoma
Borders	Ill-defined margins
Size	> 2 cm on trunk or extremities; ≥ 0.6 cm on ears, temples, periorbital, perinasal and perioral areas (facial H zone); genitalia, hands and feet
Growth	Rapid growth
Setting	Arising from chronic ulcer or wounds Nerve pain or paralysis Immunosuppressed patients
Previous therapy	Recurent
Localization	Facial H zone; genitalia, feet and sun protected skin

TABLE 16-3	Low-risk factors for basal cell carcinoma and squamous cell carcinoma
Borders	Well-defined margins
Size	< 2 cm on trunk or extremities; < 0.6 cm on ears, temples, periorbital, perinasal and perioral areas (facial H zone); genitalia,hands and feet
Growth	Slow growth
Setting	Healthy patients with minimal comorbidity
Previous therapy	Primary
Localization	Trunk and extremities

TABLE 16-4	Fitzpatrick's classification of sun-reactive skin types	
Skin type	**Skin color**	**Characteristics**
I	White; very fair; red or blond hair; blue eyes; freckles	Always burns, never tans
II	White; fair; red or blond hair; blue, hazel, or green eyes	Usually burns, tans with difficulty
III	Cream white; fair with any eye or hair color; very common	Sometimes mild burn, gradually tans
IV	Brown; typical mediterranean caucasian skin	Rarely burns, tans with ease
V	Dark brown; mid-eastern skin types	Very rarely burns, tans very easily
VI	Black	Never burns, tans very easily

increase in incidence of multiple skin neoplasms including melanoma (especially superficial spreading type), BCC and SCC is seen in this disease. The syndrome is usually recognized at an early age and cutaneous malignancies may develop as early as five years of age. Management involves strict avoidance of sun exposure. Neoplasms are treated surgically. Topical 5-fluorouracil and systemic retinoic acid have been used with limited success. The prognosis is poor, with death occurring in the early 20s.

Nevoid Basal Cell Syndrome (Gorlin Syndrome)

Gorlin syndrome, or basal cell nevus syndrome, originally described by Gorlin, is a multisystemic disorder characterized by the occurrence of multiple BCC often in the hundreds, odontogenic cysts of the jaw, calcification of the falx cerebri, pitting in the palms and soles and various skeletal abnormalities (bifid ribs, brachymetacarpalism, broad nasal root and overdeveloped supraorbital rim). BCCs usually develop between the second and the third decade and are not aggressive (except in the face) and distant metastasis is rare. There is an autosomal dominant inheritance pattern. The inherited defect seems to be a defect in a tumor suppressor gene located at the long arm of chromosome 9 with 97% penetrance and variable expression (prevalence 1/56,000). Treatment is by prevention (e.g. sun avoidance and protection) and removal of the BCC. Life expectancy is normal with good prognosis. The disease can be mutilating and difficult to manage. Other genetic syndromes that predispose to skin carcinoma include (1) albinism (increased risk of SCC), (2) porokeratosis (13% chance of SCC formation) and (3) epidermodysplasia verruciformis.

Predisposing Lesions

A number of skin lesions are associated with the development of NMSC. Understanding the associated risk of malignant degeneration facilitates management of the patient and provides additional clues as to the biology of the malignant transformation.

- Nevus sebaceous of Jadassohn: Nevus sebaceous of Jadassohn is a well-circumscribed, raised, yellowish plaque that is present at birth on the scalp and face. Degeneration into BCC is seen in 10% of the cases. Elective excision with clear margins is generally recommended.
- Actinic keratoses: Actinic keratoses are the most common premalignant lesions **(Figure 16-2)**. They develop in 16% of North American Caucasians during their lifetime. The malignant transformation rate to SCC is between 10% and 13%. Treatment modalities are laser cryotherapy, 5-FU, or retinoids.

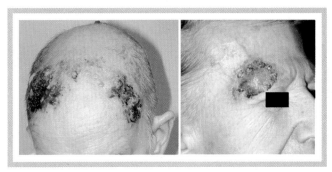

Figure 16-2: Actinic keratoses. These frequently respond well to topical therapy (5-Fluorouracil). They can clinically resemble both squamous cell carcinoma and basal cell carcinoma and the diagnosis may be confirmed by biopsy

- Cutaneous horn: The cutaneous horn is a hard keratotic growth that is longer than its base. The treatment of choice is excision. The incidence of an underlying squamous cell carcinoma is thought to be about 10%.

Immunologic Factors

Abnormalities in the host immune system have long been implicated as playing an important role in the development of cancer, although for most malignancies this role has been difficult to prove. Specifically, deficiencies of cell-mediated immunity are correlated with the development of BCC and SCC. Advanced and/or extensive NMSCs are associated with low T cell levels and apparent tumor anergy. Patients receiving chronic immunosuppressive therapy have a 50% risk of developing SCC within 20 years of transplantation; 30% of such cancers are highly aggressive.

Ultraviolet Radiation

Ultraviolet (UV) radiation causes most cases of NMSC. Eighty percent of a person's lifetime sun exposure occurs in the first 20 years of life. The skin is the organ most susceptible to damage by UV light because it is directly exposed. UV (e.g. UVA, UVB and UVC) exposure of the skin has a number of biologic effects, many of which are detrimental. UVC is more carcinogenic and might be expected to become a more relevant factor in the epidemiology of cutaneous malignancies, including melanoma and NMSC.

The acute response of skin to UV radiation is vasodilatation followed by clinical erythema. The time course of UVA erythema in humans differs from UVB, being maximal at 72 hours, compared with 24-48 hours for UVB. Adaptive changes are observed in the skin after exposure to UV light. These include increased vascularization, skin thickening (due to epidermal hyperplasia and increased thickness of the stratum corneum) and melanogenesis (tanning).

Ionizing Radiation

Ionizing radiation causes skin cancer in humans and experimental animal models. The risk is proportional to cumulative dose. Occupation of the patient may be an important factor because radiologists, uranium miners and airline pilots have a demonstrated increased incidence of skin cancer. Radiation therapy to the face, a practice formerly advocated for the treatment of acne, has been associated with an increased incidence of SCC.

Chemicals

Important hazardous chemicals include the polycyclic aromatic hydrocarbons and arsenic. The former can be found in coal tars, soot, asphalt, paraffin waxes and lubricating oils. Chronic exposure to arsenic leads to BCC and SCC, usually after a period of 18 to 45 years. Hands are often involved. Education programs and improved industrial safety will limit the number of these types of cases.

Prevention of Nonmelanoma Skin Cancer

Sunscreen

Sunscreen use in childhood (after six months of age) will encourage a lifetime behavior of sun protection and reduce skin cancer risk. Para-aminobenzoic acid is one of the most common active ingredients in sunscreens. This substance penetrates the stratum corneum and absorbs UV radiation. Titanium dioxide and zinc oxide act as physical barriers and provide the best protection. A sunscreen should have at least a sun protection factor (SPF) of 15.

Clothing

Normal light clothing provides limited protection against UV radiation. A plain white cotton T-shirt has a SPF of 10, which decreases when wet.

Chemoprevention

Chemoprevention of NMSC will ultimately be the most helpful for patients with skin cancers. Systemic retinoids that are derivatives of vitamin A have a proven chemo-preventative effect in reducing the risk of developing SCC and BCC. The mechanism of action is thought to occur via induction of apoptosis, impedance of tumor proliferation, or stimulation of differentiation during the tumor promotion phase of carcinogenesis. Oral retinoids might decrease the morbidity associated with multiple primary tumors and might reduce the risk of death in patients with high-risk cancers. Alfa difluoromethylor-nithine is the other possibility for the prevention of nonmelanoma skin cancers.

Clinical Diagnosis

A useful diagnostic tool has not yet been validated for nonmelanoma skin cancers. Over 60% of nonmelanoma skin cancers occur on the face and neck and these areas bear careful inspection. Lesions behind the ear, at the medial canthus and within the nasolabial folds are most easily missed.

As clinical diagnosis is not always reliable, a biopsy is usually performed on suspicious lesions, although some clinicians prefer to excise the entire lesion rather than perform an initial biopsy. Lesions that are raised can often be biopsied using a shave technique. If the area is flat or depressed, as with morpheaform BCC, a punch biopsy can be used, as a shave biopsy is unlikely to sample sufficient tumor cells. Sampling to the base of the lesion is especially important with SCC, where the architecture and depth are important diagnostic and treatment parameters.

Basal Cell Carcinoma

Basal cell carcinoma (BCC) is the most common malignancy among whites. This cancer causes considerable morbidity for patients and a financial burden on the health care system. Metastasis and death are rare.

Epidemiology

The incidence of BCC shows clear geographic variation. Per 100,000: Northern Europe 40-80; South Wales 114; Minnesota, USA 146; Southern USA 300; and Australia 726-1600).* This variation presumably reflects the likelihood of significant sun exposure. Among Caucasians in North America, the incidence has increased at more than 10% a year, leading to a lifetime risk of 30% of developing BCC. The incidence continues to increase with the aging population. The incidence of BCC increases after age 40. BCC is more common in men (30% to 80%) and is rare in dark-skinned people. Although 85% to 93% of BCC occurs in the head and neck area, a trend toward involvement of the trunk and extremities has been reported in Australia. Patients with BCC have an increased risk of developing a second BCC of the skin (35% at 3 years, 50% at 5 years), which increases with number of previous skin cancers, solar damage and skin sensitivity.

Differential Diagnosis

The differential diagnosis for basal cell carcinoma includes superficial basal cell carcinoma, pigmented basal cell carcinoma, infiltrating basal cell carcinoma, tricoepithe-

---

* Data obtained from: Holmes SA, Malinovszky K, Roberts DL. Changing trends in non-melanoma skin cancer in South Wales, 1988-1998. Br J Dermatol 2000;143:J224-9 and Marks R, Staples M. Trends in non-melanocytic skin cancer treated in Australia: the second national survey. Int J Cancer 1993;53:585-90

lioma, keloid, molluscum contagiosum and dermato-fibromas. There is good evidence for using the American Cancer Society's ABCDE criteria as a clinical diagnostic test to rule out malignant melanoma (see Melanoma section of this text).

Histologic Types

Although various dermatopathologic types of BCC exist, a mixed histology is often seen. These include nodular, micronodular, superficial, cystic, infiltrative and morpheaform. Histologic subtypes usually match the clinical picture. Histologic type correlates with malignant potential and recurrence and suggests clinical margins of resection. Nodular and cystic lesions are relatively indolent in contradistinction to the superficial, infiltrative, morpheaform and micronodular subtypes, which are biologically more aggressive. Superficial BCC has an increased risk of recurrence due to an increased tendency of incomplete primary excision. Infiltrative and morpheaform BCCs can be associated with aggressive local invasive behavior, with an increased tendency to recur. Both are characterized microscopically by irregular groups of tumor cells with a spiky appearance. Ulcerative and infiltrative types are more aggressive forms.

Clinical Types

Nodular Basal Cell Carcinoma

Nodular or nodulocystic BCC is the most common subtype (50% to 55%). It presents as a small solitary nodule or papule on the surface of the face skin. It has a shiny, pearly, translucent appearance and often has small or large telangiectatic vessels traversing throughout. The nodule is round or oval and the depth is usually similar to the width. Over time, the clinical picture may be dominated by ulceration in the center of the nodule surrounded by a rolled pearly border and bleeding, thus masking the nodularity ("rodent ulcer"). Although they are mostly red or flesh colored, they may show variable amounts of pigmentation mimicking or even masking melanoma.

Superficial

Superficial BCC is the second most common subtype (10%) and presents as an erythematous, flaking lesion frequently containing superficial ulcerations or crusting. The borders are usually round or oval, although they may be irregular. The lesions tend to occur mostly in the trunk. They are indolent and may be confused with a variety of benign disorders, including psoriasis, eczematous dermatitis and Bowen disease (*in situ* SCC; see below). Excision may be incomplete because the tumor may extend beyond the clinical margin or because the margin may be obfuscated by erythema arising from associated inflammation. Mohs

micrographic surgery (see treatment options) may be a valuable management option. Typically, the tumor is confined to the epidermis and growth is more radial than vertical.

Morpheaform (Sclerosing)

Morpheaform BCC is a rare subtype (2% to 5%) but aggressive variant that presents as a tan, white or yellowish atrophic plaque with ill-defined borders leading to difficulty in diagnosis and late presentation. Inflammatory induration is almost always present. The extent of the tumor is usually not apparent on clinical examination and the surgical specimen frequently has involved margins. Mohs micrographic surgery (see treatment options) is valuable in the management of these lesions. The growth pattern is radial and ulceration infrequent.

Pigmented

Pigmented BCC is a rare subtype (6%) and may be confused with melanoma. The pigment is melanin and can render the lesion a variety of colors ranging from tan to black **(Figure 16-3)**.

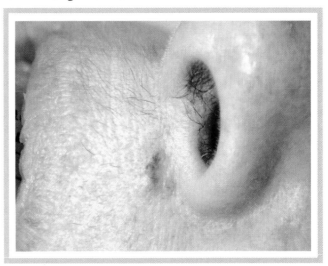

Figure 16-3: Pigmented basal cell carcinoma of the nasal sill. These lesions may be confused with nodular melanoma

Squamous Cell Carcinoma (SCC)

SCC is the second most common skin cancer after BCC **(Figure 16-4)**. SCC usually arises in damaged skin and is often preceded by sun damage, leukoplakia, actinic keratoses, or radiation damage. SCC may occur in chronic or unstable wounds and should be considered in the differential diagnosis of any chronic wound **(Figure 16-5)**.

Epidemiology

The incidence of SCC seems to be increasing. Incidence rates in Australia increased by 51% from 166 per 100,000

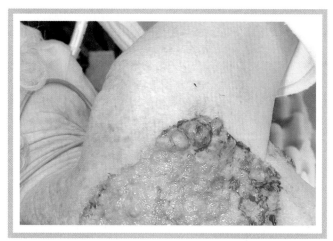

Figure 16-4: Locally advanced squamous cell carcinoma. Nodal involvement was clinically evident in this patient

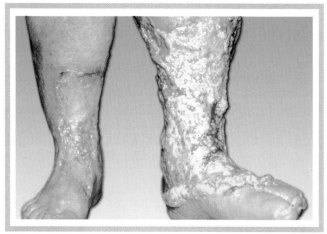

Figure 16-5: Squamous cell carcinoma arising in the setting of a chronic venous stasis ulceration. Chronic wounds that fail to heal merit biopsy.

people in 1985 to 250 per 100,000 in 1990. Whether this represents increased awareness and therefore an acquisition bias or reflects changing environmental risks remains speculative.

Histologic Types

Histologically, SCC is characterized by varying degrees of keratinocyte dysplasia. Classically, keratin pearls and intercellular bridging are seen. The grade of the tumor is determined by the degree of differentiation. High-grade tumors are marked by increased cellular atypia and loss of keratinization. High-grade tumors are biologically more aggressive and are associated with a worse prognosis.

Clinical Course

SCC presents as a painless, erythematous, poorly defined lesion with elevated borders. They may resemble an

actinic keratosis. Compared with BCC, these tumors are more aggressive and nodal metastases are more common.

Squamous Cell Carcinoma Variants

Squamous cell carcinoma can be associated with long-standing wounds, irritation or inflammation. Long-standing wounds have a 2% risk of harboring an SCC. Originally described in the setting of burn wounds (e.g. Marjolins ulcer), malignant degeneration may occur in any chronic wound including venous stasis ulcers, decubitus ulcers, hidradenitis and chronic osteomyelitis. The possibility of malignancy should be considered in any chronic wound and a biopsy should be performed. Wound or scar-associated SCC is generally more aggressive than its UV-induced counterpart and metastases more frequently (20% to 30%). The overall prognosis for patients with metastatic disease is dismal.

Bowen's Disease

Bowen's disease is an SCC *in situ* with epidermal and follicular involvement. Only 10% of cases become locally invasive; the rest remain localized for long periods. The lesion is erythematous with sharp and irregular borders. There may be superficial scaling and crusting. Lesions involving glans penis are termed erythroplasia of Queyrat.

Verrucous Carcinoma

Verrucous carcinoma is a well-differentiated variant of SCC so named due to its wart-like appearance **(Figure 16-6)**. Local invasion is common. Underlying bone involvement may occur; however, metastases are rare. Involvement of the palmar and plantar skin is common. Surgical excision is appropriate. Because recurrence after primary resection is common, Mohs surgical technique

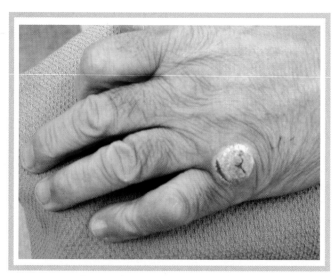

Figure 16-6: Verrucous carcinoma

may be appropriate. Radiotherapy is not advocated because it may induce anaplastic transformation.

Differential Diagnosis of Squamous Cell Carcinoma

For squamous cell cancer, the differential includes squamous cell carcinoma, keratoacanthoma, eczema and atopic dermatitis, contact dermatitis, psoriasis, pseudoepitheliomatous hyperplasia, bowenoid papulosis and seborrheic dermatitis.

Other Skin Tumors

Merkel Cell Carcinoma

Merkel cell carcinoma (MCC) is one of the most aggressive primary malignant tumors of the skin. MCC is a rare tumor; therefore, no prospective, statistically significant data are available to verify or validity of any prognostic features or treatment outcomes. Several large reviews document the development of local recurrence in 25-33% of all cases of MCC, regional disease in 25% of all cases and distant metastatic disease in 33% of cases. The overall 5-year survival rates range from 30-64%. It usually arises after the sixth decade and presents as a solitary nodule on a sun-exposed area (up to 75% in the head and neck area). It originates from the pluripotent basal cells in the epithelium. Aggressive excision with 3-5 cm margins is the treatment of choice because it is highly aggressive, locally invading subcutaneous planes, fat, lymphatics and blood vessels. Excision can be performed with surgical or Mohs surgery. This malignancy metastasizes early. The utility of sentinel node mapping and biopsy followed by selective lymphadenectomy has been documented. The other treatment options are postoperative radiotherapy for primary tumor, draining lymphatics and /or regional lymph node basins; and adjuvant chemotherapy (e.g. cisplatin or carboplatin, etoposide, topotecan and doxorubicin) for regional disease.

Dermatofibrosarcoma Protuberans

Dermatofibrosarcoma protuberans (DFSP) is rare fibrohistiocytic sarcoma that manifests clinically as a distinctive, raised and hard lesion which begins as a plaque or small nodule. Most patients are 20-40 years old. DFSP is uncommon, low grade sarcoma and the incidence rate of 0.8 cases per million persons per year. The local recurrence rate for DFSP in studies ranges from 0% to 60%, whereas the rate of development of regional or distant metastatic disease is only 1% and 4-5%, respectively. Biopsy should be made to achieve clear surgical margins. Two to four centimeter margins to investing fascia of muscle or pericranium with clear pathologic margins are advised when clinically feasible. Tumor characteristics include long, irregular and subclinical extensions. Biopsy

options are surgical excision or Mohs surgery. Radiation can be considered as primary therapy and/or postoperatively if ideal surgical margins are not achieved. Clinical trials, chemotherapy (including Imatinib mesylate), radiation or re-resection as feasible under specific clinical circumstances should all be considered in the rare event of metastatic disease.

Treatment Options for NMSC

Overview

Treatments for nonmelanoma skin cancer include surgical excision, Mohs micrographic surgery, curettage and electrodesiccation, cryosurgery, fractionated radiotherapy, topical chemotherapy, carbon dioxide laser, photodynamic therapy, intralesional interferon and retinoids **(Flow chart 16-1)**. Some of these therapies are untested or not widely available. Immunotherapy and photodynamic therapy remain experimental. Laser treatment offers theoretical advantages for certain patients, such as those taking anticoagulants. However, safety hazards and inconvenience limit their use even by dermatologists. Standard excision was recommended for nodular-ulcerative and superficial basal cell carcinoma < 2 cm in diameter and away from the face. Consideration of Mohs surgery was recommended for larger lesions, sclerosing lesions with morpheaform histology and for cosmetically sensitive areas where large tissue loss or

Flow chart 16-1: Management of nonmelanoma skin cancer. Abbreviations: BCC, basal cell carcinoma; C and E, curettage and electrodesiccation; MMS, Mohs micrographic surgery; SCC, squamous cell carcinoma; RT, radiation therapy (Reprinted by permission from Macmillan Publishers Ltd: Neville AN, Welch E, Leffel D. Management of melanoma skin cancer in 2007. Nature Clin Practice 2007;4: 462-9.)

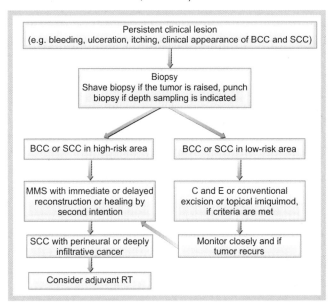

TABLE 16-5 Five-year cure rate by treatment modality for primary and recurrent basal cell (BCC) and squamous cell carcinomas (SCC). Reported by percent cure.

	Electrodesiccation and curettage	Cryotherapy	Excision	Radiation alone	Mohs	Non-Mohs methods (combined)
Primary BCC	92	93	90	91	99	91
Recurrent BCC	60	87	83	91	94	—
Primary SCC	96	96	92	90	97	92
Recurrent SCC	—	—	77	—	92	—

recurrence would be disfiguring (e.g. eyelid, ear, nose, lips). It should be noted that lack of uniformity in the method of reporting prohibited direct comparison of recurrence rates for different treatments. No similar meta-analysis reviews of treatment for all NMSC types were found (**Table 16-5**).

Surgery: Primary Excision

Oncologic cure requires that a tumor be removed completely, preferably by the simplest method. Primary excision is the most common treatment for BCC. SCC is treated more aggressively than BCC. The 5-year cure rates should exceed 95%. Treatment options and 5-year cure rates by treatment modality for two NMSC types, which are most frequent, are listed in **Table 16-5**. Recurrent NMSC, however, carries a very poor prognosis, with only a 50% cure rate. Cure rates approach 99% when surgical margins are negative. Because the goal of surgery is curative, achieving negative margins is important. When planning the excision the size of the tumor, the clinical type, grade, depth of invasion, the location, the ramifications of local recurrence and patient factors (e.g. age, general health, aesthetic considerations, etc.) should be taken into consideration.

As margin size increases, recurrence rates decrease. The appropriate margin of resection is not set in stone; rather, the surgeon must balance the risk of recurrence with loss of function or diminished cosmesis. Excision with 5 mm margins has been recommended by numerous authors as a general guideline, although smaller lesions and low-risk tumors may be managed with a 4 mm margin excision and still have a 95% cure rate. Nodular and superficial BCCs are definitively managed with surgical excision in 95% of the cases. The chance of residual tumor in micronodular, infiltrative and morpheaform are 18.6%, 26.5% and 33.3%, respectively (positive surgical margins). With the latter types, up to 1 cm margin excision is recommended. Large lesions may require wider margins because margin positivity and recurrence rates increase with size. Excisions of recurrent BCC should be avoided because of the high-failure rates. Recurrence rates are highest in the head and neck, especially the nose. Recurrent tumors should be referred for Mohs micro-

graphic surgery. Curettage prior to excision has been recommended, as a 26% improved cure rate for BCC was documented in lesions that were curetted before excision compared with noncuretted excisions in one study.

Definitive surgical margins for the management of SCC are unclear and dependent on tumor and host characteristics. For lesions smaller than 2 cm, a 4 mm margin is probably adequate, whereas lesions larger than 2 cm may be better managed with a 1 cm margin. The size of the margins may be modified depending on the differentiation, size and the invasion of surrounding structures. Some authors advocate wider margins (e.g. 3.5 cm margin for a 3 cm tumor) to achieve a 95% cure rate. For high risk SCC, the margin should be 6 mm and the excision should be into the subcutaneous fat. Early re-excision is recommended in the event of positive resection margins. The goal is to minimize risk of recurrence and metastasis. In general, local recurrence rates are around 5%.

Resected tissue is sent to the pathology laboratory for histologic examination and the defect reconstructed. Most excisions may be performed under local anesthesia in an outpatient setting. Postoperative lifestyle restrictions (on alcohol, weight lifting and exercise) should optimize wound healing.

Mohs Micrographic Surgery

Mohs micrographic surgery (MMS) aims to completely remove the tumor via consecutive excisions of the tumor, spatially orienting the specimen, histologically examining the margins, re-excising the residual tumor and repeating the cycle until the area is tumor free. It is also known as microscopically oriented histologic surgery (MOHS). The procedure is the gold standard for treating NMSC. The technique is based on the premise that the tumor spreads by contiguous growth and that removal of all tumor cells results in cure. Mohs micrographic surgery provides a higher probability of cure (reaching 99% for both BCC and SCC) and limits the defect size, promoting an improved aesthetic outcome for BCC, SCC and other NMSCs. MMS remains the most-effective method for removing NMSC, with a 5-year recurrence rate of 1% for BCC and 3% for SCC, compared with recurrence rates of 5.3% and 8%, respectively, for standard excision.

It is clearly superior for treatment of locally recurrent squamous cell carcinoma, with a 5-year cure rate of up to 90%, compared with 76.7% obtained with standard excision. The cure rate for Mohs micrographic surgery ranges from 94% to 97% (well-differentiated primary tumors) **(Table 16-5)**.

Indications for Mohs surgery in the management of primary BCC include lesions occurring at sites with high rates of treatment failure (e.g. periorbital, preauricular, nasal and nasolabial areas-typically fusion planes), lesions having poorly delineated tumor borders, aggressive malignant features, tumors involving sensitive aesthetic or functional locations (e.g. eyelid and canthus) and histologic subtypes associated with increased recurrence rates (e.g. morpheaform, sclerosing, infiltrative and basosquamous). Mohs micrographic surgery is useful in the management of the recurrent lesion where the tumor has demonstrated a more aggressive phenotype. Other indications for the technique are evolving. Disadvantages of the technique include expense and time. The Mohs surgery's process may require several hours to a full day. Large tumors may be managed using a single-stage excision with a modified frozen section technique. Additively, discontiguous or multifocal tumors are inappropriate indications because complete margin control cannot be ensured.

MMS is conducted under local anesthesia and in an outpatient setting. The surgeon curettes the visible tumor, excises a circular rim of tissue with 1-2 mm margins and maps and orients the tissue so that a tangential section reveals epidermal and deep margins. The cycle is repeated until clear margins are achieved. The defect is then reconstructed or heals by second intention.

Nonsurgical Ablation

Destructive methods (e.g. cryotherapy, electrodesiccation, curettage and laser) are appropriate methods for the management of smaller lesions that have recurrence rates comparable to primary excision. Cure rates decrease with increasing tumor size when nonsurgical ablative techniques are used. Another significant drawback is the lack of a specimen for histologic analysis. This can be disastrous in the event that the clinical diagnosis is incorrect.

Cryotherapy

Cryotherapy, at -195.6°C, with liquid nitrogen (LN) is a versatile, convenient and inexpensive modality that can treat skin cancers within minutes. Local anesthesia is not usually used but is an option because prolonged cryotherapy is painful and the freezing nonselective. Five-year cure rates for BCC and SCC treated by this method 93% and 96% **(Table 16-5)**. Most effectively delivered as a cryogen spray, LN destroys tissue through rapid freeze and slow thaw cycles. Wounds after cryotherapy of NMSC heal within 4-6 weeks by secondary intention, depending on the size, site and level of tumor destruction. Recurrent and other high-risk NMSC are inadequately destroyed by cryotherapy. Cryotherapy with LN is inexpensive and requires minimal equipment. An outpatient office procedure performed in minutes, cryotherapy is cost effective for properly selected tumors.

Electrodesiccation and Curettage

Electrodesiccation and curettage (EDC) should be rearranged to "CED" because the curettage process is the most critical and the first step before electrosurgery. Normal dermis does not curette well; a firm resistance to curettage is the usual endpoint. The curette in experienced hands delineates tumor margins and maximizes cure rates. Overall, the 5-year cure rates for primary BCC and SCC treated with C and E are 92% and 96%, respectively.

The EDC cycle should be repeated at least two to three times for maximal cure. Histologic margins are not examined with EDC. Healing is by secondary intention within 4-6 weeks. A stellate, firm, white scar is predictable. Morpheaform BCC and deep infiltrative SCC or other high-risk tumors should not be treated with EDC. Tumors that have been punch biopsied are unsuitable for EDC because there is no firm dermal plane available at the base for curettage. Soft tissues such as the lip, eyelids or atrophic skin cannot be curetted effectively. Laser may replace electrodesiccation as part of curettage. The CO_2 laser permits greater controlled tissue destruction than does electrodesiccation but requires more experience for effective use and expensive equipment. Other advantages of CO_2 laser includes excellent hemostasis, less pain during healing and possibly better cosmetic outcomes. Similar to cryotherapy, there is no margin control with EDC.

Incompletely Excised Basal Cell Carcinoma

A positive surgical margin suggests incomplete excision. Recurrence rates vary between 33% and 67% after presumed incomplete excision. Recurrence rates are higher with a positive deep margin compared with positive lateral margins (33% vs 17%). Fifty-four percent of the re-excised scars show residual tumor. Treatment options for patients having a positive margin include observation, reexcision and radiation.

Although supported by some authors, observation alone may be a poor choice. Patients may not be compliant with appropriate follow-up. It may be difficult to differentiate clinically between recurrent tumor growth and normal postsurgical induration. Considerable tumor regrowth may occur by the time that the recurrence is clinically accepted. Most authors advocate early re-excision for the management of patients having positive margins. Radiotherapy can be a second-line option in the event that re-excision is not desired.

Recurrent Basal Cell Carcinoma

Recurrent tumors are more difficult to treat and higher risk for tissue destruction and metastases. Although the results of primary excision overall are excellent, recurrences of BCC occur and their management can be challenging. Recurrence rates as high as 25% may be observed in certain anatomic locations, especially in periorbital, perinasal and periauricular regions. There is thought to be something unique about these embryonic fusion planes. Recurrence rates vary with the clinical subtype. Infiltrative, morpheaform and superficial types have the highest recurrence rates. It may be difficult to differentiate between an exuberant scar and recurrent tumor. Recurrence rates also vary with size of the primary. Recurrences of small lesions are less frequent (e.g. 4.3% for lesions < 9 mm compared with 13.7% for lesions > 10 mm). Ulceration, bleeding or erythema may be signs of recurrence. The time to recurrence may be protracted. Cumulative recurrences of 30%, 50% and 66% are observed within one, two and three years, respectively. Approximately 20% occur between five and ten years later, underscoring the need for long-term follow-up. Recurrence rates after primary surgical ablation are lowest for Mohs surgery (1%) compared with standard surgical technique. Mohs surgery is the most reliable technique for the management of recurrent lesions to reduce further recurrence.

Metastatic Basal Cell Carcinoma

Metastasis of BCC is rare (< 0.1%). Metastases may occur via lymphatic and hematogenous routes. Regional nodes, lungs and bones may be sites of involvement. The differential diagnosis of BCC includes trichoepithelioma, desmoplastic trichoepithelioma, eccrine epithelioma and microcystic adnexal carcinoma. These latter lesions are relatively uncommon.

Microcystic adnexal carcinoma is a locally invasive tumor mostly found on the lip, nose and periorbital area. Histologically, it may resemble BCC. Perineural invasion and recurrence are common. Wide local excision or Mohs surgery is the treatment of choice.

Trichoepithelioma is a benign, flesh-colored lesion that resembles BCC. Desmoplastic trichoepithelioma are benign lesions occurring mostly in women. Excision is appropriate. These lesions may be confused with morpheaform BCC histologically. Eccrine epithelioma mimics BCC in clinical behavior with aggressive local invasion. It tends to occur in the scalp and the treatment is wide local excision and possible Mohs surgery because recurrence is common.

Recurrent Squamous Cell Carcinoma

Predictors of recurrence after surgical ablation include degree of differentiation, depth of invasion and perineural invasion. The likelihood of recurrence in well, moderately and poorly differentiated sees are 7%, 23% and 28%, respectively. Seventy-eighty percent of all SCC recurrences develop within two years of initial therapy. The risk of recurrence increases with depth of invasion of the primary. Perineural invasion with or without clinical symptoms (e.g. paresthesias, pain, tingling, numbness) suggest increased recurrence rates, which may be as high 10%. For recurrent tumors or where the primary excision was inadequate or showed perineural invasion, wide excision via Moh's surgery may be reasonable.

Metastatic Squamous Cell Carcinoma

SCC has the propensity to metastasize most frequently to the regional lymph nodes and then systemically, to the lungs, bone and brain. Phenotypic correlates include location, depth of invasion, differentiation and size of the tumor. Identified factors that may increase the risk of metastasis include a tumor > 2 cm, depth of invasion > 4 mm, poor differentiation, scar carcinoma, perineural invasion, immunosuppression and history of previous treatments. Lesions on the face and dorsum of hand metastasize more commonly (10% to 20%) than lesions on the trunk and extremities (2% to 5%). The 5-year survival rate for patients having metastatic cutaneous SCC is 34%.

Medical Methods

Surgical ablative methods are in general highly effective, relatively inexpensive and well tolerated. Nonablative methods therefore must exceed these high benchmarks before being accepted as reasonable alternative therapies. These standards have not been exceeded and medical methods remain a second choice but one that may be reasonable in certain clinical settings. The use of medications may particularly be germane to the management of some of the hereditary syndromes characterized by the simultaneous occurrence of large numbers of lesions (e.g. Gorlin syndrome).

Immunotherapy

Recognition of the relevant role of the host immune system in the development of NMSC has suggested a potential indication for immune modulators as a therapeutic modality.

Interferon (IFN) is a naturally occurring antiviral biologic that may act by stimulating T-cell-mediated antitumor immune response. Intra- or peritumoral injection of interferon has been associated with complete regression rates of 50-80%. Treatment with IFN can cause flu-like symptoms including headache, myalgia and fever, which can be alleviated by taking acetaminophen. A disadvantage of IFN therapy, aside from the low cure rate, is the need for multiple intralesional injections. A common regimen is three injections per week for three weeks. This approach is now used only under specific circumstances such as when a patient is not an operative candidate because of his debilitated health or when surgery might result in disfigurement. The more aggressive forms of basal cell carcinoma do not seem to have a durable response to interferon and recurrence rates are high.

Imiquimod (Aldara, Graceway Pharmaceuticals, Malvern, PA, USA) is a topical immune-response modulator that is effective against superficial BCCs, small nodular BCCs and SCCs *in situ*. It demonstrated that patients with Bowen's disease located on the legs and shoulder, a 93% clearance rate was achieved with Imiquimod. It is an exciting, novel, topically applied immune agent with a variety of potential antiviral and antineoplastic indications. Generally, Imiquimod is associated with lesion regression rates between 70% and 100%. Superficial tumors seem to respond better than the nodular type, although long-term recurrence rates have not been assessed. The clinical effects of Imiquimod are primarily localized to the skin and percutaneous absorption into healthy skin is minimal. In addition to its original indication for external genital warts, it has been approved by the FDA for use in actinic keratoses and superficial BCC. The recommended dosing for superficial BCC is five days per week for six weeks and studies have demonstrated that this regimen provides an 88% histologic clearance rate. Reactions are similar to that of 5-FU in causing erosions and inflammation. Rare systemic complaints associated with extensive topical application include fatigue, myalgia, arthralgia and lymphadenopathy.

Photodynamic therapy (PDT) is a nonsurgical modality that may be promising. Appropriate lesions (e.g. premalignant actinic keratosis and superficial BCC and SCC *in situ*) are sensitized with various topical photosensitizers (most commonly delta-5-aminolevulinic acid—a photoporphyrin) and exposed to UVA or broad spectrum visible light. The photochemical reaction theoretically has direct and indirect tumoricidal effects. Although effective for actinic keratosis, PDT results with NMSCs do not have comparable cure rates for superficial BCC and SCC. Photodynamic treatment of nodular BCC using methyl aminolevulinate (mALA) has demonstrated complete responses in 90% of patients, with 74% remaining clear after 2 years.

Chemotherapy

Topical treatment using 5-fluorouracil may be used to treat multiple, small and superficial BCC on the trunk and limbs but seems to be ineffective for the invasive subtypes. Patient self-treat by applying the topical cream for four to six weeks. All lesions should be biopsy confirmed as superficial before 5-FU therapy. Contact dermatitis may occur with 5-FU or its components and is suspected with intense pruritus. Irritation is expected but erosions may become painful, necessitating early cessation. Topical 5-FU is also used for the treatment of actinic keratoses (SCC precursors) and is not generally as effective in the treatment of established SCC. A new form of 5-FU (Carac 0.5% 5-FU in acrylic polymer; Microsponge Enhanced Derm Technologies, Redwood City, CA, USA) may be as effective as older formulations (5-FU 5%) but with shorter treatment periods and less irritation and discomfort.

Chemotherapy administered systemically is reserved for the rare inoperable or metastatic NMSC. Temporary regression and palliation can be achieved using cisplatin.

Radiation

Radiation therapy may achieve excellent cure rates and cosmesis in properly selected tumors. Basal cell carcinomas and SCC are sensitive to radiation and a cure rate of 92% may be expected. Radiation is a noninvasive method usually reserved for elderly patients who are poor surgical candidates or for patients having residual or recurrent tumors. Adjuvant radiotherapy may be indicated after regional lymph node dissection when there is concern about extracapsular nodal extension or evidence of residual microscopic disease. Radiotherapy renders effective palliation of metastatic disease.

As a primary treatment, radiation can achieve similar cure rates as excision for properly selected tumors (< 2 cm, well-defined primaries). As adjunctive therapy, radiation combined with surgery may improve tumor control. Morpheaform (scar-like) BCC or infiltrative tumors do not respond well to radiotherapy. NMSC on hands, feet and genitalia should not be treated with radiation. The long-term cosmetic outcome following radiation therapy was reported to be good or excellent by 63% of patients, in contrast to 91% of patients after curettage and electrodesiccation and 84% after surgical excision. Disadvantages include expense, time and radiation-related complications.

Summary

NMSC continues to increase in prevalence. Each year, there are as many cases of NMSC as all other cancers combined. Although there is relatively low attributable mortality, the morbidity and expense of treatment is significant. Unlike many other malignancies, host and environmental factors relevant to the pathophysiology have clearly been demonstrated. Surgical ablation remains the mainstay of treatment. Nonsurgical options such as radiation therapy and cryosurgery, the newer additions of immunotherapy methods (e.g. imiquimod) and photodynamic therapy can be used in select tumors and can reduce morbidity.

Landmark Papers

1. Arons MS, Lynch JB, Lewis SR. Scar tissue carcinoma I: a clinical study with reference to burn scar carcinoma. Ann Surg 1965;161:170-88.
2. Der Berker D, Ibbotson S, Simpson NB, et al. Reduced experimental contact sensitivity in squamous cell but not basal cell carcinomas of skin. Lancet 1995;345: 425-6.
3. Fleming ID, Amonette R, Monaghan T, et al. Principles of management of basal and squamous cell carcinoma of the skin. Cancer 1995;75:699-704.
4. Gloster HM Jr, Brodland DG. The epidemiology of skin cancer. Dermatol Surg 1996; 22:217-26.
5. Jacobs GH, Rippey JJ, Altini M. Prediction of aggressive behavior in basal cell carcinoma. Cancer 1982;49:533-7.
6. Karagas MR, Stukel TA, Greenberg ER, et al. Risk of sub-sequent basal cell carcinoma and squamous cell carcinoma of the skin among patients with prior skin cancer. Skin cancer prevention study group. JAMA 1992;267:3305-10.
7. Kraemer KH. Xeroderma pigmentosum-A prototype disease of environmental-genetic interactions. Arch Dermatol J 1980;116:541-2.
8. Logan G. Ultraviolet injury as an experimental model of the inflammatory reaction. Nature 1963;198:968-9.
9. Marks R, Rennie G, Selwood TS. Malignant transformation of solar keratoses to squamous cell carcinoma. Lancet 1988; 1:795-7.
10. Miller SJ. Aetiology and pathogenesis of basal cell carcinoma. Clin Dermatol 1995;13:527-36.
11. Neville AN, Welch E, Leffel D. Management of melanoma skin cancer in 2007. Nature Clin Practice 2007;4: 462-9.
12. Nguyen TH, Ho DQ. Nonmelanoma Skin Cancer. Current Treatment Options in Oncology 2002;3:193-203.
13. Preston DS, Stem RS. Nonmelanoma cancers of the skin. N Engl Med 1992; 327:1649-62.
14. Preston Sr DS. Nonmelanoma cancers of the skin. N Engl J Med 1992;327: 1649.
15. Urbach F. Geographic distribution of skin cancer. J Surg Oncol 1971;3:219-34.
16. Wagner JD, Evdokimow DZ, Weisberger E, et al. Sentinel node biopsy for high-risk nonmelanoma cutaneous malignancy. Arch Dermatol 2004;140:75-9.
17. Wolf OJ, Zitelli JA. Surgical margins for BCC. Arch Dermatol 1987; 123:340-4.

Level of Evidence Table			
Recommendation	**Grade**	**Best level of evidence**	**References**
Excisional biopsy is the best initial method for evaluation of suspected skin malignancy.	B	4	1,2
For BCC with favorable histology (nodular, etc.), standard excision with 4 mm margins is recommended for lesions <2 cm in diameter in low risk areas.	A	1a	3-10
For SCC, 4 mm margins are likely adequate for low risk lesions < 2 cm. Higher risk and larger SCC treated with excision warrant wider margins (6 mm-1 cm) with excision into the subcutaneous fat.	B	3	3, 11-13
Mohs surgery is the preferred treatment for high-risk primary non-melanoma skin cancer and esthetically sensitive areas (eyelid, ear, nose, lips). It should be the primary therapy for locally recurrent SCC to achieve cure rates approaching 90%.	A	2	14, 15, 8-10
Radiation therapy provides acceptable cure rates for small (< 2 cm) tumors of favorable histology in cosmetically sensitive areas or a primary therapy in poor surgical candidates.	B	2	16-21

References

1. Garner KL, Rodney WM. Basal and squamous cell carcinoma. Prim Care 2000;27:447–58.
2. Bruce AJ, Brodland DG. Overview of skin cancer detection and prevention for the primary care physician. Mayo Clin Proc 2000;75:491–500.
3. Hochman M, Lang P. Skin cancer of the head and neck. Med Clin North Am 1999;83:261–82.
4. Thissen MR, Neumann MH, Schouten LJ. A systematic review of treatment modalities for primary basal cell carcinomas. Arch Dermatol 1999;135:1255–9.
5. Rowe DE. Comparison of treatment modalities for basal cell carcinoma. Clin Dermatol 1995;13:617–20.
6. Wolf DJ, Zitelli JA. Surgical margins for basal cell carcinoma. Arch Dermatol 1987;123:340–4.
7. Silverman MK, Kopf AW, Bart RS, Grin CM, Levenstein MS. Recurrence rates of treated basal cell carcinomas. Part 3: Surgical excision. J Dermatol Surg Oncol 1992;18:471-6.
8. Cullen FJ, Kennedy DA, Hoehn JE. Management of basal cell carcinoma: current concepts. Adv Plast Surg 1993; 10:187.
9. Wolf DJ, Zitelli JA. Surgical margins for basal cell carcinoma. Arch Dermatol 1987; 123:340–4.

10. Goldberg DP. Assessment and surgical treatment of basal cell skin cancer. Clinics in Plast Surg 1997; 24:673–86.

11. Martinez JC, Otley CC. The management of melanoma and nonmelanoma skin cancer: a review for the primary care physician. Mayo Clin Proc 2001;76:1253–65.

12. Brodland DG, Zitelli JA. Surgical margins for excision of primary cutaneous squamous cell carcinoma. J Am Acad Dermatol 1992;27:241–8.

13. Rowe DE, Carroll RJ, Day CL Jr. Prognostic factors for local recurrence, metastasis, and survival rates in squamous cell carcinoma of the skin, ear, and lip. J Am Acad Dermatol 1992;26:976–90.

14. McGovern TW, Leffell DJ. Mohs surgery: the informed view. Arch Dermatol 1999;135:1255–9.

15. Lovett RD, Perez CA, Shapiro SJ, Garcia DM. External irradiation of epithelial skin cancer. Int J Radiat Oncol Biol Phys 1990; 19:235–42.

16. Lee WR, Mendenhall WM, Parsons JT, Million RR. Radical radiotherapy for T4 carcinoma of the skin of the head and neck: a multivariate analysis. Head Neck 1993; 15:320–4.

17. Ashby MA, Smith J, Ainslie J, McEwan L. Treatment of nonmelanoma skin cancer at a large Australian center. Cancer 1989; 63:1863–71.

18. Avril MF, Auperin A, Margulis A, Gerbaulet A, Duvillard P, Benhamou E, et al. Basal cell carcinoma of the face: surgery or radiotherapy? Results of a randomized study. Br J Cancer 1997; 76:100–6.

19. Fitzpatrick PJ, Thompson GA, Easterbrook WM, Gallie BL, Payne DG. Basal and squamous cell carcinoma of the eyelids and their treatment by radiotherapy. Int J Radiat Oncol Biol Phys 1984; 10:449–54.

20. Wilder RB, Kittelson JM, Shimm DS. Basal cell carcinoma treated with radiation therapy. Cancer 1991; 68:2134–7.

21. Alam M, Ratner D. Primary care: cutaneous squamous-cell carcinoma. N Engl J Med 2001;344:975–83.

17

Melanoma

Bulent Unal, A Serhat Gur, Atilla Soran, Howard Edington

In the year 2008, an estimated 62,480 new cases of melanoma will be diagnosed. There were an estimated 7700 melanoma related deaths (4800 male and 2900 female) in 2000 and about 8,420 patients will die of the disease in United States in 2009. While the reported incidence of cutaneous melanoma has been increasing rapidly during the past 25 years, the rate of rise is slowing and the mortality rate is falling in young women, plateauing men and rising in older men and women. There is a 17 fold higher incidence of melanoma in whites than in blacks. The lifetime risk of developing melanoma for someone born in the United States in the year 2000 may be as high as one in 41 for men and one in 61 for women.

The outcome of melanoma initially depends on the stage at presentation. It is estimated that 82-85% of melanoma patients presents with localized disease and primary tumors 1 mm or less in thickness, with long-term survival achieved in more than 90% of patients. For patients with melanomas more than 1 mm in thickness, survival rates range from 50% to 90%, while patients with advanced inoperable melanoma have a long-term survival of less than 5%. Unfortunately, despite an improved case fatality rate, the overall mortality from melanoma continues to increase at a rate of 2% annually.

Risk Factors for Melanoma

While the pathogenesis of melanoma remains incompletely understood, it is generally accepted that both environmental and genetic factors are relevant. A number of lesions that clinically resemble melanoma may or may not be associated with the development of the disease. Some of these lesions and their biologic potential are enumerated below. **Table 17-1** summarizes these relationships and importantly attempts to further define them according to relative risk.

TABLE 17-1	Risk factors for malignant melanoma
Risk factors	**RR**
Atypical nevus syndrome with personal and family history of melanoma	500
Changing mole	> 400
Atypical nevus syndrome with family history of melanoma	148
Age ≥ 15	88
Dysplastic moles	7-70
History of melanoma before age 40	23
Large congenital nevus (≥15 cm)	17
Caucasian race	12
Lentigo maligna	10
Atypical nevi	7-27
Regular use of tanning bed before age 30	7.7
Multiple nevi	5-12
Personal history of melanoma	5-9
Immunosuppression	4-8
Family history (first degree) of melanoma	3-8
Nonmelanoma skin cancer	3-5
Sun sensitivity or tendency to burn	2-3

Melanocytic Lesions

Melanocytic Nevus (e.g. Junctional, Compound and Intradermal)

Melanocytic nevi mainly develop during childhood and adolescence. The most important risk factor for the development of melanoma is the number of melanocytic nevi on the body. Numerous epidemiological risk-factor studies, from various countries with Caucasian populations, have assigned a risk of 1 fold to individuals with 0-10 melanocytic nevi but an 8-10 fold increase in relative risk for those with 100 or more melanocytic nevi. Congenital melanocytic nevi occur in 1% of newborns. Although generally small (< 1.5 cm) and singular in the majority of cases, they may range to sizes greater than 9.9 cm. The lifetime risk is estimated to be 5% to 15% and varies with size of the congenital nevus **(Figure 17-1)**.

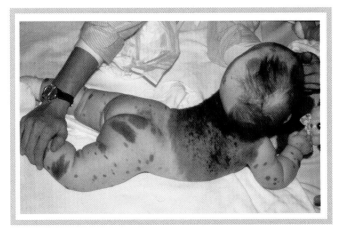

Figure 17-1: Giant congenital melanocytic nevus (bathing trunk nevus). The risk of malignant degeneration is thought to be as high as 15%. Removal at an early age although oncologically ideal, but technically it is difficult

Dysplastic Melanocytic Nevus (e.g. Junctional, Compound, Intradermal) and Atypical Melanocytic Nevi (e.g. Atypical Mole Syndrome)

Dysplastic melanocytic nevi develop throughout life in those who are predisposed genetically and are often evident within the first decade. It may resemble melanoma because it has indistinct or irregular margin, variegated and/or dark coloration and macular surface component. The risk of developing melanoma associated with dysplastic nevi is increased markedly with associated family history (100-400 fold).

An important risk factor for melanoma development is the presence of atypical melanocytic nevi. The atypical mole syndrome has been defined as: ≥ 100 melanocytic nevi, one or more melanocytic nevi that are ≥ 8 mm in size and more than one melanocytic nevi with clinical atypia. If a certain number of these atypical lesions are

present then there is a 4-6 fold increase of the relative risk for melanoma development. These risk factors interact with each other in a multiplicative fashion. This means that persons having 100 melanocytic nevi or more, among which five or more are atypical melanocytic nevi, have an about 50 fold relative risk for melanoma development.

Lentigines (e.g. Lentigo Simplex, Solar Lentigo and Lentigo Maligna)

A simple lentigo is usually less than 5 mm in diameter and isolated macule. It is usually acquired, rarely congenital and generally located in sun-protected or sun-exposed sites. Solar lentigenes also known as freckles appear as lightly pigmented tan macules in sun-exposed areas **(Figure 17-2)**. Common sites include the face, chest, back and hands. Presence of heavy sun-induced freckling appears to be an independent risk factor for developing melanoma, with estimated increased risk of 2-4 fold. Lentigo maligna (LM) is regarded by some as a melanoma *in situ* and by others as a "variety" of intraepidermal melanocytic dysplasia in sun-damaged skin.

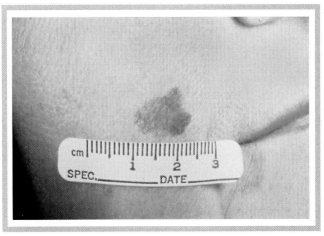

Figure 17-2: Actinic keratoses. Solar lentigo occurring on the face. The pigment usually appears homogenous

Melanoma *in situ*

Melanoma *in situ* is a purely intraepidermal process of malignant melanocytic proliferation. The three types of melanoma *in situ* (based on pattern of intraepidermal spread and architectural characteristics) are lentigo maligna, superficial spreading and acral lentiginous, which will each be discussed in detail.

Sunscreen, Clothing and Pigment Traits

The most important risk factor for the development of melanocytic nevi was the number of weeks on holiday in sunny climates. Freckling after exposure to sunlight is associated with a 1.9 times relative risk. This refers to the type of intermittent sun exposure that can cause sunburn in a certain percentage of children.

Clothing habits are significantly associated with protection from nevus development. The more clothes children wear in the sun, the fewer nevi they develop. Other risk factors for nevus development include pigment traits. The "typical" melanoma patient has sandy hair, blue eyes and fair skin. A child's skin type indicates the reaction to sun exposure and is a significant risk factor. Individuals with an inability to tan and fair skin that sunburns easily have a greater risk of developing melanoma.

Hereditary Factors

Positive family history of melanoma and inherited genetic mutations contribute to the development of melanoma. The numbers of melanocytic nevi in both fathers and mothers were significantly associated to nevus development in their children. Additionally, melanoma can occur in any ethnic group and also in areas of the body without substantial sun exposure.

Melanoma Growth Patterns

Pathologists generally describe melanoma as being in one of two growth patterns which seems to correspond with biologic behavior. The radial or horizontal growth phase seems to be associated with a more indolent clinical course as compared to the vertical growth phase which is related to a more aggressive phenotype. This growth phase difference is in some sense reflected in the staging syetem, in which a deeper level of invasion is associated with a worse prognosis and higher likelihood of metastasis.

Superficial Spreading Melanoma

Superficial spreading melanoma (SSM) is the most common variety of melanoma seen in about 70% of cases and occurs more frequently in younger adults. Posterior trunk is the most common site for men and women. Commonly (but not always) SSM shows irregular and asymmetric borders with color variegation **(Figure 17-3)**.

Nodular Melanoma

Nodular melanoma exhibits rapid growth (weeks to months) into a uniformly blue-black, dome-shaped nodule, but may appear pink or red. These account for about 10% to 30% of reported melanomas. The nodular variety is a more aggressive tumor with a shorter clinical onset than SSM. Nodular melanomas are more common in men than in women. The lesions appear most often in middle-aged patients on the trunk or head and neck **(Figure 17-4)**.

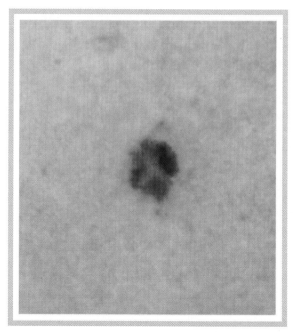

Figure 17-3: Superficial spreading melanoma. The most common phenotypic pattern. Border irregularity, asymmetry and color variegation are clinical clues.

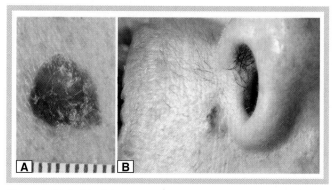

Figure 17-4: Nodular melanoma. (A) Nodular appearance clinically evident. (B) Pigmented basal cell carcinoma of the nasal sill. These lesions may be confused with nodular melanoma

Lentigo Maligna Melanoma

Lentigo maligna (LM) melanoma occurs in older adults and accounts for only 15% of cases. LM arises in elderly patients from pre-existing LM over a period that may be years in duration. Locations include sun-exposed areas such as the head, neck, upper torso and arms. They may reach large sizes (> 3 cm), appearing as tan with variegations of brown and black, but lesions may also be small (1 cm in diameter). LM is believed to be induced by ultra-violet B radiation, possibly arising initially in a solar lentigo.

Acral Lentiginous Melanoma

By definition, acral lentiginous melanoma appears on palmar, plantar and subungual skin, with a unique histopathologic appearance of intradermal radial growth phase characterized by a contiguous and continuous proliferation of pleomorphic hyperchromatic melanocytes along the basal cell layer of a hyperplastic epithelium.

Diagnosis of Melanoma

In light of the increasing incidence of melanoma, public awareness has improved. Patients with pigmented skin lesions are seeking attention with increased frequency. The vast majority of these pigmented skin lesions are benign and normally would not require treatment. The decision about which skin lesions require biopsy is clinically challenging and can sometimes be difficult because of the wide range and variety. The following steps are useful for early diagnosis for melanoma:

1. Patient history of new or changing nevus, prior personal history, family history of melanoma and number and types of nevi.
2. History and physical examination including skin for every three months.
3. Total skin examination: appearance of primary lesion, detection of subcutaneous metastases and discovery of atypical nevi and other primary melanomas (2% of melanoma patients have a synchronous primary tumor).
4. Review of systems for symptoms and signs of metastatic disease for patients who have melanoma.
5. Physical examination including palpation of inguinal, axillary, supraclavicular and head and neck lymph nodes.
6. Biopsy of the suspected primary lesion with microstaging.
7. Laboratory evaluation for signs of distant metastases from invasive melanoma such as chest X-ray, dermoscopy and lactate dehydrogenase (LDH).

Findings Suspicious of Melanoma

The clinical criterion that is currently used in the evaluation of a suspected melanoma is the American Cancer Society's "ABCDE" algorithm.

Asymmetry: One half of the lesion not identical to the other

Border: Lesion has an uneven or ragged border

Color: Lesion has more than one color (i.e. black, blue, pink, red or white)

Diameter: Lesion has a diameter greater than 6 mm

Elevation or **E**nlargement: Elevation of lesion above skin surface or enlargement by patient report

This rule was validated in four dermatology clinics, studying a total of 1,118 lesions, although the studies were not homogenous for strength of recommendation. Although the algorithm is a simple and easy to remember guide it is by no means comprehensive nor infallible. Ideally the primary should be identified before it reaches 6 mm in diameter. Another potentially useful diagnostic test is the revised 7-point checklist developed in the United Kingdom **(Table 17-2)**. This test was found to have a high sensitivity, but low specificity. Therefore, it has a low false-negative rate and is useful for ruling out the diagnosis of melanoma when negative. However, the test yields a significant number of false-positive results, leading to possibly of unnecessary biopsies and increased patient anxiety.

TABLE 17-2	Revised 7-point checklist for assessing risk of melanoma
Suspect melanoma if there are 1 or more major signs	**3 or 4 minor signs without a major sign can also indicate a need to biopsy suspicious moles**
1. Change in size 2. Change in shape 3. Change in color	4. Inflammation 5. Crusting or bleeding 6. Sensory change 7. Diameter (≥ 7 mm)

The differential diagnosis for the pigmented lesion is extensive and includes, but is not limited to, compound nevi, junctional nevi, pigmented basal cell carcinoma and an array of kerasotes. Melanoma can present in an amelanotic form and can be mistaken for a benign lesion. Therefore, it has become customary practice to perform a biopsy on any lesion in which there has been a change in appearance or behavior. Changes in appearance may include changes in border irregularity, tone, color and size. Changes in behavior may include bleeding, itching and altered texture.

Dermoscopy and Computer Dermoscopy have made significant progress in the early diagnosis of cutaneous melanoma. The characteristic features of cutaneous melanoma can be detected more easily by epiluminescence microscopy with 10-20 fold magnification and fluid immersion. Computer Dermoscopy should also be able to take microscopic and macroscopic pictures and digital analysis. A high picture resolution is an important quality standard of these devices.

If a skin lesion is suspected clinically to be malignant melanoma, it is recommended to use the ABCDE criteria and the revised 7-point checklist to guide biopsy decisions.

Biopsy of the Suspected Melanoma

Various biopsy techniques are used including incisional, punch, excisional and shave. The indications for each are based on the clinical characteristics and location of the

TABLE 17-3	Breslow thickness and current recommended margins of excision for melanoma	
Breslow thickness	**Margin of excision**	**5 years survival**
< 1 mm	1 cm	95-100%
1-2 mm	1-2 cm	80-96%
2.1-4 mm	2 cm	60-75%
> 4 mm	> 2 cm	50%

TABLE 17-4	Clark's level of invasion
Level 1:	Confined to epidermis *(in situ)*; never metastasizes; 100% cure rate
Level 2:	Invasion into papillary dermis; invasion past basement membrane (localized)
Level 3:	Tumor filling papillary dermis (localized) and compressing the reticular dermis
Level 4:	Invasion of reticular dermis (localized)
Level 5:	Invasion of subcutaneous tissue (regionalized by direct extension)

lesion. Complete excision of the tumor allows for the most precise estimates of prognosis based on histologic features, including Breslows depth—the most important histologic prognostic factor for cutaneous melanoma **(Table 17-3)**, ulceration, angiolymphatic invasion or vascular involvement, Clark level **(Table 17-4)**, mitotic rate and host response. Narrow excisional biopsy, with 2 mm to 3 mm margins around the visible borders of the lesion and into the subcutaneous fat, should be performed when possible. Wider margins (> 1-2 cm) may disrupt afferent cutaneous lymphatic flow and affect the ability to accurately identify the sentinel lymph nodes (SLN) in patients eligible for this procedure. For the same reason, orientation of the excisional biopsy should be parallel to lymphatic drainage; that is, longitudinally on the extremities.

Shave biopsies of suspected melanomas are discouraged, as partial removal of the primary tumor may preclude accurate measurement of Breslow's depth.

Multiple-punch biopsies are appropriate for large lesions, such as LM and acral lentiginous subtypes and should include the most suspicious areas (darkly pigmented or nodular). Wood's lamp examination is extremely useful in delineating clinical borders of LM and superficial spreading subtypes, by identifying hypopigmented areas of regression that may be contiguous with the pigmented portion of the cutaneous melanoma.

Prognostic Factors

The single most valuable prognostic factor for patients having a diagnosis of melanoma is the status of the sentinel node.

Other relevant prognostic data include stage **(Table 17-5)**, age (older age has decreased survival), gender

TABLE 17-5	Staging classification of melanoma and 5 years survival rates.
Classification	

Stage 0: Melanoma *in situ* (Clark Level I), 100% Survival

Stage I/II: Invasive Melanoma, 85-95% Survival
- T1a: Less than 1.00 mm primary, w/o Ulceration or Clark Levels II-III
- T1b: Less than 1.00 mm primary, w/o Ulceration or Clark Levels IV-V
- T2a: 1.00-2.00 mm primary, w/o Ulceration

Stage II: High Risk Melanoma, 40-85% Survival
- T2b: 1.00-2.00 mm primary, w/o Ulceration
- T3a: 2.00-4.00 mm primary, w/o Ulceration
- T3b: 2.00-4.00 mm primary, w/o Ulceration
- T4a: 4.00 mm or greater primary, w/o Ulceration
- T4b: 4.00 mm or greater primary, w/o Ulceration

Stage III: Regional Metastasis, 25-60% Survival
- N1: Single Positive Lymph Node
- N2: 2-3 Positive Lymph Nodes or Regional Skin/In-Transit Metastasis
- N3: 4 Positive Lymph Nodes or Lymph Node and Regional Skin/In-Transit Metastases

Stage IV: Distant Metastasis, 9-15% Survival
- M1a: Distant Skin Metastasis, Normal LDH
- M1b: Lung Metastasis, Normal LDH
- M1c: Other Distant Metastasis or Any Distant Metastasis with Elevated LDH

Stage		
I	=	T1-2a, N0, M0
II	=	T2b-4b, N0, M0
III	=	Any T, N1-3, M0
IV	=	Any T, any N, M1

TNM Melanoma Staging System (used with the permission of the American Joint Committee on Cancer (AJCC), Chicago, Illinois. The original source for this material is the AJCC Cancer Staging Manual, Sixth Edition (2002) published by Springer-Verlag, New York)

(females have an improved survival) and anatomical localization (head, neck and truncal melanomas have a worse prognosis than lesions of the extremities). Stage of disease is the most important determinant of survival in melanoma and is best established pathologically by SLN assessment in patients with primary tumor thickness > 1 mm. LN metastases significantly decrease the 5-year survival rate compared with patients who have no LN metastases and also macroscopic disease confers a worse prognosis than microscopic LN disease. SLN status is an independent prognostic factor as important as tumor thickness. Interestingly, less invasive melanomas even with lymph node metastases carry a better prognosis than deep melanomas without regional metastasis at the time of staging. Local recurrences tend to behave similarly to a primary unless they are at the site of a wide local excision (as opposed to a staged excision or punch/shave excision) since these recurrences tend to indicate lymphatic invasion. The number of metastatic sites is associated with median survival (1 site: 7 months; 2 sites: 4 months; ≥ 3 sites: 2 months). Additionally, duration of remission is associated with survival with longer remission associated with improved survival.

Important histological prognostic factors include: tumor thickness in millimeters (Breslow's depth), depth related to skin structures (Clark level), type of melanoma, presence of ulceration, presence of lymphatic/perineural invasion, angiogenesis, presence of tumor infiltrating lymphocytes (if present, prognosis is better), microsatellites, location of lesion, presence of satellite lesions and presence of regional or distant metastasis. Certain types of melanoma may have worse prognoses, but this is predominantly explained by their thickness. Others cytogenetic and molecular markers of tumor progression are presented in **Table 17-6**.

Treatment

Excision of the Melanoma

Diagnostic punch or excisional biopsies may appear to excise (and in some cases may indeed actually remove) the tumor, but further surgery is often necessary to reduce the risk of recurrence. Complete surgical excision with adequate margins and assessment for the presence of detectable metastatic disease along with short- and long-term follow-up is standard. The margin of excision is based on the thickness of the melanoma. Until 15 years ago all primary melanomas were excised with 3-5 cm margin, but multiple studies have shown that there is no advantage to margins more than 2 cm. The WHO Melanoma Group performed the first surgical trial to compare lower safety margins of 1 cm and 3 cm in primary melanomas with less than 2 mm of tumor thickness. The group found no differences in survival and only slightly increased local recurrence rates in the patients with narrower excision margins. Therefore, 1 cm margins in patients with primary melanomas with less than 1 mm tumor thickness were recommended based on these results. Later comparisons of 5 cm and 2 cm safety margins in thick primary melanomas revealed no significant advantages for the 5 cm margins. However, a recent trial comparing 1 cm and 3 cm safety margins in thick primary melanoma with 2 mm and more tumor thickness showed an increased rate of local recurrence in those with the small safety margins and a simultaneous trend towards decreased survival rates. These findings indicate that safety margin cannot be reduced to zero in melanoma. Different national guidelines now give uniform recommendations for the excision of primary melanoma. The safety margins recommended are summarized in **Table 17-3**.

The role of Mohs micrographic surgery in the surgical management of melanoma has generated controversy. The risks of tumor implantation, false-negative margins due to suboptimal melanocytic staining and inadequate margins limit the use and benefit of this technique. Advocates of the Mohs technique argue that it has the benefit of limiting the margin of excision. This limitation is especially important in critical areas with aesthetic importance, such as the face. However, the current recommendations for margins of excision, based on years of investigation and prospective studies, do not support the concept of minimal margins.

Recommendations for safety margins are now widely evidence based. The question of whether general reduction of safety margins to 1 cm is justified remains open.

TABLE 17-6	Cytogenetic and molecular markers of tumor progression and other unfavorable prognostic factors	
Cytogenetic and molecular	**Other unfavorable prognostic factors**
<ul><li>Mitotic rate</li><li>Absence of lymphocyte infiltration into tumor</li><li>Tyrosinase mRNA level in peripheral blood</li><li>DNA aneuploidy</li><li>Tumor cell type</li><li>Nuclear organizer regions</li><li>Tumor angiogenesis</li><li>Mutation in ras and other oncogenes</li></ul>	<ul><li>With equivalent thickness, melanomas of the scalp, palms and soles</li><li>Presence of a vertical phase of growth</li><li>Presence of microscopic satellites around the tumor and DNA aneuploidy of the primary tumor</li><li>High mitotic activity and regression in the primary tumor</li><li>Non-brisk lymphohistiocytic response in the primary tumor</li></ul>

Elective Regional Lymph Node Dissection

Elective regional lymph node dissection (ELND) in the absence of clinically detectable nodal metastases is a controversial procedure. Only 20% of highly selected patients undergoing ELND are found to have microscopic metastases. Prospective randomized trials in clinical stage I melanoma find no overall survival advantage for ELND in patients with intermediate-thickness melanoma (1-4 mm). ELND is currently not recommended in patients with thick melanoma (> 4 mm), because of the high risk for regional and distant metastatic disease (60-70%). In addition, ELND without lymphoscintigraphy in the head and neck region may be misdirected in up to 50% of cases, because of the variability in lymphatic pathways. When it has been done on the basis of anatomic guidelines (Sappe's lines), ELND may be misdirected in up to 30% when compared with SLN mapping with lymphoscintigraph. The possible advantages of ELND include providing staging information where SLN mapping is not feasible, while the disadvantages of ELND are increased morbidity, false-negative results, increased hospitalization and surgical costs and absence of proof of surgical benefit. The technique of lymphadenectomy varies based on the anatomic location. The principal lymphatic basins are located in the cervical neck, axillary and inguinal territories. The number of lymph nodes removed ranges from 10 to 50 and is dependent on the anatomic location.

Sentinel Lymph Node Biopsy

Currently, minimally invasive techniques (e.g. preoperative lymphoscintigraphy and intraoperative SLN mapping) are available to identify occult lymph node metastases and select patients at higher risk who may benefit from adjuvant therapy. The SLN is defined as the first LN in a lymphatic basin that receives afferent lymph flow from the primary tumor site. SLN dissection is a diagnostic procedure for identification of regional nodal micrometastases. Sentinel lymph node biopsy (SLNB) is currently recommended for patients with invasive melanoma with a thickness that ranges from 1 mm to 4 mm. The principal advantage of SLNB is that it significantly reduces the incidence of lymphedema, because a total lymphadenectomy is usually not necessary.

Preoperative lymphoscintigraphy can assess drainage patterns, thereby identifying the regional nodal basin at risk for metastases. This technique is particularly useful for identification of areas with ambiguous drainage. A Tc-99 colloid-tagged material is injected at the melanoma site. Radiolabeled material drains to the metastatic nodal groups and is measured with a gamma counter at time intervals up to 2 hours post-injection. Intraoperative SLN mapping and SLNB are used to identify the first node in drainage basin. Blue dye and radioactive material are

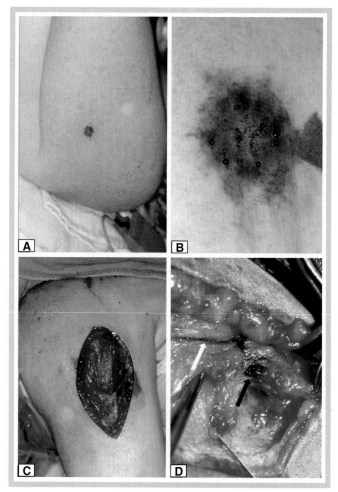

Figure 17-5: An intermediate thickness melanoma. Wide excision and sentinel node mapping and biopsy to be performed (A). The primary lesion has been injected preoperatively with radiocolloid and intraoperatively with isosulfan blue vital dye (intradermally) (B). Wide excision of the primary performed to fascia (C). Draining nodal basin is explored. Isosulfan blue dye nicely demonstrates both the afferent lymphatic (white arrow) and draining (sentinel) node (black arrow) (D)

injected at the site of melanoma. The first nodes that stain blue and exhibit radioactive uptake are removed for biopsy **(Figure 17-5)**.

The sentinel node procedure has radically impacted the management of the melanoma patient. Currently the procedure is used clinically to select patients who are at increased risk of failing primary surgical therapy and may be offered additional surgical and/or adjuvant therapy. The role and efficacy of both additional surgery and adjuvant therapy remain however somewhat controversial. It remains standard of care to treat patients having a positive sentinel node with a completion lymphadenectomy. This recommendation is based partly on the observation that about 20% of patients undergoing completion lymphadenectomy are found to have additional nodal disease.

Although a reasonable and testable assumption that these patients should benefit from the procedure, hard data to prove it is not available. Several studies have certainly suggested a clinical benefit both in terms of disease free and overall survival from this approach and early detection and aggressive surgical treatment of nodal disease seems to be logical.

Recognition of Local Recurrence, In-transit or Metastases of Melanoma

Melanoma can metastasize locally (e.g. skin and subcutaneous tissue) and regionally to one or more draining lymph nodes, or distantly to skin/soft tissue or to visceral organ sites, primary the lung, liver, brain, bone and gastrointestinal tract. Cutaneous metastases appear as red, brown, bluish, black or nonpigmented nodules, papules or plaques. These metastases may also present as subcutaneous nodules, which are often small and well-defined or associated with ecchymosis. Lymph node (LN) metastases are often palpable as firm masses. Satellites are metastases located in the dermis or subcutaneous tissue within 2 cm from the primary tumor **(Figure 17-6)**. Microscopic satellites are aggregates of malignant melanocytes in the reticular dermis, panniculus or blood and/or lymphatic vessels that are distinct and separated from the primary tumor, but observed in the same tissue section.

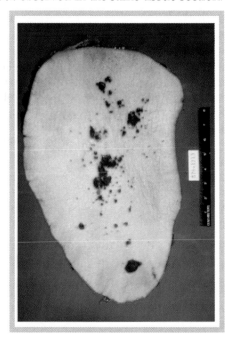

Figure 17-6: Extensive satellitosis evident. Note discontinuous involvement in a "shotgun" pattern

Lymph node metastases that are clinically suspected should be confirmed histopathologically to determine the extent of nodal involvement. Initial evaluation of suspected metastatic disease should be comprised of the following steps:
1. History
2. Physical examination
3. Chest X-ray or computed tomography (CT) scans of the chest
4. CT scan of the abdomen and pelvis for those patients who have signs or symptoms of CNS involvement
5. Blood LDH level as an overall prognostic factor and to detect early liver disease.

New imaging techniques recently introduced include spiral computed tomography (CT), whole-body magnetic resonance imaging (MRI) and positron emission tomography (PET) combined with CT (PET-CT). These imaging techniques have a high resolution and a high sensitivity for the detection of metastatic disease. Additively these techniques clearly improve identification of patients suitable for surgical metastasectomy.

In-transit metastases for melanoma are a type of stage III regional metastatic disease which are characterized by intradermal or subcutaneous nodules growing within lymphatics. The American Joint Committee on Cancer (AJCC) defines in-transit metastases as any skin or subcutaneous metastases that are more than 2 cm from the primary lesion (which distinguishes them from satellite lesions, which are within 2 cm) but are not beyond the regional nodal basin. Optimal treatment for in-transit melanomas depends on the number of lesions. If 1-3 nodules are present, the optimal management is surgical excision with minimal negative margins and appropriate staging to look for any distant metastases. Wide local excision is not indicated, as the entire anatomic region is at risk for metastases. Those patients with a high number of lesions or rapidly recurring lesions are candidates for isolated limb perfusion (ILP). ILP is a regional administration of high-dose chemotherapeutics within an extremity following cannulation of the specific artery and vein. Melphalan, a nitrogen mustard alkylating agent, is the drug of choice and is dosed per limb volume (e.g. 10 mg/L for lower extremities and 13 mg/L for upper extremities) with mild hyperthermia for 60 minutes. Overall response rates between 80% and 90% and complete response rates between 55% and 65% can be obtained. Twenty to twenty-five percent of patients can exhibit a complete response, while the remaining 80% partially respond with a duration to next recurrence of 9-12 months. Major toxicities include skin erythema, myopathy and peripheral neuropathy.

Adjuvant Treatment of Melanoma

Different treatment modalities have been examined in the adjuvant setting in patients with cutaneous melanoma. Most of the patients included in the adjuvant melanoma trials have stage III disease (e.g. locoregional metastases) or stage II disease (e.g. thick primary melanomas according to the old AJCC classification with > 1.5 mm tumor thickness). Multiple approaches to adjuvant therapy for resected high risk stages II-III melanoma have been studied. Interferon (IFN) alfa-2b is the only adjuvant therapy shown in randomized trials to significantly prolong disease free and overall survival in patients with stages IIB and III melanoma. The ability of IFN alfa-2b to improve continuous relapse free survival of high risk melanoma has been corroborated in several published trials. Other methods of treatment for patients with metastatic melanoma and as potential adjuvant therapy for patients with operable stages II and III disease hold promise for the future.

Systemic Chemotherapy, Chemotherapy and Immunotherapy (Chemobiotherapy)

Dacarbazine (also termed DTIC) is the accepted treatment of choice for metastatic malignant melanoma. A systematic review found no randomized controlled trials comparing systemic therapy with supportive care or placebo. Several trials used dacarbazine as the control agent and found response rates varying from 9.1% to 29% (no test agent was found superior).

Various *chemotherapy* agents are used, including *dacarbazine, immunotherapy* [with *interleukin-2* (IL-2)] or IFN as well as local perfusion is used by different centers. They can occasionally show dramatic success, but the overall success in metastatic melanoma is quite limited. IL-2 is the first new therapy approved for the treatment of metastatic melanoma in 20 years. Studies have demonstrated that IL-2 offers the possibility of a complete and long-lasting remission in this disease, although only in a small percentage of patients. A number of new agents and novel approaches are under evaluation and show promise.

Hormones

Although there was little evidence to suggest a benefit for any adjuvant hormone therapy, some hormones such as megestrol acetate, retinoids and coumarin are studied in several published studies.

Vaccines

Vaccine therapy has shown preliminary benefit in several case-control studies but needs to be investigated further before it can be recommended. Various types of vaccines are summarized as follows:

- Irradiated autologous or allogenic whole cell vaccines
- Partially purified antigens shed from melanoma cells in culture
- Viral oncolysates

- Vaccines that represent defined tumor antigens
- Anti-idiotype antibodies.

Radiation Therapy

Melanoma is not considered a radiation-sensitive tumor; therefore, radiation therapy (RT) has a limited role in this disease. The established uses of RT in patients with melanoma include palliative treatment of brain and bone metastases. The use of adjuvant radiation for nodal disease in melanoma remains controversial. Although nonrandomized trials of postoperative radiation to the nodal basin for melanoma have suggested improved local control, the only randomized trial reported of adjuvant radiation for localized melanoma had negative results. An attempt by the RT Oncology Group to test postoperative radiation in patients with regional neck node metastases from melanoma was closed because of poor accrual. This issue remains unresolved and considering the increased incidence of postoperative complication of lymphedema with radiation, should be used sparingly, if at all.

Postsurgical Management

Follow-up Management of Stage I (Low Risk, < 1 mm) Melanoma

- Following surgery, patients should be seen at least every 6 months for 2 years.
- A history and physical examination, including skin examination, should be done at each visit.
- Follow-up is for detection of both new primary melanomas and recurrence of original tumor.

Follow-up Management of Stage II (Intermediate Risk) Melanoma

History and physical including skin examination on every 3 months for 1 year, then on every 4 months for 1 year, then on every 6-12 months for 3 years; consider clinical trial.

- If tumor is < 4 mm thick, consider clinical trial or observation.
- If tumor is > 4 mm thick without ulceration or > 2 mm thick with ulceration (e.g. stage IIB), risks higher and adjuvant therapy with interferon alfa (IFN-alfa-2b) or clinical trial for higher-risk disease should be considered. If tumor is > 4 mm thick and ulcerated (e.g. stage IIC), the risk is further increased and adjuvant therapy with IFN-alfa-2b or a clinical trial should be considered.

Follow-up Management of Node Metastatic Stage III (High Risk) Melanoma

- Surgical excision of the primary tumor and nodal dissection (complete).

- History and physical including skin examination on every 3 months for 1 year, then on every 4 months for 1 year, then on every 6 months for 3 years, then on every 12 months from 5th year.
- Chest X-ray and LDH work on every visit (optional).
- Abdominal/pelvic/chest/brain CT scan (optional, but consider especially if planning to treat with IFN-alfa-2b).

Adjuvant Treatment of Stage III (High Risk) Melanoma

- Consider IFN-alfa-2b therapy or clinical trial of experimental agents vs IFN-alfa-2b.
- If gross extracapsular extension, consider clinical trial or RT.
- For stage III in-transit metastases, consider IFN alfa-2b therapy or clinical trial for high-risk patients, if lesions have all been rejected and no disease remains.

Management of Local Recurrences and In-transit Disease

- Local recurrence: re-excise tumor
- In-transit recurrence: if there is 1 lesion; re-excise lesion to clear margin (not wide excision margin). If there are ≥ 2 lesions, options include: excision, clinical trial for metastatic disease, hyperthermic perfusion with melphalan, investigational regional therapy and if disease-free after treatment IFN-alfa-2b or clinical trial for high-risk patients.

Adjuvant Treatment of Node Metastatic (Pathological Stage III) Melanoma

If lymph node is positive after lymphatic mapping or ELND: Do complete LN dissection then consider IFN-alfa-2b and clinical trial.

Management of Patients with Regional Lymph Node Recurrence

- No previous LN dissection: consider nodal dissection.
- Previous complete LN dissection: excise recurrence to negative margins.
- Previous incomplete dissection: complete dissection; consider RT trial if gross extracapsular extension.
- If no prior adjuvant therapy, consider IFN-alfa-2b or clinical trial for high-risk disease.

Management of Patients with Distant Recurrence

- Solitary skin or subcutaneous metastasis: resect, then observe or enroll in clinical trial for very high-risk patients.
- Solitary lung metastasis: resect if no other disease or observe for 3 months, then repeat scans. If no other disease present, resect and consider clinical trial for very high-risk patients. If other evidence of distant disease is present, treat as disseminated melanoma.

Landmark Papers

1. Antoch G, Vogt FM, Freudenberg LS, Nazaradeh F, Goehde SC, Barkhausen J, et al. Whole-body dual-modality PET/CT and whole-body MRI for tumor staging in oncology. JAMA 2003;290 3199-3206.
2. Balch CM, Buzaid AC, Soong SJ, et al. Final version of the American Joint Committee on Cancer Staging System for Cutaneous Melanoma. J Clin Oncol 2001; 19 (16): 3635-48.
3. Balch CM, Soong SJ, Gershenwald JE, Thompson JF, Reintgen DS, Cascinelli N, et al. Prognostic factors analysis of 17,600 melanoma patients: validation of the American Joint Committee on Cancer Melanoma Staging System. J Clin Oncol 2001; 19: 3622-34.
4. Barth A, Morton DL. The role of adjuvant therapy in melanoma management. Cancer 1995; 75: 726-34.
5. Breslow A. Thickness, cross-sectional areas and depth of invasion in the prognosis of cutaneous melanoma. Ann Surg 1970; 172: 902-8.
6. Cascinelli N, Morabito A, Santinami M, Mackie RM, Beli F. WHO Melanoma Programme. Immediate or delayed dissection of regional nodes in patients with melanoma of the trunk: a randomized trial. Lancet 1998; 351: 793-96.
7. Chan AD, Essner R, Wanek LA, Morton DL. Judging the therapeutic value of lymph node dissections for melanoma. J Am Coll Surg 2000;191(1):16-23.
8. Clark WH Jr, Elder DE, Guery D, IV, et al. Model predicting survival in stage I melanoma based on tumor progression. J Natl Cancer Inst 1989;81:1893-904.
9. Crosby T, Fish R, Coles B, Mason MD. Systemic treatments for metastatic cutaneous melanoma. The Cochrane Library. 2002; 2:CD001215.
10. Garbe C, Buttner P, Weiss J, Soyer HP, Stocker U, Kruger S, et al. Risk factors for developing cutaneous melanoma and criteria for identifying persons at risk: multicenter case-control study of the Central Malignant Melanoma Registry of the German Dermatological Society. J Invest Dermatol 1994;102: 695-9.
11. Grob JJ, Dreno B, de la Salmoniere P, Delaunay M, Cupissol D, Guillot B, et al. Randomised trial of interferon alpha-2a as adjuvant therapy in resected primary melanoma thicker than 1.5 mm without clinically detectable node metastases. French Cooperative Group on Melanoma. Lancet 1998; 351(9120):1905-10.
12. Heaton KM, Sussman JJ, Gershenwald JE, et al. Surgical margins and prognostic factors in patients with thick (>4 mm) primary melanoma. Ann Surg Oncol 1998; 5(4): 322-8.
13. Higgins EM, Hall P, Todd P, Murthi R, Du Vivier AWP. The application of the seven-point check-list in the assessment of benign pigmented lesions. Clin Exp Dermatol 1992; 17: 313-5.
14. Holly EA, Kelly JW, Shpall SN, Chiu SH. Number of melanocytic nevi as a major risk factor for malignant melanoma. J Am Acad Dermatol 1987; 17: 459-68.
15. Kelemen PR, Essner R, Foshag LJ, et al. Lymphatic mapping and sentinel lymphadenectomy after wide local excision of primary melanoma. J Am Coll Surg 1999; 189: 247-52.
16. Kirkwood JM, Manola J, Ibrahim J, Sondak V, Ernstoff MS, Rao U. Eastern Cooperative Oncology Group. A pooled

analysis of eastern cooperative oncology group and intergroup trials of adjuvant high-dose interferon for melanoma. Clin Cancer Res. 2004; 10: 1670-7.

17. Koh HK. Cutaneous melanoma. N Engl J Med 1991;325:171-82.

18. Kopf AW, Salopek TG, Slade J, Marghoob AA, Bart RS. Techniques of cutaneous examination for the detection of skin cancer. Cancer 1995; 75(2 Suppl): 684-90.

19. McMasters KM, Reintgen DS, Ross MI, et al. Sentinel lymph node biopsy for melanoma: controversy despite wide-spread acceptance. J Clin Oncol 2001; 19: 2851-5.

20. Morton DL, Wanek L, Nizze JA, Elashoff RM, Wong JH. Improved long-term survival after lymphadenectomy of melanoma metastatic to regional nodes. Analysis of prognostic factors in 1,134 patients from the John Wayne Cancer Clinic. Ann Surg 1991; 214(4):491-501.

21. Ringborg U, Anderson R, Eldh J, Glaumann B, Hafstrom L, Jacobsson S, et al. Resection margins of 2 versus 5 cm for cutaneous malignant melanoma with a tumor thickness

of 0.8 to 2.0 mm: randomized study by the Swedish Melanoma Study Group. Cancer 1996; 77: 1809-14.

22. Sahin S, Rao B, Kopf AW, Lee E, Rigel DS, Nossa R, et al. Predicting ten-year survival of patients with primary cutaneous melanoma: corroboration of a prognostic model. Cancer 1997; 80: 1426-31.

23. Thomas JM, Newton-Bishop J, A'Hern R, Coombes G, Timmons M, Evans J, et al. Excision margins in high-risk malignant melanoma. N Engl J Med 2004; 350: 757-66.

24. Thompson JF, Kam PC, Waugh RC, Harman CR. Isolated limb infusion with cytotoxic agents: a simple alternative to isolated limb perfusion. Semin Surg Oncol 1998;14(3): 238-47.

25. Thompson JF. The Sydney melanoma unit experience of sentinel lymphadenectomy for melanoma. Ann Surg 2001; 8(9S): 44-7.

26. Veronesi U, Cascinelli N, Adamus J, Balch C, Bandiera D, Barchuk A, et al. Thin stage I primary cutaneous malignant melanoma. Comparison of excision with margins of 1 or 3 cm. N Engl J Med 1988;318: 1159-62.

Level of Evidence Table			
Recommendation	**Grade**	**Best level of evidence**	**References**
A narrow excision margin (1-2 cm) is adequate for cutaneous melanoma compared to a wide margin (> 2 cm)	A	1a	1-4
Elective lymph node dissection in the absence of clinically positive nodes should generally NOT be performed	A	1a	5, 6
Sentinel lymph node biopsy provides important staging and prognostic information and should be offered to patients with cutaneous melanoma > 1 mm thick. It should also be considered for ulcerated thin melanomas and melanomas 0.75 to 1 mm thick.	A	1b	7-9
Immediate completion lymphadenectomy after finding a positive sentinel lymph node is recommended. There may be subsets of patients who derive greater benefit than others. Additional randomized trial data is pending	B	1b	10-16
Isolated limb perfusion/infusion should be considered as first-line therapy for unresectable recurrent and in-transit extremity melanoma	B	4	17-21
Adjuvant interferon for resected high-risk melanoma (Stage IIB/III) improves recurrence free survival. Clear overall survival benefit is less evident	A	1a	22-29

References

1. Lens MB, Dawes M, Goodacre T, Bishop JA. Excision margins in the treatment of primary cutaneous melanoma: a systematic review of randomized controlled trials comparing narrow vs wide excision. Arch Surg 2002; 137(10):1101-5.

2. Lens MB, Nathan P, Bataille V. Excision margins for primary cutaneous melanoma: updated pooled analysis of randomized controlled trials. Arch Surg 2007;142(9):885-91; discussion 891-3.

3. Haigh PI, DiFronzo LA, McCready DR. Optimal excision margins for primary cutaneous melanoma: a systematic review and meta-analysis. Can J Surg 2003;46(6): 419-26.

4. Sladden MJ, Balch C, Barzilai DA, et al. Surgical excision margins for primary cutaneous melanoma. Cochrane Database Syst Rev 2009:4:CD004835.

5. Lens MB, Dawes M, Goodacre T, Newton-Bishop JA. Elective lymph node dissection in patients with melanoma: systematic review and meta-analysis of randomized controlled trials. Arch Surg 2002;137(4):458-61.

6. Doubrovsky A, De Wilt JH, Scolyer RA, McCarthy WH, Thompson JF. Sentinel node biopsy provides more accurate staging than elective lymph node dissection in patients with cutaneous melanoma. Ann Surg Oncol 2004; 11(9): 829-36.

7. Morton DL, Thompson JF, Cochran AJ, et al. Sentinel-node biopsy or nodal observation in melanoma. N Engl J Med 2006;355(13):1307-17.

8. Kesmodel SB, Karakousis GC, Botbyl JD, et al. Mitotic rate as a predictor of sentinel lymph node positivity in patients with thin melanomas. Ann Surg Oncol 2005;12(6):449-58.

9. Ranieri JM, Wagner JD, Wenck S, Johnson CS, Coleman JJ, 3rd. The prognostic importance of sentinel lymph node biopsy in thin melanoma. Ann Surg Oncol 2006;13(7):927-32.

10. Wong SL, Morton DL, Thompson JF, et al. Melanoma patients with positive sentinel nodes who did not undergo completion lymphadenectomy: a multi-institutional study. Ann Surg Oncol 2006;13(6):809-16.

11. Ollila DW, Ashburn JH, Amos KD, et al. Metastatic melanoma cells in the sentinel node cannot be ignored. J Am Coll Surg 2009;208(5):924-29; discussion 929-30.

12. van der Ploeg IM, Kroon BB, Antonini N, Valdes Olmos RA, Nieweg OE. Is completion lymph node dissection needed in case of minimal melanoma metastasis in the sentinel node? Ann Surg 2009;249(6):1003-7.

13. Sabel MS, Griffith K, Sondak VK, et al. Predictors of nonsentinel lymph node positivity in patients with a positive sentinel node for melanoma. J Am Coll Surg 2005; 201(1):37-47.

14. Balch CM, Soong S, Ross MI, et al. Long-term results of a multi-institutional randomized trial comparing prognostic factors and surgical results for intermediate thickness melanomas (1.0 to 4.0 mm). Intergroup Melanoma Surgical Trial. Ann Surg Oncol 2000;7(2):87-97.

15. Cascinelli N, Morabito A, Santinami M, MacKie RM, Belli F. Immediate or delayed dissection of regional nodes in patients with melanoma of the trunk: a randomised trial. WHO Melanoma Programme. Lancet 1998;351(9105): 793-6.

16. Kretschmer L, Hilgers R, Mohrle M, et al. Patients with lymphatic metastasis of cutaneous malignant melanoma benefit from sentinel lymphonodectomy and early excision of their nodal disease. Eur J Cancer 2004;40(2):212-8.

17. Noorda EM, Vrouenraets BC, Nieweg OE, van Geel BN, Eggermont AM, Kroon BB. Isolated limb perfusion for unresectable melanoma of the extremities. Arch Surg 2004; 139(11):1237-42.

18. Beasley GM, Caudle A, Petersen RP, et al. A multi-institutional experience of isolated limb infusion: defining response and toxicity in the US. J Am Coll Surg 2009; 208(5):706-15; discussion 715-7.

19. Sanki A, Kam PC, Thompson JF. Long-term results of hyperthermic, isolated limb perfusion for melanoma: a reflection of tumor biology. Ann Surg 2007;245(4):591-6.

20. Beasley GM, Petersen RP, Yoo J, et al. Isolated limb infusion for in-transit malignant melanoma of the extremity: a well-tolerated but less effective alternative to hyperthermic isolated limb perfusion. Ann Surg Oncol 2008;15(8):2195-2205.

21. Cornett WR, McCall LM, Petersen RP, et al. Randomized multicenter trial of hyperthermic isolated limb perfusion with melphalan alone compared with melphalan plus tumor necrosis factor: American College of Surgeons Oncology Group Trial Z0020. J Clin Oncol 2006;24(25):4196-4201.

22. Kirkwood JM, Manola J, Ibrahim J, Sondak V, Ernstoff MS, Rao U. A pooled analysis of eastern cooperative oncology group and intergroup trials of adjuvant high-dose interferon for melanoma. Clin Cancer Res 2004;10(5):1670-7.

23. Kirkwood JM, Strawderman MH, Ernstoff MS, Smith TJ, Borden EC, Blum RH. Interferon alfa-2b adjuvant therapy of high-risk resected cutaneous melanoma: the Eastern Cooperative Oncology Group Trial EST 1684. J Clin Oncol 1996;14(1):7-17.

24. Verma S, Quirt I, McCready D, Bak K, Charette M, Iscoe N. Systematic review of systemic adjuvant therapy for patients at high risk for recurrent melanoma. Cancer 2006; 106(7):1431-42.

25. Agarwala SS, Neuberg D, Park Y, Kirkwood JM. Mature results of a phase III randomized trial of bacillus Calmette-Guerin (BCG) versus observation and BCG plus dacarbazine versus BCG in the adjuvant therapy of American Joint Committee on Cancer Stage I-III melanoma (E1673): a trial of the Eastern Oncology Group. Cancer 2004;100(8): 1692-8.

26. Garbe C, Radny P, Linse R, et al. Adjuvant low-dose interferon (alpha)2a with or without dacarbazine compared with surgery alone: a prospective-randomized phase III DeCOG trial in melanoma patients with regional lymph node metastasis. Ann Oncol 2008;19(6):1195-1201.

27. Cascinelli N, Belli F, MacKie RM, Santinami M, Bufalino R, Morabito A. Effect of long-term adjuvant therapy with interferon alpha-2a in patients with regional node metastases from cutaneous melanoma: a randomised trial. Lancet 2001;358(9285):866-9.

28. Eggermont AM, Suciu S, MacKie R, et al. Post-surgery adjuvant therapy with intermediate doses of interferon alfa 2b versus observation in patients with stage IIb/III melanoma (EORTC 18952): randomised controlled trial. Lancet 2005;366(9492):1189-96.

29. Eggermont AM, Suciu S, Santinami M, et al. Adjuvant therapy with pegylated interferon alfa-2b versus observation alone in resected stage III melanoma: final results of EORTC 18991, a randomised phase III trial. Lancet 2008;372(9633): 117-26.

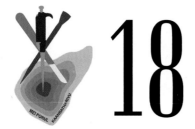

18

Soft Tissue Sarcoma

Marco A Alcala, Rahul Narang, Haroon A Choudry

Background

Soft tissue sarcomas are rare tumors of mesenchymal origin that account for < 1% of adult malignancies and 15% of childhood tumors. In 2008, there were approximately 9,400 new cases of soft tissue sarcoma in the United States, with a mortality of 3,400 patients. They present in all age groups but usually occur in the fifth or sixth decade of life, with a slight male predominance in a ratio of 1.4:1. Soft tissue sarcomas most frequently arise in the extremities (60%), followed by trunk (20%), retroperitoneum and abdomen (15%) and head and neck (5-10%). There are over 50 histologic sub-types of soft tissue sarcomas **(Figure 18-1)** that widely differ from each other in biology, aggressiveness, location, patterns of recurrence and spread and ultimately treatment and prognosis **(Table 18-1)**. Overall, the most common types are malignant fibrous histiocytoma (28%), liposarcoma (15%), leiomyosarcoma (12%), synovial sarcoma (10%), malignant peripheral nerve sheath tumor (6%) and rhabdomyosarcoma (5%). However, the frequency of histologic sub-types also varies by anatomic site of origin. The most common soft tissue sarcoma in the extremities is malignant fibrous histiocytoma, whereas, liposarcomas are the predominant sarcoma in the retroperitoneum and rhabdomyosarcomas comprise the majority of childhood soft tissue sarcomas. In the distal extremities epithelioid sarcomas are the most common sub-type in the hands, while synovial sarcoma and clear cell sarcoma comprise the majority in the feet.

Etiology

Risk factors associated with soft tissue sarcomas include genetic predisposition, environmental factors and

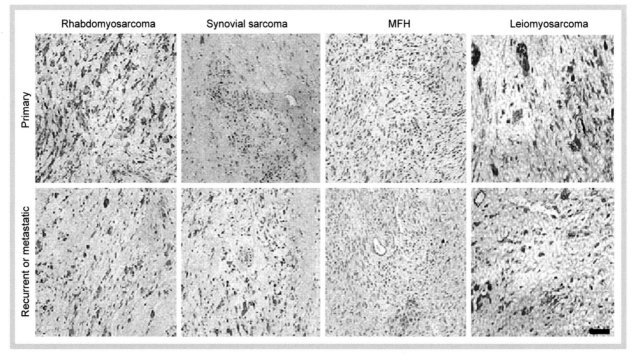

Figure 18-1: Representative histological images from various types of sarcoma

TABLE 18-1	Major histologic sub-types of soft tissue sarcomas	
Tissue	**Sarcoma**	**Incidence**
Fibrous tissue	Malignant fibrous histiocytoma	28%
	Fibrosarcoma	3%
Adipose tissue	Liposarcoma	15%
Smooth muscle	Leiomyosarcoma	12%
Skeletal muscle	Rhabdomyosarcoma	5%
Peripheral nervous system	Malignant peripheral nerve sheath tumor	6%
Blood and Lymph vessels	Angiosarcoma	2%
	Epithelioid hemangioendothelioma	1%
	Hemangiopericytoma	0.4%
	Kaposi's sarcoma	1%
Miscellaneous	Synovial sarcoma	10%
	Alveolar sarcoma	1%
	Unclassified sarcoma	11%

infectious agents. Genetic diseases including Neurofibromatosis (NF-1 gene), Li-Fraumeni syndrome (p53-mutation), Gardner syndrome (FAP-mutation) and Retinoblastoma (RB-1 mutation) have been associated with these tumors. Examples of genetic predisposition to soft tissue sarcoma include oncogene activation (e.g. MDM2, N-myc, c-erbB2 and ras), chromosomal translocations (EWS-ATF1 fusion in clear-cell sarcoma) and tumor-suppressor gene mutation (e.g. Rb-gene and p53-gene). Trauma, radiation exposure, chronic irritation/inflammation, immune-suppression and chemical exposure (e.g. polyvinyl chloride, arsenic, thorotrast, asbestos and phenoxyacetic acid) have been implicated. HIV has been linked to Kaposi's sarcoma and chronic lymphedema is associated with lymphangiosarcoma (e.g. Stewert-Treves syndrome). A better understanding of the molecular determinants of this disease is vital to identify "at risk" individuals early on and to develop targeted therapies.

Clinical Presentation

Soft tissue sarcomas predominantly present as asymptomatic masses, although up to 30% of patients suffer symptoms from visceral or neurovascular obstruction impingement. Tumors in the proximal extremities, trunk and retroperitoneum tend to present late, when they are large, as compared to those occurring in the distal extremities or head and neck, simply based on anatomic considerations. About 10% of patients present with synchronous metastatic disease and between 25% and 70% develop metachronous metastases, with tumor grade being the most significant predictor of systemic spread. Metastasis predominantly occurs hematogenously to the

lungs (30-35%), liver (25%), bone (20%) and brain (5%). Retroperitoneal soft tissue sarcomas have a predilection for liver metastasis, whereas, extremity sarcomas tend to spread to the lung, with the exception of myxoid liposarcoma of the extremity which tends to spread to the liver. Lymph node metastasis is uncommon (< 5%), except for a few histologic sub-types including epithelioid sarcoma, synovial sarcoma, rhabdomyosarcoma, clear-cell sarcoma and angiosarcoma.

Diagnosis

There is a vast differential that must be entertained when dealing with presumed soft tissue tumors. In the extremity, benign soft tissue tumors outnumber malignant masses by a ratio of 100:1, whereas, 80% of retroperitoneal soft tissue tumors are malignant of which 1/3rd are sarcomas. The differential diagnosis includes benign masses (e.g. lipoma, leiomyoma and fibroma) and other cancers (e.g. lymphoma, germ cell tumors, desmoids, adrenal tumors, renal tumors, pancreatic tumors, gastrointestinal stromal tumors and melanoma). The diagnosis and staging of soft tissue sarcomas involves a thoughtful application of imaging modalities and biopsy techniques to prevent compromising subsequent therapeutic approaches, as well as to rule out other differentials. Relevant investigations including history, physical examination, imaging, endoscopy, tumor markers and biopsy can help make a diagnosis.

In general, MRI is considered the imaging modality of choice for extremity soft tissue sarcomas, whereas, CT scans are more commonly used in retroperitoneal sarcomas **(Figure 18-2)**. A number of retrospective studies have compared contrast-enhanced CT scans and MRI in

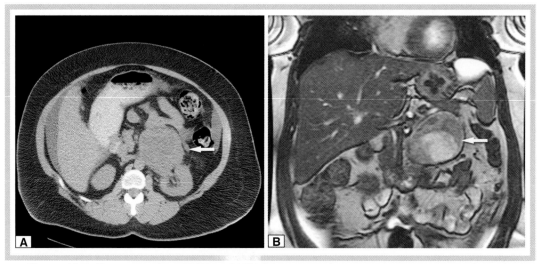

Figure 18-2: Representative CT (A) and MRI (B) images of a retroperitoneal sarcoma (arrow)

assessing tumor delineation and predicting respectability. Despite MRI being the prevailing popular choice for staging soft tissue sarcomas, there is no convincing evidence to support this bias. The Radiation Diagnostic Oncology Group (RDOG) prospectively compared CT versus MRI and found no difference in determining tumor involvement of muscle, bone, joint and neurovasculature. The role of PET scan in soft tissue sarcomas is still investigational and has been of particular interest in quantifying response rates to chemoradiation therapy.

In the extremities, image-guided core-needle biopsy or incisional biopsy is recommended. Care must be taken to orient biopsy incisions along the length of the extremity so as not to compromise subsequent surgical resection. Similarly, meticulous hemostasis is essential to prevent tumor seeding of surrounding tissue planes. Fine-needle aspiration cytology is not recommended given the inadequacy in assessing tumor grade and histology. In the retroperitoneum, biopsy is not required if the differential diagnoses can be excluded based on the history, physical examination and laboratory tests. Biopsy may

be indicated for unresectable disease, especially when considering neoadjuvant therapy, or when there is a high suspicion for lymphoma, germ cell tumor or metastasis.

Staging work up should include a chest X-ray or chest CT scan, based on the patient's perceived risk for metastatic disease. Brain and bone imaging are considered in symptomatic patients. Sentinel lymph node biopsy should be reserved for those few histologic sub-types that have a propensity for lymphatic spread.

Prognosis

A number of prognostic factors have been identified in soft tissue sarcomas **(Table 18-2)**. In general, favorable prognostic features include tumor size < 5 cm, low-grade tumors, tumors superficial to the muscular fascia, extremity sarcomas, particularly those located distally on the extremity and absence of invasion of vessels, bones and nerves. Local recurrence rates of < 10% are routinely achieved after multimodality limb-sparing resection in the extremities, whereas local recurrence approaching 50% is

TABLE 18-2	Major prognostic variables in soft tissue sarcomas	
Prognostic variable	**Favorable prognostic variables**	**Unfavorable prognostic variables**
Tumor size	Size < 5 cm	Size > 5 cm
Tumor depth	Superficial tumor location (Superficial to fascia)	Deep tumor location (Deep to fascia)
Tumor grade	Low grade tumor	High grade tumor
Tumor location	• Extremity tumor • Distal extremity	• Retroperitoneal, Trunk, Head and Neck • Proximal extremity
Local invasion (Vessels, Bones, Nerves)	Absent	Present
Resection margin	Negative	Positive
Recurrent tumor	Late recurrence	Early recurrence

commonly seen with retroperitoneal sarcomas. Patients with retroperitoneal soft tissue sarcomas are more likely to die from local recurrence, whereas with extremity sarcomas metastatic disease is the predominant cause of mortality. The 5-year survival rate for extremity soft tissue sarcomas approaches 50-60%, with 80% of deaths occurring in the first 2-3 years due to metastatic disease. Conversely, 5-year survival after treatment of retroperitoneal soft tissue sarcomas is generally < 50%, usually around 25-35%.

Factors associated with local recurrence in extremity soft tissue sarcomas include positive margins after resection, presentation with locally recurrent disease, high-grade tumors, intraoperative tumor-violation, age > 50 years and specific histologic sub-types including fibrosarcoma and malignant peripheral nerve sheath tumor. Distant metastases in extremity soft tissue sarcomas are more common in locally recurrent, high-grade, large (> 5 cm), deep tumors and non-liposarcoma histology. Predictors of mortality in extremity sarcomas include large (> 10 cm), deep, high-grade tumors, positive margins after resection and locally recurrent tumors.

Local recurrence in retroperitoneal sarcomas is associated with high-grade tumors, liposarcoma histology and contiguous organ resection. Metastasis is associated with incomplete resection of high-grade tumors. Poor survival in retroperitoneal sarcomas is associated with incomplete resection, high-grade tumors, locally recurrent and metastatic disease.

Overall, late recurrences are more favorable than early recurrences and large, high-grade tumors are more predictive of earlier mortality. Clinical, radiographic and pathologic responders to neoadjuvant therapy may have improved outcomes.

Prospectively collected data from a large cohort of patients with soft tissue sarcoma seen at Memorial Sloan-Kettering Cancer Center was used to develop a nomogram for estimating disease-specific probability of death at 12 years following complete tumor resection. Such nomograms improve our ability to more accurately quantify individual patient risk and may prove useful for patient counseling, follow-up scheduling, measuring efficacy of treatment and determining clinical trial eligibility **(Figure 18-3)**.

Staging

The revised American Joint Committee on Cancer (AJCC) staging system **(Table 18-3)** reflects the importance of

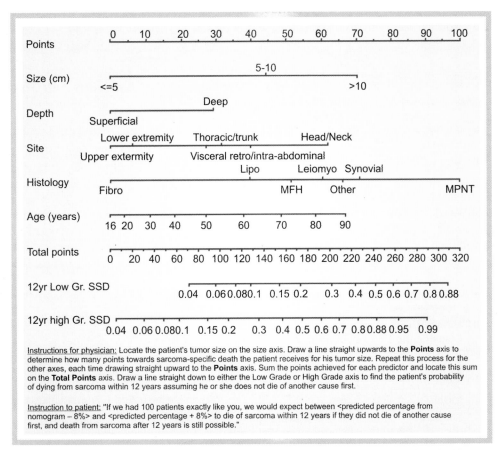

Figure 18-3: Nomogram for disease-specific probability of death. Reproduced with permission from Kattan MW, et al. J Clin Oncol 2002; 20:791-6

TABLE 18-3	AJCC staging for soft tissue sarcoma				
Primary Tumor (T)					
T1		Tumor ≤ 5 cm			
	T1a	Superficial tumor (above superficial fascia)			
	T1b	Deep tumor (invading fascia, retroperitoneal, visceral)			
T2		Tumor > 5 cm			
	T2a	Superficial tumor (above superficial fascia)			
	T2b	Deep tumor (invading fascia, retroperitoneal, visceral)			
Regional Lymph Nodes (N)					
N0		No regional lymph node metastasis			
N1		Regional lymph node metastasis			
Distant Metastasis (M)					
M0		No distant metastasis			
M1		Distant metastasis			
Histologic Grade (G)					
G1		Well differentiated			
G2		Moderately differentiated			
G3		Poorly differentiated			
G4		Undifferentiated			
Stage Grouping and 5 year survival					
Stage I	T1T2	N0	M0	G1-2	86% 5y survival
Stage II	T1T2	N0	M0	G3-4	72% 5y survival
Stage III	T2b	N0	M0	G3-4	52% 5y survival
Stage IV	Any T	N1	M1	Any G	15% 5y survival

Adapted with permission from the AJCC Cancer Staging Manual, 6th edition

tumor size, depth and grade in soft tissue sarcomas. This staging system does not apply to retroperitoneal sarcomas, visceral sarcomas, Kaposi sarcoma, dermatofibrosarcomas and desmoids. It has only been validated in extremity soft tissue sarcomas to reflect higher metastatic potential and relative risk of death with consecutive stage progression. For retroperitoneal sarcomas locoregional recurrence, rather than distant metastasis determines prognosis. For sarcomas in this location the Dutch/Memorial Sloan-Kettering Cancer Center staging system **(Table 18-4)** distributes patients more evenly and predicts outcomes more accurately.

Management of Extremity Soft Tissue Sarcomas

Surgery

Complete surgical resection is the cornerstone of treatment and the only chance for cure in soft tissue sarcomas. The surgical strategy is influenced by the anatomical location of the tumor, size, depth of invasion, proximity to vital neighboring structures, the need for vascular or soft tissue reconstruction and the patient's performance status.

Surgical resection with gross and microscopic negative margins is the most important prognostic factor influencing locoregional recurrence, however, the effect

TABLE 18-4	Dutch/ Memorial Sloan-Kettering Cancer Center classification system		
Classification	**Definition**		
Stage I	Low grade	Complete resection	No metastasis
Stage II	High grade	Complete resection	No metastasis
Stage III	Any grade	Incomplete resection	No metastasis
Stage IV	Any grade	Any resection	Metastasis

Reproduced with permission from Van Dalen T, Hennipman A, Van Coevorden F, et al. Ann Surg Oncol 2004; 11(5): 483-90

of locoregional tumor control on metastasis and survival is still controversial. Distant metastatic disease develops in 30-40% of patients regardless of improved local control strategies. Therefore, the extent of surgical resection must be tempered against its inherent effects on functional ability and quality of life issues.

Amputation used to be the standard of care in order to ensure complete tumor resection. The development of more accurate imaging modalities to better assess surgical margins preoperatively, the application of multimodality therapeutic options, including chemotherapy, radio-therapy, isolated limb-perfusion and the advancements in reconstructive surgical strategies including soft-tissue grafts/flaps and vascular prostheses has made less radical limb-sparing surgery applicable in greater than 90% of patients with equivalent local control, survival and quality of life.

Strict adherence to several principles of oncologic surgery is vital. Microscopic tumor extension beyond the pseudocapsule is commonly found, therefore, "wide" excision with a rim of normal tissue is ideal. Resection-margin width of at least 1 cm is associated with optimal local control rates. If a positive margin is obtained, re-resection to negative margins has been shown to optimize local control, metastasis-free survival and disease-specific survival, despite the use of adjuvant radiotherapy. Biopsy site/tract must be included in the resection specimen. Incisions and JP sites should be oriented so as to be included in radiation fields without necessitating excessive surrounding healthy tissue exposure to radiation. *En bloc* resection with reconstruction of contiguous vascular structures can ensure negative margins.

Retrospective studies have also shown favorable outcomes after resection of pulmonary metastases, provided complete tumor clearance is achieved. Three year survival rates range from 30-42% after complete resection. This ability to achieve complete metastatic tumor resection is the most important determinant of long-term survival, irrespective of other prognostic factors including number of metastases, unilateral versus bilateral disease and disease-free interval. Similarly, liver resection for metastatic sarcoma has demonstrated 31% 5-year survival and 32 months median survival in one study. Radio-frequency ablation of pulmonary metastases has shown good local control with minimal morbidity.

Based on current recommendations, "low-risk" soft tissue sarcomas including small (< 5 cm), low-grade and superficial-tumors are amenable to conservative limb-sparing surgery alone. All other "high-risk" soft tissue sarcomas, including large (> 5 cm), intermediate-high-grade, deep, positive/close post-resection margins, locally recurrent tumors and metastatic tumors to the skin, lymphatic system and lung, should be considered for conservative function-sparing surgery, combined with multimodality therapy, to achieve R0 resection. Amputation should be considered for those few (< 10%) patients in whom all gross tumor cannot be resected by conservative multimodality therapy or when local resection would lead to severe functional disability.

Radiation Therapy

The majority of soft tissue sarcomas are at significant risk for local recurrence (50-70%) after surgical resection alone, since most patients present with "high-risk" features. The addition of radiation therapy to surgical resection for such high-risk tumors has improved local control rates to > 90%. In general, radiation therapy improves local control without influencing distant metastasis or overall survival.

Radiation may be administered in the form of External-Beam Radiation Therapy (EBRT), Brachytherapy (BCT) or Intraoperative Radiation Therapy (IORT) alone or in combination. The timing (e.g. preoperative, perioperative and postoperative), dose-fraction, field-margin and the use of concomitant radio-sensitizers or hyperthermia have been investigated. EBRT is delivered 5 days a week for 6-7 weeks, whereas BCT is usually delivered over several hours or days. Neoadjuvant radiation allows lower radiation doses due to better tumor oxygenation, application to smaller undisturbed tissue-fields, prevents delays related to postoperative complications, reduces tumor spread during surgery and makes the surgery easier by increasing the likelihood of negative margins for large tumors or those close to vital structures. Conversely, neo-adjuvant radiation may be associated with increased wound complications, prevents histological interpretation of tumor variables and subjects all patients to radiation regardless of tumor biology.

Two landmark randomized trials support the use of adjuvant EBRT after surgery. Rosenberg, et al demons-trated that local recurrence, disease-free survival and overall survival were equivalent when comparing ampu-tation to adjuvant radiation after limb-sparing R0/R1 resection of extremity soft tissue sarcomas. Similarly, Yang, et al conducted a randomized trial comparing surgical resection with or without adjuvant-EBRT after R0/R1 resection in extremity soft tissue sarcomas. They demonstrated improved local control in low-grade and high-grade sarcomas but no benefit in disease-free or overall survival after adjuvant EBRT. There were no differences in complication rates, functional disability or quality of life associated with radiation therapy. This led to a general consensus that radiotherapy given after wide local excision or limb-preserving surgery provides a significant benefit in local disease control but no benefit in distant metastasis or overall survival. Importantly, radiotherapy does not compensate for inadequate surgical resection, demonstrated by higher local recurrence despite radiation in patients with positive post-resection margins. Certain subgroups of patients with low-risk soft tissue sarcomas, especially with wide post-resection margins (> 1 cm), may not benefit from adjuvant-EBRT, although this is still controversial and currently radiation is recommended for low-grade tumors that are > 5 cm or have close or positive margins of resection.

A single randomized trial comparing neoadjuvant EBRT and adjuvant EBRT demonstrated improved overall survival, but not local control or disease-free survival, after neoadjuvant EBRT. Although postoperative wound complications were higher after neoadjuvant EBRT, functional outcomes were better due to lower late-toxicity including fibrosis, joint stiffness and edema. Similarly, a large non-randomized study from M.D. Anderson Cancer Center demonstrated improved local control rates with neoadjuvant EBRT. Neoadjuvant radiation may be preferred when healthy wound closure is expected and close margins are anticipated. Surgical resection should be performed 3-6 weeks post-radiation. Conversely, adjuvant radiation is considered in situations where sarcoma is incidentally diagnosed on post-resection pathology or the tumor is upgraded post-resection, or negative margins are not achieved, or a more aggressive lesion is encountered than preoperatively anticipated.

Randomized trials of adjuvant BCT, after surgical R0/R1 resection of extremity and trunk soft tissue sarcomas, have demonstrated improved local control in high-grade, but not low grade, tumors without effecting disease-free or overall survival rates. Increased wound complications were seen when BCT was infused prior to postoperative day 5. In patients with positive resection margins, the additional use of adjuvant EBRT after BCT was shown to be essential for optimal local control rates. Nonrandomized studies comparing EBRT and BCT have shown equivalent local control rates of greater than 90% with equivalent morbidity and functional/quality of life measures.

Radiation-field margin encompassing 5 cm of normal surrounding tissue for EBRT and 2 cm for BCT has been recommended to reduce local recurrence, although intact intrinsic compartmental boundaries like bone, interosseous membrane or fascial planes may curtail tumor growth, thus allowing smaller radiation fields. Recommended radiation doses include 50 Gy for neoadjuvant-EBRT, 65-70 Gy for adjuvant EBRT and 40-60 Gy for adjuvant BCT infusion. Hyperfractionation and accelerated hyperfractionation techniques have shown no consistent benefit over conventional radiation therapy. Hyperthermia in combination with radiation improves local control rates with the inherent risk of severe burns.

Currently, additional radiation therapy is recommended for all high-risk tumors, including intermediate-high-grade tumors, close or positive margins, recurrent tumors, large tumors (> 5 cm). Neoadjuvant radiation is preferred over adjuvant EBRT for large, marginally resectable lesions to improve the chance of negative margins, while preserving limb function. For patients in whom the risk of wound complications is high, especially with smaller lesions, postoperative EBRT is preferred. For patients with small, low-grade, superficial lesions, with adequate post-resection margins, radiation may not be beneficial.

Chemotherapy

Metastatic spread continues to occur in 30-40% of patients with soft tissue sarcoma resulting in poor survival. The use of chemotherapy has extensively been investigated and remains controversial due to inconsistent results. The efficacy of conventional chemotherapy is limited, with response rates of 30%, without improvement in overall survival. The most commonly used drugs include Doxorubicin/Epirubicin, Ifosfamide/Cyclophosphamide, Dacarbazine (DTIC) and more recently Docetaxel and Gemcitabine. The combination of Doxorubicin and Ifosfamide provides response rates of 34% and is considered the standard of care. Although the addition of DTIC to this regimen has shown improved response rates of 47%, the additional toxicity is substantial.

A meta-analysis of 14 randomized trials of Doxorubicin-based adjuvant chemotherapy for soft tissue sarcomas published by the Sarcoma Meta-Analysis Collaboration demonstrated improved time to local and distant recurrence, recurrence-free survival, but no benefit in overall survival. This prolongation in disease-free survival was mostly due to a delay in distant metastasis and the largest benefit of adjuvant chemotherapy was evident in extremity sarcomas. Side effects were not excessive and compliance with chemotherapy remained acceptable. This comprehensive meta-analysis can be criticized for the heterogeneity of patient and tumor characteristics and the lack of inclusion of Ifosfamide in the chemotherapy regimens, which may prevent the identification of sub-sets of high-risk patients that may truly benefit from adjuvant chemotherapy. Three subsequent randomized trials using dose-intensive Doxorubicin, Ifosfamide or Epirubicin have shown inconsistent outcomes with respect to distant metastasis-free interval, disease-free survival and overall survival. A more recent update of the SMAC meta-analysis, including four additional randomized trials, demonstrated an overall survival benefit to adjuvant chemotherapy in addition to improved local and distant recurrence as well as recurrence-free survival. However, interim analysis of an ongoing randomized phase III trial conducted by the EORTC (Woll, et al 2008) failed to show any survival benefit with adjuvant chemotherapy. A large observational study by Cormier, et al has also shown that the beneficial effect of chemotherapy may not be sustained beyond one year. The use of Gemcitabine and Docetaxel in combination for patients with locally advanced unresectable and metastatic soft tissue sarcomas showed favorable results in a phase II study with response rates of 16% and overall survival of 17.9 months. However, adjuvant chemotherapy is associated with significant short- and long-term toxicity, therefore, the decision to treat must be on an individual patient basis.

Currently, patients with small (< 5 cm), low-grade soft tissue tumors should not receive chemotherapy. Intensive Doxorubicin/Ifosfamide combination adjuvant chemotherapy can be reasonably considered for adult patients with resected soft tissue sarcomas of the extremities at high risk for recurrence (deep, high-grade, > 5 cm) and at low risk for adverse effects (no underlying diseases, particularly cardiovascular), since this may delay distant metastasis and potentially improve survival. Molecular targeted therapies including Sorafenib, Bevacizumab, Sunitinib, Thalidomide, TRAIL-inhibitors and mTOR-inhibitors are under investigation.

Neoadjuvant CTX aims to maximize local control, minimize amputation rates and provide early systemic treatment of potential micrometastatic disease, while at the same time identifying responders who would benefit from adjuvant chemotherapy. A phase II randomized trial by the EORTC (Gortzak, et al 2001) did not show any benefit in terms of disease-free and overall survival using three cycles of neoadjuvant Doxorubicin/Ifosfamide prior to resection in patients with high-risk soft tissue sarcomas. A retrospective review of similar high-risk patients with soft tissue sarcomas failed to show any benefit of neo-adjuvant chemotherapy over standard adjuvant chemotherapy, regardless of response to chemotherapy, whereas a similar study showed disease-free survival benefit in patients with sarcomas > 10 cm in size.

Neoadjuvant chemoradiation has shown encouraging results in high-risk soft tissue sarcomas. The Massachusetts General Hospital piloted the use of three cycles of neoadjuvant MAID-chemotherapy (e.g. Mesna, Doxorubicin, Ifosfamide and Dacarbazine) with interdigitated preoperative radiotherapy and three cycles of adjuvant chemotherapy in high-risk soft tissue sarcoma patients. The updated results of this regimen demonstrated improved local and metastasis-free survival as well as overall survival when compared to historical controls. This prompted the Phase II RTOG 9514 Trial in which promising survival outcomes were tempered by significant major toxicity. Further clinical trials with less toxic neoadjuvant strategies are needed.

Hyperthermia and Radiation

A randomized trial comparing chemotherapy in combination with regional hyperthermia with chemotherapy alone demonstrated a significant improvement in tumor response, disease-free survival and local progression with this combined approach.

Hyperthermic Isolated Limb Perfusion

Hyperthermic Isolated limb perfusion may be used to treat unresectable extremity limb sarcoma as primary therapy or to allow limb-salvage resection. Isolated limb perfusion using TNFα, Melphalan and INFγ has shown increased respectability and local control with acceptable complications. TNFα is used at a dose of 1 mg for the upper extremity and 1-2 mg for the lower limb. Mild hyperthermia (38.5-40°C) is considered optimal. Complete response rates of 20%, partial response rates of 33% and objective response or stable disease in 40% can be achieved, although median time to progression is usually less than 6 months. Short-term limb salvage rates of 70-90% and 10 year limb salvage rates of 60% can be achieved. Furthermore, the addition of EBRT to isolated limb perfusion is feasible and increases local tumor control without increasing morbidity.

Management of Retroperitoneal Soft Tissue Sarcomas

Surgery

The principles and goals of resection are the same as for extremity sarcomas and much of the current recommendations have been extrapolated from clinical trials of extremity soft tissue sarcomas. Surgical resection of retroperitoneal sarcomas is challenging due to their large size at presentation, high rates of unresectability, frequent inability to achieve R0 resection (> 30% R1/R2 resection) and high rates of local recurrence (20-50%). Despite a 40% rate of distant disease at 10 years, most patients with retroperitoneal soft tissue sarcomas succumb to local recurrence in the absence of distant disease. Therefore, a thoughtful multimodality approach in order to achieve R0 resection is essential. Aggressive *en bloc* resection of the tumor with involved contiguous organs and vessels, followed by vascular and soft-tissue reconstruction has demonstrated local control rates of over 80% and 5-year survival rates of 67% provided that negative margins are achieved.

Radiation

The principles and goals of radiation therapy in retroperitoneal soft tissue sarcomas mirror those of extremity sarcomas. The challenges to radiation are greater given the proximity of vital gastrointestinal and neural structures.

Adjuvant EBRT has been the traditional strategy for local control after surgical resection based on retrospective studies and one randomized trial showing an almost 50% reduction in local tumor recurrence when compared to historical controls or surgery alone. Radiation doses of greater than 55 Gy are more effective but lead unacceptable collateral tissue toxicity. Improved radiation targeting using three-dimensional radiation therapy (3D-RT), intensity-modulated radiation therapy (IMRT) and tomotherapy techniques has shown promising results.

The use of intraoperative radiation therapy via brachytherapy catheters or directed electron beam radiation, especially as an adjunct to EBRT, has been advocated in order to escalate the dose of radiation at the site of resection. The biological effectiveness of single-dose IORT is equivalent to 1.5-2.5 times the same total dose of fractionated EBRT. Therefore, adding 15 Gy of IORT to 45 Gy of EBRT is equivalent to an EBRT dose of 75-87.5 Gy, which is the dose range believed to be most effective at controlling microscopic residual disease. In a randomized trial IORT in addition to adjuvant EBRT was associated with better local control rates compared to adjuvant EBRT alone but at the expense of higher toxicity especially peripheral neuropathy. High-dose rate IORT using brachytherapy catheters combined with adjuvant EBRT has also shown improved local control rates after resection.

The support for neoadjuvant radiation came from the combination of two long-term prospective trials of preoperative radiation followed by surgery in patients with resectable retroperitoneal soft tissue sarcomas. The R0/R1 resection rate was 95%, 5-year local recurrence-free survival was 60% and median overall survival was greater than 60 months, an improvement over historical controls undergoing resection alone. This lead to the ACOSOG Z9031 Phase III randomized trial comparing neoadjuvant radiation followed by surgery to surgery alone for retroperitoneal soft tissue sarcomas. Unfortunately, this trial was closed due to poor accrual.

Neoadjuvant approach to radiation is theoretically considered optimal due to the lower radiation doses required (45-50 Gy) and decreased exposure of normal surrounding tissues. Although no randomized trials are available to support this recommendation, the routine use of adjuvant EBRT should be avoided, in favor of neoadjuvant and intraoperative radiation strategies. Currently, neoadjuvant radiation is recommended for intermediate to high-grade sarcomas, especially when positive post-resection margins are anticipated.

Chemotherapy

Since most of the data regarding the use of chemotherapy in patients with retroperitoneal soft tissue sarcomas is an extrapolation of the available literature for extremity sarcomas, the same controversies exist. Similarly, the use of neoadjuvant chemotherapy to down-stage retroperi-

toneal soft tissue sarcomas is still uncertain, although limited data has shown improved local control, local recurrence-free survival and overall survival in responders versus nonresponders. A phase I trial using neoadjuvant chemoradiation in resectable high-risk retroperitoneal soft tissue sarcomas proved such an approach to be tolerable, although the benefits of this strategy are still unknown.

Follow-up

Routine follow-up is recommended in order to proactively identify tumor recurrence early on while still resectable. Current National Comprehensive Cancer Network (NCCN) surveillance guidelines recommend history and physical examination on every 3-6 months for the first 2-3 years, then on every 6 months for the subsequent 2 years, then annually. Chest imaging should be performed on every 6-12 months for stage I and on every 3-6 months for stage II/III tumors for the first 5 years and then annually. Primary site surveillance imaging with CT scan or MRI is advisable for anatomically deep seated tumors not amenable to physical examination. Soft tissue sarcoma recurrence is rare after 10 years, therefore, further surveillance is not essential at this time.

Landmark Papers

1. Badellino F, Toma S. Treatment of soft tissue sarcoma: a European approach. Surg Oncol Clin N Am 2008;17:649-72.
2. Ballo MT, Zagars GK, Pollock RE, Benjamin RS, et al. Retroperitoneal soft tissue sarcoma: an analysis of radiation and surgical treatment. Int J Radiat Oncol Biol Phys 2007;67:158-63.
3. Cormier JN, Pollock RE. Soft tissue sarcomas. Cancer J Clin 2004;54:94-109.
4. Delaney TF, Spiro IJ, Duit HD, et al. Neo-adjuvant chemotherapy and radiotherapy for large extremity soft tissue sarcomas. Int J Radiat Oncol Biol Phys 2003;56:1117-27.
5. Fadul D, Fayad LM. Advanced modalities for the imaging of sarcoma. Surg Clin N Am 2008;88:521-37.
6. Gronchi A, Casali PG, Fiore M, Mariani L, et al. Retroperitoneal soft tissue sarcomas: patterns of recurrence in 167 patients treated at a single institution. Cancer 2004;100:2448-55.
7. Kane JM. Surveillance strategies for patients following surgical resection of soft tissue sarcomas. Curr Opin Oncol 2004;16:328-32.
8. Kraybill WG, Harris J, Sprio IJ, et al. Phase II study of neoadjuvant chemotherapy and radiation therapy in the management of high-risk, high-grade, soft tissue sarcomas of the extremities and body wall: RTOG Trial 9514. J Clin Oncol 2006;24:619-25.
9. Mendenhall WM, Zlotecki RA, Hochwald SN, Hemming AW. Retroperitoneal soft tissue sarcoma. Cancer 2005;104:669-75.

10. Meric F, Hess KR, Varma DGK, Hunt KK, et al. Radiographic response to neo-adjuvant chemotherapy is a predictor of local control and survival in soft tissue sarcomas. Cancer 2002;95:1120-26.

11. O'Sullivan B, Davis AM, Turcotte R, Bell R, Catton C, Chabot P, et al. Preoperative versus postoperative radiotherapy in soft tissue sarcoma of the limbs: a randomized trial. The Lancet 2002;359:2235-41.

12. Pawlik TM, Pisters PWT, Mikula L, Feig BW, et al. Long-term results of two prospective trials of preoperative external beam radiotherapy for localized intermediate- or high-grade retroperitoneal soft tissue sarcoma. Ann Surg Oncol 2006;13:508-17.

13. Pervaiz N, Colterjohn N, Farrokhyar TR, et al. A systematic meta-analysis of randomized controlled trials for adjuvant chemotherapy for localized resectable soft tissue sarcoma. Cancer 2008;113:573-81.

14. Pisters PWT, Ballo MT, Fenstermacher MJ, Feig BW, et al. Phase I trial of preoperative concurrent Doxorubicin and radiation therapy, surgical resection and intraoperative electron-beam radiation therapy for patients with localized retroperitoneal sarcoma. J Clin Oncol 2003;21:3092-7.

15. Pisters PWT, Ballo MT, Patel SR. Preoperative chemoradiation treatment strategies for localized sarcoma. (Educational Review) Ann Surg Oncol 2002;9:535-42.

16. Pisters PWT, Harrison LB, Leung DHY, Woodruff JM, Casper ES, Brennan MF. Long-term results of a randomized trial of adjuvant brachytherapy in soft tissue sarcomas. J Clin Oncol 1996;14:859-68.

17. Pisters PWT, Leung DHY, Woodruff J, Shi W, Brennan MF. Analysis of prognostic factors in 1401 patients with localized soft tissue sarcomas of the extremities. J Clin Oncol 1996;14:1679-89.

18. Pisters PWT, Patel SR, Prieto VG, et al. Phase I trial of pre-operative Doxorubicin-based concurrent chemoradiation and surgical resection for localized extremity and body wall soft tissue sarcomas. J Clin Oncol 2004;22:3375-80.

19. Rosenberg SA, Tepper J, Glatstein E, Costa J, Baker A, Brennan M, et al. The treatment of soft tissue sarcomas of the extremities: prospective randomized evaluations of (1) limb-sparing surgery plus radiation therapy compared with amputation and (2) the role of adjuvant chemotherapy. Ann Surg 1982;196:305-15.

20. Sarcoma Meta-analysis Collaboration. Adjuvant chemotherapy for localized resectable soft tissue sarcoma of adults: meta-analysis of individual data. The Lancet 1997;350:1647-54.

21. Sindelar WF, Kinsella TJ, Chen PW, DeLaney TF, et al. Intraoperative radiotherapy in retroperitoneal sarcomas: final results of a prospective randomized clinical trial. Arch Surg 1993;128:402-10.

22. Stoeckle E, Coindre JM, Bonvalot S, Kantor G, et al. Prognostic factors in retroperitoneal sarcoma: a multivariate analysis of a series of 165 patients of the French Cancer Center Federation Sarcoma Group. Cancer 2001; 92:359-68.

23. Strander H, Turesson I, Cavallin-Stahl E. A systematic overview of radiation therapy effects in soft tissue sarcoma. Acta Oncologica 2003;42:516-31.

24. VanDalen T, Hennipman A, VanCoevorden F, Hoekstra HJ. Evaluation of a clinically applicable post-surgical classification system for primary retroperitoneal soft tissue sarcoma. Ann Surg Oncol 2004;11:483-90.

25. Yang JC, Chang AE, Baker AR, Sindelar WF, Danforth DN, Topalian SL, et al. Randomized prospective study of the benefit of adjuvant radiation therapy in the treatment of soft tissue sarcomas of the extremity. J Clin Oncol 1998;16:197-203.

26. Zlotecki RA, Katz TS, Morris CG, Lind DS, et al. Adjuvant radiation therapy for resectable retroperitoneal soft tissue sarcoma: the University of Florida experience. Am J Clin Oncol 2005;28:310-16.

Level of Evidence Table			
Recommendation	Grade	Best level of evidence	References
Radiotherapy improves local control of retroperitoneal sarcoma. Timing (pre-op vs post-op) and method of delivery (e.g. EBRT, IORT and brachytherapy) should consider potential morbidities, tumor factors (e.g. grade and histology) and potential for complete resection	B	1b	1-6
Adjuvant radiotherapy improves local control of high grade and marginally resected extremity and trunk sarcoma	A	1a	7-13
Preoperative radiotherapy of extremity sarcoma increases wound complications with unclear oncologic benefit	A	1b	14-16
Adjuvant chemotherapy for resected soft-tissue sarcoma improves disease control and disease-free survival. Best responses are seen in high-grade and large tumors as well as sarcoma subtypes with known greater sensitivity (e.g. synovial sarcoma)	A	1a	17-22
Neoadjuvant chemotherapy for high-risk sarcoma (high-grade, T2b) is feasible but with unclear benefits	C	2b	23-29

References

1. Sindelar WF, Kinsella TJ, Chen PW, et al. Intraoperative radiotherapy in retroperitoneal sarcomas. Final results of a prospective, randomized, clinical trial. Arch Surg 1993; 128:402-10.

2. Pawlik TM, Pisters PW, Mikula L, et al. Long-term results of two prospective trials of preoperative external beam radiotherapy for localized intermediate- or high-grade retroperitoneal soft tissue sarcoma. Ann Surg Oncol 2006; 13:508-17.

3. Tzeng CW, Fiveash JB, Popple RA, et al. Preoperative radiation therapy with selective dose escalation to the margin at risk for retroperitoneal sarcoma. Cancer 2006; 107:371-9.

4. Krempien R, Roeder F, Oertel S, et al. Intraoperative electron-beam therapy for primary and recurrent retroperitoneal soft-tissue sarcoma. Int J Radiat Oncol Biol Phys 2006; 65:773-9.

5. Stoeckle E, Coindre JM, Bonvalot S, et al. Prognostic factors in retroperitoneal sarcoma: a multivariate analysis of a series of 165 patients of the French Cancer Center Federation Sarcoma Group. Cancer 2001; 92:359-68.

6. Gieschen HL, Spiro IJ, Suit HD, et al. Long-term results of intraoperative electron beam radiotherapy for primary and recurrent retroperitoneal soft tissue sarcoma. Int J Radiat Oncol Biol Phys 2001; 50:127-31.

7. Cahlon O, Spierer M, Brennan MF, et al. Long-term outcomes in extremity soft tissue sarcoma after a pathologically negative re-resection and without radiotherapy. Cancer 2008; 112:2774-9.

8. Alektiar KM, Velasco J, Zelefsky MJ, et al. Adjuvant radiotherapy for margin-positive high-grade soft tissue sarcoma of the extremity. Int J Radiat Oncol Biol Phys 2000; 48:1051-8.

9. Alektiar KM, Brennan MF, Healey JH, et al. Impact of intensity-modulated radiation therapy on local control in primary soft-tissue sarcoma of the extremity. J Clin Oncol 2008; 26:3440-4.

10. Khanfir K, Alzieu L, Terrier P, et al. Does adjuvant radiation therapy increase loco-regional control after optimal resection of soft-tissue sarcoma of the extremities? Eur J Cancer 2003; 39:1872-80.

11. Strander H, Turesson I, Cavallin-Stahl E. A systematic overview of radiation therapy effects in soft tissue sarcomas. Acta Oncol 2003; 42:516-31.

12. Pisters PW, Harrison LB, Leung DH, et al. Long-term results of a prospective randomized trial of adjuvant brachytherapy in soft tissue sarcoma. J Clin Oncol 1996; 14:859-68.

13. Yang JC, Chang AE, Baker AR, et al. Randomized prospective study of the benefit of adjuvant radiation therapy in the treatment of soft tissue sarcomas of the extremity. J Clin Oncol 1998; 16:197-203.

14. Davis AM, O'Sullivan B, Bell RS, et al. Function and health status outcomes in a randomized trial comparing preoperative and postoperative radiotherapy in extremity soft tissue sarcoma. J Clin Oncol 2002; 20:4472-7.

15. O'Sullivan B, Davis AM, Turcotte R, et al. Preoperative versus postoperative radiotherapy in soft-tissue sarcoma of the limbs: a randomised trial. Lancet 2002; 359:2235-41.

16. Davis AM, O'Sullivan B, Turcotte R, et al. Late radiation morbidity following randomization to preoperative versus postoperative radiotherapy in extremity soft tissue sarcoma. Radiother Oncol 2005; 75:48-53.

17. Pervaiz N, Colterjohn N, Farrokhyar F, et al. A systematic meta-analysis of randomized controlled trials of adjuvant chemotherapy for localized resectable soft-tissue sarcoma. Cancer 2008; 113:573-81.

18. Adjuvant chemotherapy for localised resectable soft tissue sarcoma in adults. Sarcoma Meta-analysis Collaboration (SMAC). Cochrane Database Syst Rev 2000; CD001419.

19. Cormier JN, Huang X, Xing Y, et al. Cohort analysis of patients with localized, high-risk, extremity soft tissue sarcoma treated at two cancer centers: chemotherapy-associated outcomes. J Clin Oncol 2004; 22:4567-74.

20. Petrioli R, Coratti A, Correale P, et al. Adjuvant epirubicin with or without Ifosfamide for adult soft-tissue sarcoma. Am J Clin Oncol 2002; 25:468-73.

21. Frustaci S, De Paoli A, Bidoli E, et al. Ifosfamide in the adjuvant therapy of soft tissue sarcomas. Oncology 2003; 65 (Suppl 2):80-4.

22. Adjuvant chemotherapy for localised resectable soft-tissue sarcoma of adults: meta-analysis of individual data. Sarcoma Meta-analysis Collaboration. Lancet 1997; 350:1647-54.

23. Kraybill WG, Harris J, Spiro IJ, et al. Phase II study of neoadjuvant chemotherapy and radiation therapy in the management of high-risk, high-grade, soft tissue sarcomas of the extremities and body wall: Radiation Therapy Oncology Group Trial 9514. J Clin Oncol 2006; 24:619-25.

24. Wendtner CM, Abdel-Rahman S, Krych M, et al. Response to neoadjuvant chemotherapy combined with regional hyperthermia predicts long-term survival for adult patients with retroperitoneal and visceral high-risk soft tissue sarcomas. J Clin Oncol 2002; 20:3156-64.

25. Issels RD, Abdel-Rahman S, Wendtner C, et al. Neoadjuvant chemotherapy combined with regional hyperthermia (RHT) for locally advanced primary or recurrent high-risk adult soft-tissue sarcomas (STS) of adults: long-term results of a phase II study. Eur J Cancer 2001; 37:1599-608.

26. Gortzak E, Azzarelli A, Buesa J, et al. A randomised phase II study on neo-adjuvant chemotherapy for 'high-risk' adult soft-tissue sarcoma. Eur J Cancer 2001; 37:1096-103.

27. Grobmyer SR, Maki RG, Demetri GD, et al. Neo-adjuvant chemotherapy for primary high-grade extremity soft tissue sarcoma. Ann Oncol 2004; 15:1667-72.

28. Pisters PW, Patel SR, Varma DG, et al. Preoperative chemotherapy for stage IIIB extremity soft tissue sarcoma: long-term results from a single institution. J Clin Oncol 1997; 15:3481-7.

29. Meric F, Hess KR, Varma DG, et al. Radiographic response to neoadjuvant chemotherapy is a predictor of local control and survival in soft tissue sarcomas. Cancer 2002; 95:1120-6.

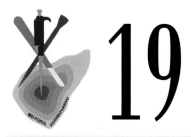

19

Noninvasive and Benign Breast Tumors

Atilla Soran, A Serhat Gur, Bulent Unal, Marguerite Bonaventura

Introduction

A breast mass or lump may be reported by a patient or detected by a physician on routine clinical examination. Breast lesions may also be detected by a screening mammography. Whether a mass is actually present can be very difficult to determine. In the absence of a surgical scar, a mass associated with skin dimpling is malignant until proven otherwise. A mass that changes with the menstrual cycle or has been present and stable for years is more likely to be benign. A change in the overall size of the breast is usually not a sign of cancer.

Whether a mass is solid or cystic cannot be determined by clinical examination alone. Only an ultrasound (not a mammogram) can determine whether a mass is cystic or solid, which is why palpable masses must be evaluated by both mammogram and ultrasound.

Retrospective and prospective studies have shown a relative risk of breast cancer of 1.5 to 1.6 for women with benign breast disease as compared with women in the general population. The College of American Pathologists categorized the benign breast diseases according to the relative risk of breast cancer **(Table 19-1)**.

Fibroepithelial Lesions

Fibroadenoma

Fibroadenoma is a common, usually single lesion, typically seen in patients between the ages of 20 and 40. This lesion may enlarge during pregnancy, but usually becomes smaller as patients age. Clinically, fibroadenomas are usually sharply demarcated, with well-circumscribed smooth borders. They may also be painful. They are

TABLE 19-1	Categories of the College of American Pathologist Classification of benign breast disease*	
Pathology category	Level of increased risk for invasive breast cancer	Pathological types included in the category
1	No increase	Adenosis (other than sclerosing adenosis) Ductal ectasia Fibroadenoma without complex features Fibrosis Mastitis Mild hyperplasia without atypia Ordinary cyst (microscopic or gross) Simple apocrine metaplasia (no associate hyperplasia or adenosis) Squamous metaplasia
2	Slightly increased	Fibroadenoma with complex features Moderate or florid hyperplasia without atypia Sclerosing adenosis Solitary papilloma without coexistent atypical hyperplasia
3	Moderately increased	Atypical ductal hyperplasia Atypical lobular hyperplasia
4	Markedly increased	Ductal carcinoma *in situ* Lobular carcinoma *in situ*

*Adapted with permission from Wang J, Costantino JP, Tan-Chiu E, Wickerham DL, Paik S, Wolmark N. Lower category benign breast disease and the risk of invasive breast cancer. J Natl Cancer Inst 2004; 96:616-20

somewhat rubbery, although fibroadenomas in older patients may have varying degrees of fibrosis, making them firmer. A palpable mass not seen radiographically should be biopsied to rule out malignancy. If a mass can be imaged, it should be biopsied using image guidance. With a pathologic diagnosis of fibroadenoma, this lesion can be followed clinically and removed if it enlarges. The patient should be examined and the ultrasound should be repeated on every 6 months. Once stability has been documented by two consecutive ultrasounds, the patient can be followed annually.

Several authors have opted for conservative management of the fibroadenomas in patients younger than a certain age. Twenty-five, thirty-five and forty years of age have been suggested as thresholds. Another study demonstrated that a large proportion of fibroadenomas in women younger than 20 years will resolve. In the management of fibroadenoma, two concerns need to be acknowledged: first, the stroma and epithelium of the fibroadenoma itself can undergo malignant transformation and second, carcinoma *in situ* arising within a fibroadenoma. Therefore, excision of fibroadenoma in women under the age of thirty-five may eliminate the problem of epithelial progression.

When pathologists cannot distinguish fibroadenoma from phyllodes tumor, the mass should completely be removed. Of the women with fibroadenomas, 10-15% have multiple, distinct, smooth, mobile masses and core biopsy of one or two of these masses is reasonable. If pathology indicates a fibroadenoma, the other masses may be presumed to be the same and these women can be followed clinically and with ultrasound. Giant or juvenile fibroadenomas may enlarge quickly and can become large enough to visibly distort the breast. An enlarging fibroadenoma should surgically be excised (enucleated). If the breasts are not fully developed, care should be taken to preserve the breast bud. Other benign, less-common adenomas include tubular adenomas and lactating adenomas seen during pregnancy.

The risk of cancer in patients with fibroadenomas has been reviewed in multiple studies. Although initial work by Dupont, et al, pointed to a slight increase in risk of cancer, the risk of invasive breast cancer was 2.17 times higher among the patients with fibroadenoma than among the controls (95% CI, 1.5 to 3.2). They have since concluded that when family history and adjacent proliferative changes are factored out, the relative risk approaches 1. Furthermore, atypia found within fibroadenomas did not seem to increase the risk for cancer as only 1 patient out of 13 went on to develop cancer. In the subgroup analysis of the National Surgical Adjuvant Breast and Bowel Project's Breast Cancer Prevention Trial (BCPT), Protocol P-1 they found 50 patients with fibroadenomas in the cohort patient group and 2 of 50 patients developed

invasive breast cancer. They could not determine the relative risk rate for fibroadenoma because of the small number of patients. Complete excision is recommended for fibroadenoma especially in patients over thirty-five years of age.

Phyllodes Tumor

Phyllodes tumors (formerly called cystosarcoma phyllodes) are typically seen in the same age group as breast carcinoma (median age, 45 years). However, phyllodes tumors can occur in young adults and occasionally adolescents. Grossly, typical phyllodes tumors are well rounded and well circumscribed but more firm than fibroadenomas. They may be of any size, but many are large, reaching 10 cm or greater **(Figure 19-1)**. Microscopically, phyllodes tumors show stromal hypercellularity with interspersed benign glandular/ductal elements. The appearance of the stromal components is important in determining whether some lesions should be classified as fibroadenomas or phyllodes tumors. Typically, phyllodes tumors have a leaf-like pattern and a more cellular stroma than fibroadenomas.

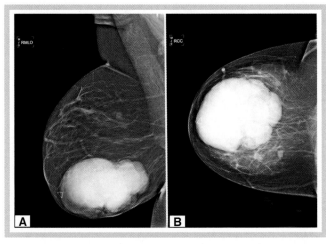

Figure 19-1: Mammographic view of a large phyllodes tumor. (A) Mediolateral oblique view, (B) Craniocaudal view

These lesions are categorized as benign, borderline or malignant based on a combination of histological features including: stromal cellular atypia, mitotic activity, stromal overgrowth, type of tumor margin (circumscribed vs infiltrative) and tumor necrosis. Reported incidences of each subtype have varied widely in the literature. Phyllodes tumors are categorized as benign in 5-92%, as borderline in 2-40% and as malignant in 25-45% in the literature. Despite these classifications, histological grade has been found to correlate poorly with biologic behavior.

Many studies have attempted to identify histological and clinical prognostic factors implicated in the risk for local and distant recurrence. This is difficult because of the rarity of this tumor, differences in pathologic interpretation and selection bias for the type of treatment provided in various series. Despite these impediments, several important observations have been made. The literature does not suggest a correlation between tumor size and increased risk for local recurrence, although size has been implicated in the risk for developing distant disease. A positive surgical margin is the most powerful predictor of local recurrence. Local recurrence does not correlate with an increased risk for distant disease and does not seem to affect survival. The literature is divided on the relationship between histological grade and risk for local recurrence. Some series suggest an increase in local recurrence among borderline and malignant lesions, but this has not been found in other large series. In contrast, the development of metastatic disease has been shown to correlate with grade and experts have estimated that 20% of patients with malignant tumors will develop metastatic disease. Stromal overgrowth has been identified as an important independent histological predictor of distant recurrence.

Local recurrence occurs in approximately 15% of patients with phyllodes tumors and is more frequent after inadequate excision. Distant failure occurs in approximately 5-10% of cases overall and in approximately 20% of malignant lesions. Wide local excision with margins of greater than 1 cm is the preferred primary treatment. Simple enucleation of the tumor, as is commonly used in the treatment of fibroadenoma, is inadequate treatment for phyllodes tumors. In a series of 101 patients, most of whom (99%) had pathologically negative margins after surgery, Chaney, et al reported a low actuarial 10-year rate of local recurrence (8%), suggesting that the risk for local recurrence can significantly be decreased but not eliminated when negative margins are obtained. The management algorithms of phyllodes tumors and recurrent phyllodes tumors, which were based on National Comprehensive Cancer Network (NCCN) guidelines, are shown in **Figures 19-2 and 19-3**.

Hamartoma

Mammary hamartoma has a reported incidence of 0.1-0.7%. Hamartoma has the typical mammographic appearance of lucent lesions containing fat, varying radiodense fibrous and adenomatous elements, a sharp

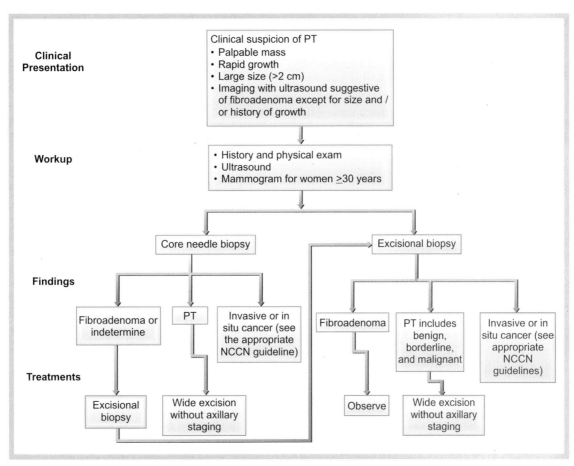

Figure 19-2: The NCCN clinical practice guidelines for the treatment of phyllodes tumors (PT) (Adapted with permission from the NCCN Breast Cancer Guidelines v1.2010)

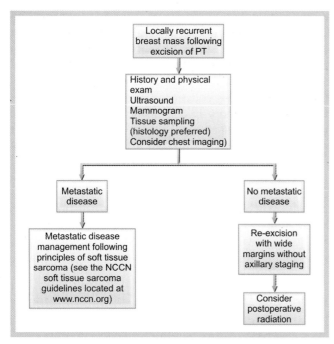

Figure 19-3: The NCCN clinical practice guidelines for the treatment of recurrent phyllodes tumors (adapted with permission from the NCCN Breast Cancer Guidelines v1.2010)

margin and sometimes a thin capsule. Lobulated densities are dispersed within the encapsulated fat, described as a "slice of salami". MRI shows the presence of internal fat density in addition to the smooth well defined hypo-intense rim and internal heterogeneous enhancement, which are characteristic of breast hamartoma. The pathology of hamartoma remains poorly defined; the original definition was used for a clinically discrete nodule composed of a variable amount of epithelial elements in a fibrofatty stroma. The presence of lobules within a fibrotic stroma, which surrounds and extends to between individual lobules and obliterates the usual interlobular specialized loose stroma, is most characteristic. The correct identification of hamartoma is important because of recurrence and coincidental epithelial malignancy. Diagnosing hamartoma of the breast is difficult, especially in core biopsy or fine-needle aspiration cytology. The diagnosis of hamartoma may be an incidental finding after biopsy or total excision of the mass. The pathologist, who sees fibrous tissue within the lobules, or fibrous tissue and fat in the stroma with or without pseudoangiomatous changes, should be alerted to the possibility of a hamartoma.

Adenoma

Ductal adenoma of the breast was described as a benign adenomatoid lesion by Azzopardi and Salm in 1984 and often occurs in older women. It involves small to medium sized breast ducts, but rarely involves large sized ducts.

They rarely exceed 2 cm in greatest dimension. The mean age of the patients in the literature was 51 years. Most cases showed intraductal growth but a fibrotic component sometimes involves the extraductal region, demonstrating a pseudoinvasive appearance. Therefore, it is important to differentiate this lesion from carcinoma. Page and Anderson stated that this disease is an undefined disease with mixed characteristics of sclerosing adenosis, fibroadenoma with ductal structure and intraductal papilloma. Apocrine metaplasia of the ductal epithelium is present in over half of the cases and occasional cells with foamy cytoplasm may be seen. Epithelial cells infrequently manifest nuclear pleomorphism and large nucleoli, possibly attributable to apocrine metaplasia. Microcalcifications are occasionally present and may coalesce to form large densities. Ductal adenomas are benign lesions with no tendency for recurrence after complete excision and no evidence of an increased risk of subsequent carcinoma. Therefore, the treatment of adenomas is surgical excision. However, since ductal adenoma is an uncommon breast lesion that can clinically and histologically mimic carcinoma, surgeons and pathologists should familiarize themselves with this lesion.

Infiltrative Pseudomalignant Lesions

Radial Scars

Radial scars have caused much confusion in the management of breast disease. These lesions are easily confused with invasive cancers mammographically as they form radiating spicules similar to cancer. They differ from cancer in the lack of a central mass and the common characteristic of a "black star". Also, pathologically, radial scars are difficult to differentiate from an invasive cancer as they demonstrate proliferative changes surrounding a fibroelastic core. This appearance mimics a well-differentiated invasive ductal carcinoma. It has been suggested that the entire lesion be excised to make the correct pathologic diagnosis. However, it appears that an 11-gauge vacuum core biopsy may be adequate to diagnose radial scars. In a comparison between 11- and 14-gauge biopsy techniques, there were no missed cancers in the 11-gauge group but a 5% missed cancer rate in the 14-gauge biopsies. The Vanderbilt group has published a retrospective cohort study of 880 cases of radial scar with an average follow-up of 20 years. In this study, 7% of patients developed breast cancer at 10 years, a relative risk of 1.82 (95% CI, 1.2-2.7) compared with controls. Interestingly, this increased risk was seen only in those lesions with coexistent proliferative disease (92% of total number of lesions), while the small percentage without proliferative disease was identical to controls. There may be an association between tubular cancer and radial scars since tubular neoplasms have often been identified with radial scars.

Sclerosing Adenosis

Adenosis refers to an increased number of milk ducts. The best known and most clinically apparent form of adenosis is sclerosing adenosis, which refers to a proliferation of ducts with poorly formed lumina (ductular spaces). Sclerosing adenosis is a pathologic finding that can be confused with invasive cancer. One study reported that 4 out of 12 pathologists misdiagnosed sclerosing adenosis as invasive cancer. Sclerosing adenosis usually has a relatively circumscribed border, although it may slightly be irregular. When cut, it may have a firm and gritty feel, mimicking carcinoma. If cancer is suspected, immuno-histochemical stains such as smooth muscle myosin, calponin or p63 are used to evaluate myoepithelial cells. An intact myoepithelial cell layer in breast ducts is characteristic of a benign lesion. Loss of the myoepithelial cell layer is a feature of malignancy. Sclerosing adenosis usually presents mammographically as microcalcifications. As in radial scars, there may be a central radiolucent area rather than the opaque center found with cancer. The accuracy of core biopsy in the diagnosis of sclerosing adenosis appears adequate. In one study, 8% of core biopsies demonstrating sclerosing adenosis were associated with cancer, mostly intraductal, with 86% accuracy rate (6 out of 7 patients). Core biopsies were obtained using 11- and 14-gauge biopsy devices. With regard to breast cancer risk, sclerosing adenosis carries a 1.5-3.7 times relative risk of developing invasive cancer. This relative risk might increase to 5.5, translating to a 1.2% risk per year of cancer, if atypia is associated with the sclerosing adenosis. In the subgroup analysis of the National Surgical Adjuvant Breast and Bowel Project's Breast Cancer Prevention Trial (BCPT), Protocol P-1, there were 12 patients with sclerosing adenosis and none of them has developed invasive breast cancer with a mean follow-up time of 79 months.

Cystic Lesions

Cysts

Cysts may be palpable or nonpalpable; simple or complex. If a palpable mass is a simple cyst on ultrasound, it does not need to be aspirated, unless the patient is having discomfort. Simple cysts found incidentally on ultrasound (e.g. nonpalpable or asymptomatic) do not require aspiration. Cystic fluid should be submitted for cytologic analysis only if the fluid is bloody. Simple cysts that resolve sonographically and clinically after aspiration require no further treatment. Cysts that do not resolve either clinically or on ultrasound, or ones that recur, should undergo core biopsy or be surgically removed. Complex cysts, even those that are not palpable, require aspiration and cytologic evaluation of the fluid or core biopsy to rule out malignancy. In the National Surgical Adjuvant Breast and Bowel Project's Breast Cancer Prevention Trial (BCPT), Protocol P-1 study, cysts were the most common lesions diagnosed, occurring in 674 (49%) of patients diagnosed with a benign breast lesion. Even if the study has limitations, the crude and adjusted relative risk for breast cancer in patients diagnosed with cysts were 1.79 (95% CI, 1.20-2.68) and 1.60 (95% CI, 1.07-2.40), respectively.

Fibrocystic Changes

Fibrocystic changes are commonly seen in the breast. Several terms have been applied to the condition of fibrocystic changes including: mammary dysplasia, fibrocystic disease, cystic mastopathy and cystic hyperplasia. The term describes pathologic changes seen under the microscope and should not be used to describe clinical findings. The histological changes include varying amounts of fibrosis and cyst sizes. Biopsy reveals microcysts, adenosis, apocrine metaplasia or gross cysts. If fibrosis is the predominant process, the condition may be referred to as "fibrous mastopathy". Calcification can be seen in association with fibrocystic changes. Fibrocystic changes, as a histological entity, do not convey an increased risk of breast cancer unless moderate to severe hyperplasia, with or without atypia, is present. Usual follow-up are recommended for fibrocystic breast disease after the diagnosis.

Hyperplastic Epithelial Lesions

Intraductal Papilloma

Intraductal papillomas may be located in large or small ducts and project into the duct lumen. Florid papillomatosis of the nipple duct (nipple adenoma) can have a very complex architecture but is a benign lesion. Clinically, papillomas usually present with bloody nipple discharge.

Due to a marked variation in papillary lesions, a clear strategy toward their management has not been developed. Excision is usually curative, although some patients may have multiple papillomas. Pathology reports of papillomas may include anything from single, solitary benign papillomas to malignant papillary invasive cancers. To better define these lesions, pathologists have tried to classify them according to two characteristics: the number of lesions and the presence or absence of atypia. Papillomas usually present as either a large, solitary, central papilloma or multiple, peripheral micropapillomas.

The presence of atypia and the number of lesions plays a role in determining future breast cancer risk. When atypical hyperplasia, within or surrounding the papilloma, is excluded, a solitary papilloma carries a relative risk of 2.04 to 2.1 compared to 3.01 to 3.54 with micropapillomas. When atypia is associated with the papilloma, this risk increases from 5.1 to 13.1 for solitary papillomas and from 4.4 to 7.0 for micropapillomas. The presence of papillomas does not predict laterality in future breast cancer cases. The risk of finding invasive cancer on an excisional biopsy, after finding a papilloma by a core biopsy, increases with the presence of atypia and the number of papillomas present.

Hyperplasia without Atypia

Hyperplasia exists on a spectrum from hyperplasia without atypia, to atypical hyperplasia, to *in situ* carcinoma, which may either be ductal or lobular. In cases of hyperplasia without atypia, an increased risk for subsequent breast cancer has been demonstrated in many studies. The relative risk with moderate or florid ductal hyperplasia ranges from 1.5 to 2.0 and the risk is independent of other risk factors such as family history. Even though these patients are at increased risk, the need for chemoprevention and heightened screening has not been supported. Furthermore, surgical excision is not required after core biopsy unless there is a concern for additional disease or a question of concordance between pathology and the clinical picture (e.g. mammogram findings, ultrasound findings and physical examination).

Inflammatory Disorders

Fat Necrosis

Fat necrosis is usually a result of bleeding caused by trauma. Bleeding into the breast can occur after needle biopsy or surgery or as a result of blunt trauma. Core needle biopsy results in ecchymosis or hematoma in up to 50% of women. Most resolve spontaneously. A rapidly expanding hematoma requiring surgical exploration is rare. Intraoperative blood loss during lumpectomy is usually not significant; however, postoperative bleeding occurs in approximately 2% of patients. It typically develops within the first 24 hours but may begin days later, especially if the patient is taking anticoagulants. A significant volume of blood can accumulate in a lumpectomy cavity and many patients require surgical exploration and evacuation of hematoma.

Blunt trauma to the breast, such as occurs with seat belt injury, can also result in significant blood loss. Unlike post-lumpectomy bleeding, blunt trauma almost always causes diffuse bleeding that cannot be managed surgically. A large volume of blood can be lost in the breast

parenchyma, resulting in hypotension and anemia and the treatment is supportive. In the days after injury, patients may develop impressive ecchymosis as the blood percolates along the tissue planes to the dependent areas of subcutaneous fat and skin. Months later, a mass may develop as a result of traumatic fat necrosis. It may simulate malignancy; however, unlike a malignant mass, fat necrosis is typically very tender and has a specific mammographic appearance. Fat necrosis may be seen after a surgical procedure and in mammary duct ectasia, as both may produce fibrosis and calcification. In some cases, microscopic examination is necessary to rule out malignancy. Unlike surgery for nonspecific mastalgia, surgical removal of a painful area of fat necrosis is usually therapeutic. Inflammatory and malignant conditions can coexist in the same breast, sometimes side by side.

Other Inflammatory Disorders

Other inflammatory disorders include lymphocytic mastitis, sometimes seen in diabetics as the so-called "diabetic mastopathy" and granulomatous mastitis, which may be seen in association with foreign body reaction, infection by organisms such as mycobacterial and fungal organisms, sarcoidosis and systemic inflammatory disorders. These patients should routinely be followed up with magnetic resonance imaging or ultrasonography and core biopsy if the lesions become clinically or radiologically suspicious. Lesions can be excised for cosmetic reasons or if malignancy cannot be excluded.

Miscellaneous Lesions

The miscellaneous benign lesions of the breast include lipomas, vascular lesions, pseudoangiomatous stromal hyperplasia, chondromatous tumors, leiomyoma, neural lesions, adenomyoepithelioma, myofibroblastoma, mucocele-like lesion and collagenous spherulosis. Excisional biopsy may be recommended for nonconcordant biopsy results or increase in size.

Lipoma of the breast often causes diagnostic and therapeutic uncertainty. Clinically, it may be difficult to distinguish a lipoma from other conditions. Fine-needle aspiration cytology is often not helpful. Both mammography and ultrasound scanning are often negative.

Vascular tumors of the breast are uncommon and may be diagnosed at any age.

They may be variants of hemangioma or angiosarcoma. Benign vascular lesions of the breast are categorized into six major groups: perilobular hemangioma, hemangioma, angiomatosis, venous hemangioma, subcutaneous nonparenchymal hemangioma and aneurysm. The term atypical hemangioma has been used to describe benign vascular lesions with atypical cytologic features, including rare mitoses and/or nuclear pleomorphism, in the absence of endothelial growth characteristic for angiosarcoma.

Pseudoangiomatous stromal hyperplasia (PASH) is a benign proliferative lesion of breast stroma first described in 1986. Clinically, PASH usually presents as a mass which may grow rapidly and may be associated with other benign or malignant lesions. The clinical and radiological appearance is similar to that of a fibroadenoma. PASH may be diagnosed preoperatively by imaging techniques including ultrasound, mammography or magnetic resonance imaging. Excision of PASH after CNB may be considered for patients with symptoms, enlarging lesions, or lesions classified as Breast Imaging Reporting and Data System (BI-RADS) 4 or 5. PASH diagnosed by CNB allows selected patients to avoid excision.

Chondromatous tumors of the breast are exceedingly rare and are a benign, cartilage-containing breast tumor. Cartilage-containing lesions of the breast are unusual and most are malignant tumors such as stromal sarcomas, phyllodes tumors or adenocarcinomas.

Leiomyomas are benign smooth muscle neoplasms that can occur anywhere in the body. When they occur in the breast they are more commonly seen in the subareolar position and have been reported in both men and women. Intraparenchymal leiomyomas of the breast are described exclusively in women and are extremely rare. The treatment for leiomyoma of the breast is simple excision.

Neural lesions such as Schwannoma are extremely rare benign tumors of the breast. It usually appears as a breast lump having clinical and radiological characteristics suggestive of kindness. Its diagnosis is histological while treatment is surgical.

Adenomyoepithelioma is a rare primary tumor of the breast. Pathologically, the tumor consists of epithelial cells accompanied by myoepithelial cells, normally present in the glandular tissue of the breast. Adenomyoepithelioma is a benign tumor that can be treated by a local excision. Recurrence, though rare, usually occur more than two years after the initial excision and may be attributed to an incomplete excision.

Myofibroblastoma is a rare benign tumor of the breast predominantly seen in men in their sixth to seventh decades. Malignant neoplasms, such as stromal sarcoma, malignant fibrous histiocytoma and spindle-cell sarcoma, or metaplastic carcinoma should not be confused with a myofibroblastoma. The clinical significance of this entity lies primarily in its recognition as a distinctive benign neoplasm.

Mucinous lesions of the breast are more common. In a retrospective histologic review, mucin-filled ducts were found in approximately 3% of breast specimens, while the incidence of mucocele-like lesions was 2%. Since most mucinous lesions of consequence result in imaging abnormalities, the greater use of screening mammography will result in increased detection of these lesions. Cases of symptomatic mucocele-like lesions characteristically present as masses in premenopausal women.

Collagenous spherulosis of the breast is a rare incidental finding frequently associated with benign and preinvasive lesions of the breast, including sclerosing adenosis, radial scar, intraductal papilloma, fibroadenoma, atypical ductal hyperplasia, ductal carcinoma in situ and lobular carcinoma in situ. Collagenous spherulosis has an estimated incidence of less than 1% in excisional specimens and about 0.2% in cytologic material. It is important to correctly diagnose collagenous spherulosis, not only because it is innocuous, requiring no therapeutic intervention, but also because of its close cytologic resemblance to certain malignancies such as adenoid cystic carcinoma.

Noninvasive Breast Cancers (Precursor and Preinvasive Lesions)

Precursors and preinvasive lesions of the breast include atypical ductal hyperplasia (ADH), atypical lobular hyperplasia (ALH), ductal carcinoma in situ (DCIS) and lobular neoplasia (LN). These lesions represent a heterogeneous group with problems associated with their definition, classification, diagnosis and management. The diagnosis of these lesions represents a clinical dilemma for the patient and the physicians. Following a diagnosis of atypical hyperplasia, LN or DCIS, a patient is immediately considered at high risk for future development of invasive breast carcinoma (IBC). There is no "atypical lobular hyperplasia (ALH)."

The classic model of breast cancer progression (**Figure 19-4**) is seen as a *linear multistep process* manifesting as a sequence of pathologically defined stages. Molecular alterations within normal breast epithelium give rise to ADH, the first premalignant stage of breast cancer progression. Progressive molecular alterations give rise to DCIS, the second premalignant stage of the disease.

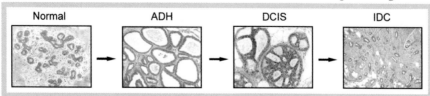

Figure 19-4: Classical linear model of human breast cancer proliferation (Adapted with permission from Moulis S, Sgroi DC. Re-evaluating early breast neoplasia. Breast Cancer Res 2008; 10:302)

Additional molecular alterations in DCIS are thought to give rise to the malignant stages of invasive and metastatic carcinoma.

Distinct molecular events occur in normal breast epithelium giving rise to two divergent molecular pathways within which *linear* and *horizontal* progression occurs. The first pathway is characterized by genetic alterations that include gain of 1q and loss of 16q and this pattern of genetic alteration is seen predominantly in low grade DCIS and invasive ductal carcinoma (IDC) and in a subset (low grade-like) of intermediate grade tumors. The second pathway is characterized by amplification of 11q13 and 17q12 in high grade tumors and 11q13 in a subset (high grade-like) of intermediate grade tumors. Additional support for the divergent of two pathway models is provided by gene expression profiling data (depicted as a gene expression heatmap) generated from ADH, DCIS and IDC. More specifically, low grade tumors express a unique set of genes that is rarely seen in high grade tumors and vice versa. Intermediate grade tumors express either "low grade-like" gene expression signatures or "high grade-like" gene expression signatures. These results together support a modified model of breast cancer progression **(Figure 19-5)**.

Atypical Ductal Hyperplasia (ADH)

Atypical ductal hyperplasia (ADH) is considered a high risk lesion and falls between benign hyperplasia and DCIS when examined on breast cancer models of tumor progression. Page, et al described the diagnostic criteria of ADH which are based on the cytological and architectural features of the lesion. Although some studies have suggested that ADH is a direct precursor to cancer, it is generally believed that ADH is a marker for an increased risk of breast cancer, usually reported at 4 to 5 times that of the general public. In those with a family history, the risk is 11 times that of the general public. In the classic study by Page, et al 12% of 150 women with ADH developed IBC in an average period of 16 years. Forty-four percent of these cancers occurred in the contralateral breast, suggesting that ADH is not a direct precursor. In a study from the Mayo Clinic, approximately 20% of patients with ADH developed cancer over a follow-up period of 13.7 years. The investigators did not find an association with family history in this study.

Nonetheless, just as there are different levels of severity of invasive or non-invasive cancer, there exists a way to "grade" ADH into mild, moderate and marked categories **(Table 19-2)**. This classification scheme does not imply

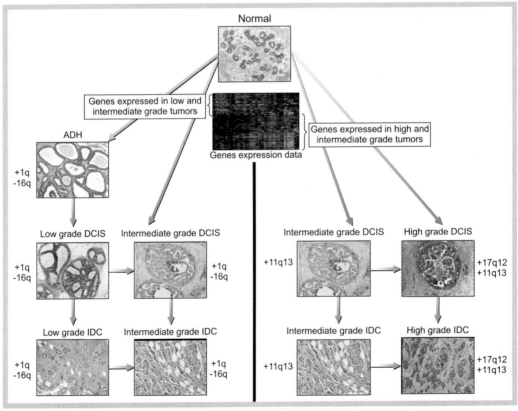

Figure 19-5: Contemporary model of breast cancer progression based on genetic and gene expression data (Adapted with permission from Moulis S, Sgroi DC. Re-evaluating early breast neoplasia. Breast Cancer Res 2008; 10:302)

TABLE 19-2	Pathological grades of ADH*
Mild ADH	• Monomorphic epithelial cell proliferation without myoepithelial cells • Mild increase in nuclear-cytoplasmic ratio and nuclear hyperchromasia • Less than ¼ of the circumference of the duct
Moderate ADH	• Monomorphic proliferation of epithelial cells that project into and at times bridge across the ductal lumen • Some loss of polarity • ¼ to ½ the ductal circumference
Marked ADH	• Monotonous population of epithelial cells that partially or completely fill ductal lumen as sheets of epithelial cells and there may be a few acinar spaces • There is < 2 mm of involvement • Greater than ½ the ductal circumference

* Adapted with permission from Doren E, Hulvat M, Norton J, et al. Predicting cancer on excision of atypical ductal hyperplasia. Am J Surg 2008; 195:358-62.

that ADH is a direct precursor of cancer, but it may enable clinicians to stratify patients into different *"levels of risk"* which can be useful when discussing a diagnosis of ADH and explaining the need for further surgical excision. Indeed, Degnim, et al showed that another pathologic factor of ADH, the number of foci, conferred a much higher risk of developing cancer over long-term follow-up. The relative risks of breast cancer increases in a dose-response fashion for women with one, two and three or more foci of atypia, with a statistically significant test for trend. With a single focus, the cumulative incidence of breast cancer reached 18% at 25 years. For women with two or more foci of atypia, the cumulative risk of breast

cancer was greater than 40% at 25 years. Moreover, in the highest risk subgroup of women with three or more foci and histological calcifications, the cumulative incidence exceeded 50% over 25 years.

Management

With the advent of both breast screening programs and the directional vacuum-assisted biopsy (DVAB) technique, ADH diagnosis is associated with a rate of carcinoma ranging from 11% to 35% in subsequent excisions. Generally authors have recommended a mandatory surgical biopsy while others have discussed options including surgery or follow-up. Surgical decision-making is usually based on personal or family history of breast cancer, palpable or ultrasonographic associated mass, incomplete removal of calcifications with DVAB, or difficult mammographic follow-up. More recently some authors have used pathological criteria to identify a subset of patients who would not benefit from surgery. They assessed the extent of ADH within ducts and demonstrated that underestimation does not occur when ADH is confined to 1-2 ducts on biopsy. In a retrospective study, which included 300 ADH patients, published in 2008, the authors defined three criteria that can help in choosing between "surgery" or "follow-up". These criteria include lesion size, complete removal of microcalcifications with DVAB and extent of ADH. From these data, they deduced a schema **(Figure 19-6)** of management for patients with ADH on DVAB.

Ductal Carcinoma In Situ

Ductal carcinoma *in situ* (DCIS) is a proliferation of abnormal epithelial cells confined by the basement membrane of the mammary ductal system. Screening

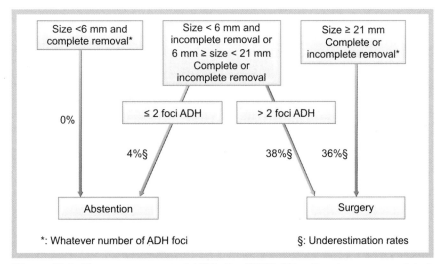

Figure 19-6: The management of ADH after DVAB (Directional vacuum-assisted biopsy)(Adapted with permission from Forgeard C, Benchaib M, Guerin N, et al. Is surgical biopsy mandatory in case of atypical ductal hyperplasia on 11-gauge core needle biopsy? A retrospective study of 300 patients. Am J Surg 2008; 196:339-45)

mammography has led to a significant increase in the incidence of DCIS over the last two decades. DCIS accounts for 18% of all newly diagnosed breast cancers in the USA. The incidence of DCIS increased from 2.4 cases per 100,000 women in 1981 to 27.7 cases per 100,000 women by 2001. During 1992-2001, there was a 236% increase in the number of women diagnosed with DCIS.

Diagnosis

Similar to IBC, DCIS is more common in the upper-outer breast quadrant, which supports the notion that DCIS is a precursor to IBC. In the current hypothesis, almost all cases of IDC arise from DCIS. Therefore, detection of DCIS reduces the subsequent incidence of IDC.

Historically, DCIS has been diagnosed in a small proportion of patients presenting with a palpable mass, pathologic nipple discharge or occasionally, as an incidental biopsy finding. In modern practice, DCIS is most frequently identified in asymptomatic women with screen detected microcalcifications.

To standardize radiological terms and reports, the American College of Radiology has established the Breast Imaging Reporting and Data System (BI-RADS). Based on this system, microcalcifications seen in a segmental distribution, linear pattern and pleomorphic shapes are most predictive of malignancy. This calcification constellation is typical for high-grade DCIS with comedo type necrosis. The intraductally spreading DCIS generally leads to coarse pleomorphic and branching calcifications **(Figure 19-7)**. The presence of unclear grouped calcifications, common in the BI-RADS 4 category, permits an opportunity of detecting DCIS in its early stages. These lesions are associated with a malignancy rate of 20-35%.

Technological advances in breast imaging are likely to be associated with further increases in the incidence of

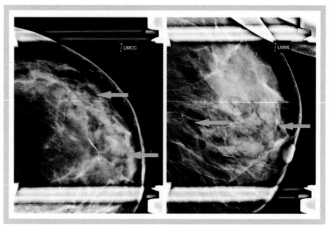

Figure 19-7: Typical appearance of DCIS on mammography. These magnification views show pleomorphic calcifications (arrows) in a segmental distribution, typical of DCIS

DCIS. Full-field digital mammography (FFDM) combined with computer aided detection (CAD) is more effective than analogue film mammography in screening pre- and perimenopausal women and those with dense breasts. Magnetic resonance imaging (MRI) has a higher sensitivity for breast cancer than mammography and is emerging as the best modality for screening young women at high risk. MRI may have particular utility in assessing the extent and distribution of disease in the breast **(Figure 19-8)**. Even if there is a debate in the effectiveness of MRI on DCIS, a prospective observational study has demonstrated MRI to be significantly more sensitive than mammography for the diagnosis of DCIS (92% vs 56%). Interestingly, cases missed by one imaging modality were detected by the other, suggesting that MRI would function best as an adjunct to screening mammography.

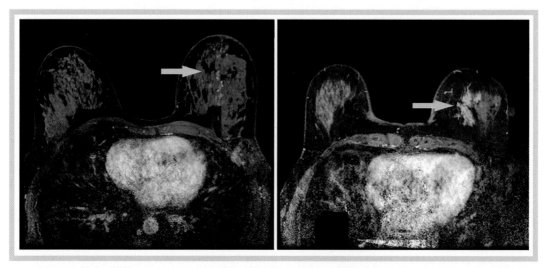

Figure 19-8: MRI appearance of DCIS. This T1 weighted MRI shows clumped non-mass-like enhancement in a ductal distribution, typical of DCIS (arrows)

Biopsy

Most of the DCIS is identified on screening mammography as indeterminate microcalcifications. In a study of 23,810 patients with DCIS, data available on 6,212 patients, revealed a median tumor size of 0.9 cm. Because of this, mammographic or stereotatic guidance is required to biopsy this lesion. Appropriate biopsy tools include core needle biopsy (CNB) and DVAB. Fine needle aspiration has no role in the diagnosis of DCIS because of the low sensitivity and specificity.

CNB allows a tissue cylinder to be excised. Histopathological diagnoses including prognostic criteria such as tumor grading and hormone receptor status can be obtained. CNB is associated with a relatively low morbidity and low equipment costs. However, CNB has recognized limitations. CNB may miss microcalcifications because the lesion is not reliably sampled. Thus, the patient may not be spared a surgical procedure. The failure of CNB to spare the patient a surgical procedure is higher for calcifications than for masses. DVAB was introduced to circumvent these problems. DVAB removes a greater tissue volume and minimizes sampling error. When targeting microcalcifications at percutaneous biopsy, removal of calcification-containing tissue is mandatory to allow a reliable histopathological diagnosis. During DVAB, removal of the microcalcifications can be documented under direct vision. DVAB has been shown to increase the diagnostic yield and upgrade ADH to DCIS in approximately 25% of cases. Stereotactic DVAB has been established as the procedure of choice in diagnosing DCIS.

Pathologic Classification and Natural History

Numerous classification schemes have been proposed for DCIS; all of them are based on tumor features and are designed to predict the risk of recurrence/progression to IBC. The traditional classification of DCIS is based on architectural pattern (e.g. comedo, cribriform, micropapillary, papillary, or solid), cell polarization (orientation of the apical cell border toward the ductal lumen), cell necrosis and nuclear grade (e.g. low, intermediate, or high). Consensus conferences held in 1997 and 2000 generated comprehensive classification schema for DCIS. They determined that the following key features must be assessed by the pathologists: nuclear grade, cell necrosis, cell polarization and architectural pattern. They also recommended that margin status, tumor size and the presence or absence of calcification should be noted in the pathology report.

The biological diversity of DCIS lesions corresponds with variable malignant potential and consequently an elusive natural history. Though DCIS is defined as a pre-invasive condition, not all lesions will progress to IBC. The natural history of small, non-comedo low grade DCIS treated by biopsy alone has been evaluated in studies with long-term follow-up. After a median of 31 years, 39% of patients developed IBC, all of which occurred in the same breast quadrant as the DCIS and 45% of these patients died of metastatic disease. The overall progression of DCIS to IBC has been reported to range from 14% to 75%. Hence, it would seem that patients who receive no treatment beyond a diagnostic biopsy remain at significant risk of ipsilateral IBC. Increased risk has been demonstrated in lesions of low, intermediate and high nuclear grade, however, the onset interval seems to be longest for low nuclear grade lesions.

Prognosis

Tumor size has been correlated with local recurrence (LR) in patients with DCIS treated by breast conserving surgery (BCS) ± radiation therapy (RT). DCIS treated by BCS alone was associated with 10-year LR rates of 11% and 48%, respectively, for lesions smaller and larger than 10 mm. On the contrary, the French study reported LR rates of 30% and 31% in the BCS group for lesions under or over 10 mm, respectively and 11% and 13% for the same subgroups in the BCS + RT group.

Studies have shown significant differences in LR based upon negative margin width in patients treated by BCS alone or treated by BCS + RT. The incidence of residual tumor was found to be related to margin width, with 41% at < 1 mm, 31% at 1-2 mm and 0% with at least 2 mm of clearance. In addition to clear surgical margins, total excision volume has also been associated with LR. The Joint Centre Experience reported LR rates at 5 years of 9% and 0% for volumes < 60 and > 60 cm^3, respectively. Excision volumes < 60 cm^3 have been shown to increase the relative risk of LR in women under 45 years of age.

High grade DCIS is associated with a greater risk of LR and IBC. This has been illustrated in several studies of DCIS treated by BCS alone, with LR rates ranging from 6% to 31.5%, for low-grade and high-grade lesions, respectively. High nuclear grade has consistently been associated with poor prognosis and LR in DCIS. The combination of high nuclear grade and comedonecrosis was reported to correlate with the increased risk of LR after BCS. Similarly, the combination of nuclear grade and cellular polarization has been associated with the increased risk of LR.

Histological type, in particular comedo DCIS, has been identified as a risk factor for LR. Favorable prognostic types include clinging and micropapillary.

The National Surgical Adjuvant Breast and Bowel Project (NSABP) study B-17 evaluated nine pathologic features and found four to be independently related to a higher risk for LR on univariate analysis: the presence of comedonecrosis, solid (rather than cribriform) histologic

TABLE 19-3	Van Nuys prognostic index*		
Score	1	2	3
Size (mm)	<15	16-40	> 41
Margin width (mm)	>10	1-9	< 1
Pathologic classification	Nonhigh grade without necrosis (nuclear grades 1 or 2)	Nonhigh grade with necrosis (nuclear grades 1 or 2)	High grade with or without necrosis (nuclear grade 3)
Age (year)	>60	40-60	< 40

*Adapted with permission from Silverstein MJ. The University of Southern California/Van Nuys prognostic index for ductal carcinoma in situ of the breast. Am J Surg 2003; 186:337-43.

One to three are awarded for each of four different predictors of local breast recurrence (size, margin width, pathologic classification, age)

type, presence of lymphoid infiltrate and focality. On multivariate analysis, however, only comedonecrosis remained a statistically significant predictor of recurrence. A similar analysis in the European Organization for Research and Treatment of Cancer (EORTC) study 10853 reviewed 863 patients over a median follow-up of 5.3 years. The investigators found presence of symptoms in young age (< 40 years) that led to the detection of DCIS, growth pattern (e.g. cribriform and solid), presence of disease at the surgical margins and treatment by local excision alone were the most important factors associated with a higher risk for LR.

The Van Nuys Prognostic Index (VNPI) **(Table 19-3)** is a combination of parameters (e.g. patients' age, tumor's size, surgical margin width, nuclear grade and the presence/absence of comedonecrosis) which has predictive utility for LR after BCS (with or without adjuvant RT) and can facilitate clinical decision-making.

The hormone receptor profile of DCIS has prognostic and therapeutic implications. High grade DCIS lesions which are estrogen receptor (ER) and progesterone receptor (PR) negative are significantly associated with HER2 and p53 positivity. ER positivity in low and intermediate grade DCIS was significantly more common than in high grade DCIS. ER negative lesions tend to be PR negative and high grade lesions with microinvasion tend to be HER2 positive and hormone receptor negative. HER2 positivity and ER/PR negativity are individually associated with risk of recurrence.

Management and Treatment

Historically, the gold-standard surgical approach to DCIS management was mastectomy and resulted in nearly 100% disease control. However, BCS+RT has been found to yield excellent local control in IBC, leading to the question of why a more radical surgical procedure should be required for this noninvasive form of breast carcinoma. It is paradoxical that in some cases DCIS will be treated more radically than confirmed IBC. At present it is not possible to reliably predict which lesions will progress,

however, DCIS is curable and successfully treated patients do not develop IBC. In practice this means that all patients should be offered treatment, but in view of the disease heterogeneity, the optimal treatment of DCIS remains controversial.

Silverstein MJ published the recurrence rates according to VNPI. Patients with VNPI scores of 4, 5 and 6 do not show a local disease-free survival benefit from RT. Patients with an intermediate rate of LR (VNPI 7-9) are benefited by RT. There is a statistically significant decrease in LR rate, averaging about 12% to 15% throughout the curves, for irradiated patients with intermediate VNPI scores compared with those treated by excision alone.

Surgical Managements

Mastectomy

The primary intention of surgical treatment is to comple-tely remove DCIS, reducing the risk of LR and IBC. Mastectomy is the procedure which provides greatest local control, approximately 98% at 7 years, with an overall recurrence rate of 1.4%. Indications for mastectomy include: large tumors (> 4 cm depending on breast size), multicentric lesions, inadequate margins, recurrence after BCS and patient preference. Silverstein, et al recommend mastectomy for the patients who have 10-12 VNPI scores because conservatively treated DCIS patients with a VNPI of 10-12 recur at an extremely high rate even with RT. In women requiring or requesting mastectomy for DCIS, skin-sparing mastectomy can facilitate immediate breast reconstruction with an implant and/or autologous flap resulting in an excellent cosmetic outcome.

Breast conserving surgery

The increasing incidence of smaller, mammographically detected lesions has been associated with changes in management strategy. Complete local excision can often be achieved without mastectomy. However, the oncolo-gical adequacy of breast conserving surgery (BCS) alone remains controversial. Despite the overall good prognosis, a significant number of patients undergoing BCS for DCIS develop LR, of which approximately half are invasive cancers. One-fifth of these develop metastatic disease. The NSABP B-17 trial randomized 818 patients after lumpectomy with complete excision of DCIS, to either whole breast RT or no further treatment. After a median follow-up of 129-months, among 403 women treated by lumpectomy alone, LR rate was 31.7%. In the study EORTC-10853 with a 126-month median follow-up, LR rate was 26% for the patients treated with BCS without RT. However, Silverstein MJ recommends excision alone for the patients who had 4-6 VNPI scores (LR rate was 1%).

Adjuvant radiotherapy

The combination of BCS with adjuvant RT has been advocated to address issues of oncologic adequacy, particularly with regard to LR. RT has demonstrated local recurrence risk reduction in the three large randomized controlled trials **(Table 19.4)**. Silverstein MJ recommends RT in patients with USC/VNPI score of 7-9. There was a statistically significant decrease in LR rate, averaging about 12% to 15% throughout the curves, for irradiated patients with 7-9 USC/VNPI scores compared with those treated by excision alone.

Axilla in DCIS

Pure DCIS, by definition, is limited by the basement membrane, without risk of lymphatic or vascular invasion. However, extensive DCIS can harbor foci of microinvasive disease. For this reason, lymph node involvement has been identified in 1-3% of patients. The low rate of nodal metastases, the high survival rate of DCIS and the significant morbidity of an axillary lymph node dissection are reasons why its routine application in the management of pure DCIS is no longer recommended. However, the evaluation of axillary nodes by sentinel lymph node biopsy (SLNB) may be considered, in certain situations, such as larger lesions (> 4 cm), palpable lesions, high-grade disease, CNB-proven microinvasive disease, when suspicious nodes are evident on axillary sonograms and with mastectomy.

Multivariate analysis demonstrated that the presence of a palpable lesion was the only predictive factor for positive SLNB in DCIS. Julian TB, et al evaluated the invasive nodal recurrence (INR) rates of the patients which included the NSABP B-17 and B-24 trials. In the NSABP B-17 study, the rate of INR was 0.83/1000 patient-years. In the NSABP B-24 study, 6 of the 1,799 patients developed INR (0.36/1000 patient-years), 3 in the excision + RT group (0.37/1000 patient-years) and 3 in the excision + RT + tamoxifen group (0.35/1000 patient-years). They concluded that if the long-term INR rate is used as a surrogate for the initial status of the axilla in patients with DCIS who are treated conservatively, then the likelihood of nodal disease seems to be extremely rare at the time a patient is diagnosed with DCIS. These very low INR rates could indicate that SLNB at the time of diagnosis would have a low yield and would subject patients to unnecessary morbidities associated with SLNB. If we assume that microinvasive disease was missed at the initial pathology review in 5-10% of the cases, the need and the utility of SLNB is also questioned. It may be that the only indication to perform an SLNB in DCIS patients is when a mastectomy is required. In that case, if an IBC is found at final pathology, it would technically be impossible to perform an SLNB. Based on the current literature, a selective approach of SLNB can be advised in patients with an excisional biopsy diagnosis of high grade DCIS as well as in patients undergoing mastectomy.

TABLE 19-4	The randomized controlled trials for the treatment of DCIS with radiotherapy					
Study name	N	Median follow-up (month)	BCS (LR/n) (%)	BCS+RT (LR/n) (%)	p	
[1]NSABP B-17	813	129	124/403 (31.7%)	61/410 (15.7%)	0.001	
[2]EORTC 10853	1010	126	132/503 (26%)	75/507 (15%)	<0.0001	
[3]UK/ANZ	1694	53	119/544 (22%)	22/267 (8%)	0.04	

[1] NSABP: National Surgical Adjuvant Breast and Bowel Project (Fisher ER, Dignam J, Tan-Chiu E, et al. Pathologic findings from the National Surgical Adjuvant Breast Project (NSABP) eight-year update of Protocol B-17: Intraductal carcinoma. Cancer 1999; 86:429-38.

[2] EORTC: European Organization for Research and Treatment of Cancer (Bijker N, Peterse JL, Duchateau L, et al. Risk factor for recurrence and metastasis after breast conserving therapy for ductal carcinoma in situ: analysis of European Organisation for Research and Treatment of Cancer trial 10853. J Clin Oncol 2001;19:2263-71.

[3] UK/ANZ: United Kingdom Coordinating Committee on Cancer Research (UKCCCR) (Houghton J, George WD, Cuzick J, Duggan C, Fentiman IS, Spittle M. Radiotherapy and tamoxifen in women with completely excised ductal carcinoma in situ of the breast in the UK, Australia and New Zealand: randomized controlled trial. Lancet 2003; 362:95-102).

BCS: Breast Conserving Surgery
RT: Radiotherapy
LR: Local Recurrence

Systemic Therapy in DCIS

Hormone therapy

In the NSABP B-24 trial, women treated with BCS + RT were subsequently randomized to placebo or tamoxifen (10 mg twice a day for 5 years). After 7-years median follow-up, the LR rates were 11.1% and 8% in the placebo and tamoxifen groups, respectively (P = 0.02). The absolute reduction was significant for invasive LR. No significant benefit was observed in the following groups: age >50 years, *in situ* LR, complete local excision and absence of necrosis.

The UK/ANZ DCIS trial showed that for patients not receiving RT, adjuvant tamoxifen did not significantly reduce the incidence of ipsilateral IBC or DCIS. However, the total number of DCIS events (ipsilateral and contralateral) was significantly reduced by tamoxifen (6% vs 10%, P = 0.03). Tamoxifen had no significant effect for patients receiving adjuvant RT. The use of adjuvant tamoxifen should be restricted to patients who are likely to benefit, such as young women who are receptor positive, in the absence of risk factors which may exacerbate the potential side effects.

Tamoxifen is not the only hormonal therapy available and it is unclear which hormonal therapy is optimal for hormone receptor-positive DCIS. To help answer this question, the NSABP conducted B-35, a phase III trial to compare the effectiveness of anastrozole (an aromatase inhibitor; 1 mg daily) with that of tamoxifen (20 mg daily) in preventing subsequent breast cancer (e.g. local, regional and distant recurrences and contralateral breast cancer) in postmenopausal women with primary DCIS treated with lumpectomy and breast irradiation. The results of this trial, which closed in 2006, are pending and, when available, will help to guide the management of hormone-receptor positive DCIS.

Chemotherapy

The NSABP is developing a phase III randomized trial of trastuzumab for patients with HER-2/neu-overexpressing DCIS treated with BCS yielding negative margins. Patients will be randomized to receive six weeks of whole-breast irradiation with or without concurrent trastuzumab. The M.D. Anderson Cancer Center has begun a trial of neoadjuvant trastuzumab for DCIS. They hypothesize that trastuzumab will have substantial activity against DCIS, perhaps even more than it has against IBC, because the volume of disease in DCIS patients is normally much lower than in IBC patients. The results of these trials may change the future systemic treatment of DCIS.

Vaccines

Several trials in the neoadjuvant setting are already under-way and may reflect an emerging paradigm in the management of DCIS. The relatively long latency between the appearance of DCIS and the development of IBC provides an opportunity to test novel therapies that may affect the natural history of breast cancer and possibly reduce the morbidity resulting from current treatments. One novel avenue of investigation focuses on the use of cancer vaccines. DCIS patients are good candidates for testing therapeutic and preventative vaccines because they are generally otherwise healthy. Additionally, induced immune responses in these patients have greater potential efficacy because DCIS progresses slowly and the disease burden is relatively small. Vaccination in this setting represents a strategic shift away from the treatment of advanced disease in which vaccines have had limited success.

The NCCN guidelines for the treatment and the proposed treatment algorithm of DCIS is shown in **Figures 19-9 and 19-10**, respectively.

Lobular Neoplasia

Lobular neoplasia (LN) represents the spectrum of changes within the lobule, ranging from atypical lobular hyperplasia (ALH) to lobular carcinoma in situ (LCIS) and is associated with increased risk for developing subsequent IBC. In 1978, Haagensen, et al published their series of 211 patients and reviewed the literature on "LCIS" not associated with other forms of breast cancer. Their conclusions were largely in agreement with those of Foote and Stewart, who considered the term "LCIS" a misnomer when not associated with invasive cancer. The evidence available at that time suggested that the lesions were in fact a "benign, noninfiltrating, special microscopic form of lobular proliferation of the mammary epithelium". They suggested the use of the term "LN" instead. This term was subsequently widely accepted and played an important role in changing the management of the lesion, from mastectomy to follow-up.

Although LN is a relatively uncommon diagnosis, its incidence has been increasing, especially among post-menopausal women. Overall, the age-adjusted, age-specific LCIS rates increased fourfold in the United States from 0.90 per 100,000 persons in 1978-80 to 3.19 per 100,000 persons in 1996-98, based on data from the Surveillance, Epidemiology and End Results (SEER) Program.

Clinical Evaluation

LCIS is most frequently diagnosed in women between the ages of 40 and 55 years (fewer than 10% of patients with LN are postmenopausal). Generally, LCIS and ALH are asymptomatic and clinically occult. Unlike IBC, LCIS rarely (if ever) forms a palpable mass. This is the primary reason that LCIS and ALH are most commonly diagnosed as incidental findings among women undergoing breast biopsy for another reason, such as a benign palpable mass

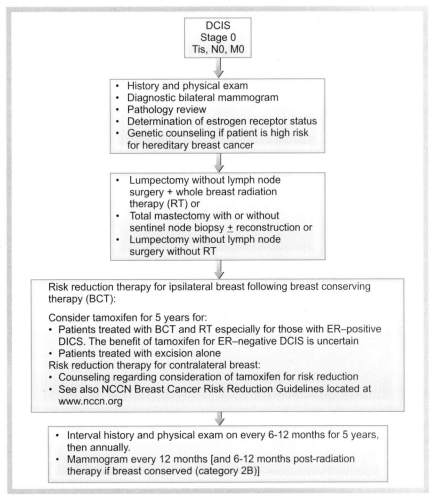

Figure 19-9: The NCCN clinical practice guidelines for the treatment of ductal carcinoma in situ (DCIS) (Adapted with permission from the NCCN Breast Cancer Guidelines v1.2010)

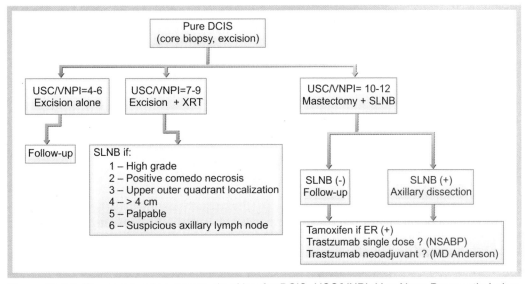

Figure 19-10: The proposed treatment algorithm for DCIS. USC/VNPI: Van Nuys Prognostic Index; SLNB: Sentinel lymph node biopsy; XRT: Radiation therapy; ER: Estrogen receptor

or an indeterminate mammographic finding. Some evidence shows that pleomorphic LCIS, a subset of LCIS, is not completely incidental but is associated with mammographic calcifications. However, this represents a small group of patients. With the exception of the rarer forms of LCIS with necrosis and associated microcalcification, LCIS is in general radiologically coverted.

Multifocality and multicentricity are often confused but conceptually distinct terms. *Multifocality* is a microscopic finding in which disease is sprinkled in a discontinuous fashion in one region of the breast, whereas *multicentricity* refers to how disease is grossly distributed in the breast in multiple distinct regions or LCIS may exhibit both of these features and also bilaterality.

The original publications by Foote, Stewart and Muir described the multifocal nature of LCIS. These investigators observed that when patients underwent mastectomy after surgical biopsy showing LCIS, the mastectomy specimen commonly had residual disease in areas outside the biopsy cavity, tending to show a speckled, microscopic distribution in multiple lobules of a given breast region. In contrast, multicentricity with LCIS is more difficult to prove. Rosen, et al provided the most convincing data, observing LCIS in multiple quadrants of the breast in 24 of 50 (48%) mastectomy specimens. Regarding the bilaterality of LCIS, Swain's review of 15 studies shows bilaterality rates varying from 9% to 69%. Beute, et al reviewed mammography and pathology of 104 patients with LCIS identified from biopsies and mastectomy specimens. Among these patients, 82 underwent sampling of both breasts either through mirror-image biopsy or contralateral mastectomy. Bilateral LCIS was found in half of these patients (41/82). The subgroups analysis of 182 women with LCIS who were enrolled in the National Surgical Adjuvant Breast Project (NSABP) Protocol B-17 but received no treatment other than lumpectomy showed that the number of ipsilateral breast tumor recurrence and contralateral breast tumor recurrence observed in this large cohort of patients with LCIS is markedly less than that noted by others after a comparable period of follow-up. A retrospective chart review of the University of Michigan's Cancer Registry revealed 105 patients with LCIS as a histologic component of invasive cancer. They found that LCIS is not associated with an increase in contralateral or ipsilateral recurrence for an invasive cancer.

Histopathology

According to the latest World Health Organization classification of breast tumors, LN is defined as a "proliferation of generally small and often loosely cohesive cells originating in the terminal duct-lobular unit, with or without pagetoid involvement of terminal ducts." Architecturally, these lesions are characterized by a variable enlargement of the acini, which are filled by a monomorphic population of small, rather discohesive, round, cuboidal or polygonal cells, with inconspicuous cytoplasm. The cells of classic LN can be classified into two subtypes, according to criteria laid down by Haagensen and revised by Sneige, et al. Type A is characterized by bland and mildly discohesive cells, with scant cytoplasm and nuclei approximately (1.5 × the size of a lymphocyte nucleus); and type B, which characteristically have more abundant cytoplasm, slightly bigger nuclei (2 × the size of a lymphocyte nucleus), mild to moderate nuclear atypia (still falling into nuclear grade 1 or 2) and indistinct or absent nucleoli. The term ALH is used to refer to a partial involvement of acini by LN cells. According to Page, et al, to diagnose LCIS, more than half of the acini in an involved lobular unit must be filled and distended by the characteristic cells, leaving no central lumina.

Pleomorphic LCIS (PLCIS) was first identified as a distinct entity by Eusebi, et al in 1992. Cells are remarkably larger than those of classic LN and have more abundant, pink and finely granular cytoplasm. PLCIS frequently displays features of apocrine differentiation and harbor more pleomorphic atypical nuclei with conspicuous nucleoli.

Prognosis

Early epidemiological studies suggested that a diagnosis of LN would confer an increased risk of developing IBC but IBC was not necessarily of lobular histology. The absolute risk for developing ipsilateral breast cancer after LCIS has been detected is 17% with the relative risk of 8.0 in the first 15 years of follow-up when compared with the general population. However, it has recently been shown that this risk is higher in the ipsilateral breast and mainly at the site of the biopsied LN.

Mathematic modeling suggests that during the first 15 years after biopsy, women with LCIS have 10.8 times the risk for breast cancer compared with women of comparable age without proliferative changes on breast biopsy. The reported incidence of IBC in patients with LCIS has ranged from 2% to 38%. In reported series of patients diagnosed with LCIS through surgical biopsy and then followed up without further intervention, 2-20% of patients developed ipsilateral IBC and 1-18% developed contralateral IBC. The NSABP published the 12 year follow-up study of the patients with LCIS. They evaluated the frequencies and average annual rates per 100 patient-years according to the grades of LCIS for all ipsilateral breast tumor recurrences (IBTRs). The grade of LCIS combined grade 2-3 LCIS versus grade 1 LCIS were predictive for the endpoint of IBTRs that consisted of invasive carcinoma and DCIS with or without a component of LCIS. The rates for all IBTRs were statistically significant when patients who had grade 2-3 LCIS together were compared with patients who had grade 1 LCIS ($P = 0.023$). The grade of LCIS was not significantly related to invasive IBTR, *per se*; however, all grades of LCIS ($P = 0.037$) and combined grade 2-3 LCIS versus grade 1 LCIS ($P = 0.010$) were predictive for the endpoint of invasive IBTR and for IBTR consisting of DCIS with or without a component of LCIS. None of the other pathologic variables were significantly related to IBTR; and none of those variables, including grades of LCIS, were related to all contralateral breast tumors or to contralateral breast tumors consisting of invasive carcinoma or its total with IBTR consisting of DCIS.

Surgical Management

Because classic LCIS generally does not require surgical treatment, surgical biopsy showing LCIS should not demand further intervention. The implication is that surgical margins for LCIS are not clinically relevant. Therefore, surgical removal of more breast tissue simply because the excised tissue had LCIS at the edge is not necessary. A possible exception to this is in patients with pleomorphic LCIS, although the long-term follow-up data are not adequate to make definitive recommendations.

Liberman, et al retrospectively reviewed the Memorial Sloan-Kettering experience of 1315 consecutive stereotactic biopsies, of which 16 were found to have LCIS on percutaneous CNB (1.2%). Based on their findings and most authors agree that excision should be performed in cases of LN diagnosed on a CNB in the following instances:

i. Another lesion, which would itself be an indication for surgical excision, is also present on the core biopsy (such as ADH or a radial scar).
ii. There is a discordance between clinical, radiological and pathological findings.
iii. There is an associated mass lesion or an area of architectural distortion.
iv. ALH or LCIS showed mixed histological features with difficulty in distinguishing the lesion from DCIS, or shows a mixed E-cadherin staining pattern.
v. The morphology is consistent with that of the pleomorphic variant of lobular neoplasia.

In general, LCIS is not a contraindication for breast conserving surgery. Most studies have not shown an increased risk for ipsilateral breast cancer recurrence after breast conservation for IBC coincident with LCIS. The extent of LCIS did not seem to affect the risk for recurrence. Furthermore, the risks for contralateral disease and distant failure were not affected by the presence or extent of LCIS within the ipsilateral breast.

Prophylactic endocrine therapy

After tamoxifen had been shown to decrease the risk for contralateral breast cancer, it was initially chosen for breast cancer prevention trials. Of the 3 worldwide tamoxifen prevention trials published, only the NSABP P-01 specifically evaluated participants with LCIS. The NSABP study shows a statistically significant benefit from tamoxifen in the prevention setting, although the patient populations enrolled in each trial have important differences. The NSABP P-01 trial is a randomized, double blind trial. Participants in this trial were randomized to tamoxifen, 20 mg daily, versus a placebo for a planned duration of 5 years. Of the women with a history of LCIS, 411 were randomized to the placebo arm and 415 to the tamoxifen arm. The results showed that 18 cases of IBC occurred in the placebo arm and 8 cases occurred in the tamoxifen arm. These numbers translated to a 56% reduction in risk for IBC among patients with LCIS who used tamoxifen. Thus, tamoxifen's benefits were seen whether subjects had pre-existing LCIS or atypical hyperplasia. In addition, no difference in survival was observed or expected between the two arms, primarily because only short-term follow-up was conducted. The FDA has approved tamoxifen for breast cancer prevention.

Recent evidence suggests a similar magnitude of benefit from the related drug, raloxifene. In the NSABP P-2 Study of Tamoxifen and Raloxifene (STAR) trial, the two drugs had equivalent effects in reducing risk of IBC in all examined high-risk women, including women with a history of atypical hyperplasia or LCIS, who had the highest annual rates of IBC. In this initial report of the STAR trial, raloxifene and tamoxifen were equivalent in efficacy for lowering the risk of invasive breast cancer. The cumulative incidence rates were 25.1 per 1000 women (raloxifene) versus 24.8 per 1000 (tamoxifen) ($P = 0.83$). In contrast to tamoxifen, raloxifene does not reduce the risk of noninvasive breast cancer. In the STAR trial, tamoxifen and raloxifene had equivalent effects in reducing risk of invasive breast cancer in all examined subgroups, including women with a history of atypical hyperplasia or LCIS, who had the highest annual rates of invasive breast cancer. The LCIS subgroup rates of 9.83 (tamoxifen) and 9.61 (raloxifene) per 1000 women are about 2.5 times higher than those for women who participated in the study and had no history of LCIS (3.76 [tamoxifen] and 3.86 [raloxifene] per 1000). Raloxifene has been then approved by the FDA for postmenopausal women with high risk for breast cancer.

Prophylactic Mastectomy

A prophylactic mastectomy of both breasts with immediate reconstruction may be an option for women with LCIS and a very strong family history of breast cancer. Prophylactic total mastectomy in women with BRCA gene mutations significantly reduces the risk of breast cancer by approximately 90%. If this option is being

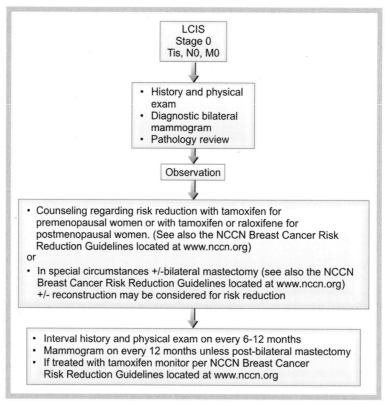

Figure 19-11: The NCCN clinical practice guidelines for the treatment of lobular carcinoma *in situ* (LCIS) tumors (Adapted with permission from the NCCN Breast Cancer Guidelines v1.2010)

considered, evaluation should include consultation with a genetics counselor and both oncologic and reconstructive surgeons. Psychological consultation should also be considered because of the impact of a prophylactic mastectomy on body image and sexuality.

Follow-up

Women diagnosed with LCIS should undergo yearly mammography. Digital mammography with additional screening ultrasound should be considered in women who have dense breasts. Currently, there is no evidence that MRI should be used for intensified surveillance as has been recommended in women with a genetically increased risk. Ductal lavage (DL) is a new method for the sampling of breast epithelium. Data regarding its sensitivity in the detection of epithelial abnormalities, including carcinoma in situ, remain limited. The use of DL remains investigational and close follow-up should be continued for all patients undergoing DL even if the results are benign.

The treatment algorithm for LN, which is based on NCCN guidelines, is shown in **Figure 19-11**.

Acknowledgments

The authors wish to thank Oya Andacoglu, MD, Marie Ganott, MD, Margarita Zuley, MD and Ryan Kelley, BA for their assistance with designing and preparing the Figures and Tables.

Landmark Papers

1. Houghton J, George WD, Cuzick J, et al. Radiotherapy and tamoxifen in women with completely excised ductal carcinoma in situ of the breast in the UK, Australia and New Zealand: randomised controlled trial. Lancet 2003; 362:95-102.
2. Fisher B, Dignam J, Wolmark N, et al. Tamoxifen in treatment of intraductal breast cancer: National Surgical Adjuvant Breast and Bowel Project B-24 randomised controlled trial. Lancet 1999; 353:1993-2000.
3. Goodwin A, Parker S, Ghersi D, et al. Post-operative radiotherapy for ductal carcinoma in situ of the breast. Cochrane Database Syst Rev 2009; CD000563.
4. Julien JP, Bijker N, Fentiman IS, et al. Radiotherapy in breast-conserving treatment for ductal carcinoma in situ: first results of the EORTC randomised phase III trial 10853. EORTC Breast Cancer Cooperative Group and EORTC Radiotherapy Group. Lancet 2000; 355:528-33.

5. Fisher B, Dignam J, Wolmark N, et al. Lumpectomy and radiation therapy for the treatment of intraductal breast cancer: findings from National Surgical Adjuvant Breast and Bowel Project B-17. J Clin Oncol 1998; 16:441-52.
6. Jeruss JS, Vicini FA, Beitsch PD, et al. Initial outcomes for patients treated on the American Society of Breast Surgeons MammoSite clinical trial for ductal carcinoma-in-situ of the breast. Ann Surg Oncol 2006; 13:967-76.
7. Tan JC, McCready DR, Easson AM, et al. Role of sentinel lymph node biopsy in ductal carcinoma-in-situ treated by mastectomy. Ann Surg Oncol 2007; 14:638-45.
8. Vogel VG, Costantino JP, Wickerham DL, et al. Effects of tamoxifen vs raloxifene on the risk of developing invasive breast cancer and other disease outcomes: the NSABP Study of Tamoxifen and Raloxifene (STAR) P-2 trial. Jama 2006; 295:2727-41.
9. Fisher B, Costantino JP, Wickerham DL, et al. Tamoxifen for the prevention of breast cancer: current status of the National Surgical Adjuvant Breast and Bowel Project P-1 study. J Natl Cancer Inst 2005; 97:1652-62.

Level of Evidence Table

Recommendation	Grade	Best level of evidence	References
Adjuvant tamoxifen for ER-positive DCIS reduces subsequent breast-cancer events.	B	1b	1, 2
Ipsilateral whole-breast radiation reduces invasive and non-invasive recurrences after breast-conserving therapy of DCIS.	A	1a	3-5
Partial breast irradiation after excision of DCIS is safe but has unknown efficacy.	C	1b (early results)	6
Routine sentinel node biopsy is indicated during mastectomy for DCIS.	A	2b	7, 8
Selective sentinel node biopsy should be considered during breast-conserving therapy of DCIS in patients younger than 55 years, high grade lesions, lesions > 4 cm, palpable DCIS, mammographic mass or diagnosed by core-needle biopsy.	B	2b	9,10
Neoadjuvant hormone therapy of ER-positive DCIS remains experimental.	C	1b	11,12
Neither screening MRI nor sentinel node biopsy is indicated in the setting of prophylactic mastectomy.	B	2b	13-15
Hormone therapy is effective for women desiring risk reduction for breast cancer.	A	1b	16-19
Routine surgical biopsy of lobular neoplasia (e.g. ALH, LCIS) diagnosed by core-needle biopsy is indicated to rule-out invasive cancer.	C	3a	20-24
The addition of contrast-enhanced MRI to screening women at high-risk for breast cancer increases the sensitivity of mammography and should be considered.	B	1a	25-27
Wide excision alone is adequate for phyllodes tumors.	B	2b	28, 29

References

1. Houghton J, George WD, Cuzick J, et al. Radiotherapy and tamoxifen in women with completely excised ductal carcinoma in situ of the breast in the UK, Australia and New Zealand: randomised controlled trial. Lancet 2003; 362:95-102.
2. Fisher B, Dignam J, Wolmark N, et al. Tamoxifen in treatment of intraductal breast cancer: National Surgical Adjuvant Breast and Bowel Project B-24 randomised controlled trial. Lancet 1999; 353:1993-2000.
3. Goodwin A, Parker S, Ghersi D, et al. Post-operative radiotherapy for ductal carcinoma in situ of the breast. Cochrane Database Syst Rev 2009; CD000563.
4. Julien JP, Bijker N, Fentiman IS, et al. Radiotherapy in breast-conserving treatment for ductal carcinoma in situ: first results of the EORTC randomised phase III trial 10853. EORTC Breast Cancer Cooperative Group and EORTC Radiotherapy Group. Lancet 2000; 355:528-33.
5. Fisher B, Dignam J, Wolmark N, et al. Lumpectomy and radiation therapy for the treatment of intraductal breast cancer: findings from National Surgical Adjuvant Breast and Bowel Project B-17. J Clin Oncol 1998; 16:441-52.
6. Jeruss JS, Vicini FA, Beitsch PD, et al. Initial outcomes for patients treated on the American Society of Breast Surgeons MammoSite clinical trial for ductal carcinoma-in-situ of the breast. Ann Surg Oncol 2006; 13:967-76.

7. Dominguez FJ, Golshan M, Black DM, et al. Sentinel node biopsy is important in mastectomy for ductal carcinoma in situ. Ann Surg Oncol 2008; 15:268-73.

8. Tan JC, McCready DR, Easson AM, et al. Role of sentinel lymph node biopsy in ductal carcinoma-in-situ treated by mastectomy. Ann Surg Oncol 2007; 14:638-45.

9. Yen TW, Hunt KK, Ross MI, et al. Predictors of invasive breast cancer in patients with an initial diagnosis of ductal carcinoma in situ: a guide to selective use of sentinel lymph node biopsy in management of ductal carcinoma in situ. J Am Coll Surg 2005; 200:516-26.

10. Goyal A, Douglas-Jones A, Monypenny I, et al. Is there a role of sentinel lymph node biopsy in ductal carcinoma in situ?: analysis of 587 cases. Breast Cancer Res Treat 2006; 98:311-4.

11. Chen YY, DeVries S, Anderson J, et al. Pathologic and biologic response to preoperative endocrine therapy in patients with ER-positive ductal carcinoma in situ. BMC Cancer 2009; 9:285.

12. Hwang ES, Esserman L. Neoadjuvant hormonal therapy for ductal carcinoma in situ: trial design and preliminary results. Ann Surg Oncol 2004; 11:37S-43S.

13. Black D, Specht M, Lee JM, et al. Detecting occult malignancy in prophylactic mastectomy: preoperative MRI versus sentinel lymph node biopsy. Ann Surg Oncol 2007; 14:2477-84.

14. Soran A, Falk J, Bonaventura M, et al. Is routine sentinel lymph node biopsy indicated in women undergoing contralateral prophylactic mastectomy? Magee-Womens Hospital experience. Ann Surg Oncol 2007; 14:646-51.

15. McLaughlin SA, Stempel M, Morris EA, et al. Can magnetic resonance imaging be used to select patients for sentinel lymph node biopsy in prophylactic mastectomy? Cancer 2008; 112:1214-21.

16. Land SR, Wickerham DL, Costantino JP, et al. Patient-reported symptoms and quality of life during treatment with tamoxifen or raloxifene for breast cancer prevention: the NSABP Study of Tamoxifen and Raloxifene (STAR) P-2 trial. Jama 2006; 295:2742-51.

17. Vogel VG, Costantino JP, Wickerham DL, et al. Effects of tamoxifen vs raloxifene on the risk of developing invasive breast cancer and other disease outcomes: the NSABP Study of Tamoxifen and Raloxifene (STAR) P-2 trial. Jama 2006; 295:2727-41.

18. Fisher B, Costantino JP, Wickerham DL, et al. Tamoxifen for the prevention of breast cancer: current status of the National Surgical Adjuvant Breast and Bowel Project P-1 study. J Natl Cancer Inst 2005; 97:1652-62.

19. Cuzick J, Forbes JF, Sestak I, et al. Long-term results of tamoxifen prophylaxis for breast cancer—96-month follow-up of the randomized IBIS-I trial. J Natl Cancer Inst 2007; 99:272-82.

20. Menon S, Porter GJ, Evans AJ, et al. The significance of lobular neoplasia on needle core biopsy of the breast. Virchows Arch 2008; 452:473-9.

21. Bowman K, Munoz A, Mahvi DM, et al. Lobular neoplasia diagnosed at core biopsy does not mandate surgical excision. J Surg Res 2007; 142:275-80.

22. Sohn VY, Arthurs ZM, Kim FS, et al. Lobular neoplasia: is surgical excision warranted? Am Surg 2008; 74:172-7.

23. Elsheikh TM, Silverman JF. Follow-up surgical excision is indicated when breast core needle biopsies show atypical lobular hyperplasia or lobular carcinoma in situ: a correlative study of 33 patients with review of the literature. Am J Surg Pathol 2005; 29:534-43.

24. Cangiarella J, Guth A, Axelrod D, et al. Is surgical excision necessary for the management of atypical lobular hyperplasia and lobular carcinoma in situ diagnosed on core needle biopsy?: a report of 38 cases and review of the literature. Arch Pathol Lab Med 2008; 132: 979-83.

25. Leach MO, Boggis CR, Dixon AK, et al. Screening with magnetic resonance imaging and mammography of a UK population at high familial risk of breast cancer: a prospective multicentre cohort study (MARIBS). Lancet 2005; 365:1769-78.

26. Lord SJ, Lei W, Craft P, et al. A systematic review of the effectiveness of magnetic resonance imaging (MRI) as an addition to mammography and ultrasound in screening young women at high risk of breast cancer. Eur J Cancer 2007; 43:1905-17.

27. Warner E, Messersmith H, Causer P, et al. Systematic review: using magnetic resonance imaging to screen women at high risk for breast cancer. Ann Intern Med 2008; 148:671-9.

28. Pezner RD, Schultheiss TE, Paz IB. Malignant phyllodes tumor of the breast: local control rates with surgery alone. Int J Radiat Oncol Biol Phys 2008; 71:710-3.

29. Macdonald OK, Lee CM, Tward JD, et al. Malignant phyllodes tumor of the female breast: association of primary therapy with cause-specific survival from the Surveillance, Epidemiology and End Results (SEER) program. Cancer 2006; 107:2127-33.

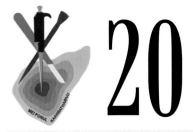

20 *Invasive Breast Cancer*

Yewching Teh, Ronald Johnson, Gretchen Ahrendt

History of Breast Cancer and Therapy

Breast cancer has been described as early as 3,500 years ago by the Egyptians who documented bulging tumors in the breast which had no cure. Hippocrates wrote of his theory that breast cancer is a humoral disease. This perception changed in the 19th century when Dr. William Halsted theorized that breast cancer was a localized disease. This brought about the practice of radical mastectomy to treat breast cancer by surgical removal. This procedure left women with chest wall deformities, chronic pain and lymphedema. Dr Bernard Fisher put forth an alternative hypothesis that breast cancer is not a localized disease, but that it has the potential to spread through lymphatics and blood. Through rigorous clinical trials, Dr Fisher revolutionized breast cancer treatment to our current practice of breast-conserving surgery and multimodality treatment. In the 21st century, we are moving on to the molecular basis of breast cancer, recognizing various genes that predispose women and men to developing breast cancer, genes that are responsible for various phenotypes of breast cancer and therefore, paving a way for development of targeted therapy to combat this disease.

Epidemiology

Breast cancer remains the most commonly diagnosed cancer in American women with an estimated 182,460 new cases for 2008. One in eight women will be diagnosed with breast cancer in their lifetime. The widespread application and improvements in screening mammography have contributed to an increase in the diagnosis of nonpalpable, early stage breast cancer since the 1980s. The mortality has declined due to early diagnosis, improvements in multimodality treatment including appropriate use of surgery, adjuvant systemic therapy and radiation and the introduction of biologic therapy. Despite these advances, breast cancer is the second most common cause of US cancer deaths in women with an estimate of 41,730 deaths in 2008. There is a difference in breast cancer incidences in women of different ethnic backgrounds. **Table 20-1** shows this difference based on the SEER data.

TABLE 20-1	Incidence rates by ethnicity
Ethnicity	**Rate (per 100,000 women)**
White	130.6
Black	117.5
Hispanic	90.1
Asian/Pacific Islander	89.6
American Indian/Alaska Native	75

Risk Factors and Risk Assessment

For clinicians to make appropriate decisions for screening, genetic testing and preventative strategies, it is necessary to recognize breast cancer risk factors and stratify patients into different risk levels of developing breast cancer.

The most important risk factor is **gender**. The ratio of female to male breast cancer is 100:1. With gender aside, **age** is the major risk factor. Based on SEER data from 2001 to 2005, < 16 cases of breast cancer occurred in women under the age of 20 years. The incidence increased to 1/1130 in the 20-49, 1/392 in the 50-64, 1/250 in the 65-74 and 1/238 in the over 75-year old age groups. The median age at diagnosis is 61 years.

Women who have a **family history** of breast cancer, specifically first-degree relatives are at an increased risk of developing breast cancer. It is important to distinguish between sporadic postmenopausal breast cancers in first-degree relatives from a pattern that is more suspicious for a genetic predisposition. Most women with the former association will not develop breast cancer. Conversely, women who have a family history suggestive of a hereditary breast cancer syndrome are at a higher risk. (See Genetic Predisposition section).

Exposure to both endogenous and exogenous **hormones** increases the risk of developing breast cancer. Endogenous factors include a long menstrual history, i.e.

early menarche before age 11 years, late menopause, nulliparity and being > 35 years old at first full-term birth. The Women's Health Initiative Study highlighted the role of exogenous hormone exposure in breast cancer risk. It showed that women with prolonged use of combination estrogen-progesterone hormonal replacement therapy (HRT) are at increased risk of breast cancer compared to non-users. Cessation of HRT resulted in a return of breast cancer risk to baseline levels after five years. Some evidence exists for a decrease in metastatic breast cancer incidence since implementation of recommendations for more stringent exogenous HRT. HRT use in postmenopausal women to manage menopausal symptoms must be balanced with the increased risk of breast cancer. Long-term use of HRT solely for management of perimeno-pausal symptoms is no longer advised.

A **personal history** of unilateral breast cancer confers a risk of developing contralateral breast cancer of 0.5-1% per year following the initial diagnosis. A history of **biopsy-proven proliferative breast disease** also increases the risk of developing breast cancer. Those with a history of papillomas have a 1.5-2 fold risk, with atypical ductal or lobular hyperplasia (AH) a 4-5 fold risk and with lobular carcinoma in situ (LCIS) a 8-10 fold risk than the general population. The risk associated with these histologies applies equally to both breasts.

Women who received **radiation** to the thoracic area (e.g. Hodgkin's Disease) have a 20-30% risk of developing breast cancer 10-30 years after treatment. This risk increases with increased dose and younger age of exposure, especially before age 30.

There is increasing evidence that **modifiable lifestyle factors** can increase a woman's risk for developing breast cancer. These include obesity in postmenopausal women, lack of physical activity and moderate amount of alcohol consumption.

Breast cancer risk assessment tools are available to assist clinicians and patients in quantifying the short-term and long-term personal risk of developing breast cancer. These tools provide objective data to reassure patients who overestimate their risk and to assist in decision-making regarding risk reduction strategies. For the general population, the modified Gail Model is commonly used. An online version can be found on the National Cancer Institute website (**http://www.cancer.gov/bcrisktool**). This tool provides the projected 5-year and lifetime risk for developing breast cancer for women older than age 35 years. It incorporates the patient's age, age at menarche, age at first livebirth, presence of first-degree relative with breast cancer, personal history of breast biopsy and if so, whether pathology showed atypical hyperplasia. The limitations are that there are no adjustments for strong family history of breast cancer or for genetic mutations. It is also based on data from Caucasian females and

therefore does not account for racial differences. The Claus Model takes into account both strong family history of breast cancer as well as ovarian cancer.

Patients are considered high risk for breast cancer development if they have a history of thoracic radiation, an estimated 5-year risk of invasive breast cancer > 1.7 in women > 35 years old or lifetime risk > 20% as defined by risk assessment models, strong family history or genetic predisposition, or a biopsy-proven diagnosis of LCIS or AH.

Genetic Predisposition and Counseling

Five to ten percent of all breast cancers are caused by an inherited gene mutation. About two thirds of hereditary breast cancers are due to mutations that have not been discovered. Twenty-five percent are due to BRCA1 and 2 mutations. Less that 10% are due to other known genes that cause Li-Fraumeni Syndrome, Muir-Torre Syndrome, Cowden disease and Peutz-Jegher's Syndrome, Bannayan-Riley-Ruvalcaba Syndrome which are of autosomal dominant inheritance and Ataxia Telangiectasia which is of autosomal recessive inheritance.

Certain characteristics of the woman and her family history should heighten the clinician's suspicion for a pattern of genetic inheritance. These include early-onset breast cancer (prior to age 40), multiple cases of breast and/or ovarian cancer in the same individual or first degree/close relatives affecting more than one generation, male breast cancer, a family member with a known gene mutation and Ashkenazi Jewish descent. Evaluation of family history should include paternal and maternal lineage as genetic predisposition can be inherited through either side of the family.

BRCA1&2 gene mutations account for 3% of all breast cancer cases and 80% of inherited breast cancer with a known mutation. The highest incidence of BRCA carrier status is in people of Ashkenazi Jewish descent. The lifetime risk of breast cancer is 60-80% and these women are typically 10-20 years younger at diagnosis when compared to women without mutations.

BRCA1 gene is found on the long arm of chromosome 17q12-21. It has a high penetrance and accounts for 45% of hereditary breast cancer. The type of breast cancer that develops in BRCA1 mutation carriers tend to be poorly differentiated, estrogen and progesterone receptor negative and HER2/neu nonexpressing. There is also a greater incidence of medullary histologic subtype. Patients have a 20-40% risk of developing ovarian cancer and are also at risk of developing prostate, colon and pancreatic cancers.

BRCA2 gene is found on chromosome 13q12.3. It accounts for 35% of hereditary breast cancer. It is associated with male breast cancer. The type of breast cancer found in BRCA2 mutation carriers is more heterogeneous. There is a 10-20% risk of developing ovarian cancer and a higher risk for prostate, pancreatic, stomach, melanoma and colon cancers.

The probability that an individual has a germline mutation of the BRCA1/2 gene can be assessed by the statistical software, *BRCAPRO*. The software is based on the individual's family history of breast and ovarian cancer, the age at onset of cancer and the total number of family members who have never developed breast or ovarian cancer.

Recognition of a familial pattern of hereditary breast cancer should prompt discussion on genetic counseling and testing. The goals for genetic counseling are to educate patients on their risk for hereditary cancer, assess their risk, explain the benefits and limitations of genetic testing, interpret the genetic test results, explain the available medical management options based on the test results and to provide referrals to support resources and research opportunities.

Genetic testing should be performed on the affected individual. When there are multiple individuals, the family member with the highest likelihood of being tested positive (early-onset disease, bilateral disease, or multiple primaries) should be tested first.

Prevention

Women should be educated on preventable risk factors which can be decreased by lifestyle modifications. This includes limiting the use of HRT to those whose symptoms cannot be alleviated by non-hormonal treatments and if absolutely necessary, limiting the dose and duration. Women should also be counseled regarding limiting alcohol consumption, weight control and increasing physical activity.

Bilateral oophorectomy is recommended in women with a known or strongly suspected BRCA1/2 mutations. It decreases the risk of ovarian cancer, although mutation carriers remain at risk for primary peritoneal carcinoma. Bilateral oophorectomy also decreases the risk of breast cancer by 50%. The timing of this procedure should be between 35-40 years of age or upon completion of childbearing. It should be performed after addressing issues of reproductive plans, menopausal symptoms and osteoporosis and the consequences of hormonal changes on quality of life.

Prophylactic bilateral mastectomy can reduce the risk of developing breast cancer by at least 90% in women who are at moderate risk. It is most commonly considered in patients with BRCA1/2 mutations. When counseling women who are contemplating prophylactic mastectomy, other alternatives of risk reduction, the risks and benefits of the procedure, the reconstructive options and recovery process should be addressed. Importantly, the psychological effects of losing the breasts should be discussed including the potential negative body image and interference with new or existing relationships.

Both tamoxifen (20 mg/day) and raloxifene (60 mg/day) can be used as hormonal chemoprevention. The NSABP Breast Cancer Prevention Trial (P-1) was a randomized controlled chemoprevention trial that included healthy premenopausal and postmenopausal women aged 35 years or older who had > 1.7% 5-year risk of developing breast cancer. The women were randomized to either tamoxifen or placebo. At 7-year follow-up, this study showed that tamoxifen decreased the risk of breast cancer by 43% in this group of women. The maximum risk-reduction benefit was seen in women with a history of AH or LCIS. There was no difference in survival.

A subset evaluation revealed the risk reduction was 62% for BRCA2 carriers but there was no risk reduction in BRCA1 carriers. The NSABP Study of Tamoxifen and Raloxifene (STAR) (P-2) trial was a randomized trial of postmenopausal women aged 35 years or older who had > 1.7% 5-year risk of developing breast cancer. The women were randomized to either tamoxifen or raloxifene. Raloxifene was found to be as effective as tamoxifen in reducing the risk of invasive cancer; however, it was not as effective in reducing the risk of noninvasive cancer. In women considering chemoprevention, the contraindications and the potential side effects of tamoxifen and raloxifene must be considered. Tamoxifen is frequently associated with undesirable quality of life side effects including hot flashes and vaginal discharge. Less common but serious side effects include venous thromboembolism and endometrial cancer. Many women with only a modest increased risk of breast cancer decline tamoxifen due to this unfavorable risk/benefit ratio. Raloxifene has a more favorable side-effect profile and fewer uterine cancers and thromboembolic events. There are ongoing trials evaluating the effectiveness of aromatase inhibitors as breast cancer prevention drugs.

Presentation

In the past, more than 50% of patients presented with palpable breast cancers that were detected on self-examination. Since the introduction of screening mammography, most patients present with screening detected breast cancers that are clinically occult. Clinical findings at presentation can include a palpable discrete breast mass, asymmetric parenchymal thickening, skin changes such as thickening, erythema and peau d'orange appearance and nipple changes such as inversion, discharge, eczema and crusting and axillary lymphadenopathy. All clinical findings need to be evaluated with a complete history and physical examination followed by breast imaging. Less

TABLE 20-2	Screening guidelines for high risk patients
Risk group	**Screening method**
Prior thoracic radiation, Now age < 25 years	BSE – monthly CBE – annually
Prior thoracic radiation, Now age > 25 years	Mammogram annually – begin 8-10 years after radiation or age 40 yrs, whichever first Consider MRI as adjunct to mammogram CBE – annually
5-year risk of invasive breast cancer ≥ 1.7 in women > 35 years or Lifetime risk > 20% or LCIS or Atypical hyperplasia	Mammogram annually CBE – every 6-12 months Consider MRI as adjunct to mammogram Consider risk reduction strategies
Strong family history or genetic predisposition, age < 25 years	CBE – annually
Strong family history or genetic predisposition, age > 25 years	Mammogram annually – starting at age 25 years or 5-10 years prior to youngest breast cancer case CBE – every 6-12 months Consider MRI as adjunct to mammogram

For all age groups and regardless of level of risk for developing breast cancer, women are encouraged to perform monthly BSE

than 10% of patients present with distant metastases at presentation.

Screening

For all age groups and regardless of level of risk for developing breast cancer, women are encouraged to perform monthly breast self-examination (BSE). While BSE does not decrease breast cancer mortality it enables a woman to become familiar with her breasts and may detect interval breast cancers that develop between screenings. Premenopausal women may find BSE most informative when performed at the end of menses.

For an average risk patient who is between the ages of 20-39 years old, the recommendation for screening is a clinical breast examination (CBE) every 1-3 years. Women who are > 40 years of age should undergo annual CBE and annual mammogram.

For high risk patients, screening guidelines are based upon the type of risk factor(s). **Table 20-2** summarizes the recommendations.

The decision to continue screening for breast cancer in the elderly population is based on clinical judgment. Patients who have severe comorbidities that will limit life expectancy and the ability to perform interventions based on screening results should not be required to undergo screening. Patients who have at least five years of life expectancy should probably undergo screening.

Diagnostic Modalities

Mammography

Screening mammography includes standard cranial-caudal and medial-lateral oblique views. Screening mammogram is performed annually and used in asymptomatic patients. When abnormalities are detected on screening mammography, patients are asked to undergo diagnostic mammography.

Diagnostic mammography entails additional views including true lateral and tangential views and magnified and spot compression views that focus on the area of abnormality. Diagnostic mammography is also indicated to evaluate patients who present with signs and symptoms of breast problems.

When evaluating mammograms, it is important to compare current to old mammograms. Tissue density, calcifications, asymmetry, nodularity and architectural distortions should be noted **(Figure 20-1)**.

The American College of Radiology Imaging Network (ACRIN) and Digital Mammographic Imaging Screening Trial (DMIST) showed that the accuracy of digital mammography is equivalent to film screen mammography for the general screening population. Digital mammography detected significantly more cancer than film screen mammography in women less than age 50, pre- and perimenopausal women and women with dense breasts.

Ultrasound

Ultrasound is useful as a complementary diagnostic study to confirm size and position of any breast mass. It is useful in patients with dense breasts who present with palpable masses not visualized on mammography. Ultrasound characteristics suspicious for malignancy include lesions that are taller than wide, posterior acoustic shadowing and irregular or ill-defined borders. Ultrasound is also useful for evaluation of axillary lymph nodes (ALNs) prior to surgery. Metastatic ALNs appear abnormally rounded

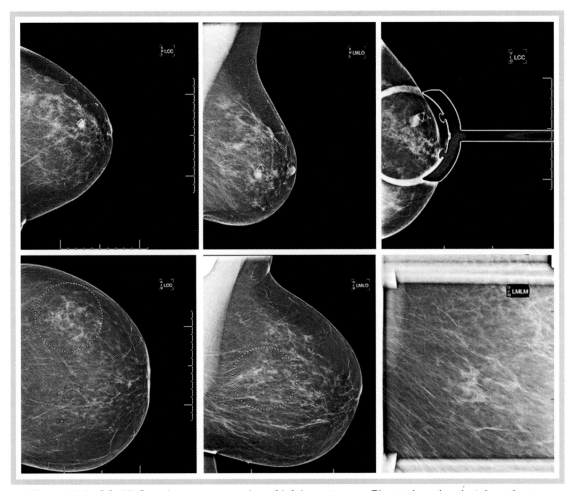

Figure 20-1: CC, MLO and spot compression of left breast mass. Biopsy: Invasive ductal carcinoma. CC, MLO and magnification of calcifications left breast. Biopsy: DCIS

with a thickened cortex and loss of normal fatty hilum **(Figure 20-2)**. Ultrasound-directed fine needle aspiration or core needle biopsy of abnormal LNs is useful to determine the approach for axillary staging.

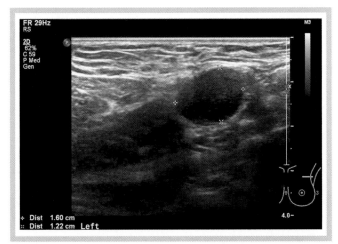

Figure 20-2: Ultrasound of axillary lymph node with thickened cortex and loss of fatty hilum

Magnetic Resonance Imaging (MRI)

Dynamic contrast-enhanced breast MRI is used with increasing frequency to locally stage primary breast cancer and assist with operative planning. Breast images are acquired before and after administration of intravenous gadolinium. Malignant lesions demonstrate rapid contrast enhancement due to neovascularity and abnormal permeability of neoplastic vessels **(Figure 20-3)**. Benign breast findings may also show enhancement and there can be considerable overlap in the pattern of enhancement between benign and malignant lesions. Therefore, biopsy of abnormal lesions detected by MRI is essential prior to surgical decision-making.

In patients with a diagnosis of breast cancer, MRI is used as a staging evaluation to define extent of cancer and presence of multifocal or multicentric cancer in the ipsilateral breast and as screening for contralateral breast cancer at time of initial diagnosis. One systematic review and meta-analysis showed MRI detected additional disease in 16% of women with breast cancer. Occult contralateral disease was found in 3% of women. MRI

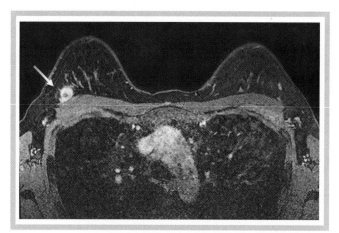

Figure 20-3: Breast MRI with enhancing mass UOQ right breast, marked by yellow arrow

findings altered surgical management from wide local excision to mastectomy in 8.1% patients and from wide local excision to more extensive surgery in 11.3% patients. There is limited data that the use of MRI to affect the choice of local therapy improves outcome in local recurrence or survival.

In patients who are being treated with neoadjuvant chemotherapy, MRI evaluation before and after treatment helps define the extent of disease prechemotherapy, the response to chemotherapy and the potential for breast-conserving surgery. MRI is also used to identify occult primary breast cancer in women who present with Paget's disease of the nipple or with biopsy-proven adenocarcinoma in the axilla who have normal mammogram, ultrasound and physical examination.

The use of MRI as an adjunct to mammography for screening is indicated in certain high risk women **(Table 20-2)**.

Management of Imaging Results

The BI-RADS classification is a standardized method of reporting final assessment of breast imaging findings. **Table 20-3** summarizes this classification.

For lesions that are categorized as BI-RADS 4 and 5, tissue biopsy should be performed. Appropriate

radiologic-pathologic correlation is indicated following percutaneous needle biopsy. Radiologic-pathologic discordance (e.g. a finding of benign histology with a category 5 lesion) mandates further evaluation. The options would be repeated imaging with additional percutaneous tissue sampling or surgical excision.

Tissue Biopsy

Tissue diagnosis is essential prior to surgical treatment to guide patient counseling and multimodality treatment planning. Tissue can be obtained by using percutaneous core needle biopsy (CNB), fine-needle aspiration (FNA) or wire-localized excisional biopsy.

CNB is the preferred approach because it is the least invasive method that will provide specimens suitable for histology and immunohistochemical receptor studies. It can be performed using 14-, 11- or 9-gauge needles under stereotactic, ultrasound or MRI guidance. Clip placement should be part of this procedure to mark the area of biopsy.

FNA requires cytopathology expertise that may not be available in every institution. The specimen obtained is inadequate to confirm invasion.

Wire-localized excisional biopsy as the initial method for tissue diagnosis should be reserved for lesions that are not amenable to percutaneous needle biopsy. These lesions include faint calcifications that are not well-visualized for stereotactic biopsy, lesions too close to the chest wall or nipple, or lesions in breasts that are too thin following compression for stereotactic biopsy. Wire-localized excisional biopsy is sometimes required following percutaneous biopsy if there is radiologic-pathologic discordance and if the results reveal high risk lesions (e.g. papilloma, AH, radial scar and LCIS).

Pathology and Histology

The identification of mammary stromal invasion differentiates in situ from invasive carcinoma. Invasive carcinoma has the potential to metastasize to regional LNs or to distant sites, most commonly bone, lung, liver and brain.

Standard pathology reporting for breast cancer tissue specimens should provide information on the histo-

TABLE 20-3	BI-RADS classification	
Category	**Description**	**Action**
0	Incomplete	Obtain additional imaging and/or prior imaging for comparison
1	No abnormality detected	Routine annual screening
2	Benign finding(s)	Annual screening
3	Probably benign finding	6-month follow-up for 1-2 years to document stability.
4	Suspicious abnormality	Biopsy should be considered
5	Highly suggestive of malignancy	Biopsy should be performed
6	Known biopsy-proven malignancy	Appropriate action should be taken

pathologic subtype and grade, tumor size, surgical margin status, lymphovascular space invasion, estrogen receptor (ER) and progesterone receptor (PR) status, HER2/neu status and LN status. At our institution, Ki-67 a proliferative indicator is also routinely reported. All these factors have important prognostic implications and also help guide treatment recommendations.

The Nottingham Grading system describes the histologic grade. It incorporates the degree of tubule formation, nuclear pleomorphism and mitotic count. The score ranges from 3 to 9, with 3-5 being low, 6-7 intermediate and 8-9 high grade.

Pathology report on nodal status should include the number of LNs harvested, the number of metastatic LNs, the size of metastatic deposit in the LN and the presence or absence of extracapsular extension.

At the time of detection, approximately 70-85% of breast cancers are invasive breast cancers while the rest are noninvasive breast cancers. Invasive ductal carcinoma nothing-otherwise-specified (NOS), accounts for 75% of all invasive breast cancer. Ten percent are invasive lobular carcinoma and the remainders are metaplastic carcinoma and special histologic variants of invasive carcinomas of ductal origin: tubular carcinoma, mucinous carcinoma, medullary carcinoma and papillary carcinoma. It is recognized that the histologic variants of invasive carcinoma have different metastatic potential, however, local and adjuvant therapy are not primarily influenced by histologic classification.

Patients with Paget's disease of the breast usually present with eczematous rash of the areola with bleeding, ulceration and /or itching of the nipple. This presentation is often confused with a dermatologic condition resulting in diagnostic delay. Histologically it is characterized by neoplastic cells in the epidermis of the nipple-areolar complex (NAC). Invasive and noninvasive breast cancer that is not necessarily adjacent to the NAC can be found in 80-90% of patients. Therefore, complete imaging workup to detect cancer should be performed in addition to a skin biopsy of the NAC. If cancer is found, breast-conserving therapy with NAC excision is an option if the cosmetic outcome is acceptable. If no breast lesion is found, excision of the NAC is still required.

Other less common types of cancer that may be found in the breast include lymphoma, sarcoma and metastatic.

Prognostic Factors

Adjuvant treatment decisions following surgery are strongly based on the individual prognostic discriminants of the primary breast cancer. Historically, in the absence of distant metastases, the most important prognostic factor is the LN status followed by tumor size. Other prognostic factors are the ER/PR status, HER2/neu status, age at diagnosis, histopathologic type and grade, proliferative rate and gene expression profile.

Prognosis is generally better for the special histologic types of invasive breast cancer compared to invasive ductal carcinoma NOS. Prognosis is worse with a higher histopathologic grade and when lymphovascular invasion is present.

Estrogen receptors are expressed by 70-80% of breast cancers and are more common in postmenopausal breast cancer. ER/PR expression is measured by semiquantitative immunohistochemical staining. Hormonal receptor expression is frequently associated with a better prognosis and predictive of response to endocrine therapy, although some controversies exist about the role of ER in prognosis, as the ER status appears to affect the timing but not the rate of recurrence. However, tumors that overexpress HER2/neu gene, which is identified in about 25% of all breast cancer, exhibit the opposite effect and are associated worse prognosis. HER2/neu status can be determined by immunohistochemistry or by fluorescence *in situ* hybridization (FISH). Immunohistochemistry detects the protein product. A score of 0 or 1+ is nonexpression; 2+ is indeterminate and 3+ is overexpression of the gene. When an indeterminate immunohistochemistry score is obtained, FISH for the amplified gene is performed. It is reported as a HER2 gene-chromosome 17 ratio. A ratio of < 1.8 is negative, a ratio of > 2.2 is amplification of the gene and 1.8-2.2 is borderline.

Staging of Disease

Breast cancer staging is based on the American Joint Committee on Cancer (AJCC) TNM classification system. This classification system includes the primary tumor characteristics (T), regional LN status (N) and distant metastases status (M). The sixth edition of the AJCC breast cancer-staging manual introduced substantial modifications to incorporate the detailed LN information obtained from sentinel LN staging (Table 20-4). Isolated tumor deposits identified with immunohistochemical stains for cytokeratin can be identified and remain of uncertain clinical significance. The current staging classification standardizes the reporting of these findings to permit prospective evaluation of the impact of isolated tumor cells on relapse-free and overall survival.

Management

The preoperative evaluation, neoadjuvant chemotherapy option and the specifics of surgical approach will be discussed in detail, followed by a stage-by-stage description of the management of breast cancer.

TABLE 20-4	TNM classification for breast cancer
Classification	**Definition**
Primary tumor (T)	
TX	Primary tumor cannot be assessed
T0	No evidence of primary tumor
Tis	Carcinoma in situ
Tis (DCIS)	Ductal carcinoma in situ
Tis (LCIS)	Lobular carcinoma in situ
Tis (Paget)	Paget disease of the nipple with no tumor (Paget disease associated with a tumor is classified according to the size of the tumor)
T1	Tumor $\leq$ 2 cm in greatest dimension
T1mic	Microinvasion $\leq$ 0.1 cm in greatest dimension
T1a	Tumor > 0.1 cm but $\leq$ 0.5 cm in greatest dimension
T1b	Tumor > 0.5 cm but $\leq$ 1 cm in greatest dimension
T1c	Tumor > 1 cm but $\leq$ 2 cm in greatest dimension
T2	Tumor > 2 cm but $\leq$ 5 cm in greatest dimension
T3	Tumor > 5 cm in greatest dimension
T4	Tumor of any size with direct extension to chest wall or skin, only as described below
T4a	Extension to chest wall, not including pectoralis muscle
T4b	Edema (including peau d'orange) or ulceration of the skin of the breast, or satellite skin nodules confined to the same breast
T4c	Both T4a and T4b
T4d	Inflammatory carcinoma
Regional lymph nodes (N)	
NX	Regional lymph nodes cannot be assessed (e.g. previously removed)
N0	No regional lymph node metastasis
N1	Metastasis in movable ipsilateral axillary lymph node(s)
N2	Metastases in ipsilateral axillary lymph nodes fixed or matted, or in clinically apparent ipsilateral internal mammary nodes in the absence of clinically evident axillary lymph-node metastasis
N2a	Metastasis in ipsilateral axillary lymph nodes fixed to one another (matted) or to other structures
N2b	Metastasis only in clinically apparent ipsilateral internal mammary nodes and in the absence of clinically evident axillary lymph-node metastasis
N3	Metastasis in ipsilateral infraclavicular lymph node(s), or in clinically apparent ipsilateral internal mammary lymph node(s) and in the presence of clinically evident axillary lymph-node metastasis; or metastasis in ipsilateral supraclavicular lymph node(s) with or without axillary or internal mammary lymph-node involvement
N3a	Metastasis in ipsilateral infraclavicular lymph node(s) and axillary lymph node(s)
N3b	Metastasis in ipsilateral internal mammary lymph node(s) and axillary lymph node(s)
N3c	Metastasis in ipsilateral supraclavicular lymph node(s)
Regional lymph nodes (pN)	
pNX	Regional lymph nodes cannot be assessed (e.g. previously removed or not removed for pathologic study)
pN0	No regional lymph node metastasis histologically, no additional examination for isolated tumor cells
pN0(i-)	No regional lymph node metastasis histologically, negative immunohistochemical staining
pN0(i+)	Isolated tumor cells identified histologically or by positive immunohistochemical staining, no cluster > 0.2 mm
pN0 (mol-)	No regional lymph-node metastasis histologically, negative molecular findings (RT-PCR)

Contd...

Contd...

Classification	Definition
pN0 (mol+)	No regional lymph-node metastasis histologically, positive molecular findings (RT-PCR)
pN1	Metastasis in one to three axillary lymph nodes and /or in internal mammary nodes with microscopic disease detected by sentinel lymph node dissection but not clinically apparent
pN1mi	Micrometastasis (> 0.2 mm, none > 2.0 mm)
pN1a	Metastasis in one to three axillary lymph nodes
pN1b	Metastasis in internal mammary nodes with microscopic disease detected by sentinel lymph-node dissection but not clinically apparent
pN1c	Metastasis in one to three axillary lymph nodes and in internal mammary lymph nodes with microscopic disease detected by sentinel lymph-node dissection but not clinically apparent
pN2a	Metastasis in four to nine axillary lymph nodes (at least one tumor deposit > 2.0 mm)
pN2b	Metastasis in clinically apparent internal mammary lymph nodes in the absence of axillary lymph-node metastasis
pN3	Metastasis in 10 or more axillary lymph nodes, or in infraclavicular lymph nodes, or in clinically apparent ipsilateral internal mammary lymph nodes in the presence of one or more positive axillary lymph nodes; or in more than three axillary lymph nodes with clinically negative microscopic metastasis in internal mammary lymph nodes; or in ipsilateral supraclavicular lymph nodes
pN3a	Metastasis in 10 or more axillary lymph nodes (at least one tumor deposit > 2.0 mm), or metastasis to the infraclavicular lymph nodes
pN3b	Metastasis in clinically apparent ipsilateral internal mammary lymph nodes in the presence of one or more positive axillary lymph nodes; or in more than three axillary lymph nodes and in internal mammary lymph nodes with microscopic disease detected by sentinel lymph-node dissection but not clinically apparent
pN3c	Metastasis in ipsilateral supraclavicular lymph nodes
Distant metastasis (M)	
MX	Distant metastasis cannot be assessed
M0	No distant metastasis
M1	Distant metastasis

Adapted with permission from the AJCC Cancer Staging Manual, 6th Edition"

Preoperative Evaluation of the Patient

Evaluation of a patient with breast cancer should include an assessment of breast cancer risk factors, a history of the presentation of disease and a review of systems to detect possibility of distant metastases. A detailed gynecological history, medical history, previous breast procedures, family history and medications should be obtained. Based on identified risk factors, if there is a suspicion for hereditary breast cancer, genetic counseling is indicated.

Diagnostic breast imaging should be reviewed in each case. Extent of disease is evaluated to determine the candidacy for breast-conserving therapy. Attention should be given to the contralateral breast to rule out synchronous disease. Additional studies are ordered as indicated. The pathology results including ER/PR status and HER2/neu status should also be reviewed as this might influence neoadjuvant chemotherapy recommendations.

Comprehensive breast examination starts with the patient in an upright position. The patient is examined with arms at her side and raised above her head. Both breasts are inspected for symmetry, skin changes (e.g. indentation, thickening, edema and peau d'orange appearance) and nipple changes (e.g. retraction, eczema and discharge). Skin indentation is caused by tethering of skin to the breast by Cooper's ligaments. Breast edema, skin thickening and peau d'orange are caused by lymphatic obstruction by the tumor. Palpation of the breast parenchyma is then performed with patient in upright and supine position with her arms raised above her head. The breast parenchyma is palpated in a systematic fashion to include each quadrant, the subareolar tissue and the axillary tail. Masses are evaluated for location, size, shape, consistency and mobility. Examination of the LNs includes the supraclavicular, infraclavicular and axillary nodal regions. The lymph nodes are characterized in terms of number, size, mobility and whether they are matted.

In general, staging for metastatic disease in patients presenting with Stages I and II breast cancer is guided by the presence of symptoms or findings on physical examination suggestive of metastatic disease. Routine CT scans of the chest, abdomen and pelvis and bone scan is indicated in patients who present with Stage III disease.

Neoadjuvant Therapy

Neoadjuvant chemotherapy (NACtx) is indicated in patients who present with inoperable locally advanced breast cancer (LABC) and inflammatory breast cancer. It is increasingly used for patients with operable disease who have unfavorable tumor:breast size ratio to convert a mastectomy-only option to a breast-conserving surgery (BCS) option following response to NACtx. Administration of chemotherapy prior to surgery also provides important information about *in vivo* response of the tumor to the agents utilized and treats potential systemic disease without delay.

NSABP B-18 compared disease-free and overall survival among patients with operable breast cancer randomly assigned to four cycles of preoperative adriamycin/cyclophosphamide (AC) versus postoperative AC. The trial demonstrated that NACtx is equivalent to adjuvant chemotherapy in terms of disease-specific and overall survival. NSABP B-27 showed a higher rate of complete pathological response in patients treated with preoperative AC followed by docetaxel compared to AC alone. High-grade, ER-negative cancers with high proliferative rates are more likely to have a complete pathologic response than low-grade ER-positive cancer. Although tumor response to NACtx is high for ER-negative cancers, disease-free survival is significantly higher in ER-positive disease.

Chemotherapy regimens that are used in the adjuvant setting can be used in the neoadjuvant setting. Tumors that overexpress HER2/neu should also be treated with trastuzumab. However, due to the cardiotoxicity of trastuzumab and anthracycline agents, trastuzumab is commonly given with docetaxel and cisplatin.

Prior to initiating NACtx, pretreatment tumor size and extent should be documented by clinical exam and breast imaging including mammography and breast MRI. Intralesional clip placement is essential in the event there is complete clinical response. Close follow-up during therapy by the medical and surgical oncologist is essential. If there is minimal response or disease progression after several cycles of NACtx, an alternative regimen should be considered followed by local therapy.

Follow-up with the surgeon mid-chemotherapy is recommended for evaluation of clinical response and to discuss surgical treatment plan. Following completion of chemotherapy, repeat breast imaging is performed to assess radiographic response and finalize surgical management. Surgery can be performed safely 3-4 weeks

after the last chemotherapy cycle provided absolute neutrophil count is > 1500 and platelet count is > 100,000. Tumors that respond well to NACtx can potentially be treated with BCS if the criteria for this procedure are met.

Axillary staging in patients receiving NACtx is controversial. ALNs should be evaluated by clinical examination and ultrasound at the time of initial diagnosis. In the circumstance where the axilla is clinically negative prior to initiating NACtx, there are differences of opinion on the timing of axillary staging. One option is to perform a sentinel lymph node dissection (SLND) prior to NACtx to enable treatment based on the stage at presentation. The second option is to perform SLND after NACtx to provide post-therapy prognostic information and potentially spare some women with microscopic nodal involvement the need for axillary lymph node dissection (ALND). For patients with ALN metastases at presentation, ALND post-chemotherapy is appropriate for axillary staging. However, approximately 30% of patients with positive ALN(s) will be downstaged to node-negative disease at completion of NACtx. No consensus exists on how to manage node-positive patients who have a complete clinical response and convert to clinically node-negativity after NACtx. In selected cases post-chemotherapy SLN staging may be appropriate. Retrospective single-institution studies report a false-negative rate of 11% for SLND following NACtx. In the absence of prospective clinical trial data, the decision to utilize SLND for staging post-NACtx should be made after review of the tumor response and shared decision-making with the patient.

Neoadjuvant therapy can also be in the form of endocrine therapy in postmenopausal women with ER-positive breast cancer. Two randomized trials have proven that neoadjuvant anastrozole or letrozole result in higher rates of BCS compared to tamoxifen.

Surgical Approach

Surgical Procedure Selection

When counseling a woman regarding options for surgical treatment for breast cancer, several factors need to be taken into consideration. The tumor:breast size ratio and the type of breast cancer may preclude BCS. LN status should be evaluated to decide whether to proceed with SLND or ALND. Importantly, the patient's treatment preference should be taken into account.

Randomized clinical trials with up to 20 years of follow-up have shown that for early stage breast cancer, overall survival is equivalent for total mastectomy (TM) and breast-conserving therapy (BCT), which comprises wide local excision (WLE) followed by whole breast irradiation (WBI). NSABP B-06 was a landmark randomized prospective clinical trial to compare WLE+ALND with or without WBI and TM+ALND. The trial began in 1976 and women with tumors up to 4 cm were eligible to participate. Twenty-year rate of ipsilateral tumor recurrence was 39% in patients who did not receive WBI versus 14% in the radiated arm. No significant differences were observed in rates of distant metastasis or overall survival. NSABP B-21 built upon the findings of B-06. One thousand and nine (1009) women with node-negative invasive breast cancer that were ≤ 1 cm underwent WLE+ALND. They were then randomly assigned to tamoxifen, radiation, or radiation and tamoxifen. The 8-year cumulative ipsilateral breast tumor recurrence was 16.5%, 9.3% and 2.8% respectively for the three arms. These findings were confirmed by additional European trials establishing the safety and efficacy of BCT for early stage breast cancer. Compared to TM, BCT is associated with a higher ipsilateral breast recurrence rate but has equivalent survival rates. Therefore, for women with stage I or II breast cancer who desire breast conservation, BCT is an appropriate form of local control as long as free margins and acceptable cosmetic results are attainable.

Breast-Conserving Surgery

Breast-conserving surgery is also known as wide local excision, lumpectomy, segmental mastectomy, or partial mastectomy. It is imperative that margins of all BCS specimens be evaluated. This requires orientation of the specimen by the surgeon and description of the margin status by the pathologist. There is no standard definition for what constitutes a negative surgical margin. In general, invasive cancer less than 2 mm from the inked specimen edge is considered a close margin. Patients with close or positive surgical margins are advised to have additional surgery to exclude residual disease. Most patients can be managed with re-excision to achieve clear margins. Mastectomy may be indicated if margins remain positive after re-excision, if there are multiple positive margins, or if re-excision will not allow an acceptable cosmetic outcome.

BCS must be followed by WBI to decrease the risk of local recurrence. For breast cancers that are detected by mammographic calcifications or are associated with extensive ductal carcinoma in situ (DCIS), postexcision mammogram is obtained to document complete excision of all calcifications prior to initiating radiation therapy. BCS is not recommended in patients who have contraindications to radiation, multicentric breast cancer, large tumor:breast size ratio that will result in an unacceptable cosmetic outcome, in general tumors ≥ 5 cm, inflammatory breast cancer, inoperable LABC and ipsilateral recurrence in patient who previously had BCT.

Mastectomy

Earlier detection of breast cancer and the use of neoadjuvant therapy have enabled more women to undergo breast conservation. Total mastectomy (TM), which involves removing the entire breast tissue and NAC, remains an alternative to BCT for surgical management of invasive carcinoma. Mastectomy is indicated in patients with large tumors that are poorly responsive to systemic therapy, inflammatory carcinomas and inoperable stage III breast cancer following neoadjuvant chemotherapy, tumors associated with extensive malignant microcalcifications not amenable to surgical excision with an acceptable cosmetic deformity, failure to achieve negative resection margins after attempts at breast conservation and patients who have contraindications to radiation therapy. Patients recommended to undergo mastectomy must be informed about their options for breast reconstruction.

When reconstruction is desired, a decision must be made regarding the possibility of immediate versus delayed reconstruction (see Breast Reconstruction section). If immediate reconstruction is planned, a skin-sparing mastectomy (SSM) is performed. This form of mastectomy preserves the natural skin envelope which provides a template for reconstructing a breast that has a more natural contour with remarkable symmetry to the normal contralateral breast. Rates of locoregional recurrence following SSM are comparable to TM.

Modified radical mastectomy (MRM) removes the entire breast tissue, NAC and ipsilateral axillary contents *en bloc*. It is indicated in patients who have pathologically involved ALNs.

Nipple-sparing mastectomy preserves the NAC and is gaining in popularity. Selection criteria and long-term outcomes for these procedures are emerging.

Axillary Staging

NSABP B-04 compared radical mastectomy to TM with or without axillary radiation. The results showed that axillary recurrence was 1% in patients with ALND compared to 18% in patients without ALND. Radiation to the axilla was less effective than ALND in preventing recurrence. However, there was no difference in survival. In the patients who had ALND, 40% with clinically negative axilla had positive LNs.

Although axillary clearance has not been associated with a survival benefit, ALN status remains the most important prognostic factor in breast cancer and is important for local control.

ALND has been the standard procedure for axillary staging until the late 20th century when the SLN mapping and biopsy was introduced. Randomized clinical trials have shown that this procedure is associated with less morbidity and is an accurate reflection of the axillary LN status. It is now the preferred method for axillary staging in patients presenting with a clinically negative axilla.

Sentinel Lymph Node Mapping and Biopsy

The SLN(s) represent(s) the first node(s) to receive lymphatic drainage from the breast. The SLN accurately reflects the status of the axilla with a false-negative rate of < 10%. Patients with a negative SLN can be spared complete ALND with its attendant morbidities.

SLND is an appropriate form of axillary staging in clinically node-negative breast cancer. This procedure should also be performed in patients undergoing TM for DCIS or extensive local resections in the upper outer quadrant of the breast. Surgery in the upper outer quadrant divides lymphatic channels to the axilla and could preclude an SLND in the event invasive cancer is found on final pathology. Contraindications for this procedure are clinically node-positive patients, previous ALND and inflammatory breast cancer. This procedure is feasible in patients with multifocal or multicentric disease, prior breast surgery, previous minor axillary surgery and following NACtx.

Pathological assessment of SLNs can be performed intraoperatively by frozen section or touch preparation cytology. At our institution, intraoperative assessment is performed only if the suspicion for metastases is high based on tumor characteristics, or with identification of an enlarged firm SLN. Final pathological analysis is by multilevel node sectioning and hematoxylin-eosin stain. The role of routine immunohistochemistry analysis of SLNs is still not defined.

Patients who have SLN metastases are recommended to have completion level I and II axillary lymph node dissection. Approximately 50% of patients will have no additional metastases identified in the remaining axillary nodes (non-SLN) following ALND. Intense efforts have been applied to identify factors that predict non-SLN metastases. In general, the risk of non-SLN metastases increases with the primary tumor size, SLN metastasis size and the number of positive SLN. A web-based nomogram developed at Memorial Sloan Kettering Cancer Center is available at **www.mskcc.org/mskcc/html/15938.cfm** to provide an estimate of the probability of non-SLN metastasis. The predicted probability of additional positive nodes can be used to guide discussions regarding further axillary surgery or alternatives such as axillary radiation or observation. No cohort of SLN-positive patients has been identified where the risk of non-SLN involvement is < 5%.

A learning curve is associated with performing SLND. The American Society of Breast Surgeons guidelines for performing SLND recommend surgeons should perform twenty SLND procedures validated by an ALND (or mentored by an experienced colleague) before performing SLND alone.

Axillary Node Dissection (Figure 20-4)

The ALNs are divided into three levels. Levels I, II and III are the nodes located lateral, deep and medial to the pectoralis minor muscle respectively. Levels I and II ALND are indicated when patients present with pathologically positive LNs, if SLN mapping fails to identify the SLN and following positive SLN findings. Removal of level III ALN provides little further benefit as only 1-3% of stage I and II patients have level III involvement in the absence of level I or II disease.

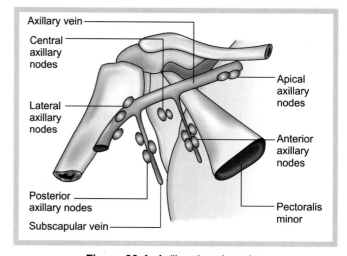

Figure 20-4: Axillary lymph nodes

Breast Reconstruction

Mastectomy is a figure-deforming procedure with potential psychosocial effects on patients, including their body image, ability to maintain pre-existing relationships and ability to form new relationships. Therefore, it is extremely important for all women undergoing mastectomy to be informed of their options for breast reconstruction, which include autologous tissue, synthetic implants or a combination of both. The timing and type of breast reconstruction are influenced by patient's preference, patient's comorbidities, previous surgeries, smoking history and their need for postmastectomy radiation therapy (PMRT). Regardless of the type of reconstruction, patients must be counseled that secondary procedures are required for revisions, nipple reconstruction and tattooing of the NAC. When immediate reconstruction is planned, SSM is preferred to preserve the skin envelope and provide a superior cosmetic outcome.

Implant-based reconstruction involves placement of a tissue expander under the pectoralis major muscle. The expander is gradually expanded over time to the desired size before being replaced by a permanent implant. Implant-alone reconstruction is contraindicated in previously irradiated breast due to a high incidence of complications. In such circumstances, it can be combined with autologous tissue, commonly a latissimus dorsi flap. Implant-alone reconstruction does not involve donor site morbidity and has a faster recovery than autologous tissue reconstruction. Complications associated with implant-based reconstruction include capsular contracture, implant malposition, rupture, infection and extrusion.

There are a number of donor sites that provide combinations of skin, muscle and fat that can be used for autologous tissue reconstruction. The transverse abdominis muscle (TRAM) flap is one of the most common flaps used. It can be performed as a pedicle or free flap. The deep inferior epigastric perforator (DIEP) flap is a muscle-sparing variation of the TRAM flap that decreases the morbidity of decreased abdominal wall strength. The latissimus dorsi muscle flap as mentioned is an option that is usually used in combination with an implant. It is a good option for patients who do not have adequate abdominal adipose tissue. The gluteal artery flap is another option for patients without adequate abdominal adipose tissue who prefer autologous tissue reconstruction.

When PMRT is indicated, immediate reconstruction is generally not recommended. The long-term cosmetic and functional outcome for the reconstructed breast following radiation is generally inferior to the non-radiated reconstruction. Although autologous tissue flaps may tolerate radiation therapy better than implant-based reconstructions, achieving good symmetry and minimizing fibrosis in the reconstruction cannot be guaranteed. There is increasing interest in the delayed-immediate reconstruction strategy which involves placement of a tissue-expander at the time of mastectomy as a temporizing measure. Once the final pathology results are available, a determination can be made as to the indications for PMRT. Patients who do not require radiation can proceed with implant-based or autologous tissue reconstruction. If radiation is recommended, the tissue expander can be removed or left in place throughout treatment. Once radiation is complete, a decision regarding the most suitable reconstruction can be made.

Management by Stage of Breast Carcinoma

Early Stage (Stage I or II: T1/2 + N0/1)

About 75% of breast cancers are detected early with tumors < 5 cm and without clinical findings of matted nodes. As previously discussed, local control of breast cancer by BCT is equivalent to TM in terms of overall breast cancer survival. Evaluation of the ALN status by SLND is preferred provided patient has a clinically-negative axilla and the surgical team has the appropriate experience in performing the procedure. ALND is indicated in clinically node-positive patients, patients who have metastases in the SLNs, or patients in whom the SLN identification was unsuccessful.

Locally Advanced (Stage III: T3 + N1/2/3; T4 + any N; any T + N2/3)

About 10% of patients present with tumors ≥ 5 cm, tumors fixed to the chest wall or with fixed axillary lymphadenopathy and are considered to have locally advanced breast cancer (LABC). Patients judged inoperable at diagnosis require neoadjuvant therapy before operative intervention. The success of BCT in this population is not established although it could be entertained in patients who experience complete clinical and radiographic response to chemotherapy. Most patients who present with LABC will ultimately require a mastectomy for definitive surgical management. The decision for postmastectomy radiation therapy (PMRT) is based on disease stage at presentation. For this reason, patients with LABC who undergo mastectomy are advised to delay breast reconstruction. Management of the axilla is as for early stage disease.

Inflammatory Breast Cancer

Inflammatory breast cancer comprises 1-5% of all breast cancers. It is a clinical diagnosis characterized by an erythematous, warm and enlarged breast with thickened skin and *peau d'orange* appearance. There is often no discrete palpable mass. Symptoms usually have a rapid onset and can often be mistaken for an infectious process, resulting in a delay in diagnosis and treatment. This clinical presentation is due to the presence of tumor in the dermal lymphatic system and/or the result of significant lymphatic obstruction in the breast from tumor or ALN involvement. Skin biopsy may demonstrate tumor emboli in the subdermal lymphatics. However, a negative skin biopsy does not negate the diagnosis of inflammatory cancer.

Inflammatory cancer is judged inoperable at diagnosis due to the extensive skin involvement with tumor and these patients are initially managed with NACtx. Patients who have disease progression while on chemotherapy should receive preoperative radiation therapy. For patients who have poor response on chemotherapy, a second chemotherapy regimen should be considered.

The vast majority of cases will have resolution of the underlying skin changes although there may be residual microscopic or macroscopic disease in the breast. Due to the extensive skin involvement at presentation, MRM is the recommended surgical management. These patients are advised to forego immediate breast reconstruction because PMRT is necessary to minimize locoregional recurrence risk.

Axillary Metastasis

Patients who present with axillary lymphadenopathy and occult breast cancer make up 3-5% of all breast cancer cases. These patients should undergo standard breast imaging including diagnostic mammography and breast ultrasound. MRI will identify a primary breast lesion in 70% of these patients. When a primary lesion is not identified, treatment should include ALND. WBI is recommended as local failures are reported in the absence of breast treatment. Mastectomy is not mandatory, but a reasonable alternative to WBI.

Special Situations

Invasive Breast Cancer during Pregnancy

Breast cancer is detected during pregnancy in 1.2/10,000 live births. This makes up 2.8% of all breast cancers. Diagnosis of breast cancer during pregnancy is often delayed due to glandular changes in the breast and the low level of suspicion for breast cancer in the younger population.

If breast cancer is suspected, mammography with shielding of the gravid uterus can be performed safely. Ultrasound can be performed to supplement the imaging work-up.

When breast cancer diagnosis is confirmed, consultation with maternal-fetal medicine must be obtained to document fetal development and age. Knowledge of the estimated date of delivery is important to aid surgical and chemotherapy planning.

Cancer detected during the first trimester is best treated with TM as radiation is contraindicated at anytime during pregnancy. BCS is possible for cancers diagnosed during the third trimester as radiation therapy can be administered after delivery. Cancers diagnosed after the first trimester, when fetal organogenesis is complete, can be treated with chemotherapy if this modality will be part of the postsurgical therapy. This will allow surgery to be delayed until the third trimester or after delivery and may make BCS feasible.

Axillary staging can be achieved with SLND using ^{99m}Tc-sulfur colloid injection. The estimated fetal dose from the radioactive substance is ≤ 0.014 mGy and this level is far less than the limit for pregnant women as determined by the National Council on Radiation Protection and Measurements. Isosulfan blue dye is contraindicated due to the potential harm to the fetus from an allergic/anaphylactic reaction.

The criteria for systemic chemotherapy in pregnant women are the same as in non-pregnant women. Chemotherapy cannot safely be administered during the first trimester, as fetal malformation risk is high. It can safely be given in the second and third trimester but should be stopped after the 35th week or within 3 weeks

of planned delivery. Anthracycline-based regimens are preferred. There are very limited data on the safety of taxanes or trastuzumab in pregnancy. Endocrine therapy and radiation therapy must not be given during pregnancy.

Pregnant patients who undergo TM and wish to have breast reconstruction are advised to delay reconstruction until pregnancy-related breast changes resolve to allow symmetry to be achieved to the contralateral breast.

Male Breast Cancer

The incidence of male breast cancer is 1% of all breast cancers. It is higher in BRCA2 mutation carriers. Breast cancers in men typically present as palpable lumps as men are not routinely screened for disease. Evaluation should include diagnostic mammography and ultrasound. The staging work-up is the same as for female patients. Genetic testing should be performed. The standard surgical treatment is TM with SLND if clinically node-negative. Radiation and chemotherapy indications are the same as for female patients. Stage for stage, the prognosis for breast cancer in men is the same when compared to women.

Anatomic and Technical Considerations

Breast-Conserving Surgery (Lumpectomy/ Segmental Mastectomy/Partial Mastectomy)

Breast-conserving surgery (BCS) entails wide local excision of breast cancer that includes the tumor and a margin of surrounding normal breast tissue. Lesions that are nonpalpable require wire-localization under mammography- or ultrasound-guidance to accurately localize the area of excision. Intraoperative ultrasound can be used to localize nonpalpable masses and facilitate incision placement. This procedure is favored as it avoids the need for preoperative wire-localization and is associated with higher rates of negative margins on initial excision. In most cases, the incision should be made directly above the lesion. In the superior hemisphere of the breast, incisions along the lines of resting skin tension should be made. In the inferior hemisphere of the breast, radial incisions should be made to avoid displacement of the nipple-areolar complex **(Figure 20-5)**. The success of BCS is dependent on the ability to obtain histologically negative margins. Intraoperative orientation of the specimen is performed to guide pathological analysis of margins. At our institution, specimen radiograph is obtained in anterior-posterior and medial-lateral views to confirm the lesion and biopsy clip are within the specimen and to help determine whether the margins are clear of the mass or calcifications. Specimen ultrasound is an alternative tool to assess margins for mass lesions. Irrigation of the wound bed is performed. Wound closure is performed in two layers, an intradermal layer of interrupted 3-0 absorbable

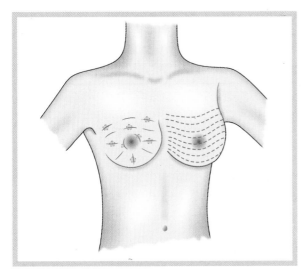

Figure 20-5: Skin incisions for breast-conserving surgery

suture, followed by a subcuticular layer of running 4-0 absorbable suture.

Simple/Total Mastectomy

Simple or total mastectomy (TM) removes the entire breast glandular tissue and NAC. An elliptical incision is made to encompass the NAC which is removed with the specimen. The extent of the ellipse should leave skin flaps that will lay flat against the chest wall without folds. Skin flaps are raised superiorly and inferiorly. Care must be taken to preserve the inframammary crease. The boundaries of resection are the clavicle superiorly, the external oblique muscle inferiorly, the lateral border of the sternum medially and the latissimus dorsi muscle laterally. The breast tissue is then excised from the pectoralis major muscle taking the pectoralis fascia with the specimen. Laterally, the dissection stops at the clavipectoral fascia to preserve the axillary contents. The axillary tail is marked for orientation. A drainage catheter is placed in the wound bed to prevent seroma formation. The skin is closed in two layers as for BCS. Patients are admitted overnight. They receive instructions for postoperative physical therapy **(Figure 20-6)**.

Modified Radical Mastectomy

Modified radical mastectomy (MRM) is the removal of the breast tissue, NAC and axillary contents *en bloc* . It is performed in patients who have pathologically involved ALNs. Levels one and two ALNs are removed, preserving the level three ALNs.

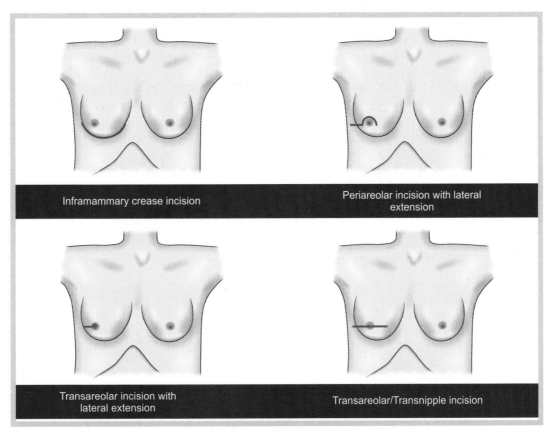

Inframammary crease incision

Periareolar incision with lateral extension

Transareolar incision with lateral extension

Transareolar/Transnipple incision

Figure 20-6: Mastectomy incisions

Skin-Sparing Mastectomy and Nipple-Sparing Mastectomy

Skin Sparing Mastectomy

Skin-sparing mastectomy (SSM) is performed when breast reconstruction is planned immediately following a mastectomy. The boundaries of dissection are identical to those for a TM and the NAC is also sacrificed. However, dissection is performed through a periareolar incision to preserve the natural skin envelope and inframammary crease. This dissection is technically more challenging as the periareolar incision is relatively smaller than the traditional elliptical incision. In rare circumstances, a clear plane of dissection cannot be developed due to the presence of cancer in the most anterior breast tissue and skin excision overlying the breast parenchyma is necessary. SLND can be performed via the periareolar incision or, if necessary, via a separate axillary incision.

Nipple-sparing mastectomy is gaining acceptance for the management of breast cancer and in the prophylactic setting despite the absence of prospective trials to evaluate efficacy. A retrospective review from M.D. Anderson on the incidence of occult NAC involvement in patients undergoing SSM found occult tumor in 5-6% of specimens. Occult NAC involvement was more common in patients with multicentric disease, centrally located tumors and with extensive DCIS. Nipple-sparing mastectomy is technically more demanding than conventional SSM due to the need to preserve blood supply to the NAC. In carefully selected patients with early stage breast cancer who desire mastectomy NAC can be considered **(Figure 20-7)**.

Oncoplastic Surgery

Oncoplastic breast-conserving surgery refers to local tissue rearrangement following wide segmental excision of breast cancer to improve cosmetic outcome. As an alternative to mastectomy, large volume full thickness segmental excisions combined with local breast flap advancement can increase the options for breast conservation in patients with extensive segmental breast cancer. These procedures include use of a parallelogram skin incision, batwing mastopexy, donut mastopexy and reduction mastopexy methods. Preoperative consultation with radiology to plan tumor localization with multiple localizing wires for extensive areas of calcification will increase the chances for negative surgical margins. Patients benefit from consultation with plastic surgery to discuss contralateral symmetry procedures. It is advisable to await final pathology results to determine margin status before proceeding with any contralateral procedures. Positive resection margins following large-volume oncoplastic resection are generally an indication for mastectomy.

Surgical Staging of the Axilla

Sentinel Lymph Node Mapping and Biopsy

Sentinel lymph node mapping is achieved by injection of radiolabeled tracer and/or vital blue dye into the breast prior to the planned procedure. The dual technique of radioisotope and blue dye yields the highest SLN localization rates with the fewest false-negative SLNs. The patient receives an injection of ^{99m}Tc-sulfur colloid into the breast prior to surgery. Isosulfan blue dye (Lymphazurin 1%, US Surgical Corp, Norwalk, CT) is injected intraoperatively. At our institution, injection is performed at the subareolar location and we do not routinely obtain preoperative lymphoscintigrams. Dilute methylene blue can be used as an alternative to isosulfan blue. Intradermal injections of methylene blue are to be avoided due to the risk of skin necrosis. At our institution, a 1.25 mg/ml dilution is injected in the subareolar tissue. The SLN can be localized with a hand-held gamma probe and with direct visualization of blue-stained lymphatics or node(s). Assessment of the axillary bed by digital examination for enlarged, firm nodes is also performed. If performed during BCS, a separate small incision is made in the inferior axillary hairline. If performed during TM, the procedure can be performed through the lateral portion of the mastectomy incision. An average of 2-3 SLNs is found. If SLN mapping fails to identify an SLN, the surgeon should proceed with an ALND.

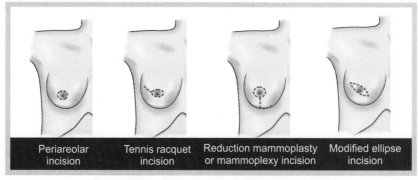

| Periareolar incision | Tennis racquet incision | Reduction mammoplasty or mammoplexy incision | Modified ellipse incision |

Figure 20-7: Skin sparing mastectomy incisions

Axillary Lymph Node Dissection

As mentioned previously levels I and II ALND are standard for adequate staging of breast cancer. Recommendations for incision placement are as for SLND. The area of dissection is an inverted triangle with the axillary vein superiorly, the latissimus dorsi muscle laterally and the chest wall medially. Several important structures must be identified during this procedure. The medial pectoral neurovascular bundle must be identified as it emerges between the pectoralis major and minor muscles. The axillary vein must be identified superiorly and the dissection should not exceed this boundary to avoid brachial plexus injury. The thoracodorsal nerve is always accompanied by its vascular bundle that originates from the axillary vein and artery. At the same level as the thoracodorsal nerve, the long thoracic nerve is found on the chest wall. Injury to the thoracodorsal nerve will cause weakness of the latissimus dorsi muscle and interfere with arm abduction. Injury of the long thoracic nerve will cause winging of the scapula. Intercostobrachial nerves are sometimes divided during surgery causing medial arm numbness. Other possible complications include axillary vein injury or thrombosis.

Adjuvant Chemotherapy

The goal of administering adjuvant chemotherapy is to treat occult micrometastatic disease to prevent future overt clinical presentation.

Decisions for systemic therapy are based on prognostic and predictive factors including age, LN status, tumor size and grade, ER/PR status and HER2/neu status. Patients with ≥ 10% risk of systemic relapse are recommended to receive adjuvant treatment. Therefore, adjuvant chemotherapy is offered to the majority of patients with invasive breast cancer except for those with the most favorable disease (node-negative and < 1 cm tumor). Another group of patients whom chemotherapy may not be indicated are those over 70 years and those with comorbid conditions. In this group of patients, the decision to treat with chemotherapy should be individualized.

Based on evidence from randomized clinical trials, patients with node-positive breast cancer benefit from receiving adjuvant chemotherapy even in the setting of ER-positive disease. The clinical challenge is to identify patients with the highest risk of relapse who have the most benefit. Several risk assessment tools are now available to the clinician to aid in the decision-making for chemotherapy.

Gene-expression profiling has demonstrated that differential expression of certain genes is a more powerful prognostic indicator than traditional factors such as tumor size and LN status. There are two FDA-approved gene assays that can stratify patients at different risk levels for relapse. Oncotype DX (Genomic Health, Redwood City, California) is a 21-gene assay using reverse transcription polymerase chain reaction technique on RNA isolated from paraffin-embedded breast cancer tissue. It has been validated to accurately predict risk of relapse as well as response to chemotherapy and endocrine therapy in ER/PR-positive, node-negative invasive breast cancer. It is reported as a continuous score called the Recurrence Score. A score of < 18 is low, 18-30 is intermediate and > 30 is high risk. There is also data to indicate that this assay can be used reliably in postmenopausal node-positive patients. MammaPrint is a microarray test that analyzes 70 genes from DNA extracted from fresh frozen breast tumor tissue. It is also used in early stage node-negative breast cancer patients. The need for fresh frozen tumor tissue limits the use of this assay.

Adjuvant! Online (**www.adjuvantonline.com**) is a computer-based algorithm that incorporates clinical and pathological prognostic factors (e.g. patient age, comorbidities, tumor size, tumor grade, number of involved axillary lymph nodes etc.). It has been validated to accurately estimate the absolute and relative 10-year disease-free and overall survival with or without chemotherapy. It does not take into consideration HER2/neu status.

Combination chemotherapy regimens are more effective than single agent regimens in treating breast cancer. The Early Breast Cancer Trialists' Collaborative Group reported in their 2005 overview analysis that anthracycline-based polychemotherapy results in a reduction in the risk of death of 38% for patients < 50 years old and 20% in the 50-69 year-old age group. These reductions are independent of the use of endocrine therapy (tamoxifen), ER status, nodal status, or other tumor characteristics.

Endocrine Therapy

For years, tamoxifen was the endocrine therapy of choice for patients with ER-positive invasive breast cancer to reduce ipsilateral recurrence, contralateral breast cancer and distant metastases.

Recently, the aromatase inhibitor (AI) alone or as a sequential therapy following tamoxifen have been shown to be superior to tamoxifen in disease-free survival and in reducing the number of contralateral breast cancer events in postmenopausal women. AIs block the peripheral conversion of estrogen precursors from the adrenal glands to estrogen but do not block ovarian estrogen production. Therefore, they are only effective in post-menopausal women. The three commonly used AIs are anastrozole and letrozole which are nonsteroidal AIs and exemestane, a steroidal AI. All three are equivalent in efficacy and side effect profile.

Tamoxifen is a selective estrogen receptor modulator. Tamoxifen use for five years has been shown to reduce breast cancer recurrence by 47% and reduce the risk of death by 26% regardless of age or menopausal status. The Early Breast Cancer Trialists' Collaborative Group overview analysis showed that, for ER-positive patients, the use of tamoxifen for five years reduced the annual recurrence rate by 39% and the annual breast cancer death rate by 31%. These findings were independent of age, menopausal status, use of chemotherapy, PR status or axillary LN status. Five years of tamoxifen is superior to two years and the survival benefit persists after treatment is discontinued. This overview underscores the importance of systemic endocrine therapy in the multimodality approach to breast cancer treatment.

All patients with ER/PR-positive cancer should be considered for adjuvant endocrine therapy. Premenopausal women should receive tamoxifen. If menopausal status is confirmed, the patient should be switched over to an AI. In postmenopausal women, the firstline therapy should be an AI alone or sequentially with tamoxifen. Tamoxifen can be given to patients who decline or have intolerable side effects from AIs. Treatment should be continued to five years. Periodic assessments should be performed to ensure tolerance and compliance to the drug.

AIs are associated with fewer adverse events compared to tamoxifen including fewer endometrial cancers, thromboembolic events, vaginal discharge and hot flashes. However, AIs are associated with more musculoskeletal symptoms, osteoporosis and an increased risk of fracture compared to tamoxifen.

Targeted Therapy—Trastuzumab

The era of targeted therapies for breast cancer is rapidly emerging. The drug trastuzumab, or Herceptin, has emerged as a major advance in the systemic treatment of breast cancer. It is a humanized mouse monoclonal antibody, targeting the HER2/neu protein which is overexpressed in 25-30% of breast cancers. Initially used for the treatment of metastatic breast cancer, recent studies have confirmed the efficacy of this drug in the adjuvant and neoadjuvant setting. With short-term follow-up, one year of trastuzumab (combined with conventional chemotherapy) reduces the risk of local, regional or systemic relapse by 50% in patients with HER2/neu positive breast cancer. For high-risk HER2/neu positive breast cancer patients, the addition of trastuzumab is now a standard option.

Radiation Therapy

Adjuvant whole breast radiation is routinely recommended following BCS to decrease the risk of local recurrence. It is also required following mastectomy in certain circumstances and for occult breast cancer presenting with axillary LN involvement treated with ALND without mastectomy.

Although all patients with invasive breast cancer have lower rates of local recurrence following breast radiation, the magnitude of benefit is proportional to the level of local recurrence risk. The risk of local recurrence in patients over 70 years old with small, histologically favorable, node-negative, ER-positive tumors may sufficiently be low to consider omission of adjuvant radiation. It is important to evaluate comorbidities and life expectancy in elderly breast cancer patients to compare their risk of breast cancer recurrence with competing causes of mortality.

CT-based treatment planning is used to delineate the target to limit the amount of radiation exposure to the heart and lungs.

Radiation Therapy following Breast-Conserving Surgery

Radiation therapy following breast-conserving surgery can be delivered as whole breast irradiation or partial breast irradiation.

Whole Breast Irradiation

When whole breast irradiation (WBI) is planned, the excisional wound is given 4-6 weeks to heal before treatment begins. If chemotherapy is a part of the treatment plan, radiation is administered after completion of chemotherapy. A total dose of 50 Gy is delivered in 25 fractions to the entire breast for five days per week for five weeks. This is often followed by a local boost to the surgical site given at 2 Gy per fraction for a total of 10 Gy.

Radiation therapy is generally well tolerated. Side effects include skin changes ranging from the more common sunburn to the rare necrosis and breast parenchymal changes including radiation-associated calcifications that may interfere with future mammograms. Rarely pneumonitis, ischemic heart disease and radiation-induced carcinogenesis may occur. Importantly, the skin and breast parenchymal changes have implications on breast reconstruction planning.

Radiation is contraindicated in patients who have prior radiation to the breast or chest wall, patients who are pregnant or have active connective tissue disease involving the skin (especially scleroderma and lupus).

Partial Breast Irradiation

Partial breast irradiation (PBI) is an alternative to whole breast radiation and is increasingly being utilized. PBI can be delivered using multiple interstitial catheters, a balloon catheter that is placed in the lumpectomy cavity or with conformal external beam radiation. The target is the tumor bed and a surrounding 1 cm margin. Treatment begins soon after surgery and is given twice a day for five days. The advantages of partial breast radiation include the ability to target the radiation dose directly to the primary tumor bed which represents the area at highest risk for true local recurrence and a short duration of treatment. Most series of PBI are single institution phase I/II studies and include highly selected patients with limited follow-up. The American Society of Breast Surgeons Mammosite Breast Brachytherapy Registry Trial has enrolled over 1,400 patients with a median follow-up of 43 months. Local recurrence rates are reported to be less than 5% with good to excellent cosmetic outcomes achieved in 90% of patients. The long-term local recurrence risk following PBI is unknown and patients are encouraged to participate in available clinical trials comparing PBI to WBI. Patients considering PBI outside of a clinical trial should be age ≥ 45, have ductal cancer histology, have tumor size ≤ 3 cm, have negative surgical margins and are node-negative.

Radiation Therapy following Mastectomy

The accepted indications for post-mastectomy radiation therapy (PMRT) include pathologic tumor size ≥ 5 cm, ≥ 4 pathologically positive LN and positive surgical margins. Relative indications include patients with multicentric disease with total tumor volume approaching 5 cm and close surgical margins. Clinical trials have reported a survival advantage with PMRT in premenopausal women with 1-3 positive axillary nodes. Although these trials were criticized for inadequate axillary clearance and high rates of regional recurrence, the 2005 Oxford overview analysis confirmed a survival advantage with the administration of PMRT. At our institution, patients with >20% risk of locoregional relapse are considered for PMRT. As the indications for PMRT expand, it is increasingly difficult to advise patients undergoing mastectomy whether to have immediate reconstruction. Planning targeted radiation therapy to the chest wall is complicated by the presence of a reconstructed breast mound and higher doses of radiation may be administered to the underlying lungs or heart. Preoperative consultation with radiation oncology and a preoperative evaluation of the ALNs can help guide the decision for immediate or delayed reconstruction.

Regional Lymph Node Radiation

At our institution, routine internal mammary or supra-clavicular LN irradiation is not performed. It is reserved for patients who have node involvement. ALN irradiation is indicated in patients who have incomplete axillary clearance or who have bulky disease prior to ALND.

Recurrence and Management of Metastatic Disease

Recurrence

The incidence of local and locoregional recurrence following BCT is 5-10% at 10 years. The most common site for local recurrence is the tumor bed. Local recurrence is associated with systemic metastases < 10% of the time. Following mastectomy, local chest wall recurrence usually occurs within the first 2-3 years. It is associated with distant metastases in up to two thirds of patients.

Recurrence must be documented by tissue biopsy. The patient should be restaged following a diagnosis of recurrence. Most local recurrences following BCT can be managed successfully with mastectomy. Chest wall recurrences following mastectomy should undergo local excision if feasible, followed by chest wall irradiation if not previously given. Unresectable chest wall recurrence should receive radiation therapy if no prior radiation was given.

Endocrine therapy and chemotherapy should be given as indicated in the adjuvant setting.

Metastatic Disease

Breast cancer may metastasize to bone, soft tissue, distant LNs, lung, liver and less commonly, the brain, meninges, stomach or adrenal glands. High grade, ER/PR-negative cancers are more often responsible for visceral organ metastases, while the slower-growing, low grade, ER/PR-positive cancers are more often associated with bone and soft tissue metastases. There is currently no cure for metastatic breast cancer; however, long-term disease control is possible especially for bony metastases in ER/PR-positive cancers.

In patients who present with symptomatic visceral metastases, chemotherapy should be the firstline of treatment. Unlike in the adjuvant or neoadjuvant setting, single-agent chemotherapy is indicated. Chemotherapy is also used in patients who have disease progression after several regimens of endocrine therapy or who are intolerant to endocrine therapy. Trastuzumab should be considered if the metastatic disease is HER2/neu overexpressing.

Patients with ER/PR-positive metastatic disease and who do not have symptomatic visceral disease should be treated with endocrine therapy. Premenopausal women should also undergo ovarian ablation or suppression in addition to endocrine therapy. Patients are maintained on endocrine therapy until disease progression or unacceptable side effects occur. Options for endocrine therapy include AIs which are the firstline therapy, fulvestrant, tamoxifen, toremifene, megestrol acetate, fluoxymesterone and ethinyl estradiol.

Bisphosphonate is indicated if patients have bone metastases and have an expected survival of greater than three months. Both pamidronate and zoledronate are approved for this purpose. Calcium and vitamin D should be taken concurrently. One of the side effects of bisphosphonate is osteonecrosis of the jaw. Patients should undergo dental examination with preventive measures undertaken prior to starting therapy.

In the patient presenting with metastatic disease on initial diagnosis, there is growing evidence that local control of the primary tumor either with BCS or with mastectomy may improve survival. It is appropriate to first initiate systemic therapy to monitor response and assess for disease progression. Patients who respond to systemic therapy with regression or remission of metastases are most likely to benefit from surgical removal of the primary tumor.

Follow-up and Surveillance

Most recurrences occur within the first five years after initial treatment. However, recurrences more than twenty years later have also been reported. Therefore, it is essential that breast cancer survivors undergo routine surveillance.

A thorough history and physical examination should be performed every four months for two years, followed by every six months for the next three years, then yearly. Following BCS, a mammogram is recommended six months after treatment as a new baseline mammogram to document surgical and radiation changes. Mammograms should then be performed yearly. If patients received chemotherapy, biochemical evaluation and chest radiograph should be performed annually. In an asymptomatic patient, routine bone scan or CT of the chest, abdomen or brain is not necessary.

Patients who still have a uterus and are taking tamoxifen should undergo annual gynecological assessment. Those with visual problems should undergo ophthalmology examination for cataracts. Patients on an AI should undergo bone health monitoring in the form of a bone mineral density scan periodically. Assessing for tolerance during follow-up visit is essential to ensure compliance to endocrine therapy. Patients who experience side effects can be counseled on ways to minimize their symptoms.

Outcomes

While the incidence of breast cancer has remained relatively stable, the death rate has declined. This is due to the improvement of multimodality treatment for breast cancer.

One of the biggest improvements is with the development of trastuzumab to increase survival in HER2/neu

TABLE 20-5	5-Year survival rate by stage
Stage	**Rate (%)**
Stage 0	100
Stage I	100
Stage IIA	92
Stage IIB	81
Stage IIIA	67
Stage IIIB	54
Stage IV	20

overexpressing breast cancers, which in the past was associated with poorer outcome. Currently, only 20% of women with breast cancer are expected to die of the disease. The 5-year relative survival rates by stage are shown in **Table 20-5**.

New Frontiers

The recent years have seen tremendous discovery and development in the multimodality management of breast cancer. With molecular gene profiling, the heterogeneity of breast cancer is increasingly being recognized and molecular classification of breast cancer has been made possible. Five major subtypes have been identified using DNA microarray gene assay. Based on retrospective analysis, these subtypes are associated with different relapse-free and overall survival rates. The Luminal A and B subtypes express ER-related genes but not HER2/neu gene. The Basal subtype does not express ER-related genes or HER2/neu gene. The next subtype is the HER2/neu expressing subtype and lastly, the normal breast-like subtype that has characteristics similar to normal breast tissue. With a better understanding of the various phenotypes of breast cancer, we can treat breast cancer more effectively.

Improved understanding of molecular signaling pathways and cellular growth and death has contributed greatly to the development of targeted therapy. For example, bevacizumab, an angiogenesis inhibitor, is currently being studied in neoadjuvant and adjuvant therapy clinical trials. It is only one of many targeted therapy agents that is being studied including other growth factor inhibitors, intracellular signaling inhibitors, protease inhibitors and vaccines. Another area of development is the use of serum tumor markers and circulating tumor cells in assessing response to treatment and surveillance of patients following adjuvant treatment or in the metastatic setting.

Feasibility of *in situ* tumor ablation techniques (e.g. cryoablation, radiofrequency ablation, focused ultrasound, laser-induced thermal therapy, microwave ablation, etc.) and use of intraoperative radiotherapy are also being investigated.

PET Mammography, mammoscintigraphy and tomosynthesis are breast imaging technologies that are being explored as adjuncts to mammography for screening and detection, delineating extent of disease to aid BCS and monitoring response to treatment.

Summary

- For clinicians to make appropriate decisions for screening, genetic testing and preventative strategies, it is necessary to recognize breast cancer risk factors and stratify patients into different risk levels of developing breast cancer.
- Patients are considered high risk for breast cancer development if they have a history of thoracic radiation, an estimated 5-year risk of invasive breast cancer > 1.7 in women > 35 year-old or lifetime risk > 20% as defined by risk assessment models, strong family history or genetic predisposition, or a biopsy-proven diagnosis of LCIS or AH.
- Mammography, ultrasound and breast MRI provide effective screening and diagnosis for breast cancer. Surgical planning based solely on MRI findings should not be performed without prior surgical biopsy to confirm malignancy.
- CNB is the preferred approach for tissue biopsy because it is the least invasive method that will provide specimens suitable for histology and immunohistochemical receptor studies. Excisional biopsy as the initial method for tissue diagnosis should be reserved for lesions that are not amenable to percutaneous needle biopsy.
- Neoadjuvant chemotherapy (NACtx) is indicated in patients who present with inoperable locally advanced breast cancer (LABC) and inflammatory breast cancer. It is increasingly used for patients with operable disease who have unfavorable tumor:breast size ratio to convert a mastectomy-only option to a breast-conserving surgery (BCS) option following response to NACtx. Administration of chemotherapy prior to surgery also provides important information about *in vivo* response of the tumor to the agents utilized and treats potential systemic disease without delay.
- Randomized clinical trials with up to twenty years of follow-up have shown that for early stage breast cancer, overall survival is equivalent for total mastectomy and breast-conserving therapy. Therefore, for women with stage I or II breast cancer who desire breast conservation, BCT is an appropriate form of local control as long as free margins and acceptable cosmetic results are attainable. Mastectomy is indicated in patients with large tumors that are poorly responsive to systemic therapy, inflammatory carcinomas and inoperable

stage III breast cancer following neoadjuvant chemotherapy. Women undergoing mastectomy should be informed of their options for breast reconstruction.
- Randomized clinical trials have shown that sentinel lymph node dissection is associated with less morbidity and is an accurate reflection of the axillary LN status. It is now the preferred method for axillary staging in patients presenting with clinically negative axilla.
- Adjuvant therapy for breast cancer may include chemotherapy and endocrine therapy. Radiation therapy must follow breast-conserving surgery to decrease the risk of local recurrence.
- Gene-expression profiling has demonstrated that differential expression of certain genes is a more powerful prognostic indicator than traditional factors such as tumor size and LN status. Two FDA-approved gene assays that stratify patients at different risk levels for relapse are available to guide treatment decision-making.
- Most recurrences occur within the first five years after initial treatment. However, recurrences more than 20 years later have also been reported. Therefore, it is essential that breast cancer survivors undergo routine surveillance.
- There is currently no cure for metastatic breast cancer; however, long-term disease control is possible especially for bony metastases in ER/PR-positive cancers. In the patient presenting with metastatic disease on initial diagnosis, there is growing evidence that local control of the primary tumor either with BCS or mastectomy may improve survival.

Landmark Papers

1. Fisher B, Anderson S, Bryant J, et al. Twenty-year follow-up of a randomized trial comparing total mastectomy, lumpectomy and lumpectomy plus irradiation for the treatment of invasive breast cancer. N Engl J Med 2002;347:1233-41.
2. Veronesi U, Cascinelli N, Mariani L, et al. Twenty-year follow-up of a randomized study comparing breast-conserving surgery with radical mastectomy for early breast cancer. N Engl J Med 2002;347:1227-32.
3. Veronesi U, Paganelli G, Viale G, et al. Sentinel-node-biopsy as a staging procedure in breast cancer: Update of a randomised controlled study. Lancet Oncol 2006;7:983-90.
4. Mansel RE, Fallowfield L, Kissin M, et al. Randomized multicenter trial of sentinel node biopsy versus standard axillary treatment in operable breast cancer: the ALMANAC Trial. J Natl Cancer Inst 2006;98:599-609.
5. Krag D, Weaver D, Ashikaga T, et al. The sentinel node in breast cancer: a multicenter validation study. N Engl J Med 1998;339:941-6.
6. Early Breast Cancer Trialists' Collaborative Group. Effects of radiotherapy and of differences in the extent of surgery

for early breast cancer on local recurrence and 15-year survival: an overview of the randomised trials. Lancet 2005;366:2087-2106.

7. Houssami N, Ciatto S, Macaskill P, et al. Accuracy and surgical impact of magnetic resonance imaging in breast cancer staging: systematic review and meta-analysis in detection of multifocal and multicentric cancer. J Clin Oncol 2008;26:3248-58.

8. Sorlie T, Perou CM, Tibshirani R, et al. Gene expression patterns of breast carcinomas distinguish tumor subclasses with clinical implications. Proc Natl Acad Sci USA 2001; 98:10869-74.

Level of Evidence Table			
Recommendation	**Grade**	**Best level of evidence**	**References**
Breast-conserving therapy (lumpectomy + radiation) versus mastectomy is appropriate for early stage breast cancer	A	1b	1-6
Axillary staging with sentinel lymph node biopsy in clinically node-negative patients is an acceptable and preferred method compared to axillary dissection	A	1b	7-10
Axillary staging with sentinel node biopsy may be performed before or after neoadjuvant therapy with equivalent accuracy for early clinically node-negative cancers	B	1a	11-14
Completion axillary lymph node dissection may potentially be omitted if only sentinel node micrometastases are identified	B	2b	15-18
Postmastectomy—postchemotherapy radiation should be considered for node positive disease (particularly $\geq$ 4 positive axillary nodes), larger tumors (> 5 cm) and/or positive margins	A	1b	19-26
Neoadjuvant therapy is indicated for inflammatory breast cancer, locally advanced cancers and early cancers in women who could undergo and desire breast conservation except for tumor size	A	1b	27-33
Breast MRI during the preoperative staging of breast cancer will detect additional lesions in the ipsilateral and contralateral breast that require workup and potentially altering therapy. Long-term clinical benefit (survival) as well as cost-effectiveness has not been demonstrated	B	3a	34-38
Breast MRI should be performed for the detection of occult breast cancers presenting as axillary adenopathy if standard imaging is negative	A	3a	39
Breast MRI for monitoring response to neoadjuvant chemotherapy may alter surgical therapy particularly with respect to breast-conservation options	B	4	40, 41
Breast MRI for screening high risk women in addition to mammography, ultrasound and clinical breast exam will detect additional cancers. Screening efficacy (improved survival, earlier stage detection) has not been demonstrated	B	3a	42-44
Gene expression profiling should be considered to help prognosticate recurrence risk and guide adjuvant therapy in node-negative, hormone receptor-positive breast cancer patients	B	2b	45-49
Resection of the primary tumor should be considered for patients presenting with metastatic disease.	B	2b	50-52

References

1. Arriagada R, Le MG, Rochard F, Contesso G. Conservative treatment versus mastectomy in early breast cancer: patterns of failure with 15 years of follow-up data. Institut Gustave-Roussy Breast Cancer Group. J Clin Oncol 1996; 14(5):1558-64.

2. Blichert-Toft M, Rose C, Ersen JA, et al. Danish randomized trial comparing breast conservation therapy with mastectomy: six years of life-table analysis. Danish Breast Cancer Cooperative Group. J Natl Cancer Inst Monogr 1992;11:19-25.

3. Fisher B, Erson S, Bryant J, et al. Twenty-year follow-up of a randomized trial comparing total mastectomy, lumpectomy and lumpectomy plus irradiation for the treatment of invasive breast cancer. N Engl J Med 2002; 347(16):1233-41.

4. Poggi MM, Danforth DN, Sciuto LC, et al. Eighteen-year results in the treatment of early breast carcinoma with mastectomy versus breast conservation therapy: the National Cancer Institute Randomized Trial. Cancer 2003;98(4):697-702.

5. van Dongen JA, Voogd AC, Fentiman IS, et al. Long-term results of a randomized trial comparing breast-conserving therapy with mastectomy: European Organization for Research and Treatment of Cancer 10801 trial. J Natl Cancer Inst 2000;92(14):1143-50.

6. Veronesi U, Cascinelli N, Mariani L, et al. Twenty-year follow-up of a randomized study comparing breast-conserving surgery with radical mastectomy for early breast cancer. N Engl J Med 2002;347(16):1227-32.

7. Krag D, Weaver D, Ashikaga T, et al. The sentinel node in breast cancer—a multicenter validation study. N Engl J Med 1998;339(14):941-6.

8. Mansel RE, Fallowfield L, Kissin M, et al. Randomized multicenter trial of sentinel node biopsy versus standard axillary treatment in operable breast cancer: the ALMANAC Trial. J Natl Cancer Inst 2006;98(9):599-609.

9. Veronesi U, Paganelli G, Viale G, et al. Sentinel-lymph-node biopsy as a staging procedure in breast cancer: update of a randomised controlled study. Lancet Oncol 2006;7(12): 983-90.

10. Veronesi U, Paganelli G, Viale G, et al. A randomized comparison of sentinel-node biopsy with routine axillary dissection in breast cancer. N Engl J Med 2003;349(6):546-53.

11. Gimbergues P, Abrial C, Durando X, et al. Sentinel lymph node biopsy after neoadjuvant chemotherapy is accurate in breast cancer patients with a clinically negative axillary nodal status at presentation. Ann Surg Oncol 2008; 15(5): 1316-21.

12. Hunt KK, Yi M, Mittendorf EA, et al. Sentinel lymph node surgery after neoadjuvant chemotherapy is accurate and reduces the need for axillary dissection in breast cancer patients. Ann Surg 2009.

13. Kelly AM, Dwamena B, Cronin P, Carlos RC. Breast cancer sentinel node identification and classification after neoadjuvant chemotherapy-systematic review and meta analysis. Acad Radiol 2009;16(5):551-63.

14. van Deurzen CH, Vriens BE, Tjan-Heijnen VC, et al. Accuracy of sentinel node biopsy after neoadjuvant chemotherapy in breast cancer patients: a systematic review. Eur J Cancer 2009.

15. Fournier K, Schiller A, Perry RR, Laronga C. Micrometastasis in the sentinel lymph node of breast cancer does not mandate completion axillary dissection. Ann Surg 2004; 239(6):859-63; discussion 863-5.

16. Hwang RF, Gonzalez-Angulo AM, Yi M, et al. Low locoregional failure rates in selected breast cancer patients with tumor-positive sentinel lymph nodes who do not undergo completion axillary dissection. Cancer 2007; 110(4):723-30.

17. Langer I, Guller U, Viehl CT, et al. Axillary lymph node dissection for sentinel lymph node micrometastases may be safely omitted in early-stage breast cancer patients: long-term outcomes of a prospective study. Ann Surg Oncol 2009.

18. Reed J, Rosman M, Verbanac KM, Mannie A, Cheng Z, Tafra L. Prognostic implications of isolated tumor cells and micrometastases in sentinel nodes of patients with invasive breast cancer: 10-year analysis of patients enrolled in the prospective East Carolina University/Anne Arundel Medical Center Sentinel Node Multicenter Study. J Am Coll Surg 2009;208(3):333-40.

19. Clarke M, Collins R, Darby S, et al. Effects of radiotherapy and of differences in the extent of surgery for early breast cancer on local recurrence and 15-year survival: an overview of the randomised trials. Lancet 2005; 366(9503): 2087-2106.

20. Killander F, Anderson H, Ryden S, Moller T, Hafstrom LO, Malmstrom P. Efficient reduction of locoregional recurrences but no effect on mortality twenty years after postmastectomy radiation in premenopausal women with stage II breast cancer: a randomized trial from the South Sweden Breast Cancer Group. Breast 2009.

21. Nielsen HM, Overgaard M, Grau C, Jensen AR, Overgaard J. Study of failure pattern among high-risk breast cancer patients with or without postmastectomy radiotherapy in addition to adjuvant systemic therapy: long-term results from the Danish Breast Cancer Cooperative Group DBCG 82 b and c randomized studies. J Clin Oncol 2006;24(15): 2268-75.

22. Overgaard M, Hansen PS, Overgaard J, et al. Postoperative radiotherapy in high-risk premenopausal women with breast cancer who receive adjuvant chemotherapy. Danish Breast Cancer Cooperative Group 82b Trial. N Engl J Med 1997; 337(14):949-55.

23. Overgaard M, Jensen MB, Overgaard J, et al. Postoperative radiotherapy in high-risk postmenopausal breast-cancer patients given adjuvant tamoxifen: Danish Breast Cancer Cooperative Group DBCG 82c randomised trial. Lancet 1999;353(9165):1641-8.

24. Overgaard M, Nielsen HM, Overgaard J. Is the benefit of postmastectomy irradiation limited to patients with four or more positive nodes, as recommended in international consensus reports? A subgroup analysis of the DBC G 82 b&c randomized trials. Radiother Oncol 2007;82(3): 247-53.

25. Ragaz J, Olivotto IA, Spinelli JJ, et al. Locoregional radiation therapy in patients with high-risk breast cancer receiving adjuvant chemotherapy: 20-year results of the British Columbia randomized trial. J Natl Cancer Inst 2005;97(2):116-26.

26. Taghian A, Jeong JH, Mamounas E, et al. Patterns of locoregional failure in patients with operable breast cancer treated by mastectomy and adjuvant chemotherapy with or without tamoxifen and without radiotherapy: results from five National Surgical Adjuvant Breast and Bowel Project randomized clinical trials. J Clin Oncol 2004; 22(21):4247-54.

27. Kim T, Lau J, Erban J. Lack of uniform diagnostic criteria for inflammatory breast cancer limits interpretation of treatment outcomes: a systematic review. Clin Breast Cancer 2006;7(5):386-95.

28. Liauw SL, Benda RK, Morris CG, Mendenhall NP. Inflammatory breast carcinoma: outcomes with trimodality therapy for nonmetastatic disease. Cancer 2004;100(5):920-8.

29. Smoot RL, Koch CA, Degnim AC, et al. A single-center experience with inflammatory breast cancer, 1985-2003. Arch Surg 2006;141(6):567-72.

30. Gajdos C, Tartter PI, Estabrook A, Gistrak MA, Jaffer S, Bleiweiss IJ. Relationship of clinical and pathologic response to neoadjuvant chemotherapy and outcome of locally advanced breast cancer. J Surg Oncol 2002;80(1):4-11.

31. Olson JA, Jr., Budd GT, Carey LA, et al. Improved surgical outcomes for breast cancer patients receiving neoadjuvant aromatase inhibitor therapy: results from a multicenter phase II trial. J Am Coll Surg 2009;208(5):906-14; discussion 915-6.

32. Deo SV, Bhutani M, Shukla NK, Raina V, Rath GK, Purkayasth J. Randomized trial comparing neo-adjuvant versus adjuvant chemotherapy in operable locally advanced breast cancer (T4b N0-2 M0). J Surg Oncol 2003;84(4):192-7.

33. Kaufmann M, von Minckwitz G, Smith R, et al. International expert panel on the use of primary (preoperative) systemic treatment of operable breast cancer: review and recommendations. J Clin Oncol 2003; 21(13): 2600-8.

34. Brennan ME, Houssami N, Lord S, et al. Magnetic Resonance Imaging Screening of the Contralateral Breast in Women With Newly Diagnosed Breast Cancer: Systematic Review and Meta-Analysis of Incremental Cancer Detection and Impact on Surgical Management. J Clin Oncol 2009.

35. Houssami N, Ciatto S, Macaskill P, et al. Accuracy and surgical impact of magnetic resonance imaging in breast cancer staging: systematic review and meta-analysis in detection of multifocal and multicentric cancer. J Clin Oncol 2008;26(19):3248-58.

36. Lehman CD, DeMartini W, Anderson BO, Edge SB. Indications for breast MRI in the patient with newly diagnosed breast cancer. J Natl Compr Canc Netw 2009;7(2):193-201.

37. Bilimoria KY, Cambic A, Hansen NM, Bethke KP. Evaluating the impact of preoperative breast magnetic resonance imaging on the surgical management of newly diagnosed breast cancers. Arch Surg 2007;142(5):441-5; discussion 445-7.

38. Siegmann KC, Baur A, Vogel U, Kraemer B, Hahn M, Claussen CD. Risk-benefit analysis of preoperative breast MRI in patients with primary breast cancer. Clin Radiol 2009;64(4):403-13.

39. de Bresser J, de Vos B, van der Ent F, Hulsewe K. Breast MRI in clinically and mammographically occult breast cancer presenting with an axillary metastasis: a systematic review. Eur J Surg Oncol 2009.

40. Chen JH, Feig BA, Hsiang DJ, et al. Impact of MRI-evaluated neoadjuvant chemotherapy response on change of surgical recommendation in breast cancer. Ann Surg 2009; 249(3):448-54.

41. Chen JH, Feig B, Agrawal G, et al. MRI evaluation of pathologically complete response and residual tumors in breast cancer after neoadjuvant chemotherapy. Cancer. 2008; 112(1):17-26.

42. Lord SJ, Lei W, Craft P, et al. A systematic review of the effectiveness of magnetic resonance imaging (MRI) as an addition to mammography and ultrasound in screening young women at high risk of breast cancer. Eur J Cancer 2007; 43(13):1905-17.

43. Plevritis SK, Kurian AW, Sigal BM, et al. Cost-effectiveness of screening BRCA1/2 mutation carriers with breast magnetic resonance imaging. JAMA. May 24 2006;295(20):2374-84.

44. Warner E, Plewes DB, Hill KA, et al. Surveillance of BRCA1 and BRCA2 mutation carriers with magnetic resonance imaging, ultrasound, mammography and clinical breast examination. JAMA 2004;292(11):1317-25.

45. Buyse M, Loi S, van't Veer L, et al. Validation and clinical utility of a 70-gene prognostic signature for women with node-negative breast cancer. J Natl Cancer Inst 2006; 98(17):1183-92.

46. Paik S, Shak S, Tang G, et al. A multigene assay to predict recurrence of tamoxifen-treated, node-negative breast cancer. N Engl J Med 2004;351(27):2817-26.

47. Paik S, Tang G, Shak S, et al. Gene expression and benefit of chemotherapy in women with node-negative, estrogen receptor-positive breast cancer. J Clin Oncol 2006;24(23):3726-34.

48. van de Vijver MJ, He YD, van't Veer LJ, et al. A gene-expression signature as a predictor of survival in breast cancer. N Engl J Med 2002;347(25):1999-2009.

49. Zujewski JA, Kamin L. Trial assessing individualized options for treatment for breast cancer: the TAILORx trial. Future Oncol 2008;4(5):603-10.

50. Bafford AC, Burstein HJ, Barkley CR, et al. Breast surgery in stage IV breast cancer: impact of staging and patient selection on overall survival. Breast Cancer Res Treat 2009;115(1):7-12.

51. Blanchard DK, Shetty PB, Hilsenbeck SG, Elledge RM. Association of surgery with improved survival in stage IV breast cancer patients. Ann Surg 2008;247(5):732-8.

52. Fields RC, Jeffe DB, Trinkaus K, et al. Surgical resection of the primary tumor is associated with increased long-term survival in patients with stage IV breast cancer after controlling for site of metastasis. Ann Surg Oncol 2007;14(12): 3345-51.

Section 5

Endocrine Organs

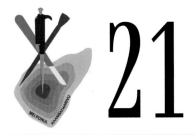

21

Thyroid Cancer

Ibrahim Yazji, Jennifer B Ogilvie

History

Prior to the beginning of the twentieth century, the surgical treatment of thyroid cancer was associated with extremely poor outcomes. Thyroid tumors were often diagnosed late and patients typically presented with dysphagia, vocal cord paralysis or invasion into surrounding soft tissue structures. Perioperative mortality in patients undergoing surgery for thyroid cancer was 60% in Butlin's 1887 review of 50 patients and there were no long-term cures. Technical advances in thyroid surgery by Billroth, Kocher, Halsted, Crile, Mayo, Lahey and others in the late nineteenth and early twentieth centuries reduced mortality from over 25% to under 5%.

Administration of thyroid extract to prevent myxedema after total thyroidectomy was developed in 1891 by Murray. The importance of parathyroid preservation to prevent postoperative tetany was identified by Mikulicz and refined by Halsted in the early twentieth century. Mikulicz also focused attention on the preservation of the recurrent laryngeal nerves during thyroid surgery and was a proponent of an operative technique that left the posterior aspect of the thyroid lobes intact to protect the recurrent nerve. The effects of injury to the external branch of the superior laryngeal nerve was widely recognized after the Italian opera singer Amelita Galli-Curci lost the upper register of her voice after thyroidectomy in 1935. Continued refinement of surgical technique by experienced endocrine surgeons continued throughout the twentieth century so that total thyroidectomy and cervical lymph node dissection for thyroid cancer is now a safe and well-tolerated procedure.

Epidemiology

Thyroid nodules are widely prevalent worldwide. The prevalence of palpable thyroid nodules in areas of iodine sufficiency is approximately 1% in men and 5% in women. The widespread use of ultrasonography for a variety of clinical indications has resulted in a striking increase in the prevalence of thyroid nodules, up to 50% or greater in women, to match the rates obtained from autopsy studies.

Thyroid carcinoma is the most common endocrine malignancy, comprising 1% of all malignant tumors. The prevalence of thyroid carcinoma varies worldwide from 0.5 to 10 per 100,000 of the population. The incidence of thyroid carcinoma in the United States was 37,000 in 2008, with 1,300 yearly cancer-related deaths. Over the past 30 years this incidence has increased from 3.6 to 8.7 per 100,000 per year and almost all new cases are small papillary thyroid cancers.

Thyroid tumors can be categorized by cellular origin into two major groups **(Table 21-1)**. The first group is derived from thyroid follicular cells, which includes five histologically distinct types: papillary thyroid carcinoma (PTC), follicular thyroid carcinoma (FTC), oncocytic (Hürthle cell) carcinoma (HCC), poorly-differentiated thyroid carcinoma (PDTC) and anaplastic thyroid carcinoma (ATC). PTC and FTC represent approximately 95% of all malignant thyroid lesions and are identified as the well-differentiated subtypes of thyroid carcinomas (WDTC). The second group of thyroid tumors is derived from non-follicular cells and encompasses medullary thyroid carcinoma (MTC), derived from parafollicular (C) cells, primary thyroid lymphoma, metastatic lesions to the thyroid and other rare tumors, including sarcoma, paraganglioma, teratoma and plasmacytoma.

TABLE 21-1	Thyroid cancer — Frequency and Survival	
Type	**Relative frequency (%)**	**10-year survival rate (%)**
Follicular cell origin		
Papillary	80-85	90-95
Follicular	8-10	70-95
Hürthle	3-5	70
Anaplastic	1-2	Less than 5
Non-follicular cell origin		
Medullary	3-5	70-90
Lymphoma	1-5	50-85

Risk Factors

Radiation Exposure

One of the most important non-hereditary risk factors for the development of well-differentiated thyroid carcinoma is radiation exposure (XRT). This association has clearly been identified and reconfirmed in multiple studies analyzing different groups of patients that were exposed to XRT for various reasons. Thyroid cancer is more prevalent amongst individuals that were exposed to radiation secondary to nuclear accidents, including Hiroshima, Nagasaki and Chernobyl. In addition, individuals that were exposed to therapeutic head and neck XRT for malignancy, such as Hodgkin's lymphoma, or for non-malignant conditions such as acne, tonsillitis or thymic enlargement, have also been found to be at higher risk of developing WDTC. The lifetime risk of developing thyroid cancer amongst individuals exposed to high-dose radiation is reported to be 5-9 times that of those with no radiation exposure. The lag time between exposure to XRT and diagnosis of thyroid cancer is on the order of 2-3 decades.

Genetic Factors

Hereditary factors may play a role in the development of both PTC and MTC. Patients presenting with a thyroid nodule should be screened for a family history of first degree relatives with thyroid carcinoma or familial thyroid cancer syndromes, including Multiple Endocrine Neoplasia type II (MEN II), Cowden's syndrome, Carney Complex, familial polyposis and Werner syndrome.

RET is a proto-oncogene encoding a tyrosine kinase receptor. When altered by a mutation, the RET oncogene has been implicated in the development of MTC, via the uncontrolled activation of intracellular pathways. Sporadic and germline RET mutations are associated with somatic and familial cases of MTC, respectively. Germline RET mutations are inherited in an autosomal dominant fashion. Hereditary forms of MTC account for 20-25% of all reported MTC cases. Depending on the codon site of RET mutation, the disease occurs either alone as familial medullary thyroid cancer (FMTC), or in association with other endocrine tumors as MEN II.

Somatic mutations which activate the MAPK signaling pathway are found in over 70% of sporadic PTC. The most common genes affected are the serine-threonine kinase BRAF, the GTP-binding protein RAS and the receptor tyrosine kinase RET-PTC rearrangements. BRAF point mutations, especially V600E (T1799A), are the most common mutations in sporadic PTC, occurring in at least 40% and are associated with extrathyroidal extension, advanced stage, increased recurrence and decreased survival. RET/PTC rearrangements, particularly RET/

PTC1 and RET/PTC3, are found in 20-40% of sporadic PTC and are more prevalent in young patients or patients with a history of XRT exposure. RAS mutations are seen in up to half of all FTC and more recently have been associated with encapsulated follicular variant PTC. However, RAS mutations are also found in benign follicular adenomas. BRAF, RET/PTC and RAS can be identified in FNA biopsy specimens and are becoming important adjuncts in the diagnosis of thyroid cancer.

Only 5% of PTC cases are familial in origin. A variety of genes, including APC and PTEN, have been implicated in the development of hereditary forms of PTC in conjunction with other tumors. However, no gene has yet been associated with isolated familial PTC. There is no convincing evidence so far to suggest a familial form of FTC.

Gender

For unclear reasons, women are more likely than men to develop WDTC by a ratio of 3:1; however, both genders are equally likely to develop MTC and ATC.

Low-iodine Diet

Although this risk factor is negligible in the United States, it has been shown that a diet low in iodine can be associated with an increased risk of developing PTC, especially in combination with radiation exposure.

Presentation

The majority of patients diagnosed with thyroid cancer have no signs or symptoms of the disease; an incidental finding of a thyroid nodule detected on neck imaging, such as carotid ultrasound, MRI or PET CT, is what often prompts their evaluation. Other patients are evaluated for a palpable neck mass, either self-recognized or found on routine physical exam. It is important to note that 5-10% of all thyroid nodules are malignant and that palpable nodules harbor the same risk of malignancy as their non-palpable counterparts. Patients may present with symptoms of enlarging neck mass, such as neck pain, hoarseness, dysphagia or supine dyspnea, which may indicate locally advanced tumors with invasion into surrounding structures.

A thorough history and physical examination is the initial step in the work up of thyroid mass. Important high-risk features include history of head and neck irradiation, exposure to radiation from nuclear events, family history of thyroid cancer or MEN II syndrome, rapid thyroid enlargement and symptoms of hoarseness, dysphagia, or dyspnea. In addition, thyroid nodules in patients less than 20 years of age or patients above 65 raise the clinical suspicion of malignancy. On physical examination, findings suggestive of malignancy include firm thyroid nodules larger than 1 cm, fixation to the surrounding tissue, enlarged supraclavicular or cervical lymph nodes, or evidence of vocal cord paralysis on fiberoptic laryngoscopy.

Diagnosis

Although nondiagnostic for malignancy, a thyroid function panel should be obtained to determine the functional status of the thyroid gland. A calcitonin level is indicated in the workup of thyroid nodule when the diagnosis of MTC is considered based on additional features of MEN II such as hypercalcemia or pheochromo-cytoma, or in the setting of a positive family history for FMTC or MEN II. Baseline calcium level is not part of the diagnostic laboratory workup of thyroid nodule but should be considered preoperatively when surgery is indicated, to rule out concurrent parathyroid disease.

Thyroid scintigraphy with I123 has recently fallen out of favor because it has failed to adequately differentiate benign from malignant lesions. Cold (lower uptake) and warm (normal uptake) nodules are more likely to be benign, however still have a significant chance of harboring malignancy and should be biopsied; on the other hand, hot (higher uptake) nodules are rarely malignant. Therefore, the use of thyroid scintigraphy is only useful in the evaluation of a solitary nodule in a hyperfunctional thyroid. If the radionuclide scan demonstrates a hot (higher uptake) region that corresponds to the known nodule, then no further cytologic evaluation of this nodule is necessary.

Thyroid ultrasonography (US) is the imaging modality of choice in the evaluation of thyroid nodules. Non-palpable thyroid nodules visualized on US are found in up to 50% or more of the population; therefore, US should not be used as a screening tool on low risk patients in order to avoid the detection of clinically irrelevant nodules. However, US is indicated as a screening tool for patients with risk factors such as history of head and neck irradiation or familial thyroid cancer syndromes. US should be the first step in the diagnostic workup of a palpable thyroid nodule in conjunction with thyroid function tests. US is used to exclude the presence of other nodules, to determine the size, location, extension, appearance (e.g. solid, cystic or mixed) and echogenic and vascular characteristics of all nodules and to rule out suspicious cervical lymphadenopathy. It is important to note that the overall risk of malignancy is the same in solitary nodules versus multinodular goiter (MNG), whether palpable or discovered on US.

US features of thyroid nodules suspicious for malignancy include hypoechogenicity, hypervascularity, irregular or multilobulated shape and the presence of microcalcifications **(Figure 21-1)**. It is important to note that these suspicious US features have high positive predictive value and low negative predictive value for the diagnosis of thyroid carcinoma secondary to low sensitivity and high specificity. Therefore, the absence of these features on a nodule larger than 1 cm should not preclude patients from undergoing the next step in the evaluation, i.e. fine-needle aspiration biopsy.

Fine-needle aspiration (FNA) biopsy is widely recognized as the most accurate and cost-effective method in the preoperative evaluation of thyroid nodules **(Figures 21-2A to D)**. FNA is most accurate in nodules between 1 and 4 cm in size. To improve the sampling accuracy, all

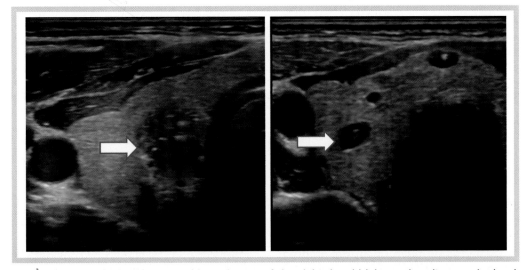

Figure 21-1: (Left) Papillary thyroid carcinoma of the right thyroid lobe under ultrasound, classic appearance as a heterogeneous nodule with microcalcifications. (Right) Colloid cysts of the right thyroid lobe under ultrasound, typically hypoechoic, smooth bordered nodules with 'comet tail artifact.' *Provided by Mitchel Tublin, MD; Department of Radiology, University of Pittsburgh Medical Center*

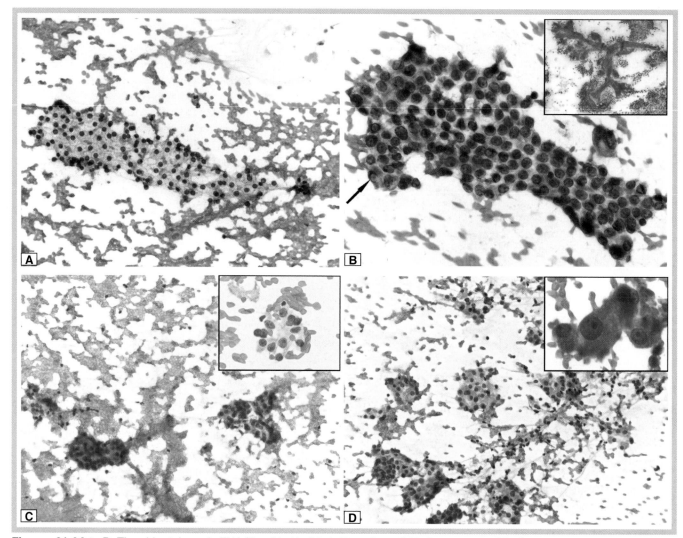

Figures 21-2A to D: Thyroid cytology via FNA (Provided by Marie Dvorakova, MD; Department of Pathology, University of Pittsburgh Medical Center)

A. Benign colloid nodule: the cytologic preparations have typically low to moderate cellularity and abundant colloid. Follicular cells are uniform, regularly spaced and arranged in macrofollicles or cohesive two dimensional sheets (Papanicolaou stain).

B. Papillary thyroid carcinoma: the cytologic preparations have typically high cellularity with neoplastic cells arranged in crowded sheets; occasionally, fibrovascular cores can be appreciated (inset, Diff-Quick stain). The follicular cells have pale powdery chromatin, irregular nuclear contours, nuclear grooves and pseudoinclusions (arrow, Papanicolaou stain).

C. Suspicious for a follicular neoplasm: the cytologic preparations have typically high cellularity and scant to absent colloid. Follicular cells are arranged in trabeculae or microfollicles (inset, Diff-Quick stain) and show crowding, nuclear enlargement and mild pleomorphism (Papanicolaou stain).

D. Suspicious for a Hürtle cell neoplasm: the cytologic preparations are composed of a relatively pure population of oncocytic (Hürtle) follicular cells with voluminous granular cytoplasm, enlarged nuclei and prominent nucleoli in microfollicular arrangement (Papanicolaou stain)

FNA biopsies should be performed under US guidance. In the evaluation of thyroid nodules under 4 cm in size, FNA biopsy, performed by an experienced physician under US guidance and interpreted by an experienced cytopathologist, has at least 90% accuracy and false-negative rates of 5% or less. FNA of thyroid nodules greater than 4 cm in size, however, have been shown to have a higher false-negative rate of up to 13%.

Low-risk patients with a subcentimeter thyroid nodule are not routinely sent for FNA, but are followed clinically with a US every 6-12 months. However, certain sub-centimeter nodules should be considered for evaluation with FNA if the patient is at high risk, or if the nodule has suspicious features on US. Nodules greater than 4 cm in size have been found to have a higher overall rate of malignancy, as well as an increased false-negative rate on FNA and should definitively be evaluated with diagnostic lobectomy or total thyroidectomy.

In the setting of multinodular goiter, the nodule most suspicious for malignancy based on its US features and not simply the dominant largest nodule should be aspirated preferentially. However, if multiple nodules larger than 1 cm in size exist but none have suspicious US features, then the largest one should be targeted preferentially with FNA.

Suspicious US features of cervical lymph nodes include increased size, cystic degeneration, microcalcifications and loss of the normal fatty hilum. Any suspicious cervical lymph nodes identified on US should be evaluated with FNA biopsy. FNA aspirates should also be sent for thyroglobulin, which, if positive, is diagnostic for metastatic WDTC.

FNA cytology results are typically divided into at least four categories **(Table 21-2)**. The first category is non-diagnostic representing 10-15% of cases and indicates that the aspirate does not meet adequacy criteria (at least 6 follicular cell groups, each containing 10-15 cells from at least 2 separate aspirates of a thyroid nodule). In non-diagnostic cases the FNA should be repeated. If repeated FNA cytologic evaluation yields a non-diagnostic result, then diagnostic lobectomy or total thyroidectomy should be considered, especially in the setting of solid nodules.

The second FNA cytologic category is benign, the most common finding on FNA representing 70% of all cases. Benign lesions diagnosed on FNA include colloid nodule, follicular or oncocytic (Hürthle cell) adenoma, lympho-cytic thyroiditis, granulomatous thyroiditis or benign cyst. Serial US on every 6-12 months should be used to monitor growth in asymptomatic benign nodules less than 4 cm in diameter. If nodular growth (> 50% in volume or > 2 mm in at least 2 dimensions) is detected, then a repeat FNA biopsy is indicated.

The third diagnostic category of FNA cytology is indeterminate, also termed follicular (or oncocytic) lesion or neoplasm and is reported in 10-15% of cases. The differential of a follicular (or oncocytic) lesion includes follicular (or oncocytic) adenoma, hyperplastic nodule, lymphocytic thyroiditis, FCC, HCC and follicular or Hürthle cell variant of PTC. The overall rate of malignancy is approximately 20% and patients with indeterminate FNA should undergo at least a diagnostic thyroid lobectomy. Patients with additional risk factors should be considered for total thyroidectomy. Molecular testing for the detection of BRAF and RAS mutations or RET/PTC rearrangements has recently been shown to increase the diagnostic accuracy of indeterminate FNA cytology and is under investigation.

The final FNA cytologic category is malignant or suspicious for malignancy, which accounts for approximately 5% of all thyroid FNA. In these cases total thyroidectomy and appropriate cervical lymph node dissection is indicated.

Histopathology and Pathophysiology

PTC

PTC is the most common form of thyroid carcinoma, accounting for at least 80% of all cases. PTC is derived from thyroid follicular cells that produce thyroid hormone. PTC is typically diagnosed on FNA cytology, which demonstrates hypercellularity with cell clusters occasionally arranged in a papillary formation. These cells have enlarged nuclei with intranuclear cytoplasmic pseudoinclusions and nuclear grooves.

The histological appearance of PTC is that of a complex network of papillae comprised of a fibrovascular core with surrounding follicular thyroid cells that are larger than normal with cuboidal to low columnar shape. Psammoma bodies, which represent calcified necrotic tumor papillae, are a fairly specific diagnostic feature and can be seen in 40-60% of PTC cases. Multinucleated giant-cell hysticoes are also a frequent histological feature of PTC. PTC lesions are often sharply circumscribed. Multifocal tumors are seen in 18-87% of PTC.

There are several histopathological variants of PTC. The follicular variant of PTC (FVPTC) is characterized by more follicular rather than papillary architecture, but has similar cellular and nuclear features to classical PTC. FVPTC lesions are commonly encapsulated. Well-encapsulated FVPTC with no infiltrative components are typically

TABLE 21-2	Diagnostic categories for reporting interpretation of thyroid fine-needle aspiration		
Cytologic interpretation	**Frequency (%)**	**Possible diagnoses**	**Notes**
Non-diagnostic	10-15		Insufficient or bloody aspirate
Benign	70	Colloid nodule, hyperplastic nodule, thyroid cyst, Hashimoto's thyroiditis	False-negative 3%
Indeterminate	10-15	Follicular adenoma, Hürthle-cell adenoma, FTC, HCC and follicular or Hürthle cell variant of PTC	Rate of malignancy 20%
Malignant	5	PTC, MTC, ATC, PTL, Metastatic carcinoma	False-positive 1%

indolent tumors, with a low incidence of lymph node involvement or distant metastases. Tall cell variant is a more aggressive form of PTC and is characterized by frequent angiolymphatic invasion and extrathyroidal extension. Other rare and aggressive variants of PTC include the columnar cell and diffuse sclerosing variants.

Patients with PTC usually present in their third to fifth decade of life and the 10-year survival rates of PTC are excellent at 90-95%. Cervical lymph node involvement, most commonly to the central compartment (level VI-VII), tends to occur early in PTC and is reported in 30-90% of all patients. Hematogenous spread is uncommon in PTC but does occur in up to 5% of cases to the lungs, bone and brain.

FTC

FTC is the second most common thyroid carcinoma, constituting approximately 10% of all thyroid carcinomas and is also derived from thyroid follicular cells. Its malignant potential is solely based on the histologic demonstration of capsular or vascular invasion. On cytologic evaluation, FTC is hypercellular, with benign-appearing follicular cells and scant colloid and no malignant nuclear features. Therefore, the only way to distinguish FTC from follicular adenoma is via careful histopathological examination of a surgically removed lesion to identify capsular or vascular invasion.

Patients with FTC tend to present in their fifth to sixth decade of life. In contrast with PTC, cervical lymph node involvement is uncommon in FTC and is only reported in 5-10% of patients at the time of diagnosis. However, distant metastases are more common in FTC than PTC and can be found in 10-30% of patients at initial presentation. The 10-year survival rate of FTC is 70-95% and stage for stage is similar to PTC. Minimally invasive FTC appears to have a very indolent course with low rates of metastasis and excellent long-term survival.

HTC

Hürthle (oncocytic) cells are also derived from thyroid follicular cells. They are large, polygonal cells characterized by increased mitochondrial content which gives a characteristic granular, eosinophilic cytoplasm. Hürthle cell neoplasms are considered variants of follicular neoplasms, containing greater than 75% dominance of Hürthle cells. Like follicular lesions, Hürthle cell lesions can either be benign or malignant and only histological demonstration of capsular and vascular invasion can confirm malignancy.

HCC comprises 5% of all thyroid carcinomas. The mean age of presentation is 50 years. At the time of initial presentation, the rate of cervical lymph node involvement in HCC is 10-25% and that of distant metastasis is 10-20%. HCC is considered to be more aggressive than the more common well-differentiated carcinomas of the thyroid. The overall 10-year survival rate of HCC is approximately 70%. It is important to note that only 10% of Hürthle cell carcinomas take up I131, which reduces diagnostic and therapeutic options for recurrent or metastatic HCC.

MTC

MTC comprises less than 5% of all thyroid carcinomas. Tumors arise from the parafollicular (C) cells of the thyroid gland. C cells are derived from the neural crest and produce calcitonin. MTC can readily be diagnosed on FNA via characteristics such as hypercellularity and hyperchromatic nuclei in elongated "plasmacytoid" cell bodies. Amyloid appears as amorphous background material that can be recognized with Congo red staining. In equivocal cases, immunohistochemical staining for calcitonin can be used for definitive diagnosis. MTC stains positively for CEA and negatively for thyroglobulin. When the diagnosis of MTC is made, basal calcitonin and CEA levels should be measured and patients should be screened for pheochromocytoma and hyperparathyroidism to rule out MEN II. Serum calcitonin levels directly correlate with tumor size. The incidence of positive cervical lymph node involvement in MTC correlates with the size of the lesion at the time of diagnosis and is up to 80% for lesions greater than 1 cm in size and 100% in the setting of capsular invasion. Distant metastases are present in nearly 15% of patients with MTC at initial presentation.

MTC are 75% sporadic and 25% hereditary. Hereditary cases are commonly multifocal and bilateral, whereas sporadic cases are usually unifocal. The hereditary MTC syndromes include MEN IIA, MEN IIB and FMTC; all have autosomal dominant inheritance and 100% penetrance. MEN IIA consists of MTC, pheochromocytoma (in 40% of patients) and hyperparathyroidism (20% of patients). MEN IIB consists of MTC, pheochromocytoma (in 70% of patients), marfanoid habitus and ganglioneuromatosis. FMTC is characterized by MTC alone. MTC in MEN IIB is associated with the most aggressive phenotype and usually develops by the age of 10, with a high propensity for rapid growth and distant metastasis. MTC in MEN IIA may appear in the first decade of life, but it almost always develops by the second decade. MTC in FMTC is typically diagnosed in adulthood.

When MTC is confined to the thyroid gland, the overall 10-year survival rate is excellent at 90%, but survival decreases to 70% when cervical lymph nodes are involved and is only 20% when distant metastases are present.

ATC

The incidence of ATC is less than 300 cases per year in the United States, or 1.5-2% of all thyroid carcinomas diagnosed annually. These tumors are highly aggressive and usually present as a rapidly growing neck mass, typically with associated mass-like effects, such as hoarseness, dysphagia, dyspnea and cervical tenderness. Other manifestations include superior vena cava syndrome, ball-valve tracheal obstruction and hyperthyroidism due to necrosis of normal thyroid tissue and release of thyroid hormone. Ultrasonography and FNA biopsy are the diagnostic procedure of choice for any rapidly enlarging thyroid mass.

Cytologically, ATC is characterized by high mitotic activity and highly atypical appearing cells. Occasionally, ATC is difficult to distinguish from metastatic carcinoma to the thyroid gland. Cytokeratin is the best histochemical marker of ATC. Although ATC typically does not stain positive for thyroglobulin, positive thyroglobulin staining if present confirms thyroid origin.

Histologically, there are three predominant patterns of ATC: spindle cell, giant cell and squamoid cell. Common features of ATC include large foci of necrosis and invasion into adjacent muscular or vascular structures. On gross examination, ATC is tan-white, fleshy and large with areas of necrosis and hemorrhage.

ATC primarily occurs in older age-groups, most commonly after the fifth or sixth decades of life. At the time of diagnosis, the primary tumor is larger than 5 cm in 80% of patients and likely to be multifocal and bilateral. Fifty percent of patients will already have extrathyroidal extension, direct local invasion of adjacent structures, regional lymph node involvement or distant metastasis to the lung, brain, or rarely to skin and bowel. The 5-year survival rate for anaplastic thyroid carcinoma, all of which are considered stage IV disease, is less than 10%.

PTL

Primary thyroid lymphoma (PTL) is a rare malignancy of the thyroid gland. It typically presents as rapidly enlarging thyroid mass, which makes it difficult to distinguish clinically from ATC. However, a significant portion of PTL arises within a background of Hashimoto's thyroiditis. The majority of thyroid lymphomas are diffuse large B-cell lymphomas (DLBCL), extranodal marginal zone of mucosa-associated lymphoid tissue (MALT) lymphomas or mixed types. PTL may be difficult to diagnose by FNA but flow cytometry (confirming the clonal origin of the tumor) and atypical lymphocytes often help distinguish PTL from Hashimoto's thyroiditis.

The diagnosis of PTL is typically made between the ages of 50 and 80, with a peak incidence in the sixth decade. An older patient with a rapidly enlarging neck mass and history of Hashimoto's thyroiditis should raise the suspicion for primary thyroid lymphoma.

Staging

Multiple classification systems have been developed for WDTC to identify patients of low, intermediate and high risk. Risk-stratification systems include: AMES (age, presence of distant metastases or extrathyroidal extension and size of tumor), AGES (age, grade, extrathyroidal extension and size of tumor), MACIS (metastases, age, completeness of resection, invasion and size of tumor) and others depicted in **Table 21-3**. The TNM staging system by the American Joint Committee on Cancer (AJCC) incorporates three essential components: the size and extent of the primary tumor (T), lymph node involvement (N) and evidence of distant metastasis (M)

TABLE 21-3	Risk-stratification systems for patients with well-differentiated thyroid carcinoma						
Prognostic factors	**Risk-Stratification Systems**						
	EORTC (1979)	**AGES (1987)**	**AMES (1988)**	**U OF C (1990)**	**MACIS (1993)**	**OSU (1994)**	**MSKCC (1995)**
Age	x	x	x		x		x
Sex	x		x				
Size		x	x	x	x	x	x
Multicentricity						x	
Histological grade		x					x
Histological type	x	x	x		x		x
Extrathyroid invasion	x	x	x	x	x	x	x
Nodal involvement				x		x	x
Distant metastasis	x	x	x	x	x	x	x
Incomplete resection					x		

EORTC: European Organization for Research and Treatment of Cancer; AGES: Age, Grade, Extent, Size; AMES: Age, Metastasis, Extent, Size; U of C: University of Chicago; MACIS: Metastasis, Age, Completeness of Resection, Invasion, Size; OSU: Ohio State University; MSKCC: Memorial Sloan-Kettering Cancer Center

TABLE 21-4	Thyroid cancer staging system*

T categories for thyroid cancer:

TX:	Primary tumor cannot be assessed
T0:	No evidence of primary tumor
T1:	The tumor is 2 cm (slightly less than an inch) across or smaller
T2:	Tumor is between 2 cm and 4 cm (slightly less than 2 inches) across
T3:	Tumor is larger than 4 cm or has begun to grow into nearby tissues outside the thyroid
T4a:	Tumor of any size and has grown extensively beyond the thyroid gland into nearby tissues of the neck
T4b:	Tumor has grown either back toward the spine or into nearby large blood vessels

For anaplastic thyroid cancers:

T4a:	Tumor is still within the thyroid and may be resectable (removable by surgery)
T4b:	Tumor has grown outside of the thyroid and is not resectable

N categories for thyroid cancer:

NX:	Regional (nearby) lymph nodes cannot be assessed
N0:	No spread to nearby lymph nodes
N1:	Spread to nearby lymph nodes
N1a:	Spread to lymph nodes around the thyroid in the neck (cervical)
N1b:	Spread to lymph nodes in the sides of the neck (lateral cervical) or the upper chest (upper mediastinal)

M categories for thyroid cancer:

MX:	Presence of distant metastasis (spread) cannot be assessed
M0:	No distant metastasis
M1:	Distant metastasis is present, involving distant lymph nodes, internal organs, bones, etc.

Stage Grouping:

Stage Grouping for Papillary or Follicular Thyroid Carcinoma (Differentiated Thyroid Cancer)

Patients younger than 45 years:
Stage I (any T, any N, M0)
Stage II (any T, any N, M1)

Patients 45 years and older:
Stage I (T1, N0, M0)
Stage II (T2, N0, M0)
Stage III (T3, N0, M0 or T1-3, N1a, M0)
Stage IVA (T4a, N0-1a, M0 or T1-4, N1b, M0)
Stage IVB (T4b, any N, M0)
Stage IVC (any T, any N, M1)

Stage Grouping for Medullary Thyroid Carcinoma
Stage grouping for medullary thyroid carcinoma in people of any age is the same as for papillary or follicular carcinoma in people older than age 45.

Stage Grouping for Anaplastic/Undifferentiated Thyroid Carcinoma
All anaplastic thyroid cancers are considered stage IV, reflecting the poor prognosis of this type of cancer.
Stage IVA (T4a, any N, M0)
Stage IVB (T4b, any N, M0)
Stage IVC (any T, any N, M1)

*Adapted with permission from the American Joint Committee on Cancer Staging Manual, 6th edn.

(Table 21-4). Subsequent staging takes into account the histological subtype, the TNM classification, as well as the patient's age. Future risk stratification systems will likely incorporate molecular characteristics of the primary tumor, as the prognosis associated with various tumor mutations becomes better understood.

In general, WDTC is considered low risk if all tumor is resected with no local or vascular invasion, there are no local or distant metastases and no aggressive histological or molecular subtypes (e.g. tall cell variant or BRAF-positive tumors). Intermediate risk WDTC is characterized by aggressive histological or molecular subtypes, microscopic extrathyroidal extension, vascular invasion or positive cervical lymph node metastases. High risk WDTC has macroscopic local invasion, incomplete resection or distant metastases.

Management

Preoperative Evaluation

In addition to a complete history and physical examination, a focused neck exam is an integral part of the preoperative evaluation of patients undergoing surgery for biopsy-proven thyroid cancer or high risk lesions. Any suspicion on history or physical examination of vocal cord paralysis should prompt evaluation via fiberoptic laryngoscopy. Preoperative neck US of the entire thyroid with bilateral cervical lymph node mapping is highly recommended. In addition, US-guided FNA of palpable or sonographically suspicious lymph nodes should be performed to detect lymph node metastases for preoperative staging and surgical planning. Other radiographic modalities, such as CT, MRI, PET, are not necessary as part of the initial preoperative evaluation of thyroid cancer. A neck and chest CT scan may be obtained preoperatively for patients with large goiters, ATC and PTL to assess the extent of the disease and rule out substernal component. A routine preoperative thyroglobulin measurement is not recommended.

Role of Neoadjuvant Therapy

Neoadjuvant chemotherapy has no role in the current management of WDTC or MTC. Neoadjuvant radiation therapy (XRT) in the form of external beam radiation (EBRT) can be considered for patients with inoperable, locally invasive PDTC. However, neoadjuvant EBRT should be restrictively and judiciously utilized, as it often complicates subsequent operations due to the development of fibrosis and adhesions.

On the other hand, multimodal neoadjuvant therapy does have a role in the treatment of ATC. Some studies have shown combined neoadjuvant chemotherapy and radiation therapy may have a positive effect on local control and may allow subsequent palliative resection of previously inoperable tumors. The widely used combination chemotherapeutic agents are Adriamycin and Cisplatin. However, neoadjuvant therapy in ATC has not been shown to improve survival.

Successful treatment of PTL is based on accurate identification of the histological subtype and staging. Both diffuse large B-cell and mixed lymphomas are best treated with multimodality therapy consisting of CHOP (Cyclophosphamide, Adriamycin, Vincristine and Prednisone) combined with XRT. MALT lymphomas with their more indolent course may be amenable to single modality XRT or total thyroidectomy alone if diagnosed at an early stage.

Surgical Treatment

PTC

Total thyroidectomy for PTC > 1 cm has been shown on multivariate analysis to significantly reduce recurrence rates and improve survival. PTC is frequently a multifocal disease. Total thyroidectomy provides the most complete cancer clearance, more effective postoperative radioactive iodine ablation and identification of distant metastases and enables the use of thyroglobulin as a marker to monitor for recurrence postoperatively.

For suspicious or indeterminate unilateral, unifocal lesions less than 4 cm in size, whose malignant potential has not been determined by FNA, an ipsilateral thyroid lobectomy with isthmusectomy is considered the minimal initial surgical procedure until further pathology is confirmed. For unilateral, unifocal PTC that are subcentimeter in size, without evidence of metastasis, capsular extension or angiolymphatic invasion in low-risk patients, lobectomy alone may be sufficient, although the patient should undergo regular surveillance of the remaining lobe to screen for recurrence.

Most surgeons agree that total thyroidectomy is the best surgical approach for all patients with unilateral and unifocal suspicious lesions greater than 4 cm in size, or suspicious lesions of any size in high risk patients. Total thyroidectomy is also recommended for all documented PTC > 1 cm, all PTC associated with local or distant metastasis and all PTC in high risk patients.

The extent of cervical lymph node dissection in PTC is a controversial topic. Multiple studies have shown that nodal involvement increases the risk of local recurrence but has little effect on survival in otherwise low risk patients. The rate of lymph node involvement in PTC is at least 20-50%. Prophylactic lymph node dissections have identified lymph node micrometastases in up to 80%, the significance of which is unknown. Cervical lymph node metastases are detected either via palpation pre- and intraoperatively, or via US and FNA preoperatively.

Cervical lymph node compartments are depicted in **Figure 21-3**. Most experienced thyroid surgeons recommend complete central compartment (level VI-VII) lymph node dissection for PTC with clinically involved lymph nodes. Prophylactic central compartment lymph node dissection should be considered in patients with large or high risk tumors (T3 or T4). If nodal metastases are clinically present laterally, then the surgeon should perform a functional or modified radical lymph node dissection (levels II-V) on the affected side.

FTC and HCC

In contrast to PTC, most FTC and HCC tend to be larger (greater than 2 cm), solitary and unilateral. As it is impossible to differentiate malignant from benign

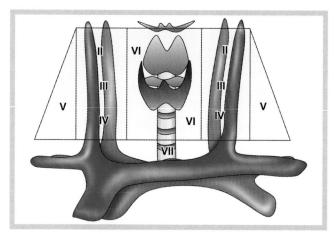

Figure 21-3: Cervical lymph node (LN) compartments. Level I: submandibular and submental LN (not depicted in this figure). Levels II, III and IV: upper, middle and lower jugular LN. Level V: posterior triangle LN (posterior to the SCM). Level VI: From the hyoid bone superiorly, to the upper border of the manubrium inferiorly, between the carotid arteries laterally. Level VII: From the upper border of the manubrium superiorly, to the innominate artery inferiorly, between the carotid arteries laterally

follicular or Hürthle cell lesions on FNA, a diagnostic thyroid lobectomy and isthmusectomy is the recommended initial procedure for all follicular and oncocytic (Hürthle cell) lesions. If the lesion is benign on final pathology, no further surgical intervention is needed. However, if the lesion is malignant with capsular or vascular invasion, then the recommended approach is to perform a completion thyroidectomy. Low risk patients who are found on permanent pathology to have FTC with minimal or limited capsular invasion may not require completion thyroidectomy. Only 10% of FTC and about 25% of HCC have nodal metastases at the time of diagnosis. Compartment-oriented lymph node dissection is indicated only if there is clinical evidence of nodal involvement (palpable or via US and confirmed on FNA). When lymphadenopathy is extensive in a patient with a follicular neoplasm, the tumor is likely an invasive follicular variant of PTC.

MTC

A complete family history is essential of patients diagnosed with MTC. Any family history of thyroid cancer, pheochromocytoma or hyperparathyroidism should raise the suspicion for hereditary MTC syndrome. All patients with MTC should undergo biochemical screening for pheochromocytoma, with 24-hour urine collection for metanephrines, followed by CT or MRI for localization if metanephrines are positive. A baseline calcium level should be obtained to rule out primary hyperparathyroidism. Finally, all patients should undergo genetic testing for germline RET proto-oncogene mutations. If an MTC patient is diagnosed with pheochromocytoma, adrenalectomy should precede thyroidectomy, after appropriate fluid resuscitation and alpha blockade.

Surgical resection is the only effective treatment for MTC. Parafollicular (C) cells do not take up iodine, thus radioiodine ablation is not an effective adjuvant treatment. Patients with MTC should undergo total thyroidectomy with central compartment lymph node dissection. Ipsilateral modified radical lymph node dissection should be considered if central compartment nodes are positive. Contralateral modified radical lymph node dissection is also warranted if abnormal contralateral lymph nodes are noted via preoperative US or intraoperative examination, or if bilateral tumors are present.

Patients with MTC and a germline RET mutation should have family members undergo genetic counseling and testing for the same mutation. Guidelines have been developed for the management of family members with a hereditary form of MTC (e.g. FMTC, MEN IIA and IIB) based on their specific RET codon mutation. Although all are high risk mutations with penetrance of close to 100%, RET codons are classified into three risk levels, which are used to determine the appropriate timing of prophylactic thyroidectomy **(Table 21-5)**.

TABLE 21-5	RET codon mutations, risk levels and management in hereditary MTC	
Risk level	**Mutational codons**	**Recommended management**
Level 1 (high risk)	768, 790, 791, 804, 891	Controversial; some advocate for prophylactic thyroidectomy by age 5 years, others by age 10 years, while some recommend periodic calcitonin testing with surgery at first abnormal level
Level 2 (higher risk)	609, 611, 618, 620, 630, 634	Prophylactic thyroidectomy before the age of 5 years
Level 3 (highest risk)	883, 918, 922	Prophylactic thyroidectomy within the first 6 months of life
Type of hereditary MTC	**Mutational codons**	
FMTC	609, 611, 618, 620, 630, 634, 768, 790, 791, 804, 891	
MEN IIA	609, 611, 618, 620, 634, 790, 791	
MEN IIB	883, 918, 922	

ATC

Surgery plays a limited and more palliative role in the treatment of ATC. However, it remains an important component of the multimodal approach to this disease. Although, radical resection of ATC is often discouraged secondary to significant morbidity, debulking thyroidectomy should be considered for symptomatic patients as it provides a form of palliation when combined with adjuvant chemotherapy and radiation. On the other hand, neoadjuvant chemotherapy and radiation followed by debulking have been shown to achieve good local control and avoid tracheostomy for some patients with ATC.

PTL

Multiple studies have shown no difference in survival in patients with PTL who were treated with surgical debulking plus adjuvant chemotherapy and radiation versus those who received chemotherapy and radiation alone. However, when FNA and flow cytometry fail to diagnose PTL in an enlarging or symptomatic goiter, surgical resection should be performed for diagnostic and therapeutic purposes.

Lymph Node Dissection

Cervical lymph nodes are grouped into seven levels **(Figure 21-3)**. Complete central compartment lymph node dissection (level VI-VII) includes the removal of all lymphatic and fibrofatty tissue between the two carotid arteries laterally, from the hyoid bone superiorly, down to the innominate vessels inferiorly. The most common locations for involved lymph nodes in the central compartment are the prelaryngeal (Delphian), pretracheal and bilateral paratracheal lymph nodes.

Functional or modified radical lymph node dissection (Levels II, III, IV and V) involves the removal of all lymphatic and fibrofatty tissue along the jugular chain from the angle of the mandible superiorly to the innominate vessels inferiorly, from the anterior border of the trapezius muscle laterally to the common carotid artery medially and to the anterior scalene muscle posteriorly. The jugular vein, sternocleidomastoid muscle, phrenic, spinal accessory, vagus, cervical sensory and brachial plexus nerves are preserved intact.

Parathyroids

If the blood supply to the parathyroid glands is compromised or if they cannot be preserved *in situ* during a total thyroidectomy, then resection and biopsy should be performed to confirm the presence of normal parathyroid tissue, followed by auto-transplantation, typically into the sternocleidomastoid, strap or non-dominant brachioradialis muscle.

Anatomical and Surgical Considerations (Figure 21-4)

Nonrecurrent Laryngeal Nerve

The course of the recurrent laryngeal nerve (RLN) differs on the right and left sides of the neck. The left RLN branches from the vagus at the level of the aortic arch. It then passes below the arch and reverses its course to continue superiorly, posterior to the aortic arch and into the visceral compartment of the neck. It travels near or in the tracheoesophageal groove until it enters the larynx just behind the cricothyroid articulation. The right RLN branches from the vagus more superiorly than does the left, at the level of the subclavian artery. It loops behind the right subclavian artery and ascends superiomedially toward the tracheoesophageal groove. It then continues superiorly until entering the larynx behind the cricothyroid articulation. In approximately 5 of 1000 patients, a nonrecurrent laryngeal nerve is found on the right side. This arrangement typically occurs when a retroesophageal right subclavian artery arises from the dorsal side of the aortic arch. The nonrecurrent laryngeal nerve branches from the vagus at approximately the level of the cricoid cartilage and directly enters the larynx without looping around the subclavian artery. A left-sided nonrecurrent laryngeal nerve is even more rare and occurs when a right-sided aortic arch and ligamentum arteriosum are concurrent with a left retroesophageal subclavian artery.

Reoperative Neck

Reoperative thyroid surgery may be performed for a variety of reasons, such as completion thyroidectomy for well-differentiated thyroid cancer (WDTC), recurrence of thyroid cancer in the cervical lymph nodes or thyroid bed, or a new primary tumor in the thyroid remnant after a previous neck operation for benign disease.

Attention should be paid to anatomical changes that may be encountered during reoperative thyroid surgery. The carotid sheath is a very important landmark for lymph node dissection; however, it may medialize following thyroidectomy and be located directly adjacent to the trachea. In addition, fibrosis from prior surgery may cause increased difficulty in identifying and preserving the recurrent laryngeal nerve and parathyroid glands.

Substernal Goiter

Substernal goiter is generally defined as a thyroid mass that has 50% or more of its volume located below the thoracic inlet. It remains a significant consideration in the differential diagnosis of mediastinal masses, particularly those located in the anterior mediastinum. Most surgeons consider the presence of a substernal goiter to be an indication for surgical resection in an acceptable surgical candidate. The rationale is primarily related to the risk of

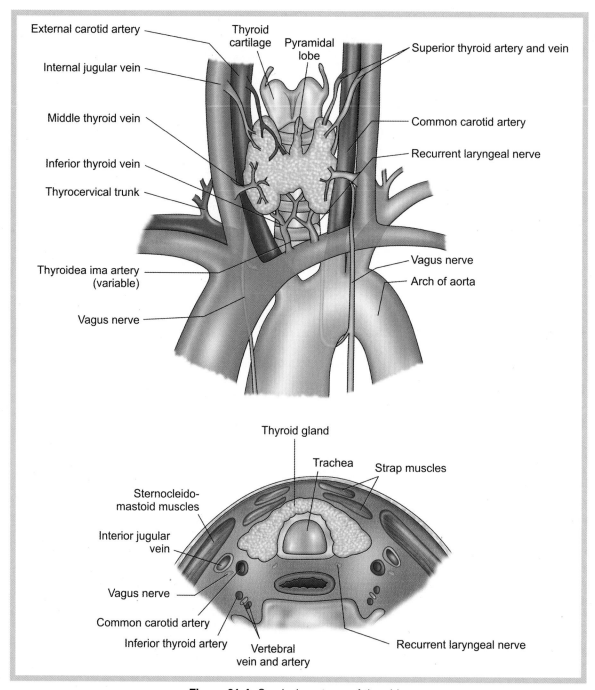

Figure 21-4: Surgical anatomy of thyroid

serious complications that can occur because of compression of visceral or vascular structures within the bony thoracic cavity, most importantly airway compromise. Additional reasons include the relative ineffectiveness of thyroid hormone suppressive therapy and concerns that delaying surgery until compressive symptoms develop may render the operation more technically difficult. Finally, malignancy has been reported in 5-15% of substernal goiters and FNA biopsy for definitive diagnosis may be dangerous or impossible.

Substernal goiters most commonly descend into the anterosuperior mediastinum. The great vessels may be near the capsule of the gland or displaced anteriorly or inferiorly, although the predominant vascular supply typically remains in a cervical location, allowing the surgeon to mobilize the goiter out of the superior mediastinum through a standard cervical incision without the need for sternotomy. Typically, substernal goiters descend to one side of the trachea or the other, causing tracheoesophageal deviation to the contralateral side.

Centrally located substernal goiters may compress the trachea between the sternum and spine, displacing the esophagus. When goiters are located in the anterosuperior mediastinum, the recurrent laryngeal nerve is usually not displaced from the tracheoesophageal groove, but it may on occasion be wrapped tightly around the goiter. Occasionally, substernal goiters may extend into the posterior mediastinum between the trachea and esophagus, significantly displacing these structures and distorting the normal relationship of the recurrent laryngeal nerve with the trachea. Goiters located in the posterior mediastinum or posterior thoracic cavity may also be complicated by a relatively normal location of the great vessels, making anterior exposure more difficult. Finally, goiters extending into the posterior thoracic cavity are extrapleural and behind the lung, which also makes anterior exposure more difficult.

Surgical Complications

Although thyroid surgery is generally considered a safe procedure, it has a host of potential complications that must be discussed with the patient preoperatively.

Injury to the Recurrent Laryngeal Nerve

The recurrent laryngeal nerve (RLN) innervates all of the intrinsic muscles of the larynx with the exception of the cricothyroid muscle, which is innervated by the superior laryngeal nerve (SLN). Deliberate identification of the course of the RLN during thyroidectomy minimizes the risk of injury. When the nerve is visualized and preserved, the reported RLN injury rate during thyroidectomy is 0-2.1%. This rate is reportedly higher in a reoperative neck (2-12%), or if the nerve is not clearly identified (4-6.6%).

The RLN is classically identified as it crosses the inferior thyroid artery in a cephalad direction to enter the larynx, however, the most common site of nerve injury is at the ligament of Berry, where the RLN enters the larynx, just below the cricoid cartilage. The RLN may run deep to the ligament of Berry, pass through it, or even penetrate the thyroid gland a short distance at this level. Although the RLN is described to ascend in the tracheoesophageal groove, the RLN may in fact be more lateral, especially on the right. The course of the right RLN is relatively oblique and lateral, whereas the course of the left RLN is more medial. The nerve may branch several times before entering the larynx and the anterior branch contains the critical motor fibers.

Mechanisms of injury to the RLN include complete or partial transection, traction, contusion, crush, burn, ligation and compromised blood supply. The consequence of such injury is vocal fold paresis or paralysis. Patients with unilateral vocal fold paralysis typically present with postoperative hoarseness. Other potential sequelae of unilateral vocal fold paralysis are dysphagia and aspiration. Bilateral vocal fold paralysis usually manifests acutely after extubation. Both vocal folds are typical in a paramedian position, causing partial airway obstruction. Patients with bilateral vocal fold paralysis present with stridor, respiratory distress or both.

When suspected, injury to the RLN after thyroidectomy should be evaluated via fiberoptic laryngoscopy to assess vocal fold mobility. Laryngeal electromyography (EMG) may be useful to distinguish vocal fold paralysis from cricoarytenoid joint dislocation secondary to intubation. Furthermore, EMG may yield information concerning the prognosis of the patient with RLN injury. Patients with bilateral vocal fold paralysis who present with symptoms of airway compromise require emergency reintubation or tracheostomy. Fiberoptic laryngoscopy may be performed to confirm the diagnosis when the patient is clinically stable.

Indications for treatment of unilateral vocal fold paralysis include dysphonia, aspiration and ineffective cough. Permanent corrective procedures for unilateral vocal fold paralysis are not performed until at least 6 months after thyroidectomy because a reversible injury will improve by that time. However, if aspiration is present, temporary treatment with an absorbable vocal fold injection should be performed. Temporary injections often allow for immediate return of glottic competence while the nerve recovers. If laryngeal EMG after 6 months shows no chance for meaningful RLN recovery, then a permanent injection or medialization laryngoplasty can be offered.

The principal goal for surgery in bilateral vocal fold paralysis is to improve airway patency. Cordotomy and arytenoidectomy are the most common procedures. These procedures enlarge the airway and may permit decannulation of a tracheostomy. However, the patient must be counseled that his or her voice will likely worsen after surgery.

Hypoparathyroidism

Hypoparathyroidism is the most common complication after total thyroidectomy. Hypoparathyroidism and resulting hypocalcemia, may be permanent or transient. The rate of permanent hypoparathyroidism after thyroidectomy is 0.4-13.8%, and is usually caused by direct trauma, devascularization, or inadvertent removal of the parathyroid glands during surgery. The rate of temporary hypoparathyroidism is reported at 2-53% and it is likely due to reversible ischemia of the parathyroid glands during surgery.

Symptoms and signs of hypocalcemia from hypo-parathyroidism include perioral paresthesias, carpopedal spasm, mental status changes, tetany, laryngospasm, seizures, QT prolongation on ECG and cardiac arrest. The Chvostek and Trousseau signs may be elicited at bedside in the setting of hypocalcemia. The Chvostek sign is elicited by tapping the facial nerve in the preauricular area and observing perioral or facial contractions. The Trousseau sign is the induction of carpal spasm upon inflation of a blood pressure cuff. If iatrogenic hypoparathyroidism is a concern, a serum-calcium level should be obtained and supplemental calcium, occasionally with 1,25-OH vitamin D, should be administered until return of normal parathyroid function.

The best way to preserve parathyroid function is to identify all four parathyroid glands and maintain their blood supply. The inferior thyroid artery typically supplies all 4 parathyroid glands, but they often receive collaterals from the superior thyroid artery. The parathyroid glands appear in various shapes and have a caramel-like color, but turn dusky when they lose their blood supply. All parathyroid vessels that are not able to be spared should be ligated as close to the thyroid as possible during thyroidectomy to preserve collaterals. If a devascularized parathyroid gland is identified or a gland is inadvertently removed with the thyroid specimen, then it should be biopsied to confirm normal parathyroid tissue, cut into 1-2 mm pieces and reimplanted in the SCM or strap muscle. The location should be marked with a permanent suture or a clip applier.

Neck Hematoma

The incidence of neck hematoma after thyroid surgery is low (0.3-1%), but it is a devastating complication that all surgeons must be aware of. An unrecognized or rapidly expanding hematoma can impede venous return in the neck and lead to swelling and airway compromise. Such patients should be evaluated immediately. If airway compromise is present, the surgical incision must first be opened to evacuate the hematoma. The airway must be secured either by expedient intubation or if necessary tracheostomy and the patient must then be taken back to the operating room emergently for wound exploration. If the hematoma is not rapidly enlarging and the airway is not compromised, the patient may then be taken to the operating room directly for evacuation and neck exploration.

Complications of Neck Dissection

The neck harbors multiple important structures that can be injured during modified radical lymph node dissection. Injury to the spinal accessory nerve (CN XI) causes paralysis of the ipsilateral SCM and trapezius muscle, cervical sensory nerve injury causes ipsilateral neck numbness, vagus nerve injury may cause postvagotomy syndrome and ipsilateral vocal cord paralysis, phrenic nerve injury may cause ipsilateral hemidiaphragm paralysis and sympathetic ganglion injury may cause an ipsilateral Horner's syndrome. Injuries can also occur to the jugular vein, carotid artery and thoracic duct, causing a chyle leak or chylothorax.

Adjuvant Therapy

Retrospective cohort studies have demonstrated multimodal adjuvant therapy to be beneficial in reducing local recurrence rates of WDTC, with a positive effect on cause-specific long-term survival, particularly in high risk patients. Adjuvant treatment has not been proven to improve outcomes in low risk patients with WDTC.

Following total or near total thyroidectomy for WDTC, the most important component of adjuvant therapy is radioactive iodine (RAI) ablation via the use of I-131. In general, adjuvant treatment with radioactive iodine ablation is recommended for all patients with large (> 4 cm) or locally invasive WDTC, distant metastases and selected patients with smaller tumors and additional intermediate or high risk factors. Patients are given a low dose of I-131 4-6 weeks after total thyroidectomy in order to determine the presence of residual thyroid tissue in the thyroid bed, as well as to identify undiscovered metastatic lesions for staging. The goal of RAI is to maximize iodine uptake by remnant thyroid tissue, under TSH stimulation (goal TSH > 30 mU/L). To achieve that purpose, patients are prepared for RAI with thyroid hormone withdrawal for three weeks. Alternatively, patients can be given an intramuscular injection of Thyrogen™, recombinant human thyrotropin, prior to RAI and avoid thyroid hormone withdrawal symptoms. Approximately one week after the treatment dose of RAI, patients undergo whole body scan to evaluate for distant metastases.

Following thyroidectomy and RAI, all patients with WDTC are treated with thyroid hormone to appropriately suppress TSH. The rationale beyond thyroid hormone suppressive treatment is to prevent stimulation and growth of any remnant cancer cells that are TSH responsive. Patients with high risk WDTC are treated with thyroid hormone to suppress TSH < 0.1 mU/L. Low and intermediate risk WDTC patients are typically suppressed to a goal TSH of 0.1-0.5 mU/L.

RAI and TSH-suppression are of no benefit in the treatment of MTC because these tumors do not take up radioiodine and parafollicular (C) cells do not have TSH receptors for TSH suppression.

External-beam radiation therapy (EBRT) is generally not an effective adjuvant treatment for thyroid cancer, but has been found in some retrospective studies to improve local control for WDTC patients with unresectable advanced local disease or those at high risk for recurrence. MTC patients with unresectable disease may also be candidates for adjuvant EBRT to improve locoregional control. EBRT can also be considered as a palliative treatment for distant metastatic lesions and for patients with ATC.

Chemotherapy is not an effective adjuvant therapy for most thyroid cancers. It has a very limited role in the treatment of WDTC. It has been used with very limited and inconsistent success for symptomatic advanced disease that is surgically unresectable, irresponsive to RAI and not amenable or unresponsive to EBRT. In contrast, chemotherapy, usually CHOP, in combination with radiation is routinely used for the treatment of PTL. The combination of EBRT and doxorubicin-based chemotherapy can improve locoregional control and may prolong survival in small number of patients with ATC.

Recurrence and Management of Metastatic Disease

Surgical resection is the treatment of choice for locally recurrent WDTC. Surgery is less effective for the treatment of distant metastases, but can be used to remove resectable lung nodules or bony metastases that are unresponsive to RAI.

If locally recurrent, iodine-avid WDTC is detected on surveillance RAI-scanning, then additional I-131 can be used to treat small nodal metastasis not large enough for surgical resection. Follow-up whole body scan may demonstrate other metastatic lesions not seen on the surveillance scan. FDG PET and PET-CT imaging **(Figure 21-5)** has evolved as an effective measure to evaluate for recurrent WDTC in patients with elevated serum thyroglobulin (Tg) and negative RAI scans.

EBRT can be used for recurrent WDTC if there is evidence of unresectable local disease that is unresponsive to RAI, although it is of limited efficacy. EBRT may also

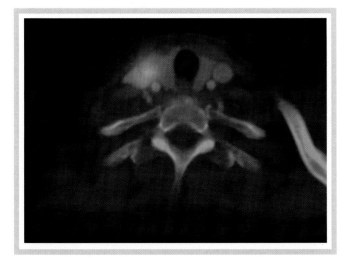

Figure 21-5: FDG-avid 2-cm right thyroid nodule on PET-CT scan, an incidental finding in a 75-year-old female on a follow-up study for possible recurrence of colorectal adenocarcinoma. (*Provided by Mitchel Tublin, MD; Department of Radiology, University of Pittsburgh Medical Center*)

be considered in the treatment of metastatic WDTC, particularly localized or painful bony metastases. Doxorubicin-based chemotherapy may sensitize WDTC metastases to EBRT. EBRT is a component of multimodal therapy for ATC and PTL.

Chemotherapy has a limited role in the treatment of advanced radioiodine-resistant thyroid cancers, such as PDTC, MTC and ATC. Patients with advanced or metastatic thyroid cancer should be considered for clinical trials of new agents such as tyrosine kinase inhibitors, antiangiogenesis agents and growth modulators.

Follow-up and Surveillance

WDTC

The majority of recurrent WDTC is diagnosed in the first 5 years; however, recurrence may also occur decades later. PTC is more likely to recur in the thyroid bed or cervical lymph nodes, while FTC is more likely to recur as distant metastases. WDTC sites of metastasis include the lungs, bone, brain, liver and adrenal glands. Patients with WDTC are usually followed every 6 months for 1-3 years and then yearly after that. Follow-up testing for recurrence includes TSH-stimulated serum Tg measurements and RAI scan, either after thyroid hormone withdrawal or recombinant human thyrotropin. Anti-Tg antibodies, present in about 25% of patients, produce a falsely reduced level of Tg, thus, anti-Tg antibodies are measured simultaneously with serum Tg.

All patients with WDTC should also undergo complete neck ultrasound to screen for recurrence. In low risk patients with undetectable TSH-stimulated Tg and negative RAI scan after remnant ablation, subsequent follow-up can be limited to yearly TSH suppressed Tg measurement, physical exam and ultrasound as indicated. Patients at high risk for local recurrence (e.g. residual microscopic disease, positive nodal disease and extra–thyroidal local invasion) should be followed more closely with TSH-stimulated Tg, ultrasound and RAI scans. Recurrent cervical lymph nodes should be biopsied under ultrasound guidance and the aspirate sent for Tg measurement. FDG PET is helpful in detecting metastases in Tg-positive, RAI-negative patients with WDTC and, if positive, predicts an increased disease specific mortality.

MTC

Neither serum Tg nor RAI scanning are useful in the follow-up of MTC. Calcitonin and CEA levels are followed as tumor markers and can be compared to basal post-operative levels to monitor for recurrence. Routine neck ultrasound is also important for local surveillance and suspicious cervical lymph nodes should be biopsied under ultrasound guidance.

ATC

There are no tumor markers available for ATC, but frequent physical examination and various imaging modalities (US, CT, FDG PET) helps to determine the extent of disease.

New Frontiers and Controversies

The extent of lymph node dissection in the initial surgical treatment of WDTC and the management of recurrent micrometastases remains a controversial topic. Multiple studies have shown that nodal involvement increases the risk of local recurrence but has little effect on survival in otherwise low or intermediate risk patients. Minimizing the risk of local recurrence must be balanced against the potentially increased morbidity of aggressive cervical lymphadenectomy.

The use of RAI in low risk patients is another controversial topic in the treatment of WDTC. Additionally, the dose of I-131 administered varies among different treatment centers. Traditionally, a high-dose regimen of 100-200 mCi has been used routinely in many centers. However, more recently, a lower-dose regimen of 30 mCi has been shown to produce equally effective remnant ablation and should be considered for low risk patients. The long-term risks of secondary malignancy after RAI are low but deserve further study in patients who have been treated with high cumulative doses of I-131.

Novel treatments for WDTC currently under investigation include tyrosine kinase inhibitors, angiogenesis inhibitors and growth modulators. Phase II trials of axitinib, motesanib, sorafenib and thalidomide have documented some clinical efficacy in patients with metastatic thyroid cancer. Other clinical trials are ongoing.

Risk stratification of WDTC continues to evolve. Early identification of molecular markers that appear to correlate with biologic tumor behavior of PTC may help stratify patients into appropriate treatment groups. RET/PTC, RAS or BRAF kinase inhibitors may form the basis of effective new treatment options for WDTC.

Landmark Papers

1. Bonnet S, Hartl D, Leboulleux S, Baudin E, Lumbroso J, Ghuzlan A, et al. Prophylactic lymph node dissection for papillary thyroid cancer less than 2 cm: implications for radioiodine treatment.Journal of Clinical Endocrinology and Metabolism 2009;94:1162-7.
2. Cobin R, Gharib H, Bergman D, Clark O, Cooper D, Daniels G, et al. AACE/AAES medical/surgical guidelines for clinical practice: management of thyroid carcinoma. Endocrine Practice 2001;7.
3. Cooper D, Doherty G, Haugen B, Kloos R, Lee S, Mandel S, et al. Management guidelines for patients with thyroid nodules and differentiated thyroid cancer. Thyroid 2006;16.
4. Gharib H, Papini E, Valcavi R, Baskin HJ, Crescenzi A, Dottorini M, et al. AACE/AME medical guidelines for clinical practice for the diagnosis and management of thyroid nodules. Endocrine Practice 2006;12.
5. Greenblatt H, Herbert C. Palliation of advanced thyroid malignancies. Surgical Oncology 2007;16:237-47.
6. Lang B, Lo C. Surgical options in undifferentiated thyroid carcinoma. Word J Surg 2007;31:969-79.
7. Mazzaferri E. A vision for the surgical management of papillary thyroid carcinoma: extensive lymph node compartmental dissections and selective use of radioiodine. Journal of Clinical Endocrinology and Metabolism 2009; 94:1086-8.
8. Pinchot S, Sippel R, Chen H. Multi-targeted approach in the treatment of thyroid cancer. Therapeutics and Clinical Risk Management 2008;4:935-47.

Level of Evidence Table			
Recommendation	**Grade**	**Best level of evidence**	**References**
Ultrasonography is the initial imaging modality of choice in the workup of a palpable thyroid nodule.	A	3a	1-4
FNA should be performed on all suspicious thyroid nodules.	A	3a	5-8
Total thyroidectomy decreases local recurrence and improves survival compared to thyroid lobectomy in well-differentiated thyroid cancers.	B	2b	9-16
Complete thyroidectomy is associated with greater morbidity than unilateral lobectomy.	B	2c	17-19
Prophylactic central lymph node dissection for papillary thyroid cancer is safe and may reduce recurrence and increase survival.	B	2b	20-24
Complete node dissection of the lateral neck compartment after identification of cervical metastasis reduces recurrence compared to selective dissection.	B	4	25-27
The TNM staging system is the most generalizable and useful staging system for differentiated thyroid carcinoma.	B	1b	28-31
The use of radioiodine after total and near-total thyroidectomy in well-differentiated thyroid cancer decreases recurrence and may improve overall survival.	B	2a	9, 32-34
Adjuvant TSH suppression decreases recurrence and mortality after thyroidectomy for well-differentiated cancer.	B	2a	35-37
The primary modalities of surveillance for recurrence after thyroidectomy and ablation of differentiated thyroid cancer are serum thyroglobulin level and neck ultrasound.	B	2b	38-40
Selective resection of metastases (as part of multimodal therapy with radioiodine and external beam radiation) from differentiated thyroid cancer potentially improves survival.	B	4	41-44
Total thyroidectomy is indicated in anticipation of radioiodine therapy for differentiated thyroid cancer metastatic at presentation.	B	2b	45
Testing for *RET* mutations should be performed in patients with MEN II, medullary thyroid cancer and primary C cell hyperplasia. Prophylactic thyroidectomy is indicated for identified carriers.	A	1c	46
Patients with localized medullary thyroid cancer should undergo total thyroidectomy with prophylactic central compartment dissection.	B	2b	47, 48
Pheochromocytoma must be excluded prior to operation for MTC in MEN II. If present, surgical resection then takes precedence.	A	1c	46

References

1. Morris LF, Ragavendra N, Yeh MW. Evidence-based assessment of the role of ultrasonography in the management of benign thyroid nodules. World J Surg 2008; 32:1253-63.
2. Stulak JM, Grant CS, Farley DR, et al. Value of preoperative ultrasonography in the surgical management of initial and reoperative papillary thyroid cancer. Arch Surg 2006; 141:489-94; discussion 494-6.
3. Tan GH, Gharib H, Reading CC. Solitary thyroid nodule. Comparison between palpation and ultrasonography. Arch Intern Med 1995; 155:2418-23.
4. Kouvaraki MA, Shapiro SE, Fornage BD, et al. Role of preoperative ultrasonography in the surgical management of patients with thyroid cancer. Surgery 2003; 134:946-54; discussion 954-5.
5. Lundgren CI, Zedenius J Skoog L. Fine-needle aspiration biopsy of benign thyroid nodules: an evidence-based review. World J Surg 2008; 32:1247-52.

6. Tee YY, Lowe AJ, Brand CA, et al. Fine-needle aspiration may miss a third of all malignancy in palpable thyroid nodules: a comprehensive literature review. Ann Surg 2007; 246:714-20.

7. Braga M, Cavalcanti TC, Collaco LM, et al. Efficacy of ultrasound-guided fine-needle aspiration biopsy in the diagnosis of complex thyroid nodules. J Clin Endocrinol Metab 2001; 86:4089-91.

8. Alexander EK, Heering JP, Benson CB, et al. Assessment of nondiagnostic ultrasound-guided fine needle aspirations of thyroid nodules. J Clin Endocrinol Metab 2002; 87:4924-7.

9. Mazzaferri EL, Jhiang SM. Long-term impact of initial surgical and medical therapy on papillary and follicular thyroid cancer. Am J Med 1994; 97:418-28.

10. Mazzaferri EL, Kloos RT. Clinical review 128: Current approaches to primary therapy for papillary and follicular thyroid cancer. J Clin Endocrinol Metab 2001; 86:1447-63.

11. Kebebew E, Duh QY, Clark OH. Total thyroidectomy or thyroid lobectomy in patients with low-risk differentiated thyroid cancer: surgical decision analysis of a controversy using a mathematical model. World J Surg 2000; 24:1295-302.

12. Grant CS, Hay ID, Gough IR, et al. Local recurrence in papillary thyroid carcinoma: is extent of surgical resection important? Surgery 1988; 104:954-62.

13. Hay ID, Grant CS, Bergstralh EJ, et al. Unilateral total lobectomy: is it sufficient surgical treatment for patients with AMES low-risk papillary thyroid carcinoma? Surgery 1998; 124:958-64; discussion 964-6.

14. Esnaola NF, Cantor SB, Sherman SI, et al. Optimal treatment strategy in patients with papillary thyroid cancer: a decision analysis. Surgery 2001; 130:921-30.

15. Wanebo H, Coburn M, Teates D, et al. Total thyroidectomy does not enhance disease control or survival even in high-risk patients with differentiated thyroid cancer. Ann Surg 1998; 227:912-21.

16. Bilimoria KY, Bentrem DJ, Ko CY, et al. Extent of surgery affects survival for papillary thyroid cancer. Ann Surg 2007; 246:375-81; discussion 381-4.

17. Zerey M, Prabhu AS, Newcomb WL, et al. Short-term outcomes after unilateral versus complete thyroidectomy for malignancy: a national perspective. Am Surg 2009; 75:20-4.

18. Rosato L, Avenia N, Bernante P, et al. Complications of thyroid surgery: analysis of a multicentric study on 14,934 patients operated on in Italy over 5 years. World J Surg 2004; 28:271-6.

19. Rafferty MA, Goldstein DP, Rotstein L, et al. Completion thyroidectomy versus total thyroidectomy: is there a difference in complication rates? An analysis of 350 patients. J Am Coll Surg 2007; 205:602-7.

20. Chisholm EJ, Kulinskaya E Tolley NS. Systematic review and meta-analysis of the adverse effects of thyroidectomy combined with central neck dissection as compared with thyroidectomy alone. Laryngoscope 2009; 119:1135-9.

21. Moo TA, Umunna B, Kato M, et al. Ipsilateral versus bilateral central neck lymph node dissection in papillary thyroid carcinoma. Ann Surg 2009; 250:403-8.

22. Koo BS, Choi EC, Yoon YH, et al. Predictive factors for ipsilateral or contralateral central lymph node metastasis in unilateral papillary thyroid carcinoma. Ann Surg 2009; 249:840-4.

23. Shah MD, Hall FT, Eski SJ, et al. Clinical course of thyroid carcinoma after neck dissection. Laryngoscope 2003; 113:2102-7.

24. Scheumann GF, Gimm O, Wegener G, et al. Prognostic significance and surgical management of locoregional lymph node metastases in papillary thyroid cancer. World J Surg 1994; 18:559-67; discussion 567-8.

25. Cognetti DM, Pribitkin EA, Keane WM. Management of the neck in differentiated thyroid cancer. Surg Oncol Clin N Am 2008; 17:157-73, ix.

26. Davidson HC, Park BJ, Johnson JT. Papillary thyroid cancer: controversies in the management of neck metastasis. Laryngoscope 2008; 118:2161-5.

27. Kupferman ME, Patterson M, Mandel SJ, et al. Patterns of lateral neck metastasis in papillary thyroid carcinoma. Arch Otolaryngol Head Neck Surg 2004; 130:857-60.

28. Lang BH, Chow SM, Lo CY, et al. Staging systems for papillary thyroid carcinoma: a study of 2 tertiary referral centers. Ann Surg 2007; 246:114-21.

29. Lang BH, Lo CY, Chan WF, et al. Staging systems for papillary thyroid carcinoma: a review and comparison. Ann Surg 2007; 245:366-78.

30. Brierley JD, Panzarella T, Tsang RW, et al. A comparison of different staging systems predictability of patient outcome. Thyroid carcinoma as an example. Cancer 1997; 79:2414-23.

31. Loh KC, Greenspan FS, Gee L, et al. Pathological tumor-node-metastasis (pTNM) staging for papillary and follicular thyroid carcinomas: a retrospective analysis of 700 patients. J Clin Endocrinol Metab 1997; 82:3553-62.

32. Mazzaferri EL. Thyroid remnant 131I ablation for papillary and follicular thyroid carcinoma. Thyroid 1997; 7:265-71.

33. Sawka AM, Brierley JD, Tsang RW, et al. An updated systematic review and commentary examining the effectiveness of radioactive iodine remnant ablation in well-differentiated thyroid cancer. Endocrinol Metab Clin North Am 2008; 37:457-80, x.

34. Toniato A, Boschin I, Casara D, et al. Papillary thyroid carcinoma: factors influencing recurrence and survival. Ann Surg Oncol 2008; 15:1518-22.

35. Cooper DS, Specker B, Ho M, et al. Thyrotropin suppression and disease progression in patients with differentiated thyroid cancer: results from the National Thyroid Cancer Treatment Cooperative Registry. Thyroid 1998; 8:737-44.

36. McGriff NJ, Csako G, Gourgiotis L, et al. Effects of thyroid hormone suppression therapy on adverse clinical outcomes in thyroid cancer. Ann Med 2002; 34:554-64.

37. Jonklaas J, Sarlis NJ, Litofsky D, et al. Outcomes of patients with differentiated thyroid carcinoma following initial therapy. Thyroid 2006; 16:1229-42.

38. Kloos RT Mazzaferri EL. A single recombinant human thyrotropin-stimulated serum thyroglobulin measurement predicts differentiated thyroid carcinoma metastases three to five years later. J Clin Endocrinol Metab 2005; 90: 5047-57.

39. Rosario PW, Borges MA, Fagundes TA, et al. Is stimulation of thyroglobulin (Tg) useful in low-risk patients with thyroid carcinoma and undetectable Tg on thyroxin and negative neck ultrasound? Clin Endocrinol (Oxf) 2005; 62:121-5.

40. Pacini F, Molinaro E, Castagna MG, et al. Recombinant human thyrotropin-stimulated serum thyroglobulin combined with neck ultrasonography has the highest sensitivity in monitoring differentiated thyroid carcinoma. J Clin Endocrinol Metab 2003; 88:3668-73.

41. Zettinig G, Fueger BJ, Passler C, et al. Long-term follow-up of patients with bone metastases from differentiated thyroid carcinoma — surgery or conventional therapy? Clin Endocrinol (Oxf) 2002; 56:377-82.

42. Niederle B, Roka R, Schemper M, et al. Surgical treatment of distant metastases in differentiated thyroid cancer: indication and results. Surgery 1986; 100:1088-97.

43. Pak H, Gourgiotis L, Chang WI, et al. Role of metastasectomy in the management of thyroid carcinoma: the NIH experience. J Surg Oncol 2003; 82:10-8.

44. Stojadinovic A, Shoup M, Ghossein RA, et al. The role of operations for distantly metastatic well-differentiated thyroid carcinoma. Surgery 2002; 131:636-43.

45. Sampson E, Brierley JD, Le LW, et al. Clinical management and outcome of papillary and follicular (differentiated) thyroid cancer presenting with distant metastasis at diagnosis. Cancer 2007; 110:1451-6.

46. Kloos RT, Eng C, Evans DB, et al. Medullary thyroid cancer: management guidelines of the American Thyroid Association. Thyroid 2009; 19:565-612.

47. Moley JF, DeBenedetti MK. Patterns of nodal metastases in palpable medullary thyroid carcinoma: recommendations for extent of node dissection. Ann Surg 1999; 229:880-7; discussion 887-8.

48. Pelizzo MR, Boschin IM, Bernante P, et al. Natural history, diagnosis, treatment and outcome of medullary thyroid cancer: 37 years experience on 157 patients. Eur J Surg Oncol 2007; 33:493-7.

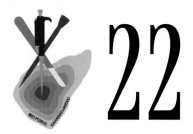

22

Parathyroid

Michael T Stang, Sally E Carty

Hyperparathyroidism (HPT) is the clinical manifestation of a functional parathyroid neoplasm causing parathormone (PTH) excess. PTH can be overproduced in several complex settings which are termed primary (PHPT), secondary (SHPT) and tertiary hyperparathyroidism (THPT). PHPT can arise sporadically or from inherited syndromes that include multiple endocrine neoplasia type 1 (MEN1), multiple endocrine neoplasia type 2A (MEN2A), isolated familial hyperparathyroidism (FHPT) and familial hyperparathyroidism-jaw tumor syndrome (FHJT). SHPT is caused by renal insufficiency, hypocalcemia, hyperphosphatemia and/or severe vitamin D deficiency. THPT occurs by definition with a history of renal failure, and is diagnosed when long-standing SHPT becomes autonomous and results in hypercalcemia.

Overall, the neoplastic enlargement of two or more parathyroid glands is dubbed multiglandular disease (MGD). The rate of MGD varies widely by HPT disease type. Although in SHPT hyperplasia is always present, in PHPT and THPT the neoplastic process governing PTH excess can be a solitary enlarged gland (adenoma), two enlarged glands (double adenomata), diffuse enlargement of all glands (hyperplasia) or a malignant growth (carcinoma). Therefore, the dual issues in successful treatment of HPT are correct identification of the HPT type which determines the likelihood of MGD, and correct surgical management to achieve biochemical cure.

Epidemiology

The incidence of PHPT is reported to be increasing in recent decades but this trend is very likely due to improved disease recognition. Prior to the mid 1970s, PHPT was considered a relatively rare disorder diagnosed only with development of late clinical manifestations (e.g. renal, neural or osteal end organ damage). The introduction of routine automated calcium measurement by multichannel analyzer profoundly changed HPT diagnosis and recently published data place the overall incidence at 27-28 cases per 100,000 people annually.

PHPT is two to three times more common in women and for both sexes the incidence increases with age so that the incidence of PHPT increases to 0.2% for Caucasian women age > 60. Despite the relatively high rate in the general population, PHPT mortality is low accounting for an estimated 0.3 deaths per million per year in the US. To date the morbidities of PHPT and their costs to the US health care system remain incompletely characterized.

Risk Factors

Most cases of PHPT are sporadic and arise without an identifiable etiologic factor other than female sex, age and associated inherited endocrine tumor syndromes. Radiation exposure to the head and neck, particularly in childhood, is also known to increase PHPT risk; children who received external beam radiation for the treatment of tonsillar disease were 2.9 times more likely to develop HPT during their lifetime. The observed increased radiation risk also includes environmental exposure, e.g. Japanese survivors of atomic blasts demonstrated a 4-fold increase in the incidence of parathyroid tumors with an average latency period of 50 years between the point of exposure and the development of detectable parathyroid disease. After childhood irradiation, the onset of PHPT (which arises almost exclusively from parathyroid adenoma in this setting) occurs about a decade later than the onset of radiation-related papillary thyroid cancer.

Because estrogen acts to lower serum calcium, the onset of menopause can uncover mild PHPT. The use of exogenous estrogen after menopause can also delay the diagnosis of mild PHPT; with the recent profound decreases in the use of supplemental estrogen, it will be interesting to observe if there is an increase in the age-related incidence of PHPT in coming years. Although PHPT is notably more prevalent in vitamin D-deficient geographical areas (e.g. in northern latitudes) chronic vitamin D deficiency is not yet a recognized etiologic factor in PHPT.

Presentation and Features of HPT

The clinical features of longstanding PHPT are directly related to the physiologic effects of excess parathormone and hypercalcemia upon end organ function. In patients with normal renal function, a chronically high level of PTH causes an increase in renal reabsorption of filtered calcium, phosphaturia, increased reabsorption of bone and increased synthesis of 1,25-dihydroxyvitamin D_3 [1,25 $(OH)_2D_3$], which in turn augments intestinal calcium absorption.

Historically, patients with advanced PHPT presented with nephrolithiasis, osteitis fibrosa cystica, peptic ulcer, muscle atrophy and even coma. In the modern era, the most common PTHP presentation is by routine biochemical screening, which is widely performed specifically to allow HPT diagnosis prior to the onset of severe symptoms. Most patients with incidentally-diagnosed PHPT are by no means asymptomatic. In order of frequency, the subtler sequelae of HPT include: bone mineralization deficits (osteoporosis or osteopenia), neuromuscular complaints (e.g. fatigue, lethargy, muscle and/or bone aches), neuropsychiatric dysfunction (e.g. insomnia, memory loss, depression and mood disturbance), hypertension, gastrointestinal complaints (e.g. gastroesophageal reflux, dyspepsia and pancreatitis) and polyuria/polydipsia. Many patients with PHPT manifest several of these clinical features as well as general malaise. The subtler features of PHPT are not specific to PHPT however, and so were not described in the early HPT literature and are still underreported in some studies today.

The *degree* of hypercalcemia can influence the presentation of PHPT. Many patients with mild hypercalcemia (10.5-11.0 mg/dL) are minimally symptomatic or asymptomatic but patients with moderate hypercalcemia (11-14 mg/dL) are more often symptomatic and the risk of significant disability rises sharply when calcium levels climb above 12 mg/dL. Severe hypercalcemia (> 14 mg/dL) is associated with progressive lethargy, altered mental status and even coma and should be regarded as a medical emergency requiring hospital admission. The *rate* of rise in serum calcium can also influence PHPT presentation; chronically hypercalcemic patients may function relatively normally whereas patients with calcium levels that rise abruptly often experience symptoms at lesser absolute calcium levels. Elderly and/or debilitated patients can be more adversely affected by hypercalcemia compared to patients without medical disability.

PHPT affects the renal system in several interdependent ways. Elevated calcium inhibits antidiuretic hormone (ADH) secretion, promoting a state of relative dehydration (nephrogenic diabetes insipidus) with the oft-reported polydipsia and polyuria. A more distal consequence of PHPT is nephrolithiasis, although this occurs less frequently in the modern era. Early studies reported renal stones in up to 40% of patients but with routine screening for abnormal calcium, this percentage has declined to 15-20% of modern patients with PHPT. The renal calcifications observed in PHPT are typically composed of calcium oxalate or calcium phosphate and likely result from compensatory hypercalciuria which eventually leads to calcific disease of the renal parenchyma (nephrocalcinosis). If left uncorrected, nephrocalcinosis can ultimately result in renal insufficiency, an end organ disease that is not reversed by curative parathyroid surgery.

Excess PTH induces abnormally high bone turnover particularly at sites rich in cortical bone, such as the distal radius. By contrast, postmenopausal women with osteoporosis have the greatest deficiencies in cancellous bone at sites such as the vertebral spine. The classic dramatic PHPT sequelae of brown tumors, osteoporotic fractures and osteitis fibrosa cystica are relatively rare now in industrialized countries, but even in mild PHPT, dual-energy X-ray absorptiometry (DEXA) bone scans routinely show reduced cortical bone density. The diminished bone density of PHPT predisposes to fractures of the distal forearm, vertebrae, ribs and pelvis and with curative surgery, PHPT patients demonstrate improvement in vertebral and hip bone mineralization.

With respect to the cardiovascular system, PTH is vasodilatory and has chronotropic and inotropic effects, while hypercalcemia is associated with vascular and valvular calcification, hypertension, left ventricular hypertrophy and diastolic dysfunction. With surgical correction of HPT, ventricular hypertrophy will improve along with concurrent stabilization of valvular sclerosis, but hypertension does not reverse postoperatively. PHPT is reportedly associated with an increased risk of cardiovascular related mortality and myocardial infarction, which *does* normalize within one year following curative parathyroid surgery.

Patients with PHPT often report a sensation of early fatigue. Classically, advanced PHPT was associated with proximal muscle weakness affecting the lower extremities and was characterized by neuropathic atrophy of type-2 muscle fibers. In the modern era, this degree of neuromuscular dysfunction is rare but over half of PHPT patients will report some degree of muscle cramping or myoneuralgia. Fatigue symptoms are quite common and resolve in 80% of PTHP patients with operative cure. The neuropsychiatric symptoms of PHPT, including depression, anxiety, malaise and impaired cognition, also demonstrably improve with normalization of PTH and calcium levels.

As with PHPT, the clinical spectrum of SHPT has changed over time with more astute detection and with earlier treatment of patients on renal replacement therapy.

Historically, symptoms of bone pain, myopathy, tendon rupture and extraskeletal calcifications were common but today most patients with SHPT are less frequently symptomatic. Some complications of SHPT can require close attention including early coronary artery calcification, debilitating bone pain, cardiomyopathy, pruritis, uremic calcific arteriolopathy (calciphylaxis) and neuropsychiatric issues.

Pathology and Histology

Parathyroid adenomas are benign neoplasms composed of chief cells, oncocytic cells or transitional oncocytic cells and are typically separated from an adjacent rim of normocellular parathyroid tissue by a fibrous capsule. The cells of adenomas are usually arranged in sheets but can occasionally be observed in trabecular or follicular patterns. The nuclei are generally rounded with dense chromatin and are larger than those of the adjacent normal parathyroid cells. Mitotic figures may be present in up to 70% of cases; however, the proliferative fraction as assessed with Ki-67 is generally less than 4%. Tumor cells are positive for cytokeratins, PTH and chromogranin A. Occasionally, parathyroid adenomas may have a follicular architecture difficult to differentiate from thyroid neoplasm.

Parathyroid adenomas represent a mono- or oligoclonal expansion resulting from loss of growth inhibition. A well described molecular abnormality involves the cyclin D1 (CCND1/PRAD1) oncogene, which produces a protein in parathyroid adenoma that inactivates the tumor suppressor retinoblastoma (Rb) protein to promote cell cycle progression. CCND1 gene rearrangements result in placement of the 5' regulatory domain of the PTH gene in proximity to the CCND1 gene and thus overexpression of cyclin D1 protein. This specific rearrangement is present in only about 5% of adenomas; however, 20-40% overexpress CCND1 by at least one of several mechanisms. The MEN1 tumor suppressor gene, with its protein product *menin* which is involved in transcriptional regulation of JunD, also plays a role in the pathogenesis of parathyroid adenomas. A significant proportion (13 - 20%) of parathyroid adenomas are associated with LOH at or near the MEN1 location, or associated with a somatic mutation of the MEN1 gene.

The distinction between asymmetric hyperplasia and adenoma may be extremely difficult, if not impossible, to make by pathologic assessment alone. Hyperplasia is represented by an increase in parenchymal cell mass and occurs as a result of the proliferation of all parathyroid cell types in multiple parathyroid glands. The enlargement of the glands is symmetric in only half of cases and the weight of individual hyperplastic glands can vary from 150 mg to more than 10 gm. In hyperplasia, cells are distributed in diffuse and/or nodular patterns and the amount of stromal fat is usually noticeably decreased. In some instances, however, there may be abundant stromal fat (lipohyperplasia).

Evaluation and Management

Biochemical Diagnosis

As with any surgical disease process the history and physical examinations are of utmost importance, but in PHPT it is unfortunately also a fact that at least 10% of initial operative failures arise from incorrect diagnosis. The initial clinical evaluation is thus directed at recognizing signs or symptoms of PHPT (above), confirming the biochemical diagnosis and identifying inherited forms of PHPT (below).

When hypercalcemia is identified either as a result of investigation for recognized HPT symptoms or incidentally on routine biochemical screening, the next step is confirmation. Calcium level should be measured in the fasting state since false-positive elevations are associated not only with food but also with prolonged tourniquet time, high-dose calcium supplementation and use of thiazide diuretics (which should be discontinued for one week prior to retesting). Most patients have a normal albumin level so measurement of ionized calcium offers minimal diagnostic advantage. Other serum studies that should be performed include serum phosphorus, which is often low to low-normal in PHPT and serum creatinine to evaluate renal function.

Following confirmation of hypercalcemia, the intact PTH level should be measured. Biologically active PTH circulates mostly as an 84 amino acid peptide but biologically inactive carboxyterminal degradation fragments of varying lengths are also present and may be spuriously detected depending on the assay type chosen. Accurate PTH measurement currently requires use of a sandwich immunochemiluminescent (ICMA) assay which uses antibodies directed simultaneously at both the amino- and carboxy-terminal regions of the intact molecule. The demonstration of an elevated calcium level together with an elevated or inappropriately high-normal serum PTH level confirms the diagnosis of HPT **(Figure 22-1)**.

Secondary elevation of PTH, for example by bisphosphonate use and/or chronic vitamin D deficiency, is frequent and often confounds the diagnosis of PHPT. Vitamin D deficiency is currently endemic in the US. Determination of a low vitamin D level indicates deficiency and should prompt endocrinologic correction. Today many patients with PHPT actually have a subclinical initial presentation with a high-normal serum calcium level that rises to hypercalcemia only when appropriate vitamin D therapy is initiated. Other conditions causing PHPT

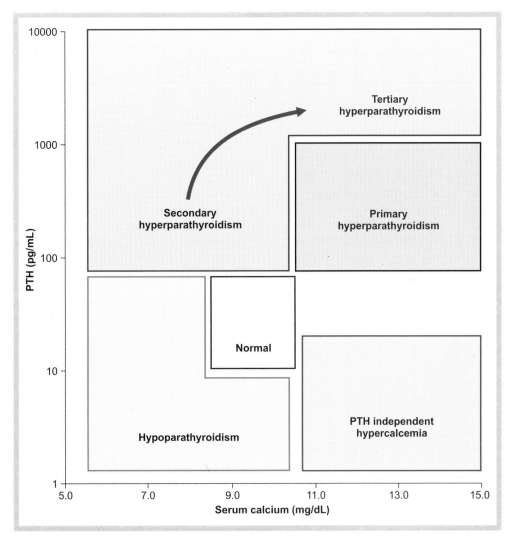

Figure 22-1: Biochemical determination of HPT. This schematic illustrates an approximate correlation of serum calcium levels and PTH along with the expected disease expression of primary hyperparathyroidism (PHPT), secondary hyperparathyroidism (SHPT), tertiary hyperparathyroidism (THPT), hypoparathyroidism and PTH independent hypercalcemia

diagnostic uncertainty include hypercalcemia of malignancy, vitamin D toxicity and chronic granulomatous disease, and these can usually be identified by thorough history, measurement of 25-hydroxyvitamin D level and/or measurement of PTH related-peptide level (PTHrp).

Another diagnostic pitfall in the evaluation of PHPT is the rare autosomal dominant disorder of familial benign hypocalciuric hypercalcemia (FBHH) which results from an inactivating mutation in the calcium-sensing receptor of the parathyroid glands and kidneys, causing a higher set point for renal calcium excretion. FBHH is associated with mild hypercalcemia and minor elevation of PTH. It also produces a low 24-hour urine calcium excretion (generally < 100 mg) and a Ca/Cr clearance ratio < 0.01. Because the only identified morbidity of FBHH is unnecessary parathyroid surgery, it is vital to ask about a

family history of early-onset asymptomatic hypercalcemia and to measure urine calcium excretion in patients with mild biochemical PHPT.

PHPT is not uncommonly seen in association with inherited endocrine tumor syndromes. It is essential to identify inherited forms of PHPT preoperatively because the surgical and clinical management of such patients is different. In a recent study, 1.6% of patients referred for surgery of apparent sporadic PHPT actually had undiagnosed MEN 1 and a simple 6-question panel was observed to be highly effective in identifying such patients preoperatively **(Table 22-1)**.

Decision for Surgery and Localization in PHPT

Parathyroid exploration provides the only cure of PHPT, is cost effective and is the current standard of care for

TABLE 22-1	Six-question panel for MEN1 screening

Do you have any blood relatives with a history of:
- Neck surgery?
- Kidney stones?
- Brain tumors?
- Ulcers?
- High calcium levels?
- Pancreatic tumors?

symptomatic patients. As discussed above the definition of *symptomatic* has varied over time and is still incompletely defined. The goal of surgery for PHPT is to prevent progression to renal failure, osteoporotic fracture and cardiac mortality. At one year after curative surgery, improvements in fatigue, weakness, bone pain, joint pain, forgetfulness, mood swings, thirst, irritability and depression are reported by patients and correspond to a 60% increase in general health.

For PHPT patients without any symptoms at all, certain risk factors forecast disease progression and affect the decision for surgical exploration. The National Institutes of Health 1990 Consensus Conference recommended that surgical treatment of PHPT be offered not only to patients with nephrolithiasis, osteitis fibrosa cystica, overt neuromuscular symptoms (documented proximal muscle weakness, atrophy, hyperreflexia, gait disturbance) or a life-threatening episode of hypercalcemia, but also to asymptomatic patients with: age < 50, serum calcium level 1-1.6 mg/dL above the normal range, 30% reduction in creatinine clearance compared to age-matched controls, 24 hour urine calcium excretion > 400 mg, or forearm bone density reduced more than two standard deviations below that of age-, gender- and race-matched controls (z-score) **(Table 22-2)**. Summary statements of subsequent international workshops in 2002 and 2009 advised broader criteria for surgery that include a calcium level 1.0 mg/dL above the normal range or a bone mineral density at any site reduced by more than 2.5 standard deviations (t-score) **(Table 22-2)**. The 2009 workshop removed elevated urinary calcium as an indication for surgery and advocated the use of z-scores for premenopausal women and men < 50 years of age. All three conferences stressed the importance of careful long-term follow-up for patients being managed with observation only, and cited unwillingness to participate in vigilant follow-up as an independent indication for surgery. For asymptomatic patients being observed nonoperatively, the current surveillance recommendations are summarized in **Table 22-3**.

Systematic prospective analysis of the NIH criteria for surgery versus surveillance has not yet been performed. However, it is known that approximately one-third of asymptomatic PHPT patients who do not meet NIH criteria at presentation will progress to meet criteria for surgery and that progression is more likely for patients diagnosed at < 50 years. Cost efficacy studies favor operative management for asymptomatic patients. The emerging consensus nationally is that all patients with asymptomatic PHPT should undergo consultation with an endocrine surgeon before settling on a specific management course.

Parathyroid imaging does not have a role in the diagnosis of PHPT. False-positive imaging results are quite common, and there is currently no imaging study that accurately distinguishes adenoma from MGD. Imaging

TABLE 22-2	NIH criteria for parathyroid exploration		
	Original (1990)	**Updated (2002 & 2009)**	
Age	< 50	< 50	
Serum level of calcium	1.0-1.6 mg/dL above normal	1.0 mg/dL above normal	
Creatinine clearance	Reduced by 30% compared to normal age-matched	Reduced to < 60 ml/min	
24-hour urinary calcium excretion	> 400 mg	Not indicated	
Bone mineral density	z-score < -2.0 in forearm	Premenopausal women Men age < 50 years	z-score < -2.5 any site
		Postmenopausal women Men age > 50 years	t-score < -2.5 any site

TABLE 22-3	Recommendations for observation in asymptomatic PHPT
Serum calcium	Biannually to annually
Serum creatinine	Annually
Bone mineral density	Every 1-2 years (3 sites)

results can be very useful in planning the operative strategy since enlarged parathyroid glands vary widely in location and number throughout the neck and upper mediastinum. Once a decision has been made for surgery, the routine use of preoperative imaging has been shown to increase the success rate, decrease the operative time and decrease the complications of parathyroid exploration. Among the imaging modalities available, the most sensitive, specific and cost effective are cervical ultrasonography and single photon emission computed tomography (SPECT) ^{99m}Technetium sestamibi. Neither modality alone has sensitivity much better than 85% in detecting abnormal parathyroid glands. Even with a single bright "light bulb" focus of activity on sestamibi SPECT imaging, MGD can be expected in at least 8.4% of patients with PHPT. Concurrent use of ^{99m}Tc-sestamibi nuclear imaging and ultrasound can synergistically improve correct localization by 10-14% (see **Figure 22-2** for schematic of localization techniques). Routine use of ultrasound in preoperative planning is also very helpful in identification of concurrent thyroid pathology.

Surgical Approach in PHPT

Surgical cure of PHPT is defined as durable normalization of serum calcium level, most commonly reported at 6 months postoperatively. The operative failure rate is 1-4% among experienced surgeons but can be much higher among inexperienced surgeons. Operative failure carries with its high costs in both morbidity and health care dollars. The therapeutic intent of surgery in PHPT is to resect the source(s) of PTH overproduction, and the central tasks of parathyroid exploration are thus identifying the presence or absence of MGD (adenoma versus hyperplasia) and locating the abnormal gland(s) for removal.

Currently only two techniques are proven to reliably exclude MGD in PHPT and these are bilateral four-gland exploration and intraoperative PTH monitoring. Four-gland exploration is the "gold standard" approach and involves dissection, visualization and comparison of all parathyroid glands. An essential component of any type of parathyroid exploration is the ability to estimate visually the size of identified parathyroid tissue with accuracy. Normal parathyroid glands are tiny, flat, discrete, tan/pink in color and 35-50 mg in weight, although in PHPT they can be suppressed to even smaller size. Enlarged parathyroid glands on the other hand vary widely in size (e.g. 100 mg -20 gm), in shape (e.g. round, long/thin, bilobed) and in color (e.g. red/brown, tan-red, pink, pale pink, white) and not uncommonly have a cystic component (3% in a recent series). Enlarged parathyroid glands < 100 mg frequently indicate MGD, but when single are termed "microadenoma."

The second proven technique to identify MGD is intraoperative quick PTH monitoring. This method is widely used because it facilitates focused dissection, short operative time and optimization of postoperative calcium supplementation. PTH, which has a short half-life of 3-5 minutes in most patients, is measured just prior to and after resection of an enlarged parathyroid gland using a modified rapid assay first developed at the University of Miami. In the event the PTH does not drop with resection of an enlarged gland, the presence of other hyperfunctional parathyroid glands is deduced and further exploration is performed. Although nationally the most prevalent criterion for an adequate PTH drop is a 50% decrease at 10 minutes postresection, stricter criteria are in use in several centers and we require that the PTH also fall into the normal range to diagnose an appropriate response to resection. Intraoperative PTH monitoring is especially useful in successfully managing reexploration, double adenomata, hyperplasia, intrathyroidal adenoma, supernumerary adenoma, inherited forms of PHPT, lithium-associated PHPT and parathyroid cancer.

During parathyroid exploration the surgeon needs to be familiar with all the normal and ectopic locations for parathyroid glands and needs to employ meticulous dissection and logical thought progression. Glands of inferior embryologic origin derive from the third branchial pouch, reside anteromedial to the junction of the recurrent laryngeal nerve and the inferior thyroid artery and can reside in the cervical thymus, undescended at the carotid bulb, within the thyroid lobe, or inside the carotid sheath. Parathyroid glands of superior embryologic origin derive from the fourth branchial pouch, reside posterolateral to the neurovascular junction, and are frequently found in the tracheoesophageal groove, retropharyngeal space or hyperdescended in the upper mediastinum. Supernumerary parathyroid glands are common (13% of people have > 4 parathyroid glands). Focused (minimally invasive) and/or video-assisted parathyroidectomy are currently validated and accepted practices when supported by intraoperative PTH monitoring. For enlarged parathyroid glands localized deep within the mediastinum on preoperative imaging (which occurs in only 1/1000 patients at first exploration) video-assisted thoracoscopic resection with intraoperative PTH monitoring is the preferred approach.

Intraoperative weight assessment of all resected parathyroid tissue is obligatory and standard. Frozen section examination is useful in excluding false-positive resection, example of brown fat, lymph node, or pedunculated thyroid tissue, but histologic criteria alone are simply not reliable in distinguishing adenoma from MGD. Intraoperative findings can be used to deduce the presence and location of missing or supernumerary enlarged parathyroid glands. Should the anatomy reveal > 2 enlarged parathyroid glands (more than double adenomata) the patient is considered to have hyperplasia

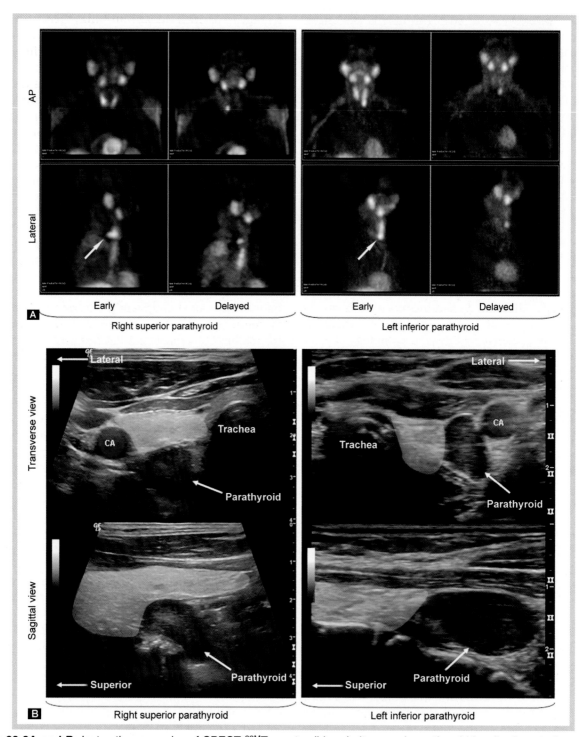

Figures 22-2A and B: Instructive examples of SPECT [99M]Tc-sestamibi and ultrasound parathyroid localization studies.

A. Demonstrates paired early and delayed SPECT images with anteroposterior and lateral reconstructions of right posterior and left inferior parathyroid adenomas. Retained radiotracer uptake in the suspected adenomas is clearly illustrated on the delayed images following expected thyroid washout. Notice also the posterior projection seen with superior parathyroid adenoma compared to an anterior position of inferior adenoma.

B. Concordant transverse and sagittal ultrasound images of the parathyroid adenomas presented in Part A. The parathyroid adenomas are clearly detectable as solid hypoechoic lesions. The surrounding thyroid gland (tan shading), carotid artery (CA) and tracheal structures are highlighted for demonstration purposes. Again notice the posterior and descended position along the tracheoesophageal groove of a superior parathyroid adenoma compared to anterior positioning of an inferior parathyroid adenoma along the thyrothymic tract and subtotal parathyroidectomy is performed leaving a viable 50-100 mg parathyroid remnant *in situ* and marked with a small metal clip. In dissection, it is important to circumferentially mobilize identified glands to avoid missing an adenoma whose superficial portion appears normal in size (i.e. "tip of the iceberg"). The hilar blood supply of a normal parathyroid gland is variable in origin but is always visible, so that during exploration a normal parathyroid gland can be mobilized without devascularization by gentle reflection away from the thyroid gland. Capability for cryopreservation of resected parathyroid tissue is also considered standard, although permanent hypoparathyroidism complicates initial exploration < 1% of the time for most endocrine surgeons today.

Diagnosis and Management of SHPT and THPT

SHPT characteristically evolves in the setting of renal insufficiency but also can be due to any cause of chronic hypocalcemia and/or vitamin D deficiency such as sprue, cystic fibrosis, intestinal bypass surgery or vitamin D resistance. The more clinically ubiquitous etiology is renal replacement therapy as most patients on dialysis have some degree of SHPT. This is particularly pronounced if $1,25(OH)_2D_3$ is not adequately replaced and/or phosphate levels are not controlled. Renal origin HPT is a complex process rooted in a deficiency of the biologically active form of cholecalciferol, the resulting diminished intestinal absorption of calcium and hyperphosphatemia. These physiologic conditions combine to provoke a persistent hypocalcemic state and serve as a constant stimulus for PTH production and parathyroid gland hyperplasia. The biochemical diagnosis of SHPT involves demonstration of normal or low-normal serum calcium levels, elevated PTH **(Figure 22-1)** and high phosphorus levels in cases of renal HPT.

The prolonged and constant stimulation of SHPT may in due course transform diffuse parathyroid hyperplasia into a monoclonal neoplasm with autonomous function. The point at which normal feedback regulation diminishes is designated THPT and is typified as hypercalcemia in a patient with a history of renal failure. THPT can occur at any stage of renal failure and may persist even after renal transplantation. As with PHPT, it is marked biochemically by elevation of *both* serum calcium and PTH **(Figure 22-1)**.

The goal of medical treatment in SHPT is to postpone the evolution of diffuse MGC into irreversible autonomous tumor. This is managed by reducing serum phosphorous and providing biologically active cholecalciferol. Antiquated phosphate binding medications included aluminum which was toxic or calcium which caused hypercalcemia. Currently, in addition to limiting dietary phosphorus, it is recommended that patients with hyperphosphatemia use calcium and aluminum-free phosphate binders such as sevelamer HCl and lanthanum carbonate; treatment with these agents is effective in lowering serum phosphorus but has little effect in reducing PTH levels. Calcitriol is used in SHPT to lower PTH levels, though it can also induce hypercalcemia and hyperphosphatemia, whereas contemporary vitamin D analogues such as paricalcitol and doxercalciferol have been shown to reduce PTH levels with less toxicity. The Kidney Disease Outcomes Quality Initiative (KDOQI) guidelines for patients on renal replacement therapy are summarized in **Table 22-4**. In most cases, standard treatment with phosphate binders and vitamin D sterols is only able to achieve target serum PTH levels in about a quarter of hemodialysis patients and is able to achieve all KDOQI parameters for less than 10% of patients.

The best treatment for SHPT is restoration of normal renal function by kidney transplantation. When this is not possible or is delayed, standard treatment in addition to the calcimimetic agent cinacalcet, improves outcomes with a decreased risk of need for parathyroidectomy, bone fracture and cardiovascular hospitalization. Cinacalcet treatment is generally well tolerated but limiting adverse side effects can include nausea, vomiting or diarrhea. Parathyroidectomy is indicated for SHPT when medical management fails to meet treatment goals. Additionally, the KDOQI guidelines recommend parathyroidectomy for SHPT patients meeting more specific criteria as outlined in **Table 22-4**.

TABLE 22-4	The kidney disease outcomes quality initiative (KDOQI) clinical practice guidelines
	Goal of Maintenance
Serum calcium	between 8.4-9.5 mg/dL
Serum phosphorous	between 3.5-5.5 mg/dL
Calcium phosphorous product (Ca × P)	Less than 55
PTH level	between 150-300 pg/mL
KDOQI Guideline Indications for Parathyroidectomy in SHPT	
Hyperphosphatemia refractory to medical management with PTH > 800 pg/mL	
Extraosseous calcifications (calciphylaxis) with PTH > 500 pg/mL	
Progressive renal osteodystrophy	
Intractable pruritis	

THPT may occur in patients who are dialysis dependent as well as those who have received renal transplantation. Development of THPT in patients who are expected to remain dialysis dependent indefinitely indicates parathyroidectomy. The majority of patients who undergo renal transplant with THPT, however, will demonstrate slow correction in serum calcium and PHT to near normal levels over the first 12 months post-transplant with only about 12% remaining hypercalcemic at 48 months after transplantation. Therefore, THPT patients who have recently received or who anticipate renal transplantation soon should be managed non-operatively if at all possible.

There are two varieties of parathyroidectomy in the treatment of SHPT and THPT: total parathyroidectomy (with or without autotransplantation) and subtotal parathyroidectomy. These procedures have equally been validated and choice is largely left to the discretion of the informed patient as advised by the endocrine surgeon. As a general rule, a balance needs to be struck between removing sufficient parathyroid tissue to achieve a normal PTH level, while guarding against permanent hypoparathyroidism. All parathyroid glands should be identified and enough tissue resected to leave the patient with a remnant representing approximately 40-80 mg either *in situ* (performed commonly) or at the site of autotransplantation (performed less commonly). In THPT arising after successful renal transplantation, up to 10% of patients are found at exploration to have only one single enlarged parathyroid gland, which may simply be resected.

Complications, Follow-up and Surveillance

Immediately after parathyroid exploration patients require particular attention to the airway and to monitoring for cervical hematoma, which is the most preventable cause of poor outcome. Prevention requires meticulous hemostasis before closure of the incision. An expanding cervical hematoma can lead to profound venous congestion and glottic closure with secondary airway compromise. When observation suggests a hematoma, the patient should be calmly and immediately transported to the operating room in the presence of the surgical team and judiciously re-intubated by an experienced anesthesiologist. Preparations should be made to evacuate the hematoma to facilitate re-intubation, but this or/and emergent tracheostomy is/are rarely necessary today. The expected rate of hematoma is about 1/300 cases while delayed hematoma occurs much less commonly. At our center, patients who have a focused parathyroid exploration and show no signs of bleeding following surgery can safely be discharged after 6 hours of observation.

We routinely give one dose of intravenous prophylactic antibiotic within 1 hour prior to the incision, using a first-line agent such as cefazolin (or clindamycin as a second choice in the event of allergy). With this regimen, cervical wound infection is exceedingly rare, occurring in about 1/1000 patients.

After initial parathyroid exploration the risk of permanent unilateral recurrent laryngeal nerve (RLN) paralysis is low with experienced endocrine surgeons, on the order of 0-0.8% in larger series. Routine preoperative laryngoscopy or routine intraoperative RLN monitoring is therefore of little benefit unless the patient is hoarse preoperatively or is undergoing reoperation of any type; as an example, prior anterior cervical discectomy is a strong risk factor for occult RLN deficit in our experience. Approximately 80% of apparent RLN nerve deficits presenting immediately after surgery will resolve within six months, but all patients with persisting hoarseness in the postoperative setting should have laryngoscopy and counseling from a voice specialist.

Cure after parathyroid exploration for PHPT is assessed by serum calcium at ≥ 6 months following surgery. Confirmed documentation of hypercalcemia occurring less than 6 months after parathyroidectomy is termed *persistent HPT* and usually represents unsuccessful search for a missed adenoma. Hypercalcemia that is first documented at greater than 6 months following parathyroid surgery is defined as *recurrent HPT* and generally indicates multiglandular disease that was unrecognized at exploration, but more rarely can also represent parathyroid carcinoma (see below) or parathyromatosis. Although it can also occur embryologically, parathyromatosis is usually a technical problem arising from capsular rupture during resection of a parathyroid gland, which then seeds tissue which can result in recurrence in a locally widespread pattern. Thus, it is important not to breach the capsule while resecting enlarged parathyroid glands.

Six months after surgery for PHPT about 35% of normocalcemic patients will have an elevated PTH level, which is thought to be secondary response to bone remineralization and/or to chronic vitamin D deficiency. This pattern occurs much less frequently (15%) when patients routinely take calcium and vitamin D supplements for six months postoperatively. Because this biochemical pattern can also be the earliest indicator of recurrent PHPT (1-3%) we recommend that all normocalcemic patients take maintenance calcium and vitamin D supplementation for six months postoperatively and that patients with elevated PTH be followed long-term.

The causes of failed initial parathyroid exploration include surgeon inexperience, ectopic or supernumerary parathyroid gland location(s), MGD, error in biochemical diagnosis and parathyroid carcinoma. Because the risks of remedial surgery are higher across the board and include bilateral recurrent nerve paralysis, reoperation is reserved for patients with nephrolithiasis, worsening bone mineralization, worsening renal function, or significant hypercalcemia (calcium level ≥ 12 mg/dL). The management of patients with persistent or recurrent HPT is complex. The initial step is to reconfirm the biochemical diagnosis of HPT including a 24 hour urinary calcium excretion and review of all prior records and a careful family history are essential. All tissue specimens removed at the initial exploration should be reexamined histologically for the presence or absence of parathyroid tissue. With any type of prior anterior neck surgery, laryngoscopy should be performed to assess current vocal cord function. If preoperative localization is positive in the reoperative setting, the cure rate can be as high as 95% but this success is based upon patient selection and a minimum of two imaging studies showing concordant findings is recommended. Should sestamibi and cervical ultrasonography provide equivocal results, more advanced localization procedures including ^{99m}Tc-sestamibi SPECT-CT, four-dimensional CT (4D-CT), MRI or selective venous sampling can be employed. When bilateral foci are identified, to avoid the risk of bilateral vocal cord paralysis experts now deliberately "stage" the laterality of re-exploration and also may use recurrent laryngeal nerve monitoring. Ultimately, a frank discussion with the patient of the higher risks and expected benefits is central to the decision-making process prior to parathyroid re-exploration.

Parathyroid Surgery in Inherited Syndromes, Cysts and Carcinoma

The setting of a germline genetic mutation causing parathyroid gland enlargement and hyperfunction has a significant impact on both the surgical approach and its outcomes. Hereditary HPT patients also need to be screened for other potentially confounding clinical manifestations of the respective inherited syndrome.

The MEN1 syndrome is secondary to autosomal dominant genetic alteration of a chromosome 11q13 tumor suppressor gene that encodes the ubiquitously expressed nuclear protein product *menin*. The penetrance of PHPT in MEN1 is close to 100% while pancreatic islet and pituitary tumors occur in about 65% and 40% of patients, respectively. Multiglandular parathyroid disease is assumed in all patients. If MEN1 is missed on family history, or in a patient who represents as a new mutation, persistent HPT is likely and recurrent HPT is certain. The successful diagnosis of MEN1 in patients presenting with apparent sporadic PHPT is greatly facilitated by use of a simple 6-question panel **(Table 22-1)**. In a recent study, MEN1 accounted for about 26% of patients found to have parathyroid hyperplasia at exploration for presumed sporadic PHTP and was more likely in males < 30 years at presentation with PHPT. A patient suspected to have MEN1 should undergo *menin* mutational analysis, but the test is costly, can take time, requires genetic counseling for the proband and due to genetic heterogeneity does not identify the disorder in about 15% of affected patients.

MEN1 PHPT is currently treated by either total parathyroidectomy and non-dominant forearm autotransplantation, or by subtotal parathyroidectomy. Patients require extensive counseling preoperatively to assist in decision-making because these operations have different morbidity rates. Supernumerary parathyroid glands are reported common in MEN1 and bilateral cervical thymectomy has been widely recommended and performed, but more recently its value has been called into question. Capability for cryopreservation of parathyroid tissue resected during parathyroid surgery is essential in allowing future autografting in the event of permanent hypoparathyroidism.

MEN2A is an autosomal dominant disorder expressed as medullary thyroid cancer (MTC), pheochromocytoma and PHPT. MEN2A results from mutation of the gene encoding the tyrosine kinase RET. The penetrance of PHPT in MEN2A is approximately 30% and it usually results in mild HPT presenting in adulthood. Parathyroid gland enlargement is asymmetrical and not all patients require subtotal parathyroidectomy. Intraoperative PTH assessment helps to ensure appropriate hormone reduction into the normal range and to identify ectopic or supernumerary glands. In MEN2A at least 90% of patients will develop MTC prior to PHPT, thus total thyroidectomy for MTC can be followed decades later by a difficult remedial parathyroid exploration. If not already performed, total thyroidectomy is mandated at the time of parathyroid exploration for MEN2A.

Familial hyperparathyroidism-jaw tumor syndrome (FHJT or HPT-JT) arises from mutation of the tumor suppressor gene HRPT2 which encodes the *parafibromin* product. The primary clinical features are HPT, fibro-osseus lesions of the mandible and maxilla and renal lesions including cysts, hamartoma and even Wilms tumor. PHPT is expressed in 80% of patients affected with HPT-JT, tends to present at a relatively young age (mean 32 years) and is associated with asymmetric gland enlargement that can be cystic in nature. The surgical approach is the same as that for MEN2A: resection of enlarged glands. An important feature of HPT-JT management is that parathyroid carcinoma may be present in as many as 15% of cases.

Parathyroid cysts are not uncommon lesions of the neck and mediastinum. They are found in roughly 3% of routine parathyroid explorations, either incidentally or by presentation as a symptomatic neck mass. The majority (85%) of parathyroid cysts are functional and likely represent cystic change of a functional parathyroid adenoma. The cystic fluid is clear or colorless in the majority of cases but turbid or straw-colored fluid occurs nearly as often; all parathyroid cyst fluid is pathognomonically discernible by elevated PTH levels > 1000 pg/mL and not uncommonly > 10,000 pg/mL. For PHPT patients with functional parathyroid cysts, surgical excision is done in

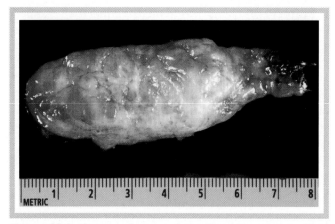

Figure 22-3. Gross pathology of parathyroid carcinoma. Note should be made of white/grey appearance in this parathyroid tumor which was found to be fibrotic, firm and densely adherent to the surrounding mediastinal structures

conjunction with intraoperative PTH assessment to exclude MGD, and meticulous care must be taken to avoid rupture of the cyst into the operative field.

Parathyroid carcinoma occurs in 1% or fewer patients with sporadic PHPT but definitely deserves specific consideration. The diagnosis can be made intraoperatively, histologically or both. Preoperative features which raise suspicion of malignancy include a serum calcium > 14 mg/dL, a PTH level > 5 times normal, the presence of a palpable neck mass or hoarseness (signifying involvement of the recurrent laryngeal nerve). Parathyroid carcinoma can occur in patients with MGD. Features which suggest parathyroid carcinoma to the alert surgeon at exploration include a white or grey, firm and locally adherent gland **(Figure 22.3)** and these features mandate *en bloc* resection to offer the best chance of cure. Resection should include meticulous preservation of the parathyroid capsule, removal of the ipsilateral thyroid lobe when adherent and excision of associated components of the central neck compartment. Molecular analysis assessing loss of heterozygosity (LOH) can improve the discrimination between benign, atypical and malignant parathyroid neoplasms. Notably, between 80-100% of parathyroid carcinomas demonstrate LOH at one of the loci for HRPT2, PTEN, retinoblastoma, or HRAS while benign cases show only 8-13% loss of the same alleles. With incomplete resection the recurrence rate is > 50% and the average interval to disease recurrence is 41 months. The prognosis of those with recurrent disease is poor as patients develop the life-threatening complications of uncontrolled hypercalcemia. PC can metastasize, usually to lungs, bone and/or liver, but with adequate and appropriate initial *en bloc* resection PC recurs infrequently. Patients should be surveyed annually for life with concurrent serum calcium and PTH measurement.

Landmark Papers

1. Potts JT Jr, Fradkin JE, Aurbach GD, Bilezikian JP, Raisz LG (Eds). Proceedings of the NIH consensus development conference on diagnosis and management of asymptomatic primary hyperparathyroidism. J Bone Miner Res 1991; 6: S1-S166.
2. Bilezikian JP, Potts JT Jr, Fuleihan Gel-H, Kleerekoper M, Neer R, Peacock M, et al. Summary statement from a workshop on asymptomatic primary hyperparathyroidism: a perspective for the 21st century. J Clin Endocrinol Metab 2002; 87: 5353-61.
3. Bilezikian JP, Khan AA, Potts JT Jr. Third International Workshop on the Management of Asymptomatic Primary Hyperthyroidism. Guidelines for the management of asymptomatic primary hyperparathyroidism: summary statement from the third international workshop. J Clin Endocrinol Metab 2009; 94: 335-9.
4. National Kidney Foundation. K/DOQI clinical practice guidelines for bone metabolism and disease in chronic kidney disease. Am J Kidney Dis 2003; 42: S1-201.
5. Irvin GL 3rd, Deriso GT 3rd. A new, practical intraoperative parathyroid hormone assay. Am J Surg 1994;168: 466-8.
6. Chen H, Sokoll LJ, Udelsman R. Outpatient minimally invasive parathyroidectomy: a combination of sestamibi-SPECT localization, cervical block anesthesia and intraoperative parathyroid hormone assay. Surgery 1999; 126: 1016-21.
7. Reeve TS, Babidge WJ, Parkyn RF, Edis AJ, Delbridge LW, Devitt PG, Maddern GJ. Minimally invasive surgery for primary hyperparathyroidism: systematic review. Arch Surg 2000; 135: 481-7.
8. Carty SE, Worsey J, Virji MA, Brown ML, Watson CG. Concise parathyroidectomy: the impact of preoperative SPECT 99mTc sestamibi scanning and intraoperative quick parathormone assay. Surgery 1997; 122: 1107-14.
9. Carty SE, Roberts MM, Virji MA, Haywood L, Yim JH. Elevated serum parathormone level after "concise parathyroidectomy" for primary sporadic hyperparathyroidism. Surgery 2002; 132: 1086-92.
10. Yip L, Seethala RR, Nikiforova MN, Nikiforov YE, Ogilvie JB, Carty SE, Yim JH. Loss of heterozygosity of selected tumor suppressor genes in parathyroid carcinoma. Surgery 2008; 144: 949-55.
11. Yip L, Ogilvie JB, Challinor SM, Salata RA, Thull DL, Yim JH, Carty SE. Identification of multiple endocrine neoplasia type 1 in patients with apparent sporadic primary hyperparathyroidism. Surgery 2008; 144: 1002-6.
12. AACE/AAES Task Force on Primary Hyperparathyroidism. The American Association of Clinical Endocrinologists and the American Association of Endocrine Surgeons position statement on the diagnosis and management of primary hyperparathyroidism. Endocr Pract 2005; 11: 49-54.
13. Wells SA Jr, Debenedetti MK, Doherty GM. Recurrent or persistent hyperparathyroidism. J Bone Miner Res 2002; 17(Suppl 2): N158-62.
14. Carty SE, Norton JA. Management of patients with persistent or recurrent primary hyperparathyroidism. World J Surg 1991;15(6): 716-23.

Level of Evidence Table

Recommendation	Grade	Best level of evidence	References
Curative surgery for symptomatic PHPT is indicated to improve neuropsychiatric and cognitive deficits as well as bone mineral density	A	2b	1-5
PHPT is associated with an increased risk of cardiovascular related mortality which normalizes following curative parathyroid surgery	B	2c	6
Parathyroid surgery is recommended for asymptomatic patients meeting certain criteria for age, serum calcium, creatinine clearance reduction and bone mineral density loss	B	2a	7-9
Parathyroid surgery should be considered even for patients with asymptomatic PHPT who do not meet NIH criteria for exploration based on their risk for progression, quality of life improvement and cost-effectiveness	B	1b	10-13
Routine cervical ultrasound, sestamibi scan and intraoperative PTH assay should be performed to maximize the success of targeted parathyroid exploration	B	2b	14-17
Guided unilateral neck exploration for PHPT provides successful outcomes equivalent to bilateral neck exploration	A	1b	18-22
The calcimemetic agent cinacalcet should be considered as first-line therapy for secondary HPT	B	1a	23, 24
Tertiary HPT can adequately be treated by renal transplantation before requiring parathyroidectomy	B	3a	25, 26
Total parathyroidectomy (+/- autotransplantation) versus subtotal para-thyroidectomy have equivalent results for the treatment of SHPT and THPT	B	2b	27-29

References

1. Silverberg SJ, Shane E, Jacobs TP, Siris E, Bilezikian JP. A 10-year prospective study of primary hyperparathyroidism with or without parathyroid surgery. N Engl J Med 1999; 341(17):1249-55.
2. Pasieka JL, Parsons LL, Demeure MJ, et al. Patient-based surgical outcome tool demonstrating alleviation of symptoms following parathyroidectomy in patients with primary hyperparathyroidism. World J Surg 2002;26(8): 942-9.
3. Quiros RM, Alef MJ, Wilhelm SM, Djuricin G, Loviscek K, Prinz RA. Health-related quality of life in hyperparathyroidism measurably improves after parathyroidectomy. Surgery 2003;134(4):675-81; discussion 681-73.
4. Roman SA, Sosa JA, Mayes L, et al. Parathyroidectomy improves neurocognitive deficits in patients with primary hyperparathyroidism. Surgery 2005;138(6):1121-28; discussion 1128-29.
5. Sheldon DG, Lee FT, Neil NJ, Ryan JA, Jr. Surgical treatment of hyperparathyroidism improves health-related quality of life. Arch Surg 2002;137(9):1022-6; discussion 1026-8.
6. Hedback G, Oden A. Increased risk of death from primary hyperparathyroidism—an update. Eur J Clin Invest 1998; 28(4):271-6.
7. Bilezikian JP, Khan AA, Potts JT, Jr. Guidelines for the management of asymptomatic primary hyperparathyroidism: summary statement from the third international workshop. J Clin Endocrinol Metab 2009;94(2):335-9.
8. Rao DS, Phillips ER, Divine GW, Talpos GB. Randomized controlled clinical trial of surgery versus no surgery in patients with mild asymptomatic primary hyperparathyroidism. J Clin Endocrinol Metab 2004;89(11):5415-22.
9. Udelsman R, Pasieka JL, Sturgeon C, Young JE, Clark OH. Surgery for asymptomatic primary hyperparathyroidism: proceedings of the third international workshop. J Clin Endocrinol Metab 2009;94(2):366-72.
10. Ambrogini E, Cetani F, Cianferotti L, et al. Surgery or surveillance for mild asymptomatic primary hyperparathyroidism: a prospective, randomized clinical trial. J Clin Endocrinol Metab 2007;92(8):3114-21.
11. Rubin MR, Bilezikian JP, McMahon DJ, et al. The natural history of primary hyperparathyroidism with or without parathyroid surgery after 15 years. J Clin Endocrinol Metab 2008;93(9):3462-70.
12. Sejean K, Calmus S, Durand-Zaleski I, et al. Surgery versus medical follow-up in patients with asymptomatic primary hyperparathyroidism: a decision analysis. Eur J Endocrinol 2005;153(6):915-27.
13. Zanocco K, Angelos P, Sturgeon C. Cost-effectiveness analysis of parathyroidectomy for asymptomatic primary hyperparathyroidism. Surgery 2006;140(6):874-81.
14. Chen H, Sokoll LJ, Udelsman R. Outpatient minimally invasive parathyroidectomy: a combination of sestamibi-SPECT localization, cervical block anesthesia and

intraoperative parathyroid hormone assay. Surgery 1999; 126(6):1016-21.

15. Arici C, Cheah WK, Ituarte PH, et al. Can localization studies be used to direct focused parathyroid operations? Surgery 2001;129(6):720-9.

16. Carty SE, Worsey J, Virji MA, Brown ML, Watson CG. Concise parathyroidectomy: the impact of preoperative SPECT 99mTc sestamibi scanning and intraoperative quick parathormone assay. Surgery 1997;122(6):1107-14.

17. Irvin GL, 3rd, Sfakianakis G, Yeung L, et al. Ambulatory parathyroidectomy for primary hyperparathyroidism. Arch Surg 1996;131(10):1074-8.

18. Haciyanli M, Lal G, Morita E, Duh QY, Kebebew E, Clark OH. Accuracy of preoperative localization studies and intraoperative parathyroid hormone assay in patients with primary hyperparathyroidism and double adenoma. J Am Coll Surg 2003;197(5):739-46.

19. Miccoli P, Berti P, Materazzi G, Ambrosini CE, Fregoli L, Donatini G. Endoscopic bilateral neck exploration versus quick intraoperative parathormone assay (qPTHa) during endoscopic parathyroidectomy: a prospective randomized trial. Surg Endosc 2008;22(2):398-400.

20. Russell CF, Dolan SJ, Laird JD. Randomized clinical trial comparing scan-directed unilateral versus bilateral cervical exploration for primary hyperparathyroidism due to solitary adenoma. Br J Surg 2006;93(4):418-21.

21. Siperstein A, Berber E, Mackey R, Alghoul M, Wagner K, Milas M. Prospective evaluation of sestamibi scan, ultrasonography and rapid PTH to predict the success of limited exploration for sporadic primary hyperparathyroidism. Surgery 2004;136(4):872-80.

22. Westerdahl J, Bergenfelz A. Unilateral versus bilateral neck exploration for primary hyperparathyroidism: five-year follow-up of a randomized controlled trial. Ann Surg 2007; 246(6):976-80; discussion 980.

23. Cunningham J, Danese M, Olson K, Klassen P, Chertow GM. Effects of the calcimimetic cinacalcet HCl on cardiovascular disease, fracture and health-related quality of life in secondary hyperparathyroidism. Kidney Int 2005; 68(4):1793-1800.

24. Garside R, Pitt M and erson R, et al. The effectiveness and cost-effectiveness of cinacalcet for secondary hyperpara-thyroidism in end-stage renal disease patients on dialysis: a systematic review and economic evaluation. Health Technol Assess 2007;11(18):iii, xi-xiii, 1-167.

25. D'Alessandro AM, Melzer JS, Pirsch JD, et al. Tertiary hyperparathyroidism after renal transplantation: operative indications. Surgery 1989;106(6):1049-55; discussion 1055.

26. Triponez F, Clark OH, Vanrenthergem Y, Evenepoel P. Surgical treatment of persistent hyperparathyroidism after renal transplantation. Ann Surg 2008;248(1):18-30.

27. Gagne ER, Urena P, Leite-Silva S, et al. Short- and long-term efficacy of total parathyroidectomy with immediate autografting compared with subtotal parathyroidectomy in hemodialysis patients. J Am Soc Nephrol 1992;3(4):1008-17.

28. Hargrove GM, Pasieka JL, Hanley DA, Murphy MB. Short- and long-term outcome of total parathyroidectomy with immediate autografting versus subtotal parathyroidectomy in patients with end-stage renal disease. Am J Nephrol 1999; 19(5):559-64.

29. Takagi H, Tominaga Y, Uchida K, et al. Subtotal versus total parathyroidectomy with forearm autograft for secondary hyperparathyroidism in chronic renal failure. Ann Surg 1984;200(1):18-23.

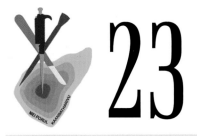

23

Adrenal Tumors

Linwah Yip

An incidental adrenal lesion is any adrenal mass > 1 cm that is identified on cross-sectional imaging obtained for unrelated reasons. Incidental adrenal lesions can be identified in up to 5% of patients and the prevalence increases with age; in patients > 70 years old, there is a 7% probability of having an incidental adrenal lesion. The majority are benign adrenal adenomas; however, ~ 10% of incidental lesions demonstrate hormonal hyper-secretion (functional) and up to 5% are malignant. The malignancy rate can be as high as 25-35% in patients with a prior history of cancer. It is not unusual for patients to be referred to a surgeon for evaluation of an incidental adrenal lesion and a systematic outcomes-based approach should be used to determine if adrenalectomy is ultimately necessary.

The signs and symptoms associated with a functional adrenal mass can be elicited with a careful history and physical and are shown in **Table 23-1**.

Primary Aldosteronism

Primary aldosteronism (PA) can be identified in up to 10% of hypertensive patients. Familial PA is rare (< 1% of cases) and should be suspected if the patient is < 20 years and

TABLE 23-1	Signs and symptoms of hormonal excess			
Condition	**Hormone**	**Common chief complaint**	**Symptoms**	**Exam findings**
Primary aldosteronism	Aldosterone	Hypertension resistant to appropriate use of ≥ 3 medications	Muscle weakness and palpitations usually associated with hypokalemia	Hypertension (rarely malignant), hypokalemia (< 30%), mild hypernatremia, hypomagnesemia
Cushing's syndrome	Cortisol	Change in physical appearance	Bruising, proximal muscle weakness, reddish-purple striae > 1 cm wide, weight gain, dorsocervical and supraclavicular fat pads, facial rounding, hirsutism, balding, acne, poor healing, cognitive changes (e.g. depression, fatigue, decreased concentration, impaired memory and irritability)	Hypertension, osteoporosis, type 2 diabetes, hypokalemia, hyperlipidemia, kidney stones
Pheochromocytoma	Norepinephrine and epinephrine	Paroxysmal symptoms either spontaneous or triggered by postural changes, procedures, tyramine-containing foods, or medications	Palpitations or tachycardia, severe headache, diaphoresis, anxiety, panic symptoms, pallor, tremor	Hypertension, orthostasis, cardiomyopathy, blurry vision, papilledema, constipation, hyperglycemia

there is a family history of PA, early onset hypertension and/or strokes. Much more commonly, PA is sporadic and secondary to either bilateral adrenal hyperplasia or an adrenal adenoma (Conn's syndrome). Hypokalemia is seen in only 9-30% of patients with primary aldosteronism and should not be used as a screening criterion. The initial screening test should be a plasma aldosterone and plasma renin activity obtained with the patient seated and in the morning. An aldosterone to renin ratio (ARR) of > 20 prompts additional confirmatory testing. A suppressed renin can result in an elevated ARR, even with a normal aldosterone. An aldosterone of > 15 ng/dL in conjunction with an elevated ARR is considered by some as another criterion for PA. Age > 65 years and renal failure are common reasons for false-positive results.

Prior to obtaining ARR, hypokalemia should be corrected and patients should not restrict their sodium intake. Spironolactone, amiloride, triamterene, potassium-wasting diuretics and licorice-root based products such as authentic licorice or chewing tobacco should be avoided for at least 4 weeks prior to testing. Alternatively, verapamil, hydralazine and alpha-adrenergic blockers can be used for blood pressure control.

Following an abnormal ARR, one of the following four confirmatory tests should be performed. A positive oral sodium loading test is a 24-hour urinary aldosterone of > 12 µg/24 hours following 3 days of oral sodium intake at 6 gm/day. A positive saline infusion test occurs if plasma aldosterone levels are > 10 ng/dL after a 2 L normal saline infusion over 4 hours. An upright plasma aldosterone > 6 ng/dL 4 days after receiving fludrocortisone 0.1 mg q6h with KCl supplementation to keep potassium levels close to 4 mmol/L and NaCl supplements to keep urinary sodium excretion adequate is a positive fludrocortisone suppression test. A positive captopril challenge test is a persistently elevated plasma aldosterone despite captopril 25-50 mg administered 1 hour previously.

After confirming the diagnosis of PA, the source of excess aldosterone secretion needs to be determined. The indication for adrenalectomy is PA secondary to a solitary adrenal adenoma or unilateral adrenal hyperplasia. Bilateral adrenal disease is treated medically. An adrenal CT or MRI scan should be obtained but ultimately, adrenal venous sampling (AVS) is used to differentiate between unilateral versus bilateral disease and to also lateralize the unilateral site. Even with a clear unilateral adrenal mass on CT, studies have demonstrated that up to 25% could have bilateral disease or aldosterone hypersecretion from the contralateral gland. Some advocate the selective use of AVS and forego the procedure among patients < 40 years with a solitary adenoma.

AVS requires a fair amount of technical expertise and proficiency. The right adrenal vein, in particular, can be difficult to cannulate. A continuous cosyntropin infusion at 50 µg/hour initiated 30 minutes prior to sampling can help minimize stress-induced fluctuations in aldosterone and augment the cortisol gradient between the adrenal vein and the inferior vena cava (IVC). After catheterization of the femoral vein, cortisol and aldosterone levels are obtained from blood in both adrenal veins and a background location such as the periphery, IVC or external iliac vein. An adequate sample is confirmed if the adrenal vein to background cortisol ratio is > 10:1 with cosyntropin infusion and > 3:1 without cosyntropin infusion. Unilateral aldosterone hypersecretion is confirmed if the aldosterone to cortisol ratio is at least four times higher than the ratio on the contralateral side. The complication rate of AVS is 2.5% and includes groin hematoma, adrenal hemorrhage and adrenal vein dissection. If AVS is unsuccessful, it can be repeated, the patient can be treated medically, or alternative methods to determine laterality can be considered. The posture stimulation test is associated with 85% accuracy and can be helpful.

Following adrenalectomy, hypokalemia resolves in 98% of patients usually within 1 month. Although improved hypertensive control occurs in 90%, only 1/3 have complete resolution and normalization can take up to 6 months. A recent study identified factors that can increase the likelihood of resolution and include requiring ≤ 2 antihypertensive medications, duration of hypertension ≤ 6 years, BMI ≤ 25 and female gender. Younger age and negative family history for hypertension have also been shown in some studies to increase the likelihood of hypertension resolution postoperatively.

Cushing's and Subclinical Cushing's Syndrome

Cushing's syndrome is the clinical manifestation of prolonged exposure to inappropriately high levels of glucocorticoids. The most common cause is prescribed (exogenous) steroids. An abnormal hypothalamic-pituitary-adrenal (HPA) axis can lead to physiological hypercortisolism secondary to conditions such as physical stress, psychiatric conditions, morbid obesity, uncontrolled diabetes mellitus, or pregnancy or pathologic hypercortisolism that should be evaluated and treated. Pathologic hypercortisolism can be either ACTH-dependent (pituitary, i.e. Cushing's disease or ectopic ACTH-producing tumor) or ACTH-independent (adrenal).

The most significant sequela of Cushing's syndrome is the increased cardiovascular mortality. Other important consequences include decreased bone mineral density, cognitive dysfunction and diminished quality of life. Although many of these symptoms improve following treatment, studies have shown that the effects do not completely normalize when compared to age-matched controls.

Subclinical Cushing's syndrome is diagnosed when an abnormal HPA axis is biochemically apparent, but the patient does not have any obvious signs of Cushing's syndrome. It is usually unmasked during the evaluation of an incidental adrenal lesion and with routine screening can be seen in 5-20% of patients. The majority do not progress to Cushing's, however there is an association between subclinical Cushing's with insulin resistance and hypertension. Although several small series have shown improvements in glucose and blood pressure control after adrenalectomy, a causative association has been difficult to definitively determine. Even with subclinical Cushing's, suppression of the contralateral gland can still occur (75%) resulting in Addisonian crisis after adrenalectomy if preventive treatment is not appropriately given.

Initial testing for Cushing's can include either 24-hour urine free cortisol (UFC) or late night salivary cortisol or overnight 1 mg (low dose) dexamethasone suppression test. A suppressed plasma ACTH level will confirm the presence of ACTH-independent Cushing's but may not always be present in patients with subclinical Cushing's. In order to be valid, the urine collection for the 24-hour UFC should have adequate volume and creatinine. A result above the upper limit of normal, which can vary between testing laboratories, is considered a positive test. Because of normal variability, the test should be repeated for validation. One of the advantages of a 24-hour UFC is that medications that increase cortisol-binding globulin, such as oral contraceptives and other estrogen containing medications, will not affect the levels. Up to 30% of obese patients can have a false-positive result. A late night salivary cortisol evaluates for the loss of cortisol fluctuation that is seen with normal circadian rhythm. Two salivary samples are obtained on separate nights between 2300-2400 h. Salivary cortisol levels > 145 ng/dL are abnormal with a comparable sensitivity and specificity to UFC measurements. False-positives can be seen in smokers and in patients who chew tobacco. Patients who work in the evenings or alternate shifts will need to have the collection time adjusted accordingly.

In addition to testing for Cushing's, the 1 mg overnight dexamethasone test is also the most sensitive test for subclinical Cushing's and should be obtained in all patients with an incidental adrenal lesion. Between 2300-2400 h, dexamethasone 1 mg is ingested and a serum cortisol is obtained between 0800-0900 h the next morning. A cortisol that does not suppress to < 1.8 µg/dL is abnormal. Phenytoin, phenobarbitol, carbamazepine, rifampin and alcohol can accelerate the hepatic clearance of dexamethasone reducing the amount of available dexamethasone and potentially cause a falsely elevated cortisol level. Increased cortisol-binding globulin is seen in patients taking estrogen, oral contraceptive medications and mitotane that can also result in a falsely elevated serum cortisol level. In contrast, liver and renal failure reduce dexamethasone clearance increasing the effective concentration and potentially resulting in a falsely lowered morning cortisol level.

Perioperative management of Cushing's and subclinical Cushing's should include stress-dose steroids. Prednisone is continued postoperatively at 10-15 mg/day until recovery of the HPA axis occurs, usually 6-9 months after surgery, but may take as long as 2 years. Mineralocorticoid replacement is not necessary after unilateral adrenalectomy.

Other

Hypersecretion of sex hormones are rare. Unless the patient presents with virilizing or feminizing features, routine screening (e.g. DHEA, DHEA-S, testosterone, estrogen, etc.) is not necessary.

Pheochromocytoma

Pheochromocytomas are tumors of the catecholamine-secreting chromaffin cells in the adrenal medulla. Asymptomatic pheochromocytoma is diagnosed in 5-10% of patients with incidental adrenal lesions and if unrecognized, can be lethal during adrenalectomy. It is highly recommended that all patients with adrenal masses undergo biochemical screening for pheochromocytoma.

Norepinephrine and epinephrine are metabolized in chromaffin cells to normetanephrine and metanephrine. Typically, extra-adrenal pheochromocytomas (i.e. paragangliomas) produce mostly norepinephrine while pheochromocytomas in patients with multiple endocrine neoplasia type 2 (MEN2) or neurofibromatosis type 1 (NF1) produce predominantly epinephrine. Measuring 24-hour urine fractionated metanephrines or plasma free metanephrines gives the best diagnostic sensitivity. There is no consensus which test is best. Urine metanephrine testing is a well-established test and does not require a separate office visit. However, obviously, it cannot be performed in patients with renal failure. On the other hand, plasma metanephrine testing is not always widely available and requires medical staff trained for the blood collection. An intravenous line for blood draw is placed and the patient then lies in a quiet room for 30 minutes prior to sample collection. Plasma reference levels are not adjusted for age which may make plasma metanephrine testing more appropriate for children. An elevation of at least two-fold is considered positive; a four-fold elevation is associated with a near 100% diagnostic accuracy. The possibility of a false-positive result should be considered with only mild elevations. Patients should be counseled prior to testing to avoid interfering substances and medication lists thoroughly reviewed (**Table 23-2**). The clonidine suppression test is another diagnostic test but is rarely used.

TABLE 23-2	Metanephrine testing and interfering medications	
Medication class	**Generic**	**Brand-name**
Tricyclic anti-depressants	Amitriptyline Nortriptyline Protriptyline Imipramine	Elavil Aventyl, Pamelor Vivactil Topfranil
MAO-inhibitors	Tranylcypromine Isocarboxazid	Parnate Marplan
Other anti-depressants	Venlafaxine Bupropion Befazodone Quetiapine	Effexor Wellbutrin, Zyban Serzone Seroquel
ADHD	Atomoxetine Methylphenidate	Strattera Ritalin, Concerta, Metadate
Stimulants	Caffeine Nicotine Theophylline Sibutramine	 Theo-Dur, Slo-bid Meridia
Alpha-blockers	Phenoxybenzamine Doxazosin Terazosin Reserpine	Dibenzyline Cardura Hytrin Serpasil
Beta-blockers	Atenolol Metoprolol Propranolol Labetalol Nebivolol	Tenormin Lopressor Inderal Normadyne Bystolic
Calcium-channel blockers	Nifedipine Amlodipine Diltiazem Verapamil	Procardia Norvasc Cardizem Calan, Verelan
Vasodilators	Hydralazine Isosorbide Minoxidil	Apresoline Isordil Loniten
Sympathomimetics	Pseudoephedrine Amphetamines	Sudafed
Antibiotics	Chloramphenicol Tetracycline Erythromycin	Chloromycetin Sumycin, Tetracyn Erythrocin
Other	Acetaminophen Prochlorperazine Levodopa	Tylenol Compazine Laradopa

Either a CT or MRI scan is usually adequate for localization (**Figure 23-1**). A ^{123}I labeled MIBG scan is useful if the lesion is large (> 5 cm) and there is concern for metastatic disease or despite positive biochemical results and strong clinical suspicion, no adrenal lesions are seen on cross-sectional imaging. The routine use of MIBG has been shown to be unnecessary.

Inadequate or inappropriate perioperative management of pheochromocytoma patients can cause life-threatening hypertensive crisis and cardiac arrhythmias.

All patients should receive preoperative blockade, but there are no randomized studies and no clear consensus on the optimal management algorithm. At our institution, the endocrine surgeon initiates treatment at least 2 weeks prior to the planned surgical procedure. Phenoxybenzamine is administered at a starting divided daily dose of 1 mg/kg. Patients are counseled to maintain aggressive fluid hydration (> 64 ounces/day) to help prevent the symptomatic postural hypertension that is an otherwise common side effect. Other side effects that

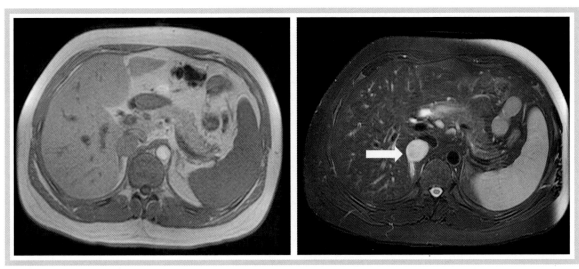

Figure 23-1: On MRI axial T1 imaging (L), a 4 cm right adrenal mass is seen that is hyperintense (arrow) on axial T2 imaging (R), characteristic of a pheochromocytoma. Biochemical evaluation confirmed a pheochromocytoma and after adequate alpha-blockade, a laparoscopic right adrenalectomy was performed

patients should be counseled about ahead of time include dizziness, syncope, nasal congestion and retrograde ejaculation. Our goal is to induce a mild reflex tachycardia of 30 beats per minute as the patient goes from supine to standing. Heart rates are monitored and medication dose-escalated by 10-20 mg 2-3 times per week as needed.

Other blockade regimens that have been used include other alpha-blockades (e.g. prazosin, terazosin and doxazosin) or calcium-channel blockers (e.g. amlodipine, nifedipine, or verapamil). The advantages of calcium-channel blockers is the avoidance of coronary spasm that can occur with alpha-blockade. Metyrosine is a tyrosine analog that inhibits the rate-limiting step in catecholamine synthesis and is routinely used by some in conjunction with alpha-blockade to help prevent excess catecholamine release perioperatively. The dose is started 1-3 weeks preoperatively at 250 mg every 8-12 hours and increased up to 1.5-2 gm/day. The medication has a number of side effects including depression, anxiety, sedation, galactorrhea and extrapyramidal signs. Diarrhea and crystalluria can occur at higher doses. If the symptoms do not improve after dose-lowering, the medication should be stopped.

Pheochromocytoma patients are admitted the evening prior to surgery. The adequacy of the alpha-blockade is assessed, a cardioselective beta 1-blocker is started if tachycardia is present (atenolol or metoprolol) and IV fluid hydration is initiated. An arterial line should be placed prior to anesthesia induction as catecholamine surge can occur even before surgical incision. A central venous catheter is helpful for intravenous access, although large bore peripheral IVs are equally effective. Intraoperatively, anesthesia should have medications readily available for treatment of both hypertension and hypotension.

Phentolamine is a short-acting intravenous alpha-blocker that can be useful. After resection of the adrenal tumor, volume expansion should be the first line of treatment for hypotension. Postoperative ICU admission is not mandatory unless the patient's hemodynamic status warrants close-observation.

Approximately 20-30% of patients with pheochromocytomas have a germline mutation in one of the five susceptibility genes: *RET, VHL, NF1, SDHD* and *SDHB*. A family history positive for manifestations of one of the susceptible genetic syndrome, age ≤ 40 years, multicentric or synchronous tumors, paragangliomas or malignant pheochromocytoma should prompt genetic testing **(Table 23-3)**. We refer all patients to our genetic counselors for discussion and appropriate counseling of the patient and affected family members.

Malignant Pheochromocytoma

The diagnosis of malignant pheochromocytoma is solely dependent on the presence of metastases. Histopathologic findings of cytologic atypia, vascular invasion, size > 5 cm, increased mitotic activity and / or increased proliferative activity by Ki-67 staining may help predict malignancy but, are not diagnostic. Malignancy is identified in 5-35% of pheochromocytomas and varies depending on genetic background. Synchronous metastases are found in ~10% of pheochromocytoma patients. *SDHB* mutations are also associated with a worse prognosis. Overall 10-year survival is 40% however, this varies widely. Metastatic lesions in the bone, in particular, can be very indolent and there are reports of > 25 years survival without adjuvant treatment. On the other hand, patients with lung and liver metastases usually have survival < 5 years.

TABLE 23-3	Genetic syndromes associated with pheochromocytoma	
Condition	**Affected gene**	**Manifestations**
Multiple Endocrine Neoplasia type 2	RET	MEN2A: Medullary thyroid carcinoma, primary hyperparathyroidism MEN2B: Medullary thyroid carcinoma, mucosal neuromas
Von Hippel-Lindau Disease	VHL	Renal cysts, retinal angiomas, CNS hemangioblastomas, renal cell carcinoma, pancreatic cysts and islet-cell tumors
Neurofibromatosis type 1	NF1	Café-au-lait spots, Lisch nodules, neurofibromas, axillary and/or inguinal freckling, skeletal and vascular anomalies
Familial pheochromocytoma paraganglioma	SDHB, SDHC, or SDHD	GIST, renal cell carcinoma, head and neck paraganglioma

Surgical debulking can help symptom palliation and theoretically decrease tumor volume to maximize subsequent medical therapy; however, a survival benefit has never been shown. External beam radiation and radiofrequency ablation are other treatment alternatives. An improvement in symptoms can be seen in 75% of patients treated with ^{131}I-MIBG. Soft tissue metastases respond best, but even in this group a complete response is seen in < 5%. Progressive bone metastases may have better response to higher doses; however, toxicities include bone marrow suppression and accompanying hematologic complications, ovarian failure and hypothyroidism. ^{131}I-MIBG is only available in a handful of specialized facilities because it is not commercially available.

Tumors that no longer take up MIBG are usually treated with a cytotoxic regimen of cyclophosphamide, vincristine and dacarbazine which can produce a complete response in 10%. In a long-term study, patients reported improvement in symptoms and some even had tumor shrinkage that facilitated surgical resection. However, there was no statistically significant benefit in survival. Side effects included bone marrow suppression, peripheral neuropathy and GI toxicity. Other chemotherapy regimens used include mesna, doxorubicin, ifosfamide, dacarbazine (MAID), gemcitabine or etoposide-cisplatin.

More recent reports of using one of the tyrosine kinase inhibitors, sunitinib, for malignant pheochromocytomas have showed promising preliminary results. Malignancies that are associated with VHL mutations, such as renal cell carcinomas and potentially pheochromocytomas, result in accumulation of hypoxia-inducible factor alpha with downstream upregulation of VEGF and PDGF. Sunitinib is an inhibitor that targets PDGFR and VEGFR, among other tyrosine kinases. A complete response was seen in 1 of 3 patients treated in one series and randomized multi-institutional trials are ongoing. Sunitinib is an oral medication and usually well-tolerated. Complications can include hypertension, hypothyroidism, bone marrow suppression and left ventricular dysfunction.

Evaluation of the Incidental Adrenal Lesion

In the absence of any obvious signs or symptoms of hormonal hypersecretion, the NIH State-of-the-Science Conference recommends an overnight 1 mg dexamethasone suppression test and 24-hour urine or plasma fractionated metanephrines for all patients with an incidental adrenal lesion **(Figure 23-2)**. Patients with hypertension should also have plasma potassium, aldosterone and renin levels determined. Functional lesions are usually resected.

If the incidental lesion is non-functional, then the risk of adrenocortical carcinoma (ACC) is considered which takes into account lesion size and radiographic characteristics. The size of the adrenal mass seen on cross-sectional imaging has been a well-studied risk factor. A large study that included the SEER database demonstrated a two-fold increased risk of malignancy among adrenal lesions ≥ 4 cm. The rate of malignancy among lesions ≥ 4 cm ranges in studies from 5-15%. As a result of these correlations, size ≥ 4 cm is considered by many to be an indication for adrenalectomy to exclude malignancy.

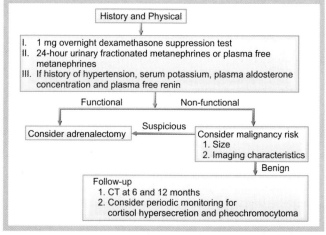

Figure 23-2: Evaluation of patients with incidental adrenal lesion

However, the majority of lesions over 4 cm are still benign and smaller malignancies can be missed. Radiographic characteristics are also an important consideration in determining malignancy risk. Benign adenomas are often composed of lipid-rich cortical cells that demonstrate characteristic findings on CT, either enhanced or unenhanced and MR with chemical shift imaging **(Table 23-4, Figures 23-3 and 23-4)**. A number of studies have shown that these imaging characteristics are associated with high sensitivities and specificities in predicting benign disease. In one study of 151 adrenal masses with histopathologic correlation, a mass that had Hounsfield units ≤10 was associated with adrenal adenoma with 100% specificity and 41% sensitivity. Chemical shift MRI that demonstrates loss of signal on out of phase images is another characteristic that is associated with benign adrenal adenoma with 96% sensitivity and 90% specificity. We recently reported a large series of 196 adrenals and the correlation of radiographic characteristics

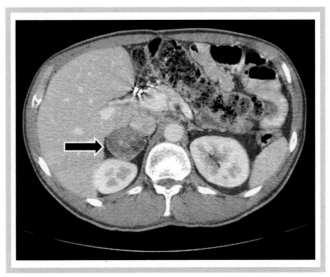

Figure 23-4: On CT scan, an incidental 4.7 cm heterogeneous right adrenal mass was seen (arrow). On final histopathology, a myelolipoma with fibrosis and hemorrhage was diagnosed

to histopathology and showed that all masses with benign imaging were confirmed benign. Equally importantly, all malignancies had non-benign imaging. Although the majority of lesions with non-benign imaging are lipid-poor adenomas, resection should strongly be considered to exclude malignancy.

Fine-needle aspiration biopsy is not recommended to evaluate for ACC and can be dangerous. Unrecognized pheochromocytoma, needle-track seeding and injury to organs in close proximity are common complications. Most importantly, biopsy cannot diagnose ACC and usually does not determine whether adrenalectomy will be necessary. Biopsy is helpful only in the clinical scenarios of a known extra-adrenal malignancy and the presence of an unresectable adrenal mass, suspicion of adrenal tuberculosis or possible adrenal lymphoma. Pheochromocytoma must always be biochemically excluded prior to the procedure.

Adrenal lesions that are not resected should be followed, however there is no universally agreed upon consensus and little data supporting duration or mode of follow-up. The NIH consensus recommends CT at 6-12 months. Long-term follow-up studies show that most lesions remain stable in size and up to 25% of lesions grow over 1 cm **(Figure 23-5)**. In studies with up to 10-year follow-up, the risk of developing ACC is exceedingly low. Hormone hypersecretion does develop in up to 10% of patients over time with the risk increasing in patients with larger (> 3 cm) lesions. The most common is hypersecretion of cortisol (either subclinical Cushing's or Cushing's) but also rarely, pheochromocytoma. These are based on small studies and not all patients were initially routinely screened for subclinical Cushing's. The NIH

TABLE 23-4	Radiographic characteristics associated with benign adenoma
Radiographic characteristics	

HU <10 on non-contrasted CT
Delayed enhanced CT:
  Relative washout ≥ 40%
  Absolute washout ≥ 60%	

Chemical shift MR with loss of signal on out-of-phase imaging	

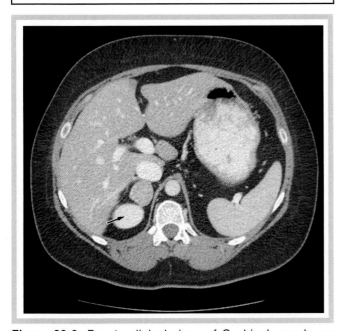

Figure 23-3: Due to clinical signs of Cushing's syndrome confirmed by biochemical testing, an adrenal protocol CT scan was obtained and showed a 3.2 cm right adrenal mass (arrow) with absolute washout of 76%, consistent with a lipid-poor adenoma. After laparoscopic right adrenalectomy, pathology confirmed an adrenal cortical adenoma

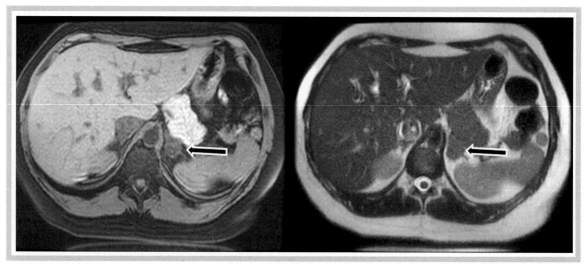

Figure 23-5: MRI to characterize an incidentally identified 2.1 cm left adrenal mass demonstrated intermediate signal intensity on T1 images (L) (arrow) with homogeneous signal dropout on out of phase imaging and no significant signal on T2 images (R) (arrow), characteristic of a benign adrenal adenoma. However, the mass grew on serial cross-sectional imaging and laparoscopic left adrenalectomy was performed. A 4 cm benign adrenal adenoma was confirmed on final histopathology

consensus recommends yearly functional screening with a 1 mg overnight dexamethasone suppression test and urine or plasma fractionated metanephrines.

Adrenocortical Carcinoma

ACC is rare with an estimated prevalence of 0.7-2 cases per million. Women are more commonly affected than men in most series. The age at presentation is either in childhood or between 40-50 years. ACC is associated with 3 hereditary syndromes: Li-Fraumeni, Beckwith-Wiedemann and Multiple Endocrine Neoplasia Type 1 **(Table 23-5)**. Overall 5-year survival is < 50%.

The molecular changes leading to ACC are not well understood. It is also not known if benign adrenal adenomas progress to ACC, although longitudinal studies of patients with benign adenomas suggest that this progression is unlikely. Sporadic ACCs are associated with mutations in the tumor suppressor genes *p53* and *MEN1*. Overexpression of IGF2 and activation of the Wnt signaling pathway have also been implicated in ACC pathogenesis.

Ongoing studies to further elucidate the underlying genetic alterations are limited by the rarity of the tumor.

Hormonal hypersecretion is seen in ~ 60% of ACC. The most frequent presentation is Cushing's syndrome associated with a rapidly progressive clinical course. Hypokalemia can be seen in association with significantly elevated cortisol levels. Simultaneous androgen or estrogen secretion is also common and cases of aldosterone secreting ACC have been reported. Non-functional ACC present with abdominal symptoms or back pain. Constitutional symptoms such as weight loss and anorexia can also be present.

The presence of distant or lymph node metastasis and local invasion are diagnostic of ACC. The Weiss criteria is most commonly used in the pathologic diagnosis of ACC. At least three of the following nine criteria should be observed: nuclear grade III or IV, mitotic rate > 5/50 high power field, atypical mitoses, ≤ 25% clear cells, diffuse architecture pattern in ≥ 1/3 of the tumor, confluent necrosis and venous, sinusoidal or capsular invasion. High mitotic rate and significant necrosis have

TABLE 23-5	Genetic syndromes associated with adrenocortical carcinoma		
Syndrome	**Affected gene**	**Risk of ACC**	**Other manifestations**
Li-Fraumeni	p53 or CHEK2	3-4%	Soft tissue sarcoma, osteosarcoma, breast cancer, brain tumor, leukemia
Beckwith-Wiedemann	11p15.5 locus (IGF2, h19, p57)	Up to 5%	Exomphalos, macroglossia, gigantism, childhood tumors including nephroblastoma, hepatoblastoma, rhabdomyosarcoma
MEN1	Menin	rare	Primary hyperparathyroidism, pancreatic islet cell tumors, pituitary adenomas

been shown to be poor prognostic indicators. Immuno-histochemical markers such as D11, inhibin-alpha, melan A and chromogranin A can be used to help verify that the cell origin is adrenocortical and overexpression of Ki-67, IGF-2 or cyclin E can be used to help make the diagnosis of malignancy.

In 2004, the UICC and WHO published their first staging system which was based on the McFarlane-Sullivan staging system used previously. Solitary ≤ 5 cm tumors (T1) confined to the adrenal (N0M0) are stage I while > 5 cm tumors (T2N0M0) are stage II. Stage III includes tumors with infiltration into surrounding tissue (T3N0M0) or ≥ 1 positive lymph node (T1-3N1M0). Stage IV includes tumors with local invasion into surrounding tissue and positive lymph nodes (T3N1M0), tumors invading into adjacent organs (T4), or distant metastases (TXNXM1). Validation of this staging system has shown variable results with some demonstrating that the prognostic difference between T3 and T4 tumors is subtle. The presence of distant metastases is an independently poor prognostic indicator and changes making M1 disease the defining criterion for stage IV disease have been proposed.

There is little debate that the long-term outcome for ACC patients is worse with poorly differentiated tumors, positive resection margins and lymph node or distant metastases. Large size (> 12 cm) and age > 55 years have been shown in some studies to also be poor prognostic indicators. Chemotherapy and radiation have not been effective adjuvant treatments for ACC and surgery remains the mainstay of therapy. Surgical intent should be for margin negative disease with *en bloc* resection of involved organs if necessary. Occasionally, IVC thrombi are encountered and may require cardiopulmonary bypass or another venous exclusion procedure for adequate resection. Open transabdominal adrenalectomy is indicated for large tumors, locally invasive tumors or those with evidence of nodal metastases **(Figure 23-6).** Smaller tumors can considered for laparoscopic resection, especially if no obvious signs of malignancy are seen on preoperative imaging. If there is invasion encountered during laparoscopic resection, conversion to an open procedure should strongly be considered to facilitate complete resection without tumor spillage or capsular disruption. Prospective studies to evaluate the long-term outcomes of laparoscopic ACC resection have not been performed and because of the low disease incidence, may be challenging to complete.

Liver and lung distant metastases are most common. With synchronous metastatic disease, median survival is < 12 months. Tumor debulking may be palliative to help ameliorate hormonal hypersecretion. Retrospective studies have shown improved survival with surgical treatment of recurrent or metachronous metastatic disease if complete resection can be achieved.

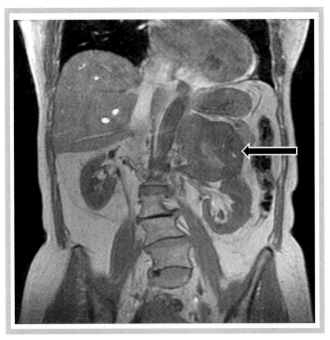

Figure 23-6: After presenting with Cushing's syndrome, an MRI showed an 8.5 cm irregular left adrenal mass displacing the kidney and pancreas (arrow). No adenopathy or renal vein invasion is seen. Open adrenalectomy was performed and final pathology confirmed an adrenal cortical carcinoma with capsular, vascular and periadrenal adipose tissue invasion.

Adjuvant radiotherapy of the adrenalectomy bed may help reduce locally recurrent disease, however there have been no differences in disease free survival or overall survival. Radiation treatment of bone and brain metastases can be palliative.

A number of cytotoxic chemotherapies have been used for adjuvant treatment of ACC with poor response rates. Combination therapy with etoposide, cisplatin, doxorubicin and mitotane has shown 20-50% response rates. A large multi-institutional trial comparing this regimen to stretozotocin with mitotane is ongoing. Treatment with mitotane alone has shown the best response and patient tolerance. In a recent retrospective, multicenter study comparing surgery to surgery with mitotane, the addition of mitotane was associated with longer recurrence-free and overall survival. Randomized prospective studies are needed before determining whether mitotane should be the standard of care. Mitotane should be started at 2 gm/day and titrated to achieve serum levels of 14-20 μg/dL which usually correlates to a dose of 4-6 gm/day. Mitotane causes adrenal suppression, thus cortisol and mineralocorticoid supplementation need to be given simultaneously. UFC, serum ACTH and electrolyte levels should be monitored. Thyroid function, lipids and testosterone levels should also be closely followed. Common adverse effects that may require dose reduction include neutropenia, GI distress (e.g. nausea, diarrhea and anorexia), abnormal hepatic function, confusion, ataxia and gynecomastia.

Surveillance for patients should include an enhanced CT of the chest and abdomen every 3 months and hormonal monitoring if the tumor was initially functional. The interval can be increased after the first year to every 6 months for 5 years, then yearly.

Metastases to the Adrenal

Metastatic lesions to the adrenal are second most common adrenal lesions **(Figure 23-7)**. Malignancies that can frequently metastasize to the adrenals include lung, kidney, colon, melanoma and breast. ^{18}F-FDG PET can be a useful screening test for patients with a history of malignancy, but up to 15% of benign adenomas can also be PET-avid. Isolated metastases to the adrenal can be resected with 5-year survival up to 30% in some series. Size of the metastatic lesion < 4.5 cm has been shown to be a prognostic factor associated with improved long-term survival. Metastases that are metachronous compared to those that are synchronous have been associated in some small studies with improved survival after adrenalectomy.

Laparoscopic metastasectomy has been shown to be oncologically equivalent to the open approach. Recurrence rates are 10-20% and long-term survival is similar regardless of operative approach. Port-site recurrence is very rare and only seen in case reports. Laparoscopic adrenalectomy is well-documented to result in decreased operative time, blood loss and hospital stay, and patients with isolated adrenal metastases should be considered for laparoscopic adrenalectomy.

Adrenalectomy

A number of approaches exist for adrenalectomy. Laparoscopic adrenalectomy was first performed in the early 1990s and is currently considered the standard approach for adrenal lesions without obvious signs of malignancy. Safe laparoscopic resection has been reported for pheochromocytomas, large lesions and solitary metastatic adrenal lesions. Masses 10-12 cm may be difficult laparoscopically but resection can be facilitated with a hand-assist device. The advantages have been well-described and most notably include a decreased length of hospital stay (mean 3 versus 7 days). Although operative charges may slightly be higher for laparoscopic surgery, cost-benefit analysis has shown reduced costs for the laparoscopic approach, predominantly due to the decreased hospital stay.

Laparoscopic adrenalectomy is most commonly performed either transperitoneal or retroperitoneal. Direct comparisons have not shown any significant advantage of one method over the other. The patient is positioned in the lateral decubitus position for the transperitoneal approach and the visualization may be more familiar to most surgeons. The retroperitoneal approach can be performed with the patient positioned laterally or prone and the anatomy may be less familiar. However, avoiding the abdomen is advantageous in patients who have had previous abdominal surgery in the same quadrant and

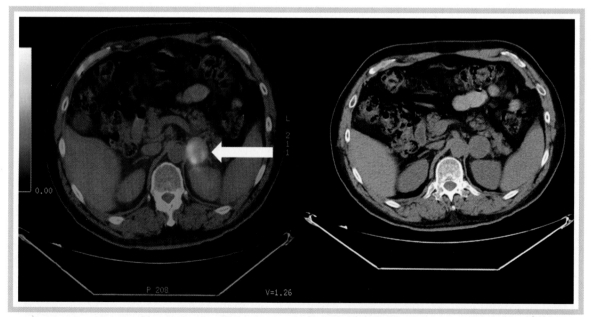

Figure 23-7: Two years after lobar resection for a right lower lobe squamous cell carcinoma (T2N1), a 4 cm PET-avid left adrenal lesion is seen (arrow). Metastatic squamous cell carcinoma is confirmed after retroperitoneoscopic left adrenalectomy

with experience, the operative times can be shorter. Repositioning the patient for bilateral adrenalectomy is not necessary if the prone positioning is used.

Laparoscopic Lateral Transperitoneal Approach

Using a beanbag support, the patient is positioned laterally at a 60° angle with the operative side up. The table is flexed to give maximal flexion between the iliac crest and the costal margin. The surgeon and assistant stand on the same side facing the patient. Typically 4-5 trocars are used with the initial 12 mm port placed at the mid-clavicular line approximately 2 cm below the costal margin. Once pneumoperitoneum is established, additional 5 mm ports are placed 2 cm below the costal margin in the posterior axillary, midaxillary and midclavicular lines. Occasionally a 5th port may be needed to help retract a large spleen or liver. On the left, the splenic flexure should be mobilized until the lienorenal ligament is identified which is then divided 1 cm lateral to the spleen cranially until the short gastrics and stomach are seen. The spleen and pancreatic tail should be gently retracted medially to expose the retroperitoneal space. The ultrasonic scalpel, hook cautery, or LigaSure™ vessel sealing system can be used to help maintain hemostasis while dissecting the lateral and anterior aspects of the adrenal gland. If the adrenal cannot be identified, an intraoperative ultrasound can be useful. The inferior phrenic vein can often be identified during this dissection which eventually joins the adrenal vein. Once the adrenal vein is identified, it should be dissected free, clipped and divided. The adrenal can then be retracted superiorly and laterally to help facilitate hemostatic division of its attachments. The adrenal parenchyma should not be manipulated to avoid tearing and bleeding. As the attachments closest to the renal hilum are divided, care must be taken to avoid transecting the medial limb of the adrenal or a superior branch of the renal artery.

The right side requires mobilization and retraction of the liver anteriorly which is facilitated with the fan retractor. The right triangular ligament and lateral attachments will most likely need to be divided to avoid tearing the liver capsule during retraction. The retroperitoneum is entered along the posterior surface of the right lobe. The superior aspect of the adrenal is identified and the attachments between the adrenal and the liver are divided using the ultrasonic, hook cautery or LigaSure™ device. The lateral border of the inferior vena cava is dissected free and the right adrenal vein identified. The right vein is much shorter than the left and care must be taken to avoid avulsing the vein off the IVC during the dissection. Once the vein is divided, the adrenal can be elevated and the remaining attachments divided as described for the left side. The adrenal is removed using an impermeable nylon laparoscopic specimen retrieval bag through the 12 mm port. The specimen should be examined to ensure that the adrenal has been removed in its entirety.

Laparoscopic Posterior Retroperitoneal Approach

The patient is placed in a prone jack-knife position with 90° flexion of the bed centered at the iliac crest. A bed support elevates the patient allowing the bulk of the abdominal contents to hang and not apply undue pressure on the retroperitoneum. The surgeon and assistant stand side by side on the operative side. A 1-1.5 cm incision is made at the initial port site lateral to the tip of the 12th rib and the retroperitoneum is entered using blunt dissection. Additional 5 mm ports are placed 4-5 cm lateral below the 11th rib and 3 cm below the 12th rib just lateral to the paraspinous muscles. Once the port sites have been established, a blunt trocar with inflatable balloon is placed in the initial port site and insufflation to 20-25 mmHg achieved. The 5 or 10 mm 30° laparoscope is placed in the middle port and under direct visualization, a working space is bluntly created in the retroperitoneum. The upper pole of the kidney is identified which facilitates identification of the adrenal gland. While retracting the kidney caudally, the adrenal is mobilized cranially and medially. As the adrenal is mobilized, it can be lifted to help identification of the adrenal vein. On the right, the IVC can be seen posteriorly and the adrenal vein is seen posterolaterally. On the left, the adrenal vein can be seen joining the inferior phrenic vein medial to the upper pole of the kidney. After dividing the vein, the remaining attachments are divided hemostatically. If additional retraction of the kidney is needed, especially on the left, a fourth trocar can be placed below the initial trocars. The pneumoperitoneum pressure should be decreased and the adrenalectomy bed carefully examined for hemostasis before removal of the trocars.

Open Adrenalectomy

Open adrenalectomy is indicated for large adrenal masses that have a high preoperative suspicion for malignancy and may involve *en bloc* resection of adjacent organs. In these cases, a transabdominal approach is preferred. A unilateral or bilateral subcostal incision is used and can be extended superiorly along the midline to the xiphoid process to help mobilize the liver, if needed. The operative approach is very similar to the laparoscopic approaches. If a splenectomy is anticipated, immunizations for pneumococci, *H. influenzae* and meningococci should be given 2 weeks preoperatively.

Other Operative Approaches

More recently, robotic surgery has been used with notable advantages for some procedures. For example, the improved dexterity with reticulating instruments has been helpful in prostatectomies. Another advantage includes better ergonomics for the surgeon. Studies have shown that robotic-assisted adrenalectomy is associated with equivalent outcomes when compared to the laparoscopic approach. Whether any advantages will justify the increased cost of the robotic equipment is still under ongoing study. Single incision laparoscopic surgery (SILS) has been described for adrenalectomy and more recently, transvaginal natural orifice translumenal endoscopic surgery (NOTES) adrenalectomy was described using cadaver and porcine models.

Bilateral Adrenalectomy

Bilateral adrenalectomy is considered in patients with ACTH-dependent Cushing's who have failed pituitary surgery and medical management, ACTH-independent macronodular adrenal hyperplasia (AIMAH), or in patients with hereditary pheochromocytoma and bilateral adrenal involvement. It can also be considered with bilateral adrenal adenomas, adrenal gland metastases and congenital adrenal hyperplasia. Often, patients with Cushing's who have failed conventional management are evaluated for surgery after prolonged excess cortisol exposure and are at high risk for perioperative complications including infection, poor wound healing, thromboembolic events and bleeding. AIMAH can be associated with asymmetric adrenal gland involvement and unilateral adrenalectomy of the largest adenoma has been shown to result in long-term resolution of the hypercortisolism. Adrenal vein sampling has also been reported to help localize the side of the predominant cortisol hypersecretion and prevent bilateral adrenalectomy if possible.

Bilateral adrenalectomy can be performed using the laparoscopic or open approach. Laparoscopic bilateral adrenalectomy is associated with a shorter hospital stay and fewer wound complications. The most common laparoscopic approach is transperitoneal however, this requires repositioning of the patient for the contralateral side. A retroperitoneal approach eliminates this step but, is anatomically less familiar and not as frequently utilized.

Following bilateral adrenalectomy, lifelong glucocorticoid and mineralocorticoid replacement will be needed. Patients need to be educated on the signs and symptoms of adrenal insufficiency which include hypotension, anorexia, nausea, abdominal pain, weakness, fatigue, lethargy or confusion. The condition can be fatal if not recognized and promptly treated. Hypoglycemia and hyperkalemia are seen and hyponatremia is also common, due to mineralocorticoid deficiency. IVF hydration should immediately be started and either dexamethasone 4 mg IV or hydrocortisone 100 mg IV needs to be administered.

Dexamethasone does not interfere with serum cortisol levels and should be used if further diagnostic tests are anticipated. Maintenance medication doses include either hydrocortisone 15-30 mg divided into two doses daily or prednisone 5-7.5 mg daily, adjusted to keep patients clinically eucortisol and fludrocortisone 0.1-0.2 mg daily, titrated to keep plasma renin activity levels in the upper range of normal. Long-term benefit has been shown after surgery with improvements in blood pressure control and diabetes.

To prevent the need for glucocorticoid and mineralocorticoid replacement as well as reduce the risk of life-threatening adrenal crisis, cortical-sparing adrenalectomy can be performed, most commonly considered in patients with bilateral pheochromocytomas. The risk of cortical-sparing adrenalectomy is recurrent or persistent disease. Most series that report low recurrence rates have follow-up less than the duration of relapse which has been reported to be ~ 10 years after initial surgery. However, these series also report high success rates in preventing steroid supplementation and adrenal crisis. After cortical-sparing adrenalectomy, recurrences are treated with completion adrenalectomy. Partial adrenalectomy has also been performed in some patients with aldosterone- and cortisol-secreting tumors.

Cortical function can be maintained with preservation of at least 1/3 of the gland and function is not dependent on maintaining a patent adrenal vein. Intraoperative ultrasound is an important adjunct to help determine the dissection margin and to also verify that the remnant has no residual disease. Both the open and laparoscopic approaches have been used successfully.

Summary

- An elevated aldosterone to plasma renin activity ratio is consistent with primary aldosteronism, but additional confirmatory testing should be performed.
- In primary aldosteronism, adrenalectomy is treatment for solitary adrenal adenoma or unilateral adrenal hyperplasia. Adrenal venous sampling can help localize the source of aldosterone hypersecretion.
- A 1 mg overnight dexamethasone suppression test can identify patients with Cushing's or subclinical Cushing's syndrome.
- All patients with adrenal lesions should undergo screening for pheochromocytoma with either a 24-hour urine fractionated metanephrine or plasma free metanephrine prior to any planned intervention, including FNA biopsy which is only rarely indicated.
- Up to 30% of pheochromocytoma patients can have a germline mutation in the *VHL, NF1, RET, SDHB* or *SDHD* genes and genetic counseling should be considered.

- Malignant pheochromocytoma is diagnosed with metastatic or recurrent disease. Histopathologic features are not confirmatory.
- Adrenocortical carcinoma is rare, but more frequent in incidental adrenal lesions over 4 cm in size. Characteristic CT and MRI findings can help determine the malignancy risk.
- Open adrenalectomy is indicated if carcinoma is suspected. Complete resection with clear margins should be the surgical intent.
- Laparoscopic surgery is associated with decreased length of hospital stay and is the standard operative approach for adrenal lesions without obvious signs of malignancy. There are no significant patient outcome differences when laparoscopic adrenalectomy is performed retroperitoneally compared to transabdominally.

Landmark Papers

1. Allolio B, Fassnacht M. Adrenocortical carcinoma: clinical update. J Clin Endocrinol Metab 2006; 91:2027-37.
2. Erlic Z, Neumann HPH. When should genetic testing be obtained in a patient with phaeochromocytoma or paraganglioma? Clin Endocrinol 2009; 70:354-7.
3. Fassnact M, Johanssen S, Quinkler M, et al. Limited prognostic value of the 2004 International Union Against Cancer (UICC) staging classification for adrenocortical carcinoma. Cancer 2009; 115:243-50.
4. Funder JW, Carey RM, Fardella C, et al. Case detection, diagnosis and treatment of patients with primary aldosteronism: an Endocrine Society clinical practice guideline. J Clin Endocrinol Metab 2008; 93:3266-81.
5. Korbkin M, Giordano TJ, Brodeur FJ, et al. Adrenal adenomas: relationship between histologic lipid and CT and MR findings. Radiology 1996; 200:743-7.
6. Lenders JWM, Pacak K, Walther MM, et al. Biochemical diagnosis of pheochromocytoma: which test is best? JAMA 2002; 287:1427-34.
7. Montori VM, Young Jr WF. Use of plasma aldosterone concentration-to-plasma renin activity ratio as a screening test for primary aldosteronism: a systematic review of the literature. Endocrinol Metab Clin N Am 2002; 31:619-32.
8. Niemann LK, Biller BMK, Findling JW, et al. The diagnosis of Cushing's syndrome: an Endocrine Society clinical practice guideline. J Clin Endocrinol Metab 2008; 93:1526-40.
9. Quayle FJ, Spitler JA, Pierce RA, et al. Needle biopsy of incidentally discovered adrenal masses is rarely informative and potentially hazardous. Surgery 2007; 142:497-504.
10. Rossi R, Tauchmanova L, Luciano A, et al. Subclinical Cushing's syndrome in patients with adrenal incidentaloma: clinical and biochemical features. J Clin Endocrinol Metab 2000; 85:1440-8.
11. Schell SR, Talamini MA, Udelsman R. Laparoscopic adrenalectomy for nonmalignant disease: improved safety, morbidity and cost-effectiveness. Surg Endosc 1999;13:30-4.
12. Sturgeon C, Shen WT, Clark OH, et al. Risk assessment in 457 adrenal cortical carcinomas: how much dose tumor size predict the likelihood of malignancy? J Am Coll Surg 2006; 202:423-30.
13. Terzolo M, Ali A, Osella G, et al. Prevalence of adrenal carcinoma among incidentally discovered adrenal masses: a retrospective study from 1989-1994. Arch Surg 1997; 132:914-9.
14. Terzolo M, Angeli A, Fassnacht M, et al. Adjuvant mitotane treatment for adrenocortical carcinoma. N Engl J Med 2007; 356:2372-80.
15. Walz MK, Alesina PF, Wenger FA, et al. Posterior retroperitoneoscopic adrenalectomy - results of 560 procedures in 520 patients. Surgery 2006; 140:943-50.
16. Young, Jr WF, Stanson AW, Thompson GB, et al. Role for adrenal venous sampling in primary aldosteronism. Surgery 2004; 135:1227-35.
17. Zarnegar R, Young Jr, WF, Lee J, et al. The aldosteronoma resolution score: predicting complete resolution of hypertension after adrenalectomy for aldosteronoma. Ann Surg 2008; 247:511-8.

Level of Evidence Table			
Recommendation	**Grade**	**Best level of evidence**	**References**
Aldosterone to plasma renin activity ratio should be the initial screening test for primary aldosteronism.	B	3a	1
Due to inaccuracy in CT/MRI imaging, adrenal venous sampling is indicated to determine laterality in primary aldosteronism.	A	1a	2, 3
Routine screening for subclinical Cushing's syndrome should be performed on incidental adrenal lesions.	B	4	4-5
Measurement of plasma free metanephrines is the test of choice for diagnosing pheochromocytoma.	B	2b	6, 7
Resection of incidental non-functioning adrenal masses >5cm should be considered due to the risk of malignancy.	B	2b	8, 9

Contd...

Contd...

Recommendation	Grade	Best level of evidence	References
Adrenal FNA biopsy is unreliable and should not be performed unless a positive result will alter surgical management.	B	2b	8, 10-13
Adjuvant mitotane should be considered to improve at least recurrence-free survival in ACC patients.	B	2b	14-16
Adjuvant radiation may also decrease local recurrence in ACC.	B	2b	17
Laparoscopic versus open adrenalectomy is acceptable for benign and malignant (primary or secondary) lesions.	B	2b	18-21

References

1. Montori VM, Young WF, Jr. Use of plasma aldosterone concentration-to-plasma renin activity ratio as a screening test for primary aldosteronism. A systematic review of the literature. Endocrinol Metab Clin North Am 2002;31(3): 619-32, xi.

2. Kempers MJ, Lenders JW, van Outheusden L, et al. Systematic review: diagnostic procedures to differentiate unilateral from bilateral adrenal abnormality in primary aldosteronism. Ann Intern Med 2009;151(5):329-37.

3. Young WF, Stanson AW, Thompson GB, Grant CS, Farley DR, van Heerden JA. Role for adrenal venous sampling in primary aldosteronism. Surgery 2004;136(6):1227-35.

4. Rossi R, Tauchmanova L, Luciano A, et al. Subclinical Cushing's syndrome in patients with adrenal incidentaloma: clinical and biochemical features. J Clin Endocrinol Metab 2000;85(4):1440-8.

5. Sippel RS, Chen H. Subclinical Cushing's syndrome in adrenal incidentalomas. Surg Clin North Am 2004;84(3): 875-85.

6. Lenders JW, Pacak K, Walther MM, et al. Biochemical diagnosis of pheochromocytoma: which test is best? JAMA 2002;287(11):1427-34.

7. Yu R. Ordering pattern and performance of biochemical tests for diagnosing pheochromocytoma between 2000 and 2008. Endocr Pract 2009;15(4):313-21.

8. Mazzaglia PJ, Monchik JM. Limited value of adrenal biopsy in the evaluation of adrenal neoplasm: a decade of experience. Arch Surg 2009;144(5):465-70.

9. Terzolo M, Ali A, Osella G, Mazza E. Prevalence of adrenal carcinoma among incidentally discovered adrenal masses. A retrospective study from 1989 to 1994. Gruppo Piemontese Incidentalomi Surrenalici. Arch Surg 1997; 132(8):914-19.

10. Lumachi F, Borsato S, Brandes AA, et al. Fine-needle aspiration cytology of adrenal masses in noncancer patients: clinicoradiologic and histologic correlations in functioning and nonfunctioning tumors. Cancer 2001; 93(5):323-9.

11. Quayle FJ, Spitler JA, Pierce RA, Lairmore TC, Moley JF, Brunt LM. Needle biopsy of incidentally discovered adrenal masses is rarely informative and potentially hazardous. Surgery 2007;142(4):497-502; discussion 502-4.

12. Kebebew E, Siperstein AE, Clark OH, Duh QY. Results of laparoscopic adrenalectomy for suspected and unsuspected malignant adrenal neoplasms. Arch Surg 2002;137(8):948-51; discussion 952-3.

13. Lumachi F, Borsato S, Tregnaghi A, et al. CT-scan, MRI and image-guided FNA cytology of incidental adrenal masses. Eur J Surg Oncol 2003;29(8):689-92.

14. Icard P, Goudet P, Charpenay C, et al. Adrenocortical carcinomas: surgical trends and results of a 253-patient series from the French Association of Endocrine Surgeons study group. World J Surg 2001;25(7):891-7.

15. Kasperlik-Zaluska AA, Migdalska BM, Zgliczynski S, Makowska AM. Adrenocortical carcinoma. A clinical study and treatment results of 52 patients. Cancer 1995;75(10): 2587-91.

16. Terzolo M, Angeli A, Fassnacht M, et al. Adjuvant mitotane treatment for adrenocortical carcinoma. N Engl J Med 2007; 356(23):2372-80.

17. Fassnacht M, Hahner S, Polat B, et al. Efficacy of adjuvant radiotherapy of the tumor bed on local recurrence of adrenocortical carcinoma. J Clin Endocrinol Metab 2006; 91(11): 4501-4.

18. Brunt LM, Doherty GM, Norton JA, Soper NJ, Quasebarth MA, Moley JF. Laparoscopic adrenalectomy compared to open adrenalectomy for benign adrenal neoplasms. J Am Coll Surg 1996;183(1):1-10.

19. Moinzadeh A, Gill IS. Laparoscopic radical adrenalectomy for malignancy in 31 patients. J Urol 2005;173(2):519-25.

20. Adler JT, Mack E, Chen H. Equal oncologic results for laparoscopic and open resection of adrenal metastases. J Surg Res 15 2007;140(2):159-64.

21. Schell SR, Talamini MA, Udelsman R. Laparoscopic adrenalectomy for nonmalignant disease: improved safety, morbidity and cost-effectiveness. Surg Endosc 1999; 13(1):30-4.

Gastrointestinal Tract

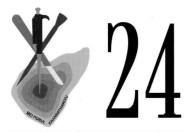

24

Esophageal Cancer

Edward Cheong, Farzaneh Banki, Arjun Pennathur, James D Luketich

Incidence

Esophageal cancers are aggressive tumors with an increasing incidence in the western world. In fact, the rate of increase in the incidence of esophageal adenocarcinoma (EAC) has been higher than any other cancer in the United States. Historically, squamous cell carcinoma (SCC) of the esophagus was the most common esophageal malignancy internationally, accounting for more than 90% of esophageal cancers. In the last three decades, there has been a rapid rise in the incidence of EAC in the western world, with a reported increase in white males of 563% from 1.01 per 100,000 person-years in 1975-1979 to 5.69 per 100,000 person-years in 2000-2004. A similar rapid increase was also apparent among white women, in whom the adenocarcinoma rate increased 435% from 0.17 to 0.74 per 100,000 person-years over the same time period. The National Cancer Institute reported 13,900 new cases and 13,000 deaths from esophageal adenocarcinoma in 2003 and anticipated 16,470 new cases and 14,539 deaths in 2009. EAC is now the predominant esophageal cancer in the western world.

Worldwide, the incidence of SCC varies considerably with geographic location and the highest rates occur in northern China and northern Iran, where incidence exceeds 100 in 100,000 individuals. In the United States, the incidence is less than 2 per 100,000, although rates are nearly quadruple for African Americans. SCC predominates in African Americans over Caucasians by a ratio of 6:1 and EAC has the opposite preponderance, occurring in Caucasians over African Americans at a ratio of 4:1. In the western world, there is less impact on the incidence of SCC from dietary factors, such as nitrosamines, due to different food preservation techniques and the primary etiology of esophageal SCC is the use of tobacco and alcohol with tobacco exposure being associated with a ten-fold higher risk for esophageal SCC in heavy smokers relative to nonsmokers. There is a greater than multiplicative effect between smoking and alcohol consumption that occurs in SCC; for EAC, the effect is only additive. Prior aerodigestive tract malignancies predispose to a higher risk for

esophageal cancer. Ten to fifteen percent of second primary cancers in patients with prior oropharyngeal cancer or lung cancer occur in the esophagus. Chronic inflammation and stasis, which occur with strictures caused by caustic injury and achalasia, are long-term risks for esophageal SCC; in addition, patients with tylosis, which is inherited in an autosomal dominant fashion, and Plummer-Vinson syndrome have a greater risk for esophageal SCC.

Other cancers of the esophagus are rare and include small cell carcinoma and benign and malignant smooth muscle tumors, such as leiomyoma and leiomyosarcoma. Small cell carcinoma of the esophagus may account for 0.8-2.4% of esophageal malignances. Esophageal small cell carcinoma occurs most commonly in the 6th to 8th decades of life and has a very poor prognosis, regardless of treatment. Smooth muscle tumors make up ~ 1% of all esophageal primary tumors. It has been estimated that up to 50% of smooth muscle tumors in the gastrointestinal tract occur in the esophagus. Esophageal smooth muscle tumors occur most frequently in the lower 1/3 of the esophagus and dysphagia is the most common symptom. In patients with leiomyosarcoma, the 5-year survival rate is estimated to be ~ 20%, although this data was obtained from review of only 58 patients. Leiomyoma is the most common benign esophageal lesion, accounting > 50% of benign esophageal tumors. The peak incidence is between 39-59 years of age, well below the average age at diagnosis for EAC, SCC and malignant smooth muscle tumors.

In this chapter we will review the pathogenesis, prevention, surveillance, diagnostic and staging modalities, treatment options and palliation of esophageal carcinoma, with a focus on esophageal adenocarcinoma. Much of the information presented is also applicable to other types of esophageal tumors.

Pathogenesis of Esophageal Adenocarcinoma

Gastroesophageal Reflux Disease

Patients with recurring symptoms of reflux have an eight-fold increase in the risk of esophageal adenocarcinoma. Other markers of gastroesophageal reflux disease (GERD), such as hiatal hernia, esophageal ulcer and frequent use of antacid or histamine-H2 blockers, are associated with an increased risk but do not appear to be independent risk factors.

Barrett's Esophagus

Barrett's esophagus (BE) is the condition in which columnar epithelium replaces the squamous epithelium that normally lines the distal esophagus. BE develops when GERD damages the squamous esophageal mucosa and the injury heals through a metaplastic process in which columnar cells replace squamous ones. The abnormal columnar epithelium that characterizes Barrett's esophagus (called specialized intestinal metaplasia) predisposes patients to adenocarcinoma. Esophageal adenocarcinoma develops in approximately 0.5% of patients with BE per year and GERD is the main recognized risk factor. However, in 10-30% of patients with EAC, BE is not found. It is unclear in these cases whether the segment of intestinal metaplasia was short or the tumor overgrew the metaplastic epithelium. In a case-control study linking GERD to EAC, people with long-standing, severe reflux symptoms (symptoms > 5 years prior to cancer diagnosis) had an odds ratio of 43.5 for EAC. It is now generally accepted that Barrett's epithelium can progress through a metaplasia-dysplasia-carcinoma progression but the natural history of dysplasia in Barrett's esophagus is not well defined. In a recent study of 76 patients with high-grade dysplasia who had no evidence of cancer on an extensive initial evaluation, the 5-year cumulative incidence of esophageal cancer was 59%. In another study of 100 such patients, esophageal adenocarcinoma was found in 32% during eight years of follow-up. Identification of high-grade dysphasia (HGD) has been considered as an indication for an esophagectomy or aggressive endoscopic treatment, since occult invasive cancer has frequently been identified at the time of resection. Without treatment, invasive cancer develops within three years in up to half of patients with HGD.

Obesity

The increasing prevalence of obesity in the western world is thought to add to the rising incidence of esophageal adenocarcinoma. It has been postulated that obesity increases intra-abdominal pressure and gastroesophageal reflux contributing to the increased risk of adenocarcinoma. In a nationwide, population-based, case-control study in Sweden by Lagergren et al, 189 patients with adenocarcinoma of the esophagus were compared to 820 controls (randomly selected from a continuously updated population register). Odds ratios estimated the relative risk for esophageal adenocarcinoma. The adjusted odds

ratio was 7.6 among persons in the highest body mass index (BMI) quartile compared with persons in the lowest. Obese persons (persons with a BMI > 30 kg/m^2) had an odds ratio of 16.2 compared with the leanest persons (persons with a BMI < 22 kg/m^2). These results suggest a strong association between BMI and esophageal adenocarcinoma.

Genetic Findings

The molecular pathogenesis of BE and EAC includes the accumulation of multiple genetic alterations over time. In BE, loss of heterozygosity of such tumor suppressor genes as p53, the adenomatous polyposis coli gene (APC), the gene deleted in colorectal cancer (DCC) and p16 is correlated with progression from metaplasia to dysplasia to adenocarcinoma. Reflux of acidic gastric contents and bile acids into the lower esophagus has been identified to have a role in esophageal malignancy and upregulates caudal-related homologue 2 (CDX2), a regulatory gene involved in embryonic development and axial patterning of the alimentary tract. Lipocalin 2 and Cyclin D1 are specifically expressed by the Barrett's epithelial cells. In addition, the pathogenesis of Barrett's esophagus may occur via bile-stimulated cell signaling through the epidermal growth factor receptor (EGFR).

Prevention

Despite excellent control of symptoms with aggressive anti-acid therapy, including use of antacids, antireflux surgery and surveillance programs, the incidence and number of deaths from esophageal adenocarcinoma are increasing and prevention of this cancer remains challenging. Many patients whose GERD symptoms have been resolved with antisecretory therapy continue to have acid reflux. In fact, up to 80% of patients treated with twice daily proton pump inhibitors (PPIs) continue to demonstrate nocturnal gastric acid reflux. Combination regimens employing PPIs and H2-blockers can produce gastric achlorhydria, leading investigators to speculate that such medical therapy might impact favorably on the natural history of BE. However, achlorhydria is also a known risk factor for developing adenocarcinoma of the stomach and is thought to promote the propagation of bacteria that produce carcinogenic nitrosamine compounds. Acid suppression also increases serum gastrin levels, which are associated with increased proliferative markers and mucosal hyperplasia in patients with BE. No medical or surgical therapy has been definitively proven to promote the regression of BE, prevent the progression of BE or eliminate the risk of EAC. Though not substantiated by prospective, randomized studies, to date, several larger non-randomized series have suggested a possible reduction in the overall risk of cancer progression in patients undergoing fundoplication. In a comprehensive review of the outcomes in 97 patients with BE treated with fundoplication and a median follow-up of five years, regression of low-grade dysplasia to a nondysplastic Barrett's epithelium occurred in 44% of patients. No patient developed HGD or cancer in 410 patient-years of follow-up. In another randomized study of 59 patients with BE, comparing medical (H2-blockers or omeprazole) and surgical therapy, a decrease in the length of BE was noted in the surgical arm. Six patients developed dysplasia (5 low-grade, 1 high-grade with early EAC) in the medical arm, compared to only one (HGD with early EAC) in the surgical arm. Interestingly, the patient with progression in the surgical arm had evidence of failure of the antireflux procedure documented by 24 hr pH monitoring. Patients with successful antireflux surgery, as documented by 24 hr pH studies, had no dysplastic changes or progression to adenocarcinoma. Independent predictors of regression from low-grade dysplasia to BE were the presence of a short segment of Barrett's and successful antireflux surgery. Additionally, the new modality of radiofrequency ablation has shown encouraging results with near-complete regression of dysplasia and BE and is discussed further in this chapter.

Surveillance

The major challenge in treating esophageal adenocarcinoma is that half the patients are unresectable at the time of diagnosis due to the presence of systemic disease. If a screening program could detect the disease at an earlier stage, there could be a greater possibility of cure. In patients with BE, the incidences of low grade dysplasia, HGD and esophageal adenocarcinoma are approximately 4%, 1% and 0.5% per year, respectively. This increasing awareness of BE as a precursor to EAC has led to the development of surveillance programs, which have allowed earlier detection of EAC in the metaplasia-dysplasia-adenocarcinoma sequence. Therefore, patients found to have BE are candidates for regular endoscopic surveillance. Unfortunately, the survival benefits and cost-effectiveness of endoscopic surveillance for esophageal cancers have not been demonstrated. In 11 studies with 1,127 patients with BE; only 3.5% actually progressed to cancer. Proponents argue that productive screening should focus on patients with multiple risk factors (e.g. GERD, Caucasian race, male gender, age greater than 50 years and long duration of symptoms) and small studies have suggested that surveillance can identify early stage, potentially curable neoplasms. However, few patients with esophageal cancer are diagnosed via surveillance programs. Less than 5% of patients with esophageal cancer were known to have had BE before they sought help for

symptoms of cancer and up to 40% had no prior history of GERD. Currently, the American College of Gastroenterology recommends that the presence of dysplasia guide surveillance endoscopy for BE because dysplasia is currently the best pathological predictor of cancer development. If dysplasia is not present, endoscopy is recommended every 3 years and if low-grade dysplasia is present, surveillance endoscopy is recommended every 6 months for 1 year and yearly thereafter, if no progression is seen. If HGD is present, it should be confirmed by an experienced pathologist. There is a high incidence of invasive cancer already present in patients with HGD (about 40%) and a high risk of invasive cancer developing in these patients, which supports the recommendation and our opinion that patients with HGD should be offered esophagectomy for treatment. If the patient is unfit for surgery or refuses surgery, endoscopic treatment with ablative therapies or intensive surveillance (endoscopy every 3 months with four-quadrant biopsies taken at every 1 cm of BE segment) can be offered to identify occult carcinoma, which can be present in about 40% of cases.

Clinical Presentations

Most patients with esophageal adenocarcinoma have dysphagia (74%), weight loss (57%) and odynophagia (17%) at the time of diagnosis. If weight loss exceeds more than 10% of body mass, it is an independent indicator of poor prognosis. Dyspnea, cough, hoarseness and pain (e.g. retrosternal, back or right upper abdomen) occur less often but may reflect the presence of extensive, unresectable disease. The physical examination is usually unremarkable. Lymphadenopathy, particularly in the left supraclavicular fossa (Virchow's node), hepatomegaly and pleural effusion may indicate metastatic disease.

Staging of Esophageal Cancer

TNM Classification

The TNM classification system is traditionally used to stage esophageal carcinoma (**Table 24-1 and Figure 24-1**). The American Joint Committee on Cancer (AJCC) classification does not distinguish tumors that have invaded the mucosa (T1a) and submucosa (T1b). T1a lesions have lesser chance of nodal spread with most series showing lesser than 10% incidence, while about 30% of T1b lesions will have nodal metastases. In addition, the number of lymph nodes involved, histology, degree of differentiation and location seem to have an impact on survival of patients with esophageal cancer. These issues are being considered and addressed in the next AJCC revisions for staging.

TABLE 24-1	TNM classification for staging of esophageal carcinomas		
T	**Primary Tumor**		
TX	Tumor cannot be assessed		
T0	No evidence of tumor		
Tis	High-grade dysplasia		
T1	Tumor invades the lamina propria, muscularis mucosae or submucosa. It does not breach the submucosa		
T2	Tumor invades into, but not beyond, the muscularis propria		
T3	Tumor invades the paraesophageal tissue but does not invade adjacent structures		
T4	Tumor invades adjacent structures		
N	**Regional lymph nodes**		
NX	Regional lymph nodes cannot be assessed		
N0	No regional lymph node metastases		
N1	Regional lymph node metastases		
M	**Distant metastasis**		
MX	Distant metastases cannot be assessed		
M1a:	Upper thoracic esophagus metastatic to cervical lymph nodes		
	Lower thoracic esophagus metastatic to celiac lymph nodes		
M1b	Upper thoracic esophagus metastatic to other nonregional lymph nodes or other distant sites		
	Midthoracic esophagus metastatic to either nonregional lymph nodes or other distant sites		
	Lower thoracic esophagus metastatic to other nonregional lymph nodes or other distant sites		
Stage groupings			
Stage 0	Tis	N0	M0
Stage I	T1	N0	M0
Stage IIA	T2	N0	M0
	T3	N0	M0
Stage IIB	T1	N1	M0
	T2	N1	M0
Stage III	T3	N1	M0
	T4	Any N	M0
Stage IVA	Any T	Any N	M1a
Stage IVB	Any T	Any N	M1b

Adapted from Greene FL, Page DL, Fleming ID, et al (Eds): Digestive system: esophagus. In AJCC Cancer Staging Manual, 6th edn. New York, Springer 2002;91-98.

Diagnostic Modalities

Upper endoscopy: Upper endoscopy is the gold standard for the diagnosis of esophageal carcinoma. While the presence of a mass or a nodule is diagnosed via an upper endoscopy (and presence of cancer proven by biopsy), the depth of the tumor and lymph node involvement cannot be assessed with this modality. Many fungating masses may largely be protruding in the esophageal lumen and, surprisingly, not be transmural. Therefore, other modalities are required to assess the depth of penetration and involvement of periesophageal lymph nodes.

Computed tomography (CT) scan: The sensitivity and specificity of CT scan in diagnosing locoregional nodal involvement are 84% and 67%, respectively. For distant organ metastases, the sensitivity is 81% and the specificity is 82%. Obliteration of the fat plane between the esophagus and the aorta, trachea and bronchi, pericardium and an angle of contact between the esophagus and the aorta extending more than 90 degrees may indicate T4 disease. Pericardial invasion is suspected if pericardial thickening, effusion or indentation of the heart with loss of the pericardial fat plane is seen.

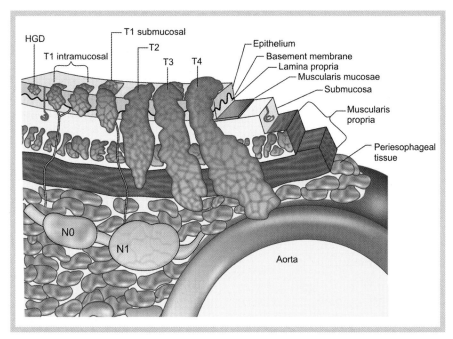

Figure 24-1: Esophageal tumor classifications. Reprinted with permission, Cleveland Clinic Center for Medical Art & Photography © 2000-2009. All Rights Reserved

¹⁸F-fluoro-2-deoxy-D-glucose positron emission tomography (FDG-PET): FDG-PET scanning has recently been introduced into esophageal cancer staging and is more accurate than conventional CT imaging, particularly in the detection of distant metastases. A systematic review has shown a moderate sensitivity and specificity of 0.51 and 0.84, respectively, for the detection of locoregional lymph node metastases and a sensitivity and specificity of 0.67 and 0.97, respectively, for detection of distant metastases. The broad implementation of FDG-PET in staging esophageal cancer was questioned by Van Westreenen, et al. In their large prospective study, no substantial benefit was detected for FDG-PET over 'conventional' diagnostic modalities (e.g. endoscopic ultrasound and CT scan). We have reported an increased accuracy of minimally invasive surgical staging compared with PET scans. In an analysis of 100 consecutive PET scans from the University of Pittsburgh, we found that although PET scanning was more accurate than CT scanning for detection of distant metastases, its sensitivity was only 69% compared with minimally invasive surgical staging.

False-negative results on PET scan generally pertain to lesions that are less than 10 mm in size. However, the fused PET-CT modality, which combines metabolic and anatomic information, improves the accuracy of staging to 90%. Integrated PET-CT has a significant incremental value over conventional staging methods, mainly in the detection of distant metastases and synchronous tumors and frequently impacts patient management. Although convincing evidence of stage IV disease can be surmised on the basis of a widely positive PET scan, patients with solitary metastases on PET scan generally warrant tissue diagnostic proof of unresectability.

Endoscopic ultrasound (EUS): Endoscopic ultrasound (EUS) is the most accurate noninvasive test for locoregional staging of the cancer (T and N classification), though distinguishing the early lesions (T1a or T1b) remains problematic. The overall accuracy of EUS for T classification is 84%. The accuracy varies with each T classification, with an accuracy of 83% for T1 cancer; 73% for T2 cancer; 89% for T3 cancer and 89% for T4 cancer. One limitation of EUS is the inability to pass the endoscope through tumor strictures, which occur in one-third of patients. Dilatation and use of mini-ultrasound probes have lessened this problem. Rounded, sharply demarcated, homogeneous and hypoechoic features of a lymph node on EUS indicate malignancy. The overall accuracy of EUS staging of locoregional nodal disease is 77%. The addition of fine-needle aspiration (FNA) to EUS further refines the staging of nodal disease, bringing the accuracy up to 85%. We routinely assess the depth of the tumor and, more importantly, the nodal involvement by EUS and FNA, since in our center, patients who present with nodal metastasis may be considered for neoadjuvant therapy.

Diagnostic endoscopic mucosal resection: Endoscopic mucosal resection (EMR) has been investigated as a diagnostic method to differentiate mucosal (T1a) from submucosal (T1b) tumors. In addition to its use as a diagnostic modality, it is also used as a therapeutic modality for treatment of superficial esophageal cancer in selected patients. We do not routinely perform diagnostic EMR in patients with diagnoses of esophageal cancer. In patients who are not fit to undergo esophagectomy, EMR as a therapeutic modality, in combination with other endoscopic treatments, is used at our center for a selected group of patients and is discussed further in this chapter.

Flexible bronchoscopy: Flexible bronchoscopy should be performed for tumors located in the upper and middle thirds of the esophagus to look for tumor infiltration. Thickening or indentation of the normally flat or slightly convex posterior membranous wall of the intrathoracic trachea or left main bronchus is suggestive of airway invasion. However, confirmation by bronchoscopy with biopsy is necessary.

Neck ultrasound: According to the current staging systems, lymph node metastases in the cervical region are considered M1b disease in patients with a mid- or distal esophageal tumor. Several studies investigated ultrasound of the neck (with FNA if indicated) as a diagnostic tool for detecting supraclavicular lymph node metastases. The sensitivity and specificity are 75% and 91%, respectively, for ultrasound alone and 72% and 100%, respectively, for ultrasound with FNA. This modality is not routinely used in our center, in the absence of clinical or other radiological evidence of supraclavicular lymphadenopathy.

Minimally invasive staging: The use of minimally invasive staging (laparoscopy or thoracoscopy) is not widely practiced, given the improving accuracies of non-invasive methods. However, we have found laparoscopic staging very useful in patients with cancer of the distal esophagus and gastroesophageal junction. Staging laparoscopy can also be performed prior to performing an MIE or definitive resection. Thoracoscopy, though rarely used, can be useful in very selected group of patients to assess suspicious lung nodules or invasion of adjacent structures by lesions that appear to be T4 lesions on radiologic imaging. In our experience, MIS staging is more accurate than EUS for the diagnosis of lymph node metastases and more accurate than PET scanning for detection of distant metastases.

Laparoscopy is useful for detecting and confirming nodal involvement and distant metastatic disease that potentially would alter treatment and prognosis in patients with esophageal cancer. Laparoscopy has been reported to change the planned therapeutic approach in 10-17% of patients. In a study with 59 subjects, only 78% of patients with regional celiac lymph nodes that appeared normal were proven by biopsy to be tumor free. Similarly, 76% of patients with lymph nodes that were abnormal in appearance were confirmed by biopsy to have node-positive disease. We found the overall staging accuracy of EUS to be only 72% compared with laparoscopy. The

sensitivity of laparoscopy to detect peritoneal metastases is 71% and the sensitivity for liver metastases is 86%.

The liver, omentum, small bowel mesentery and all peritoneal surfaces are examined during the staging laparoscopy for assessment of the resectability of cancer. Further, the extent and fixation of the tumor, invasion of the celiac axis and aorta, and perigastric lymph node involvement are assessed. We believe MIS with laparoscopy is particularly valuable in detection of occult distant metastases and exclusion of these patients from definitive surgical resection. In our practice, we do not refuse an esophagectomy until we have biopsy-proven diagnoses of bulky locoregional nodal involvement or distant metastasis. Therefore, staging laparoscopy allows us to select patients for appropriate therapy. In addition, a jejunostomy tube and a vascular access for chemotherapy can be placed at the time of laparoscopy, if required. Finally, some investigators have incorporated ligation of the left gastric artery to potentially precondition the stomach during the staging laparoscopy.

Treatment

Esophagectomy remains the main therapy for patients with resectable esophageal cancer. Surgical strategies in the treatment of esophageal cancer aim to improve prognosis by achieving the best possible local tumor control by *en bloc* resection (R0) and lymphadenectomy. Patients should be selected carefully following adequate staging and functional status assessment.

Preoperative Evaluation

The patient's physiologic status should thoroughly be evaluated to assess the risks of esophagectomy. This evaluation should include assessments of the patient's performance status, cardiovascular function, pulmonary function and nutritional status. Pulmonary complications, particularly pneumonia, are important determinants of early postoperative outcome. In a study of preoperative risk assessment by Ferguson and colleagues, pulmonary complications were associated with a > 4-fold increase in mortality. Avendano and colleagues similarly identified increased age, decreased pulmonary function and pre-operative chemoradiation as risk factors for development of pneumonia.

Complete abstinence from cigarette smoking for a minimum of 2-3 weeks prior to surgery is mandatory. Baseline pulmonary function tests with arterial blood gas values are obtained in those with suspected or documented chronic lung disease. A forced expiratory volume in 1 second (FEV_1) of less than 1 L (approximately 40% of that predicted for an average man) suggests a higher likelihood of serious pulmonary complications. Wright et al, recently used the Society of Thoracic Surgeons (STS)

General Thoracic Database for all patients treated with esophagectomy (n = 2315) for esophageal cancer and created a multivariable risk model for mortality and major morbidity. Important predictors of major morbidity were: age (P = 0.005), black race (P = 0.08), congestive heart failure (P = 0.015), coronary artery disease (P = 0.017), peripheral vascular disease (P= 0.009), hypertension (P = 0.029), insulin dependent diabetes (P = 0.009), American Society of Anesthesiology rating (P = 0.001), smoking status (P = 0.022), decrease in FEV1 < 60% of predicted and steroid use (P = 0.026).

Evaluation of the patient's functional capacity is vital in the overall risk assessment. Noninvasive stress testing is widely used to help predict risk of perioperative complications, but the poor predictive power of these tests hampers their usefulness. Stress myocardial perfusion imaging can be used for nearly all patients, even those whose medical conditions preclude exercise. Although a negative perfusion test result can offer substantial reassurance to patients and physicians, the predictive power of a positive test is poor. After estimating the risk of cardiac complications, measures should be taken to reduce this risk. Our approach is to obtain consultation from an expert cardiologist and cardiac surgeon in selected patients to develop a treatment plan that balances the risks of cardiac complications with the risks-benefits of cardiac intervention, the need for anticoagulation or antiplatelet therapy with some interventions and the risk-benefits of esophagectomy.

Surgical Approach

The surgical approaches for the treatment of esophageal cancer include an open, three-field (e.g. cervical, thoracic and abdominal) approach, a two-field approach (e.g. thoracic and abdominal), a transhiatal approach and a minimally invasive approach. The important factors affecting survival of patients who undergo esophagectomy are completeness of resection, achievement of an R0 resection and the stage of the disease. Other potential factors include the extent of lymphadenectomy and morbidity of the operation.

Transthoracic esophagectomy and transhiatal esophagectomy: Transthoracic esophagectomy (TTE) consists of mobilizing the esophagus through a thoracic approach and can be performed via an Ivor Lewis esophagectomy with an intrathoracic anastomosis or a McKeown esophagectomy with cervical anastomosis. In contrast to TTE, transhiatal esophagectomy (THE) does not require transthoracic mobilization of the esophagus. The esophagectomy is performed via an abdominal approach and the anastomosis is performed in the neck. Both procedures have their advantages and disadvantages and have traditionally been used for the treatment of patients

with esophageal cancer. In the past 30 years, THE, popularized and refined by Orringer, has become an accepted operation that has substantially reduced the morbidity and mortality that have historically been associated with transthoracic esophageal resection. A meta-analysis of 7527 patients undergoing either THE or TTE for carcinoma documented statistically significant differences in hospital mortality, blood loss, pulmonary complications, chylothorax, ICU stay and hospital stay favoring THE over TTE. However, TTE had lower anastomotic leak rates and a lower incidence of vocal cord paralysis than THE. In a recent report of 2000 THE, Orringer et al reported an in-hospital mortality of 1% and good to excellent late functional results in 73% of patients. Very few randomized trials have compared transthoracic versus transhiatal esophagectomy. Hulscher, et al conducted a randomized trial comparing TTE and THE in patients with distal and gastroesophageal junction neoplasms and found no statistical difference in survival at 5 years. In a retrospective study, Johansson, et al studied patients with T3N1 esophageal cancer who had an R0 resection alone with 20 or more lymph nodes removed and found that survival benefit of TTE was limited to patients fewer than 9 involved nodes with no difference in outcome between TTE and THE when 9 or more lymph nodes were involved. Other studies have shown that locoregional recurrence after THE occurs in approximately 23-47% compared with 1-10% after TTE. The most likely explanation for potential improved survival after TTE is better removal of locoregional disease, since unrecognized microscopic disease is removed when using *en bloc* lymph node dissection but is left behind when using transhiatal lymph node dissection. Indeed, in clinical trials, neoadjuvant chemoradiation has been added to THE in an effort to control locoregional disease, but without great success. The approach which we favor is a transthoracic resection to control locoregional disease and neoadjuvant or adjuvant therapy to address systemic disease. In our experience and others, there is clearly a relationship between the extent of nodal involvement and the survival. DeMeester's experience with the *en bloc* resection has shown almost a direct relationship between the number of involved nodes and the probability of systemic disease 2 years later. When a patient had 9 or more involved nodes, the incidence of systemic recurrent disease was 100% during follow-up. In our prospective, phase II study of neoadjuvant chemotherapy followed by esophagectomy, lymph node involvement was an independent predictor of survival and the hazard ratio gradually increased as the number of positive lymph nodes increased.

Minimally invasive esophagectomy: Minimally invasive esophagectomy (MIE) was first described by DePaula, et al in a series that included many patients with end stage achalasia from Chagas disease. Swanstrom's series of totally laparoscopic esophagectomy in 9 patients was the first report of MIE in North America. Subsequently, multiple studies have examined use and outcomes of MIE. We reported our data on 222 patients who underwent MIE at UPMC from 1996 to 2002 with an operative mortality of 1.4%, non-emergent conversion to an open procedure in 7.2% and a median intensive care unit stay of 1 day. Nguyen, et al reported their experience with 104 MIE with an in-hospital mortality of 2.9% and a median ICU stay of 2 days. Zingg, et al with 56 patients in their MIE series, reported an in-hospital mortality of 3.6% and mean ICU stay of 3 days. The use of MIE is rapidly expanding and the outcomes of this procedure are becoming more promising. This procedure can be done via two common approaches, a combined laparoscopic and thoracoscopic approach with cervical anastomosis and a laparoscopic and thoracoscopic approach with an intrathoracic anastomosis (Ivor-Lewis approach). Initially, we used a laparoscopic and thoracoscopic approach with cervical anastomosis, but as our experience increased, we adopted a minimally invasive Ivor-Lewis approach which in our hands, results in fewer complications and better functional outcomes. The indications for and technique of Ivor-Lewis MIE are discussed in detail in this chapter.

MIE with Ivor-Lewis Anastomosis — Operative Technique at UPMC

MIE by Ivor-Lewis Approach

Laparoscopic and thoracoscopic Ivor-Lewis esophagectomy is indicated for cancer of the distal esophagus and gastroesophageal junction. Tumors located proximal to the mid-esophagus are best managed by total esophagectomy with a neck anastomosis to ensure a negative proximal margin of resection. We have evolved our MIE technique from a cervical anastomosis to an intrathoracic anastomosis. As thoracic surgeons, we find that this approach is easier, allows a better thoracic lymph node dissection, results in a tension-free anastomosis, provides better perfusion to the gastric conduit, results in less (or no) vocal cord paralysis and reduces the risk of aspiration, a major morbidity of esophagectomy.

MIE with Ivor-Lewis Anastomosis — Operative Technique at UPMC

In our experience with MIE over the last one and half decades, we have developed a systematic, stepwise approach which has resulted in minimal mortality and morbidity. We believe all these steps need to be followed meticulously and patiently by the operating surgeon and precise performance of each step will optimize the

outcome of MIE. These steps are summarized in **Table 24-2.**

On-table Esophagogastroscopy

The initial step in MIE is an on-table upper endoscopy to confirm the tumor's location and the suitability of the stomach as a conduit for reconstruction.

Diagnostic Laparoscopy

After the insertion of the camera, the liver, peritoneal surfaces, omentum, small bowel mesentery and the celiac axis are examined to assess resectability.

Laparoscopic Construction of the Gastric Conduit

The five abdominal ports used for gastric mobilization are in the same configuration we use for benign esophageal operations, although they are placed somewhat lower so we can visualize the entire stomach **(Figure 24-2A)**. The gastrohepatic ligament is divided and the right and the left crura are dissected. Unlike other foregut operations, we do not divide the phrenoesophageal ligament until the conclusion of laparoscopy. This maintains the pneumoperitoneum for the duration of the procedure.

The stomach is mobilized by dividing the gastrocolic omentum. The right gastroepiploic arcade is carefully preserved. The stomach is retracted superiorly and the lymph nodes around the left gastric artery and celiac axis are dissected. The left gastric artery is ligated using a vascular stapler. The laparoscopic mobilization of the pyloroantral area must be meticulous. During this part of the procedure, we periodically grasp the antrum, near the pylorus and carefully lift it toward the diaphragmatic hiatus. When sufficiently mobilized, the pylorus should easily be elevated to the right crus in a tension-free manner. If this cannot be accomplished, or there is tension during this maneuver, further Kocher maneuver is needed. A gastric tube 5-6 cm in width is created by dividing the stomach at the lesser curve using a stapler, preserving the right gastric vessels. During this step, we have found it beneficial to have the first assistant grasp the tip of the fundus and gently stretch it toward the spleen, while a second grasper is placed on the antral area with a slight downward retraction applied. This places the stomach on slight stretch and facilitates straight staple line application, which should be parallel to the gastro-epiploic arcade **(Figure 24-2B)**. Next, the most superior portion of the gastric tube is attached to the resection specimen using two endostitches. These stitches maintain the correct orientation of the stomach as it is delivered into the mediastinum **(Figure 24-2C)**. Recently, we have included a 5 cm wide, 8-10 cm long omental pedicle,

TABLE 24-2	Steps of an Ivor-Lewis minimally invasive esophagectomy at the University of Pittsburgh

Assessment of the length of the conduit and resectability of the tumor
　　On table endoscopy and diagnostic laparoscopy

Gastric mobilization
a.　The stomach is mobilized by dividing the gastrocolic omentum. The right gastroepiploic arcade is preserved
b.　The mobility of the conduit is assessed by the ability of the antrum to reach the hiatus (Kocher maneuver if needed).

Harvest of an omental flap
　　A long omental pedicle, originating from the upper greater curvature is mobilized to further buttress the anastomosis in the chest

Left gastric artery lymphadenectomy and division
a.　The stomach is retracted superiorly and the lymph nodes around the left gastric artery and celiac axis are dissected.
b.　The left gastric artery is ligated using a vascular stapler.

Pyloroplasty
　　A pyloroplasty is created by opening the pylorus with the ultrasonic shears and closing it transversely using the endostitch.

Construction of the conduit and delivery to the mediastinum
a.　A gastric tube of 5-6 cm diameter is created by dividing the stomach parallel to the gastroepiploic arcade, preserving the right gastric vessels
b.　The most superior portion of the gastric tube is attached to the resected specimen using endostitches
c.　Stitches need to be placed adequately to maintain the correct orientation of the stomach which is delivered into the mediastinum

Laparoscopic feeding jejunostomy
a.　Using the Seldinger technique, the jejunostomy catheter is inserted with the guidewire into the introducer needle and into the efferent limb of jejunum
b.　An antitorsion stitch(es) is placed by suturing the distal jejunum

Thoracic esophageal mobilization
a.　Double lumen intubation
b.　The lung lobes are retracted laterally and the mediastinal pleura is divided
c.　The azygos vein is dissected and divided. The right vagus nerve is transected right above the azygos vein
d.　The esophagus is mobilized circumferentially from the esophageal hiatus to a level above the azygos vein
e.　All the thoracic duct branches are clipped along the lateral side of the esophagus to prevent chyle leak
f.　The gastroesophageal specimen is pulled with the preconstructed gastric conduit is pulled into the chest
g.　The esophagus is divided immediately above the level of the azygos vein

Mediastinal lymphadenectomy
a.　Complete mediastinal lymph node dissection is performed

Ivor- Lewis anastomosis
a.　A 28 mm anvil is inserted into the esophageal stump and secured with 2 purse-string sutures
b.　A gastrotomy is performed along the staple-line of the gastric conduit for placement of the circular stapler
c.　The circular stapler is inserted through the limited thoracotomy incision and advanced through the gastric conduit until its tip exits through the wall of the gastric conduit. The cartridge on the circular stapler is attached to the anvil placed in the esophageal stump and a circular stapled anastomosis is created
d.　A nasogastric tube is inserted through the anastomosis under direct visualization

Irrigation and drainage
a.　Right chest is irrigated with antibiotics
b.　A JP is placed under the omental flap and lateral to the anastomosis
c.　A chest tube is placed and the lung is expanded under direct vision

Single lumen intubation and on-table bronchoscopy
a.　Flexible bronchoscopy is performed to clear secretions

originating from the upper greater curve of the gastric conduit to further buttress the anastomosis in the chest, in selected patients. We applied this technique following a personal communication with Dr. Earl Wilkins, at Massachusetts General Hospital, who has used the omental flap around the esophageal anastomosis for many years to prevent anastomotic leak with excellent results.

This pedicle is brought up into the chest with the new conduit and at the time of the anastomosis and is subsequently wrapped around the anastomosis.

Laparoscopic Pyloroplasty

After gastric mobilization, a pyloroplasty is created by opening the pylorus with the ultrasonic shears and closing

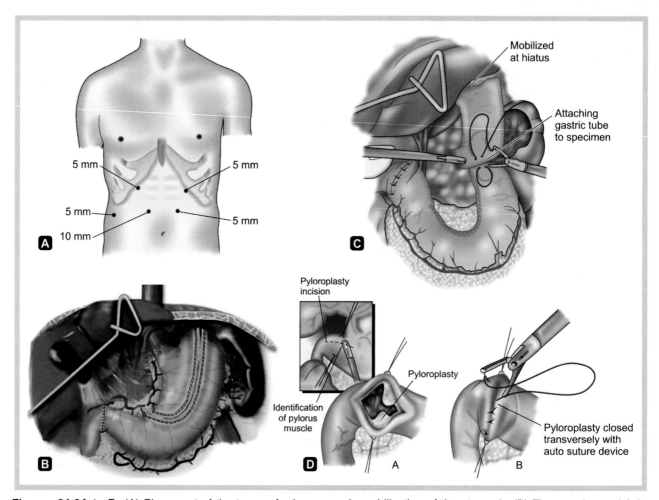

Figures 24-2A to D: (A) Placement of the trocars for laparoscopic mobilization of the stomach. (B) The gastric conduit is created by dividing the stomach parallel to the gastroepiploic arcade, preserving the right gastric vessels. (C) The most superior portion of the gastric tube is attached to the resection specimen using two endostitches. These stitches maintain the correct orientation of the stomach which is delivered into the mediastinum. (D) Pyloroplasty is created by opening the pylorus with the ultrasonic shears and closing it transversely using the endostitch

it transversely using the endostitch **(Figure 24-2D)**. We perform a pyloroplasty in all patients who undergo MIE for the esophageal carcinoma. Gravity is a major determinant of drainage for the gastric conduit. Pyloroplasty is essential during esophagectomy to prevent delayed gastric emptying in the vagotomized gastric conduit and to prevent gastric dilatation, which may lead to aspiration pneumonia during the recovery period. In a meta-analysis of 9 randomized controlled trials (553 patients), Urschel, et al demonstrated a significant reduction in early postoperative gastric outlet obstruction and post-pyloric drainage procedures when a pyloroplasty or pyloromyotomy was employed.

Laparoscopic Feeding Jejunostomy Placement

We place a feeding jejunostomy in all patients who undergo MIE for esophageal cancer. We perform a laparoscopic needle catheter jejunostomy (7 French needle catheter, Compat Biosystems, Minneapolis, USA) using a totally intracorporeal suturing technique performed via three abdominal trocars. The laparoscopic ports are the same as those used for the abdominal phase. With the patient in a 30 degree reverse Trendelenburg position, the greater omentum is reflected superiorly over the stomach to expose the transverse mesocolon. The proximal jejunum is identified 30 cm distal to the ligament of Treitz and is sutured to the left lower quadrant anterior abdominal wall using the Endostitch device (US Surgical Corporation, Norwalk, Connecticut, USA). A 2 mm skin incision is made on the anterior abdominal wall above the suspended jejunal limb. An introducer needle is placed into the peritoneal cavity close to the jejunal loop and is inserted into the jejunal lumen. Using the Seldinger technique, the jejunostomy catheter is inserted with a guidewire into the introducer needle and into the efferent limb of jejunum. The guidewire and introducer needle are removed and

10 ml of air is injected into the catheter. Distension of the jejunum as air is insufflated into the needle catheter confirms the intraluminal position of the catheter. A single intracorporeal purse-string is sutured between the jejunal loop and the anterior abdominal wall to create a seal around the catheter. An antitorsion stitch is placed by suturing the distal jejunum to the anterior abdominal wall about 4 cm distal to the site of the catheter (**Figure 24-3A**). We start the enteral feeding 24 hours after placement. The catheter is left in position for a minimum of 3 weeks or until the patient can tolerate adequate oral nutrition. The tube is flushed with 20 ml water every 8 hours to prevent clogging of the catheter.

Thoracoscopic Ivor-Lewis Gastroesophageal Anastomosis

After the patient is positioned in a left lateral decubitus position, five thoracic ports are introduced in the right chest (**Figure 24-3B**). The lung lobes are retracted laterally to expose the mediastinal esophagus. The mediastinal pleura overlying the esophagus is divided to expose the intrathoracic esophagus. The azygos vein is dissected and divided with a vascular linear stapler. The vagus nerve is transected just above the azygos vein. The esophagus is mobilized circumferentially from the esophageal hiatus to a level above the azygos vein. All the thoracic duct branches are clipped along the lateral side of the esophagus to prevent chyle leak. A complete mediastinal lymph node dissection is performed to achieve an *en bloc* resection of the tumor. The esophagus is divided immediately above the level of the azygos vein. The gastroesophageal specimen is pulled into the thoracic cavity together with the preconstructed gastric conduit. The esophageal surgical specimen is detached from the gastric conduit and removed through a limited thoracotomy incision (4 cm), which is protected with a plastic hand port. A 28 mm anvil is inserted into the esophageal stump and secured with two purse-string sutures. A gastrotomy is performed along the staple-line of the gastric conduit for placement of the circular stapler. The circular stapler is inserted through the limited thoracotomy incision and advanced through the gastric conduit until its tip exits through the wall of the gastric conduit (**Figure 24-3C**). The cartridge on the circular stapler is attached to the anvil placed in the esophageal stump and a circular stapled anastomosis is created. A nasogastric tube is inserted through the anastomosis under direct visualization. The gastrotomy is closed with either a running suture or a linear stapler (**Figure 24-3D**). The omental pedicle is subsequently wrapped around the anastomosis. A JP drain is placed lateral to the anastomosis under the omental flap (the drain will stay until postoperative day

10). The chest cavity is irrigated with antibiotic irrigation. A 28-F chest tube is placed and the lung is expanded under direct vision.

Extent of lymphadenectomy and impact on survival: There is increasing evidence that the number of lymph nodes removed is associated with improved survival after esophagectomy for cancer, although it is debated whether improved results are related to a therapeutic benefit or stage migration, due to better staging. Altorki, et al conducted a retrospective review of 264 patients with esophageal cancer treated by esophagectomy without neoadjuvant therapy. The association between overall survival and the total number of dissected lymph nodes was evaluated using multivariable Cox regression models. When the total number of resected nodes was examined as a categorical variable based on quartiles (category 1: £ 16, category 2: 17-25, category 3: 26-40 and category 4:>40), there was a reduced hazard of death with increasing number of examined nodes. Compared with those in category 1 (£ 16 resected nodes), the death hazard was reduced by 34% for patients with 17-25 resected nodes) ($P = 0.08$), by 48% for patients with 26-40 resected nodes ($P = 0.001$) and by 49% for patients with > 40 resected nodes ($P = 0.001$). For node-negative patients, death hazard was reduced significantly only when more than 40 nodes were resected (HR = 0.23, $P = 0.01$). For node-positive patients, the death hazard was significantly reduced patients with > 17 resected node as compared to those in category 1 (category 2, HR = 0.53, P = 0.03; category 2, HR = 0.39, $P = 0.001$; category 3, HR= 0.49; $P = 0.02$). They concluded that higher nodal count favorably influences survival. Peyre, et al at the University of Southern California, studied the impact of number of lymph nodes removed on survival of patients with esophageal cancer in 2303 esophageal cancer patients from 9 international centers (1381 had adenocarcinoma) who had R0 esophagectomy alone and were followed at regular intervals for 5 years or until death. Cox regression analysis showed that the number of lymph nodes removed was an independent predictor of survival. The optimal threshold predicted by Cox regression analysis for this survival benefit was removal of a minimum of 23 nodes. Other independent predictors of survival were the number of involved nodes, depth of invasion, presence of nodal metastasis and cell type.

At the University of Pittsburgh we prefer an *en bloc* removal of the tumor which involves complete abdominal and thoracic lymphadenectomy (2-field lymph node dissection). In a recent, multicenter trial of MIE (ECOG 2202), the mean number of lymph nodes removed was 20. It is highly recommended that all centers that perform MIE spend extra time and effort to perform a complete

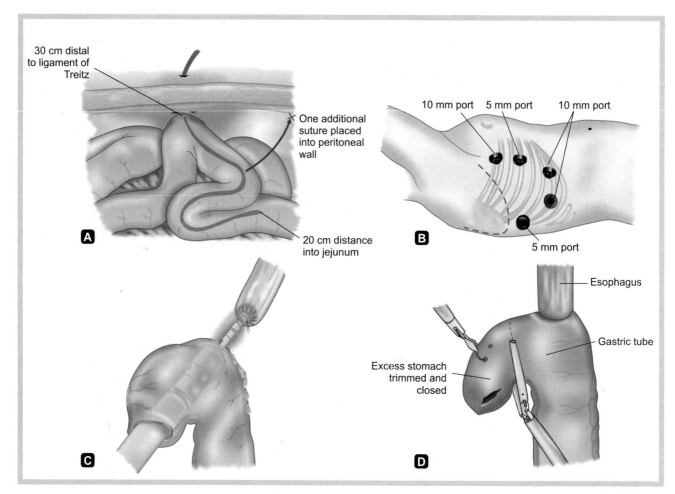

Figures 24-3A to D: (A) A loop of jejunum is tacked to the abdominal wall. A needle and feeding tube are then passed into the jejunum under laparoscopic vision. The jejunum is tacked up around the feeding tube and a stitch placed distally to prevent torsion around the feeding tube. (B) The patient is positioned in a left lateral decubitus position. Five thoracic ports are introduced in the right chest. (Operative Techniques in Thoracic and Cardiovascular Surgery, Vol. 14(3), Tsai, Levy and Luketich, Technique of minimally-invasive Ivor-Lewis esophagectomy, in press, © Elsevier (2009), used with permission). (C) A 28 mm anvil is inserted into the esophageal stump and secured with 2 purse-string sutures. A gastrotomy is performed along the staple-line of the gastric conduit for placement of the circular stapler. The circular stapler is inserted through the limited thoracotomy incision and advanced through the gastric conduit until its tip exits through the wall of the gastric conduit. The cartridge on the circular stapler is attached to the anvil placed in the esophageal stump and a circular stapled anastomosis is created. (D) The gastrotomy is closed with a linear stapler

lymphadenectomy to improve staging and possibly survival of patients who undergo minimally invasive esophagectomy.

Minimally invasive vs open esophagectomy: Nguyen and colleagues compared outcomes of patients who underwent thoracoscopic and laparoscopic esophagectomy with patients who underwent transhiatal or transthoracic esophagectomy. In this retrospective analysis, thoracoscopic and laparoscopic esophagectomy was associated with shorter operative times, less blood loss, fewer blood transfusions and shortened intensive care unit and hospital stays than transthoracic or blunt transhiatal esophagectomy. Smithers, et al studied the morbidity and

cancer survival outcomes of patients who underwent esophagectomy comparing to open thoracotomy and laparotomy (open, n = 114), with a thoracoscopic/laparotomy approach (thoracoscopic-assisted, n = 309) and a completely thoracoscopic and laparoscopic approach (total MIE, n = 23). They showed less median blood loss in the thoracoscopic-assisted (400 ml) and total MIE (300 ml) groups versus the open group (600 ml), a longer time for total MIE (330 minutes) versus thoracoscopic-assisted (285 minutes) and open (300 minutes), a longer median hospital stay for open (14 days) versus thoracoscopic-assisted (13 days) and total MIE (11 days) and less stricture formation in the open (6.1%) versus thoracoscopic-assisted (21.6%) and total MIE (36%). There

with PDT. RFA may be the ideal addendum to EMR for ablation of remaining nondysplastic Barrett's epithelium after successful resection of all localizable HGD and adenocarcinoma. A removal of all neoplastic lesions by EMR provides a specimen that can be evaluated by the pathologist for assessment of depth and other risk factors such as lymphovascular invasion. In addition, ablation of the nondysplastic Barrett's mucosa can significantly reduce the rate of metachronous neoplasia or recurrences.

Appropriate use of endoscopic treatments: We believe that endoscopic treatment of patients with HGD and esophageal adenocarcinoma need to be individualized. While endoscopic ablation techniques are potentially less morbid than esophagectomy and have shown encouraging results, their oncologic efficacy needs to be proven by further investigation and longer follow-up. A concern is that subsquamous Barrett's epithelium remains at risk for progression to adenocarcinoma and requires continued surveillance endoscopy. Therefore, our opinion at this time is that endoscopic therapies for high-grade dysplasia and early stage adenocarcinoma should only be considered appropriate for those patients who are unwilling to undergo esophagectomy or who are poor surgical candidates. We believe esophagectomy should be considered in all patients who are physiologically fit to undergo resection. Patient should be informed of all the possible therapeutic options including the risk and benefits of each treatment modality and should be involved in the decision-making process. It is crucial that surgeons be able to offer all the treatment modalities and discuss all these options in details with patients with the diagnosis of esophageal cancer.

Palliation for Esophageal Cancer

Many patients with esophageal cancer present during the later stages of the disease and more than 50% of patients have metastatic disease or are unresectable at presentation. Patients with unresectable esophageal carcinoma have a poor prognosis and the goal of therapy is to improve symptoms and quality of life while minimizing morbidity and hospital stay. The modalities that are currently available for palliation of symptoms include esophageal bypass surgery, PDT, esophageal dilation, external beam radiation, stents, neodymium:yttrium-aluminum-garnet (Nd:YAG) laser therapy and brachytherapy. Each of these modalities has their specific advantages and drawbacks. Surgical esophageal bypass for palliation is rarely used. In this chapter, we will discuss the common modalities for palliation, which include esophageal stents, PDT and lasers.

Esophageal stenting: Stents are a relatively safe and effective method of palliation for obstructing esophageal cancer. Current stent delivery systems often allow successful deployment without exposing the patient to the risks of mechanical dilation and risk of esophageal perforation. Esophageal stenting in combination with chemoradiation therapy may provide palliation and some improvement in the quality of life of patients with locally unresectable or metastatic esophageal carcinoma. Malignant endoluminal obstruction and extra-luminal compression by enlarged lymph nodes or the tumor are common indications for stenting of the esophagus. The two major types of stents used are expandable metal stents (EMS) and silicone-based stents. EMS are constructed using corrosion-resistant, biologically inert materials, such as cobalt alloys, stainless steel and nitinol (a nickel-titanium alloy). The wire stents can be woven (Wallstent), knitted (Ultraflex), bent into a zigzag (Gianturco) or coil (Esophacoil) configuration. The stent's design influences its retraction (i.e. shortening) properties. Retraction percentage is highest with the coil and lowest with the zigzag configuration. EMS can also be partially covered with polyurethane or silicone. Covered designs help reduce tumor ingrowths, but increase the risk of migration. Esophageal stents are available in a wide range of lengths (60-150 mm) but most have a similar maximal internal diameter (17-23 mm). EMS can be deployed from the proximal end, the center, or the distal end of the esophagus. Proximal delivery is better suited for proximal strictures and distal delivery is best for strictures of the gastroesophageal junction. EMS placement can be performed with the patient under conscious sedation or under general anesthesia. The stricture is identified endoscopically and measured. If the opening of the stricture is too small to accept the endoscope, the lumen may require dilation and or laser ablation before length can be assessed accurately. Radioopaque markers, applied either to the skin or to the submucosa, are used to delineate the edges of the stricture and measure the tumor length. Once the measurement of the tumor length is completed, the appropriate stent is selected. In general, we use an 18- to 23-mm-diameter stent that is 1-2 cm longer than the stricture to avoid crimping and infolding of the proximal and distal ends. A guidewire is passed through the stricture and the endoscope is withdrawn. Under fluoroscopic guidance, the delivery system is inserted over the guidewire through the stricture and aligned with the skin or mucosal markers. The stent is deployed and expands within the lumen. Proper positioning and deployment are confirmed fluoroscopically and endoscopically. Minor adjustments are possible immediately post-deployment by grasping the proximal end of the stent with endoscopic grasping forceps and pulling the stent back for repositioning. It is difficult to push the stent further once it is deployed. A post-procedure chest radiograph and barium esophagram are obtained to assess patency and serve as a reference for later assessment.

EMS are popular, as they are easier to insert than their silicone counterpart and do not require expertise in rigid endoscopy. Silicone stents are more challenging to place but are preferable for patients with benign strictures. Both silicon-based stents and EMS are susceptible to tumor growth above and below the stent, leading to recurrence of esophageal obstruction. Additionally, tumor ingrowth through stent interstices can occur with uncovered metal stents. In the absence of a tracheoesophageal fistula, the decision to use a covered stent is influenced by the potential for recurrent obstruction by tumor ingrowth and the likelihood of stent migration. When tumor overgrowth or ingrowth occurs, further restenting (i.e. placing a stent within a stent) may be of additional palliative benefit.

A few prospective randomized trials have compared silicone and metal stents for malignant esophageal obstruction. The trials included comparable groups of patients and technical success (95-100%), improvement in dysphagia (91-100%) and the need for re-intervention were similar regardless of stent type. However, the use of silicone stents was associated with a higher rate of complications and a prolonged hospital stay and poststenting survival was not significantly different. Despite a higher purchase price, EMS are more cost-effective because of shorter hospital stays and lower complication rates. At the University of Pittsburgh, a review of 100 patients treated with self-expandable metal stents demonstrated relief of dysphagia in 85% with a low perforation rate (0.8%) and no fatalities. Sixteen stents were placed in patients undergoing neoadjuvant therapy for a possible esophagectomy at a later time. At the time of esophagectomy, dissection of the periesophageal planes was more difficult but no operative complications could directly be attributed to preoperative stenting. Patients receiving chemotherapy and/or radiation following placement of EMS may be prone to perforation or fistuliza-tion, so alternatives to stenting should be sought in this subgroup of patients. In other large series of patients undergoing stenting (> 100 patients), successful placement and improvement of dysphagia were achieved in 90-100% of patients. Procedure-related mortality was low (0-2.5%). We have also reported our experience with covered plastic stents, which are also effective in relieving dysphagia, but have a high migration rate.

Photodynamic therapy: Photodynamic therapy (PDT) is an effective method for palliation and has proven beneficial in improving the common esophageal cancer-related symptoms of dysphagia and bleeding. The ideal candidate for PDT is a patient who has an obstructing endoluminal cancer. PDT offers some advantages over stenting in certain clinical situations. It is particularly useful in tumors of the proximal esophagus and the gastroesophageal junction. It may prevent the globus sensation associated with stents in the proximal esophagus and the reflux symptoms observed with stenting of the gastroesophageal junction.

In a large series from the University of Pittsburgh, Litle and colleagues reported their experience in 215 patients with bleeding, obstructing or bleeding and obstructing esophageal cancer who were treated with PDT. We evaluated the dysphagia scores, duration of palliation, reinterventions, complications and survival. We noted an improvement in dysphagia in 85% of the patients with a mean dysphagia-free interval of 66 days. In addition, bleeding was controlled in 93% of patients with one PDT course. Esophageal stents were placed following PDT in 35 patients, with a mean interval to reintervention of 58.5 days. The following complications occurred: perforation (2% of courses), stricture (2%), candida esophagitis (2%), symptomatic pleural effusions (4%) and sunburn (6%). In this study, we concluded that PDT offers effective palliation in patients with obstructing esophageal cancer in 85% of treatment courses. However, in some patients, reintervention and a multimodality approach are required to maintain palliation.

Nd-YAG laser: The most commonly used laser in thoracic surgery is the Nd-YAG laser. The Nd-YAG laser can be delivered through a small-caliber endoscope and adjusting the power level allows for a combination of coagulation (low power, defocused beam) and vaporization (high power, focused beam) of tissue. Candidates for laser therapy include patients with minimal extrinsic compression and a primarily endoluminal tumor burden with a distal patent lumen. Experienced centers have established simple rules to increase the safety of laser use and communication between the members of the operating team is essential.

In an interesting study, Lightdale and colleagues reported the results of a prospective randomized multicenter trial to compare the efficacy and safety of PDT (porfimer sodium) versus Nd:YAG laser in the treatment of patients with obstructing esophageal cancer. A total of 236 patients were randomized from 24 institutions, of which 110 patients were treated with PDT and 108 patients with Nd:YAG laser. Objective tumor response was equivalent at 1 week, but was significantly better at 1 month in the PDT group. Symptomatic improvement of dysphagia was equivalent in the two groups and there was trend toward improved response with PDT in tumors located in the upper and lower third of the esophagus, long tumors and in patients who had received prior therapy. Termination of the treatment session due to adverse reaction occurred more frequently in the Nd:YAG group (19% vs 3%; P < 0.05). Similarly, perforations from the treatment or associated dilation occurred significantly more often in the Nd:YAG group (7%) compared to the

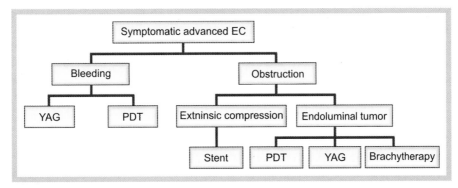

Figure 24-4: Treatment algorithm for endoscopic palliation of locally advanced esophageal carcinoma. (*EC* = esophageal cancer; *PDT* = photodynamic therapy; *YAG* = neodymium:yttrium-aluminum garnet laser) (Litle V, Luketich J, et al. Photodynamic therapy as palliation for esophageal cancer: experience in 215 patients. Annals of Thoracic Surgery, 76: 1687-93 used with permission)

PDT group (1%)($P < 0.05$). These authors concluded that PDT and Nd:YAG laser ablation resulted in equal relief of dysphagia, however, the objective tumor response was equal or better in the PDT group. Further, PDT was associated with fewer acute perforations when compared to Nd:YAG.

A proposed treatment algorithm for palliation of locally advanced esophageal carcinoma is shown in **Figure 24-4**.

Quality of Life After Esophagectomy

Esophageal carcinoma is being detected both at an earlier stage and in younger patients. Therefore, quality of life (QOL) after esophagectomy is important to patients with esophageal carcinoma and should be considered while planning for the treatment of esophageal cancer. QOL data can be used to tailor treatment and improve clinical outcomes by detecting patients' physical or psychological problems that otherwise might be overlooked, but which have profound implications for the effective delivery of care. In general, most aspects of QOL significantly deteriorate early in the postoperative phase. The only aspect of QOL that does not dramatically deteriorate after open esophagectomy is emotional function, likely due to the patients' relief that the tumor is removed. Dysphagia scores are generally improved or stable after surgery; however, dysphagia is replaced with other symptoms such as anorexia, change in taste, nausea and diarrhea. QOL scores gradually recover within 9 months of open esophagectomy. The best long-term QOL data was reported from Mayo Clinic using the SF36 questionnaire to measure health-related QOL in 105 patients who had survived 5 years or more after open esophagectomy. The median survival was 10.2 years. At the time of follow-up, 60% of the patients complained of reflux, 53% had dumping and 25% had dysphagia to solid food. Only 17% were completely asymptomatic. A cervical anastomosis

was associated with less reflux ($P < 0.05$); dumping was more frequent in younger patients and women ($P < 0.05$). Physical function scores were less than national norms; however, scores measuring the ability to work, social interaction, daily activity, emotional dysfunction and health perception were similar to national norms. This illustrates that most aspects of QOL are preserved in the long-term survivors of esophageal cancer, even though they have gastrointestinal symptoms.

Although most patients report reduced QOL in the early postoperative period, certain clinical factors are associated with poorer QOL after surgery. In a population study from Sweden by Viklund, et al QOL was examined in 100 patients 6 months after surgery. The main predictor of poor global QOL, after adjusting for the potentially confounding variables of age, sex and disease stage, was surgery-related complications. Each morbidity (e.g. anastomotic breakdown, sepsis, cardiopulmonary complications and operative technical complications) contributed to decreased QOL. Other factors, such as degree of nodal dissection, resection margins, blood loss or hospital type, did not significantly affect the QOL scores.

QOL measures can also be used to when deciding which treatment approach and surgical technique should be employed for esophageal cancer patients. In some studies, patients who have had a cervical esophagogastric anastomosis seem to have better physical and social functions and less problems with insomnia and vomiting after surgery compared with those with an intrathoracic anastomosis, whereas patients who had a pyloroplasty have fewer problems with psychosocial functions, indigestion and dysphagia. In a well-designed randomized study that compared transthoracic with transhiatal esophagectomy, de Boer, et al used the validated Rotterdam Symptom Checklist in combination with the Medical Outcomes Study Short Form-20 to assess QOL. Patients were randomized to receive a transhiatal or transthoracic esophagectomy and were followed for three years. Three months after surgery, patients in the transhiatal group (*n* = 96) reported fewer physical symptoms (*P* = 0.01) and better activity levels (*P* < 0.01) than patients in the transthoracic group (*n* = 103). However, in patients with lower esophageal tumors, there was a trend toward a survival advantage after transthoracic surgery (and extended mediastinal lymphadenectomy) which needs to be considered against the significantly decreased QOL in the first year after surgery. At longer follow-up, there was no significant difference between the two treatment groups.

Minimally invasive surgery can reduce the short-term detrimental impact on QOL that is experienced after open surgery. This is mainly achieved by reducing postoperative pain and length of stay and an earlier return to daily activity. In our series of 222 patients, at a mean follow-up of 19 months, only 4% of the patients had significant reflux. SF36 scores were compared with age-matched norms and were similar to preoperative levels 3 months after MIE. The mean dysphagia score was 1.4 (0 = no dysphagia; 5 = severe dysphagia). These QOL improvements were preserved in a cohort of 41 patients older than 75 years of age who had of MIE for esophageal cancer. In addition, we have also reported preservation of QOL after esophagectomy for T1 esophageal cancers. We believe that MIE in high volume centers experienced in minimally invasive esophageal surgery offers a good therapeutic option with acceptable morbidity and a preserved QOL.

Future Directions

It is clear that nodal metastasis is one of the most important prognostic factors in outcome. However, even in node-negative patients, the reported survival ranges from 50% to 90% at 5 years and up to 50% of these patients develop recurrent disease despite complete resection. With the inherent inaccuracies of clinical staging modalities and the limitations of the current staging system, molecular staging of esophageal cancer is an area of active investigation. Additionally, the potential implications of micrometastatic disease in patients with lymph nodes determined to be negative by routine histopathological examination is an area of active investigation. Previous studies have shown that micrometastases are associated with adverse outcome. In studies at the University of Pittsburgh, we have identified novel markers using quantitative reverse transcription polymerase chain reaction to detect occult micrometastatic disease in patients with esophageal adenocarcinoma. The presence of micrometastases in these initial studies was associated with significantly worse outcome in patients who were determined to be node-negative by routine pathological examination. Further work is ongoing in our center and others to validate these findings in a larger cohort of patients.

Summary

Esophageal cancers are an aggressive tumors and despite advances in both medical and surgical therapies, the incidence of esophageal adenocarcinoma has increased more than any other cancer in the United States. BE remains the major risk factor for esophageal adenocarcinoma. The overall survival outcome of patients who undergo esophagectomy has improved from 10% to 50% at 5 years. This improvement in survival is due to earlier detection, refinement of surgical techniques, more aggressive surgical resection including extended lymphadenectomy, advances in minimally invasive approaches, use of neoadjuvant and adjuvant therapy in selected patients and improvement of perioperative and postoperative care.

Esophagectomy remains the main treatment for esophageal adenocarcinoma, but in reality, half of patients with esophageal carcinoma are unresectable at the time of diagnosis due to the presence systemic disease. We believe that developing better screening and surveillance programs, applying an aggressive multidisciplinary approach and developing minimally invasive techniques, such as MIE, to decrease the morbidity of esophagectomy will result in an improvement in survival and in the quality of life of patients with esophageal cancer.

Landmark Papers

1. Akiyama H, Tsurumaru M, Kawamura T, Ono Y. Principles of surgical treatment for carcinoma of the esophagus: analysis of lymph node involvement. Ann Surg 1981;194:438-46.
2. Hagen JA, DeMeester SR, Peters JH, et al. Curative resection for esophageal adenocarcinoma: analysis of 100 en bloc esophagectomies. Ann Surg 2001;234:520.
3. Altorki N, Skinner D. Should en bloc esophagectomy be the standard of care for esophageal carcinoma? Ann Surg 2001;234:581-7.
4. Kelsen DP, Ginsberg R, Pajak TF, et al. Chemotherapy followed by surgery compared with surgery alone for localized esophageal cancer. N Engl J Med 1998;339:1979.
5. Medical Research Council Oesophageal Cancer Working Party. Surgical resection with or without preoperative chemotherapy in oesophageal cancer: a randomized trial. Lancet 2002; 359:1727-33.
6. Urschel JD, Vasan H. A meta-analysis of randomized controlled trials that compared neoadjuvant chemoradiation and surgery to surgery alone for resectable esophageal cancer. Am J Surg 2003;185:538.
7. Malthaner RA, Collin S, Fenlon D. Preoperative chemotherapy for resectable thoracic esophageal cancer. Cochrane Database Syst Rev 2006;3:CD001556.

8. Cunningham D, Allum WH, Stenning SP, et al. Perioperative chemotherapy versus surgery alone for resectable gastroesophageal cancer. N Engl J Med 2006; 355:11.

9. Lerut T, Nafteux P, Moons J, et al. Three-field lymphadenectomy for carcinoma of the esophagus and gastroesophageal junction in 174 R0 resections: impact on staging, disease-free survival and outcome: a plea for adaptation of TNM classification in upper-half esophageal carcinoma. Ann Surg 2004;240: 962-72.

10. Pennathur A, Luketich JD, Landreneau RJ, et al. Long-term results of a phase II trial of neoadjuvant chemotherapy followed by esophagectomy for locally advanced esophageal neoplasm. Ann Thorac Surg 2008;85: 1930-6.

11. Luketich JD, Alvelo-Rivera M, Buenaventura PO, et al. Minimally invasive esophagectomy: outcomes in 222 patients. Ann Surg 2003;238:486.

12. Smithers BM, Gotley DC, Martin I, et al. Comparison of the outcomes between open and minimally invasive esophagectomy. Ann Surg 2007;245:232.

13. Orringer MB, Marshall B, Chang AC, et al. Two thousand transhiatal esophagectomies: changing trends, lessons learned. Ann Surg 2007;246:363.

14. Nguyen NT, Hinojosa MW, Smith BR, et al. Minimally invasive esophagectomy: lessons learned from 104 operations. Ann Surg 2008;248:1081.

15. Peyre CG, Hagen JA, DeMeester SR, et al. The number of lymph nodes removed predicts survival in esophageal cancer: an international study on the impact of extent of surgical resection. Ann Surg 2008;248:549.

16. Wright CD, Kucharczuk JC, O'Brien SM, et al. Predictors of major morbidity and mortality after esophagectomy for esophageal cancer: a Society of Thoracic Surgeons General Thoracic Surgery Database risk adjustment model. J Thorac Cardiovasc Surg 2009;137:587.

17. Hulscher JB, van Sandick JW, de Boer AG, et al. Extended transthoracic resection compared with limited transhiatal resection for adenocarcinoma of the esophagus. N Engl J Med 2002;347: 1662-9.

18. Enzinger PC, Mayer RJ. Esophageal cancer. N Engl J Med 2003; 349(23):2241-52

Level of Evidence Table

Recommendation	Grade	Best level of evidence	References
Endoscopic ultrasound with EUS-FNA is the test of choice for initial local/regional staging of esophageal cancer but has lower accuracy after neoadjuvant therapy	A	1a	1, 2
PET/CT should also be considered in the staging and restaging of esophageal cancer if neoadjuvant therapy is used	A	1a	3-6
Neoadjuvant therapy improves survival compared to surgery alone for resectable esophageal cancer. Neoadjuvant chemoradiation appears more effective than chemotherapy alone	A	1a	7-10
Adjuvant chemotherapy improves postresection disease-free survival, particularly for node-positive patients, but has not demonstrated clear benefit for overall survival. No trial has compared neoadjuvant to adjuvant therapy	A	1b	11,12
Local therapies (ablation, endoscopic resection) adequately treat esophageal cancer with mucosal involvement (T1a) in medically inoperable patients	B	2b	13-16
Transhiatal compared to transthoracic approaches to esophagectomy demonstrate non-significant differences in long-term survival	A	1b	20
En bloc lymphadenectomy trends to better survival and a greater number of resected lymph nodes are associated with better survival	A	1b	17-19, 25
Minimally invasive esophagectomy for cancer is feasible and has perioperative advantages over open surgery. Long-term survival appears equivalent	B	2b	21-24

References

1. Puli SR, Reddy JB, Bechtold ML, et al. Staging accuracy of esophageal cancer by endoscopic ultrasound: a meta-analysis and systematic review. World J Gastroenterol 2008; 14:1479-90.

2. Kalha I, Kaw M, Fukami N, et al. The accuracy of endoscopic ultrasound for restaging esophageal carcinoma after chemoradiation therapy. Cancer 2004; 101:940-7.

3. Rebollo Aguirre AC, Ramos-Font C, Villegas Portero R, et al. 18F-fluorodeoxiglucose positron emission tomography for the evaluation of neoadjuvant therapy response in esophageal cancer: systematic review of the literature. Ann Surg 2009; 250:247-54.

4. Westerterp M, van Westreenen HL, Reitsma JB, et al. Esophageal cancer: CT, endoscopic US and FDG PET for assessment of response to neoadjuvant therapy—systematic review. Radiology 2005; 236:841-51.

5. van Vliet EP, Heijenbrok-Kal MH, Hunink MG, et al. Staging investigations for oesophageal cancer: a meta-analysis. Br J Cancer 2008; 98:547-57.

6. Kato H, Miyazaki T, Nakajima M, et al. The incremental effect of positron emission tomography on diagnostic accuracy in the initial staging of esophageal carcinoma. Cancer 2005; 103:148-56.

7. Gebski V, Burmeister B, Smithers BM, et al. Survival benefits from neoadjuvant chemoradiotherapy or chemotherapy in oesophageal carcinoma: a meta-analysis. Lancet Oncol 2007; 8:226-34.

8. Malthaner RA, Wong RK, Rumble RB, et al. Neoadjuvant or adjuvant therapy for resectable esophageal cancer: a systematic review and meta-analysis. BMC Med 2004; 2:35.

9. Malthaner RA, Collin S Fenlon D. Preoperative chemotherapy for resectable thoracic esophageal cancer. Cochrane Database Syst Rev 2006; 3:CD001556.

10. Urschel JD Vasan H. A meta-analysis of randomized controlled trials that compared neoadjuvant chemo-radiation and surgery to surgery alone for resectable esophageal cancer. Am J Surg 2003; 185:538-43.

11. Ando N, Iizuka T, Ide H, et al. Surgery plus chemotherapy compared with surgery alone for localized squamous cell carcinoma of the thoracic esophagus: a Japan Clinical Oncology Group Study—JCOG9204. J Clin Oncol 2003; 21:4592-6.

12. Lee J, Lee KE, Im YH, et al. Adjuvant chemotherapy with 5-fluorouracil and cisplatin in lymph node-positive thoracic esophageal squamous cell carcinoma. Ann Thorac Surg 2005; 80:1170-5.

13. Ishihara R, Tanaka H, Iishi H, et al. Long-term outcome of esophageal mucosal squamous cell carcinoma without lymphovascular involvement after endoscopic resection. Cancer 2008; 112:2166-72.

14. Shimizu Y, Tsukagoshi H, Fujita M, et al. Long-term outcome after endoscopic mucosal resection in patients with esophageal squamous cell carcinoma invading the muscularis mucosae or deeper. Gastrointest Endosc 2002; 56:387-90.

15. Manner H, May A, Pech O, et al. Early Barrett's carcinoma with "low-risk" submucosal invasion: long-term results of endoscopic resection with a curative intent. Am J Gastroenterol 2008; 103:2589-97.

16. Pech O, Behrens A, May A, et al. Long-term results and risk factor analysis for recurrence after curative endoscopic therapy in 349 patients with high-grade intraepithelial neoplasia and mucosal adenocarcinoma in Barrett's oesophagus. Gut 2008; 57:1200-6.

17. Peyre CG, Hagen JA, DeMeester SR, et al. The number of lymph nodes removed predicts survival in esophageal cancer: an international study on the impact of extent of surgical resection. Ann Surg 2008; 248:549-56.

18. Greenstein AJ, Litle VR, Swanson SJ, et al. Effect of the number of lymph nodes sampled on postoperative survival of lymph node-negative esophageal cancer. Cancer 2008; 112:1239-46.

19. Rizzetto C, DeMeester SR, Hagen JA, et al. En bloc esophagectomy reduces local recurrence and improves survival compared with transhiatal resection after neoadjuvant therapy for esophageal adenocarcinoma. J Thorac Cardiovasc Surg 2008; 135:1228-36.

20. Omloo JM, Lagarde SM, Hulscher JB, et al. Extended transthoracic resection compared with limited transhiatal resection for adenocarcinoma of the mid/distal esophagus: five-year survival of a randomized clinical trial. Ann Surg 2007; 246:992-1000; discussion 1000-1.

21. Luketich JD, Alvelo-Rivera M, Buenaventura PO, et al. Minimally invasive esophagectomy: outcomes in 222 patients. Ann Surg 2003; 238:486-94; discussion 494-5.

22. Biere SS, Cuesta MA van der Peet DL. Minimally invasive versus open esophagectomy for cancer: a systematic review and meta-analysis. Minerva Chir 2009; 64:121-33.

23. Zingg U, McQuinn A, DiValentino D, et al. Minimally invasive versus open esophagectomy for patients with esophageal cancer. Ann Thorac Surg 2009; 87:911-9.

24. Verhage RJ, Hazebroek EJ, Boone J, et al. Minimally invasive surgery compared to open procedures in esophagectomy for cancer: a systematic review of the literature. Minerva Chir 2009; 64:135-46.

25. Hulscher JB, van Sandick JW, de Boer AG, et al. Extended transthoracic resection compared with limited transhiatal resection for adenocarcinoma of the esophagus. N Engl J Med 2002;347(21):1662-69.

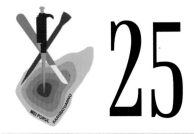

25

Gastric Cancer

Patricio M Polanco, Steven Hughes

Introduction

Gastric cancer is one of the most common causes of cancer mortality worldwide. Although its incidence has declined in developed countries, it remains a major cause of cancer-related death in the United States of America (USA). This chapter will cover gastric cancer epidemiology, clinical presentation, diagnostic modalities, staging algorithms and surgical and other therapeutic approaches. Palliative options will also be reviewed. Our discussion will be divided into discrete sections that correspond to the three major histologic subtypes of gastric neoplasms: adenocarcinomas, lymphomas and gastrointestinal stromal tumors (GIST). We will devote the majority of our discussion to gastric adenocarcinomas as this lesion represents more than 95% of neoplasms arising in the stomach.

Gastric Adenocarcinoma

Epidemiology

Gastric adenocarcinoma is the fourth most prevalent malignancy worldwide after lung, breast and colorectal cancer. Gastric cancer was the leading cause of cancer-related death until the 1980s when the mortality from lung cancer surpassed it. Importantly, the incidence of gastric cancer is in decline worldwide. Although speculative, this is largely due to the recognition of the role of *Helicobacter pylori* in the pathophysiology of the disease and improvements public health issue of drinking water source, however, dietary influences also clearly play an important role in the epidemiology of gastric adenocarcinoma.

In support of this statement, the incidence of gastric cancer has significant geographical variation. Eastern Asia (e.g. Japan, China, Korea and Taiwan), Central and South America (e.g. Costa Rica, Peru, Brazil and Chile) and Eastern Europe (e.g. former Soviet Union) have the highest rates of gastric cancer per population, while Northern Europe, North America and Africa experience the lowest incidence **(Figure 25-1).** It has been observed that the risk for gastric cancer decreases in populations migrating from high to low risk communities, especially in the second and third generations. Thus, the etiology of this geographical distribution lies predominantly upon environmental factors.

The age-adjusted incidence of gastric cancer in the USA is 8 cases per 100,000 people. There were approximately 21,500 new cases (14th most commonly diagnosed cancer) resulting in 10,880 deaths (11th most common cause of cancer-related death) in 2008. There are gender, ethnic and socio-economic variations in the incidence of gastric cancer; it is more common in men, African Americans and individuals of low socioeconomic status. While the overall incidence of gastric cancer is declining, the incidence of gastric cancer arising from the cardia is increasing, correlating with the increasing incidence of esophageal adenocarcinoma. Most experts believe that these two neoplasms likely share a common pathophysiology that differs from that of gastric cancers arising from the fundus or antrum and may be related to achlorhydria and bile reflux. Along these same lines, the histological pattern of gastric cancer is changing. Of the two histology patterns described by Lauren (expanded upon below), the *diffuse* or *infiltrative* types are encountered more frequently as the incidence of the *intestinal* type steadily decline.

Etiology and Risk Factors

As in the majority of gastrointestinal cancers, there is no single etiologic factor associated with gastric cancer.

Population characteristics: As above, USA epidemiologic studies show that male gender, black race and low socioeconomic status represent a higher risk of distal gastric carcinoma. On the other hand, obesity and high economic status are associated with risk for proximal gastric cancer. Some studies have shown an association between gastric cancer and early menopause and/or decreased years of fertility supporting the notion that reproductive hormones may provide a protective role. Interestingly, the blood-type A population has 20% increased risk for gastric cancer with a particular risk for the diffuse type of gastric cancer.

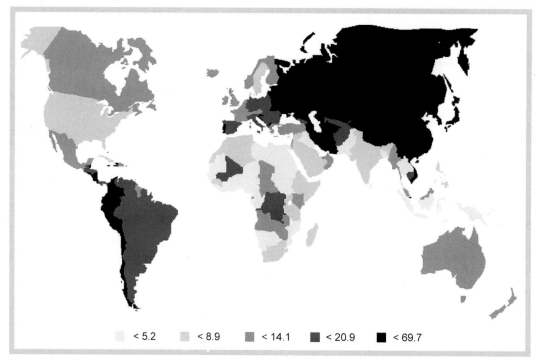

Figure 25-1: World distribution of gastric cancer. With permission, Ferlay J, Bray F, Pisani P, Parkin DM (2004). GLOBOCAN 2002: Cancer incidence, mortality and prevalence worldwide. IARC Cancer Base No. 5. Press, Lyon, France

Dietary and environmental factors: The consumption of a high salt diet, fried foods, processed meat and fish have been associated with increased rates of gastric cancer. Most of these foods contain high levels of nitrates that subsequently react with amino acids, amines and amides to produce N-nitrosocompounds or nitrosamines—all of which have been found to be carcinogenetic in animal models. High salt intake has been shown to cause repetitive mucosal damage thus favoring carcinogenesis. In contrast, diets high in vegetables, milk and vitamin A and C may have a protective role. Vitamin C has the potential benefit of reducing the formation of N-nitroso compounds in the gastric mucosa. Cereal fiber might also be a protective factor of diffuse type of gastric cancer.

Smoking is a well described risk factor for several cancers. Based on a large meta-analysis of 40 prospective studies, the risk of gastric cancer increases 1.5 to 1.6-fold in smokers, mainly in men. There is no clear association between alcohol consumption and gastric cancer.

Infectious risk factors: One of the greatest recent medical discoveries was the identification of infection with *H. pylori* as the etiology behind most benign peptic ulcer disease. *H. pylori* infection often leads to gastritis and may result in atrophy and metaplasia. Infection with this bacterium induces a 6-fold increased risk of developing gastric cancer and it is estimated to be responsible for 63%

of gastric cancer cases worldwide. The reduction of this infection through the reduced use of well water and recognition leading to treatment may largely explain the observed decrease in the incidence of gastric cancer.

Epstein-Barr virus (EBV) infection may cause gastric cancer. It is suspected that at least 5% of gastric cancers are associated with EBV infection. EBV incorporation into the host genome leads to DNA methylation including the promoter regions of many cancer-associated genes. Gastric cancers attributed to EBV are characteristically proximal (cardia) and of the diffuse type with lymphocytic infiltration.

Precursor lesions: The intestinal type of gastric cancer is thought to proceed through a sequence of precursor lesions. This begins with chronic gastritis that leads to the development of atrophy. Gastric atrophy is associated with hypochlorhydria or achlorhydria, decreased available levels of vitamin C and a compensatory increase in the trophic hormone gastrin. Importantly, hypochlorhydria favors gastric colonization by nitrose reductase-producing bacteria leading to the increased production of nitrosamines. Athrophic gastritis increases the risk of developing gastric cancer 5.7 fold. From atrophic gastritis, the sequence of intestinal metaplasia, dysplasia and eventually adenocarcinoma can ensue. In support of this sequential progression, intestinal metaplasia and dysplasia are associated with gastric cancer and have been shown to precede the development of gastric adenocarcinoma in animal models.

In addition to *H. pylori* infection, chronic gastritis may be due to pernicious anemia or previous gastric surgery. Pernicious anemia is an autoimmune disorder with antibodies directed against the hydrogen-potassium ATPase and subsequently causes chronic, atrophic gastritis. Ten percent of affected individuals develop gastric cancer, thus endoscopic surveillance is recommended in these patients. Prior gastrectomy for benign disorders is another well established risk factor for gastric cancer, typically occurring 25 or more years after the surgery. Once again, the causative agents are thought to be bilious reflux, decreased gastric pH and subsequent chronic gastritis. With the advent of medical treatment for peptic ulcer disease, this presentation has become exceptionally rare.

Familial and genetic predisposition: Currently there are robust data that supports familial predisposition to gastric cancer due to specific genetic mutations. Germline mutations of the *cdh1* gene that encodes E-cadherin are found in approximately 50% of diffuse-type gastric cancers. This mutation has also been observed in hereditary, diffuse gastric cancer. The disorder follows autosomal dominant genetics and has an accumulative risk of carcinoma development in 40-67% of males and 60-83% of females. Due to this high risk of developing gastric cancer, genetic counseling and prophylactic gastrectomy is indicated in asymptomatic carriers of *cdh1* mutation. Polymorphisms of certain molecules such as human interleukin 1 beta (IL-1β), chain 1 of IFN-gamma receptor (IFNγR1) and methylenetetrahydrofolate (MTHF) reductase have also been associated with gastric cancer. Finally, familial adenomatous polyposis (FAP) and Peutz-Jeghers syndrome kindreds are at risk for the development of gastric cancer.

Clinical Presentation

Even in early gastric cancers (EGC) the majority of patients (90%) present with vague symptoms such as non-specific pain and/or dyspepsia. Nausea, vomiting and anorexia are also common symptoms reported in EGC. Weight loss and anemia are rare (4-5%) in comparison to invasive gastric cancer. Weight loss (62%) and persistent abdominal pain (52%) are the most common symptoms of invasive gastric cancer, followed by nausea (34%), dysphagia (26%), melena (20%) and early satiety (18%). In cases of *linitis plastica*, early satiety is common. Dysphagia may occur from lesions arising in the cardia and symptoms of pseudoachalasia are reported when the myoenteric nerve plexus of Auerbach is compromised. Prepyloric lesions can produce gastric outlet obstruction. Paraneoplastic

syndromes are infrequently encountered in gastric cancer, but may include hypercoagulability, thrombophlebitis migrans (Trousseaus syndrome), microangiopathic hemolytic anemia, nephrotic syndrome and polyarthritis nodosa.

Signs of advanced disease may be identified upon physical exam and include a palpable abdominal mass, left supraclavicular adenopathy (Virchow's node), periumbilical adenopathy (Sister Mary Joseph's node), left axillary adenopathy (Irish node), ascitis or jaundice. A pelvic examination is warranted as an enlarged adenexa or ovary (Krukenberg's tumor) may be encountered, and the rectal examination facilitates the identification of a mass in the cul-de-sac (Blumer's shelf) or the presence of occult fecal blood.

Pathology

As introduced above, there are three histopathologic classifications of gastric adenocarcinoma. This original classification by Lauren includes intestinal type (53%), diffuse type (33%) and unclassified (14%). The intestinal type is found in the setting of chronic atrophic gastritis, metaplasia and dysplasia, while the diffuse type is observed in familial gastric cancer. The World Health Organization and the Japanese classifications are much more detailed, describe several histopathologic types and are useful for the prognosis base of the grade of histologic differentiation of early lesions **(Table 25-1)**.

Early gastric cancer (EGC) is defined as adenocarcinoma limited to the mucosa and submucosa of the stomach, regardless of lymph node status. The morphology of early gastric cancer can be subclassified as protruded, elevated, flat, depressed, or excavated, a relevant classification when considering endoscopic mucosal resection **(Figure 25-2)**. In Japan, where aggressive screening programs are employed, close to 50% of treated cases represent early gastric cancer. This presentation is usually well differentiated (70%); lymph node

TABLE 25-1	World Health Organization's histologic classification of gastric carcinoma

- Adenocarcinoma
  - Papillary adenocarcinoma
  - Tubular adenocarcinoma
  - Mucinous adenocarcinoma
  - Signet-ring cell carcinoma
- Adenosquamous carcinoma
- Squamous cell carcinoma
- Small cell carcinoma
- Undifferentiated carcinoma
- Others

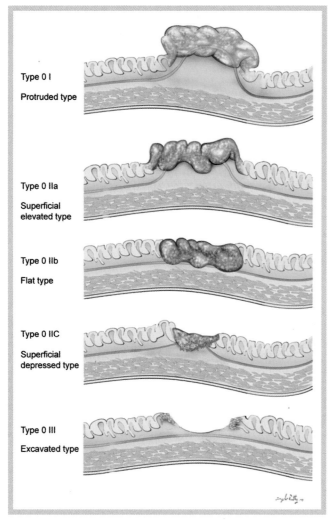

Figure 25-2: Macroscopic classification of early gastric cancer

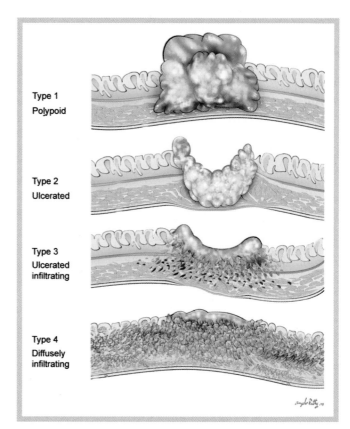

Figure 25-3: Macroscopic classification of advanced gastric cancer. Type 5, non-classifiable carcinoma, is not depicted

metastasis is present in about 10% of the cases. The overall cure rate of these neoplasms is 95% when resection and lymphadenectomy is performed.

Although misleading, advanced gastric cancer is the term use to describe tumors extending beyond the submucosa. In the USA, more than 80% of the resected gastric adenocarcinomas represent advanced lesions. The Borrmann classification characterizes the morphology of advanced gastric cancer as polypoid, ulcerative, ulcerative/infiltrating or scirrhous **(Figure 25-3)**. A fifth type is also described as nonclassifiable.

Diagnosis, Preoperative Evaluation and Staging

Any patient complaining of the symptoms described above warrants esophago-gastro-duodenoscopy (EGD). If dysphagia symptoms are reported, a barium eso-phagram prior to endoscopy is indicated. The diagnosis of gastric cancer is usually achieved and confirmed by

EGD through direct visualization, biopsy and histopatho-logical confirmation. Six to nine biopsies are required to achieve >90% sensitivity. Tumor markers in general have low sensitivity for gastric cancer. Carcinoembryonic antigen (CEA) and CA 19.9 can be elevated in about 45-50% and 20% of the cases respectively.

There are two major classification systems currently used for staging gastric cancer that predict outcome. The American Joint Committee on Cancer (AJCC) and the International Union Against Cancer (UICC) systems are used in most western countries and are based on the tumor/node/metastasis model **(Table 25-2)**. To ade-quately define the N status, at least 15 lymph nodes should surgically be obtained and analyzed. The Japanese classi-fication is a more elaborate system based on a detailed assessment of anatomic lymph node stations.

The preoperative staging workup should include com-puterized tomography (CT) of the chest, abdomen and pelvis with intravenous and oral contrast. Importantly, recent data indicates a combined positron emission tomography (PET) - CT scan is more accurate in preopera-tive staging than either PET or CT scan alone. Endoscopic ultrasonography (EUS) provides the most accurate information regarding T (accuracy 65-98%) and N stage

TABLE 25-2	**TNM staging of gastric cancer by the International Union Against Cancer and American Joint Committee on Cancer**

- T stage primary tumor
  - Tis—Carcinoma in situ, intraepithelial tumor
  - T1—Tumor extension to submucosa
  - T2—Tumor extension to the muscularis propria (T2a) or subserosa (T2b)
  - T3—Tumor penetration of the serosa
  - T4—Tumor invasion of the adjacent organs
- N stage regional lymph node
  - N0—No lymph nodes involved
  - N1—Metastasis in 1-6 regional lymph nodes
  - N2—Metastasis in 7-15 regional lymph nodes
  - N3—Metastasis in >15 regional lymph nodes
- M stage distant metastasis
  - M0—No distant metastasis
  - M1—Distant metastasis

Stage grouping:

Stage	T	N	M
0	Tis	N0	M0
IA	T1	N0	M0
IB	T1	N1	M0
	T2a	N0	M0
	T2b	N0	M0
II	T1	N2	M0
	T2a	N1	M0
	T2b	N1	M0
	T3	N0	M0
IIIA	T2a	N2	M0
	T2b	N2	M0
	T3	N1	M0
	T4	N0	M0
IIIB	T3	N2	M0
IV	T4	N1	M0
	T4	N2	M0
	T4	N3	M0
	T1	N3	M0
	T2	N3	M0
	T3	N3	M0
	Any T	Any N	M1

Reproduced with permission from AJCC Cancer Manual Staging (6th edn), Springer-Verlag, New York, 2002

(accuracy 50-70%) **(Figures 25-4 to 25-6).** Laparoscopic staging prior to resection for cure is warranted to rule out peritoneal implants and/or occult metastasis. Peritoneal cytology has been shown to be an independent predictor of recurrence by identifying otherwise occult carcinomatosis, but is rarely employed. Some authors advocate peritoneal lavage as part of preoperative evaluation (percutaneous or laparoscopic), however data in clear support of this practice is lacking. An encouraging, early literature supporting sentinel lymph node assessment for gastric adenocarcinoma exists, but this methodology currently remains investigational.

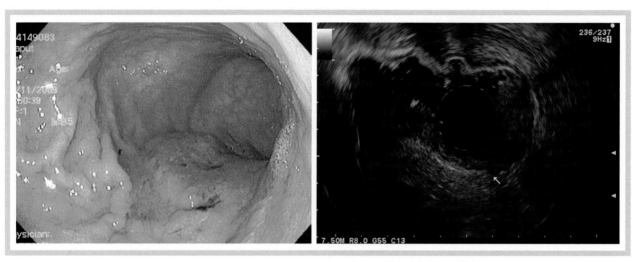

Figure 25-4: Endoscopic image (left) and endoscopic ultrasonography (right) of a T3 N1 gastric carcinoma. *Courtesy* of Scott Cooper, MD

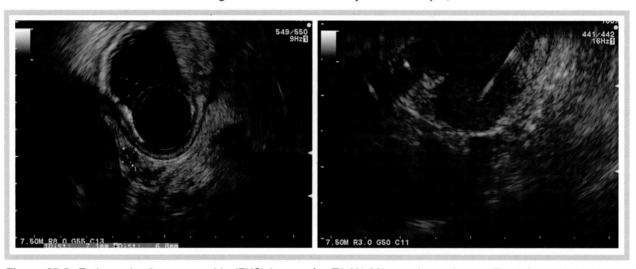

Figure 25-5: Endoscopic ultrasonographic (EUS) image of a T3 N1 M0 gastric carcinoma. The left panel depicts an enlarged lymph node suspicious for metastatic disease. On the right, fine-needle biopsy of this lymph node under EUS guidance. Courtesy of Scott Cooper, MD

Prevention and Screening Programs

Screening programs have been implemented in countries with high incidence of gastric cancer including Japan and Chile. In Japan, the screening for gastric cancer was introduced in 1960s for individuals over 40 years-of-age. Only those with abnormalities detected on barium radiographs undergo upper endoscopy. Although there is evidence that screening has contributed to detection of early asymptomatic gastric cancers, the cost-effectiveness of screening for gastric cancer in high-risk populations remains unsettled. In Western countries where the incidence of gastric cancer is low, endoscopy should be restricted to symptomatic patients and patients with identified precursor lesions or clear risk (e.g. pernicious anemia and familial gastric cancer).

Primary Treatment: Surgery

Endoscopic Mucosal Resection in Early Gastric Cancer

Endoscopic mucosal resection (EMR) was developed in high-incidence countries and should only be performed in the USA as part of a trial or in centers with large experience in this procedure. EMR should be considered in patients with Tis or T1a lesions less than 30 mm, without ulceration, or evidence of lymph node metastasis. Ten to fifteen percent of the patients with early gastric cancer have lymph node metastases and the risk of lymphatic metastasis is increased in early lesions with the following pathologic findings: increased tumor size, poor differentiation, submucosal invasion and lymphatic and vascular invasion. Thus, appropriate gastrectomy is indicated in these patients.

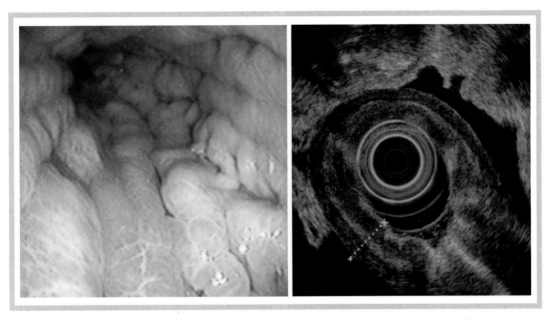

Figure 25-6: Endoscopic (left) and Endoscopic ultrasound images (right) of a diffusely infiltrating T3 gastric carcinoma (linitis plastica). *Courtesy* of Kevin McGrath, MD

Advanced Gastric Cancer

In the USA and other Western countries, advanced gastric cancer is the norm and surgery with curative intent is the mainstay of treatment. In these patients, a gastric resection with a macroscopically negative margin of 5 cm and an *en bloc* resection of the adjacent lymph nodes (D1, regional lymphadenectomy) is the standard of care. Omentectomy has also been historically performed. The overall 5-year survival in patients with gastric cancer in Western countries ranges from 10% to 21% depending on the reported experience. Stage-for-stage, the 5-year survival rate in Western countries is considerably lower as compared to the Japanese literature **(Table 25-3)**.

TABLE 25-3	5-year survival rate (%), after gastrectomy with lymphadenectomy with at least 15 lymph nodes examined		
	United States [a]		**Japan** [b]
AJCC stage	**All**	**Japanese Americans**	
IA	78	95	95
IB	58	75	86
II	34	46	71
IIIA	20	48	59
IIIB	8	18	35
IV	7	5	17
Overall	28	42	NR

[a] Hundahl, et al Cancer 2000; 88:921-32
[b] Ichikura, et al in Cancer 1999; 86:55-3

Extent of Resection

Several studies have shown that there is incongruity in the macroscopic and microscopic tumor margin. In order to assure negative margins, most authors recommend a 5 cm gross margin when performing gastric resections and intraoperative frozen section analysis. The authors do not assess the distal, duodenal margin intraoperatively. The extent of resection is dependent upon this desired margin and the location of the primary neoplasm.

Proximal tumors: As mentioned above, an increased incidence of proximal gastric adenocarcinomas is being observed in the USA. About half of the gastric carcinomas currently diagnosed are proximal. The Siewert classification describes 3 three types of gastroesophageal (GE) junction tumors based upon anatomical and topographic criteria **(Figure 25-7).** A type I Siewart lesion is associated with Barrett's esophagus or is a true esophageal adenocarcinoma growing down into the GE junction, type II lesions originate within 2 cm of the squamocolumnar junction and type III lesions are localized to the subcardia region. The recommended surgical approach of proximal, type I lesions is esophagectomy, including resection of the cardia. Total gastrectomy with Roux-en-Y anastomosis reconstruction, omentectomy and jejunostomy feeding tube placement is preferred by the authors over proximal gastrectomy with pyloroplasty for type II and III GE tumors since it prevents alkaline reflux esophagitis.

Neoplasms of the body or antrum: These represent 30-40% of all gastric adenocarcinomas. The authors recommend

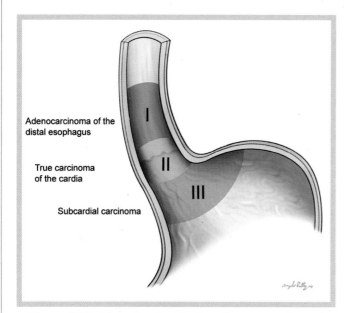

Figure 25-7: Siewert's classification of gastroesophageal (GE) junction tumors

subtotal gastrectomy with regional lymphadenectomy, omentectomy and feeding jejunostomy. Total gastrectomy for distal lesions failed to show survival benefit in two randomized trials and subtotal gastrectomy patients report a better quality of life than total gastrectomy patients.

All gastrectomy patients can be started on nutrient tube feeds in the immediate postoperative period. Once these feeds have achieved the nutritional goal (the authors provide 100% caloric needs via tube feeds for the first six postoperative weeks), they may be cycled to facilitate oral intake by day. The initiation of oral nutrition is variable and dependent upon patient factors and potential complications. Many experienced surgeons obtain water-soluble contrast upper gastrointestinal series prior to the initiation of oral intake, but this practice is not based upon data. Patients are initiated on clear liquids and then advanced to six small meals per day.

Extent of Lymphadenectomy

This remains a controversial issue between Western and Eastern gastric cancer experts. The lymphatic drainage of the stomach initially studied by Inoue in 1936 and later by Kodama and Yoshida in 1988 described 16 stations for lymphatic drainage divided in three groups: N1, N2 and N3 **(Figure 25-8)**. A D1 lymphadenectomy refers to a limited dissection of the perigastric lymph nodes (stations 1-6) whereas a D2 lymphadenectomy is extended to include lymphatics along the hepatic, left gastric, celiac and splenic arteries and thus classically includes distal pancreatectomy and spenectomy (stations 1-11) **(Figure 25-9)**. An extended D3 lymphadenectomy includes

the lymph nodes described above with removal of the porta hepatic and periaortic lymph nodes (stations 1-16).

Japanese surgeons have long recommended extended lymph node dissections based upon several studies showing survival benefits on patients undergoing radical (D2 and D3 resections) versus regional (D1) lymphadenectomy and even some of the Western literature has suggested potential benefit to extended lymphadenectomy, however this was largely attribute to an improved accuracy of staging. In fact, "stage migration" has long been alleged to be responsible for the improved long-term survival reported in the Japanese literature.

Despite these retrospective reports suggesting improved survival with radical lymph node dissection, prospective Western and Asian studies have failed to prove survival benefit from extended lymphadenectomy. The British Cooperative study of the Medical Research Council, the Dutch Gastric Cancer Group trial and the multicenter Japan Clinical Oncology Group Trial (D2 vs D3) all found that a more extensive lymphatic resection resulted in significantly higher morbidity and mortality when compared with the less extensive resection and no significant difference was found in overall survival. These studies did identify a decrease in the risk of recurrence with extended lymphadenectomy, but no long-term survival benefit was realized due to the higher operative mortality. Splenectomy and pancreatectomy are the predominate cause of increased morbidity and mortality, thus several authors have proposed modified D2 lymph node dissections limiting splenectomy or pancreatectomy to when these organs are involved by local invasion of the primary lesion. Using this approach Sierra reported a 5-year survival rate of 50.6% in D2 group versus 41.4% in D1 group, without significant differences in morbidity and mortality between groups.

In summary, this controversial topic remains unresolved. A D2 lymphadenectomy sparing the pancreas and spleen for invasive gastric cancer is currently recommended when performed by an experienced surgeon in a high volume center, but is not required to meet the Western standard of care. Routine splenectomy does not attain survival benefits and only should be performed if the tumor is adherent to the spleen or its vascular supply. Timely, preoperative vaccinations for encapsulated organisms are warranted if splenectomy is anticipated.

Sentinel Lymph Node Biopsy in Early Gastric Cancer

Since virtually no EGCs confined to the mucosa and about 20% of tumors limited to the submucosa harbor lymph node metastasis, several Japanese authors have proposed the use of sentinel lymph node biopsy (SLNB) in early gastric cancer to determine the need for lymphadenectomy. The usefulness of this approach remains questionable due to problems with the false-negative rate (0-29%)

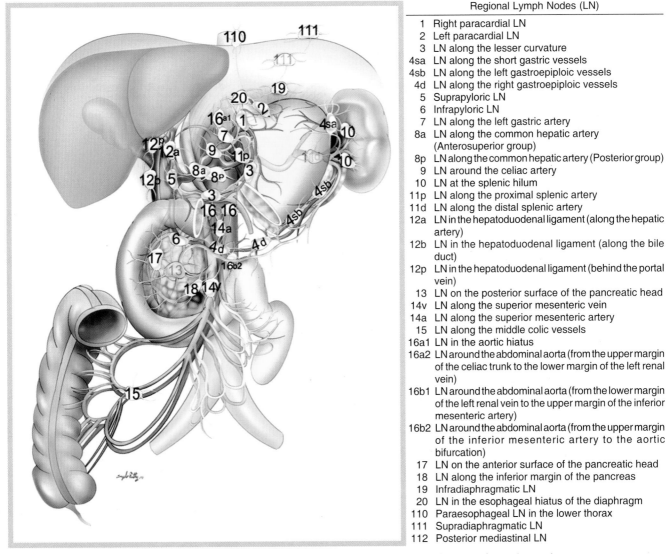

	Regional Lymph Nodes (LN)
1	Right paracardial LN
2	Left paracardial LN
3	LN along the lesser curvature
4sa	LN along the short gastric vessels
4sb	LN along the left gastroepiploic vessels
4d	LN along the right gastroepiploic vessels
5	Suprapyloric LN
6	Infrapyloric LN
7	LN along the left gastric artery
8a	LN along the common hepatic artery (Anterosuperior group)
8p	LN along the common hepatic artery (Posterior group)
9	LN around the celiac artery
10	LN at the splenic hilum
11p	LN along the proximal splenic artery
11d	LN along the distal splenic artery
12a	LN in the hepatoduodenal ligament (along the hepatic artery)
12b	LN in the hepatoduodenal ligament (along the bile duct)
12p	LN in the hepatoduodenal ligament (behind the portal vein)
13	LN on the posterior surface of the pancreatic head
14v	LN along the superior mesenteric vein
14a	LN along the superior mesenteric artery
15	LN along the middle colic vessels
16a1	LN in the aortic hiatus
16a2	LN around the abdominal aorta (from the upper margin of the celiac trunk to the lower margin of the left renal vein)
16b1	LN around the abdominal aorta (from the lower margin of the left renal vein to the upper margin of the inferior mesenteric artery)
16b2	LN around the abdominal aorta (from the upper margin of the inferior mesenteric artery to the aortic bifurcation)
17	LN on the anterior surface of the pancreatic head
18	LN along the inferior margin of the pancreas
19	Infradiaphragmatic LN
20	LN in the esophageal hiatus of the diaphragm
110	Paraesophageal LN in the lower thorax
111	Supradiaphragmatic LN
112	Posterior mediastinal LN

Figure 25-8: Lymph node (LN) stations according to Japanese classification of gastric carcinoma.

that may be related to a high frequency of skip metastasis (15-20%), the identification of several sentinel lymph nodes (generally 2-7) and the need for a transabdominal surgical procedure for lymph node detection and retrieval. Currently two large-scale, prospective multicenter trials are being performed in Japan and their results will provide a better perspective of the use of SLNB in the management or early gastric cancer.

Linitis Plastica

This is defined as a diffuse, intensively infiltrative gastric cancer that involves the majority or the entire gastric wall. *Linitis plastica* represents 5% of all gastric cancers and is associated with poorly differentiated (diffuse type) adenocarcinoma with signet ring cells on histology. It is typically diagnosed in younger patients and has an extremely poor prognosis with rapid progression causing

death, usually in less than 6 months. Thus, outside the randomized neoadjuvant trial setting, the authors consider *linitis plastica* a contraindication for attempt at curative resection. If resection is attempted, total gastrectomy is recommended resulting in an overall 7-year survival less than 8% **(Figure 25-10)**.

Laparoscopic Resection for Gastric Cancer

Laparoscopic resection of the stomach maintaining oncologic principles is feasible and has been reported to result in less blood loss, earlier return of bowel function and reduced hospital stay. Two prospective, randomized studies of 59 and 164 patients with distal gastric cancers compared laparoscopic-assisted to open subtotal gastrectomy approach have been published. No significant differences were found in morbidity, mortality, or 5-year overall and disease-free survival between the laparoscopic

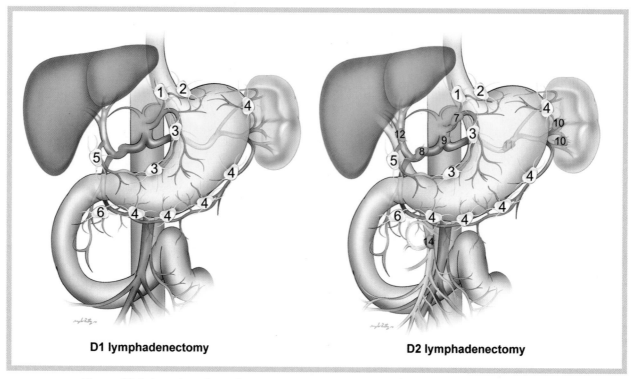

D1 lymphadenectomy   **D2 lymphadenectomy**

Figure 25-9: Lymph node stations removed in a D1 (left) and D2 (right) lymphadenectomy.
A D2 lymph node dissection includes both perigastric and perivascular lymph nodes

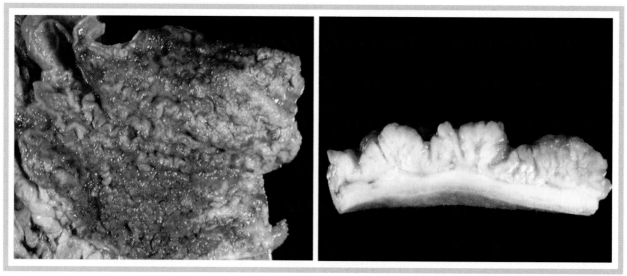

Figure 25-10: Gross pathology a diffusely infiltrative (linitis plastica) T3 gastric adenocarcinoma.
Courtesy of Kevin McGrath, MD

and open gastrectomy groups, however, the larger study did report improved quality of life in the group that received laparoscopic treatment. Less rigorously designed studies have demonstrated the feasibility of laparoscopic extended lymphadenectomy and robotic-assisted gastrectomy that also include extended lymphadenectomy. Although the viability and potential benefits of minimal-access surgery have been shown, the majority of these procedures continue to be performed through standard incisions.

Complications of Gastrectomy for Gastric Cancer

The overall morbidity and mortality of gastric resection ranges from 25% to 46% and 4% to 13% respectively and are largely dependent upon the extent of the resection. Beyond the general risks of major surgical procedures, complications specifically related to the gastrectomy include anastomotic leak, dumping syndrome, delayed gastric emptying, diarrhea, bile reflux gastritis, Roux stasis syndrome, gallstones, anemia and malnutrition/weight loss. Anastomotic leak occurs in 3-21% of patients; esophageal anastomoses are considerably more at risk. Similarly, a duodenal stump leak continues to plague gastric surgeons, although this complication should be rare in the setting of resection for neoplasm as compared to gastric surgery performed for complications of peptic ulcer disease. If a leak is uncontrolled, abdominal sepsis ensues, mandating reoperation with repair or drainage.

Five to ten percent of gastric surgery patients develop severe post-prandial symptoms referred to as dumping syndrome. Early dumping syndrome occurs within 15-30 minutes following a meal and usually presents with diaphoresis, palpitation, light-headedness, weakness, abdominal cramps and watery diarrhea. Late dumping syndrome symptoms occur 2-3 hours following a meal and are characteristic of hypoglycemia and hyperinsulinemia. Most of these symptoms can be treated medically with dietary modifications, avoidance of hyperosmotic fluids and somatostatin analogs.

Delayed gastric emptying occurs in approximately 10% of patients and either presents early and transiently delaying the initiation of oral nutrition or years after surgery when it presents as a chronic and difficult to treat condition. Obstruction or stricture from a technical error or marginal ulcer must first be excluded. If gastric atony is implicated, medical management with metoclopramide and/or erythromycin is indicated. Alkaline bile reflux may occur following Billroth II reconstructions. Conversion to a Roux-en-Y reconstruction is curative, but may lead to Roux stasis syndrome **(Figures 25-11 and 25-12)**.

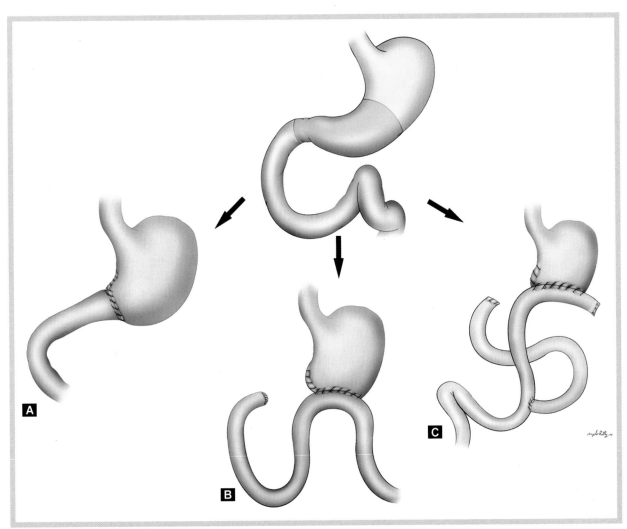

Figure 25-11: Anastomotic reconstructions after partial or subtotal gastrectomy: (A) Billroth I, (B) Billroth II or (C) Roux-en-Y gastrojejunostomy

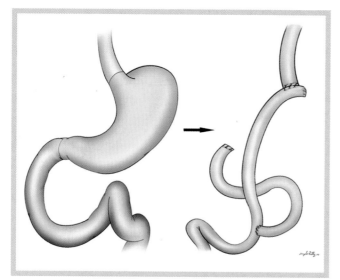

Figure 25-12: Esophagojejunostomy reconstruction after total gastrectomy

Adjuvant Therapy

Chemotherapy

Numerous randomized control trials have compared the value adjuvant systemic chemotherapy after gastric cancer resections and have produced inconsistent results. In an effort to produce a clear conclusion, at least four meta-analyses have been performed. Earle, et al in 1999 and Mari, et al in 2000 published meta-analyses of 13 Western and 19 Western and Asian trials, respectively. They both identified a small survival benefit in patients that received 5-fluorouracil-based chemo-therapy. A larger benefit was observed in the meta-analyses reported by Panzini and Janunger that included 17 and 21 randomized trials respectively, however critics recommended caution when interpreting this data due to the heterogeneity in the studies and the use of different treatment protocols that, for the most part, were based on 5-fluorouracil (5-FU). Most of these studies have design biases and other limitations that impair their interpre-tation. Importantly, when Western and Asian studies were analyzed separately, no survival benefit was observed for the treated patients in the Western groups (95% confidence interval of 0.83-1.12). Very recently, a large randomized Japanese trial reported improved overall survival in patients treated in the adjuvant setting with S-1, a novel oral fluoropyrimidine which is a combination of tegafur (a prodrug of 5-FU), 5-chloro-2,4-dihydropiridine (CDHP) and oxonic acid. However, S-1 is currently unavailable in North America. To summarize, postoperative chemotherapy in the adjuvant setting lacks strong level I evidence.

Radiation Therapy

Numerous non-randomized studies have supported a role for radiotherapy (RT) in the preoperative, postoperative and palliative management of gastric cancer, most utilizing external beam radiation therapy combined with 5-FU as sensitizing chemotherapy agent. A randomized trial of 436 patients reported by the British Stomach Cancer Group found no 5-year survival benefit in patients that received postoperative radiation or chemotherapy versus surgery alone. In a single randomized control study of preoperative radiotherapy (40 Gy/4 weeks) for adeno-carcinoma of the cardia, higher R0 resection rates were found in patients that received radiotherapy prior to surgical exploration versus those that underwent surgery alone (89.5% vs 79%). The survival rate in the preoperative radiation arm was also improved (30% vs 20%). However, despite this evidence for lesions arising in the cardia, the use of preoperative radiation alone is not routinely employed or recommended as standard management in patients with resectable gastric cancer.

Chemoradiation Therapy

Several randomized trials have studied the use of combi-ned chemotherapy and radiation therapy in the adjuvant setting after resection with curative intent for gastric adenocarcinoma. The Intergroup Trial initiated by the Southwest Oncology Group (SWOG 9008/INT-0116) assessed the use of surgery alone versus combined chemo-therapy plus radiotherapy in 556 patients that underwent curative (R0) resection. The combined adjuvant therapy consisted in five monthly cycles of bolus chemotherapy (5-FU and leucovorin) with concomitant RT (45 Gy) with the second and third cycle. Although only 65% of patients completed the adjuvant treatment, an increase in median survival (36 vs 27 months), 3-year relapse-free survival (48% vs 31%) and overall survival (50% vs 41%) with the combined adjuvant therapy was observed. The results if this study established postoperative chemoradiation as standard therapy in patients following resection of gastric adenocarcinoma.

Neoadjuvant Therapy

A number of theoretical advantages can be achieved by treating *in situ* neoplasms prior to surgery, but for gastric adenocarcinoma the most compelling reason is the rate of surgical complications and/or a rapid decline in performance status that precludes patients from receiving additional therapy. As above, gastric adenocarcinoma response rates to 5-FU-based regimens are relatively poor, but the combination of epirubicin (or doxorubicin) and cisplatin with 5-FU (ECF) can induce reasonable response rates (~ 60%). Importantly, a positive response to neoadjuvant chemotherapy has been shown to predict survival.

The British Medical Research Council reported the first well-powered multi-institutional, prospective randomized phase III trial for perioperative chemotherapy (MAGIC trial). This study included 503 patients with gastric or esophageal cancer stage II or higher that were randomized to receive either three cycles of chemotherapy with neoadjuvant ECF prior to surgery with curative intent or followed by three addition cycles of ECF and outcomes were compared to surgery alone. Seventy-four percent of the patients had gastric cancer, 13% had esophageal cancer and 11% had esophagogastric junction cancer. There was a significant improvement in the 5-year survival rate (36% vs 23%) and progression-free survival in the neoadjuvant/adjuvant therapy group versus the surgery-only group. Thus, level I evidence supports the use of neoadjuvant chemotherapy for gastric adenocarcinoma.

Intraperitoneal Chemotherapy

Gastric adenocarcinoma frequently presents or recurs in the peritoneal cavity, leading to the notion that intraperitoneal chemotherapy (IPC) should improve outcomes. Two cohort studies from Japan found such a benefit when surgery alone was compared to intraperitoneal lavage with mitomycin and 5-FU or cisplatin after curative resection in tumors with serosal exposure—a 3rd arm showed benefit to hyperthermic over normothermic IPC. Unfortunately, subsequent randomized trials have failed to show survival benefit from IPC. IPC, performed in the setting of a clinical trial at a high-volume center, remains an option for select patients with metastatic, gastric adenocarcinoma.

Palliative Management of Unresectable Gastric Cancer

Carcinomatosis, distant metastasis and regional encasement of named vessels are contraindications for gastrectomy with curative intent. However, palliative goals to reduce or eliminate pain, bleeding, obstruction and perforation may be met surgically in appropriate patients and there is some level III evidence of survival benefit from palliative gastrectomy in patients with locally advanced or metastatic disease. More recently and in addition to improvements in chemotherapeutics and external beam radiotherapies, advances in endoscopic stent technology, interventional radiology and other methodologies, such as argon laser or photodynamic therapy, have reduced the number of patients requiring palliative gastric surgery. Endoscopic placement of stents or palliative RT may be used to alleviate symptoms of obstruction. Surgical excision, external beam radiation, endoscopic treatment or angiography with selective embolization all may be appropriate in patients experiencing bleeding.

Palliative chemotherapy is not yet standard of care at most cancer centers and many unresectable or recurrent disease patients lack adequate performance status to tolerate chemotherapy. All patients with advanced, metastatic cancer should receive best supportive care and patients with a good performance status should be considered for a chemotherapy clinical trial. A recent meta-analysis of randomized trials compared the use of chemotherapy versus supportive care showing increased one year survival (20% vs 8%), longer symptom-free time and improved quality of life in the chemotherapy group. ECF (epirubicin, cisplatin, infusional 5-FU) has demonstrated improved median survival and quality of life benefits when compared to FAMTX (5-FU, adriamycin and methotrexate) and MCF (mitomycin, cisplatin, 5-FU). Recently two phase III trials (REAL 2 and ML17032) have shown the efficacy of capecitabine in lieu of continuous-infusion 5-FU in combination with epirubicin, cisplatin or oxaliplatin. Several ongoing clinical trials are studying the role of new agents like S-1 (FLAGS study) and bevacizumab (anti-VEGF antibody) in the management of advanced, unresectable gastric cancer. No first-line regimen consensus for palliative chemotherapy has been defined.

Follow-up and Surveillance

Gastric cancer patients require close monitoring of their nutritional status and gastric-resection patients require replacement of vitamin B_{12} and iron supplementation. The authors routinely maintain postoperative patients on supplemental tube feeding until completion of adjuvant therapy, slowly weaning this supplementation to ensure maintenance of body weight. As to surveillance, National Cancer Cooperative Group (NCCN) guidelines recommended a complete history and physical examination on every 4-6 months for three years and annually thereafter. Routine surveillance for asymptomatic recurrence is not currently supported by data. Thus, imaging and endoscopy are reserved for symptomatic patients.

Gastric Lymphoma

Epidemiology

Primary, localized gastric lymphoma (GL) represents the second most common malignancy after adenocarcinoma and is the most common extranodal site of lymphoma, representing 75% of all the gastrointestinal lymphomas. However, only 3% of all gastric neoplasms are lymphomas. GL are more common in older patients, having a peak incidence in the sixth and seventh decades of life being and are more common in men than women (2:1).

Some pathologic processes have been identified as risk factors that predispose to GL. Chronic gastritis due to *H. pylori* infection has been associated with low-grade mucosa associated lymphatic tissue (MALT or MALToma), while Epstein-Barr virus is related to Burkitt's lymphoma of the stomach. Autoimmune disorders like rheumatoid arthritis, Sjögren's syndrome, systemic lupus erythematous and Wegener's granulomatosis have been related to primary gastrointestinal lymphomas. Congenital immunodeficiency syndromes (i.e. Wiskott-Aldrich, severe combined immunodeficiency syndrome and X-linked agammaglobulinemia), acquired immuno-deficiency syndrome (AIDS) and long standing immuno-suppressive therapy (i.e. post-transplant) have all been identified as risk factors predisposing to GL.

Clinical Presentation

GL presents similarly to gastric adenocarcinoma with symptoms of epigastric pain, early satiety, anorexia, weight loss, nausea, vomiting, fatigue and occult GI bleeding. The physical exam is usually unremarkable unless advance disease is present were a palpable mass or peripheral lymphadenopathy can be observed.

Pathology

There are several classification systems for lymphomas (Table 25-4). The World Health Organization's (WHO's)

classification is presently favored. Most GLs diffuse large B-cell lymphomas (55%), followed by the extranodal marginal B-cell lymphomas (MALT) (40%), Burkitt's lymphomas (3%) and mantle cell and follicular lymphomas represent less the 1% each.

Diagnosis and Staging

Like in other gastric tumors, EGD is usually performed based upon presenting symptoms, typically revealing nonspecific gastritis and ulceration and/or mass. At the author's institution, endoscopic ultrasonography is routinely employed to assess depth of gastric invasion and to guide the biopsy. Histologic analysis and testing for *H. pylori* is performed. Once GL is confirmed, the preoperative staging workup should include B_2 microglobulin, CT scan of chest, abdomen and pelvis and bone marrow biopsy. Numerous staging systems have also been described, however the Ann Arbor staging system is the stratification most frequently used (Table 25-5).

Treatment and Follow-up

Treatment of extranodal, marginal B-cell lymphoma (MALT) is usually limited to eradication of *H. pylori* infection and results in remission in 75% of the cases. *H. pylori* treatment involves the classic "triple therapy", which combines an acid suppression (proton pump inhibitor or histamine blocker) with the antibiotics

TABLE 25-4	Most common histologic classifications for gastrointestinal lymphomas	
WHO	**Working**	**Real**
Extranodal marginal zone lymphoma (MALT)	Small cleaved cell type	——
Follicular lymphoma	Small cleaved cell type	Follicular center lymphoma
Mantle cell lymphoma		——
Diffuse large B-cell lymphoma	Large cleaved follicular center cell	Diffuse large B-cell lymphoma
Burkitt's lymphoma	Small noncleaved follicular center cell	Burkitt's lymphoma

TABLE 25-5	Ann Arbor classification of Hodgkin and Non-Hodgkin lymphoma
The addition of A or B will depend on the absence (A) or presence (B) of the systemic ("B") symptoms (unexplained fever, night sweats or unexplained weight loss exceeding 10% of body weight during the six months prior to diagnosis)	
Stage I	Involvement of a single lymph node region (I) or of a single extralymphatic organ or site (IE)*
Stage II	Involvement of two or more lymph node regions or lymphatic structures on the same side of the diaphragm alone (II) or with involvement of limited, contiguous extralymphatic organ or tissue (IIE)
Stage III	Involvement of lymph node regions on both sides of the diaphragm (III) which may include the spleen (IIIS) or limited, contiguous extralymphatic organ or site (IIIE) or both (IIIES)
Stage IV	Diffuse or disseminated foci of involvement of one or more extralymphatic organs or tissues, with or without associated lymphatic involvement

*The designation "E" refers to extranodal contiguous extension (i.e. proximal or contiguous extranodal disease). A single extralymphatic site as the only site of disease should be classified as IE, rather than stage IV. Reproduced with permission from Carbone PP, et al. Cancer Res. 1971; 31:1860 and Lister TA, et al. J Clin Oncol 1989; 7:1630.

clarithromycin and amoxicillin. Metronidazole can be substituted for amoxicillin in those with significant penicillin allergies and both levofloxacin and tetracycline have been utilized as part of the regimen depending on allergy profile and response to therapies. These therapies can be combined with bismuth colloid for a "quadruple therapy", and should be continued for 10-14 days with documented clearance of *H. pylori* by urease breath test or repeat biopsy. Transmural extension of gastric lymphoma, regional lymph node involvement, transformation to a large cell phenotype, chromosomal translocation (11;18) and nuclear BCL-10 expression are predictors of failure after eradication of *H. pylori*. Chemotherapy or radiotherapy should be considered in this group of patients and MALToma arising in the absence of *H. pylori* infection. Due to potential recurrence, close follow-up of these patients is recommended. Periodic EGD with biopsies is recommended 2 months after treatment to corroborate eradication and on every 3-6 months thereafter to document regression. The overall 5-year-survival of the extranodal marginal B-cell lymphoma even in those who failed eradication of *H. pylori* or lacked this etiology is above 90%.

The treatment of the other types of GL is more controversial. The most common chemotherapy regimen applied is cyclophosphamide, doxorubicin, vincristine and prednisone (CHOP) with or without external beam radiation (usually 30 Gy). Surgical resection had been historically performed either as single therapy or to prevent perforation following tumor response to chemotherapy. However, the risk of perforation has been overstated and unacceptable recurrence rates without chemotherapy have been found. A Mexican randomized control trial assigned 589 patients with primary gastric diffuse large B-cell lymphoma to either surgery alone, surgery plus radiation, surgery plus chemotherapy (CHOP) or chemotherapy alone showed that chemotherapy should be considered the treatment of choice since it has better 10 year survival and avoids postgastrectomy morbidity. Furthermore a nonrandomized German multicenter study (GIT NHL 02/96) revealed a survival rate at 42 months of 86% with surgery compared with 91% for patients with chemotherapy or radiation without surgery. Thus, surgical resection of GL should have a limited role, namely to obtain an otherwise elusive diagnosis or to manage complications (e.g. perforation, bleeding or obstruction).

Finally, Mantle cell lymphoma, usually seen in older patients, is largely considered incurable with a median survival of 3-5 years. Burkitt's lymphoma is more commonly seen in immunosuppressed patients and more typically originates in the ileocecal region. The prognosis for Burkitt's lymphoma is predominantly dependent on the patient's underlying disease and the ability to with-draw/reverse the immunosuppression. Chemotherapy is the treatment of choice for both Mantle cell and Burkitt's lymphoma.

Gastrointestinal Stromal Tumors (GIST)

Epidemiology

Gastrointestinal stromal tumors (GISTs) are the most common mesenchymal tumors arising from the stomach, but account for less than 3% of all gastric neoplasia. It is estimated that approximately 5,000 new cases of GISTs are diagnosed every year in the USA. The majority of GISTs are located in the stomach (60-70%), followed by the small intestine (20-30%) and less commonly (10%) the esophagus, colon and rectum. These lesions have a mean age of 60 years at diagnosis, but can affect any age group. The incidence is slightly higher in men than women.

Familial GISTs have been described in kindred's harboring mutations in the *c-kit* loci. Other GISTs associations have been made to familial paraganglyoma and neurofibromatosis type 1. The association of GISTs (usually multifocal), pulmonary chondromas and extra-adrenal paragangliomas has been described as the triad of Carney.

Pathology and Risk of Malignant Behavior

GISTs were initially thought to arise from the smooth muscle cells, being mistakenly classified as leiomyomas or leiomyosarcomas. Upon histologic analysis, they seem to arise from the muscularis propria and specifically from the interstitial cells of Cajal, part of the autonomic innervation that regulates intestinal motility. The cellular morphology of GISTs varies from spindle-shaped to epithelioid character. About 70% of GISTs are spindle cell type, while 20% are epithelioid and 10% are of a mixed type.

More than 80% of all GISTs are CD117 antigen positive. This antigen is part of the *c-kit* transmembrane receptor tyrosine kinase (RTK) that is the product of the *c-kit* proto-oncogene. A mutation of this gene leads to constitutively active *c-kit* protein producing oncogenic signaling. The identification for CD-117 antigen by immunohisto-chemistry can distinguished between leiomyomas or other spindle-cell tumors in the GI tract which are typically CD-117 negative. Over two thirds of GISTs are also positive for CD-34.

Current analysis of GISTs is incapable of determining biological behavior. Thus all GISTs must be considered to harbor malignant potential. Based on large retrospective studies, tumor size, site of origin and mitotic count are reliable markers of malignant potential and a consensus stratification of risk has been forwarded **(Table 25-6)**.

TABLE 25-6	Proposed approach for defining risk of aggressive behavior in GISTs	
Lowest risk	< 2 cm	Less than 5 per 50 HPF*
Low risk	2-5 cm	Less than 5 per 50 HPF
Intermediate risk	< 5 cm	6-10 per 50 HPF
	5-10 cm	Less than 5 per 50 HPF
High risk	> 5 cm	Less than 5 per 50 HPF
	> 10 cm	Any mitotic rate
	Any size	Less than 10 per 50 HPF

*HPF: High powered field.

Those patients with tumors larger than 10 cm or more than 10 mitotic counts per 50 high powered fields (HPF) have the highest risk for the aggressive behavior of the GISTs and have the worst prognosis when compared to small (< 2 cm) with less than 5 mitosis per 50 HPF. The stomach, as a site of origin, predicts a lower risk for malignant behavior.

Clinical Presentation

The clinical presentation varies according to anatomic location and tumor size. Gastric GISTs are most commonly identified in the fundus, but may arise anywhere in the stomach. Neoplasm growth can extend intraluminally (endophytic) extralumenally (exophytic) or as a combination. Most of small GISTs are asymptomatic and are usually incidentally diagnosed during evaluation of non-specific symptoms. Ulceration of overlying mucosa results in up to 60% cases presenting with gastrointestinal hemorrhage. Other common symptoms are abdominal pain, abdominal mass, nausea, vomiting, anorexia and weight loss. Symptoms typically appear when the neoplasm is large (more than 5 cm) or are when they arise in critical locations (i.e. the pylorus, thus compromising the gastric outlet). There are some case reports of spontaneous rupture and bleeding into the peritoneal cavity. The majority of GISTs metastases occur in the liver, omentum or peritoneal cavity. Lymph node metastases are rare.

Diagnosis

The evaluation of GISTs is similar to other gastric malignancies and most diagnoses are made upon EGD performed for bleeding or symptoms. Findings vary depending on the predominant growth pattern (endophytic or exophytic). Usually, the over-lying mucosa is smooth, without folds and intact unless ulceration is present. Endoscopic ultrasound is recommended for guided biopsy. Contrast enhanced computed tomography is crucial for evaluation of the primary tumor and potential metastases.

Treatment and Prognosis

Surgical resection without residual disease is the treatment of choice for resectable gastric GISTs. *En bloc* resection of the gastric tumor with the involved adjacent organs to assure negative margins of resection is sometimes necessary, but rarely encountered; large GISTs that appear by preoperative imaging to involve adjacent organs often are found at celiotomy to arise from a small stalk and lack involvement of adjacent organs. Since lymph node metastases are rare, there is no added benefit to extended lymph node dissection. Careful manipulation of these neoplasms to avoid rupture and peritoneal seeding is imperative. The 5-year survival after surgical resection ranges from 32% to 63%.

Patients with unresectable or metastatic disease should receive imanitib mesylate (Gleevec), an oral *c-kit* tyrosine kinase inhibitor. This drug blocks *c-kit* signaling as well as signaling through PDGFRα (platelet-derived growth factor receptor alpha), another RTK involve in the pathogenesis of GISTs. The initial success of imanitib mesylate in patients with advanced, unresectable disease prompted its use in borderline resectable lesions and as adjuvant therapy in patients with high risk recurrence. Just recently, the results of a double-blind, placebo-controlled, multicenter trial of the American College of Surgeons Oncology Group (ACOSOG) has been published. This study included more than seven hundred patients in 230 institutions of the US and Canada and compared the use of imanitib versus placebo in resected GISTs larger than 3 cm. It showed that the use of adjuvant imanitib therapy after resection reduces recurrence to 8% from 20% (at median follow up of 19.7 months) and significantly improves recurrence-free survival when compared to placebo (98% vs 83% at 1 year) Other studies have shown some survival benefit with cytoreductive surgery in patients with metastatic GISTs that are responding to imanitib treatment.

Summary

- The incidence of gastric cancer varies widely by location, indicating an important role of environmental factors in the pathogenesis of the disease.
- Infection with *H. pylori* induces a 6-fold increased risk of developing gastric cancer and it is estimated to be responsible for 63% of gastric cancer cases worldwide.
- Due to this high risk of developing gastric cancer, genetic counseling and prophylactic gastrectomy are indicated in asymptomatic carriers of *cdh1* mutation.
- Preoperative evaluation of a patient with suspected gastric cancer should include a PET-CT and an endoscopic ultrasound.

■ In patients with early gastric adenocarcinoma, a gastric resection with a macroscopically negative margin of 5 cm and an *en bloc* resection of the adjacent lymph nodes (D1, regional lymphadenectomy) is the standard of care.

■ The extent of regional lymphadenectomy is a topic of significant controversy. A decrease in the risk of recurrence with extended lymphadenectomy (D2/3) has been documented, but no long-term survival benefit was realized due to the higher operative mortality. Extended resections carry significant morbidity and mortality and should be performed only in high volume centers, if at all.

■ MALT lymphoma is strongly associated with *H. pylori* infection and treatment of early stage MALT is eradication of the bacteria.

■ The biological behavior of gastrointestinal stromal tumors (GISTs) can be difficult to interpret, thus all GISTs must be considered to harbor malignant potential. Based on large retrospective studies, tumor size, site of origin and mitotic count are reliable markers of malignant potential.

Acknowledgements:
Angelo Rutty, MD for the elaboration of all the illustrations of this chapter.
Scott Cooper, MD and Kevin McGrath, MD for their contribution of endoscopic and endoscopic ultrasound imaging.

Landmark Papers

1. Aviles A, Nambo MJ, Neri N, Huerta-Guzman J, Cuadra I, Alvarado I, et al. The role of surgery in primary gastric lymphoma: results of a controlled clinical trial. Ann Surg 2004;240(1):44-50.

2. Bonenkamp JJ, Hermans J, Sasako M, van de Velde CJ. Extended lymph-node dissection for gastric cancer. Dutch Gastric Cancer Group. N Engl J Med 1999;340(12):908-14.

3. Cunningham D, Allum WH, Stenning SP, Thompson JN, Van de Velde CJ, Nicolson M, et al. MAGIC Trial Participants. Perioperative chemotherapy versus surgery alone for resectable gastroesophageal cancer. N Engl J Med 2006;355(1):11-20.

4. Cuschieri A, Fayers P, Fielding J, Craven J, Bancewicz J, Joypaul V, Cook P. Impact of total lymph node count on staging and survival after gastrectomy for gastric cancer: data from a large US-population database. J Clin Oncol 2005;23(28):7114-24.

5. Dematteo RP, Ballman KV, Antonescu CR, Maki RG, Pisters PW, Demetri GD, et al. On behalf of the American College of Surgeons Oncology Group (ACOSOG) Intergroup Adjuvant GIST Study Team. Adjuvant imatinib mesylate after resection of localised, primary gastro-intestinal stromal tumour: a randomised, double-blind, placebo-controlled trial. Lancet 2009;373:1097-104.

6. Earle CC, Maroun JA. Adjuvant chemotherapy after curative resection for gastric cancer in non-Asian patients: revisiting a meta-analysis of randomised trials. Eur J Cancer 1999;35(7):1059-64.

7. Hallissey MT, Dunn JA, Ward LC, Allum WH. The second British Stomach Cancer Group trial of adjuvant radio-therapy or chemotherapy in resectable gastric cancer: five-year follow-up. Lancet 1994;343(8909):1309-12.

8. Huscher CG, Mingoli A, Sgarzini G, Sansonetti A, Di Paola M, et al. Laparoscopic versus open subtotal gastrectomy for distal gastric cancer: five-year results of a randomized prospective trial. Ann Surg 2005; 241(2):232-7.

9. Kim YW, Baik YH, Yun YH, Nam BH, Kim DH, Choi IJ, Bae JM. Improved quality of life outcomes after laparoscopy-assisted distal gastrectomy for early gastric cancer: results of a prospective randomized clinical trial. Ann Surg 2008;248(5):721-7.

10. Koch P, Probst A, Berdel WE, Willich NA, Reinartz G, Brockmann J, et al. Treatment results in localized primary gastric lymphoma: data of patients registered within the German multicenter study (GIT NHL 02/96). J Clin Oncol 2005; 23(28):7050-9.

11. Macdonald JS, Smalley SR, Benedetti J, Hundahl SA, Estes NC, Stemmermann GN, et al. Chemoradiotherapy after surgery compared with surgery alone for adenocarcinoma of the stomach or gastroesophageal junction. N Engl J Med 2001;345(10):725-30

12. Mari E, Floriani I, Tinazzi A, Buda A, Belfiglio M, Valentini M, et al. Efficacy of adjuvant chemotherapy after curative resection for gastric cancer: a meta-analysis of published randomised trials. A study of the GISCAD (Gruppo Italiano per lo Studio dei Carcinomi dell'Apparato Digerente). Ann Oncol 2000; 11(7):837-43.

13. Panzini I, Gianni L, Fattori PP, Tassinari D, Imola M, Fabbri P, et al. Adjuvant chemotherapy in gastric cancer: a meta-analysis of randomized trials and a comparison with previous meta-analyses. Tumori 2002;88(1):21-7.

14. Sakuramoto S, Sasako M, Yamaguchi T, Kinoshita T, Fujii M, Nashimoto A, et al. Adjuvant chemotherapy for gastric cancer with S-1, an oral fluoropyrimidine. N Engl J Med 2007;357(18):1810-20.

15. Sano T, Sasako M, Yamamoto S, Nashimoto A, Kurita A, Hiratsuka M, et al. Gastric cancer surgery: morbidity and mortality results from a prospective randomized controlled trial comparing D2 and extended para-aortic lympha-denectomy—Japan Clinical Oncology Group study 9501. J Clin Oncol 2004;22(14):2767-73.

16. Scharwz RE, Smith DD. Clinical impact of lymphade-nectomy extent in respectable gastric cancer of advanced stage. Ann Surg Oncol 2007;14(2):317-28.

17. Sierra A, Regueira FM, Hernandez-Lizoain JL, Pardo F, Martínez-Gonzalez MA, A-Cienfuegos J. Role of the extended lymphadenectomy in gastric cancer surgery: experience in a single institution. Ann Surg Oncol 2003; 10(3):219-26.

18. Siewert J, Feith M, Werner M, Stein HJ. Adenocarcinoma of the esophagogastric junction: results of surgical therapy based on anatomical/topographic classification in 1,002 consecutive patients. Ann Surg 2000;232(3):353-61.

Level of Evidence Table			
Recommendation	**Grade**	**Best level of evidence**	**References**
Endoscopic ultrasound should be considered as a modality particularly sensitive for T staging of gastric cancers from which to base diagnostic and therapeutic decisions (e.g. laparoscopy, endoscopic resection).	B	1a	1-3
Subtotal gastrectomy is appropriate for distal tumors compared to total gastrectomy with equivalent long-term outcomes and better quality of life.	A	1b	4-6
Laparoscopic resection of gastric cancer can achieve oncologic outcomes similar to open resection with the perioperative benefits associated with minimally invasive surgery.	B	1b	7,8
In Western patients, D2 versus D1 lymphadenectomy does not demonstrate a survival benefit and may increase morbidity.	A	1a	9-12
Neoadjuvant chemotherapy potentially improves overall and disease-free survival for resectable gastric cancers.	B	1b	13-15
Adjuvant chemotherapy with or without radiation must be considered after curative resection of node-positive cancers and those with invasion beyond the submucosa.	A	1a	16,17
Prophylactic (for transmural disease) or therapeutic (for carcinomatosis) intraperitoneal chemotherapy combined with complete resection potentially improves survival.	B	1a	1-3
Eradication of *H. pylori* should be the initial therapeutic management of *H. pylori*-positive gastric MALT lymphomas.	A	4	18-20
Chemotherapy is the treatment of choice over surgical resection for primary gastric diffuse large cell lymphoma.	A	1b	21
Complete resection without regional lymphadenectomy is appropriate for GIST.	A	2b	22-24
Adjuvant imatinib improves recurrence-free survival after curative GIST resection.	A	1b	25
Neoadjuvant imatinib should be considered for locally advanced and recurrent GIST to improve resectability.	B	4	26, 27

References

1. Puli SR, Batapati Krishna Reddy J, Bechtold ML, et al. How good is endoscopic ultrasound for TNM staging of gastric cancers? A meta-analysis and systematic review. World J Gastroenterol 2008; 14:4011-9.
2. Mouri R, Yoshida S, Tanaka S, et al. Usefulness of endoscopic ultrasonography in determining the depth of invasion and indication for endoscopic treatment of early gastric cancer. J Clin Gastroenterol 2009; 43:318-22.
3. Power DG, Schattner MA, Gerdes H, et al. Endoscopic ultrasound can improve the selection for laparoscopy in patients with localized gastric cancer. J Am Coll Surg 2009; 208:173-8.
4. Bozzetti F, Marubini E, Bonfanti G, et al. Subtotal versus total gastrectomy for gastric cancer: five-year survival rates in a multicenter randomized Italian trial. Italian Gastrointestinal Tumor Study Group. Ann Surg 1999; 230:170-8.
5. Gouzi JL, Huguier M, Fagniez PL, et al. Total versus subtotal gastrectomy for adenocarcinoma of the gastric antrum. A French prospective controlled study. Ann Surg 1989; 209:162-6.
6. Jentschura D, Winkler M, Strohmeier N, et al. Quality-of-life after curative surgery for gastric cancer: a comparison between total gastrectomy and subtotal gastric resection. Hepatogastroenterology 1997; 44:1137-42.
7. Huscher CG, Mingoli A, Sgarzini G, et al. Laparoscopic versus open subtotal gastrectomy for distal gastric cancer: five-year results of a randomized prospective trial. Ann Surg 2005; 241:232-7.
8. Strong VE, Devaud N, Allen PJ, et al. Laparoscopic versus open subtotal gastrectomy for adenocarcinoma: a case-control study. Ann Surg Oncol 2009; 16:1507-13.
9. Hartgrink HH, van de Velde CJ, Putter H, et al. Extended lymph node dissection for gastric cancer: who may benefit? Final results of the randomized Dutch gastric cancer group trial. J Clin Oncol 2004; 22:2069-77.
10. Bonenkamp JJ, Hermans J, Sasako M, et al. Extended lymph-node dissection for gastric cancer. N Engl J Med 1999; 340:908-14.

11. Cuschieri A, Weeden S, Fielding J, et al. Patient survival after D1 and D2 resections for gastric cancer: long-term results of the MRC randomized surgical trial. Surgical Co-operative Group. Br J Cancer 1999; 79:1522-30.

12. McCulloch P, Nita ME, Kazi H, et al. Extended versus limited lymph nodes dissection technique for adenocarcinoma of the stomach. Cochrane Database Syst Rev 2004; CD001964.

13. Cunningham D, Allum WH, Stenning SP, et al. Perioperative chemotherapy versus surgery alone for resectable gastroesophageal cancer. N Engl J Med 2006; 355:11-20.

14. Hartgrink HH, van de Velde CJ, Putter H, et al. Neo-adjuvant chemotherapy for operable gastric cancer: long term results of the Dutch randomised FAMTX trial. Eur J Surg Oncol 2004; 30:643-9.

15. Persiani R, Rausei S, Pozzo C, et al. 7-Year survival results of perioperative chemotherapy with epidoxorubicin, etoposide and cisplatin (EEP) in locally advanced resectable gastric cancer: up-to-date analysis of a phase-II study. Ann Surg Oncol 2008; 15:2146-52.

16. Macdonald JS, Smalley SR, Benedetti J, et al. Chemoradiotherapy after surgery compared with surgery alone for adenocarcinoma of the stomach or gastroesophageal junction. N Engl J Med 2001; 345:725-30.

17. Earle CC, Maroun J, Zuraw L. Neoadjuvant or adjuvant therapy for resectable gastric cancer? A practice guideline. Can J Surg 2002; 45:438-46.

18. Roggero E, Zucca E, Pinotti G, et al. Eradication of Helicobacter pylori infection in primary low-grade gastric lymphoma of mucosa-associated lymphoid tissue. Ann Intern Med 1995; 122:767-9.

19. Bayerdorffer E, Neubauer A, Rudolph B, et al. Regression of primary gastric lymphoma of mucosa-associated lymphoid tissue type after cure of Helicobacter pylori infection. MALT Lymphoma Study Group. Lancet 1995; 345:1591-4.

20. Chen LT, Lin JT, Tai JJ, et al. Long-term results of anti-Helicobacter pylori therapy in early-stage gastric high-grade transformed MALT lymphoma. J Natl Cancer Inst 2005; 97:1345-53.

21. Aviles A, Nambo MJ, Neri N, et al. The role of surgery in primary gastric lymphoma: results of a controlled clinical trial. Ann Surg 2004; 240:44-50.

22. Woodall CE, 3rd, Brock GN, Fan J, et al. An evaluation of 2537 gastrointestinal stromal tumors for a proposed clinical staging system. Arch Surg 2009; 144:670-8.

23. Bucher P, Egger JF, Gervaz P, et al. An audit of surgical management of gastrointestinal stromal tumours (GIST). Eur J Surg Oncol 2006; 32:310-4.

24. Pierie JP, Choudry U, Muzikansky A, et al. The effect of surgery and grade on outcome of gastrointestinal stromal tumors. Arch Surg 2001; 136:383-9.

25. Dematteo RP, Ballman KV, Antonescu CR, et al. Adjuvant imatinib mesylate after resection of localised, primary gastrointestinal stromal tumour: a randomised, double-blind, placebo-controlled trial. Lancet 2009; 373:1097-104.

26. Eisenberg BL, Harris J, Blanke CD, et al. Phase II trial of neoadjuvant/adjuvant imatinib mesylate (IM) for advanced primary and metastatic/recurrent operable gastrointestinal stromal tumor (GIST): early results of RTOG 0132/ACRIN 6665. J Surg Oncol 2009; 99:42-7.

27. Andtbacka RH, Ng CS, Scaife CL, et al. Surgical resection of gastrointestinal stromal tumors after treatment with imatinib. Ann Surg Oncol 2007; 14:14-24.

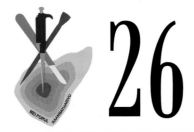

26

Small Bowel Cancer

Raymond Eid, Herbert J Zeh III

Small bowel cancer (SBC) is a rare entity that is increasing in incidence in the past few decades. The diagnosis of small intestinal tumors is often a challenge due to the rarity and diversity of these lesions, in addition to the variable and the nonspecific presenting signs and symptoms. Consequently, a majority of these tumors are discovered at a late stage with meager available therapeutic interventions.

Small intestinal tumors arise from different histological lineages; epithelial cells (e.g. adenomas, adenocarcinomas, and carcinoids), mesenchymal cells (e.g. sarcomas and gastrointestinal stromal tumors) or from lymphatic tissues (e.g. lymphomas). In addition, the small intestine can be the site of distant metastasis of other malignancies.

Epidemiology

Small bowel tumors are amongst the rarest types of cancer accounting for only 2% of all gastrointestinal cancers. Every year, there are approximately 6100 new cases of small bowel tumors with 1100 death cases per year in the USA. The National Cancer Institute estimates 6230 new cases for the year 2009 in the USA, with a corresponding 1110 deaths. SBC accounts for much lower incidence than colorectal, gastric or pancreatic malignancies. The natural history and prognosis of patients with SBC varies with different histological subtypes, with approximately overall survival of 50% for all types.

The incidence of benign small intestinal neoplasm is difficult to determine since most cases are asymptomatic and are usually discovered incidentally during radiographic or endoscopic examination, surgery or autopsy. More than 40 different histological distinct tumors have been described to arise in the small intestine; however, more than 95% of the time, it is adenocarcinoma, carcinoid, stromal tumors (GIST) or lymphomas.

SBC commonly occurs in old age, most commonly in the seventh decade of life, with a slight male and caucasian preponderance. Until recently, adenocarcinoma of the small intestine comprised the most common histologic type of malignant tumors of the small intestine in population-based registry data from the Surveillance, Epidemiology and End Results (SEER) program of the National Cancer Institute. They constituted 45% of all SBC, followed by carcinoid (29%), then lymphoma (16%) and finally sarcoma (10%). Over the last decade, the incidence of carcinoid tumors increased significantly from 29% to 44% surpassing adenocarcinoma as the most common tumors of the small intestine, with a decrease in the incidence of adenocarcinoma from 45% to 33%. The incidence of stromal tumors and lymphoma remained unchanged.

Pathogenesis

The small intestine is an organ of paramount importance, constituting ~ 75-80% of the entire length of the GI tract and owning ~ 90% of the absorptive surface. Fortunately, the incidence of cancer in the small bowel is disproportionately rare when compared to other organs and there are several hypotheses that have been proposed to explain this. The observation is more than obvious. Recurrence of cancer in colorectal cancer is 20-fold more common with colo-colic anastomoses than an ileocolonic anastomoses and recurrence of gastric cancer is 5-fold more common on the gastric side of a gastrojejunostomy compared to the jejunal side. Living between two sites of high malignancy rates (e.g. stomach and colon), small bowel is a minor site for malignancies with SBC constituting < 5% of all GI malignancies in most industrialized countries. The proposed reasons for this are listed below:

- *High levels of benzopyrene hydroxylase and folate receptors:* Benzopyrene is well known and potent mutagen that intercalates with DNA and interferes with transcription. It is present in cigarette smoke and may be found in high levels in barbecued food, canned food and charbroiled (grilled) foods. Benzopyrene hydroxylase converts this compound to a less toxic one and is found in much higher levels in the small intestine compared to the colon. Folate receptors, which are believed to play an antagonistic role in carcinogenesis, are found in high levels in the small intestine.

- *Low bacterial load:* Anaerobic bacteria, present in large quantities in the colon, are rare in the small bowel. Presence of bacteria may interact with bile salts and bile acids that may act as tumor promoters.
- *Fast transit time:* Almost 50% of the stomach's contents empty in 2.5-3 hours, which is the same amount of time it takes for the much longer small intestine to empty 50% of its contents. In contrast, the colon takes almost 30-40 hours for its entire transit. Not surprisingly, the word 'jejunum' derives itself from 'jejunus' meaning 'empty' as Galen, a historic physician almost always found this part of the intestine to be empty after death. The much faster transit time provides less exposure and less chronicity of any carcinogenic stimulus in the lumen or contents.
- *High cellular turnover:* The small intestine replaces its cellular mass at the rate of 90 gm/day. This provides less chance for a certain 'critical mass' to be reached with senescent cells, to provide any breeding ground for cancer.
- *Liquid and alkaline milieu:* Alkalinity of the small intestinal chyme renders most carcinogens less active.
- *Safe stem cells:* The small intestine has far fewer stem cells, which could be exposed to carcinogens. Moreover, the stem cells in the small intestine are located deep in the intestinal glandular crypts, where they are least exposed to the intraluminal carcinogenic stimuli.
- *Immune protection:* Small intestine has an abundance of lymphoid cells in Peyer's patches. It is also abundant in surface immunity due to the high levels of mucosal immunoglobulin (IgA). This theory is also supported by other findings such as the increased incidence of SBC in IgA deficient individuals and the remarkably low incidence of malignancy in the spleen, which is also a immune cell-rich organ.

However, the fact that SBC is rare should also make the surgical oncologist weary about another implication that, when SBC develops, it is probably the result of a failure of unknown, yet very important antitumor mechanism which places the individual at risk for other malignancies. This is supported by the fact that 30-40% of SBCs have another synchronous malignancy and that risk of SBC rises in the presence of certain other malignancies. It is for this reason that the surgeon should thoroughly explore the bowel and the abdomen before proceeding with a definitive resection.

Risk Factors

Although the etiology of small intestinal neoplasms is still largely unknown, several risk factors and genetic conditions have been recognized to predispose to an increased risk of developing SBCs. They are listed below and the most important ones are discussed further.

Risk Factors

- Hereditary nonpolyposis colorectal cancer (HNPCC)
- Familial adenomatous polyposis (FAP)
- Peutz-Jeghers syndrome (PJS)
- Crohn's disease (CD)
- Colorectal and other malignancies (Wilm's tumor, anal cancer, squamous cell skin cancer, Hodgkin's lymphoma, etc.)
- Cholecystectomy
- Peptic ulcer disease
- Cystic fibrosis
- Celiac disease (Tropical sprue)
- Lifestyle—high fat diet
- Male gender, African-American ethnicity and old age

- *Hereditary nonpolyposis colorectal cancer (HNPCC):* HNPCC, also called Lynch syndrome, is an inherited condition characterized by mutations in the DNA mismatch repair genes. Affected individuals have about 80% lifetime risk for colon cancer. In addition, patients with HNPCC are at increased risk for development of other malignancies namely SBCs that occur most commonly in the duodenum and jejunum, with a lifetime risk of 1%.
- *Familial adenomatous polyposis (FAP):* FAP is a condition caused by a germline mutation in the adenomatous polyposis coli (APC) gene, a tumor suppressor gene. Patients with FAP develop early onset of hundreds to thousands of adenomatous polyps primarily throughout the colon as well as in the small intestine largely in the duodenum. In effect, periampullary adenocarcinoma is the leading cause of death in patients with FAP following total colectomy developing in 2-5% of patients, with a lifetime risk of 330-fold over that of the general population. Periodic screening with esophagogastroduodenoscopy is hence crucial in this patient population. In addition, patients with FAP have higher incidence of desmoid tumors in the small intestine as well as the mesentery.
- *Peutz-Jeghers syndrome (PJS):* PJS is an autosomal dominant inherited disorder caused by a mutation in the STK11 (LKB1) tumor suppressor gene. It is characterized by intestinal hamartomatous polyps in association with mucocutaneous melanocytic macules on the lips and oral mucosa. Although the intestinal polyps are benign hamartomas, patients with PJS have a 15-fold increased risk of development of small as well as large intestinal adenocarcinomas compared with that of the general population.
- *Celiac disease:* Celiac disease is an autoimmune disorder characterized by villous atrophy of the small intestine caused by a reaction to gliadin, a gluten protein found in wheat. Refractory conditions are associated with lymphoma, referred to as *enteropathy-associated T-cell lymphoma* (EATL) in 39% of the cases. These lympho-

mas are primarily localized to the jejunum and are T-cell in origin. To a lesser extent, celiac disease can also be associated with adenocarcinoma mainly of the jejunum. The adherence to a gluten-free diet reduced the risk of all malignancies associated with celiac disease.

- *Chronic inflammation:* Several conditions with chronic mucosal inflammation have been associated with increased occurrence of both adenocarcinoma and lymphoma in the small intestine. Patients with inflammatory bowel disease, in particular Crohn's disease (CD) have a recognized 10-66.7 increased risk of developing small intestinal adenocarcinomas compared to the general population. In effect, CD-associated adenocarcinomas occur in approximately 2% of patients with longstanding CD for more than 10 years and are usually localized to the ileum. Both medical and surgical management appears to decrease the risk of CD-associated adenocarcinomas.

- *Immunosuppression:* Both iatrogenic following transplantation and acquired immunosuppression states have been associated with increased rates of lymphomas and sarcomas. Lymphomas in the setting of immunosuppression are termed *Post-Transplant Lymphoproliferative Disorder (PTLD)* and are usually characterized by uncontrolled proliferation of B-cell lymphocytes following infection with Epstein-Barr virus.

  Gardner's syndrome, an autosomal dominant genetic disorder, is characterized by multiple colonic polyps, multiple osteomas and skin and soft tissue tumors. Patients with this condition have higher incidence of desmoid tumors compared to the general population. The neurofibromas in von Recklinghausen disease have potential malignant transformation into paragangliomas. Patients with cystic fibrosis have been noted to have increased incidence of ileal adenocarcinomas.

- *Other malignancies:* As mentioned above, the development of SBC might signal the failure of an efficient and probably quasi-ubiquitous antitumor mechanism that may mean malignancies at other sites. Patients with other primary cancers, such as colon and breast cancers, are at a higher risk of developing SBC.

Clinical Presentation

Small bowel malignancies present in a nonspecific fashion. The most frequent presenting signs and symptoms include abdominal pain, nausea, vomiting and weight loss which are present in more than 45% of patients. Cancer of the small bowel is more likely to be symptomatic earlier in the course as opposed to benign lesions, which are more frequently discovered incidentally on a radiologic exam or at surgical exploration. Approximately 50% of all small bowel tumors present with an acute event, usually an obstruction or a perforation and that proportion tends to increase further as tumors enlarge.

The scarcity of each histological subtype makes it difficult to draw generalizations about specific signs and symptoms specific for each subtype. Adenocarcinomas tend to be associated with pain and obstruction when compared to other malignant subtypes. Sarcomas are frequently associated with acute GI hemorrhage while lymphomas appear to present more commonly with intestinal perforation. In addition, different subtypes have predilection to different regions of the small intestine. Adenocarcinomas tend to involve mainly the duodenum, while carcinoids more commonly develop in the ileum. On the other hand, sarcomas and lymphomas can affect the entire small bowel.

Diagnosis

Several factors hinder early diagnosis of small bowel tumors. The variability of symptoms along with the lack of early and specific clinical symptoms combined with the lack of physical findings contributes to a delay in diagnosis in most of the cases. In one large study, the average delay in diagnosis was from 8 to 12 months. The delay in diagnosis was accounted for by either failure to obtain a proper diagnostic test or misinterpretation of test results. On the other hand, patient's failure to report symptoms delayed diagnosis by only 2 months. Accurate preoperative diagnosis is rarely established. A high index of suspicion is crucial for the adequate evaluation of patients with suspected small bowel malignancies. No single test or testing strategy has been established in the work-up of small bowel tumors. The investigations available in the armamentarium of probing small pathology are listed below:

Work-up for SBC
- Plain abdominal radiographs
- CT scan with contrast
- Small bowel follow through (SBFT)
- CT enteroclysis
- Video capsule endoscopy (VCE)
- Enteroscopy and double balloon enteroscopy
- Retrograde ileoscopy

- *Plain abdominal radiographs:* These are simple tests of not any use in the diagnostic setting of a neoplasm, unless the presentation is that of obstruction. Plain radiographs can reliably diagnose small bowel obstruction ~ 50-60% of the time.
- *Small bowel follow through (SBFT):* This is a serial contrast exam of the small bowel that requires considerable length of time. It is well-suited for examination of luminal abnormalities and mucosal morphology.

- *CT scan:* In most centers, computed tomography (CT) has become one of the initial modalities used for the evaluation of both vague or nonspecific abdominal complaints and acute abdominal pain. CT scan allows for specific diagnosis in 70-80% of adenocarcinoma, 58% of lymphomas and 33% of carcinoids. In addition to detecting the primary tumor, CT scans are also used in the evaluation of extraintestinal involvement and distant metastasis as part of the staging process. The various histological subtypes have some characteristic findings on CT scan. Adenocarcinoma most commonly causes a discrete annular thickening with abrupt concentric or irregular "overhanging edges". Strictures are usually rigid (on fluoroscopic examinations), unlike gastrointestinal stromal tumors (GIST) or lymphomas. Proximal bowel loop dilatation is commonly noted. Duodenal adenocarcinoma frequently present as intraluminal polyps, while more distal polypoid lesions can present with intussusception **(Figure 26-1)**, which typically displays a 'target sign': low attenuation at the center with high attenuation in the periphery.

  Higher grade or more advanced lesions may ulcerate making distinction from other types of SBC, mainly lymphoma difficult. Small bowel lymphomas are commonly detected either as nodular filling defect or as segmental infiltrating mass with associated thickened bowel wall and aneurysmal dilatation of the intestinal lumen. Signs of obstruction can occasionally be seen. The absence of lymphadenopathy in other places in the body, including the superficial lymph node basins, the hilar and mediastinal lymph node basins and the retroperitoneal area is essential for diagnosis. Carcinoid tumors appear on CT scan as homogeneous masses displacing small bowel loops. Not infrequently, soft tissue stranding surrounding the lesion is seen associated with patches of mesenteric calcification. These are called 'desmoplastic reactions' **(Figures 26-2A and B)**, a very specific finding for the diagnosis of carcinoid tumors. GIST are generally discrete submucosal homogeneous masses that enhance greatly on CT scans due to their hypervascular nature. Larger GIST tumors may have central necrosis sometimes with calcifications suggestive of more aggressive behavior.

- *Small bowel enteroclysis:* 'Clysis' is derived from the greek word 'kylsis' meaning to 'flush with enema'. Enteroclysis by inference is often referred to as 'small bowel enema', although this is a misleading terminology, as the contrast, unlike an enema is not give retrograde via the anorectal route, but by a naso-duodenal tube that delivers contrast directly to the jejunum. The movement of the contrast is then seen by

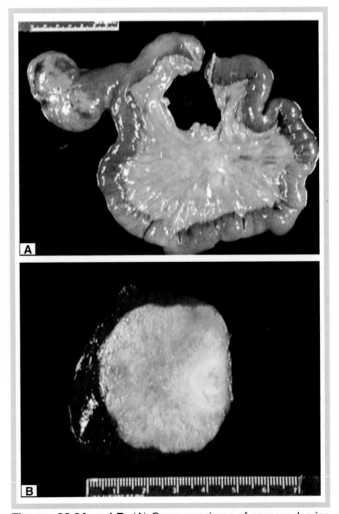

Figures 26-2A and B: (A) Gross specimen of neuroendocrine tumor of the ileum. (B) Neuroendocrine tumors demonstrate intense desmoplastic reaction and fibrosis of the abdominal wall. (*Courtesy* Steven Hughes, MD, University of Pittsburgh Medical Centre)

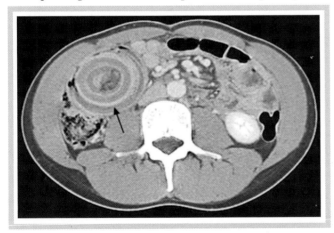

Figure 26-1: A 22-year-old man presented with chronic intermittent abdominal pain, nausea and vomiting. CT scan showed proximal jejunal intussusception. At surgery, the patient was found to have a pedunculated benign lipomatous polyp (*NEJM 2007; 357 (26):e30. Copyright 2007 Massachusetts Medical Society. All rights reserved*)

fluoroscopy. Enteroclysis is a dynamic contrast technique that uses a combination of barium and methyl-cellulose to uniformly distend the small bowel without abolishing peristalsis. Enteroclysis study results in considerable increase in sensitivity and specificity with sensitivity close to 90% in detecting small bowel tumors. Based on radiographic findings, it often provides accurate predictions for different histologic subtypes and is especially useful in investigating the small bowel beyond the ligament of Treitz. Newer enteroclysis techniques are recently developed and are achieved in combination with CT or MRI. CT enteroclysis combines the benefits of enteroclysis (luminal distention) with the benefits of CT scans, namely extraluminal examination. Multiple limited institutional studies proved CT enteroclysis to be superior to formal enteroclysis both in detecting small bowel neoplasms and for the diagnosis of CD; further studies still need to confirm the advantage of CT/MRI enteroclysis over conventional enteroclysis as the imaging of choice in the evaluation of small intestinal pathologies.

- *Small bowel enteroscopy:* Esophagogastroduodenoscopy (EGD) and extended colonoscopy are occasionally part of the diagnostic work-up of small intestinal tumors. They allow direct visualization of the duodenum or the distal ileum respectively, in addition to biopsy for a definite diagnosis. More recently, double-balloon enteroscopy, also known as push enteroscopy was developed in 2001. It allows the visualization of the entire small bowel with the ability to biopsy any suspicious lesions. However, the procedure is technically challenging with currently very limited expertise and equipments.
- *Video capsule endoscopy (VCE):* This has dramatically changed the diagnosis and management of many diseases of the small intestine such as gastrointestinal bleeding, CD, polyps and small bowel malignancies. Unfortunately, VCE does not allow tissue sampling or precise localizations of lesions. VCE has demonstrated higher sensitivity and specificity than older techniques such as UGI/SBFT. One of the main risks associated with capsule endoscopy is retention of the capsule itself, which is clinically significant in about 1% of the cases, requiring surgical laparotomy for removal of the capsules.
- *Nuclear medicine scans:* In addition to the above modalities, other radiological techniques have been developed and are useful in specific clinical situations. Radionuclide imaging using indium-11 octreotide, a radioactive somatostatin analogue, is a useful scan in diagnosing carcinoids. Octreotide scan is highly sensitive in the localization of primary and metastatic carcinoid tumors since tumor cells express high levels

of somatostatin receptor. Octreotide imaging has sensitivity greater than 90% in identifying carcinoid tumors. Angiography or technetium (^{99m}Tc) radionuclide scan used in patients with active bleeding can sometimes be helpful in the diagnosis and localization of certain small intestinal tumors. Hypervascular tumors, namely carcinoids and leiomyosarcomas, provide a specific pattern on the study that can be diagnostic of the tumor type.

Adenocarcinoma

As previously mentioned, adenocarcinoma was, until recently, the most common histological type of malignant small bowel tumor. They usually present between the sixth and eighth decade of life with slight male preponderance. Adenocarcinoma arising in the small intestine most commonly occurs in the duodenum (65%), followed by the jejunum and the ileum. Patients with CD do not follow the same trend, with more than two thirds of CD-associated adenocarcinoma occurring in the ileum. The overall 5-year disease-free survival is approximately 30% with mean survival of 20 months. Survival rates are also somewhat dependent on the primary tumor site, with duodenal tumors having the worse prognosis (28% 5-year survival) and ileal disease the best prognosis (38% 5-year survival).

Genetics

Similar to the progression of colorectal cancer, it is suggested that small intestinal adenocarcinoma develops from preexisting adenomas. Developing data are increasingly in support of the adenoma-adenocarcinoma pathway—multistep genetic alterations involving multiple sequence mutations in several germline as well as somatic genes. Several germline mutations involving the cyclooxygenase and APC genes, seen in common inherited syndromes like FAP and HNPCC, have also been described in small bowel adenocarcinoma. Larger adenomas as well as villous features, both risk factors seen in colorectal cancer, are also associated with more advanced small bowel adenocarcinoma.

Staging and Prognosis

The most commonly used staging system for the small bowel adenocarcinoma is the TNM system of the American Joint Committee on Cancer (AJCC).

Primary tumor (T) staging

Tx	tumor cannot be assessed
T0	No evidence of primary tumor
Tis	Carcinoma in situ
T1	Invasion of lamina propria or submucosa
T2	Invasion of muscularis propria

T3   Invasion through muscularis propria into subserosa or into nonperitonealized perimuscular tissue (mesentery or retroperitoneum) with extension 2 cm or less

T4   Perforation of visceral peritoneum or direct invasion of other organs or structures (includes other loops of small intestine, mesentery or retroperitoneum more than 2 cm and the abdominal wall by way of serosa; for the duodenum only, includes invasion of pancreas)

Regional lymph nodes (N)
Nx   Regional lymph nodes cannot be assessed
N0   No regional lymph node metastases
N1   Regional lymph node metastasis

Distant metastasis (M)
Mx   Distant metastasis cannot be assessed
M0   No distant metastasis
M1   Distant metastasis

Stage	*TNM*
0	Tis N0 M0
IA	T1 N0 M0
IB	T2 N0 M0
IIA	T3 N0 M0
IIB	T4 N0 M0
III	Any T N1 M0
IV	Any T Any N M1

Unfortunately, due to the nonspecific nature of symptoms, most patients present with stage III or IV with a dismal prognosis. Duodenal adenocarcinoma of the ampulla of Vater has a different staging system. In general, prognosis of intestinal carcinoma is worse compared to similarly staged other types of SBC and colon cancer. Nodal status was found to be the most important prognostic indicator for long-term survival in patients. Distant metastases also greatly affected staging and hence prognosis. Multiple additional prognostic factors were further accumulated from a number of studies. These include positive surgical margins, lymphovascular involvement and poor tumor differentiation. The depth of tumor invasion, the site of the tumor, including duodenum, jejunum and ileum, in addition to the size of the tumor of 5 cm or greater did not significantly predict survival in several recent review series.

Management

Complete surgical resection is the only potential cure for adenocarcinoma arising in the small bowel. Segmental resection of involved bowel segments along with the mesentery provides control of draining lymph nodes and improves long-term survival by controlling risk of metastasis. For those tumors arising in the duodenum, there are a variety of surgical options, including segmental duodenal resection, pancreaticoduodenectomy or pancreas-preserving duodenal resection. For duodenal tumors, several studies demonstrated improved survival in patient undergoing pancreaticoduodenectomy versus segmental resection. For tumors in the distal duodenum or in the mesenteric small bowel, segmental resection with lymphadenectomy is the treatment of choice. In the setting of FAP, isolated resection of individual polypoid lesions had high recurrence rates. More formal surgical procedures, such as pancreas-preserving duodenectomy or segmental resection, have been advocated.

Due to the scarcity of cases, few studies have addressed the role of adjuvant therapy in the management of intestinal carcinoma. Several retrospective studies examined the benefit of chemotherapy, mainly fluoropyrimidine-based regimens, in patients with small bowel adenocarcinoma. Most of these reports failed to propose any benefit in treatment groups in terms of survival or tumor recurrence. Several other chemotherapeutic agents have been used alone or in conjunction with 5-FU. These include, but not limited to, capecitabine, oxaliplatin and leucovorin. However, the optimal regimen and the degree of benefit remain to be identified. The role of radiotherapy, either as neoadjuvant therapy for large duodenal tumors or for palliative treatment of obstructing tumors consists primarily of case reports or small case series. However, the survival benefit of radiotherapy alone or in combination with chemotherapy is still largely unknown.

Carcinoid Tumors

Carcinoid tumors are rare, slow-growing neuroendocrine tumors derived from enterochromaffin cells in the intestinal tract, also known as Kulchitsky cells. They can potentially develop anywhere in the body, however, they most commonly arise in the gastrointestinal tract (75%), in addition to the lung or bronchus. Other sites such as liver, pancreas, testicles or ovaries are much less common. Within the GI tract, they commonly affect the appendix **(Figure 26-3)**, ileum (usually within 60 cm of ileocecal valve) and rectum. Carcinoid tumors are characterized by the production of more than 30 hormonal products, the most prominent being serotonin, histamine, dopamine, tachykinins and prostaglandins. Carcinoid syndrome, a constellation of symptoms including flushing and diarrhea are related to secretion of active peptide hormones from carcinoid tumors, occurs in only 5-7% of patients with small bowel carcinoid.

Carcinoid tumors affect males (52.4%) more often than females with an average age of presentation of 66 years, which is within 2 years of the average age of diagnosis for non-carcinoid small intestinal tumors. Caucasian patients (80.4%) are significantly more affected compared

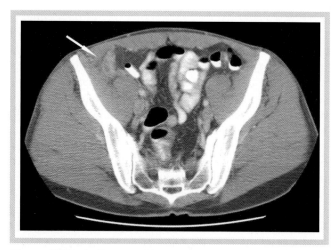

Figure 26-3: A 47-year-old man presented with evidence of acute appendicitis on CT. At surgery, the patient was found to have a primary appendiceal carcinoid tumor

to other ethnic groups. Carcinoid tumors generally follow an indolent course, with a 5-year survival rates between 52% and 77%. More than two thirds of carcinoid tumors have local-regional metastatic spread at the time of presentation. A considerable percentage (29%) of small intestinal carcinoids is associated with other non-carcinoid neoplasms. Although the meaning is still unknown, it may indicate common risk factors or predisposing factors between carcinoid and non-carcinoid tumors of the small intestine.

Incidence

Many recent studies have suggested an increase in the incidence of all small intestinal cancers. Surprisingly, the incidence of carcinoid tumors was demonstrated to have the most dramatical increase over the past 30 years. In fact, more than 4-fold increase in the incidence of carcinoid tumors was reported over the last two decades making them the most common small bowel malignancy (37.4%), followed by adenocarcinoma (36.9%).

Prognosis

For small intestinal carcinoids, size of the primary tumor in addition to depth of invasion are the best predictors of risk for local, regional and distant metastases. In a large retrospective study, a direct correlation was established between the risk of tumor spread and the tumor size as well as depth of invasion. Tumors larger than 10 mm in size have the highest rate of metastasis (73.6%), while tumors between 6 mm and 10 mm metastasized in 31.5% of the cases. Even small carcinoid tumors (less than 6 mm) were associated with significant rate of metastasis (15.8%). In addition, lesions with transmural invasion metastasize in 68.4% of the time, as opposed to tumors with limited

submucosal invasion (30.8%). The overall 5-year survival for all patients was approximately 73.3%. Survival was significantly better for patients without distant metastasis; 90.9% as opposed to 68.2% 5-year survival.

Carcinoid Syndrome

Carcinoid syndrome describes a constellation of symptoms, including cutaneous flushing, diarrhea and wheezing mediated by several tumor-derived humoral factors that are secreted into the systemic circulation. These substances include more than 30 different polypeptides, biogenic amines and prostaglandins, with the most prominent being serotonin, histamine, dopamine, tachykinins and prostaglandins. The exact contribution of every secretory molecule is still unknown. The liver usually metabolizes some of these substances preventing their release into the hepatic vein and systemic circulation. Therefore, liver metastasis is thought to be essential for the development of carcinoid syndrome. A majority (80%) of patients with carcinoid syndrome have small bowel carcinoids. On the other hand, almost 10% of patients with small bowel carcinoids present with carcinoid syndrome and two-third of these patients would develop some symptoms during the course of their disease. Symptoms of carcinoid syndrome can be precipitated by alcohol ingestion, stress and certain physical activity involving pressure to the right upper quadrant. The most effective treatment for relieving symptoms of carcinoid syndrome is the use of the long-acting somatostatin analog octreotide. Around 80% of patients report improvement of flushing and diarrhea. Besides improving and even preventing symptoms, octreotide has been found to have a role in tumor growth control, which will be discussed further in the next section. For refractory symptoms, cyproheptadine, a non-selective potent antihistamine, improved severe diarrhea in a certain percentage of patients. On the other hand, the addition of IFN-α to octreotide helped control symptoms in patients who did not respond to octreotide alone.

Management of Localized Disease

Because of potential metastasis even with small size (less than 6 mm), segmental resection with accompanying draining mesenteric lymph nodes is the treatment of choice for localized primary carcinoids arising in the small bowel. As noted previously, because of the relatively high risk for synchronous neoplasms, a thorough inspection of the bowel should be performed. Five-year survival after resection of localized disease ranges between 50% and 85%. For appendiceal carcinoids, tumor size was the most important prognostic indicator. About 30% of tumors larger than 2 cm in size were found to have distant metastasis at the time of diagnosis, while smaller tumors almost never metastasized. Based on that, appendiceal carcinoids smaller than 2 cm can be treated with a simple appendectomy while larger tumors with a right hemicolectomy. Carcinoid crisis could occasionally be precipitated during induction of anesthesia or manipulation of the tumor intraoperatively, hence pretreatment with octreotide is also recommended.

Management of Advanced Disease

In general, surgery has a limited curative role in carcinoid tumors since most tumors have metastasized by the time of diagnosis. However, given the slow indolent course of most carcinoids, several authors have advocated resection of the primary tumor along with the metastatic lymph nodes, irrespective of the presence of widespread metastatic disease. Resection is also recommended for the prevention of fibrosing mesenteritis. The decision to perform palliative resection for disseminated carcinoid tumors should then carefully balance the risks and benefits of the procedure. The goal of treatment of metastatic carcinoid tumor should be improving survival and controlling symptoms through cytoreduction. Different modes of cytoreductive treatments for metastatic carcinoid, such as surgery, hepatic arterial chemoembolization and systemic chemotherapy, will be discussed in more detail.

Surgery/Local Ablative Therapy

The liver is the most common site of metastatic disease. Unfortunately, a significant portion of patients present with bilobar liver disease. In the absence of extensive bilobar liver disease, liver failure or extensive metastatic disease, surgical debulking or formal liver resection with the associated primary tumor should be attempted with a curative intent. It has already been established in several case series that surgical debulking of patients with small number of liver nodules provided a prolonged disease-free survival. By retrospective analysis, major hepatectomy appears to be effective in symptom-control of carcinoid syndrome in 96% of patients. About 84% of patients may eventually have tumor recurrence and 59% of patients may have recurrence of their symptoms in 5 years. Liver resection markedly improves the 5-year survival rate from 36% to 61%. The role of orthotopic liver transplantation in unresectable liver disease still remains to be established with large studies. Other cytoreductive techniques for treatment of carcinoid tumors have been reported as well. These include local ablative techniques such as radiofrequency ablation (RFA) and cryoablation. Both of these procedures can be performed percutaneously or laparoscopically. They are safe and allow reduction in octreotide dosing. But long-term efficacy of these procedures still remains to be confirmed.

Chemoembolization Therapy

Hepatic arterial chemoembolization has been applied as a palliative treatment in patients with liver metastases who are not candidates for surgical resection. It is based on the assumption that most tumor cells derives their blood supply from the hepatic artery while healthy cells from the portal vein. In two large retrospective reviews of all patients treated with hepatic arterial chemoembolization at the M. D. Anderson Institute from 1992 to 2005, 150 patients with carcinoid tumor underwent hepatic chemoembolization. The median response duration was 17 months, with response rate of 67% with greater than a 50% reduction in their tumors. Progression-free survival rates were 75%, 35% and 11% at 1, 2 and 3 years. The addition of chemotherapy to hepatic artery embolization was not beneficial for metastatic carcinoid tumors. The probability of survival at 1 year was 93%, 60% at 2 years and 24% at 5 years. This demonstrates its relative safety and effectiveness as a palliative technique in patients with unresectable, symptomatic hepatic metastases. Generalized fatigue and nausea are common symptoms following the procedure. Elevation in the liver function test could be an adverse effect and should be monitored in the postoperative period. Carcinoid crisis can also be seen with chemoembolization and therefore all patients should be premedicated with octreotide.

Chemotherapy

A variety of chemotherapeutic agents have been investigated for the treatment of metastatic carcinoid tumors. Several randomized studies evaluated the efficacy of streptozocin combined with 5-FU or cyclophosphamide for advanced carcinoid tumors with only minor responses. As a result, no best systemic chemotherapy is yet recognized and the role of chemotherapy continues to be debated. Besides improving symptoms of severe flushing and diarrhea associated with metastatic carcinoid tumor, octreotide was also reported to prevent progression of metastatic carcinoid tumors in multiple small case series. The use of interferon-α has been reported to result in 40-50% biochemical responses and tumor stabilization in 20-40% of the cases. The combination of IFN-α with octreotide or with other chemotherapeutic agents has also been examined. However, it is not clear that combined treatment is superior to either agent alone. Reduced efficacy of conventional systemic chemotherapy has prompted the development of novel molecular targeted therapy for advanced carcinoid tumors. Imatinib or sunitinib, tyrosine kinase inhibitors were observed to delay tumor cell growth in preclinical studies. They demonstrated partial response in 2% of individuals while disease stability in 83% over 1-year period. Carcinoid tumors are highly vascular tumors and overexpression of vascular endothelial growth factor (VEGF) and its receptors (VEGFR type 1 and 2) have been documented in the majority of carcinoid tumors. Bevacizumab, a humanized monoclonal antibody targeting VEGF was investigated in phase II clinical trials, showing disease stability in 95% of patients when combined with octreotide compared to 68% for IFN-α and octreotide. Similar results were reported with Everolimus, a molecule inhibiting the mTOR pathway. Further studies still need to investigate the long-term benefit and safety of these novel targeted therapies.

Intestinal Lymphoma

Lymphoma accounts for the third most common neoplasm (10-15%) arising in the small intestine. Extranodal lymphoma constitutes 20-40% of all cases of lymphoma. GI lymphomas are the most extranodal form of lymphoma, accounting for up to half of all extranodal disease. The stomach harbors most GI lymphomas (75%), followed by the small intestine, the colon and then other organs like the pancreas and the liver. Specific criteria were established to differentiate primary from secondary lymphomas. No superficial lymphadenopathy should be palpated on physical examination and the absence of mediastinal lymphadenopathy should be documented on chest radiograph. Both peripheral blood smears and bone marrow biopsies should have no evidence of disease involvement. In addition, the disease should be confined to the affected small bowel segment and the regional draining mesenteric lymph nodes only. Finally, no evidence of hepatic or splenic involvement should be seen except via direct extension from the primary tumor. While uncommon in the western world, primary intestinal lymphoma comprises the most common primary gastrointestinal lymphoma in the Middle East and the Near East. Due to increased immigration of people from these areas, as well as increase in the incidence of lymphoma among immunocompromised patients, the incidence of intestinal lymphoma has doubled over the last two decades. Primary intestinal lymphoma affects patients in their seventh decade of life, with male predominance (60%) and may present with perforation **(Figure 26-4)**.

Several predisposing conditions have been associated with increased incidence of small bowel lymphoma like autoimmune diseases, all forms of immunosuppression (both iatrogenic and acquired), inflammatory bowel disease specifically CD and prior radiation exposure.

Staging

Almost all GI lymphomas are non-Hodgkin lymphoma and most of them are B-cell in origin. Much less common are T-cell primary lymphomas that commonly occur in the setting of long-term celiac disease, hence the name EATL. Unlike other solid tumors of the gastrointestinal tract, the TNM staging system does not apply to small bowel lymphoma. Rather, staging is based on the Ann Arbor staging system adapted for non-Hodgkin lymphomas. In this staging system, stage I is a lymphoma limited to a single site. Stage II tumors are confined to below the diaphragm and separated into two subgroups: those with regional (stage II 1E) and distant (stage II 2E) lymph node involvement. Stage III is when organs on both sides of the diaphragm are involved and stage IV is widespread dissemination including the liver and the spleen. Consequently, tumor spread is the most significant prognostic indicator for intestinal lymphoma.

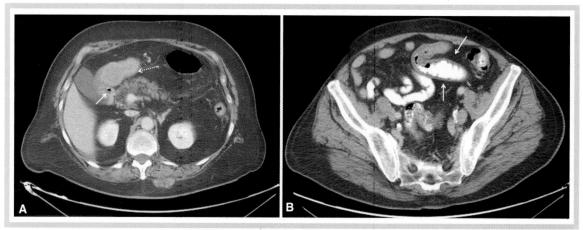

Figures 26-4A and B: Small bowel lymphoma. (A) A 66-year-old female presented with acute onset abdominal pain and peritoneal signs. She was found to have free intraperitoneal air (arrow), thickened proximal small bowel (dashed arrow). At surgery, patient was found to have small bowel lymphoma with evidence of perforation. (B) CT scan of a patient demonstrating marked thickening of the jejunum in a patient with small bowel lymphoma

Subtypes

A vast majority of lymphomas arising in the GI tract are of B-cell in origin and generally fall into one of four following categories:

- diffuse large cell lymphoma
- mucosal-associated lymphoid tissue (MALT)-associated lymphomas
- mantle cell lymphoma
- Burkitt's lymphoma.

Far less common are the T-cell intestinal lymphomas, with the EATL being the most common type.

Mucosal-Associated Lymphoid Tissue Lymphoma

Mucosal-associated lymphoid tissue (MALT) lymphomas are currently the most common primary gastrointestinal lymphomas. In the REAL/WHO classification, MALT is now called *'marginal zone B-cell lymphoma'*. MALT lymphomas occur more commonly in the stomach, followed by the small intestine (most commonly in ileocecal region), the colon and the esophagus. They occur more commonly in men in their sixth decades of life. On gross pathology, these tumors present as unifocal, ulcerated overhanging lesions. Histologically, they are characterized by cellular heterogeneity with marginal zone cells similar to those of Peyer's patch and mesenteric nodal tissue. Non-neoplastic reactive lymphoid follicles surrounded by centrocytes are characteristic, with the neoplastic marginal zone occupying the marginal zone or intrafollicular region. These tumor cells express elevated levels of IgM. They express B-cell associated antigens, including CD19, CD20, CD22 and CD79a. They are usually CD5 negative CD10 negative, CD23 negative and CD43 variable. Unlike the large diffuse B cells, they are not associated with Bcl-2 or Bcl-1 rearrangements. Clinically, these tumors are associated with chronic inflammatory conditions, including autoimmune disorders such as Sjögren's syndrome and Hashimoto's thyroiditis. Epidemiological studies demonstrate strong association with chronic *Helicobacter pylori* infection. Most of the patients present early (stage I or II) in the disease process. MALT lymphomas are considered to be antigen driven as regression has been reported with eradication of the *H. pylori* infection. Management of intestinal MALT lymphomas encompasses both surgical and medical treatment, with small intestinal lymphomas having better prognosis that tumors arising in the stomach.

Immunoproliferative small intestinal disease (IPSID), also know as 'alpha heavy chain disease' or Mediterranean lymphoma, is a subtype of MALT lymphomas that occur exclusively in the Mediterranean area. It is characterized by defective secretion of alpha heavy chain. IPSID tend to present in younger males with more diffuse involvement, predominantly of the proximal small intestine.

Similar to MALT lymphomas, IPSID are also thought to be antigen driven with association with *Campylobacter jejuni*.

Diffuse Large B-Cell Lymphoma

Diffuse large B-cell lymphoma is the second most common non-Hodgkin's lymphoma occurring in the GI tract. The ileocecal region is most commonly affected. Grossly, diffuse large B-cell lymphoma present as focal ulcerated lesions in the distal small intestine. On histology, these tumors are composed of diffuse large B cells with large nuclei that are twice the size of a normal lymphocyte. These tumor cells stain positive for CD19, CD20, CD22 and CD79a. Bcl-2 gene is rearranged in approximately 30% of the cases. Similar to other lymphomas, immunosuppression is a major risk factor. These tumors affect men more frequently, with a median age of 54-61 years. Surgery is still the mainstay treatment of localized disease followed by adjuvant radiation or chemotherapy. Overall 5-year survival has been reported to be between 50% and 70%.

Mantle Cell Lymphoma

Mantle cell lymphoma (MCL) is a rare type of primary GI lymphomas that can present either with an indolent or a very aggressive course. They have a predilection to the small intestine and the colon. They more commonly affect men (4:1) in their sixth and seventh decades of life. Grossly, mantle cell lymphoma present as multiple whitish polypoid lesions, that on histology illustrates high resemblance to nodal lymphomas. They consist of a dense CD5 positive naïve B cells within the mantle zone that surrounds germinal centers. MCL has been associated with t (11:14)(q13;q32) chromosomal translocation causing overexpression of cyclin D1. Four histologic subtypes have been described: nodular, diffuse, mantle zone and blastic. Blastic type has the worst prognosis while nodular and diffuse have the best prognosis. Sadly, most MCL present as a stage IV disease with limited response to current management.

Burkitt's Lymphoma

Burkitt's lymphoma is highly aggressive B-cell lymphomas that can arise in the GI tract, accounting less than 5% of all small intestinal lymphomas. Burkitt's lymphomas have a characteristic epidemiology. Endemic Burkitt's lymphoma is seen predominantly in Central Africa, affecting children with peak incidence at 8 years of age. The endemic type is associated with Epstein-Barr virus (EBV) infection and involved the gastrointestinal tract in only 20-30% of cases. Conversely, sporadic Burkitt's lymphoma occurs more commonly in westernized countries and affecting a broader age population. Sporadic cases have not been associated with EBV infections. Unlike endemic form, sporadic cases commonly affect the GI tract especially the ileocecal region. On the gross specimen, they present as large masses, occasionally mimicking appendicitis. On histology, cells are monomorphic medium-sized cells with multiple prominent nuclei and a rich basophilic cytoplasm. The tumor has an extremely high rate of proliferation, giving it a *'starry sky'* pattern, imparted by the numerous benign macrophages that have ingested apoptotic tumor cells. Treatment of small intestinal Burkitt's lymphoma consists primarily of chemotherapy, usually vincristine, cyclophosphamide, doxorubicin and methotrexate.

T-Cell Lymphoma

T-cell lymphomas of the small intestine are less common than previously described B-cell lymphomas accounting for 10-15% of intestinal lymphomas. Patients commonly present with distal small bowel perforation and peritonitis. On gross pathology, intestinal ulceration with transmural replacement of the intestinal wall by highly pleomorphic lymphoid cells may be seen. A large number of surrounding intraepithelial lymphocytes may also show cellular atypia. The tumor cells are positive for CD3, CD7, CD8 and CD103 while negative for CD4. The majority of T-cell lymphomas arise in the setting of long-standing enteropathy, primarily celiac disease, hence the name EATL. Multiple epidemiological studies correlated EATL with gluten consumption. EATL is described in approximately 5-10% of all patients with celiac disease. The relative risk of developing a lymphoma in the setting of celiac disease is 25- to 100-fold higher than in normal patients. T-cell lymphomas affect men and women equally. They most commonly arise in the jejunum or the proximal ileum. They tend to remain localized however dissemination is common with the progression of the disease. They typically present as large circumferential ulcers in the absence of large masses with associated mesenteric lymphadenopathy. As with other types of lymphomas, perforation is a common presentation for T-cell lymphomas, so is small bowel obstruction. T-cell lymphomas tend to have worse prognosis when compared to B-cell tumors with 5-year survival rate close to 10%.

Gastrointestinal Stromal Tumor

Gastrointestinal stromal tumors (GISTs) comprise the most common mesenchymal tumors of the small intestine. Arising from the intestinal cells of Cajal, GISTs were just recently characterized by the presence of gain-of-function *c-kit* (CD117) mutation, a tyrosine kinase receptor involved in cellular proliferation, apoptosis and differentiation. They most commonly involve the stomach and proximal small intestine. Most (80-90%) of all GISTs arise because of *c-kit* mutation. GISTs that do not have a mutated *c-kit* have a mutation in another tyrosine kinase receptor gene, platelet derived growth factor (PDGF) receptor alpha. These molecular markers have allowed the distinction of GIST from other histologically similar mesenchymal tumors such as leiomyomas, leiomyosarcomas, schwannomas and others. It is now recognized that a vast majority of the tumors that had previously been identified as leiomyomas and leiomyosarcomas are actually CD117-positive GISTs. Until recently, GISTs were notorious for being resistant to chemotherapy. The molecular discoveries have stimulated the development of targeted therapies against these moieties. Recently, the *c-kit* tyrosine kinase inhibitor Imatinib (Glivec/Gleevec), a drug initially designed to treat chronic myelogenous leukemia, was found to be useful in the treatment of GISTs. Clinical trials have found that this compound is very effective in treating GISTs without many of the side effects associated with traditional chemotherapy.

Epidemiology

Interpretation of previous epidemiological data for mesenchymal tumors is challenging since only in the last decade that molecular characterizations of these tumors was developed. The incidence of all GISTs in the GI tract is estimated at 10-20 per million of the population. There are approximately 4500-6000 cases of GISTs per year in the United States. This makes GIST the most common mesenchymal tumor of the small intestine, but in all, constitutes only 0.5-1% of all gastrointestinal tumors. GISTs are diagnosed equally in men and woman with a peak incidence in patients between 50 and 60 years of age. They are most commonly found in the jejunum, followed by the ileum and lastly the duodenum. These tumors tend to present with pain, intussusception or bleeding.

Clinicopathologic Correlates of Malignant Potential

The identification of the *c-kit* gain-of-function mutation characteristic of most GISTs has allowed better classification and understanding of the clinicopathologic correlates of these tumors. Although only approximately 30-50% of tumors are clinically malignant, all GISTs have malignant potential and it is now acknowledged that GIST tumors are no longer classified as benign or malignant. About half of resected GISTs recur within the first five years. Several criteria have been found to predict the behavior of GIST tumors and stratify them according to the risk of recurrence and metastasis.

- *Tumor size:* Tumor size is one of the major criteria in the NIH 2002 consensus for risk stratification of GISTs. Several retrospective studies have supported the idea that virtually all GISTs have malignant potential. This risk is noticeable for tumors larger than 2 cm and increases significantly for tumors larger than 5 cm in the largest dimension.

- *Mitotic rate:* Mitotic rate is the second major criteria for risk stratification of GIST tumors besides tumor size. Five or more mitoses per 50 high powered field (HPF) indicate worse outcome, while mitotic rates higher than ten per 50 HPF predict high recurrence and metastases, irrespective of tumor size or location with 5-year survival rates approximately 25%.
- *Tumor site:* Anatomic location was established to be another criteria affecting outcome in patients with GIST tumors. Small intestinal GISTs, mainly jejunal/ileal were found to have more malignant behavior when compared to duodenal tumors, followed by rectal and gastric GISTs. Risk was independent of tumor size or mitotic rate.

Other histopathological criteria of malignant behavior have been examined including cellularity and nuclear atypia, mucosal invasion, multiple genetic mutations and ulceration, but none of these have been shown to correlate well with prognosis of mesenchymal tumors.

Management

The principal treatment for localized, resectable GISTs arising in the small intestine is complete surgical excision. *En bloc* segmental resection of the tumor with grossly negative margins is usually the goal. Wider resection of surrounding uninvolved tissue did not prove to improve outcome. Considering the friable consistency of GISTs, great care should be taken to prevent tumor rupture and spillage, which has been associated with carcinomatosis. Unlike other types of small intestinal tumors, such as adenocarcinoma or carcinoids, GISTs rarely metastasize to regional mesenteric lymph nodes and therefore routine lymphadenectomy is not recommended. Progression of the disease is mainly to the peritoneum and to the liver, which should carefully be inspected at the time of surgical exploration.

Until recently, surgery was the mainstay treatment for GISTs with no data to support adjuvant chemotherapy or radiation for the management of completely resected GISTs. In significant number of patients with advanced disease, negative surgical margins may not be possible, greatly impacting disease-free survival and life expectance, with median survival ranging from 10 to 23 months. With recent understanding of molecular alterations associated with stromal tumors, tyrosine kinase inhibitors were investigated in the management of metastatic and resected GISTs. Over the last several years, several clinical trials showed significant benefit of imatinib (Gleevec) in both recurrence-free and overall survival in patient with GISTs. The overall survival at 3 years was 97%, while recurrence-free survival was 61% at 3 years. Imatinib was approved by the FDA in 2008 for the treatment of resected GIST after prior approval in 2001 for the treatment of metastatic stromal tumors. The use of imatinib as a neoadjuvant therapy for unresectable tumors is still under investigation. Sunitinib, a relatively newer multitargeted receptor tyrosine kinase inhibitor, initially approved for the treatment of renal cell carcinoma, is also now approved for the treatment of imatinib-resistant GISTs.

Other Mesenchymal Tumors

Overwhelmingly, the majority of the mesenchymal tumors that arise in the small intestine are gastrointestinal stromal tumors. A less common group of mesenchymal neoplasms, histologically similar to other soft tissue tumors, consists of leiomyomas and leiomyosarcomas, inflammatory fibroid polyps, desmoid tumors, inflammatory and myofibroblastic tumors, solitary fibrous tumors, schwannomas and peripheral nerve sheath tumors.

Leiomyomas and Leiomyosarcomas

Intestinal leiomyomas and leiomyosarcomas are very rare tumors arising in the small intestine. They arise from the muscularis propria and muscularis mucosa layers of the bowel wall. Leiomyosarcomas, the most common non-GIST mesenchymal tumors, were previously over-diagnosed before current molecular characterization of GIST. They stain positive for desmin and actin and are typically negative for CD117 (*c-kit* and CD34). Local tumor growth is common initially and usually extraluminal, hence obstruction is late. As tumor size increases, tumor ulceration and bleeding is observed. Metastasis is hematological, mainly to the liver and peritoneum. About one-third of patients have metastasis at the time of diagnosis. Prognosis of leiomyosarcomas is very poor.

Inflammatory Fibroid Polyps

Inflammatory fibroid polyps are benign submucosal lesions infrequently encountered in the small intestine. They are composed of myofibroblastic type of mesenchymal cells and inflammatory cells in a mixture of small granulation tissue-like vessels, spindle cells and inflammatory cells especially eosinophils. These lesions can stain positively for CD34; however, they do not stain for CD117 with the exception of very small areas of stroma within these tumors.

Desmoid Tumors

Desmoid tumors are histologically benign fibrous tumors originating from musculoaponeurotic structures throughout the body. These spindle cell tumors are frequently confused with GISTs. Histologically, they are characterized by fibroblastic proliferation and formation of bundles of spindle cells around blood vessels in a dense hypocellular fibrous stroma. Few mitotic figures are seen and necrosis is usually absent. They stain for vimentin, smooth muscle actin and nuclear beta catenin. Although these tumors are histologically benign with no potential for metastasis, they tend to be locally aggressive, damaging nearby structures and organs. They tend to recur even after complete resection. They occur in higher incidence in patients with familial adenomatous polyposis syndrome (FAP) and Gardner's syndrome. The main treatment consists of complete surgical resection with wide margin to assure negative microscopic margins, however this is often restricted by anatomic location and involvement of vital structures. Other treatment modalities include chemotherapy (methotrexate and vinblastine, doxorubicin), radiation therapy, NSAIDs and antiestrogens (tamoxifen).

Inflammatory and Myofibroblastic Tumors

Also known as *inflammatory pseudotumors* or *inflammatory fibrosarcomas*, these tumors are rare inflammatory mesenchymal tumors that have been described in small intestinal mesentery in young individuals. They also arise in the stomach where they can also be associated with peptic ulcer disease or chronic gastritis. Grossly, these tumors appear as solid white masses with infiltrative margins. On histology, they are characterized by spindle cells admixed with lymphocytes and plasma cells. These lesions are believed to be benign reactions to infectious processes although local recurrence has been reported. They rarely behave in a malignant fashion. On immunohistochemistry, they stain positive for desmin, muscle-specific actin and cytokeratin, but negative for CD117 and CD34. Sixty percent of these lesions stain for anaplastic lymphoma kinase, a growth factor receptor.

Schwannomas

Schwannomas of the gastrointestinal tract are also rare tumors that occur in the small intestine, stomach, colon and esophagus. On gross specimen, these lesions are rubbery yellowish trabeculated tumors that histologically are characterized by peripheral lymph nodes aggregates with prominent nuclear palisading and Verocay bodies formations along with numerous thick walled hyalinized vessels similar to schwannomas found elsewhere in the body. They stain strongly for S-100 and glial fibrillary acidic protein (GFAP) but are negative for CD117 (*c-kit*), CD34 and smooth muscle actin (SMA). These lesions almost always behave as benign lesions.

Summary

■ Small bowel cancer (SBC) is a rare, yet increasing disease.

■ Diagnosis may be difficult due to the nonspecificity of the symptoms and hence clinical suspicion is key to diagnosis.

■ Carcinoids of the small bowel are increasing and may be the most common malignancy of the small bowel, if not an equal share-holder of tumors to adenocarcinoma.

■ Lymphomas are common tumors in the small bowel and may present with perforation.

■ GISTs should be differentiated from leiomyomas and leiomyosarcomas and they possess malignant potential.

Landmark Papers

1. Soga J. Early-stage carcinoids of the gastrointestinal tract: an analysis of 1914 reported cases. Cancer 2005;103(8): 1587-95.

2. Bamboat ZM, Berger DL. Is right hemicolectomy for 2.0-cm appendiceal carcinoids justified? Arch Surg 2006;141(4): 349-52; discussion 352.

3. Moertel CG, Weiland LH, Nagorney DM, Dockerty MB. Carcinoid tumor of the appendix: treatment and prognosis. N Engl J Med 1987;317(27):1699-1701.

4. Syracuse DC, Perzin KH, Price JB, Wiedel PD, Mesa-Tejada R. Carcinoid tumors of the appendix. Mesoappendiceal extension and nodal metastases. Ann Surg 1979; 190(1): 58-63.

5. Dabaja BS, Suki D, Pro B, Bonnen M, Ajani J. Adeno-carcinoma of the small bowel: presentation, prognostic factors, and outcome of 217 patients. Cancer. 2004;101(3): 518-26.

6. Singhal N, Singhal D. Adjuvant chemotherapy for small intestine adenocarcinoma. Cochrane Database Syst Rev 2007(3):CD005202.

Level of Evidence Table

Recommendation	Grade	Best level of evidence	References
Aggressive and early resection of small intestinal carcinoid tumors is warranted for cure and to avoid complications of intestinal ischemia or bowel obstruction from mesenteric involvement.	B	4	1-3
Right hemicolectomy is indicated for localized appendiceal carcinoids > 2 cm in size, mesoappendiceal invasion, or aggressive histology.	B	4	4-6
Complete resection of small bowel adenocarcinoma offers the best chance of survival.	B	2c	7-9
Adjuvant therapy (5-FU based regimens) improves survival in advanced small bowel adenocarcinoma.	B	4	10-12

References

1. deVries H, Wijffels RT, Willemse PH, et al. Abdominal angina in patients with a midgut carcinoid, a sign of severe pathology. World J Surg 2005;29(9):1139-42.
2. Hellman P, Lundstrom T, Ohrvall U, et al. Effect of surgery on the outcome of midgut carcinoid disease with lymph node and liver metastases. World J Surg 2002;26(8): 991-7.
3. Soga J. Early-stage carcinoids of the gastrointestinal tract: an analysis of 1914 reported cases. Cancer 2005;103(8):1587-95.
4. Bamboat ZM, Berger DL. Is right hemicolectomy for 2.0-cm appendiceal carcinoids justified? Arch Surg 2006;141(4): 349-52; discussion 352.
5. Moertel CG, Weiland LH, Nagorney DM, Dockerty MB. Carcinoid tumor of the appendix: treatment and prognosis. N Engl J Med 1987;317(27):1699-1701.
6. Syracuse DC, Perzin KH, Price JB, Wiedel PD, Mesa-Tejada R. Carcinoid tumors of the appendix. Mesoappendiceal extension and nodal metastases. Ann Surg 1979;190(1): 58-63.
7. Howe JR, Karnell LH, Menck HR, Scott-Conner C. The American College of Surgeons Commission on Cancer and the American Cancer Society. Adenocarcinoma of the small bowel: review of the National Cancer Data Base, 1985-1995. Cancer 1999;86(12):2693-2706.
8. Talamonti MS, Goetz LH, Rao S, Joehl RJ. Primary cancers of the small bowel: analysis of prognostic factors and results of surgical management. Arch Surg 2002;137(5):564-70; discussion 570-1.
9. Dabaja BS, Suki D, Pro B, Bonnen M, Ajani J. Adenocarcinoma of the small bowel: presentation, prognostic factors, and outcome of 217 patients. Cancer 2004; 101(3):518-26.
10. Overman MJ, Kopetz S, Wen S, et al. Chemotherapy with 5-fluorouracil and a platinum compound improves outcomes in metastatic small bowel adenocarcinoma. Cancer 2008;113(8):2038-45.
11. Overman MJ, Varadhachary GR, Kopetz S, et al. Phase II study of capecitabine and oxaliplatin for advanced adenocarcinoma of the small bowel and ampulla of Vater. J Clin Oncol 2009;27(16):2598-2603.
12. Singhal N, Singhal D. Adjuvant chemotherapy for small intestine adenocarcinoma. Cochrane Database Syst Rev 2007(3):CD005202.

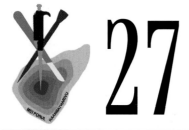

27

Colon Cancer

Amber Wooten, Pragatheeshwar Thirunavukarasu, Richard Fortunato, Wolfgang Schraut

Background

Colorectal cancer (CRC) is the fourth most common site of malignancy in the USA, ranking third among males and females, when ranked separately. The number of new cases of colon cancer in 2009 was estimated to be ~106,000. CRC occurs with a slightly high predominance in men (sex ratio, 1.4: (1) and has a higher incidence in African-Americans and lower socioeconomic groups. In the United States, there is an association between the ethnicity and the incidence of CRC for both genders in decreasing order of CRC incidence: African-Americans, Caucasians, Asian Americans, Hispanic Americans and Native Americans. It is most common in black men and least common in American-Indian/Alaska Native women.

Approximately 60% of all colon cancer is believed to be preventable if routine colonoscopic screening is complied with by men and women aged 50 or above. Overall 5-year survival rate is around 60%, as per Surveillance, Epidemiology and End Results (SEER) data. The introduction of screening techniques, especially colonoscopy, has made colon cancer a potentially preventable disease. This has been shown by the decreased death rate from colon cancer in recent years as the number of screening colonoscopies has risen. Colonoscopy is leading to detection and removal of premalignant polypoid lesions and detection of established malignancies at an earlier stage. It stands to reason that higher surveillance leads to a reduced incidence of colon cancer.

Risk Factors

The lifetime risk of developing CRC is ~ 6%. About 75% of patients diagnosed with CRC have no identifiable risk factors and are considered to be of 'average' risk.

Risk Factors for Colorectal Cancer

- Age > 50 years
- Colonic polyps and polyposis syndromes
- Genetic cancer syndromes
- Positive family history
- Inflammatory bowel disease
- Previous history of colorectal cancer
- Diabetes and insulin resistance
- Smoking
- Alcohol
- Obesity
- African-American ethnicity
- Prior pelvic radiation

Age: With more than 90% of the patients being older than 50 years, age is the most important risk factor. This risk continues exponentially with an estimated 4-fold and 7-fold increase in risk for those aged 70-74 years and 80-84 years respectively, compared to those aged 50-54 years.

Colonic polyps: The National Polyp Study revealed that colonoscopic polypectomies resulted in a lower-than-expected incidence (about 76-90% decrease) of CRC. If polyps are left untreated, invasive cancer develops in 24% of the patients within 20 years. Polyps that are multiple, large (> 1 cm) and particularly those with an unfavorable (villous or tubulovillous) histology pose an increased risk of cancer. Several polyposis syndromes which are characterized by multiple polyps throughout the colon and also elsewhere in the GI tract are especially at an increased risk for CRC and will be discussed in further detail below.

Prior history of colorectal cancer: Up to 3% of patients who have had a prior surgical resection of CRC, may present with metachronous cancers in the first 5 years after surgery. The risk of a second primary CRC is 3-fold higher in those who have had a prior CRC. Tight surveillance is necessary not only for this reason but also to detect recurrence, which is fairly common in CRC, depending on the original lesion.

Family history: A first-degree relative with confirmed CRC increases one's relative risk (RR) of developing CRC by 2.25 and by 4.25 if more than one first-degree relative has a history of CRC. In addition, a family member diagnosed with CRC before the age of 45 confers a RR of 3.87 for developing CRC on the other family members.

Cancer syndromes: Familial syndromes, such as Hereditary Non-Polyposis Colon Cancer (HNPCC), Familial Adenomatous Polyposis (FAP), etc., confer an increased risk of developing CRC relative to those without such family histories, although these special circumstances account for only 5-6% of newly diagnosed CRC cases per year. HNPCC is responsible for 3% of all new CRC, while FAP is only attributed to 0.05-1% of the cases per year. In addition, HNPCC is associated with an increase of synchronous and metachronous cancers relative to average risk patients.

Inflammatory bowel disease: Inflammatory bowel disease (IBD) is associated with roughly 1% of all new cases of CRC diagnosed annually. The risk conferred by Chronic Ulcerative Colitis (CUC) depends on the duration and extent of the disease, with a prevalence of ~ 3.7% in longstanding disease. Increased risk appears after a decade of pancolitis and is cumulatively 5-10% after 20 years, ~ 20% after 30 years and ~ 30% after 35 years. Left-sided colitis offers more risk than right-sided colitis and this increased risk appears 15-20 years after the onset of the former. A subset of patients with UC who have primary sclerosing cholangitis are at even higher risk, with predominance in the right colon. Isolated proctitis appears to offer no extra risk compared to the general population, although CUC-related CRC is most common in the rectum and sigmoid colon. Some CUC patients have areas of dysplasia called Dysplasia Associated Lesion or Mass (DALM), which in turn may be adenoma-like or non-adenoma like. Non-adenomatous DALMs are typically hard to identify on routine colonoscopy. Non-adenoma like DALMs have a 60% risk of harboring invasive carcinoma, which requires a colectomy. Adenoma-like DALMs can be differentiated from sporadic adenomas in CUC patients by the following features **(Table 27-1)**.

Although, the risk of CRC in Crohn's disease (CD) was initially believed to be less compared to CUC, it is now thought that risk may be comparable. CRC develops at an earlier age in the IBD population.

TABLE 27-1	Differential features between sporadic adenomas and adenoma-like DALM in CUC
CUC-related sporadic adenomas	**CUC-related adenoma-like DALM**
Often occurs in older patients, with short duration of disease	Often occurs in younger patients, with longstanding disease
Lamina propria mononuclear cells and neutrophils are uncommon	Lamina propria mononuclear cells and neutrophils are common
Strong/diffuse B-catenin staining and weak/negative p53 staining	Strong/diffuse p53 staining and weak/negative B-catenin staining

Race and ethnicity: In the United States, there is an ethnic association with the incidence of CRC of either gender. In decreasing order, the risk is higher for African-Americans > Caucasians > Asian Americans > Hispanic Americans > Native Americans. In addition, African-Americans have the highest mortality from CRC overall and display worse 5-year survival rates for all stages compared to Caucasians. Genetics, environmental factors and a lower socioeconomic status, screening and treatment rate may contribute to this discrepancy.

Diabetes mellitus and hyperinsulinemia: Many studies have evaluated the relationship between diabetes mellitus (DM) and CRC and found that diabetics have a 30% increased risk of CRC compared to non-diabetics. This is thought to be due to increased levels of colonocyte growth factors, insulin-like growth factor (IGF-I) and IGF binding protein-3 (IGFBP-3) stimulated by the hyperglycemia. The exact mechanism is still to be defined.

Lifestyle and body habitus: Heavy smoking (1 pack/day or more) increases the RR of developing CRC compared to non-smokers 1.4-2.0 fold. Smokers with colon cancer are known to have BRAF mutations as well. CRC is seen more in obese patients (RR: 1.5) and less in people who exercise regularly.

Colonic Polyps

Polyp is derived from Greek word *'polypous'* meaning many (poly) feet (pous) **(Figure 27-1)**. The understanding of colonic polyps, their natural history and pathophysiology is crucial to the comprehensive study of CRC. Polyps are intraluminal protuberances of the mucosa. Polyps are broadly classified as non-neoplastic and neoplastic. The further classification is as follows,

Non-neoplastic polyps
- Hyperplastic
- Mucosal
- Inflammatory
- Hamartomatous

Neoplastic polyps
- Adenomas
  - Tubular, villous, tubulovillous
  - Sessile, pedunculated, flat, depressed
  - Small (< 5 mm), medium (5-10 mm), large (>10 mm)
  - Low grade and high grade dysplasia
- Carcinomas

Hyperplastic polyps: These are the most common non-neoplastic polyps and are characterized by hyperplastic glandular epithelium, decreased cytoplasmic mucus and the lack of atypia or nuclear hyperchromatism. A hyperplastic polyp, by itself is not a precursor for cancer, although some studies have shown that the presence of a

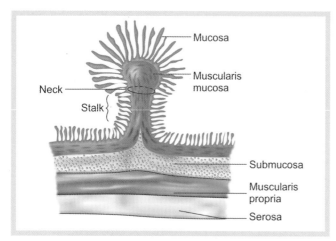

Figure 27-1: Structure of colonic polyp

abnormalities. Lesions called 'serrated adenomas' were once considered to be hyperplastic polyps, but now are considered as a separate adenoma entity due to its higher risk of CRC.

Mucosal polyps: Mucosal polyps are small tissue protuberances or excrescences and comprise of histologically normal mucosa. They are often small (< 5 mm) and confer no increased risk of CRC.

Inflammatory polyps: These polyps occur at sites of colitis and are merely postinflammatory sequelae. They do not harbor dysplasia and confer no increased CRC risk. Due to their increased vascularity and subsequent risk of post-colonoscopic polypectomy bleeding, they are best left alone when the diagnosis is certain. However, these polyps are to be viewed with suspicion in the setting of IBD at which time polypectomy may be considered to rule out carcinoma.

Hamartomatous polyps: Hamartomas are lesions of a tissue that contain the normal cellular elements but with distorted tissue architecture. The conditions commonly associated with hamartomatous polyps are Juvenile polyposis, Peutz-Jeghers syndrome, Cowden syndrome and Cronkhite-Canada syndrome **(Table 27-2)**.

Adenomatous polyps: Adenomas are benign yet dysplastic lesions. All adenomas are dysplastic and hence have malignant potential. Adenomas are fairly common and increase with age, with a prevalence of ~30% by age 50 and ~ 50% by age 70. Although only few adenomas (2%) harbor invasive cancer, almost all cancer arises from

distal hyperplastic polyp is associated with a ~ 25% risk of a proximal neoplasm and ~ 5% risk of an advanced neoplasm. Currently, the consensus is that a hyperplastic polyp found distally in a sigmoidoscopy does not warrant full colonoscopy. Features that are suspicious in hyperplastic polyps are location in right colon, large (> 1 cm) size, multiple polyps, presence of adenomatous component and hyperplastic polyposis syndrome (HPS). HPS is characterized by multiple (> 30) hyperplastic polyps throughout the colon, that are typically large, flat and present on the crests of the haustral folds. No germline mutation has yet been identified, although lesions in HPS are found to have BRAF mutations and hypermethylation

TABLE 27-2	Conditions associated with hamartomatous polyps			
Disease	**Pattern of inheritance**	**Histological features**	**Comments**	**Cancer risk**
Juvenile polyposis	Autosomal dominant	Dilated cystic glands and inflamed lamina propria	Presents as bleeding. Familial Juvenile Polyposis (FJP) is associated germline mutation of SMAD4 and PTEN genes.	<= 50%
Peutz-Jeghers syndrome	Autosomal dominant	Glandular epithelium along with smooth-muscle-cell proliferation in the muscularis mucosa	Perioral pigmentation, small bowel polyps Complications include GI bleeding, intussusception, obstruction. Associated with STK11 gene mutation	<=13%
Cowden syndrome or multiple hamar-toma syndrome	Autosomal dominant	Hamartomas of all three embryonal cell layers	Thyroid and breast cancer, intestinal polyposis. Associated with PTEN mutation	nil*
Cronkhite-Canada syndrome	Non-familial, unknown etiology	Eosinophilic infiltrate and myxoid expansion of lamina propria	Alopecia, skin hyperpigmentation, onychodystrophy, GI bleeding, high mortality rate	nil*

* No established risk.

adenomas. This process is called the adenoma-carcinoma sequence and it takes about 7 years to evolve. The risk of CRC in adenomas is cumulative: ~ 5% in 5 years and ~14% in 10 years in unresected polyps. In other words, 10% of all patients with adenomas will develop CRC. A single adenoma found on sigmoidoscopy should prompt a full colonoscopy as it could be an indication of a more proximal lesion, even in some cases an advanced neoplasm. Their malignant potential depends on their size, multiplicity, morphology and histology. Adenomas are classified in several different ways:

1. *Based on size:* Adenomas may be small (< 5 mm), medium (5-10 mm) or large (> 1 mm). Small adenomas grow at the rate of ~ 0.5 mm/year and their malignant potential increases with size. The incidence of malignancy in adenomas <1 cm is 1-2% and increases to ~10% for 1-2 cm adenomas and rockets to > 40% in adenomas > 2 cm. This risk is probably related to the increase in the villous component of the adenoma which increases with size. In general, polyps > 1 cm should be considered high-risk and removed.

2. *Based on histology:* Every adenoma can have two architectural patterns: tubular and villous. The tubular architecture is characterized by fine branching pattern of the epithelium. On the other hand, long glands that extend straight down from the surface with minimal or no branching pattern characterizes the villous type. Depending on the share of the villous or tubular component, adenomas are classified as given in **Table 27-3**.

3. *Based on morphology:* Polyps may be pedunculated (attached to the colonic wall by a mucosal stalk), sessile (no stalk, base is adherent flushed with the wall), flat (no intraluminal protuberance, defined as having height less than ½ the diameter of the lesion) or depressed. Flat lesions may contribute to 27-36% of adenomas and may not constitute a statistically significant risk of cancer. Although depressed lesions may account to < 1% of all adenomas, a large prospective study of 1000 consecutive patients found that likelihood of severe dysplasia or Duke's A adenocarcinoma is as high as 75% in depressed lesions.

4. *Based on severity of dysplasia:* Colonic polyps were initially classified as those of mild, moderate or severe dysplasia, depending on the degree of nuclear hyperchromatism, cell crowding, etc. However, this gave room for much interobserver varibility. In an attempt to reduce the above, polyps are now classified as those of 'low grade' or 'high-grade' dysplasia. The latter is present in up to 7% of adenomatous polyps. The terms 'carcinoma in situ' and 'intramucosal carcinoma' were used to signify breach of lamina propria. Since invasive malignancy in colon cancer is defined as breach of muscularis mucosa and there are no lymphatics in the lamina propria, the above-mentioned terms are currently not used. For all practical purposes, a colonic polyp with high-grade dysplasia that is completely excised with negative margins is considered to constitute definitive curative management.

5. *Serrated adenoma:* About two decades ago, polyps were classified only as either hyperplastic (no dysplasia and no cancer risk) or adenomas (with dysplasia and cancer risk). Hyperplastic polyps that had a section with jagged-edge or saw-tooth appearance were called 'serrated' polyps. They were believed to be totally innocuous. However, it has been recognized that serrated polyps have admixture of both hyperplastic and adenomatous elements and hence confer a risk of cancer. These serrated polyps (initially believed to be simply hyperplastic polyps) are now known to have adenomatous elements and hence the term 'serrated adenomas'. Longacre, in 1990 reported that there was 'significant' dysplasia in 37% and intramucosal carcinoma in 11% of serrated polyps which he then called 'Mixed Hyperplastic-Adenomatous Polyps' (MHAP). This signifies 'high-grade dysplasia' (by the current terminology), thereby warranting close surveillance, polypectomy and possibly surgical resection. Although serrated adenomas can occur anywhere in the colon and rectum, they are typically right-sided and large (> 1 cm). A subgroup of serrated adenomas, the 'sessile serrated adenomas' (SSA) are to be differentiated from the 'traditional serrated

TABLE 27-3	Classification of adenoma as per the share of villous or tubular component			
Type	Histology	Prevalence among adenomas	Location	Cancer occurrence
Tubular	>75% tubular component and < 25% villous	~ 80%	Equally distributed throughout colon	< 5%
Tubulovillous	26-75% tubular component and < 75% villous	~ 5-15%	Equally distributed throughout colon	20-25%
Villous	>75% villous component and < 25% tubular component	~ 5-15%	Predominance in rectum	35-40%

adenomas' (TSA). The former are the high-risk lesions in Hyperplastic polyposis, a disease initially thought to be completely benign, until Torlakovic and Snovic in 1996 showed the opposite. SSAs with dysplasia are now considered to be related to BRAF oncogene mutations and MSI-H (microsatellite instability-high) colon cancer.

6. *Malignant polyp:* Polyps may harbor malignancy, which in colon cancer is defined as invasion of the muscularis mucosa. The most important factor affecting treatment options for malignant polyps is the presence, absence or risk of regional lymph node spread. Haggitt's classification **(Figure 27-2)** divides malignant polyps, based on the level of invasion. Only level 4 (submucosal invasion) has shown to be of prognostic value **(Table 27-4)**.

TABLE 27-4	Haggitt's classification for malignant polyps, 1985
Level	**Location of carcinoma**
0	Confined to mucosa only
1	Confined to head of polyp
2	Confined to neck of polyp, no invasion of stalk
3	Invasion of stalk of polyp
4	Invasion of submucosa

7. Overall, ~ 25% of malignant polyps will have lymph node metastasis. Useful markers of unfavorable pathological features at high risk for lymph node metastasis are grade 3 (poorly differentiated) histology, lymphovascular invasion and positive margins. Another important factor is the depth of invasion and extent of 'lateral invasion', which has been introduce in Japanese literature by Kikuchi in 1995. Here, the level of submucosal invasion (Sm) is classified as Sm1 (upper third), Sm2 (middle third) and Sm3 (lower third). In addition, Sm1 has been subclassified into Sm1a, Sm1b and Sm1c as those with B/A ratios of 0.25, 0.25-0.5, > 0.5 respectively, wherein B is the horizontal measure of involved part (submucosal invasion) and A is the horizontal measure of the total lesion. A Mayo clinic series reported that the incidence of lymph node metastasis in Sm3 lesion is ~ 23%. For treatment purposes, any lesion at or above Sm1c must be treated surgically. Endoscopically treatable lesions are best removed by polypectomy for protruding lesions and by Endoscopic Mucosal Resection (EMR) for flat lesions.

In summary, colonic polyps should be scrutinized histologically and treated appropriately to decrease the risk of colon cancer. In general, the 'red flags' for colonic polyps are—
- Large (>1 cm) adenoma size
- Presence of high-grade dysplasia
- Villous histology
- Significant multiplicity
- Large and sessile adenomatous polyps
- 'Depressed' morphology
- Invasive carcinoma, especially with submucosal invasion.

Genetics of Colon Cancer

CRC is one of the well-studied models for the genetic carcinogenesis. Genetic alterations in the structure of a gene are called 'mutations', derived from the Latin word 'mutare', meaning 'to change'. Mutations that occur at or before the fertilization of the ovum carry the mutation to all cells in the body and are called germline mutations. In contrast, mutation may occur in a certain cell type or tissue

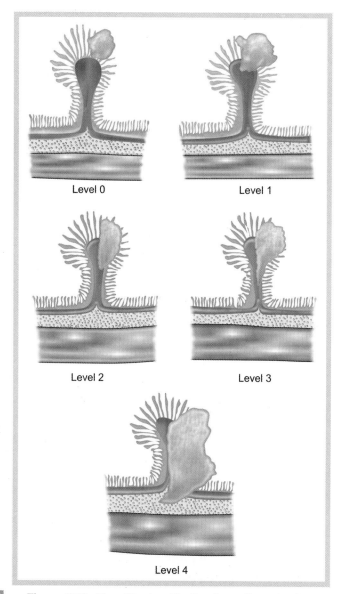

Level 0

Level 1

Level 2

Level 3

Level 4

Figure 27-2: Haggitt's classification for malignant polyps

only and are called 'somatic' mutations. Alternatively, an individual may inherit a mutation or may acquire it in a *de novo* fashion. Colon cancer can occur in one of the three epidemiological patterns:

- *Sporadic*—A pattern of occurrence of CRC that is not associated with a defined inheritance pattern or a family history. Although sporadic tumors may contain mutations in genes that are implicated in inherited syndromes, sporadic tumors are identified by the absence of inheritance of such mutations. This pattern accounts for ~ 70% of all cases of CRC.
- *Inherited*—A pattern of occurrence that is clearly identifiable by an inheritance of a mutation or defective gene. Family history, when elicited, identifies the inherited predisposition, not only to colonic but to several related extra colonic neoplasms. This pattern accounts for ~ 10% of all cases of CRC.
- *Familial*—A pattern of occurrence that is identifiable by a family history and increased predisposition to colon cancer and by the absence of a defined inheritance pattern already described in inherited cases of CRC. This accounts for ~ 25-30% of all cases of CRC.

Genes involved in CRC may either be oncogenes (those that function in cell cycle control/growth whereby mutation causes increased proliferation of cells) or tumor suppressor genes (those that normally inhibit cell proliferation and the mutation of which leads to loss of that inhibition). There are genes which are responsible for the correction of DNA mismatches—'Mismatch Repair' (MMR) genes and some more whose function is probably not directly related to carcinogenesis but have a influence in the process—called 'modifier' genes.

The molecular genetics of colon cancer were described by Vogelstein and Fearon as a 'multistep process of carcinogenesis' which theorizes that cancer is the result of accumulation of several mutations and genetic abnormalities over time that transform a normal cell via intermediate cell types to a frankly malignant cell. This is the basis of the 'adenoma-carcinoma' sequence, which delineates that invasive cancer in the colon occurs by the stepwise transformation of normal colonic mucosa to an adenoma with high-grade dysplasia to carcinoma. Roughly, the transformation of an adenoma to carcinoma is believed to occur over a span of 7 years or more. The stepwise transformation is propelled by the similarly stepwise mutations in genes, which are explained below in more detail.

APC Gene

APC stands for 'Adenomatous Polyposis coli'. It is a tumor suppressor gene located in chromosome 5. The APC gene product is believed to promote the degradation of a cell armadillo protein called 'beta-catenin'. APC mutations result in the nuclear and cytosolic accumulation of beta-catenin that binds and activates Transcription factor 4 (Tcf-4), which is the control 'switch' for the cell to either enter growth or undergo differentiation. The final common pathway of APC gene mutation coincides with what is called the Wingless type (Wnt) pathway, which is signaling cascade that also involves beta-catenin. The end result is uncontrolled cell proliferation and a resistance to apoptosis. APC mutations are significant in that they occur—

- in up to 80% of sporadic CRC
- as a germline mutation in FAP
- in 6% of all Ashkenazi Jews and in ~ 28% of people who have a personal or family history of CRC. Familial CRC in this population is attributed to a single codon (codon 1307) germline mutation of APC and hence the risk of CRC is less than those with FAP.

p53 Gene

p53 is the acronym for 'protein with a weight of 53 kDa'. This gene is called the 'guardian of the genome' or the 'master watchman' because it prevents the proliferation of cells that sustain DNA damage. It is located in chromosome 17 and operates by affecting the expression of several of its target genes, which cause cell arrest when exposed to stress or damage. p53 inactivation is believed to be a relatively late occurrence in the carcinogenic process. The significance of p53 is that—

- it is mutated in 50-70% of all CRC
- it is implicated as a germline mutation in Li-Fraumeni syndrome (very interestingly, patients with this syndrome are not at higher risk for CRC!)
- p53 mutated tumors may confer poor prognosis compared to non-p53 mutated tumors.

Ras Oncogene

Ras derives its name from 'rat sarcoma', which is where these genes were discovered. There are three main Ras variants—K-ras (Kirsten), H-ras (Harvey) and N-ras (neuroblastoma). The ras oncogenes are those that control growth signal transduction. K-ras is the most frequently mutated gene in CRC. It is significant in that:

- ras mutations are present in ~ 50% of sporadic CRC
- more common in more proximal tumors
- common in large (> 1 cm) adenomas
- present in ~100% of nondysplastic aberrant crypt foci (ACF)
- ~ 25% of hyperplastic polyps have ras mutation
- K-ras mutations predict lack of response to chemo-therapy (specially with cetuximab).

Other oncogenes that are associated with CRC are src, c-myc and c-erb-2.

Other Genes

Deleted in Colon Cancer gene (DCC) in chromosome 18 is found to be involved in ~ 70% of sporadic CRC. DCC has a significant impact in prognosis. Other tumor suppressor genes in CRC include SMAD4 and SMAD2. The mismatch repair genes (MMR) are implicated in HNPCC and in a small portion of sporadic CRC. When mismatch occurs in the genome without repairs, it leaves sequences of repetitive sequences called 'microsatellites'. These microsatellites make the cell vulnerable to further mutations and hence lead to instability of the cell—a phenomenon called 'microsatellite instability' (MSI). MSI may be in two degrees—high or low. MSI-H is what that occurs in HNPCC, an inherited form of colon cancer. MSI-L is that which occurs in sporadic CRC. Interestingly, MSI in both inherited and sporadic forms of CRC is associated with better prognosis, for reasons that are still unknown. A small subset of patients with multiple colonic adenomas suggestive of FAP are negative for APC mutations and are found to have germline mutations in the MUTY homolog gene (involved in base excision repair). This condition is still not fully characterized. The accumulating body of evidence that aspirin (and other NSAIDs) may be protective in colonic adenoma/carcinoma may implicate COX-2 as a 'modifier' gene in CRC tumorigenesis.

Hereditary Colon Cancer

Non-sporadic colon cancer has a strong genetic etiological basis, which may either be well described for its pattern of inheritance (in which case it is called 'hereditary' or 'inherited') or not described but with an increased occurrence in families (called 'familial'). Clues that raise suspicion that CRC may be non-sporadic are:

- early age at presentation
- strong family history of CRC or of other cancers
- presence of other or multiple cancers or neoplasms along with CRC
- history of cancers along with birth defects or congenital anomalies.

The purpose of identification of such inherited/familial forms of cancer is to be prompted to look for other cancers, identify family members at risk, increase surveillance, offer risk-reduction strategies and ultimately decrease cancer mortality. Hereditary colon cancer can broadly be divided into two groups—polyp associated (often called polyposis, such as FAP) and non-polyp associated such as HNPCC. Although there are many other syndromes that go along in both of these groups, attention will be paid mostly to these two disorders.

FAP, although called 'familial', technically falls under the inherited CRC category because of knowledge about its inheritance pattern. The 'classic FAP' is characterized by the presence of numerous (> 1000) polyps in the colon, which may literally 'carpet' the entire colon. FAP may be caused by one of several hundreds of germline mutations in the APC gene, that eventually result in a truncated APC gene product. It is autosomal dominant and the risk of CRC depends on the severity of polyposis. The severity of CRC (and the presence of other abnormalities) is dependent on the type of mutation in the APC gene. The APC gene has a 'hot spot', which is between codons 1250 and 1464. A mutation in the hot spot region results in profuse FAP, with the classic FAP being attributed to codon 1306. Mutations that occur on either side of the hot spot, near the 3' or 5' end of the gene result in milder forms of FAP called Attenuated FAP (AFAP), which is characterized by < 1000 adenomas. Certain associated syndromes like Gardner's syndrome have specific mutations in the APC gene. This phenomenon of varying disease manifestation with the type of genetic alteration is called 'genotype-phenotype' association and is critically important for the surgeon as it helps direct decision-making on the timing and type of surgery. For example, people who present with FAP and are found to have a mutation often associated with desmoids may be considered for a simpler procedure possibly less prone to desmoid induction. Since FAP is being a germline mutation, the risk of cancer persists even after total colectomy. It may occur in the rectum (if left behind), the anal transition zone, the ileal pouch or even in the ileostomy. This is only a reiteration of the 'two-hit' hypothesis: the germline mutation being the first hit and the presence of irritation in any of these areas being the second.

The aim of surgery in FAP is to decrease the mortality from CRC. The surgical options in FAP are grouped into two: Rectal sparing and non-rectal sparing. Rectal sparing means performance of a total colectomy with ileorectal anastomosis (IRA). This approach has been used for several decades. It is technically not demanding and avoids the potential risks of extensive pelvic surgery. The obvious downside is the risk of rectal cancer in the remnant rectum (which is often at least 15 cm in length). The two non-rectal sparing surgical options are Total proctocolectomy with ileal pouch-anal anastomosis (IPAA) and Total proctocolectomy with ileostomy. These procedures involve removal of all mucosa at risk for malignant degeneration but are more complex than IRA, especially IPAA. Several aspects must be considered when deciding on the type of operative therapy.

- *Age of the patient:* Proctocolectomy with ileostomy is a viable option in old patients, those with pre-existing poor bowel and sphincter function and in those with multiple comorbidities. Here, the simplest safest operation with the lowest risk of complications is needed.

- *Risk of rectal cancer:* The risk of rectal cancer may reach 40% after IRA. The risk is cumulative over years. A good rule to follow is the density of rectal polyps. Greater than 20 adenomas in the rectum make further endoscopic surveillance difficult and hence IRA an untenable option. The number of polyps in the anal transition zone (ATZ) is also important, as it is best to perform a hand-sewn anastomosis in this situation. If there is a rectal cancer, then it is best to perform a proctocolectomy with ileostomy.
- *Sphincter function:* Intact sphincteric function is a prerequisite for an IPAA. Even minor impairment will lead to 'accidents' as the stool is usually quite liquid. For these patients, a proctocolectomy with an ileostomy is the only option.
- *Genotype-phenotype association:* As mentioned before, it may be crucial to know the genotype of the patient. It may provide clues for the development of non-colonic problems and thus affect surgical decision-making. A young female patient with attenuated FAP with a mutation in the 3' end of the APC gene (with predilection for desmoids) and minimal rectal polyps may be offered IRA, later during her lifetime or after completing a family, in order to postpone the formation of postoperative desmoids. In contrast, an older male with a hot-spot mutation and several comorbidities may be offered proctocolectomy and ileostomy.

All patients should accept the possibility of requiring a permanent stoma. A temporaray ileostomy may be needed in IPAA to protect the anastomosis. Continent ileostomies are not performed as frequently now, due to the need for reparative surgeries.

HNPCC (Lynch syndrome) is caused by an autosomal dominant inherited germline mutation in the mismatch repair genes. Depending on the gene involved, HNPCC also displays genotype-phenotype association. Lynch II syndrome denotes patients with extracolonic cancers as well, the most common being uterine endometrial cancer. The overall risk of CRC is ~ 50-70%. The crux of the problem in HNPCC is its diagnosis. Amsterdam II criteria can easily be remembered using the "3-2-1" mnemonic: 3 or more relatives with pathologically verified Lynch cancers, in 2 successive generation wherein at least 1 of them was diagnosed before the age of 50. Another commonly used criteria is the Bethesda guidelines. The problem with both these criteria are their poor specificities. Almost 50% of those who meet the Amsterdam criteria and nearly 80% of those who meet the Bethesda guidelines do not have HNPCC! From the surgeon's standpoint, HNPCC should be thought of in the setting of other cancers, which should give the impetus to anticipate metachronous CRC and cancers in other locations.

Pathology of Colon Cancer

More than 90% of colon cancers are adenocarcinomas. Colon cancer can pathologically be classified in several ways which is summarized in the **Table 27-5**.

Broadly speaking, colon cancer may be gland-forming ('adeno' type) or non-gland forming. Some non-gland-forming types may be associated with special features, for example, the signet-ring carcinoma. Accumulation of intracellular mucin can displace or 'push' the nucleus to the periphery, giving the appearance of a signet ring and hence the name. These account for ~ 1% of all CRC and have a poor prognosis due to their tendency for rapid intramural spread. Mucin is sometimes produced in large amounts and may form > 50% of the tumor mass. These tumors are called 'mucinous' or colloid adenocarcinomas and are characterized by an increased incidence in rectum and sigmoid and a poor response to chemotherapy. Another type is the small-cell type, which is a non-gland forming and shows neuroendocrine differentiation. Recently, a medullary-type variety was included in the WHO classification of colon cancer—it is a pointer for MSI and HNPCC. Ulcerative cancers are common in the sigmoid and descending colon while the exophytic tumors seen more common in the cecum and the ascending colon. From the surgeon's standpoint, it is important to recognize the poor prognostic pathological types and the patterns

TABLE 27-5	Pathological classification of colon cancer	
By gross appearance	**By histological type (WHO)**	**By histological grade**
Ulcerative Annular/Scirrhous Exophytic Infiltrative	Adenocarcinoma in situ Adenocarcinoma Mucinous/colloid type Signet ring cell type Squamous Adenosquamous Medullary Small cell (oat cell) Other (lymphoma, Kaposi's, carcinoid, etc.)	Well differentiated Moderately differentiated Poorly or undifferentiated

of clinical progression in patients. Less than 3% of CRC have another primary at the same time ('synchronous') and another 3% develop another primary within first 5 years of surgical resection of the previous cancer ('metachronous').

Presentation of Colon Cancer

With increasing use of colonoscopic screening, colon cancer may be found at an early asymptomatic stage and thus have a good prognosis. In general, patients who present with symptoms of colon cancer have a lower 5-year survival compared to their asymptomatic counterparts. Most common symptoms include:

- abdominal pain
- alteration in bowel habits (includes frequency, consistency and caliber)
- bleeding (melena and hematochezia)
- anemia.

Unexplained and isolated anemia without any GI symptoms may be present in up to 10% of the CRC patients and for this reason, CRC should be ruled out in any male or non-menstruating female with unexplained iron-deficiency anemia. CRC may also present with perforation or obstruction, both of which confer poor prognosis. Left-sided colon cancers are often constrictive and patients may complain of constipation alternating with diarrhea or a change in the caliber of the stool. Sigmoid cancers can mimic diverticulitis and cause pain, obstruction or fistulas to the bladder or vagina. Right-sided colon cancers often present as melena or anemia and are less likely to be constrictive. An uncommon, yet interesting presentation of colon cancer is in association with *Streptococcus bovis* infection or bacteremia. Those with *S. bovis* infection have a 25-30% chance of harboring colon cancer, although colonic polyps are even more common than carcinoma. Fecal carriage rate of *S. bovis* in the CRC population is much higher than the normal population. The reason for this association is unknown.

Staging

The staging of colon cancer has undergone an evolution with several different classifications and their modifications. Still remaining are the Duke's staging system, the Astler-Coller modification of Duke's system and the TNM classification, which is used in American-Joint-Committee-on-Cancer (AJCC) staging. Duke originally designed his staging for rectal cancer, but it came to be used in colon cancer because of its simplicity.

A	Invasion of muscularis propria—'within the wall'
B	Invasion of subserosa—'through the wall'
C	Lymph node involvement

Later, he subcategorized lymph nodes into those that are near the specimen (C1—perirectal) and those that are at the mesenteric vessel ligature points (C2—apical). Stage D for distant metastasis was added. The Astler-Coller staging (MAC) differs slightly as follows,

A	Still 'within the wall' but invasion of submucosa
B	Still 'through the wall', but B1-muscularis propria, B2-subserosa, B3 (adjacent structures)
C	Lymph node involvement and C1, C2, C3 are B1, B2, B3 with nodal involvement respectively
D	Distant metastases

MAC was considered useful, in that it identified the importance of submucosal invasion, the invasion of muscularis and subserosa and the involvement of lymph nodes. The TNM/AJCC (6th edition) classification, is most widely used now:

Stage 0	T is	N 0	M 0
Stage I	T 1-2	N 0	M 0
Stage II A	T 3	N 0	M 0
Stage II B	T 4	N 0	M 0
Stage III A	T 1-2	N 1	M 0
Stage III B	T 3-4	N 1	M 0
Stage III C	Any T	N 2	M 0
Stage IV	Any T	Any N	M 1

T is	In situ carcinoma
T 1	Invading submucosa
T 2	Invading muscularis propria
T 3	Invading subserosa
T 4	Invading adjacent structures
N 1	Regional nodes 1-3
N 2	Regional nodes > 4
M 1	Metastasis

Critically important in staging of colon cancer is an accurate knowledge of what the term 'regional lymph node involvement' implies. A quick reference is given below:

Tumor site	Regional lymph nodes
Cecum	Cecal (ant/post), Ileocolic, R colic
Ascending colon	Ileocolic, right colic, middle colic
Hepatic flexure	Right colic, middle colic
Transverse colon	Middle colic
Splenic flexure	Middle colic, left colic and also inferior mesenteric
Descending colon	Inferior mesenteric, also left colic and sigmoid
Sigmoid Colon	Inferior mesenteric, sigmoidal and even superior rectal (especially when the rectosigmoid is involved)

Next to these classifications, the following terms are commonly used clinically:

- Local—confined to colon only, no lymph nodes involved
- Locoregional—colon with regional lymph node involvement
- Locally advanced—colonic tumor mass infiltrating into adjacent structures
- Advanced—implying distant metastases.

Screening

Accepting the theory of progressive transformation from a benign polyp to an invasive cancer, provides the rationale for colonoscopic evaluation which allows timely early detection of prolonged lesions and thus should potentially prevent the development of CRC. Listed below are the recommendations for CRC-screening promoted by the American Cancer Society and the Agency for Health Care Policy and Research (comprised of the American College of Gastroenterology, American Gastroenterological Association, American Society of Colon and Rectal Surgeons, American Society for Gastrointestinal Endoscopy and Society of American Gastrointestinal Endoscopic Surgeons) **(Table 27-6)**.

The National Polyp Study and American Society of Colon and Rectal Surgeons recommendations for surveillance after polypectomy are listed in **Table 27-7**.

Preoperative Work-up

The preoperative work-up of colon cancer can be done comprehensively, by keeping in mind the following facts:

- Detection of a lesion anywhere in the colon mandates the full visualization of the colon.

TABLE 27-6	Recommendations for CRC screening	
CRC risk	**Recommended screening options**	**Age to begin screening**
Average	At least one of the following: • FOBT* annually • Flexible sigmoidoscopy every 5 years • FOBT annually and flexible sigmoidoscopy every 5 years • Air contrast barium enema every 5-10 years • Colonoscopy every 10 years	50 years
Family history	At least one of the following • Air contrast barium enema every 5 years • Colonoscopy every 10 years	Whichever is earliest: • 40 years • 10 years before the age of diagnosis of the youngest affected family member
HNPCC	• Colonoscopy every 1-3 years • Genetic counseling/testing	21 years
FAP	• Flexible sigmoidoscopy or colonoscopy every 1-2 years • Genetic counseling/ testing	Puberty
Ulcerative colitis	Colonoscopy with biopsies for dysplasia every 1-2 years	Whichever is earliest: • 7-8 years after diagnosis of pancolitis • 12-15 years after diagnosis of left-sided colitis

* FOBT—Fecal occult blood testing

TABLE 27-7	Recommendations for surveillance after polypectomy	
Polyp burden	**Time to 1st follow-up colonoscopy**	**Time to next follow-up colonoscopy**
< 1 cm, single	3 years	If recurrent polyps, 1 year If normal, 5 years
> 1 cm or multiple	1 year	If recurrent polyps, 1 year If normal, 5 years
< 3 tubular adenomas or <1 cm (no family history of polyps of CRC)	5 years	If recurrent polyps, 1 year If normal, 5 years
> 3 cm sessile (completely resected)	3-6 months to 1 year	6-12 months for a year and then every year for 5 years

- Up to 20% of CRC patients present with metastases and synchronous liver lesions.
- Roughly 15% or more of liver lesions are nonpalpable intraoperatively.
- CEA functions as a useful tool in post-resection surveillance.
- Presence of accumulating evidence that genetic mutation may help identify a subset of patients who may or may not be suitable for certain treatments.

With the above in mind, the preoperative work-up of colon cancer should include the following:

- Full colonoscopy
- If full colonoscopy not done, then double contrast barium enema or CT colonography
- CT scan of the abdomen and pelvis (preferably with IV contrast)
- CT scan of the chest to rule out metastases
- Preoperative serum CEA level
- Evaluation of urinary tract with intravenous pyelogram or cystoscopy in selected cases (large bulky tumors and/or with urinary symptoms)
- K-ras genotyping for planning chemotherapy
- MRI when CT with IV contrast is not preferable
- PET or PET-CT in selected cases (routine preoperative use is not recommended).

While not considered a necessity, a preoperative CT scan has become routine practice in most centers. CT is useful for detecting lymph node involvement, metastatic liver lesions, transmural tumor spread and peritoneal implants although the sensitivity to detect these abnormalities is different for each. Although there has been a trend toward using MRI and PET, these studies are not recommended as a routine. They are more commonly used in rectal cancer, in cases of recurrence or to assess resectability in reoperative situations.

Carcinoembryonic Antigen

Carcinoembryonic antigen (CEA) is a glycoprotein (antigenic) that is secreted by the epithelial cells of the GI tract. It was found to be present in extracts from colon cancer tissue (carcino) and also found to be produced in prenatal fetal tissue (embryonic) and hence the name 'carcinoembryonic antigen'. CEA is elevated in a multitude of neoplastic and non-neoplastic conditions (including heavy smoking). Several studies have proved the utility of CEA testing in colon cancer so much that it has been recommended to be integrated to the TNM staging. CEA may or may not be increased in colon cancer and after surgery. A level above 5 ng/ml is concerning. The importance of CEA is that:

- An elevated serum CEA (> 5 ng/ml) is an independent poor prognostic indicator in colon cancer, irrespective of stage.

- In node-negative CRC, elevated preoperative CEA predicts poor 5-year survival.
- In node-positive CRC, elevated preoperative CEA predicts a short time to recurrence.
- Lack of postoperative decline in preoperative CEA suggest possible reminiscent tumor and also worse 5-year survival.
- Prognostic capacity of preoperative elevated CEA is believed to be independent of the number of histologically positive nodes.
- Elevation of CEA seems to correlate with the degree of encirclement of tumor in the colonic lumen, but unrelated to presence or absence of obstruction.
- Elevation of postoperative CEA during surveillance should prompt a search for recurrent disease.

Although there is lack of sufficient evidence to support adjuvant chemotherapy in node-negative patients with an elevated serum CEA, such therapy is still being debated. CEA has assumed so much credibility as a prognostic factor that it has been suggested to include CEA in the TNM classification wherein CRC patients would be classified as either Cx (not assessable), C0 (< 5 ng/ml) or C1 (>= 5 ng/ml).

Prognosis

Prognosis of colon cancer as in the case with other cancers depends on the stage. The 5-year survival of CRC patients, as per the SEER database, according to the AJCC sixth edition system, may be summarized as in **Table 27-8**.

It is to be noted that the prognosis of Stage IIIa tumors is better than that of stage IIb. Possibly, some patients with T4 lesions (stage IIb) underwent insufficiently radical resections or tumor biology was unfavorable. Whether these patients would benefit by adjuvant chemotherapy is a topic of debate. Prognostication of colon cancer has become more complicated with the continuing identification of new prognostic indicators, which were cleverly summarized by the College of American Pathologists

TABLE 27-8	Survival rates for colon cancer by stage
Stage	**5-year survival**
Overall	65.2%
Stage I	93.2%
Stage IIa	84.7%
Stage IIb	72.2%
Stage IIIa	83.4%
Stage IIIb	64.1%
Stage IIIc	44.3%
Stage IV	8.1%

Consensus Statement in 1999. The prognostic features were classified into several categories based on the presence of 'statistically robust' evidence **(Table 27-9)**.

Discussion here will be limited to only those factors that are of importance to the surgical oncologist. Local tumor extent can be quite variable within a stage designation. For instance, 25% of T3 tumors (invasion of the musculatis propria) will have malignant serosal cell scrapings or the T3 tumor can/may coexist with an inflammatory, hyperplastic or mesothelial reaction on the serosal surface mimicking a pT4 lesion. Identification of serosal involvement should upstage the tumor. Also, pT4 lesions are subclassified into pT4a (penetration of adjacent organ/structure) and pT4b (penetration of the peritoneum, including free perforation). The 5-year survival is worse for pT4b compared to pT4a in both metastatic (0% vs 12%) and non-metastatic (43% vs 49%) situations. Another important prognostic factor is the 'number of positive lymph nodes'. An early NSABP study showed that those with > = 4 positive lymph nodes had a significantly worse survival than those less than 4 which is reflected in the TNM classification: N1 (< 4) and N2 (> = 4). By consensus, the required number of lymph nodes in the surgical specimen to adequately stage a tumor is 12. So, the surgical specimen should carefully be inspected for 12 nodes and if unsuccessful, then special techniques such as fat clearing should be used. If < 12 nodes are found after detailed examination postoperatively, then the patient is considered to be inadequately staged requiring

closer surveillance. It is important to reiterate that nodal status (N) is determined solely by regional node involvement (or lack thereof) whereas involvement of non-regional or distant nodes constitutes metastatic disease.

It is not uncommon to find enlarged mesenteric extramural nodules during surgery. These mesenteric nodules may be lymph nodes replaced by tumor (in which case, there may be histological evidence of reminiscent lymph node architecture—pN disease) or discrete tumor nodules (pT3) themselves. The recent guidelines (AJCC 6th edition) however disregard this differentiation because mesenteric/extramural nodules uniformly confer worse survival. Hence, these nodules are now regarded as pN (nodal) disease, resulting in upstaging. Sometimes cancer 'deposits' may be found in lymph nodes. Those that are < 0.2 mm in size are detectable only by immuno-histochemistry or molecular diagnostics and are called Isolated Tumor Cells (ITC). Currently ITC are assigned pN0 status. Deposits > 0.2 mm but less than 2 mm, identifiable by routine histology, are called 'micro-metastases'—these are assigned pN status—resulting in the upstaging of tumors.

Identification of tumor in an endothelial-lined channel is termed 'angiolymphatic invasion', which has been proven to confer worse outcome in all stages of CRC, including malignant polyps.

Two other important prognostic factors from the surgeon's standpoint are Residual tumor status ('R' status)

TABLE 27-9	**Prognostic factors in colon cancer**	
Category	**Definition**	**Factors**
I	Definitely proved to be significant by statistically robust studies	• Local tumor extent • Regional lymph node involvement • Mesenteric nodules • Micrometastases • Vascular invasion • Residual tumor status • Elevated preoperative serum CEA
IIA	Extensively studied but still needs statistically robust studies	• Histological grade • Circumferential radial margins (CRM) • Post-neoadjuvant residual tumor status
IIB	Promising in many studies	• Histological type • 18q deletions • Tumor border • Microsatellite instability
III	Not yet studied well	• Ploidy status • K-ras genotyping • Focal neuroendocrine differentiation • Proliferative activity • Microvessel density
IV	Studied well and show no prognostic value	• Gross tumor configuration • Tumor size

and the tumor border. The term 'R' status indicates 'residual' tumor left behind after resection, implying that a curative resection was not achieved. The term 'positive margins' the same as there is residual disease. In contrast, 'r' is used to denote recurrent tumor in a patient with prior curative resection. This means that a temporary disease-free status had been achieved and that the tumor has now recurred. Another situation warranting special terminology is the disease status following neoadjuvant therapy, in which case 'y' is used in TNM staging. The R status, expected, can be classified as R0 (no residual disease), R1 (microscopic residual disease), R2 (macroscopic residual disease) and Rx (not assessable). Studies have shown that R status as expected affects prognosis. A study in T4 patients showed that the subset of patients who underwent incomplete resection (R+ status) had a 19% recurrence free 10 year actuarial survival compared to 58% in the node positive T4 group and 88% in the node negative T4 group.

The advancing edge of the gross tumor mass is called 'tumor border'. This may be infiltrative or expanding. Surgeons can grossly identify an infiltrative tumor border (which has a worse prognosis) by the inability to clearly define the edges of the tumor. Although many studies suggest that an infiltrative tumor border confers worse prognosis, it is still considered a category IIb factor, for want of statistically strong evidence. It is to be noted that angiolymphatic invasion and tumor border configuration are stage-independent prognostic factors in colon cancer.

Preoperative Preparation for Colorectal Surgery

Important in the preoperative preparation for colon resection would be:
- good counseling with the patient
- stoma marking
- preoperative antibiotics
- bowel preparation.

The current standard of care for preoperative preparation includes administering a bowel preparation the day before surgery to reduce the fecal load of the colon. This is believed to decrease the bacterial load of the colon and thus the risk of spillage of fecal contents with contamination of wound and abdominal cavity. The two preparations most commonly used are polyethylene glycol and sodium phosphate. Patients seem to tolerate sodium phosphate better than polyethylene glycol because it requires the consumption of significantly smaller volume and causes less bloating and nausea. The side effects of sodium phosphate are fluid and electrolyte imbalances and therefore this agent is not recommended in patients with renal failure, ascites, cirrhosis or heart failure.

The low rate of complications, mainly anastomotic leak in primary closure of traumatic injuries involving the unprepared colon has made some surgeons reconsider the need for preoperative bowel preparation in elective colon resection. Some studies have shown no difference in the rates of wound infection, intra-abdominal abscess and anastomotic dehiscence between those receiving mechanical bowel preparation and those without. A drawback of an unprepared colon might be the difficulty in handling a feces-loaded colon which can be heavy and hard to move compared to a cleansed colon, especially during laparoscopic procedures.

Preoperative antibiotics can be given orally and intravenously. The rationale behind oral antibiotics is the ability to decrease the bacterial load in the colon and, in combination with a bowel preparation, decrease the overall rate of contamination if spillage should occur. The most common combination includes three doses each of 1 gm neomycin and 1 gm erythromycin. Erythromycin can cause GI distress and thus ciprofloxacin or metronidazole may be substituted. Intravenous antibiotics are now part of the Surgical Care Improvement Project (SCIP) for colorectal surgery. It mandates that a broad-spectrum antibiotic be given prior to the skin incision and re-dosed as indicated throughout the procedure. Most surgeons use a second or third generation cephalosporin, or combination of fluoroquinolone and metronidazole for patients with a penicillin allergy. Debate regarding preoperative bowel preparation and oral antibiotics continues, but the current standard of care is the combination of mechanical bowel preparation and intravenous antibiotics, without oral antibiotics.

Any patient that may require a stoma should be seen by an enterostomal therapy (ET) nurse preoperatively for counseling, education and marking of the stoma site.

Another aspect of preoperative planning is the need for ureteral stents to facilitate ureteral identification, especially the left ureter during a sigmoid resection. The stents are placed after induction of anesthesia by cystoscopy. They are most beneficial during reoperative pelvic surgery or when significant retroperitoneal inflammation is present.

Surgical Management (Figures 27-3 and 27-4)

The principles for oncological surgery for the colon are as follows:
- Adequate proximal and distal margins (about 5 cm).
- High mesenteric ligation.
- Adequate regional lymph node clearance, with a minimum of 12 lymph nodes.
- Well perfused, tensionless anastomoses.
- Excellent tissue coaptation at the anastomosis.
- A temporary stoma when in doubt of anastomotic integrity.

The treatment strategy for the different stages of colon cancer are summarized in **Table 27-10**.

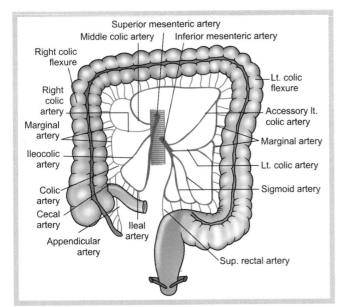

Figure 27-3: Blood supply of colon (Skandalakis JE, Colborn GL, Weidman TA, et al: Skandalakis' Surgical Anatomy: http://www.accesssurgery.com. Copyright © The McGraw-Hill Companies, Inc. All rights reserved)

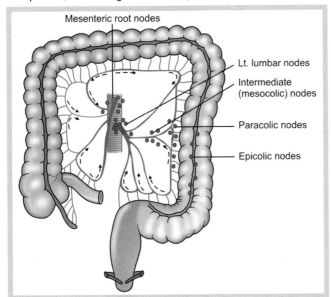

Figure 27-4: Lymphatic drainage of colon (Skandalakis JE, Colborn GL, Weidman TA, et al: Skandalakis' Surgical Anatomy: http://www.accesssurgery.com. Copyright © The McGraw-Hill Companies, Inc. All rights reserved)

Right-sided Colon Cancers

Tumors in the cecum or ascending colon are treated by a right hemicolectomy. This involves transection of distal ileum about 10 cm proximal to the ileocecal valve and of the colon at or near the hepatic flexure. The mesenteric resection begins with ligation of the ileocolic, right colic and right branch of the middle colic vessels. The dissections of the mesentery along the superior mesenteric

TABLE 27-10	Treatment strategy for the different stages of colon cancer
Stage	**Management***
Stage 0	Wide local excision (polypectomy) or segmental colon resection
Stage I	Segmental colon resection
Stage II	Segmental colon resection, chemotherapy controversial
Stage III	Segmental colon resection + adjuvant chemotherapy
Stage IV	Systemic chemotherapy, palliative surgery as needed

*The management of liver metastases in CRC is dealt with separately in another chapter.

and middle colic veins requires caution and care to avoid injury to these vessels which can be a disastrous event. The right ureter and duodenum should be identified and caution heeded while dissecting near them. Ileocolic continuity is achieved with a side-to-side anastomosis.

Left-sided Colon Cancers

For tumors of the splenic flexure or descending colon, a left hemicolectomy is required. The left branch of the middle colic and left colic vessels are ligated and the respective mesentery is removed. Mobilization of the splenic flexure is necessary. This is done cautiously so as to avoid splenic and pancreatic injury. The lesser sac is opened widely and the omentum attached to the colonic segment is removed *en bloc*. A primary anastomosis is created between the mid-transverse colon and sigmoid colon, which demands their mobilization.

Transverse Colon Cancers

Tumors of the hepatic flexure and proximal transverse colon are treated by an extended right hemicolectomy, which involves taking the middle colic artery at its origin. A primary anastomosis between ileum and distal transverse colon is created.

There are three options for approaching tumors in the mid and distal transverse colon. The most commonly performed is the extended right hemicolectomy with an anastomosis between the ileum and descending colon. Another option is an extended left hemicolectomy, which involves extending the margins of a left hemicolectomy to include the right branch of the middle colic artery and performing an anastomosis between the proximal transverse colon and the descending colon. A final option is the transverse colectomy involving ligation of the middle colic vessels with resection of the transverse colon. Both ascending and descending colon are widely mobilized so that a tension-free anastomosis can be constructed. Anastomoses can be constructed end-to-end (preferred by the authors), side-to-side or any variation.

Sigmoid Cancers

A sigmoidectomy involves ligation of the inferior mesenteric vessels and anastomosis between the descending colon and the upper rectum. Mobilization of the splenic flexure is imperative for a safe, tension-free anastomosis. The left ureter should always be identified and protected **(Figure 27-5)**.

Synchronous Colon Cancers

The incidence of synchronous colon cancers is 2-11% and synchronous adenomas occur up to 30% of the time. Adenomas can be resected at the time of colonoscopy but synchronous cancers are treated by surgical resection. If two primary cancers are widely separated then the appropriate resections with anastomoses are performed. In heeding anatomic constraints and oncologic principles, it might become necessary to perform a subtotal colectomy

with ileo-rectal anastomosis without or with a short ileal pouch to avert excessive defecatory frequency.

Surgical Details of a Right Hemicolectomy

There are several variations on any type of procedure depending on surgeons' preferences, below is a list of the essential steps of a right hemicolectomy. Acknowledging tumor-site related differences, this list is applicable to any colon resection:

1. Midline versus right transverse incision.
2. Explore the abdominal cavity for evidence of metastatic disease including good visualization and palpation of the liver possibly with ultrasound evaluation.
3. Incise along the white line of Toldt, mobilizing the colon medially.
4. Identify and protect the ureter and the duodenum.
5. Divide the colon proximally and distally.
6. Ligate the ileocolic vessel and the right branch or main trunk of the middle colic artery at their origins.

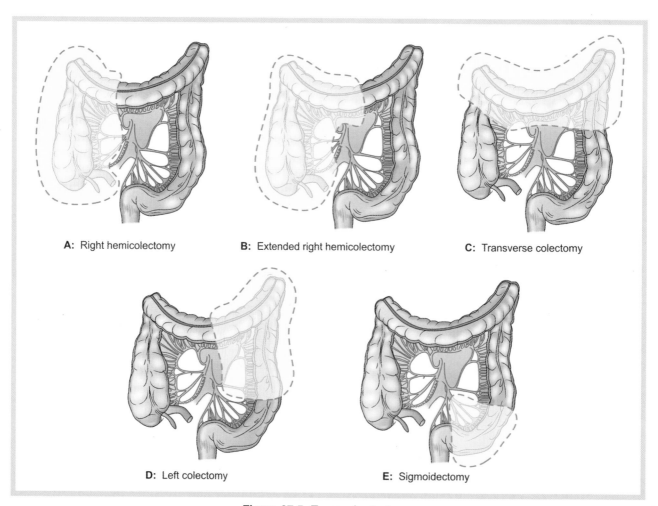

A: Right hemicolectomy **B:** Extended right hemicolectomy **C:** Transverse colectomy

D: Left colectomy **E:** Sigmoidectomy

Figure 27-5: Types of colectomy

7. Remove specimen with marked proximal and distal ends.
8. Anastomose the colon and ileum.
9. Check the anastomosis for patency and integrity.
10. Close the abdomen.

A midline incision is made and the abdomen is inspected for any signs of metastatic disease. The colon is then assessed for the location of the tumor either by visualizing a tattooed site or palpating a mass. Multiple retraction devices are available to help aid in exposure. The cecum is identified and the dissection begins along the white line of Toldt. This is an avascular plane, so bleeding is a sign of dissection in the incorrect plane. Identification of the ureter is essential. The colon is mobilized in a lateral to medial fashion. The duodenum is exposed as the colonic mesentery is carefully separated from the duodenum and pancreas.

Once the colon is fully mobilized the points of transection are selected. The distal ileum is divided 10 cm proximal to the ileocecal junction. The distal margin depends largely on the site of the lesion and should be at least 5 cm distal from the tumor. The bowel is divided using a linear cutting stapler. The peritoneum of the mesentery is then scored with electrocautery. The iliocolic vessels are identified, ligated and transected at their origin. The middle colic vessels are identified and the right branches are transected in a similar fashion. The mesentery and associated lymphatic tissue are divided and the specimen is removed. The distal and proximal margins should be marked for proper orientation.

An anastomosis between distal ileum and colon is performed. Anastomoses can be hand-sewn or stapled depending on the surgeon's preference. The anastomosis is checked for intactness, patency and viability and should be without tension. Next the mesenteric defect is closed.

The abdomen is then re-explored and the peritoneal surfaces checked for hemostasis, serosal injury and leakage. A lap, sponge, needle and instrument count is performed prior to closure of the incision.

Surgical Details of a Left Hemicolectomy or Sigmoidectomy

Left colectomies can vary depending on the site of the tumor but follow similar techniques as a right colectomy. Dissection includes mobilization of the splenic flexure and ligation of the left colic vessels and/or the inferior mesenteric vessels.

The abdominal cavity is entered and inspected as described for a right colectomy. The entire left colon is freed from its retroperitoneal attachments by incising and dissecting along the white line of Toldt. Identification and protection of the left ureter are essential.

Mobilization of the splenic flexure involves entering the lesser sac and separation of the gastrocolic omentum to the level of the middle colic artery. The transverse colon and splenic flexure are lifted off the retroperitoneum inferior to the spleen. The inferior border of the distal pancreas is identified to avoid pancreatic injury. Furthermore, the duodenum and jejunum at the ligament of Treitz may reach high onto the colonic mesentery, a variation to remember so that inadvertent injury is prevented. Once the colon is completely mobilized the sites of transection are selected and colon and mesentery are divided. The resection of splenic flexure lesions requires left colic vascular ligation and sigmoid lesions includes ligation of the inferior mesenteric vasculature. Obviously, variations in resection-extent are appropriately matched to the location of the lesion.

A colo-colonic or colorectal anastomosis is then performed as described above for a right hemicolectomy. A colorectal anastomosis requires the patient to be placed in the lithotomy position so access to the rectum from the anus is available. A circular stapling device is used to construct the anastomosis. An anvil is placed in the distal colon and connected to the stapling device that is passed through the anus to the proximal rectum. Once connected, the stapler is fired and the anastomosis is created.

Laparoscopic Surgery in Colon Cancer

Laparoscopic surgery has been an accepted approach for patients with benign disease, but surgeons were slower to adopt laparoscopic colectomy for colon cancer. This was in part due to early data concerning for port site recurrence and concern over the ability to perform sound oncologic resections laparoscopically. Several studies have since shown that implantation at port or wound sites was less than 1% for both laparoscopic and open surgeries. Multiple studies have been performed looking at the short-term and long-term data for patients undergoing laparoscopic resection for colon cancer. In 2004, the results of the Clinical Outcomes of Surgical Therapy (COST) study were reported. This was a large, multi-centered, randomized trial in North America that showed no difference in recurrence rates among patients undergoing laparoscopic versus open colectomy. In addition, the extents of resection, resection margins and lymph node harvest with laparoscopic resection of colon cancer were similar to those for open resection. The short-term outcomes from multiple randomized trials have shown that, although the operating times for laparoscopic colectomies are generally longer than open colectomies, the times to passage of flatus, first bowel movements and re-establishment of regular diet were shorter. This resulted in decreased length of stay, thereby offsetting the increased operative costs. These studies have shown that laparoscopic surgery to be an acceptable alternative to open resections for colon cancer.

Surgical Details of Laparoscopic Right Hemicolectomy

For a laparoscopic right colectomy, some surgeons may prefer patients to be in a modified lithotomy position using stirrups for anticipated intraoperative colonoscopy, but the majority of surgeons will place the patient supine on the operating table. Both arms should be tucked at the patient's side to allow both the surgeon and the assistant freedom to operate. The patient's chest should be secured to the table with tape to prevent sliding while tilting the OR table.

Trocar placement is important for any laparoscopic procedure. Some surgeons prefer entering the abdomen with a Hassan technique at the umbilicus, while others use a left upper quadrant Veress needle approach. Patients with previous abdominal surgery may warrant one approach over the other. A 10-12 mm trocar is placed in the left lower quadrant, followed by placement of a 5 mm trocar in the left upper quadrant. Additional trocars can be used if deemed necessary for assistance.

The surgery then proceeds similar as described in the open technique. The abdominal cavity is examined for evidence of metastases. Next, the patient is placed in the Trendelenburg position to begin cecal mobilization. The ureter should be identified, often easily seen at the pelvic rim. The key to laparoscopic surgery is traction and countertraction. Some surgeons prefer the standard lateral to medial mobilization; however, others use a medial to lateral dissection when performing laparoscopic colectomies. Mobilization continues to the level of the hepatic flexure.

At this point the patient should be placed in the reverse Trendelenburg position for mobilization of the hepatic flexure. The gastrocolic ligament is grasped and retracted up toward the abdominal wall. The plane between the gastrocolic ligament and transverse colon mesentery allows mobilization of the hepatic flexure. Identification and protection of the duodenum is important as dissection continues.

After mobilization of the hepatic flexure, the ileocolic vessels should be ligated. They are easily identified by applying tension on the junction of the cecum and ileum. Mesenteric windows are created in the avascular planes and the pedicle of the right colic vessels can be ligated as well.

Resection of the right colon and anastomosis can then be done extracorporeal or intra-corporeal using a linear cutting stapler. If done extracorporeally, a 4-6 cm incision is made either periumbilically or in the right lower quadrant. The wound should be protected with a plastic wound protector and the specimen is brought out of the abdomen. Resection and anastomosis is performed similar to the open technique and then the bowel is returned to the abdominal cavity. The abdomen is irrigated and

inspected for hemostasis. Trocars are removed under direct visualization. The fascia and skin are then closed.

Surgical Details of Laparoscopic Left Hemicolectomy

A laparoscopic left hemicolectomy is essentially the reverse of a right hemicolectomy with the exception of the patient being in the modified lithotomy position. The trocars are placed on the right side of the abdomen. Once access to the peritoneal cavity is accomplished, the abdomen is inspected for evidence of metastatic disease. The ureter is identified and protected followed by mobilization of the left colon up to the splenic flexure. The patient is placed in a reverse Trendelenburg position with left side up for splenic flexure mobilization. It often helps to place an additional 5 mm trocar in the left lower quadrant. The omentum is elevated anteriorly as it is separated from the colon. Once mobilized, the left colic artery is ligated and the colon is exteriorized through a periumbilical incision or left lower quadrant incision to complete the anastomosis.

Surgical Details for Laparoscopic Sigmoidectomy

For a laparoscopic sigmoidectomy the patient is always placed in lithotomy position for access to the ano-rectum. It is important to keep the thighs level with the abdomen to prevent interference with instrument manipulation. The laparoscope is introduced through a supraumbilical port and the other trocars are inserted. One is suprapubic, one is placed in the right lower quadrant and the last is placed in the left lower quadrant.

Mobilization begins with the patient in steep Trendelenburg with right side down, again following the white line of Toldt. The ureter should be identified and avoided. After mobilization of the sigmoid, dissection continues into the proximal pelvis until the proximal to mid-rectum is free along the left margin. The sigmoid is then retracted cephalad and to the patient's left to open the presacral window on the right. The superior hemorrhoidal and sigmoid vessels are then visualized and ligated. For a more extensive resection, the inferior mesenteric vessels are taken. The descending colon and splenic flexure are mobilized to gain sufficient length for a tension-free anastomosis.

Dissecting from side-to-side along the rectal wall and firing a linear cutting stapler divides the rectum. The sigmoid colon is then exteriorized through a midline or left lower quadrant incision. The proximal margin is determined and the sigmoid is resected. The anastomosis is performed using a circular stapler device. The anvil of the stapler is placed in the sigmoid and secured using a purse-string suture. The sigmoid is then returned to the abdomen and the fascia of the incision is closed.

The abdomen is re-insufflated and the anvil is attached to the shaft of the stapling device, which has been inserted into the anus and advanced across the staple line. The stapler is closed, the bowel ends are approximated and the stapler is fired. A proctoscope is then advanced to inspect the anastomosis. The pelvis can be filled with irrigation fluid air is insufflated through the proctoscope and the pelvis is inspected for air bubbles, which can signify a leak at the anastomosis. Once the anastomosis has been checked for hemostasis and air leak, the trocars are removed and fascia and skin closed.

Obstructing Colon Cancers

Malignancy is the most common cause of large bowel obstruction and treatment depends on location of the tumor and the patient's overall condition. Right-sided obstructing cancers are often treated with resection and primary anastomosis, while left sided obstructing cancers are often treated with diverting colostomy with resection of the tumor. Healthier patients with left-sided obstructing cancers may be candidates for resection with primary anastomosis and diverting loop ileostomy. Another option for obstructing left-sided or rectal cancers is colonic stenting. Stents may help avoid an emergency operation, allow time for decompression and bowel preparation and allow for colonoscopic evaluation of the proximal colon before surgical resection.

Perforated Colon Cancers

Perforated colon cancers often present with peritonitis and are associated with high rates of local recurrence and low rate of overall survival. Perforation occurs as a result of the tumor eroding through the colonic wall or due to distention of bowel proximal to an obstructing cancer. Surgery amounts to an emergency laparotomy with resection of the tumor and irrigation of the abdominal cavity. Most often an end-colostomy with Hartmann's pouch or mucous fistula is created, but some patients may be candidates for primary anastomosis and diverting loop ileostomy.

Options for Palliative Surgery

Patients with metastatic disease and poor prognosis may choose palliative care. Options for palliative surgery include diverting colostomy or ileostomy proximal to the tumor to relieve an obstruction. Alternatively, a colonic stent may be placed across the obstructing lesion. Bleeding from a tumor is a complication of advanced cancer, so patients suitable for surgery may be candidates for resection to prevent continued blood loss.

Complications

Complications of colon resections include those associated with any surgery such as bleeding, wound infection, myocardial infarction, pulmonary complications and death. Specific complications related to colon surgery include anastomotic leak, damage to the ureter or damage to adjacent organs (e.g. splenic capsule tear and small bowel enterotomy).

Anastomotic leaks may occur as a result of a compromised anastomosis from tension or inadequate blood supply. Patients can present with a wide range of symptoms including ileus, fever, abdominal pain, nausea, vomiting, leukocytosis or failure to thrive. A patient's wound should be inspected daily and wound dehiscence, development of a fistula or extensive erythema should raise concern for an anastomotic leak. If there is concern for a leak, a CT scan should be ordered to evaluate the anastomosis. Evidence of a leak includes abscess or fluid collection near the anastomosis, large amounts of fluid in the peritoneal cavity or free air. All patients with a confirmed anastomotic leak should be placed on wide-spectrum antibiotics. Leaks may be managed by drainage, which is often performed by interventional radiology or require re-operation. If the patient is spontaneously draining intestinal contents through the wound, i.e. a fistula has developed un-associated with peritonitis, then bowel rest with TPN should be instituted to allow the fistula to heal. If the anastomosis has completely separated or the leak is uncontrolled, sepsis and peritonitis are the consequence and patients require surgical intervention. In these cases, the safest and only option is to resect and to perform an end colostomy with a mucous fistula.

Damage to the ureters can occur while mobilizing the right and left colon from the lateral side walls. Repair of ureteral injuries depends on the location of the injury. Injury to the lower third of the ureter can be repaired in multiple ways. The procedure of choice is reimplantation into the bladder with a psoas-hitch procedure to minimize tension on the ureteral anastomosis. Another option is primary ureteroureterostomy. A stent should be placed to allow the ureter to heal and decrease the chance of stricture. A third option for lower ureteral injuries is transureteroureterostomy. This option is best reserved for injuries that have resulted in large urinomas and pelvic infection because it allows for an anastomosis away from the primary site of infection.

Damage to the middle-third of the ureter should be repaired by primary ureteroureterostomy. Transuretero-ureterostomy is best used when a significant portion of viable ureter is damaged. For damage to the upper third of the ureter, a primary ureteroureterostomy is the procedure of choice. If there is extensive loss of ureter preventing a primary repair, then options include autotransplantation of the kidney and transposition of bowel to replace the ureter. It is imperative to involve and have a urologist at the helm in the management and repair of these injuries.

Injuries to other organs can also occur during colon surgery including small bowel and splenic injuries. Serosal tears and small enterotomies may be repaired primarily. Larger bowel injuries should be repaired with resection and anastomosis. Injury to the spleen can occur while mobilizing the descending and transverse colon at the splenic flexure. The injury is most often a tear of the splenic capsule and may result in significant bleeding. When attempts to stop bleeding are unsuccessful, a splenectomy should be performed. These patients will need vaccinations for *Haemophilus influenzae, Neisseria meningitidis* and *Streptococcus pneumoniae* prior to discharge from the hospital.

Adjuvant Therapy for Resected Disease

Adjuvant therapy for colon cancer has seen a dynamic evolution since the finding of improved response with 5-Fluorouracil (5-FU). Most of the agents currently used were initially proven useful in metastatic disease and then employed in the adjuvant setting. The drugs and regimens commonly used in the adjuvant setting are outlined in **Table 27-11**.

Many combinations exist, but are beyond the scope of this chapter. From the surgeon's standpoint, it is important to know the following:

- Adjuvant chemotherapy is given to all stage III patients and with discretion to stage II patients.
- In stage III colon cancer, adjuvant chemotherapy after resection is the standard of care and it reduces mortality and recurrence by almost 30%. The preferred regimen is FOLFOX. In situations where oxaliplatin cannot be given, 5-FU/LV is used. Currently, FOLFIRI and Avastin are not recommended for stage III adjuvant therapy.
- In stage II disease, adjuvant chemotherapy may be used in selected patients. However, it is important to understand that poor prognostic features (as mentioned below), which are used to identify a subset of stage II patients with poor prognosis, do not necessarily mean that they would respond to adjuvant chemotherapy. So a detailed discussion with the patient and family is a must before adjuvant therapy is given. According to the ASCO guidelines, the stage II patients that are considered high-risk are:
  - T4 tumor (stage IIb)
  - Surgical specimen with 12 nodes or less
  - Lymphovascular invasion (LVI)
  - Perineural invasion
  - High grade or poorly differentiated tumor
  - Signet ring or mucinous histology.
- Adjuvant radiotherapy is still being studied in the setting of colon cancer. If the surgeon feels that the tumor cannot completely be excised, it is prudent to leave radiologically identifiable markers for postoperative radiotherapy along with chemotherapy.
  High preoperative CEA is also a poor prognostic factor in Stage II CRC, but there is insufficient evidence to support adjuvant therapy for this patient population.

Recurrent and Metastatic Disease

For patients who have undergone surgical resection of the CRC with curative intent, 20-40% will have a

TABLE 27-11	Drugs/regimen used in adjuvant setting
Drug/regimen	**Comments**
5-FU	A pyrimidine analog that inhibits thymidylate synthetase and hence thymidine synthesis
Leucovorin(LV)	Otherwise called folinic acid, which generally acts a 'rescue' agent in chemotherapy, but in colon cancer used along with 5-FU because it stabilizes the 5-FU-thymidylate synthetase complex
Levamisole (Obsolete)	An antihelminthic agent that has immunomodulatory effects, now removed from the US market for severe agranulocytosis and neutropenia
Oxaliplatin	A platinum based derivative whose exact mechanism is unknown but believed to work by inhibition of DNA synthesis. Neuropathy is the most important adverse effect
Capecitabine	A prodrug administered orally that is converted by a three step enzymatic process to 5-FU
Irinotecan	Works by inhibiting topoisomerase 1. Adverse effects include severe diarrhea and neutropenia
Cetuximab	Monoclonal antibody to EGF receptor, marketed as "Erbitux" and is known to be effective only in CRC with wild-type K-ras
Bevacizumab	Monoclonal antibody to VEGF, marketed as 'Avastin'. Adverse effects include GI complications including perforation and hypertension
MOF regimen	Semustine + vincristine + 5-FU
FLOX	5-FU/LV (bolus) + oxaliplatin
FOLFOX	5-FU/LV (infusion) + oxaliplatin
FOLFIRI	5-FU/LV + irinotecan

recurrence either locally or at a distant site. Only surgical therapy offers a chance of cure limited usually to select patients with isolated metastases. The most common sites for recurrence include peritoneum, liver and lung.

Patients with isolated local recurrence confirmed by PET scan or CT scan should undergo a wide resection of all surrounding tissue *en bloc* to ensure negative margins, if possible. Patients who present with peritoneal carcinomatosis have a much poorer prognosis. These patients respond poorly to systemic chemotherapy; however, some may have improved survival with cytoreductive surgery (debulking) and Hyperthermic Intraperitoneal Chemoperfusion (HIPEC). Patient selection is key to optimize the mortality and morbidity of HIPEC.

The most common site of distant colorectal metastases is the liver. There is a trend toward aggressive management of liver lesions. Three basic principles guide the surgical therapy of metastatic liver disease:

- The primary tumor should be completely resectable.
- Resection of all liver lesions should leave behind a functional amount of liver.
- There is no other extrahepatic tumor.

PET scanning is often used to determine the extent of extrahepatic metastases. All patients thought to be resectable should undergo operation. Neoadjuvant therapy should be considered before resection as recent studies have shown a survival benefit for patients treated with six cycles of neoadjuvant chemotherapy, followed by liver resection, and further chemotherapy.

Historically only 10-15% of patients with liver metastases were considered resectable; however, this number appears to be increasing due to better chemotherapy and aggressive surgical resections. For the patients deemed unresectable, current therapies include Radio Frequency Ablation (RFA) and Isolated Hepatic Perfusion (IHP). RFA of liver tumors may be approached laparoscopically, percutaneously, or as part of an open procedure. Results depend on many factors including the size and number of metastases. RFA has an overall local recurrence rate of 10-15%. Another option for unresectable disease is isolated hepatic perfusion, which requires isolation of the liver by performing a veno-veno bypass, accessing the gastroduodenal artery for inflow, clamping the suprahepatic IVC and porta hepatis, followed by 60 minutes of chemoperfusion. Another option would be to leave a chemoperfusion port in place—this has shown to not increase response rate compared to one time IHP, but shown to increase median survival in those who do respond. Although less common, patients with isolated lung metastases may also benefit from resection. Predictors of poor outcome in a patient with a lung metastasis include a maximum tumor size greater than 3.75 cm, a serum CEA greater than 5 ng/ml and pulmonary or mediastinal lymph node involvement. All patients with recurrent or metastatic disease regardless of location should undergo systemic chemotherapy.

Follow-up and Surveillance

Follow-up for CRC is aimed at detecting any recurrence or metachronous lesions that are potentially curable. Detection and treatment of recurrent disease may improve survival. Patients should be followed closely within the first few years after resection because 80% of recurrences occur within the first two years and 90% occur within the first four years. About 40-50% of patients will have recurrence of disease after potentially curative resection for CRC. Some advocate for intensive follow-up; however, this has never been standardized and studies have shown that intensive follow-up has not improved overall survival.

Each patient should be evaluated individually to determine proper surveillance. For instance, patients with Stage I cancers have a low likelihood of recurrence and may not need to be followed as closely as high risk patients such as those with HNPCC syndrome or T3 N+ cancers.

Imaging studies and laboratory tests, including CBC and LFTs, have not been shown to improve detection of recurrence or metastasis in asymptomatic disease and therefore are not recommended. CT scans are not recommended for primary detection of recurrence, but may be useful if CEA is elevated. The recommendations may vary depending on the organization, but the American Society of Clinical Oncology, the National Comprehensive Cancer Network and the American Society of Colon and Rectal Surgeons generally agree on the following:

1. CEA levels every 2-3 months for 2 years, then every 3-6 months for 3 years, then annually.
2. History and physical every 3-6 months for 3 years, then annually.
3. Colonoscopy 1 year after surgery, then every 3-5 years if the patient remains free of polyps and cancer.

Landmark Papers

1. Abdalla EK, Vauthey JN, Ellis LM, et al. Recurrence and outcomes following hepatic resection, radiofrequency ablation and combined resection/ablation for colorectal liver metastases. Annals of Surgery 2004;239:818-25.
2. Andre T, Boni C, Mounedji-Boudiaf L, et al. Oxaliplatin, fluorouracil and leukovorin as adjuvant treatment for colon cancer. New England Journal of Medicine 2004;350(23):2343-51.
3. Clinical Outcomes of Surgical Therapy Study Group. A comparison of laparoscopically assisted and open colectomy for colon cancer. New England Journal of Medicine 2004;350:2050-9.

4. Cohen AM. Surgical considerations in patients with cancer of the colon and rectum. Semin Oncol 1991;18:381-7.

5. Fraker DL, Soulen M. Regional therapy of hepatic metastases. Hematology Oncology Clinics of North America 2002;16:947-67.

6. Harford WV. Colorectal cancer screening and surveillance. Surgical Oncology Clinics of North America 2006; 15:1-20.

7. Joseph NE, Sigurdson ER, Hanlon AL, et al. Accuracy of determining nodal negativity in colorectal cancer on the basis of the number of nodes retrieved on resection. Annals of Surgical Oncology 2003;10:213-8.

8. Levoyer TE, Sigurdson ER, Hanlon AL, et al. Colon cancer survival is associated with increasing number of lymph nodes analyzed: a secondary survey of intergroup trial INT-0089. Journal of Clinical Oncology 2003;21:2912-9.

9. Locker GY, Hamilton S, Harris J, et al. ASCO 2006 update of recommendations for the use of tumor markers in gastrointestinal cancer. Journal of Clinical Oncology 2006;24:5313-27.

10. Registry of Hepatic Metastases. Resection of the liver for colorectal carcinoma metastases: a multi-institutional study of indications for resection. Surgery 1988;103:278-88.

11. Rex DK, Kahi CJ, Levin B, et al. Guidelines for colonoscopy surveillance after cancer resection: a consensus update by the American Cancer Society and US multisociety task force on colorectal cancer. CA Cancer J Clin 2006;56:160-7.

12. Wishner JD, Baker JW, Jr, Hoffman GC, et al. Laparoscopic-assisted colectomy: The learning curve. Surgical Endoscopy 1995;9:1179-83.

Level of Evidence Table			
Recommendation	Best level of evidence	Grade of recommendations	References
Colon cancer screening should begin at the age of 50 for people without risk factors	1	A	1-4
Increased lymph node evaluation is associated with better staging and survival in Stage II and III colon cancer. The AJCC-recommended minimum of 12 lymph nodes is otherwise less well-supported (2B)	2A	A	5-10
Laparoscopic resection of colon cancer is safe and provides equivalent oncologic results to open resection	1	B	11-16
Adjuvant treatment of Stage III colon cancer with 5-FU/leucovorin/oxaliplatin improves disease free survival and overall survival	1	A	17,18
Adjuvant treatment of Stage II colon cancer with high-risk features improves outcome	1	C	19
Hepatic resection is the treatment of choice for resectable liver metastases from colorectal cancer	2A	B	20-22, 32
Perioperative chemotherapy improves progression-free survival after resection of colorectal liver metastases	1	B	23, 24
Simultaneous resection is preferable to staged resection of synchronous colorectal liver metastases	2A	C	25-27
Cytoreduction and hyperthermic intraperitoneal chemotherapy may improve survival in colorectal carcinomatosis compared to systemic therapy alone	1	B	28, 29
Aggressive follow-up surveillance with physical exams, CEA levels and colonoscopies is indicated after curative resection	1	A	30, 31, 33,34

References

1. Mandel JS, Bond JH, Church TR, et al. Reducing mortality from colorectal cancer by screening for fecal occult blood. Minnesota Colon Cancer Control Study. N Engl J Med 1993; 328:1365-71.

2. Kronborg O, Fenger C, Olsen J, et al. Randomised study of screening for colorectal cancer with faecal-occult-blood test. Lancet 1996; 348:1467-71.

3. Newcomb PA, Norfleet RG, Storer BE, et al. Screening sigmoidoscopy and colorectal cancer mortality. J Natl Cancer Inst 1992; 84:1572-5.

4. Selby JV, Friedman GD, Quesenberry CP, Jr., et al. A case-control study of screening sigmoidoscopy and mortality from colorectal cancer. N Engl J Med 1992; 326:653-7.

5. Chang GJ, Rodriguez-Bigas MA, Skibber JM, et al. Lymph node evaluation and survival after curative resection of

colon cancer: systematic review. J Natl Cancer Inst 2007; 99:433-41.

6. Joseph NE, Sigurdson ER, Hanlon AL, et al. Accuracy of determining nodal negativity in colorectal cancer on the basis of the number of nodes retrieved on resection. Ann Surg Oncol 2003; 10:213-8.

7. Le Voyer TE, Sigurdson ER, Hanlon AL, et al. Colon cancer survival is associated with increasing number of lymph nodes analyzed: a secondary survey of intergroup trial INT-0089. J Clin Oncol 2003; 21:2912-9.

8. Tsikitis VL, Larson DL, Wolff BG, et al. Survival in stage III colon cancer is independent of the total number of lymph nodes retrieved. J Am Coll Surg 2009; 208:42-7.

9. Wang J, Kulaylat M, Rockette H, et al. Should total number of lymph nodes be used as a quality of care measure for stage III colon cancer? Ann Surg 2009; 249:559-63.

10. Wong SL, Ji H, Hollenbeck BK, et al. Hospital lymph node examination rates and survival after resection for colon cancer. Jama 2007; 298:2149-54.

11. Jayne DG, Guillou PJ, Thorpe H, et al. Randomized trial of laparoscopic-assisted resection of colorectal carcinoma: 3-year results of the UK MRC CLASICC Trial Group. J Clin Oncol 2007; 25:3061-8.

12. Bonjer HJ, Hop WC, Nelson H, et al. Laparoscopically assisted vs open colectomy for colon cancer: a meta-analysis. Arch Surg 2007; 142:298-303.

13. Kuhry E, Schwenk W, Gaupset R, et al. Long-term outcome of laparoscopic surgery for colorectal cancer: a cochrane systematic review of randomised controlled trials. Cancer Treat Rev 2008; 34:498-504.

14. Lacy AM, Delgado S, Castells A, et al. The long-term results of a randomized clinical trial of laparoscopy-assisted versus open surgery for colon cancer. Ann Surg 2008; 248:1-7.

15. Veldkamp R, Kuhry E, Hop WC, et al. Laparoscopic surgery versus open surgery for colon cancer: short-term outcomes of a randomised trial. Lancet Oncol 2005; 6:477-84.

16. Fleshman J, Sargent DJ, Green E, et al. Laparoscopic colectomy for cancer is not inferior to open surgery based on 5-year data from the COST Study Group trial. Ann Surg 2007; 246:655-62; discussion 662-4.

17. Andre T, Boni C, Navarro M, et al. Improved overall survival with oxaliplatin, fluorouracil and leucovorin as adjuvant treatment in stage II or III colon cancer in the MOSAIC trial. J Clin Oncol 2009; 27:3109-16.

18. Kuebler JP, Wieand HS, O'Connell MJ, et al. Oxaliplatin combined with weekly bolus fluorouracil and leucovorin as surgical adjuvant chemotherapy for stage II and III colon cancer: results from NSABP C-07. J Clin Oncol 2007; 25:2198-204.

19. Figueredo A, Coombes ME, Mukherjee S. Adjuvant therapy for completely resected stage II colon cancer. Cochrane Database Syst Rev 2008; CD005390.

20. Pawlik TM, Schulick RD, Choti MA. Expanding criteria for resectability of colorectal liver metastases. Oncologist 2008; 13:51-64.

21. Simmonds PC, Primrose JN, Colquitt JL, et al. Surgical resection of hepatic metastases from colorectal cancer: a systematic review of published studies. Br J Cancer 2006; 94:982-99.

22. Aloia TA, Vauthey JN, Loyer EM, et al. Solitary colorectal liver metastasis: resection determines outcome. Arch Surg 2006; 141:460-6; discussion 466-7.

23. Nordlinger B, Sorbye H, Glimelius B, et al. Perioperative chemotherapy with FOLFOX4 and surgery versus surgery alone for resectable liver metastases from colorectal cancer (EORTC Intergroup trial 40983): a randomised controlled trial. Lancet 2008; 371:1007-16.

24. Mitry E, Fields AL, Bleiberg H, et al. Adjuvant chemotherapy after potentially curative resection of metastases from colorectal cancer: a pooled analysis of two randomized trials. J Clin Oncol 2008; 26:4906-11.

25. Reddy SK, Pawlik TM, Zorzi D, et al. Simultaneous resections of colorectal cancer and synchronous liver metastases: a multi-institutional analysis. Ann Surg Oncol 2007; 14: 3481-91.

26. Hillingso JG Wille-Jorgensen P. Staged or simultaneous resection of synchronous liver metastases from colorectal cancer—a systematic review. Colorectal Dis 2009; 11:3-10.

27. Martin RC, 2nd, Augenstein V, Reuter NP, et al. Simultaneous versus staged resection for synchronous colorectal cancer liver metastases. J Am Coll Surg 2009; 208:842-50; discussion 850-2.

28. Verwaal VJ, Bruin S, Boot H, et al. 8-year follow-up of randomized trial: cytoreduction and hyperthermic intra-peritoneal chemotherapy versus systemic chemotherapy in patients with peritoneal carcinomatosis of colorectal cancer. Ann Surg Oncol 2008; 15:2426-32.

29. Elias D, Lefevre JH, Chevalier J, et al. Complete cyto-reductive surgery plus intraperitoneal chemohyperthermia with oxaliplatin for peritoneal carcinomatosis of colorectal origin. J Clin Oncol 2009; 27:681-5.

30. Desch CE, Benson AB, 3rd, Somerfield MR, et al. Colorectal cancer surveillance: 2005 update of an American Society of Clinical Oncology practice guideline. J Clin Oncol 2005; 23:8512-9.

31. Jeffery M, Hickey BE, Hider PN. Follow-up strategies for patients treated for non-metastatic colorectal cancer. Cochrane Database Syst Rev 2007; CD002200.

32. Abdalla EK, Vauthey JN, Ellis LM, Ellis V, Pollock R, Broglio KR, et al. Recurrence and outcomes following hepatic resection, radiofrequency ablation and combined resection/ablation for colorectal liver metastases. Ann Surg 2004;239(6):818-25.

33. Locker GY, Hamilton S, Harris J, Jessup JM, Kemeny N, Macdonald JS, et al. ASCO. ASCO 2006 update of recommendations for the use of tumor markers in gastrointestinal cancer. J Clin Oncol 2006;24(33):5313-27.

34. Rex DK, Kahi CJ, Levin B, Smith RA, Bond JH, Brooks D, et al. Guidelines for colonoscopy surveillance after cancer resection: a consensus update by the American Cancer Society and US Multi-Society Task Force on Colorectal Cancer. CA Cancer J Clin 2006;56(3): 160-7.

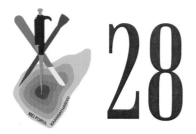

28

Cancer of the Rectum and Anus

Richard Fortunato, Linda M Farkas

Rectal Cancer

Introduction

Initial treatment for rectal cancer offered little cure and high morbidity by removing the entire rectum by means of either an abdominal or perineal approach. In 1908 Miles described the combined abdominoperineal resection (APR) technique. Later, Dixon performed a partial proctectomy for proximal tumors via a low-anterior resection (LAR). As the relationship between lymphatic removal and improved disease-free and overall survival became clear, the total mesorectal excision (TME) became the cornerstone of rectal cancer surgery. These techniques ensure tumor-free proximal, distal and radial margins and achieve the goals of an oncologically sound anatomic resection. Due to technological advances and improved understanding of tumor biology, sphincter-sparing approaches, such as an extended LAR, local excision and transanal endoscopic microsurgery (TEM), have increasingly been used to maintain functional defecation and improve patients' quality of life.

In 1990, the National Institutes of Health (NIH) recommended adjuvant chemotherapy for stage II and III rectal cancers and more recent trials have demonstrated decreased local recurrence and increased 5-year survival rates in patients receiving neoadjuvant radiation or chemoradiation (chemo-XRT) therapies. Current curative treatment for rectal cancer involves complex multidisciplinary planning combining oncologically sound surgical principles with sphincter saving techniques, neoadjuvant and adjuvant radiation and chemotherapy.

Epidemiology

Colon and rectal cancers are very similar in tumor biology and studies regarding epidemiology, risk stratification, screening and staging often combine the two entities together. As per the National Cancer Institute, there are an estimated 40,870 new cases of rectal cancer for the year 2009. Overall, 75% of patients with colorectal cancer have no identifiable risk factors and are considered to be of average risk. Specifically, the most significant risk for developing rectal cancer is having previously had a rectal cancer and 5-year recurrence rates vary between 5% and 30% depending on the preoperative stage and use of neoadjuvant or adjuvant chemo-XRT. In addition, patients with familial adenomatous polyposis (FAP) are at an increased risk of developing rectal cancer.

Presentation

The majority of patients with rectal cancer are asymptomatic, however, symptoms are more frequently seen than with colon cancer. Approximately 40% of patients will have hematochezia, melena or a change in bowel habits. Brisk bleeding from rectal tumors is rare and microcytic anemia of unknown etiology is more common with colon cancer than rectal cancer. Changes in bowel habits typically present as narrowed stool caliber and/or constipation, but loss of continence may occur if the sphincter complex is involved. Pain can occur due to tenesmus, obstruction or neuropathic pain from local invasion into the sciatic or obturator nerves. Other symptoms such as nausea, vomiting, weight loss and fatigue may occur.

Rectal Polyps

A complete review of colorectal polyps is discussed in the chapter on colon cancer (see Chapter 27); however, it is important to know that approximately 10% of patients with an endoscopically removed, malignant rectal polyp (T1) develop lymph node metastasis, even with histologically favorable characteristics. Therefore, transanal excision or radical resection is an alternative to endoscopic polypectomy and close observation. Likewise, rectal polyps with a malignant focus that are removd in piece meal fashion have undefined margin involvement, or display unfavorable histopathological characteristics (grade 3 or 4, angiolymphatic invasion or a < 2 mm margin), should undergo a full thickness transanal excision or radical resection instead of simple endoscopic resection.

Pre-therapy Staging

Accurate preoperative staging is a critical necessity for the cure of rectal cancer because treatment may change significantly depending on the stage. Radiographic staging for rectal cancer presents distinct challenges secondary to tumor location, the pelvic confines and patient tolerance. While the ideal radiographic staging modality has yet to be developed, many current technologies are able to accurately assess lymph node status, tumor depth of invasion and circumferential margins—albeit with less than perfect results. Endorectal ultrasound (ERUS), CT scan, MRI and PET scans are all being used to some degree to precisely stage rectal cancer. As such, specific prefixes are used to identify the radiographic modality used to stage the tumor; 'u'—ultrasound, 'ct'—CT scan and 'mr'—MRI scan.

Since the mid-1980s, the primary local staging device for rectal cancers has been ERUS. ERUS uses a 7.5 MHz or 10 MHz rigid transducer with a saline-filled balloon tip to accurately provide a 360-degree field of view of all five layers of the rectal wall. This affords accurate identification of the depth of tumor invasion (T) and involvement of adjacent lymph nodes (N). Tumors appear as a hypoechoic lesion invading or disrupting layers of the rectal wall. Tumors invading into the submucosa (first hypoechoic line) are uT1, those into but not beyond the muscularis propria (second hypoechoic line) are uT2, those penetrating into the adjacent perirectal fat (third hyperechoic line) are uT3 and invasion into adjacent organs represents a uT4 cancer. The overall sensitivity of ultrasound T-stage identification is 67-95% and 67-88% for N-stage status. Many consider ERUS the imaging modality of choice for early T1/T2 rectal staging because of its superior staging ability. A meta-analysis of 90 articles from 1985-2002 comparing ERUS, MRI and CT suggests that ERUS is the modality of choice for local staging of all rectal carcinomas **(Table 28-1)**.

TABLE 28-1	Radiographic accuracy for staging	
Modality	**T-stage (Mean%)**	**N-stage (Mean%)**
ERUS	85	80
MRI	79	72
CT	70	55

Newer 3-D ultrasound technology provides additional sagittal and coronal planes not visualized with standard 2-D imaging. This affords the surgeon the ability not only to visualize the extent of tumor invasion within the rectal wall but also to accurately measure the dimensions of the tumors and potentially better identify adjacent lymph nodes **(Figure 28-1)**.

Disadvantages associated with ERUS include operator dependence [overstaging (5%), understaging (10%)], the

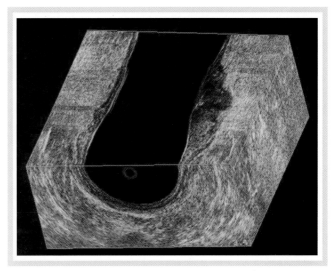

Figure 28-1: 3-D endorectal ultrasound showing a uT3uN0 rectal cancer (*Image reprinted with permission, Courtesy of B-K Medical Systems, Inc.*)

need for bowel preparation, proper positioning and patient tolerance. In addition, tumors beyond 13 cm proximal to the dentate line are difficult to stage with the fixed-length rigid probe and large tumors may block the probe from advancing proximally, thus not affording accurate tumor assessment.

CT scan for rectal tumors can identify depth of invasion (sensitivity, 61-84%) but cannot reliably detect subcentimeter lymph nodes and therefore accurately determine the lymph node status (sensitivity, 50-60%). Newer multidetector CT scans have shown a T-stage sensitivity of 95% and N-stage sensitivity of 70%, but studies are still ongoing.

MRI can be used with a surface coil detector or endorectal coil (ERC-MRI). While several studies have shown increased T-stage and N-stage accuracy with the endorectal coil with balloon insufflation, ERC-MRI can be uncomfortable for patients, difficult to position and is not universally available. For these reasons, surface coil MRI is most often used. The most recent MRI technology is a pelvic phased array coil MRI (PA-MRI), which has multiple surface coils that simultaneously detect signal, allowing for higher signal-to-noise ratios, better spatial resolution and faster imaging, affording improved detection of the degree of extramural extension, venous invasion, nodal involvement, perirectal infiltration and predicted circumferential resection margins. In fact, there is increasing evidence that the PA-MRI is superior to ERC-MRI, ERUS and CT for the staging of locally advanced extramural tumors.

Principles of Surgical Management

The treatment of rectal cancer presents many unique difficulties not encountered with colon cancer. Rectal cancer has a high risk of locoregional involvement secondary to the rectum's intrapelvic confines, lack of serosa, proximity to pelvic structures and additional circumferential margin. As such, many surgical techniques and chemo-XRT protocols have been developed to treat the various stages, locations, sizes and adjacent organ involvement presented by rectal cancers. As previously mentioned, curative treatment for rectal cancer involves a multidisciplinary approach encompassing neoadjuvant and adjuvant radiation and chemotherapy and sound oncologic resection. With such diverse methodologies complete tumor resection and good functional outcomes can be obtained.

Tumor Margins

The majority of the rectum and mesorectum are extraperitoneal and encased within the bony pelvis. Due to these tight confines, the rectum is adjacent to many vital structures affording tumor growth in many directions. Thus, in addition to the standard 5 cm proximal and 2 cm distal margins, circumferential and mesorectal margins must be completely excised. In fact, incomplete circumferential dissection is the primary reason for surgical failure and perhaps the most critical variable in determining locoregional recurrence and overall patient prognosis, especially in patients that received neoadjuvant therapy. The 6th edition of the AJCC staging manual recommends that the surgeon identify the area of deepest tumor penetration to assist the pathologist in determining the circumferential resection margin (CRM). Tumor cells < 2 mm from the margin is considered a positive CRM. In addition, it is advisable that the surgeon grade the level of resection as R0—complete resection, R1—microscopically positive margins or R2—gross residual tumor.

Lymphadenectomy

Many factors can affect the number of lymph nodes surgically retrieved including the patient's age, gender, tumor size and grade, use of neoadjuvant therapy and the surgeon's experience. Recent studies have quantified the number of lymph nodes necessary to accurately stage patients with stage II CRC as a minimum of 12. While the majority of trials grouped colon and rectal cancer together, studies looking at rectal cancer specifically report the minimal number of lymph nodes necessary to accurately diagnose stage II rectal cancer as 14 or >10. Sentinel lymph node (SLN) mapping has revolutionized the treatment of many tumors including breast carcinoma and melanoma and has been studied in both colon and rectal cancers. Unfortunately, for rectal cancer the overall mapping accuracy and sensitivity is approximately 60%, with false-negative and positive rates of about 40%. In addition, distal rectal tumors, tumor size and neoadjuvant therapy

are all independent risk factors for the inability to detect the SLN.

Surgical Techniques

To ensure complete rectal lymph node harvest and negative circumferential tumor margins, *en bloc* resection of the mesorectum is mandatory. This meticulous dissection is accomplished by a TME and has been shown to reduce LR from 12% to 4%, mandating its use for all proctectomies for cancer. The length of mesorectum that needs to be removed depends on the tumor stage and location. Several studies have failed to identify metastatic foci in the mesorectum more than 4 cm from the distal edge of the tumor or beyond 1 cm in T1 and T2 lesions. This finding, coupled with the possibility of devascularizing the anastomosis by removing entire the blood supply, has led to the recommendations that a 5 cm mesorectal margin below the level of the tumor be achieved for proximal tumors, while a complete mesorectal excision and 1-2 cm negative distal margins are required for tumors within 5 cm of the sphincter complex **(Figure 28-2)**.

Sharp dissection is begun just anterior or medial to the sympathetic nerve trunks starting at the sacral promontory and working distally along the posterior plane. The dissection is continued laterally and anteriorly, ensuring excision of Denonvillier's fascia (between the rectum and the seminal vesicles or prostate in men and rectovaginal septum in women).

Stage I-III rectal cancers located in the middle and upper rectum should be excised with a low anterior resection (LAR) and TME. In order to spare the sphincter complex and avoid a permanent colostomy, the application of a LAR is being used with increased frequency as an extended or ultra-low LAR with either a low coloproctostomy or coloanal anastomosis.

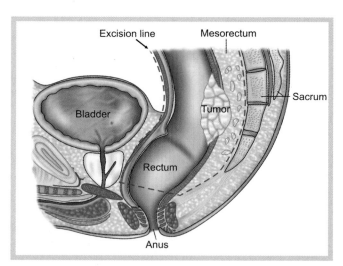

Figure 28-2: Anatomic borders for a total mesorectal excision

While laparoscopic colectomy for cancer has been shown not to be inferior to open colectomy for cancer, the data for laparoscopic proctectomy is not as clear. The use of laparoscopy within the pelvic confines affords the advantages of better visualization with magnification and improved lighting and better instrumentation; however, its role for rectal cancer is an ongoing debate. While laparoscopic proctectomy has been shown in several studies to be equivalent to open resection regarding LR, DFS and OS, the current NCCN Clinical Practice Guidelines in Oncology, only recommend a laparoscopic LAR for rectal cancers in the setting of clinical trials, due to factors regarding patient selection, surgical expertise and ability to consistently achieve negative resection margins. ACOSOG is currently accruing patients in a randomized trial comparing open versus laparoscopic proctectomy to help define the role of laparoscopy in rectal cancer therapy (see *section New Frontiers and Controversies*).

The principles of a LAR, whether open or laparoscopic, include mobilization of the sigmoid along the white line of Toldt—taking care to identify and avoid injury to the left ureter. Complete mobilization of splenic flexure may be necessary to ensure adequate mobilization for a tension free anastomosis and is the authors' recommendation. Once mobilization is sufficient, an incision is made on right side of mesosigmoid and continued superiorly to isolate the inferior mesenteric artery and inferiorly, developing an avascular plane posterior to the superior hemorrhoidal vessels but anterior to hypogastric nerve plexus. A TME dissection is then used to mobilize the rectum and after reverification of the left ureter's location, the vascular stalks of the inferior mesenteric and superior hemorrhoidal arteries are ligated. The distal rectal margin is divided and end-to-end coloproctostomy or coloanal anastomosis is fashioned.

There are many different methods of creating a coloanal sphincter sparring anastomosis: straight, transverse coloplasty, side-to-end and colonic J-pouch. Overall, the transverse coloplasty, side-to-end and colonic J-pouch techniques are similar and superior to a straight coloanal anastomosis regarding bowel frequency, urgency, fecal incontinence and use of antidiarrheal medications, with the colonic J-pouch reconstruction having the best one-year functional outcomes **(Figure 28-3)**. The decision of which technique to use is thus based upon the surgeon's experience and anatomic restrictions of the patient. It should be noted that while some patients oncologically eligible for a coloanal anastomosis may be better served with an end-colostomy or APR based on their mental, functional and continence status.

Classic teaching would recommend an APR for any rectal tumor < 8 cm from the anal verge, however, with the strong impetus for sphincter sparring procedures, neoadjuvant chemo-XRT, transanal excision of T1 tumors and the high quality of life and functional outcomes

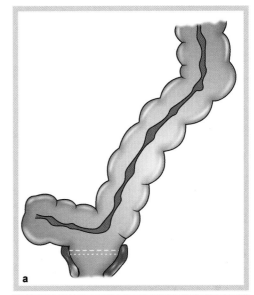

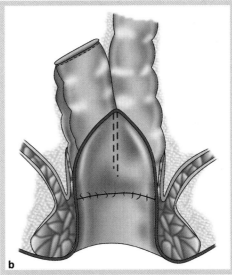

Figure 28-3: Coloanal anastomosis— side-to-end (a) and J pouch (b)

achieved with a coloanal anastomosis, current indications for an APR are for any margin negative resection that would involve the sphincter complex (i.e. any tumor within 2 cm of dentate line and potentially 1 cm from the dentate line after neoadjuvant chemo-XRT).

An APR consists of both an abdominal proctectomy (see *LAR* and *TME*) and a perineal resection. The perineal dissection starts with an elliptical excision of the anus bounded laterally by the ischioanal fossa, posteriorly by the anococcygeal ligament and anteriorly by the transverse perinei muscle. Care must be taken to avoid the urethra in males and vagina in females, unless invaded by the tumor. Intracorporeal mobilization of the sigmoid and rectum is the same as that for a LAR and an end-colostomy is created in the left lower quadrant.

In patients unable or unwilling to tolerate a major operative resection, a transanal excision may be performed in a select group of patients. The ideal candidate lesion for local excision would be:

- well to moderately differentiated lesion
- stage I adenocarcinoma
- no angiolymphatic or neural invasion
- < 5 cm from dentate line
- < 40% of rectal circumference
- < 4 cm in size

The transanal endoscopic microsurgery (TEM) procedure developed early 1980s utilizes specialized laparoscopic equipment through a 4 cm transanal cylinder to aid in exposure and resection **(Figures 28-4 to 28-7)**. Indications are identical as those for local excision with the noted exception of tumor location, whereby tumors 8 cm or further from the dentate line may be removed with these devices. Because TEM requires highly specialized skills and expensive instruments, the availability of TEM is limited. ACOSOG is in the final patient accrual phase in a trial looking at outcomes after transanal excision of T2 N0 tumors within 8 cm of the anal verge.

In the highly select cohort of T1 and T2 tumors transanally resected, patient outcomes seem comparable to that of T1 and T2 tumors removed via radical resection. Patients with T1 lesions that have favorable pathologic findings can be observed; however, as there is at least a 10% risk of local recurrence, many surgeons will include

ERUS every 3-4 months for close follow-up. T2 tumors transanally removed, in addition to ultrasound guided follow-up should undergo adjuvant chemo-XRT. Any T1 or T2 lesion that has a positive margin, poor differen-

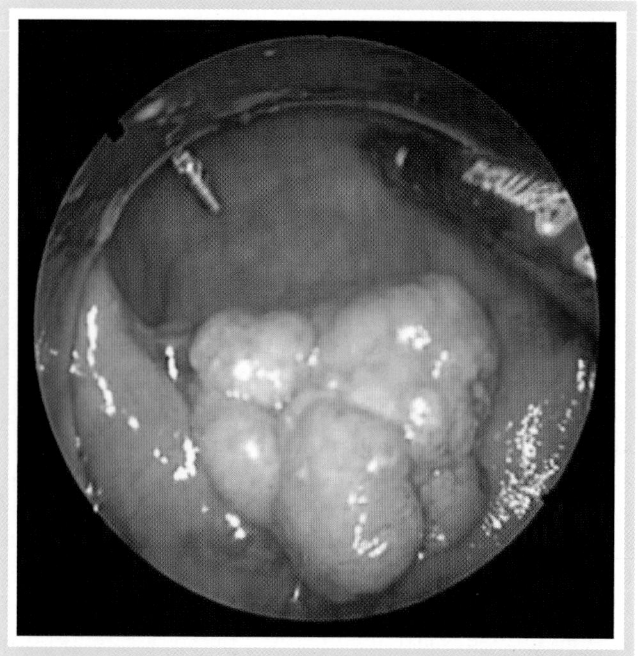

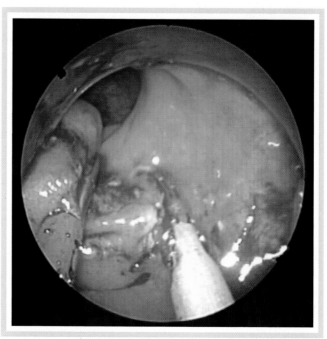

Figure 28-5: Transanal endoscopic microdissection of a T1N0 rectal tumor (*Photograph courtesy of Michael Stratton, MD, Colon and Rectal Associates, Shreveport, LA*)

Figure 28-4: Transanal endoscopic microsurgery (TEM) of a T1N0 rectal tumor 4 cm from the dentate line (*Photograph courtesy of Michael Stratton, MD, Colon and Rectal Associates, Shreveport, LA*)

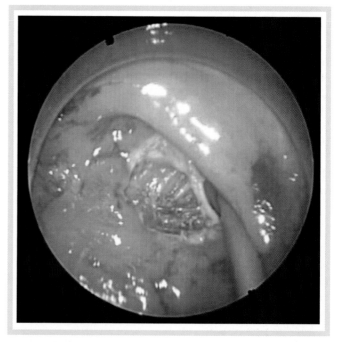

Figure 28-6: Final full-thickness rectal defect demonstrating perirectal fat after TEM of a T1N0 rectal tumor 4 cm from the dentate line (*Photograph courtesy of Michael Stratton, MD, Colon and Rectal Associates, Shreveport, LA*)

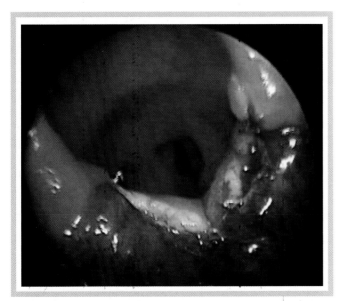

Figure 28-7: Transverse closure of a full thickness rectal defect after TEM resection of a T1N0 tumor (*Photograph courtesy of Andrew Werner, MD, Colon and Rectal Associates, Shreveport, LA*)

tiation, angiolymphatic or neural invasion should undergo an external LAR or salvage APR.

Transanal excision is performed with the patient in the prone-jack-knife position. After adequate analgesia via a pudendal nerve block or epidural spinal block is used to relax the sphincters, a self-retaining hook retractor or hand-held anal retractor is used to gain adequate exposure of the tumor. Electrocautery is then used to incise the mucosa around the tumor with 1 cm margins and continued until the perirectal fat is exposed, ensuring a full-thickness resection. As the resection continues circumferentially around the tumor, care is necessary to avoid the anterior pelvic structures such as the vagina, prostate and urethra. The resected tumor margins should be inked and the specimen oriented on cardboard with pins for pathology. Inadvertent opening of the peritoneum can safely be closed with running sutures. The rectal wall defect is closed transversely with full-thickness absorbable sutures, taking care not to narrow the rectal lumen.

Neoadjuvant Therapy

Neoadjuvant radiation or chemo-XRT offers many benefits over adjuvant therapy alone including increased tumor sensitization, lower systemic toxicity; potential tumor downstaging and size reduction and avoiding irradiation to the anastomosis—all allowing increased sphincter preservation. Current recommendations for neoadjuvant therapy are only for stage II or III disease.

In 1992, preoperative radiotherapy in France was considered the standard treatment for T3-4 rectal cancers, however, this was not adopted in the United States until 1997 when the Swedish rectal trial showed that a short-course regimen of preoperative irradiation followed by surgery within one week reduced the rates of local recurrence and improved overall survival among patients with resectable rectal cancer. A follow-up study comparing neoadjuvant short-course irradiation versus chemo-XRT followed by surgery failed to show improved overall survival but did demonstrate decreased LR for patients receiving neoadjuvant chemo-XRT. The German Rectal Cancer Study showed that preoperative chemo-XRT compared with postoperative chemo-XRT improved local control and reduced toxicity, though it did not improve overall survival. Additional studies have also demonstrated significantly decreased LR rates in patients receiving neoadjuvant and adjuvant chemo-XRT versus neoadjuvant radiation alone and as such, current recommendations endorse neoadjuvant chemo-XRT followed by adjuvant chemotherapy.

While used extensively in Europe, neoadjuvant 'short-course' radiation is only used in select patients in the United States. We will use short-course neoadjuvant radiation therapy for patients who cannot tolerate chemotherapy or cannot defer resection for the 12+ weeks that is required to receive the full chemo-XRT course. The protocol used in the Swedish rectal trial consists of 25 Gy of radiation delivered in five fractions over one week followed by surgery within one week after the last dose.

The standard neoadjuvant therapy used in the United States for patients with rectal cancer is the 'long-course; chemo-XRT regimen, which consists of chemotherapy (5-FU, leucovorin, capecitabine) combined with XRT (45-50 Gy given in fractionated doses) followed by surgery within 5-10 weeks. Current protocols include continuous 5-FU/XRT (preferred) or 5-FU plus leucovorin/XRT or capecitabine/XRT.

While the traditional practice in the United States is to use the long-course protocol, there have not been any trials directly comparing the short-course versus long-course neoadjuvant therapy to know which is better. Currently, the NSABP R-04 trial is investigating the best chemotherapy regimen to be given during the neoadjuvant period (see *section New Frontiers and Controversies*).

Adjuvant Therapy

Six months of adjuvant chemotherapy is recommended for all stage II or III disease after neoadjuvant therapy regardless of the final pathologic stage. Regimens include 5-FU ± leucovorin, FOLFOX (5-FU, leucovorin, oxaliplatin), or capeciabine.

Summary of Treatment Regimens by Location and Stage

See **Tables 28-2 and 28-3.**

Metastatic and Unresectable Rectal Cancer

In general, distant metastasis develops in 50-60% of patients diagnosed with rectal cancer and 15-25% of patients have synchronous metastasis at the time of initial diagnosis. Resectable disease is defined as the ability to achieve R0 negative margins of all local and distant metastatic tumor deposits. Unfortunately, resectable disease accounts for only about 10-20% of metastatic cases. As such, a detailed discussion of rectal metastatic disease is beyond the scope of this chapter; however, some general protocols are worth mentioning.

For stage IIb (T4) or locally unresectable disease, curative treatment consists of continuous intravenous 5-FU plus XRT or bolus 5-FU/LV plus XRT or capecitabine plus XRT. Due to increase toxicity, bolus therapy is rarely used today. The patient is then restaged and if possible, they should undergo a LAR or APR followed by adjuvant chemotherapy (5-FU ± leucovorin or FOLFOX or capecitabine). The majority of T4 lesions in women involve the vagina and can be resected *en bloc* with the rectum followed by vaginal reconstruction. Involvement with the bladder can also be treated with *en bloc* resection and reconstruction. If, however, the tumor is considered

TABLE 28-2	Treatment of stage I rectal cancer [confined to the wall (T1-2) without lymph node involvement (N0)]	
Location	**Tumor stage**	**Treatment options**
Upper rectum	T1 or T2	Low-anterior resection (LAR)
		Transanal endoscopic microsurgery (TEM)
Middle rectum	T1	Low-anterior resection (LAR)
		Transanal endoscopic microsurgery (TEM)
		Local excision
	T2	Low-anterior resection (LAR)
		Local excision/TEM with adjuvant chemo-XRT
		Neoadjuvant chemo-XRT with TEM/local excision
Lower rectum	T1	Abdominoperineal resection (APR)
		Transanal endoscopic microsurgery (TEM)
		Local excision
	T2	Abdominoperineal resection (APR)
		Local excision with adjuvant chemo-XRT
		Neoadjuvant chemo-XRT with local excision

TABLE 28-3	Treatment of Stage II [invasion into the mesorectal fat (T3) without lymph node involvement (N0)] and stage III rectal cancers [any stage with lymph node involvement (N1)]
Location	**Treatment options**
Upper rectum	Neoadjuvant chemo-XRT with LAR followed by adjuvant chemo-XRT
	LAR with adjuvant chemo-XRT
Middle rectum	Neoadjuvant chemo-XRT with LAR followed by adjuvant chemo-XRT
	LAR with adjuvant chemo-XRT
Lower rectum	Neoadjuvant chemo-XRT with an extended LAR with a low coloproctostomy or coloanal anastomosis followed by adjuvant chemo-XRT
	Neoadjuvant chemo-XRT with an abdominoperineal resection followed by adjuvant chemo-XRT
	Abdominoperineal resection with adjuvant chemo-XRT

unresectable after the initial therapy, palliative options or clinical trials may be pursued.

Patients with metastatic (M1) disease and synchronous resectable metastasis should undergo KRAS genotyping before beginning therapy because patients with this mutation are insensitive to EGFR inhibitors and should not have treatment with these biologic agents. For patients that are KRAS mutation negative, treatment protocols consist of neoadjuvant and adjuvant therapy with one of the sessions being chemotherapy (FOLFOX ± bevacizumab; FOLFIRI ± bevacizumab; CapeOX ± bevacizumab) and the other chemo-XRT (continuous IV 5-FU/pelvic XRT or bolus 5-FU plus leucovorin/pelvic XRT or capecitabine/pelvic XRT). The timing and priority in treating either the primary tumor or the metastasis depends on whether the primary lesion is symptomatic or not. Patients that are asymptomatic should undergo neoadjuvant chemo-XRT and restaged, while obstructive, bleeding or perforated primary lesions must obviously be addressed first via diversion or resection. At specialized centers, if there is no progression of the metastatic disease after neoadjuvant therapy, a combined rectal resection and liver resection can be performed simultaneously.

Patients with metastatic unresectable rectal cancer who are willing to undergo therapy should be entered into clinical trials. Palliative options to relieve obstruction or pain include stenting, creation of a diverting stoma or tumor debulking. It should be noted that stomas alleviate the obstruction, but not necessarily associated pain.

Complications, Follow-up and Surveillance

After surgery, patients should receive a history and physical, proctoscopy and CEA level every 3-6 months for the first 2 years, then biannually for 5 years. Restaging chest, abdominal and pelvic CT scans should be done annually for 3-5 years. Colonoscopy should be performed at one year and, if normal, can be repeated in 3 years and then every 5 years thereafter. If it is abnormal, it should be repeated yearly until normal, then continued as above.

The radiographic evaluation of recurrent disease is limited by the inflammation and fibrosis that result after chemotherapy, radiation and surgery and similar to preoperative staging, restaging requires multiple technologies to be confident of the results.

The majority of recurrences occur outside of the rectal wall and therefore simple proctoscopy is not as sensitive as ERUS. ERUS-guided biopsy in combination with routine ERUS surveillance is useful in the evaluation of suspicious postoperative lesions. In patients who underwent a transanal excision for T1 or T2 tumors, 31% were found to have local recurrence by ERUS despite being asymptomatic. MRI cannot reliably distinguish radiation fibrosis or post-surgical scarring from residual tumor, resulting in over-staging.

Fluoro-2-deoxy-D-glucose-positron emission tomography (FDG-PET) may offer the greatest advantage in detection of local recurrence and metastasis. FDG-PET has a sensitivity of 87-100% and specificity of 43-100% with a positive predictive value of 90-93% compared with CT, although some regions of fibrosis can still have minor radiotracer uptake and yield false-positive results. Recent studies evaluating FDG-PET versus combined FDG-PET/CT scans for metastatic surveillance/re-staging after therapy completion demonstrate a sensitivity for metastasis 78% of the time when used alone and 89% of the time when combined with CT. Currently, FDG-PET alone or in combination with CT scan is not recommended for routine surveillance but may be a useful adjunct if the CT scan result is inconclusive (see section *New Frontiers and Controversies*).

New Frontiers and Controversies

Current trials in both the United States and the Europe are evaluating some of the most difficult questions regarding rectal cancer. The majority of trials are trying to delineate the optimal neoadjuvant and adjuvant chemo-XRT therapy protocols—many of which include newer biological agents. Surgically, the role of local excision for uT2uN0 rectal cancers is being evaluated, as is laparoscopic-assisted versus open resection for rectal cancer. Several trials are evaluating the radiographic modality of choice for initial and recurrent staging. As many of these trials are completing enrollment, the next few years will define a new era of staging and treating rectal cancer.

Anal Cancer

Introduction

The vast majority of anal canal and anal margin cancers are squamous cell in origin and as such, this chapter will focus on this entity. Unless specifically mentioned, all references of anal canal or anal margin cancer refer to squamous cell cancer.

History

Historical treatment for anal canal cancer consisted of a one-stage colostomy and perianal resection while anal margin tumors were treated with local resection. In the 1940s and 1950s some began using radiation therapy in lieu of perianal resection in order to spare the sphincter complex, albeit with little success. However, by the 1960s the abdominoperineal resection (APR) largely replaced all other modalities as the primary treatment for all anal canal and large anal margin cancers, thus leaving patients with a permanent colostomy. Despite the radical resection and extended lymph node harvest, local recurrence rates ranged from 27% to 47% and 5-year survival was only about 40-70%. In 1974, Nigro, et al published their landmark paper detailing three patients with anal canal cancer treated with radiotherapy followed by 5-fluorouracil (5-FU) and mitomycin (MTC) chemotherapy without surgery. To this day, chemo-XRT remains the gold standard treatment for anal canal carcinoma and has even supplanted surgical excision for all but early stage anal margin cancer.

For almost the entire 20th century anal cancer was thought to arise from chronic perianal inflammation and it was not until the late 1990s that the association between human papilloma virus (HPV) infection and anal cancer was identified. We now know that HPV infection is necessary for the development of anal cancer, though infection alone is not the only factor required for malignancy. With the use of the HPV vaccine to prevent cervical cancer, gene therapy for anal cancer is undergoing intense research and long-term vaccination prophylaxis is yet to be determined.

Epidemiology

Cancer involving the anus, anal canal and anorectum is rare and constitutes 1.9% of all gastrointestinal cancers diagnosed annually in the United States. The National Cancer Institute estimates 5,290 new anal cancer cases for the year 2009, with 710 anal cancer attributed deaths. Anal cancers affect women 1.6:1 to men but the incidence of invasive cancers has increased approximately 1.5-1.6 fold in the last 30 years for both genders.

Risk Factors

The strongest risk factor for developing anal cancer is persistent infection with HPV. HPV is the cause of anal-genital warts and cervical cancer and the HPV-16 subtype can be detected in more than 80% of anal squamous cell cancer specimens. HPV exists throughout the female genital tract from vagina to anus and is transmitted via vaginal secretions and direct cervical contact from women and by semen from men. During intercourse the virus collects at the base of the penis and scrotum and its transmission is therefore not prevented by condom use. Many other risk factors for developing anal cancer exist and include a history of cervical, vulvar or vaginal cancer, immunosuppression after solid organ transplant, human immunodeficiency virus (HIV), receptive anal intercourse, sexually transmitted diseases, chronic local inflammation

(e.g. long-standing fistulas), prior pelvic radiation, age and smoking.

Anatomy

The classification and incidence of anal cancer are often inaccurate due to the many definitions of anal anatomy noted throughout the literature. For our discussion, we will use the standard anal anatomy defined by the American Society of Colon and Rectal Surgeons—namely, the anal canal extends from the upper border of the external anal sphincter and puborectalis muscle (anorectal ring) to the anal verge (anal orifice or introitus). The anal canal is approximately 4 cm in length contains the dentate or pectinate line and harbors tumors that cannot be visualized despite buttock retraction. The anal margin, or perianal region, comprises a 5 cm radius from the anal verge and includes tumors that can easily be visualized on examination **(Figure 28-8)**.

The anal canal includes an important histologic mucosal transition from rectal glandular epithelium to anal squamous epithelium. This change occurs within the anal canal approximately 2 cm from the anal verge, delineated by the dentate line. The anal verge represents the mucocutaneous junction of distal anal canal squamous epithelium and the hair-bearing, glandular epidermis of the perianal skin.

The anal canal above the dentate line drains superiorly via the superior rectal lymphatics to the inferior mesenteric

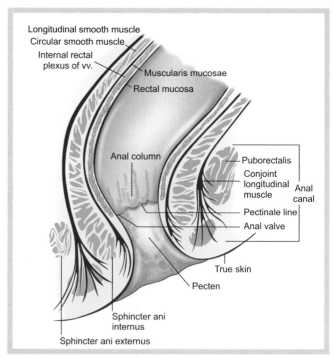

Figure 28-8: Anatomy of the anus (Reproduced with permission by O'Rahily, Muller, Carpenter and Swenson. Basic Human Anatomy, 2008;Chapter 27)

lymph nodes and laterally to the internal iliac nodes. Tumors below the dentate line drain mainly to the inguinal lymph nodes, sometimes involving the inferior and superior rectal lymphatics.

Presentation

Anal cancers typically cause bleeding (> 50%), pain (30%), sensation of a mass (30%), narrowed caliber stools or strained defecation, anal mucus discharge, pruritis and rarely, palpable inguinal lymph nodes. Fecal incontinence or malignant draining fistulas are also rare findings and occur in about 5% of patients on initial presentation. Extrapelvic metastasis is seen in 10-20% of patients, most commonly involving the liver, lung and extra-pelvic lymph nodes.

Pathology

While there are many types of anal cancer, squamous cell carcinoma comprises 75-95% of all anal canal cancers and > 95% of anal margin cancers. Previous nomenclature for anal cancer used to distinguish many subgroups of squamous cell (epithelioid) carcinoma—transitional, basaloid, cloacogenic—often leading to clinical confusion despite similar pathologic changes and prognosis. As such, the current World Health Organization (WHO) classification system makes no such pathologic distinctions and only lists squamous cell carcinoma as the head designation (**Table 28-4**).

Staging and Prognosis

The American Joint Committee on Cancer (AJCC) has designated TNM staging systems for anal canal (**Tables 28-5A and B**) and anal margin cancers (**Table 28-6A and B**). Anal margin cancer has similar tumor biology to squamous skin cancer and as such, the TNM staging used is the same as for skin cancer. Since all stages of anal canal carcinoma are treated with chemo-XRT, staging is based on microscopic examination from an incisional biopsy.

In case of multiple simultaneous tumors, the tumor with the highest T category will be classified and the number of separate tumors will be indicated in parentheses, e.g. T2(3).

While the utility of the anal cancer TNM staging systems are of debatable clinical significance, they do have prognostic implications as tumor size and lymph node involvement are directly related to the overall 5-year survival rate for all types of anal cancer. For example, a tumor < 2 cm has an 80% 5-year survival, while tumors > 5 cm have about a 50% 5-year survival. The 5-year survival with any lymph node involvement varies from 10% to 40% (**Tables 28-7 and 28-8**)

TABLE 28-4	WHO classification of anal cancer
Anal canal	
Squamous cell carcinoma	
Adenocarcinoma	
Small cell carcinoma/Neuroendocrine	
Undifferentiated/Others	
Anal margin	
Squamous cell carcinoma	
Bowen's disease	
Paget's disease	
Giant condyloma	
Basal cell carcinoma	
Others	

TABLE 28-5A	TNM staging of anal cancer	
Primary tumor (T)		
Tx	Primary tumor cannot be assessed	
Tis	Carcinoma in situ	
T0	No evidence of primary tumor	
T1	Tumor 2 cm or less in greatest dimension	
T2	Tumor more than 2 cm but not more than 5 cm in greatest dimension	
T3	Tumor more than 5 cm in greatest dimension	
T4	Tumor of any size invades adjacent organ(s), e.g. vagina, urethra, bladder (involvement of sphincter muscle(s) alone is not classified as T4)	
Lymph node (N)		
Nx	Regional lymph nodes cannot be assessed	
N0	No regional lymph node metastasis	
N1	Metastasis in perirectal lymph node(s)	
N2	Metastasis in unilateral internal iliac and/or inguinal lymph node(s)	
N3	Metastasis in perirectal and inguinal lymph nodes and/or bilateral internal iliac and/or inguinal lymph nodes	
Distant metastasis (M)		
Mx	Presence of distant metastasis cannot be assessed	
M0	No distant metastasis	
M1	Distant metastasis	

Reproduced with permission from the AJCC Staging Manual, 6th Edition

TABLE 28-5B — AJCC stage grouping for anal canal cancer

Stage	T	N	M
Stage 0	Tis	N0	M0
Stage I	T1	N0	M0
	T2	N0	M0
Stage II	T3	N0	M0
Stage IIIa	T1-3	N1	M0
	T4	N0	M0
Stage IIIb	T4	N1	M0
	Any T	N2	M0
	Any T	N3	M0
Stage IV	Any T	Any N	M1

Reproduced with permission from the AJCC Staging Manual, 6th Edition

TABLE 28-6A — TNM staging of anal margin cancer

Primary tumor (T)	
TX	Primary tumor cannot be assessed
T0	No evidence of primary tumor
Tis	Carcinoma in situ
T1	Tumor 2 cm or less in greatest dimension
T2	Tumor more than 2 cm, but not more than 5 cm, in greatest dimension
T3	Tumor more than 5 cm in greatest dimension
T4	Tumor invades deep extradermal structures (e.g. cartilage, skeletal muscle, or bone)
Regional lymph nodes (N)	
NX	Regional lymph nodes cannot be assessed
N0	No regional lymph node metastasis
N1	Regional lymph node metastasis
Distant metastasis (M)	
MX	Distant metastasis cannot be assessed
M0	No distant metastasis
M1	Distant metastasis

Reproduced with permission from the AJCC Staging Manual, 6th Edition

TABLE 28-6B — AJCC stage grouping for anal margin cancer

Stage	T	N	M
Stage 0	Tis	N0	M0
Stage I	T1	N0	M0
Stage II	T2	N0	M0
	T3	N0	M0
Stage III	T4	N0	M0
	T1-4	N1	M0
Stage IV	Any T	Any N	M1

Reproduced with permission from the AJCC Staging Manual, 6th Edition

TABLE 28-7 — Cancer stage at diagnosis

Stage at diagnosis	Frequency (%)
T1	9
T2	51
T3	30
T4	10
N1	13
M1	10 - 20

TABLE 28-8 — 5-year survival by stage

Stage	Rate (%)
T1	86
T2	86
T3	60
T4	45
N0	76
N1	54

and are therefore of limited utility for staging, screening or follow-up evaluation. While the incidence of anal cancer is low, patients with condyloma accumulate HIV-positivity and are men who have sex with men (MSM) carry the highest risk for developing anal cancer. Some centers have initiated Lugol's solution application and PAP smear preps for screening purposes, similar to gynecological colposcopy used for cervical cancer screening. These methods are only cost effective for high risk groups and some advocate screening HIV-positive MSM every 6-12 months and HIV-negative MSM every 2-3 years.

Screening

Endoanal ultrasound and pelvic CT or PET scans have high false-negative and low sensitivity rates for the detection of tumor penetration and lymph node involvement

Treatment

Evaluation of a patient with suspected anal canal or anal margin cancer involves a thorough vaginal and anal examination including a digital rectal examination (DRE), anoscopy, inguinal lymph node palpation and lesion biopsy. As previously mentioned diagnosis of anal canal or margin cancer is confirmed only via pathologic diagnosis and therefore mandates a tissue biopsy. Typically, an incisional biopsy is used for anal canal and large anal margin lesions, while small anal margin lesions may be removed by *en bloc* resection ensuring a 2 cm wide resection margin. All anal canal or anal margin cancers are treated with chemo-XRT with the sole exception of a well-differentiated stage I (T1, N0, M0) anal margin cancer, which can be treated with a 2 cm wide local resection. If the resection margins are positive, re-excision to negative margins is the preferred treatment, though local irradiation with or without 5-FU chemotherapy can be considered as an alternative treatment.

While there have been many chemo-XRT regimens studied in the literature, the most commonly used schedule involves 24 Gy of irradiation to the pelvis, external iliac, internal iliac and perirectal lymphatics administered in 12 fractions over 16 days. After a 3.5 week intermission, 28 Gy of additional radiation is administered in 14 fractions over 28 days. A 96-hour continuous infusion of 5-FU (1000 mg/m^2/24 hours, maximum 1500 mg/m^2/24 hours) with a single bolus of MTC (10 mg/m^2, no maximum) are given concomitantly on the first day of irradiation at weeks one and five.

Cisplatin has been shown to be equally efficacious in combination with 5-FU as MTC/5-FU for disease free survival (DFS) and 5-year survival; however, the colostomy rate was significantly higher in patients receiving cisplatin compared to those receiving MTC—attributed the high degree of tissue radiosensitivity noted after treatment.

The management of patients with anal canal or margin cancer that present with inguinal lymph node metastases is controversial and confers a poor prognosis. Local control can be achieved in 90% of patients receiving chemo-XRT, 65% undergoing radiation (45-60 Gy), 60% using a combined radiation/sentinel lymph node dissection and only 15% via a radical groin dissection.

Results

No matter which specific chemo-XRT regimen is administered, control of the primary cancer is achieved in 75-95% of patients, with complete regression of the tumor occurring over 6-12 weeks after treatment cessation. A fibrotic scar is typically seen after therapy and routine biopsy evaluation for residual disease is not recommended due to high false-negative rates, poor healing of the irradiated tissue and lack of benefit for long-term control or cure rates. However, lesions that are enlarging or are associated with increasing pain and new hard-edged ulcers demonstrate higher positive results when biopsied.

While long-term treatment associated injury is low (6%), mild to moderate morbidities are relatively common. Symptoms include increased fecal urgency and frequency, dyspareunia, perianal dermatitis and pruritis—all of which can be alleviated with medial therapies. Patients with HIV/AIDS have similar therapy tolerance and survival outcomes as compared to patients with anal cancer that are HIV negative and should receive the same treatment protocols.

Follow-up/Recurrence

Follow-up evaluation constitutes a DRE 8-12 weeks after treatment completion, then a DRE, anoscopy and inguinal lymph node palpation every 3-6 months for 5 years. Persistent disease is defined as biopsy proven disease present within 6 months after completing chemo-XRT and recurrent disease is that diagnosed after 6 months. Patients with persistent disease without progression can closely be followed every 4 weeks to see if remission occurs.

Locoregional persistence or recurrence occurs in about 40% of patients with anal cancer regardless of the chemo-XRT regimen administered and is correlated most directly with the T- or N-stage present at initial diagnosis. Treatment for patients with biopsy proven locoregional persistent anal canal or anal margin cancer includes a salvage APR or 5-FU/cisplatin chemotherapy followed by an APR. Five-year survival rates after a salvage APR range 39-64% and due to the irradiated perineum, a myocutaneous advancement flap should be considered in all patients undergoing a salvage APR. Isolated recurrence in the inguinal lymph nodes can be treated with either a lymph node harvest followed by XRT or chemo-XRT. Metastatic disease at presentation occurs in only 10-20% of patients and little data supports strong recommendations, however, cisplatin based chemo-therapy may be of some benefit.

Other Anal Canal Tumors

Adenocarcinoma accounts for 5-19% of all anal cancers and is more aggressive than squamous cell carcinomas. They are from three cell populations—the mucosa of the transitional zone, the base of the mucinous anal glands and from chronic anorectal fistulas. Patients are typically > 60 years old and present with a painful, draining fistula or mass. While many combinations of surgery, radiation and chemotherapy have been used, neoadjuvant chemo-XRT with an APR affords the best long-term survival (60%).

The most common gastrointestinal site of a primary melanoma is the anorectum, however, melanoma only represents 0.5-5% of all anal neoplasms. They arise at the mucocutaneous junction of the anal canal and anal margin. Patients are typically Caucasian females over the age of 60 with anal bleeding. Physical examination usually demonstrates a pigmented, polypoid or ulcerated tumor with raised borders. Melanoma is highly aggressive with 35% of patients presenting with metastatic disease at the time of diagnosis and the best long-term survival rates are less than 30%. Surgical resection affords the only possibility of cure, though major resections are controversial due to the grave prognosis. Local excision can be performed if the sphincter complex is not involved and 1-2 cm negative margins can be achieved, otherwise an APR is required. Tumors larger than 1 cm are not cured by local excision or an APR. Immunotherapy, chemotherapy and irradiation have failed to demonstrate any survival advantage.

Gastrointestinal stromal tumor (GIST) are a rare mesenchymal neoplasm of the gastrointestinal tract that abnormally expresses the tyrosine kinase (KIT) receptor, CD117, in the interstitial pacemaker cells of Cajal. They are most often located in the stomach or proximal small intestine and are only reported in the colon or rectum in 5-15% of cases. Anal GIST is very rare and represents only 3% of all anorectal mesenchymal tumors with less than 20 anal GIST cases reported in the literature. All GIST possess malignant potential and as such, surgical resection affords the only possibility for cure. Anorectal tumors have a more protracted course than other intestinal GIST and treatment favors a two-staged approach; local excision to define the risk of aggressive behavior, then a second stage APR for those declared high or very high-risk. Although surgery is the only curative treatment, recurrence is common. For patients with locally advanced, unresectable or metastatic GIST, chemotherapeutic treatment with imatinib mesylate, an oral KIT inhibitor, is recommended.

Small cell/neuroendocrine tumors make up < 1% of all colorectal malignancies and are exceedingly rare in the anal canal. Pathology classically demonstrates a high mitotic rate, hyperchromatic nuclei and pale nucleoli arranged in loose, non-cohesive sheets. Almost 80% of patients have distant metastasis at the time of diagnosis and require chemotherapy with cisplatin and etoposide. Those with tumors localized to the anal canal should undergo neoadjuvant chemo-XRT and an APR.

Other Anal Margin Tumors

Bowen's disease is a premalignant anal margin lesion also known as squamous cell carcinoma in situ (CIS), squamous intraepithelial lesion (SIL), anal intraepithelial lesion (AIN) or anal dysplasia. These lesions are usually found incidentally in a specimen removed for benign anorectal disease, such a hemorrhoid or skin tag, but may appear as a scaly, erythematous or pigmented, pruritic lesion. Although only 10% progress to cancer, there are no screening methods to determine which lesions will eventually become malignant, leading many to recommend treatment for any identified disease. Methods to identify Bowen's disease include concentric radial biopsies about the anus with frozen sections, or performing a PAP smear, whereby a characteristic hypervascularity may seen with Lugol's solution or acetic acid. Wide local excision with 1 cm margins is the most common treatment, though some have used topical 5-FU, laser or photodynamic therapy, or irradiation as therapy.

Only 20% of Paget's disease is extramammary and it is an extremely rare anorectal condition. The true etiology is unknown but it is hypothesized that an indolent intraepithelial neoplasm develops from an apocrine gland into an adenocarcinoma. Patients are usually over 70 years and present with an average of 3 years of pruritis, bleeding, weight loss and drainage. Physical examination reveals a well-demarcated palpable erythematous mass with eczema and sometimes with inguinal lymphadenopathy. It is often misdiagnosed as a condyloma, hidradenitis, rash or other condition, thus mandating biopsy for definitive diagnosis. Treatment is with wide local excision, though recurrence is common and occurs in 37-100% of patients. To ensure microscopically negative margins perianal mapping with biopsies or PAP smear should be used as is done for Bowen's disease. Re-excision yields excellent results when necessary. Tumors that demonstrate invasion should be treated with an APR and inguinal lymph node dissection if clinically palpable nodes are present. Chemo-XRT therapy remains controversial.

Verrucous carcinoma is an HPV associated neoplasm that is typically found in middle-aged men. The soft, cauliflower-like tumor can be found in both the anal canal and the anal margin and usually causes symptoms of pruritis, pain, drainage and narrowed caliber. stool. Inguinal lymphadenopathy, if present, is usually secondary to infection rather than tumor extension. Giant condyloma harbor a malignancy 58% of the time and curative treatment requires an APR. Neoadjuvant radiation has been used in some instances to shrink the tumor in order to offer the patient a less radical resection. Recurrence is high in these tumors.

Basal cell carcinoma (BCC) of the anus is very rare, accounting for only 0.2% of all anorectal cancers. They typically occur in men over the age of 65 years and most likely have a different etiology than BCC secondary to sun-exposure; however, almost one-third of patients will have a history of BCC at a different site. Physical examination is variable and they may appear as papules, plaques or ulcers, though the majority tend to be mobile and < 2 cm in size. As with BCC at other sites long-term survival is excellent and treatment is with wide local excision. Large tumors may require Mohs microsurgery or radiation followed by an APR. Recurrence occurs < 30% of the time and may be treated with re-resection.

Anal lymphoma constitutes < 1% of all anorectal neoplasms and patients often present with anal pain, pruritis and drainage in addition to classic B-constitutional symptoms of fever, chills and night sweats. Treatment is non-surgical with cyclophosphamide, actinomycin, vincristine and corticosteroids (CHOP).

Surprisingly, there have been only two document cases of anal Kaposi's sarcoma in HIV-positive patients and both were treated with chemotherapy.

New Frontiers and Controversies

Due to unique tumor biology and the rarity of the disease, the treatment for anal cancer has essentially been unchanged for the last 40 years. Nonetheless, with the advent of genotyping, the next few years may afford improved screening and the development of a preventative vaccine as has been done for cervical cancer.

Landmark Papers

1. Compton CC, Greene FL. The staging of colorectal cancer: 2004 and beyond. CA Cancer J Clin 2004;54(6): 295-308.
2. Greene F, Page D, Fleming I, Fritz A. AJCC Cancer Staging Manual. New York; Spinger-Verlag, 2002.
3. Bipat S, Glas AS, Slors FJ, Zwinderman AH, Bossuyt PM, Stoker J. Rectal cancer: local staging and assessment of lymph node involvement with endoluminal US, CT and MR imaging—a meta-analysis. Radiology 2004;232(3):773-83.
4. Heald RJ, Husband EM, Ryall RD. The mesorectum in rectal cancer surgery—the clue to pelvic recurrence? Br J Surg 1982;69(10):613-6.
5. Marr R, Birbeck K, Garvican J, Macklin CP, Tiffin NJ, Parsons WJ, et al. The modern abdominoperineal excision: the next challenge after total mesorectal excision. Ann Surg 2006;244(2):330-1; author reply 331-2.
6. Ng SS, Leung KL, Lee JF, Yiu RY, Li JC, Teoh AY, Leung WW. Laparoscopic-assisted versus open abdominoperineal resection for low rectal cancer: a prospective randomized trial. Ann Surg Oncol 2008; 15(9):2418-25.
7. Guillou PJ, Quirke P, Thorpe H, et al. JM, MRC CLASICC Trial Group. Short-term endpoints of conventional versus laparoscopic assisted surgery in patients with colorectal cancer (MRC CLASICC trial): multicenter, randomized controlled study. Lancet 2005; 365:1718-29.
8. Meyerhardt JA, Mayer RJ. Systemic therapy for colorectal cancer. N Engl J Med 2005;352(5):476-87.
9. Douillard JY, Cunningham D, Roth AD, Navarro M, James RD, Karasek P, et al. Irinotecan combined with fluorouracil compared with fluorouracil alone as first-line treatment for metastatic colorectal cancer: a multicentre randomised trial. Lancet 2000;355:1041-47.
10. Karapetis CS, Khambata-Ford S, Jonker DJ, O'Callaghan CJ, Tu D, Tebbutt NC, et al. K-ras mutations and benefit from cetuximab in advanced colorectal cancer. N Engl J Med 2008; 359(17):1757-65.
11. Adam R, Delvart V, Pascal G, Valeanu A, Castaing D, Azoulay D, et al. Rescue surgery for unresectable colorectal liver metastases downstaged by chemotherapy: a model to predict long-term survival. Ann Surg 2004;240(4):644-57.
12. Bartlett DL, Berlin J, Lauwers GY, et al. Chemotherapy and regional therapy of hepatic colorectal metastasis: expert consensus statement. Ann Surg Oncol 2006;13:1284-92.
13. Nigro ND, Vaitkevicius VK, Considine B, Jr. Combined therapy for cancer of the anal canal: a preliminary report. Dis Colon Rectum 1974;17:354-6.
14. Ajani JA, Winter KA, Gunderson LL, Pedersen J, Benson AB, 3rd, Thomas CR Jr, et al. Fluorouracil, mitomycin and radiotherapy vs fluorouracil, cisplatin and radiotherapy for carcinoma of the anal canal: a randomized controlled trial. JAMA 2008;299(16): 1914-21.
15. Flam M, John M, Pajak TF, Petrelli N, Myerson R, Doggett S, et al. Role of mitomycin in combination with fluorouracil and radiotherapy and of salvage chemoradiation in the definitive nonsurgical treatment of epidermoid carcinoma of the anal canal: results of a phase III randomized intergroup study. J Clin Oncol 1996;14(9):2527-39.
16. Faivre C, Rougier P, Ducreux M, Mitry E, Lusinchi A, Lasser P, et al. 5-fluorouracil and cisplatinum combination chemotherapy for metastatic squamous-cell anal cancer. Bull Cancer 1999;86(10): 861-5.
17. Epidermoid anal cancer: results from the UKCCCR randomised trial of radiotherapy alone versus radiotherapy, 5-fluorouracil and mitomycin. UKCCCR Anal Cancer Trial Working Party. UK Co-ordinating Committee on Cancer Research. Lancet 1996;348(9034): 1049-54.
18. Hoffman R, Welton ML, Klencke B, Weinberg V, Krieg R. The significance of pretreatment CD4 count on the outcome and treatment tolerance of HIV-positive patients with anal cancer. Int J Radiat Oncol Biol Phys 19991;44(1):127-31.
19. Cummings BJ. Metastatic anal cancer: the search for cure. Onkologie 2006;29(1-2):5-6.

Level of Evidence Table for Rectal Cancer			
Recommendation	**Best level of evidence**	**Grade of recommendation**	**References**
A single polyp with invasive cancer with favorable features and negative margins that is completely removed can be observed	2B	B	1,2
Pathologic examination of a greater number of lymph nodes (≥12) increases the likelihood of accurate rectal cancer staging to direct adjuvant therapy (see Colon Cancer recommendations)	2B	B	3,6
Preoperative radiotherapy for resectable rectal cancers decreases local recurrence and improves survival compared to surgery alone	1	A	4,7,8
Preoperative chemoradiotherapy versus radiotherapy alone improves local control and pathologic complete response rates in resectable rectal cancer but has not translated into better DFS and OS	1	B	9-12
Preoperative chemoradiotherapy improves local control and is associated with reduced toxicity and higher compliance compared to postoperative therapy	1	A	5
Total mesorectal excision improves local control regardless of additional chemotherapy or radiation	2B	B	13-16
Laparoscopic resection of rectal cancer provides equivalent oncologic outcomes in early follow-up compared to open resection while offering short-term perioperative advantages	1	B	17-20
Level of Evidence Table for Anal Cancer			
Combination chemotherapy and radiation (5-FU/mitomycin plus RT) is more effective than radiation alone for anal canal cancers	1	A	21-23, 27
Chemoradiation is appropriate initial therapy for anal canal/marg in cancers (squamous cell) compared to abdominalperineal resection.	3	A	24, 25
Salvage APR should be offered for locoregional failure of anal carcinoma.	3	B	26, 28
Well-differentiated T1N0 anal margin cancer may be managed by local excision with clear margins.	3	B	29

References

1. Seitz U, Bohnacker S, Seewald S, et al. Is endoscopic polypectomy an adequate therapy for malignant colorectal adenomas? Presentation of 114 patients and review of the literature. Dis Colon Rectum 2004; 47:1789-96; discussion 1796-7.
2. Cooper HS, et al. Endoscopically removed malignant colorectal polyps: clinicopathologic correlations. Gastroenterology 1995;108(6):1657-65.
3. Tepper JE, et al. Impact of number of nodes retrieved on outcome in patients with rectal cancer. J Clin Oncol 2001; 19(1):157-63
4. Improved survival with preoperative radiotherapy in resectable rectal cancer. Swedish Rectal Cancer Trial. N Engl J Med 1997;336(14):980-7.
5. Sauer R, et al. German Rectal Cancer Study Group. Preoperative versus postoperative chemoradiotherapy for rectal cancer. N Engl J Med 2004;351(17):1731-40.
6. Kim YW, Kim NK, Min BS, et al. The influence of the number of retrieved lymph nodes on staging and survival in patients with stage II and III rectal cancer undergoing tumor-specific mesorectal excision. Ann Surg 2009; 249:965-72.
7. Wong RK, Tandan V, De Silva S, et al. Pre-operative radiotherapy and curative surgery for the management of localized rectal carcinoma. Cochrane Database Syst Rev 2007; CD002102.
8. Kapiteijn E, Marijnen CA, Nagtegaal ID, et al. Preoperative radiotherapy combined with total mesorectal excision for resectable rectal cancer. N Engl J Med 2001; 345:638-46.
9. Bosset JF, Collette L, Calais G, et al. Chemotherapy with preoperative radiotherapy in rectal cancer. N Engl J Med 2006; 355:1114-23.
10. Gerard JP, Conroy T, Bonnetain F, et al. Preoperative radiotherapy with or without concurrent fluorouracil and leucovorin in T3-4 rectal cancers: results of FFCD 9203. J Clin Oncol 2006; 24:4620-5.

11. Bujko K, Nowacki MP, Nasierowska-Guttmejer A, et al. Long-term results of a randomized trial comparing preoperative short-course radiotherapy with preoperative conventionally fractionated chemoradiation for rectal cancer. Br J Surg 2006; 93:1215-23.

12. Sphincter preservation following preoperative radiotherapy for rectal cancer: report of a randomised trial comparing short-term radiotherapy vs. conventionally fractionated radiochemotherapy. Radiother Oncol 2004; 72:15-24.

13. Zaheer S, Pemberton JH, Farouk R, et al. Surgical treatment of adenocarcinoma of the rectum. Ann Surg 1998; 227:800-11.

14. Heald RJ, Husband EM, Ryall RD. The mesorectum in rectal cancer surgery—the clue to pelvic recurrence? Br J Surg 1982; 69:613-6.

15. Ridgway PF, Darzi AW. The role of total mesorectal excision in the management of rectal cancer. Cancer Control 2003; 10:205-11.

16. Quirke P, Steele R, Monson J, et al. Effect of the plane of surgery achieved on local recurrence in patients with operable rectal cancer: a prospective study using data from the MRC CR07 and NCIC-CTG CO16 randomised clinical trial. Lancet 2009; 373:821-8.

17. Breukink S, Pierie J, Wiggers T. Laparoscopic versus open total mesorectal excision for rectal cancer. Cochrane Database Syst Rev 2006; CD005200.

18. Ng SS, Leung KL, Lee JF, et al. Long-term morbidity and oncologic outcomes of laparoscopic-assisted anterior resection for upper rectal cancer: ten-year results of a prospective, randomized trial. Dis Colon Rectum 2009; 52:558-66.

19. Laparoscopic-assisted versus open abdominoperineal resection for low rectal cancer: a prospective randomized trial. Ann Surg Oncol 2008; 15:2418-25.

20. Lujan J, Valero G, Hernandez Q, et al. Randomized clinical trial comparing laparoscopic and open surgery in patients with rectal cancer. Br J Surg 2009; 96:982-9.

21. Epidermoid anal cancer: results from the UKCCCR randomised trial of radiotherapy alone versus radiotherapy, 5-fluorouracil and mitomycin. UKCCCR Anal Cancer Trial Working Party. UK Co-ordinating Committee on Cancer Research. Lancet 1996; 348(9034):1049-54.

22. Ajani JA, Winter KA, Gunderson LL, et al. Fluorouracil, mitomycin and radiotherapy vs fluorouracil, cisplatin and radiotherapy for carcinoma of the anal canal: a randomized controlled trial. Jama 2008; 299:1914-21.

23. Flam M, John M, Pajak TF, et al. Role of mitomycin in combination with fluorouracil and radiotherapy and of salvage chemoradiation in the definitive nonsurgical treatment of epidermoid carcinoma of the anal canal: results of a phase III randomized intergroup study. J Clin Oncol 1996; 14:2527-39.

24. Nigro ND. An evaluation of combined therapy for squamous cell cancer of the anal canal. Dis Colon Rectum 1984; 27:763-6.

25. Papillon J, Chassard JL. Respective roles of radiotherapy and surgery in the management of epidermoid carcinoma of the anal margin. Series of 57 patients. Dis Colon Rectum 1992; 35:422-9.

26. Schiller DE, Cummings BJ, Rai S, et al. Outcomes of salvage surgery for squamous cell carcinoma of the anal canal. Ann Surg Oncol 2007; 14:2780-9.

27. Bartelink H, et al. Concomitant radiotherapy and chemotherapy is superior to radiotherapy alone in the treatment of locally advanced anal cancer: results of a phase III randomized trial of the EORTC. J Clin Oncol 1997; 5:2040-9.

28. Mullen JT, et al. Results of surgical salvage after failed chemoradiation therapy for epidermoid carcinoma of the anal canal. Ann Surg Oncol 2007;4:478-83.

29. Newlin HE, et al. Squamous cell carcinoma of the anal margin. J Surg Oncol 2004;86:55-62.

Section 7

Hepatobiliary System

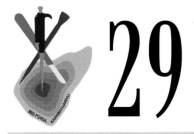

29

Liver Cancer

Tsafrir Vanounou, Kevin Tri Nguyen, T Clark Gamblin

The management of liver tumors has become increasingly more complex and consequently more multidisciplinary. Prior to embarking into liver surgery, numerous patient, tumor, liver and therapeutic factors must thoughtfully be considered in order to optimize clinical and oncological outcomes. Patient factors, such as preoperative functional status and willingness to undertake therapy, must be interpreted within the context of tumor factors, such as disease stage, speed of progression and probability of cure with intervention. Similarly, liver factors, such as degree of underlying liver or biliary dysfunction, must be taken into consideration when weighing the value of various therapeutic options spanning from aggressive surgical resection to regional or systemic therapy to palliative comfort measures. The intent of this chapter is to summarize the multidisciplinary and multimodality treatment approaches to various liver tumors.

Surgical Anatomy of the Liver

Precise anatomical knowledge of the liver and biliary tract is essential for the safe performance of surgery on this vital organ. The best way to summarize hepatic anatomy is that it is highly variable and that the details matter when it comes to successful liver surgery. That is, hepatic surgical anatomy is based on detailed knowledge of the liver's internal divisions including a functional understanding of its congenital variants. While an in-depth analysis of both is beyond the scope of this chapter, one can and should review this topic in any number of major surgical textbooks.

While classic morphological anatomy describes the external appearance of the liver and its ligamentous attachments, functional surgical anatomy focuses on the internal architecture of the liver which provides the roadmap for safe hepatic resection. In essence, functional surgical anatomy is the anatomic basis for modern day hepatic surgery and is based on the work of several pioneering authors (Cantlie, McIndoe and Counseller, Ton That Tung, Hjorstjo, Couinaud, Goldsmith, Woodburne and Bismuth).

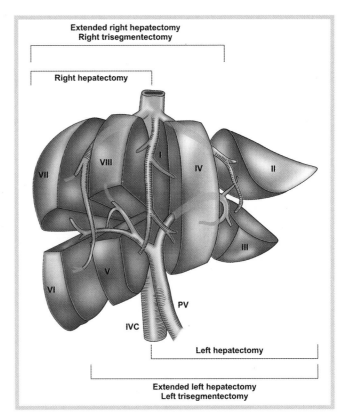

Figure 29-1: Segments of the liver

The description by Couinard in 1957 is the most complete and exact and is the most useful for the practicing surgeon. It divides the liver into eight segments based on portal segmentation such that any of the eight segments can be resected while preserving the vascular inflow, venous outflow and biliary drainage of the remaining segments **(Figure 29-1)**. The segments are numbered in a clockwise direction from an anterior view starting with the caudate lobe as segment I. These segments are combined to form sectors separated by scissurae containing the three main hepatic veins which drain directly from the upper posterior surface of the liver into the inferior vena cava.

An alternative terminology suggested by the committee of the International Hepato-Pancreato-Biliary Association (IHPBA) (http://www.ihpba.org/liver-resection-second-order-div.html) renames Couinaud's sectors into sections, particularly when describing the left liver. This Brisbane terminology is especially critical when describing the extent of hepatic resections. This chapter will predominantly use Couinaud's nomenclature when discussing surgical anatomy, while using the Brisbane terminology when describing hepatic resections.

The liver can morphologically be divided into two lobes by the falciform ligament. However, from a functional point of view, these morphological lobes have no bearing on the true internal architecture or subdivisions of the liver. Functionally, the liver is subdivided into sectors and hemilivers based on the location of its three main hepatic veins. These veins run within scissurae which divide the liver into four sectors each receiving a portal (or glissonian) pedicle. Each pedicle consists of a triad of portal vein, hepatic artery and bile duct all enveloped within a sheath formed by an extension of Glisson's capsule. This capsule is a thin fibrous covering which encases most of the liver. At the hilum, the right portal triad has a very short course before entering the substance of the liver and dividing into the right anterior and posterior pedicles. On the left side, however, the portal pedicle has a long extrahepatic course which then turns anteriorly and caudally to enter the umbilical fissure. While the anatomic variations in the branching of the portal pedicles is beyond the scope of this chapter, a thorough knowledge of these anomalies is critical for the safe performance of liver surgery.

The central scissura, containing the middle hepatic vein, corresponds to Cantlie's line which anatomically defines the right and left hemilivers. These functional right and left hemilivers are fully independent with respect to their portal and arterial vascularization and their biliary drainage. In addition, these hemilivers are asymmetrical with the right liver on average accounting for two thirds of the total liver volume and the left liver accounting for about one-third. The caudate (segment I) which is a separate anatomical unit represents 1% of the total liver volume.

The right portal scissura, comprised of the right hepatic vein, separates the right liver into two sectors—antero-medial or anterior (segments V and VIII) and posterolateral or posterior (segments VI and VII). The left portal scissura, comprised of the left hepatic vein, also separates the left liver into two sectors—anterior (segments IV and III) and posterior (segment II). Alternatively, in the Brisbane 2000 terminology of liver anatomy, the left portal scissura divides the left liver into the left medial section (segment IV) and a left lateral section (segments II and III). Of note, from an embryological and functional point of view, segment I (caudate lobe) is autonomous as its vasculature and biliary drainage is independent of the portal pedicles and the hepatic veins. The caudate lobe is supplied by portal branches from the right and left portal veins, by arterial inflow and biliary drainage from the right posterior pedicle and the left main pedicle and venous outflow draining directly into the vena cava.

While the aforementioned description outlines the 'usual' hepatic functional anatomy, it is essential that all hepatic surgery be guided by not only a thorough understanding of functional surgical anatomy but also a clear understand of the common and less common functional variants which can have a dramatic impact on the final outcome posthepatic resection. A guiding light which can help inform and direct intraoperative decision-making is the availability of high-quality pre- and intraoperative imaging. That is, preoperative cross-sectional imaging, whether CT or MRI, in conjunction with intraoperative ultrasonography permit the surgeon to identify nearly all meaningful anatomical variations such that there should be no intraoperative surprises when transecting the hepatic parenchyma thereby resulting in optimal postoperative outcomes.

Preoperative Evaluation

Preoperative assessment fundamentally begins with outlining patient comorbidities and performance status, clarifying underlying liver pathology, estimating current and future functional capacity and reserve, understanding liver anatomy and meaningful variants and finally elucidating tumor characteristics and topography. Together these elements form a roadmap which can be used to objectively assess respectability. Resectability is a complex and multifactorial inference which cannot and should not be reached until a thorough and thoughtful analysis of all the aforementioned factors are considered as a whole rather than in isolation.

Patient Factors

Assessing patient candidacy for surgical intervention begins with a thorough assessment of comorbid conditions, overall health and functional capacity. Preoperative assessment of comorbid medical illness is critical because comorbid illness has been repeatedly shown to be a major determinant of occurrence of postoperative morbidity and mortality in recent series of hepatectomy. If present, these conditions should vigorously be investigated and treated prior to considering surgical intervention. In some cases if serious or untreatable (e.g. recent myocardial infarction and advanced renal failure), these patients should not be subjected to surgery.

Comorbid illness is particularly prevalent in elderly people. While age alone should not necessarily be an exclusion criteria for surgical intervention, elderly people may be at higher risk following major hepatectomy than their younger counterparts for several reasons: their livers are relatively small because of aging; liver function is suboptimal because fatty change is not infrequently present; their costal arch is rigid causing difficulty in exposure of the upper abdomen and it is difficult to bring down their central venous pressure during liver transection without affecting the blood pressure. Therefore, elderly patients are accepted for hepatectomy only if they are free from prohibitive comorbidities.

Perhaps of greater importance than numeric age is functional status which refers to an individual's ability to perform normal daily activities required to meet basic needs, fulfill usual roles and maintain health and well-being. Decline in functional status is measured by an individual's loss of independence in activities of daily living (ADLs) over a period of time. Several tools exist to rate the ability of patients to maintain their independence in the context of their daily life and encompass dimensions of physical, emotional and cognitive well-being. The tools most often used in our practice include the Eastern Cooperative Oncology Group (ECOG) performance status, the Karnofsky Performance Scale. The ECOG scale **(Table 29-1)** is simple to determine and when used longitudinally over time allows a physician to quickly assess how a patient's disease is progressing and how the disease affects the daily living abilities of the patient thus helping to determine appropriate treatment and prognosis. For the most part, aggressive surgical or locoregional therapy should be reserved to patients with an ECOG score of 0 or 1.

Liver Pathology and Reserve

Clarifying underlying liver pathology usually starts with assessing for risk factors for liver disease such as hepatitis and alcohol intake. While it can be argued that almost all patients who develop hepatocellular carcinoma (HCC) should be tested for hepatitis exposure, for all other patients, testing can be selective based on the presence of risk factors such as intravenous drug abuse, history of tattoos or history of blood transfusion prior to 1990. All patients should specifically be asked about alcohol intake, past and present, as well as how long they have been abstinent from alcohol since these questions have a particularly important impact on whether they can be listed for liver transplantation.

Evaluation of liver functional capacity and reserve is particularly important for patients with underlying cirrhosis from chronic hepatitis or alcohol abuse. While basic liver function tests have not shown to be accurate predictors of outcomes following hepatectomy, indirect measures of liver synthetic ability (albumin, PT/INR), functional status (total bilirubin) and indicators of portal hypertension (platelet count) can all be used to formulate a more complete assessment of underlying liver pathology. Other clinical pearls which are useful to gauge the extent of underlying liver function is to ascertain whether the patient has had a history of clinical ascites, whether they have required diuretics or paracentesis to control their ascites, whether they have a history of encephalopathy or are currently taking lactulose and whether they have had a history of gastrointestinal hemorrhage from variceal disease or whether they have been noted on upper endoscopy to have esophageal varices.

While many classification systems have been proposed for the risk-stratification and selection of patients for hepatectomy, the Child-Pugh (or Child-Turcotte-Pugh) classification is perhaps the most commonly employed **(Table 29-2)**. The parameters measured in this classification score include the presence or absence of clinical ascites and encephalopathy, serum albumin and total bilirubin, as well as international normalized ratio. Together these criteria help classify patients into three classes based on a rough estimate of hepatic synthetic and detoxification capacity. Numerous studies have validated the predictive validity of the Child-Pugh score when assessing the postoperative survival in cirrhotic patients. In general, only patients with Child-Pugh class A liver function are suitable for major hepatectomy. However,

TABLE 29-1	Eastern Cooperative Oncology Group (ECOG) performance status
Grade	**ECOG performance status**
0	Fully active, able to carry on all pre-disease performance without restriction
1	Restricted in physically strenuous activity but ambulatory and able to carry out work of a light or sedentary nature, e.g., light house work, office work
2	Ambulatory and capable of all selfcare but unable to carry out any work activities. Up and about more than 50% of waking hours
3	Capable of only limited selfcare, confined to bed or chair more than 50% of waking hours
4	Completely disabled. Cannot carry on any selfcare. Totally confined to bed or chair
5	Dead

Adapted with permission from: Oken MM, Creech RH, Tormey DC, Horton J, Davis TE, McFadden ET, Carbone PP. Toxicity and response criteria of the Eastern Cooperative Oncology Group. Am J Clin Oncol 1982;5:649-55, with credit to the Eastern Cooperative Oncology Group, Robert Comis MD, Group Chair

TABLE 29-2	Child-Turcotte-Pugh classification of hepatic functional reserve			
Measure	1 point	2 points	3 points	units
Bilirubin (total)	< 2	2-3	> 3	mg/dl
Serum albumin	> 3.5	2.8-3.5	< 2.8	g/dl
INR	< 1.7	1.71-2.20	> 2.20	no unit
Ascites	None	Suppressed with medication	Refractory	no unit
Hepatic encephalopathy	None	Grade I-II (or suppressed with medication)	Grade III-IV (or refractory)	no unit

Class A: 5-6 points, Class B: 7-9 points, Class C: 10-15 points.

among patients with Child-Pugh class A liver function, the hospital mortality rate after major hepatectomy is still high, therefore both patients and surgeons must be cognizant of the postoperative morbidity and mortality in this patient subset. Patients with Child-Pugh class B liver reserve may tolerate minor resection but generally do not tolerate major hepatectomy. Patients with class C liver function are non-surgical candidate given the high risk of death from almost any invasive intervention.

Although the Child-Turcotte-Pugh scoring system was the first of its kind in stratifying the seriousness of end-stage liver disease, it is by no means the only one. While the Model for End-Stage Liver Disease (MELD) score is universally used to assess patients for liver transplantation, it has increasingly been used to predict post-operative survival in patients with cirrhosis. In fact, the MELD score has been shown to provide a complementary predictive value to the widely used Child-Pugh score. Patients with Child-Pugh class C cirrhosis and MELD scores > 14 are generally not considered for surgical intervention. Patients with Child-Pugh class B cirrhosis and MELD scores > 8-14 have an increased perioperative risk and the indication for surgery should be assessed carefully with most patients being steered toward non-surgical options. In patients with Child-Pugh class A cirrhosis and MELD scores of £ 8, perioperative mortality is low.

Addressing one of the shortcomings of the Child-Pugh and MELD classification systems is the Okuda staging system which takes into account not only functional liver reserve but also the extent of disease. The Okuda system incorporates ascites status, serum albumin and total bilirubin, as well as tumor size thus accounting for tumor extension. Several studies have evaluated the comparative accuracy of the Child-Pugh and Okuda systems with mixed results. Similarly to the Okuda system, the Cancer of the Liver Italian Program (CLIP) score, which incorporates the Child-Pugh stage, tumor morphology, alpha-fetoprotein (AFP) and portal vein thrombosis, also tries to account for both liver function and tumor characteristics. Of note however, both the Okuda and CLIP systems were intentionally developed for cirrhotic

patients with hepatocellular carcinoma while the Child-Pugh system is intended for use in all patients with cirrhosis. The Child-Pugh was originally developed to predict risk of esophageal bleeding in cirrhotic patients.

Although not routinely used in North America, dynamic tests can provide additional information on the expected residual hepatic function in patients with cirrhosis. These quantitative tests include the indocyanine green (ICG) clearance and the monoethylglycinexylidide (MEGX) clearance tests. The most commonly employed test for the assessment of liver function and functional reserve is the ICG clearance test which has been confirmed as a valuable adjunct in quantifying liver function. ICG is a dye that is cleared from the circulation by the liver and its clearance is an indicator of hepatocyte function. Studies, mostly out of Asia, suggest that an ICG retention rate at 15 minutes (ICG-R15) after intravenous administration of > 14% is the cut-off point that maximally separates patients with or without hospital mortality after major hepatectomy. One study suggested that when the ICG-R15 is below 10%, two or more segments can be resected safely, when the ICG-R15 is 10-20%, one segment can be resected safely and two or more segments may be resected with great care. However, when the ICG-R15 is > 20%, any type of hepatic resection will be associated with high postoperative risk but the patient's general condition and other liver function tests should be taken into consideration when making a decision. A caveat that must be considered when interpreting this test is that hepatic clearance of ICG depends on portal vein blood flow and bile duct patency thus falsely elevated ICG-R15 can be seen in patients with partial portal vein compression or bile duct obstruction by the tumor thereby mandating that ICG clearance results be interpreted in conjunction with imaging modalities able to rule out these confounding variables.

A final caveat regarding liver functional capacity and reserve is the concept of future liver remnant (FLR). There is no question that residual liver volume after hepatic resection is tightly correlated with postoperative liver function and with the occurrence of postoperative liver failure when the remnant is insufficient. Moreover, underlying liver disease and its associated impaired liver functional capacity mandate a larger remnant liver to achieve the same functional reserve as would be seen in a patient with a normal liver. In fact, what all the above mentioned tests (e.g. Child-Pugh, ICG-R15) try to indirectly predict is whether the future remnant liver, in light of the extent of underlying liver disease, will be sufficient to maintain hepatic synthetic function postoperatively. Studies have shown that for patients with normal livers, an FLR of > 20% is sufficient to avoid postoperative liver insufficiency. In contrast, in patients with markedly impaired baseline liver function, a 40% FLR may be required to avoid cholestasis, fluid retention and liver failure postoperatively. Patients with normal livers and a small FLR have a greater complication rate but rarely die of these complications while patients with underlying liver dysfunction and a small FLR are at high risk of dying from their postoperative complications.

Three-dimensional computed tomography (CT) can be used to accurately predict the FLR in patients with normal or mildly cirrhotic livers. The accuracy of CT volumetry suffers noticeably in the setting of moderate to severe underlying liver dysfunction. The reason for this discrepancy is that in cases of severe liver disease, volume is an inappropriate surrogate for functionality of the remnant liver. Inaccuracies can also occur when multiple or large tumors occupy a large volume of the liver to be resected. Another caveat of this test is that FLR must be interpreted within the context of patient size. That is, large patients need larger liver remnants than do smaller patients. Two options for overcoming this latter caveat exists with both formulas attempting to standardize FLR to body habitus; the first standardizes FLR by dividing it by total liver volume (FLR/TLV) which is derived from body surface area (BSA), the second divides FLR by body weight (FLR/BW). Studies have demonstrated a strong correlation between the FLR measurements standardized to BW and BSA thus highlighting that both methods are appropriate for assessing liver volume and predicting postoperative hepatic dysfunction. Overall, in noncirrhotic patients, an FLR/BW ratio of greater than 0.4 and FLR/TLV of greater than 20% provide equivalent thresholds for performing safe hepatic resection.

In patients where the FLR is deemed insufficient for safe hepatic resection, portal vein embolization or portal vein ligation can be utilized to increase the size of the remnant liver. By diverting nutrient portal flow from the segments to be resected, the remaining liver will hypertrophy thus increasing the safety of major hepatectomy in patients with normal or diseased livers. The primary difference which occurs in patients with normal and diseased underlying livers is that the resulting hypertrophy occurs quicker (within 4-6 weeks) and is more vigorous in patients with normal livers as compared to patients with cirrhosis.

Liver Anatomy and Tumor Topography

The last element critical to the complete preoperative assessment of patients planned for liver resection is to clearly illustrate the underlying liver anatomy, identify any meaningful anatomical variants as well as to outline the topography and characteristics of the hepatic tumor. Preoperative imaging is essential to this analysis.

The multidetector CT scan is the single most reliable imaging modality in outlining liver anatomy, characterizing liver pathology, gauging the extent of underlying liver disease and deciding on the resectability of the tumor based on both anatomic ground and CT volumetry of the remnant liver. CT with dynamic intravenous contrast can precisely characterize tumor pathology with a high degree of accuracy. Triphasic CT (noncontrast, arterial and portovenous phases) is the cornerstone of diagnostic imaging at our institution due to its overall accuracy, speed and relatively quick availability. Quadriphasic CT scanning (noncontrast, arterial, portovenous and delayed venous phases) is employed when the suspicion for cholangiocarcinoma (particularly hilar cholangiocarcinoma) is high. In some regions, lipiodol, an oily derivative of the poppy seed, is combined with the iodine contrast medium. Once injected intravenously, this mixture is retained by the tumor, primarily HCC and can be used with CT scanning to image small tumors.

While both CT and magnetic resonance imaging (MRI) allow for dynamic contrast-enhanced imaging, MRI tends to not add significant diagnostic value beyond that obtained with high-quality CT imaging. It is a more cumbersome test for patients and is less readily available thus is used selectively when CT imaging is contra-indicated (e.g. IV dye allergy, renal impairment) or when additional information concerning the benign or malignant nature of a hepatic lesion is needed or when additional information regarding the anatomical relationship between a tumor and major hepatic vessels is required. Ultrasound (US) is an inexpensive and quick screening tool but its sensitivity and specificity are comparatively low and thus not routinely utilized in our institution. Hepatic angiography is rarely required today. It was performed in the past for showing the arterial anatomy and served as a 'road map' for hilar dissection. Now that the arterial anatomy can be clearly and accurately shown by CT scan and intraoperative US, this test has rarely employed.

A last diagnostic complement to the work-up of liver lesions includes the use of tumor markers to help complement other diagnostics test to help establish the diagnosis as well as follow therapeutic efficacy and tumor recurrence. Tumor markers [carcinoembryonic antigen: CEA, alpha-fetoprotein (AFP) and CA19-9] are molecules occurring in blood or tissue that are associated with cancer and whose measurement or identification is useful in patient diagnosis or clinical management. In general, tumor markers can be used for one of four purposes: (1) screening a healthy population or a high risk population for the presence of cancer; (2) making a diagnosis of cancer or of a specific type of cancer; (3) determining the prognosis in a patient; (4) monitoring the course in a patient in remission or while receiving surgery, radiation or chemotherapy.

As stated before, the assessment of resectability can only be made in earnest once the aforementioned preoperative assessment has been completed. That is, the decision to resect and the choice of the extent of a hepatic resection should not solely be based on surgical judgment. In our practice we assess functional capacity using the ECOG performance score and utilize the Child-Pugh score to not only gauge liver reserve but also establish the maximum extent of surgery a patient can tolerate without undue postoperative risk. We reserve major hepatic resection for patients with an ECOG score of 0 or 1 and a Child-Pugh class A while limiting patients with impaired functional capacity and/or Child-Pugh class B to minor segmental resections. Although there is supporting data to indicate that the Child-Pugh score can be augmented by assessing tumor extent or by incorporating ICG retention testing, we do not employ this test due to the test's inherent complexity and because we believe that the nuances glimpsed from this test do not significantly augment the overall predictive ability beyond what is learned with the Child-Pugh score alone. Our institution heavily favors triphasic CT imaging augmented by thorough intraoperative ultrasonography to assess liver anatomy, detect anatomical variants and assess tumor topography. Once this data has been collected, patients are presented at our multidisciplinary conference which brings together liver surgeons, transplant surgeons, hepatologists, pathologists and radiologists. When presented with all the requisite information, this inclusive group is better able to reach treatment decisions that can maximize the patient's outcome as well as ensure adherence to best practice guidelines.

Benign and Premalignant Liver Lesions

Background

Benign liver tumors are increasingly being detected due to improvements in and routine use of imaging modalities. The most frequent benign tumors of the liver include hemangioma, hepatic adenoma (HA) and focal nodular hyperplasia (FNH). Their actual prevalence remains to be defined, with autopsy series estimating the frequency of hemangiomas at 3-20% and the frequency of FNHs at 0.4-0.8%. Present data concerning HA indicate this tumor is very rare with an estimated incidence of fewer than five cases per million persons.

The majority of patients are asymptomatic and no treatment is indicated. In fact, the natural history of hemangioma and FNH is well-documented and is typically uneventful with negligible risk of malignant degeneration or complication such as rupture or hemorrhage. Consequently, in the case of a reliable diagnosis of an asymptomatic hemangioma or focal nodular hyperplasia, elective surgery is not indicated. Surgery is reserved in these latter cases for patients with symptoms directly attributable to these benign hepatic lesions.

In contrast, the natural history of HA is not only less clear but also more treacherous with no clear consensus regarding their management. In fact, the natural history of hepatic adenomas can be complicated by life-threatening conditions, such as rupture and hemorrhage as well as the constant risk of malignant degeneration into hepatocellular carcinoma. This chapter will focus solely on hepatic adenomas given that this is the only truly premalignant liver lesion.

Pathology

Histologically, HA is characterized by sheets of monotonous hepatocytes, lacking biliary elements, surrounded by a stromal capsule with a paucity of mitotic figures. Interestingly, HA appear to maintain the normal amount and distribution of reticulin and those at high risk of malignant transformation may express high levels of nuclear β-catenin as determined by mutational analysis and real time reverse transcriptase-polymerase chain reaction (RT-PCR). Zucman-Rossi, et al also demonstrated that accompanying malignancy occurs only rarely in HA with a mutated hepatocyte nuclear factor 1α ($HNF1\alpha$) gene which is characterized microscopically by the presence of steatosis as assessed on H&E-stained sections.

Natural History

Patients diagnosed with HA are typically young women in their twenties-thirties with a history of oral contraceptive pill (OCP) use. The association between HA and the use of OCP (which also holds true for FNH) was first described during the late 1960s when Edmondson and colleagues observed that as exogenous hormone use grew in the 1960s and 1970s there was an associated increase in the reported incidence of HA.

At the heart of the dilemma surrounding HA is its uncertain natural history. That is, treatment strategies for HA remain poorly defined primarily due to the paucity of data regarding the potential for life-threatening complications such as rupture, hemorrhage and progression to malignancy. A recent multicenter analysis by Deneve, et al which analyzed 124 patients with HA over a 9 year period has helped to more clearly define the factors associated with risks of rupture and malignancy in patients with HA. Rupture occurred in 31 (25%) cases and the analysis demonstrated that ruptured tumors tended to be larger (10.5 ± 4.5 cm vs 7.2 ± 4.8 cm; $p = 0.001$) than tumors that did not rupture and that no tumor < 5 cm ruptured. Multivariate analysis highlighted the fact that tumor size > 7 cm (odds ratio, 7.8; $p < 0.01$) and recent (within 6 months) hormone use (odds ratio, 4.5; $p < 0.01$) were independent predictors of rupture risk. Five cases (4%) had evidence of underlying malignancy with an average age and tumor size of 34.6 years and 11.6 cm, respectively. All tumors harboring malignancy measured > 8 cm in diameter. In addition, three of the five patients with evidence of malignancy were actively taking OCP hormones. Therefore in this multicenter series, no ruptured tumor was < 5 cm in largest diameter and the smallest lesion harboring malignancy was 8 cm.

Diagnosis

At imaging, HAs must be unambiguously differentiated from their benign counterparts; hemangiomas and focal nodular hyperplasia **(Figures 29-2 to 29-4)**. Hepatic adenomas may appear heterogeneous, reflecting the histological nature, the complex anatomy and composition of the lesions and the mode of presentation at the time of the diagnosis. Heterogeneity is most likely associated with relatively larger lesions containing hemorrhage, necrosis, fibrosis and malignant transformation.

On US, HAs without abundant necrosis, hemorrhage or malignant degeneration will most likely have a homogeneous appearance, with somewhat variable echogenicity, which depends on the structural composition of the lesions as well as that of the surrounding liver. In general, it is often challenging—if not impossible—to diagnose HA with confidence on the basis of the US of the liver alone. Currently, CT is increasingly applied for assessment of liver lesions. However, it should be kept in mind that, in the case of monophasic CT or incorrect timing of the arterial phase, HA can easily be misdiagnosed, exposing patients to unnecessary delay in diagnosis and proper treatment.

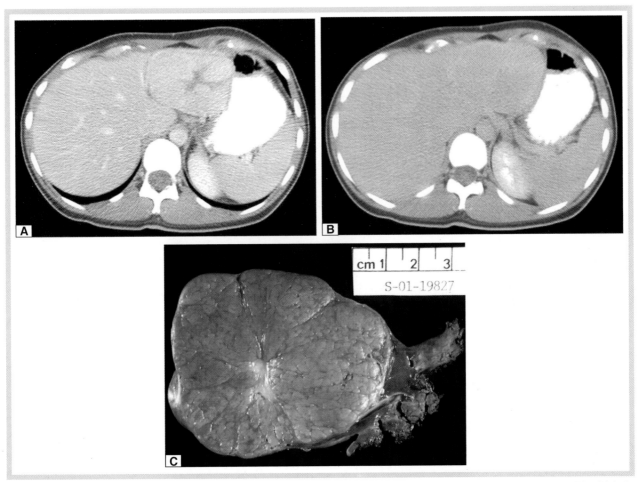

Figures 29-2A to C: CT characteristics of focal nodular hyperplasia. (A) Axial, enhanced CT shows an FNH which is hypervascular and hyperattenuating to liver on the phase scans, (B) and is isoattenuating to liver on the delayed portovenous phase scan. (C) A central scar can often be observed more readily in large lesions compared to smaller ones

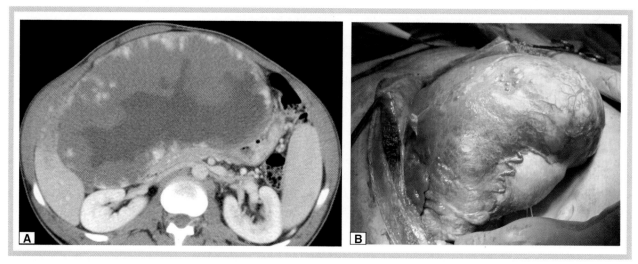

Figures 29-3A and B: CT characteristics of hepatic hemangiomas. On biphasic basic CT scan, large hemangiomas show asymmetrical nodular peripheral enhancement that is isodense with large vessels and then progressive centripetal enhancement fill-in over time

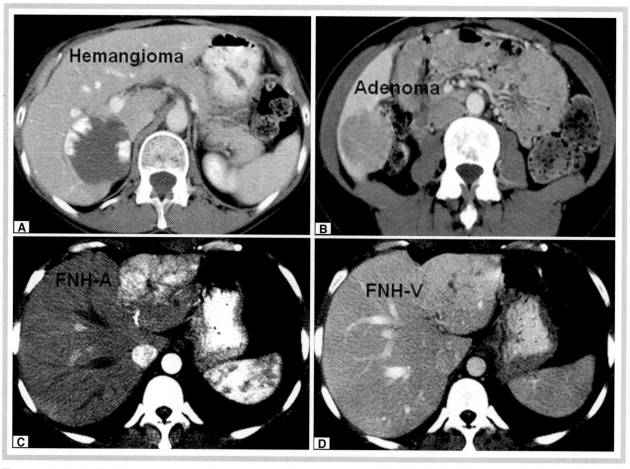

Figures 29-4A to C: CT comparisons of hemagioma, adenomas and FNH. (A) Hemangioma shows asymmetrical nodular peripheral enhancement. (B) Adenoma is hypovascular to the liver parenchyma. (C) Focal nodular hyperplasia (FNH) is hypervascular on arterial phase with a central scar and (D) isodense to the liver on venous phase

With CT, HAs without complications are likely to be isodense with the surrounding liver on unenhanced CT, become visible in the arterial phase with a homogeneous blush of contrast enhancement and then fade to isodensity in the portal or delayed phase. In cases of recent hemorrhage, HAs can often be obscured by the resulting hematoma which appears heterogeneous with predominantly high attenuation values. Calcification is present in 5-15% of cases of HAs. CT scans obtained after intravenous injection of contrast medium are central to the diagnosis of HAs with hepatic adenomas usually showing early homogeneous enhancement during the arterial phase and attenuation nearly identical to that of normal liver parenchyma on the portal venous phase. In light of the central role that the homogeneous enhancement in the arterial phase plays in the radiologic diagnosis of HA, proper timing of image acquisition is crucial. The broad availability of CT, as well as the recent development and implementation of the faster multi-slice detector machines, makes this modality an excellent tool for detection and characterization of focal liver lesions. The issue of radiation is even more important in relatively young and otherwise healthy patients with an incidental liver lesion, such as HA, that needs characterization or follow-up. One fundamental limitation of CT remains the lack of the ability to alter the intrinsic soft tissue contrast, which is useful to assess diffuse and focal liver abnormalities.

Current state-of-the-art MR imaging provides a more comprehensive and accurate workup of focal and diffuse liver disease based on the unique properties of MR imaging that possess a combination of high intrinsic soft tissue contrast combined with various distinctly different tissue characteristics at imaging and high sensitivity for the presence or absence of contrast-uptake and enhancement patterns. Dynamic gadolinium-enhanced imaging is considered essential in detection and characterization of liver lesions.

At MR imaging, these HAs often have the following characteristics: (a) almost isointense or slightly hyperintense to the surrounding liver on T1-weighted, in-phase, gradient-echo images (indicating the hepatocellular nature of the lesions); (b) compared with in-phase images, may become relatively hyperintense to the liver (due to decreased signal of the fatty liver) or hypointense as well as heterogeneous to the liver (due to decreased signal within the fatty lesion) on the T1-weighted, opposed-phase images; (c) slightly hyperintense or hypointense on fat-suppressed T2-weighted images (depending mainly on whether the HA is surrounded by fatty liver or the lesion itself contains abundant fat or fibrosis, respectively); (d) faint homogeneous enhancement (blush) in the arterial phase and (e) isointense in the delayed phase, without washout or capsular enhancement.

Treatment

The absence of clear evidence has precluded the outlining of a rational approach to hepatic adenomas. When considering the management of hepatic adenoma, the following variables are of clinical relevance: the accuracy of imaging techniques, the conclusiveness of the diagnosis, the incidence of tumor acute complications, the mortality rate after elective surgery, the mortality rate from acute tumor complications and the mortality rate after emergency surgery. Overall, the available data for these parameters is scant and of poor quality with all the studies being retrospective surgical series that are inadequate to accurately estimate the incidence of these parameters. The available data has thus done little to settle the divergence in opinion regarding the optimal management of hepatic adenomas nor has it outlined the role of surgery.

Despite the absence of level one evidence-based data, agreed upon indications for elective surgical resection of hepatic adenomas include uncertain diagnosis, inability to exclude malignancy, presence of symptoms and large size ($\geq$ 5 cm) primarily because of the risk of rupture, hemorrhage and the risk of neoplastic degeneration. In the case of small and asymptomatic hepatic adenomas, no such consensus exists regarding their optimal management resulting in a wide variation in clinical practice among liver surgeons.

On the one hand, some experts argue that the natural history and clinical behavior of asymptomatic hepatic adenomas does not justify elective surgical resection thereby advocating long-term clinical observation for these small and asymptomatic hepatic adenomas. In contrast, other experts advocate the elective resection of all hepatic adenomas provided it is done without significant morbidity or mortality because of the risk of intraperitoneal hemorrhage and the development of hepatocellular carcinoma. The factors favoring primary surgical treatment of hepatic adenomas in what tends to be a young female population include the elimination of the risk of latent malignant degeneration and hemorrhagic rupture of hepatic adenomas, the eradication of the dilemma posed by pregnancy and the avoidance of long-term radiographic follow-up with its inherent economic burden and the related public health crisis surrounding long-term exposure to radiation from screening. Moreover, while the use of the laparoscopic approach should not alter the indications for surgical resection, the advent of minimally invasive liver resection with its associated clinical benefits has nonetheless added a new dimension to this already complex debate.

Summary

- The natural history of hepatic adenoma is uncertain and can be complicated by life-threatening conditions such as rupture, hemorrhage and malignant degeneration. For these complications or when a definite histologic diagnosis is needed, surgery is advisable.

■ In clinical practice there is a wide variation concerning the use of elective surgery. Given the lack of randomized clinical trials and the inconsistent data regarding the relative merits of observation versus surgery for small, asymptomatic HA, there is no evidence to support or refute elective surgery for benign liver tumors.

Malignant Liver Lesions

Metastatic Colorectal Cancer

The liver is the main sight of metastasis of colorectal cancer. Synchronous lesions are found at presentation in 15-25% of patients and approximately 20-25% of patients will develop metachronous hepatic metastasis after resection

of the primary colon cancer. If left untreated, the median survival is 5-7.5 months with 0-2% survival at 5 years. A treatment algorithm is provided **(Figure 29-5)**.

Since the 1970s, chemotherapy for metastatic colorectal cancer was mainly with 5-fluorouracil (5-FU), either alone or in combination with other chemotherapy agents, with response rates of < 30%. The combination of 5-FU and leucovorin was the most common first-line combination in the 1990s. The addition of irinotecan (CPT-11) and oxaliplatin improved response rates to 45-51% and improved survival compared to the 5-FU/leucovorin combination. Targeted biological agents, such as cetuximab, an epidermal growth factor receptor antagonist and bevacizumab (Avastin), a monoclonal antibody against vascular endothelial growth factor, have further broaden the medical armamentarium against unresectable metastatic colorectal cancer. In the absence of surgical intervention, the current systemic therapy combinations

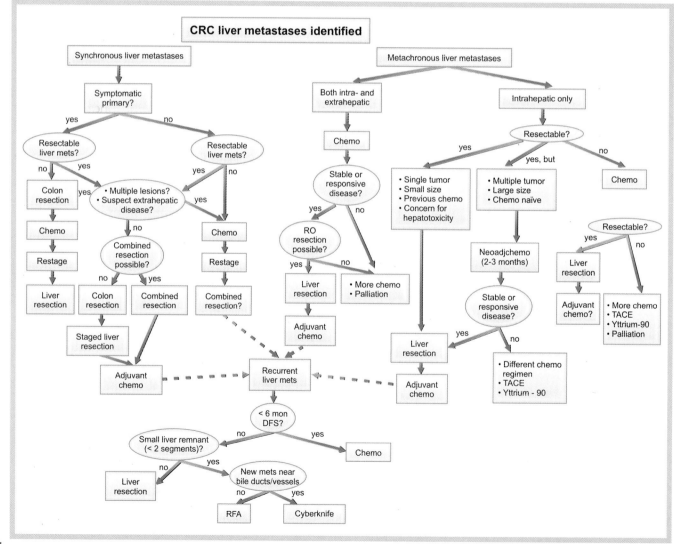

Figure 29-5: Treatment algorithm for the treatment of patients with colorectal liver metastases

provide response rates of approximately 50% with up to 20 months median survival; however, without resection, survival is rare at 5 years.

Foster, et al provided the first report in 1979 showing the superiority of liver resection for colorectal metastasis in a multi-institutional series with a 20% 5-year survival rate. More recent series have shown 5-year survival rates ranging from 32% to 71%, with the highest survival seen after hepatic resection for solitary colorectal metastasis. Ten-year survival rates of 16.7-26% and even a 15-year survival rate of 24% have been reported. One-third of patients who survive to 5 years will eventually die of cancer-related deaths, while those patients who survive to 10 years are effectively cured of their disease. Patients at 10 years with complete tumor clearance without relapse have 100% survival at 15 years.

With 15-25% of patients presenting with synchronous primary colorectal cancer and liver metastasis, the timing of resection and the administration of chemotherapy remains controversial. Reddy, et al showed that simultaneous colorectal cancer resection and minor (1-2 segments) hepatectomy appears safe, while simultaneous colorectal cancer resection and major ($\geq$ 3) hepatectomy is associated with increased mortality (8.3% vs 1.4%, p < 0.05) and severe morbidity (36.1% vs 15.1%, p < 0.05), although others have argued that simultaneous colorectal and liver resection should be undertaken, regardless of the extent of hepatectomy. Reddy, et al also found that administration of chemotherapy after, but not before, resection of synchronous colorectal liver metastasis was associated with improved recurrence-free and overall survival. However, Capussotti, et al argued that patients with synchronous liver metastases and T4 primary colon cancer, metastatic infiltration of neighboring structures and > 3 metastatic nodules should receive neoadjuvant chemotherapy before liver resection. A prospective, randomized trial is needed to further delineate the timing of chemotherapy and hepatic resection in synchronous, metastatic colorectal cancer.

Historically, 5-year survival for patients who underwent liver resection for $\geq$ 4 metastases was 18%; therefore, liver resection was recommended for patients who met strict criteria (< 4 metastatic lesions, no extrahepatic metastatic disease and ability to achieve resection margins > 1 cm). More recent studies have challenged this dogma. Altendorf-Hofmann and Scheele found that there was no survival difference in patients who underwent liver resection for < 4 colorectal metastases versus patients who underwent resection for > 4 lesions, as long as an R0 resection was achieved. Minagawa, et al showed in a series of 235 patients that the 10-year survival rate after liver resection of patients with > 4 colorectal metastases was 29%, which is comparable to the 32% survival rate of patients undergoing resection for solitary colorectal

metastasis. Pawlik, et al also demonstrated a 5-year overall and disease-free survival rates of 51% and 22%, respectively, after hepatic resection in a series of 159 patients with $\geq$ 4 metastases. Patients with certain extrahepatic metastasis also have improved survival with complete metastasectomy. Patients with liver metastasis and extrahepatic metastasis to the lung have 5-year survival rates of 30-74%, if they under complete liver and lung metastases resections. Peritoneal carcinomatosis remains a contra-indication to hepatic resection. The '1 cm rule' in hepatic resection for cancer states that anticipated resection margins of < 1 cm is an absolute or relative contra-indication to resection and have been adopted by many surgeons. Studies from the MD Anderson group showed that 5-year survival rates of patients with positive margins was significantly worse than patients with negative margins (17% vs 64%, p = 0.01); however, on multi-variant analysis, the width of the negative margin did not affect survival, as 5-year survivals of patients with sub-centimeter negative margins 1-4 mm (62%) and 5-9 mm (71%), was not significantly different from the 5-year survival in patients with > 1 cm margins (63%) (p=0.63).

The criteria of resectability have continued to evolve and expand with a paradigm shift in the definition of 'resectability' from one based on what is *removed* (number of tumors, size, extrahepatic disease) to one based on what *remains* after resection (R0 resection and sufficient functional liver reserve). The number of patients eligible for surgical intervention has increased with the more widespread use of modern chemotherapy to downstage/downsize liver tumors, portal vein embolization to improve postoperative liver reserves and combined resection with ablation and two-stage hepatectomies for multiple bilobar disease. Neoadjuvant systemic and regional chemotherapy have reportedly converted patients who were deemed unresectable to resectable at a rate of 12.5-37% with median survivals of 19-26 months and reported 2-year, 3-year, 5-year and 10-year survival rates of 100%, 54-65%, 33-40% and 23%, respectively. Portal vein embolization allows for compensatory hypertrophy of the contralateral liver lobe and should be utilized if the predicted functional liver reserve after hepatic resection is < 20% in patients with normal liver parenchyma, < 30% in patients with liver injury from chemotherapy, steatosis or hepatitis and < 40% in patients with liver cirrhosis.

For patients with multiple, bilobar hepatic metastases, combined resection with ablation and two-staged hepatectomy can be considered. Compared to surgical resection, radiofrequency ablation therapy alone for metastatic colorectal cancer to the liver is associated with higher local recurrence (9% vs 2%, p = 0.02), higher liver-only recurrence (44% vs 11%, p < 0.001) and worse overall survival (4-year 22% vs 65%, p < 0.0001). The combination of hepatic resection and ablation for the treatment of metastatic colorectal cancer to the liver is less frequently utilized (6-24%) to treat metastatic colorectal metastases; however, for multiple, bilobar disease, some of which may not be amenable to resection, then the combination of hepatic resection and ablation may expand the number of patients who can undergo liver-directed therapy and may improve long-term survival, compared to chemotherapy alone.

Two-staged hepatectomies provide an alternative management strategy for multiple, bilobar hepatic colorectal metastases. At the first operation, tumor burden in the future remnant, usually the left lobe or left lateral section, is removed with a wedge resection. This is followed by portal vein embolization of the lobe with the larger tumor burden to allow hypertrophy of the FLR and decrease postoperative liver insufficiency. In the absence of tumor progression, at the second stage, the remaining tumor burden is removed, usually with a right hepatectomy or an extended hepatectomy. Reported postoperative mortality after the first and second stage operations were 0% and 0-15%, respectively, while morbidity after the first and second stages were 15-31% and 45-56%, respectively. Three-year survival rates of 35-54% have been reported using this strategy, in otherwise, unresectable patients.

For patients with liver-only metastases that are unresectable due to either burden of disease or insufficient functional liver remnant, several palliative measures remain which are intended to prolong life while maintaining an acceptable quality of life. These measures include isolated hepatic perfusion, hepatic arterial infusion pumps and locoregional therapies such as Yittrium-90.

Summary

- Approximately 50% of patients with colorectal cancer will develop synchronous or metachronous liver metastasis.
- Chemotherapy combinations of 5-FU, leucovorin, irinotecan, oxaliplatin and targeted biologic agents (cetuximab and bevacizumab) provide increased response rates and longer survival; however, 5-year survival is rare without surgical resection.
- The criteria for resectability of colorectal liver metastases have undergone a paradigm shift toward R0 resection with adequate FLR.
- Modern chemotherapy combinations to downstage/downsize liver tumors, portal vein embolization to improve postoperative liver reserves and combined resection with ablation and two-stage hepatectomies for multiple, bilobar disease have expanded the number of patients eligible for surgical intervention for colorectal liver metastases.

Primary Liver Tumors

Hepatocellular Carcinoma

Primary liver cancer is a major concern globally. It is the sixth most common cancer worldwide (after lung, breast, colorectal, stomach and prostate cancers) with an estimated 626,000 new cases diagnosed annually as of 2002, but it is the third most common cause of death from cancer (after lung and stomach cancers). Hepatocellular carcinoma (HCC) accounts for 85-90% of the primary liver cancers.

Risk Factors

Major risk factors include infections from hepatitis B or C virus. Chronic HBV carriers have a 5-15 fold increased risk of HCC, while HCV-infected patients have 17-fold increased risk of HCC compared to the general population. Most HCC cases (> 80%) occur in the sub-Saharan Africa or Eastern Asia, with the incidence as high as 28-49/100,000 males per year and 12-15/100,000 females per year, while the incidence in the United States is 3.3/100,000 persons per year. HCC develops in background of chronic liver disease and cirrhosis in approximately 70-90% patients with HCC. The annual conversion rate of someone with cirrhosis to develop HCC is 0.26-0.6% in HBV carriers and 1-3% in HCV carriers after 25-30 years of chronic infection.

Staging

There are multiple staging classifications for HCC including the Okuda stage, French classification, Cancer of the Liver Italian Program (CLIP) classification, the Chinese University Prognostic Index (CUPI), the TNM classification, the Japanese Integrated Staging (JIS) score and the Barcelona-Clinic Liver Cancer (BCLC) staging system. There are advantages and disadvantages to each staging systems and no single classification is accepted worldwide. For example, the CLIP, CUPI and French staging systems are relevant mainly for patients with advanced HCC. The TNM system, endorsed by the American Joint Committee on Cancer (AJCC), is based on pathological findings from patients who have undergone resection. The JIS score, which incorporates the TNM system and the Child-Pugh classification, is utilized mainly in Japan and needs to be validated in the West. The BCLC staging system incorporates tumor stage, liver functional status, performance score (PS 0 - 5) and cancer-related symptoms and provide treatment algorithms based on five stages: Stage 0 (very early stage HCC: carcinoma in situ; single tumor < 2 cm, Child-Pugh A; PS 0), Stage A (early stage HCC: single tumor; 3 tumors < 3 cm; Child-Pugh A-B; PS 0), Stage B (intermediate stage: multinodular; Child-Pugh A-B; PS 0), Stage C (advanced stage: portal vein invasion; N1; M1; Child-Pugh A-B; PS 1-2) and Stage D (terminal stage: Child-Pugh C; PS >2). Stage 0 patients are optimal candidates for surgical resection. Stage A patients are candidates for liver transplantation, liver resection, or percutaneous treatments with 5 year survival rates of 50 - 70%. Stage B patients are best treated with transarterial embolization (TAE) or transarterial chemoembolization (TACE). Stage C patients should be enrolled in a clinical trial testing new therapeutic agents such as sorafenib. Stage D patients should have supportive care and treatment of symptoms.

Diagnosis

HCC is diagnosed due to symptomatic disease or with screening, using imaging modalities, such as ultrasonography, computed tomography (CT) or magnetic resonance imaging (MRI) and measurement of tumor markers, such as alpha-fetoprotein (AFP). Although not specific or sensitive, an AFP level > 400 ng/dL is highly suspicious for HCC. Due to an exclusive arterial blood supply, HCC on contrast imaging shows contrast enhancement during the early arterial phase and contrast washout during the delayed venous phase. A diagnosis of HCC can be made in a nodule > 2 cm with a background of cirrhosis if two diagnostic imaging modalities confirm tumor hypervascularity **(Figure 29-6)** or one confirmatory imaging technique with an AFP > 200-400 ng/ml. Biopsy for definitive diagnosis remains controversial. Proponents argue that biopsy establishes a diagnosis, enables the awarding of extra listing points only to those who truly have HCC, decreases the incidence of transplanting patients prematurely who do not have HCC, enables those

patients without HCC to receive a transplant without the risk of being surpassed by patients with a false-negative diagnosis based on imaging and blood work and moves beyond the current staging systems into a more equitable organ allocation policy. Opponents of biopsy before transplantation argue that biopsy will not change the indication for transplantation for HCC when it is diagnosed on the background of decompensated cirrhosis, has a 10% rate of false-negative diagnosis in nodules < 2 cm and has a risk of tumor seeding along the needle track. Patients who are resection candidates with suspected HCC should not undergo biopsy for risk of needle track seeding. On the other hand, unresectable patients who will likely undergo chemotherapy or chemoembolization should have biopsy-proven HCC before treatment.

Treatment

Patients with untreated HCC have a 5-year survival of 0-20%. Treatment options for patients with HCC should be based on stage, underlying liver function/reserve and associated comorbidities **(Figure 29-7)**. For very early stage HCC (carcinoma in situ or single tumors < 2 cm) and early stage HCC (single nodule < 5 cm or 3 nodules, each < 3 cm) in patients with Child-Pugh class A and good performance status (PS 0), treatment options include liver transplantation, hepatic resection and percutaneous ablation. Currently, there are no randomized, controlled trials comparing these three treatment options and the treatment choice depends on treatment availability, center experience and results from retrospective studies.

Transplantation offers three major advantages: resection of the primary tumor, removal of the main source

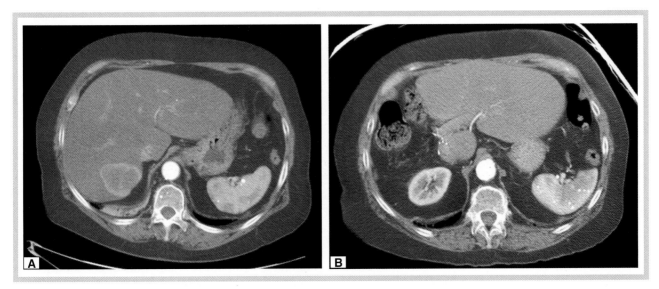

Figures 29-6A and B: Hypervascular CT characteristic and hepatic resection option for HCC. A-69-year old noncirrhotic patient with a hypervascular lesion who was not a transplant candidate due to continued alcohol use and who underwent a right hepatic lobectomy (A) with follow-up CT scan 18 months later showing no recurrence (B)

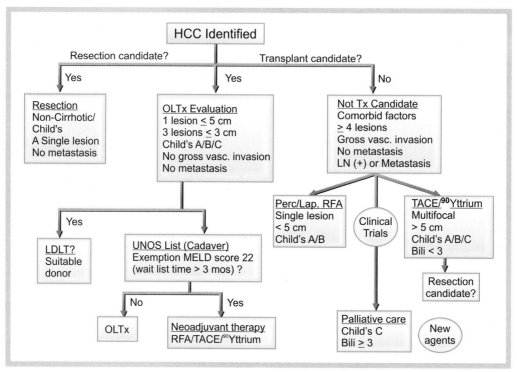

Figure 29-7: Treatment algorithm for the treatment of patients with hepatocellular carcinoma

of tumor recurrence and treatment of the background chronic liver disease. The role of transplantation in the treatment of HCC is discussed in detail later in the chapter.

Surgical resection also offers the best chance for cure in patients who are not eligible for liver transplantation **(Figure 29-7)**. The 5-year survival after surgical resection ranges from 25% to 93%, with the 93% five-year survival rate seen in very early HCC detected with screening seen in Japan. Ten year survivals have been reported between 20% and 35%. However, only 10-35% of patients are eligible for surgical resection. Contraindications to resection include extrahepatic involvement, multifocal, bilobar disease, inadequate hepatic reserve, portal hypertension or overall poor clinical condition of the patient. The use of portal vein embolization (PVE) of the planned resected liver may induce hypertrophy of the functional liver remnant and increase the boundaries of resectability. Recurrence remains the main cause of death and occurs 40-80% of the time at 5 years due to growth of occult tumor in the liver remnant, ongoing carcinogenic process in the cirrhotic remnant liver, or inadequate surgical margin. The vast majority of recurrences occur within 2 years. Tumor characteristics that have been associated with increased recurrence and poor survival include poorly differentiated tumor histology, presence of multiple nodules, liver capsule invasion, tumor size > 5 cm, as well as both macrovascular and microvascular invasion.

In light of the high recurrence following surgical resection, many groups have studied adjuvant treatments to minimize recurrent HCC after resection, with generally disappointing results. Overall, there is currently no adjuvant treatment that improves survival after HCC resection.

While still highly debatable and yet unproven, many liver units across the world are opting to resect selected patients with Child-Pugh A cirrhosis with a single small HCC and to reserve liver transplantation for those with impaired liver function (Child-Pugh B or C). For those patients who would recur after resection, the possibility would remain to be transplanted if they continued to meet eligibility criteria. While pragmatic, the equivalence of this approach compared to primary transplantation in eligible patients remains unproven and needs further evaluation before its widespread adoption.

If transplantation or resection is not an option or if the patient chooses a less invasive approach, then percutaneous ablation is a viable option and may be comparable to resection in select patients. Percutaneous ablation can be achieved by thermal ablation (radiofrequency, microwave, laser and cryoablation) or chemical ablation (alcohol, acetic acid). A number of randomized, controlled trials have compared radiofrequency ablation (RFA) to percutaneous ethanol injection (PEI) for the treatment of HCC. Lencioni, et al conducted a prospective, randomized study comparing 52 patients who underwent RFA versus 50 patients who underwent PEI for either a single

HCC < 5 cm or < 3 HCCs each < 3 cm. Complete tumor response was successful in 91% of HCCs treated with RFA with an average of 1.1 treatment sessions, but only in 82% of HCCs treated with PEI, which required an average of 5.4 treatment sessions. Local recurrence-free survival was significantly better in patients who underwent RFA than patients who underwent PEI for HCC at 1 year (98% vs 83%) and 2 years follow-up (96% vs 62%) (p = 0.002). There was a trend toward improved overall survival in patients who underwent RFA in this study, but this was not statistically significant; however, others have found improved overall and disease-free survival in patients treated with RFA versus PEI. Other ablation techniques are associated with a high rate of complications or have not proven advantageous over RFA or PEI. Cryosurgery has been associated with cryoshock (multiorgan system failure, severe coagulopathy and disseminated intravascular coagulation) in 1% of cryoablations of the liver with 28% mortality when observed. Currently, cryosurgery is rarely used. Experience with microwave technology has mainly been in Asia with a more recent introduction in the United States. Potential advantages of microwave ablation over RFA include possible larger ablation volumes, simultaneous use of multiple ablations and lack of need for ground-padding. Radiosurgery for HCC is still in the experimental phase that destroys tumors with large doses of accurately targeted megavoltage radiation.

Down-staging to meet the UNOS T2 criteria (one lesion 2-5 cm or two to three lesions < 3 cm) may be possible in patients who meet the inclusion criteria for down-staging protocol prior to liver transplantation as advocated by the UCSF group: (1) one lesion > 5 cm and < 8 cm; (2) two or three lesions, at least one > 3 cm but < 5 cm and total tumor diameter < 8 cm; (3) four or five lesions, all < 3 cm and total tumor diameter < 8 cm; and no vascular invasion by imaging studies. Down-staging treatments included TACE and laparoscopic RFA, either alone or in combination. Excellent results have been reported by the UCSF group (Yao, et al 2008) with down-staging to meet the UNOS T2 criteria in 70.5% of patients with 1- and 4-year post-transplantation survival of 96.2% and 92.1%, respectively. The Washington University group has reported a more modest down-staging rate of 24%; however, a strict down-staging inclusion criteria protocol was not used.

The past decade has also witnessed the emergence and refinement of several locoregional therapies aimed at patients with unresectable HCC. These locoregional techniques include transarterial chemoembolization (TACE) and selective internal radiation therapy (SIRT) with Yttrium-90 microspheres both of which have become the mainstay of therapy for patients with unresectable HCC. In addition, these modalities also play a selective role in the treatment of post-resection recurrence and as a bridge to transplantation. Although not curative, these promising locoregional modalities have been shown to prolong survival and impact quality of life.

Since the introduction of TACE as a palliative treatment in patients with unresectable HCC, this technique has become one of the most commonly performed image-guided procedures for HCC. Transarterial chemoembolization is a technique that exploits the preferential blood supply of HCC from the hepatic artery **(Figures 29-8 and 29-9)**. The rationale is that intra-arterial delivery of cytotoxic agents directly into the liver can preferentially achieve high intratumoral concentrations. Additionally, embolic agents are then injected to further decrease drug washout by reducing arterial inflow as well as occlude the arterial blood supply to the tumor. TACE is typically well tolerated in patients with adequate hepatic reserve. The use of TACE is supported by two randomized controlled trials as well as meta-analyses showing a survival advantage with TACE in selected patients with well-preserved liver function.

Recently, Cheng, et al (2008) reported the first randomized clinical trial involving RFA for HCC in 291 Chinese patients with 3 or fewer HCC tumors ranging in size from 3 cm to 7.5 cm. Patients were randomly assigned to treatment arms of RFA alone (n = 100), TACE alone (n = 95) or combined TACE+RFA (n = 96). With a median follow-up of 28.5 months, median survival was 22 months in the RFA group, 24 months in the TACE group and 37 months in the TACE+RFA group. Patients treated with TACE+RFA had better overall survival than those treated with TACE alone (p < 0.001) or RFA alone (p < 0.001).

Radioembolization is a minimally invasive catheter-directed therapy that delivers internal radiation via the hepatic artery that feeds HCC. Selective internal radiation therapy with Yttrium-90 (a pure beta radiation emitter) microspheres was introduced in the 1980s but the technology has significantly been refined in the past several years. The microspheres are injected directly into the hepatic arteries via a transfemoral angiographic approach and are delivered selectively to hepatic tumors **(Figure 29-10)**. SIRT can more effectively target liver disease with a higher dose of radiation compared with external-beam radiation and is associated with relatively low toxicity and a good local response. There are currently two commercially available Yttrium-90 microspheres: Therasphere® made of glass and SIR-Spheres® made of resin. While randomized studies have not been performed, several non-randomized studies have demonstrated encouraging survival results.

Although cytotoxic chemotherapy agents have been shown to achieve response rates of up to 20% in unresectable HCC, no single or combined treatment protocol has demonstrated any meaningful survival benefits. These poor results may be secondary to the high expression of

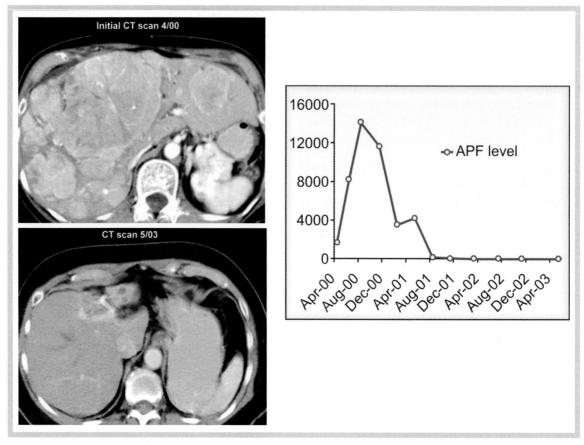

Figure 29-8: CT characteristic and chemoembolization option for unresectable HCC. A 73-year-old cirrhotic patient who underwent 12 rounds of TACE with follow-up CT scan 3 years later showing significant regression and response of AFP tumor marker

the multidrug resistance gene (MDR-1) in HCC, poor drug delivery and dose limitations from underlying liver dysfunction. Sorafenib, a multi-target tyrokinase kinase inhibitor, is the only molecular targeted agent approved for systemic therapy for advanced unresectable HCC. The SHARP trial showed that patients with advanced HCC treated with sorafenib (400 mg bid) had an improved median survival of 10.7 months compared to 7.9 months in the placebo treatment group, showing a 44% improvement (p = 0.0006) **(Figure 29-10)**. The combination of Sorafenib with Yttrium-90 and/or TACE is currently under investigation.

Patients with end-staged HCC with poor performance status and Child-Pugh class C have a 1-year survival rate of 10-20% and a median survival of < 3 months. These patients should receive supportive care and symptomatic treatment.

Summary

- Treatment of HCC requires an understanding of both the disease and the underlying liver disease process.

- Overall the treatment of HCC can broadly be characterized as potentially curative versus palliative.
- Liver resection and transplantation offer the best chance at long-term survival with recent evidence including RFA as a potentially curative intervention in carefully selected patients with small, unifocal HCC.
- In light of organ shortage and the resulting long wait times and high dropout rates, resection remains an important option for patients eligible for transplantation who have preserved liver function and early HCC.
- TACE has the greatest amount of supporting data as a palliative modality for unresectable HCC.
- In general systemic therapies except for Sorafenib offer no significant survival benefit.

Cholangiocarcinoma

Cholangiocarcinoma (CCA) is a primary hepatic malignancy originating from bile duct epithelium. The incidence of CCA has steadily increased worldwide over the past three decades with the rise unexplained by either reclassification or improved detection. Although it is the

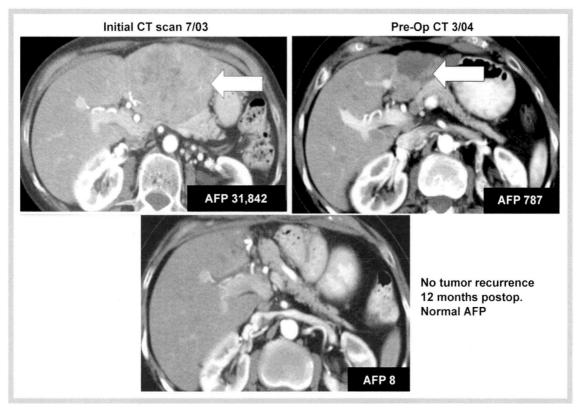

Figure 29-9: CT characteristic and chemoembolization option for unresectable HCC. A 74-year-old cirrhotic patient who underwent 4 rounds of TACE with follow-up CT scan a year later showing significant regression and response of AFP tumor marker, converting the patient to a resection candidate

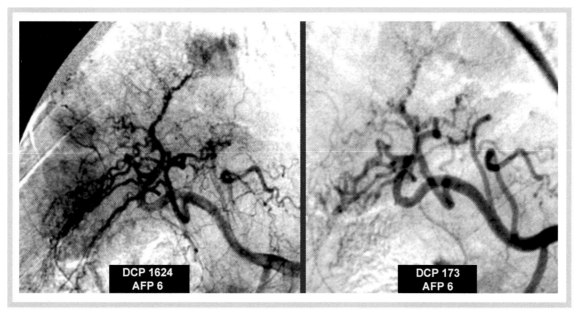

Figure 29-10: Angiographic characteristic and theraspheres (^{90}Y radiolabeled microspheres) option for unresectable HCC. A 69-year-old male cirrhotic patient who underwent one therasphere treatment with follow-up angiogram 6 months later showing significant regression of the 3 hypervascular blush and response of des-gamma-carboxyprothrombin (DCP) tumor marker

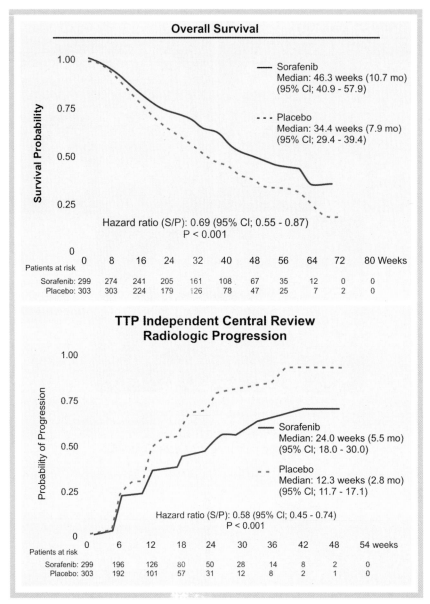

Figure 29-11: Sorafenib (Nexavar). An FDA approved oral chemotherapy treatment option for unresectable HCC that shows significantly improved overall survival and radiologic progression of HCC in patients treated with sorafenib compared to placebo control (adapted with permission from Llovet, et al, NEJM 2008; 359: 378-90. Copyright © 2008 *Massachusetts Medical Society*. All rights reserved)

second most common primary hepatic neoplasia after hepatocellular carcinoma, it remains a relatively rare and poorly understood tumor. The disease is notoriously difficult to diagnose and is usually fatal because of its late clinical presentation and the lack of effective non-surgical therapeutic modalities and the marginal survival gains with surgical resection. In general, prognosis is very poor, with a reported median survival usually below 6-9 months after diagnosis in the majority of patients with advanced disease. The overall 5-year survival, including resected patients, remains dismal at only 5-19% with a median

survival of 22 months, a rate which has not changed significantly over the past 30 years.

Classification

Although CCA can arise anywhere within the biliary tree, tumors involving the biliary confluence (e.g. hilar CCA, 'Klatskin tumor') represent the majority, accounting for 40-60% of all cases. Twenty to thirty percent of CCAs originate in the lower bile duct (extrahepatic CCA) and approximately 10% arise within the intrahepatic biliary tree (intrahepatic CCA or peripheral CCA).

While straightforward and intuitive, the latter anatomic classification is far from universally accepted. Surprisingly, there is considerable confusion as to the nomenclature and classification of this little known malignancy. Because of these inconsistencies in definition and the relatively small numbers of cases reported by each group, there is currently no consensus on the classification of CCA. For the sake of clarity, this chapter will focus solely on intrahepatic CCA which is defined as CCA arising from the epithelial cells of intrahepatic bile ducts (beyond the second order bile ducts).

Risk Factors

Although several risk factors have been identified, most patients with CCA have no identifiable risk factors. Primary sclerosing cholangitis, associated primarily with ulcerative colitis, is one of the most recognized risk factors. Patients with primary sclerosing cholangitis have a 1.5% cumulative annual risk of developing CCA and a lifetime risk of 10-20% of developing CCA. Fibropolycystic liver disease, including choledochal cysts, Caroli's syndrome and congenital hepatic fibrosis, is another commonly recognized risk factor, as are liver flukes in Asian countries (Opisthorchis viverrini, Clonorchis sinensis). Other less common risk factors include hepatolithiasis, Thorotrast (a contrast agent used from 1931 until the 1950s), Lynch syndrome II and biliary papillomatosis. The common denominator amongst these risk factors is inflammation of the biliary tract. Lastly, large epidemiological studies in the United States and Denmark have identified associations between CCA and cholangitis, cholelithiasis, choledocholithiasis, alcoholic liver disease, nonspecific cirrhosis, hepatitis C, diabetes mellitus, inflammatory bowel disease and smoking.

Pathology

In addition to anatomic classifications, intrahepatic CCA be further characterized based on specific morphology and histologic features such as nodular, massive, diffuse, sclerosing, polypoid, papillary, exophytic and infiltrating. More recently, the Liver Cancer Study Group of Japan proposed a unifying pathological classification for both intrahepatic and extrahepatic CCA consisting of mass-forming (MF), periductal-infiltrating (PI) and intraductal-growing (IG).

MF type forms a definite round-shaped mass with an expansive growth pattern but does not usually invade the major branch of the portal triad. PI type is defined as a mass extending longitudinally along the bile duct, occasionally involves the surrounding blood vessels and/or hepatic parenchyma, often resulting in dilatation of the peripheral bile duct. IG type proliferates toward the lumen of bile duct occasionally involving superficial extension.

This type of intrahepatic CCA is usually detected in a thick bile duct.

Histologically, intrahepatic CCA arises from cholangiocytes and is in most cases a moderately- to well-differentiated tubular adenocarcinoma. The most characteristic histological feature is the presence of abundant desmoplastic stroma in intrahepatic CCA compared with HCC, leading to a low diagnostic yield of random biopsies. Desmoplasia may also cause capsular retraction which can often be appreciated on cross-sectional imaging.

A number of mutations in oncogenes and tumor suppressor genes have been identified in CCA. Several studies have shown abnormal expression of the K-ras oncogene and the p53 tumor suppressor gene with these genetic alterations associated with a more aggressive phenotype. K-ras and p53 mutations have also been identified in bile and pancreatic juice of affected patients and have emerged as potential molecular markers of disease.

Staging

Because intrahepatic CCA is a rare type of primary liver cancer, accounting only for 5-10% of all primary liver cancers, the International Union against Cancer (UICC) defined the TNM staging system solely from clinical experience in treating HCC. Similarly, the American Joint Committee on Cancer (AJCC) includes intrahepatic CCA in the same category as primary liver cancers, such as HCC for staging, although extrahepatic CCA has a completely separate staging criterion. However, based on the distinct difference in the mechanism and biologic behavior between HCC and intrahepatic CCA, many organizations are in the progress of restructuring the staging system.

Diagnosis

Symptoms of CCA tend to be vague and insidious in development and therefore are often diagnosed at an advanced stage when only palliative approaches can be used. While the most common presenting symptom in patients with hilar CCA is painless jaundice, intrahepatic CCA, in contrast, is usually asymptomatic, even at advanced stages and is diagnosed incidentally on imaging studies or on evaluation of abnormal liver enzymes. When intrahepatic CCA presents with symptoms, these usually consist of abdominal pain or anemia, as well as other nonspecific constitutional symptoms such as weakness, fatigue or weight loss.

Currently, there are no tumor markers specific for CCA although the carbohydrate antigen 19-9 (CA19-9) is commonly used despite its low specificity. Although CA 19-9 is increased in benign, such as bacterial cholangitis, primary biliary cirrhosis or alcoholic liver disease, an extremely elevated CA 19-9 often denotes unresectable disease.

Although accuracy in diagnosis and staging is critical for the effective management of CCA, it is difficult to achieve in practice. A combination of noninvasive and invasive imaging studies, such as computed tomography (CT), magnetic resonance imaging (MRI), positron emission tomography (PET) scanning, endoscopic retrograde cholangiopancreatography (ERCP), endoscopic ultrasound (EUS) and optical coherence tomography, are used but have thus far not profoundly impacted the early diagnosis and accurate staging of CCA. In addition, emerging molecular diagnostic methods and new approaches to enhance the diagnostic yield and utility of biliary cytology are being examined and defined.

Computed tomography (CT) and magnetic resonance imaging (MRI) scans are commonly used noninvasive approaches for the detection and staging of CCA. Both are excellent at providing information about the morphology of the lesion, hepatic parenchyma, lymph nodes, possible dilatation of the intrahepatic and extrahepatic bile ducts, as well as vascular encasement and extrahepatic spread. Intrahepatic tumors may be identified as a large mass with satellite nodules (a characteristic finding in intrahepatic CCA) or simply as dilatation of the bile duct in the case of periductal-infiltrating or intraductal tumors not associated with an identifiable mass.

Until recently MRI/magnetic resonance cholangiopancreatography (MRCP) offered an advantage over CT scanning since the biliary tree could be visualized non-invasively. However, multi-slice three-dimensional spiral CT cholangiography (3-D CTC) with minimum-intensity projection has emerged as an accurate technique for the delineation of the biliary system and diagnosis of CCA in patients with low serum bilirubin levels (< 2 mg/dl). However, if the point of biliary obstruction is thought to be proximal to the perihilar region, then percutaneous transhepatic cholangiography (PTC) is the preferred modality for delineating the extent of biliary involvement. Lastly, CT or MRI angiography can both be used to more fully evaluate vascular involvement.

While some studies have shown that the sensitivity and specificity of the FDG-PET may be higher than that of other imaging modalites or cytological examination of bile, more data is needed before PET scanning becomes a standard diagnostic test for CCA. Recently, FDG-PET has been evaluated for the staging of CCA by Anderson et al in 31 patients. Although FDG-PET had 85% sensitivity for diagnosis of mass lesions, sensitivity for infiltrating tumors was only 18%. The overall sensitivity for metastases was 65% and the detection of unsuspected metastases by FDG-PET changed the surgical management in 30%

of patients. False-positive scans were observed in PSC and patients with biliary stents and a normal PET scan does not exclude cancer therefore PET findings should be interpreted cautiously in the setting of CCA.

Endoscopic retrograde cholangiopancreatography (ERCP) offers a distinct advantage over most radiological imaging tests in that it not only provides information about the horizontal intrabiliary spread of the tumor but tissue samples can also be obtained by brush cytology or biopsy. Unfortunately, however, the sensitivity of brush cytology for diagnosing CCA has been poor prompting the use of advanced analysis approaches such as the use of fluorescence *in situ* hybridization and digital image analysis to help increase their diagnostic yield. While both fluorescence *in situ* hybridization and digital image analysis (DIA) is more sensitive than cytology, the resulting specificity is generally lower. Sandwich enzyme-linked immunosorbent assay can show a 71% sensitivity and 90% specificity for new tumor markers in serum and bile including genomic and proteomic markers such as CA19-9, CEA and mucin5, subtypes A and C (MUC5AC). Intraductal ultrasonography (IDUS) is particularly helpful in augmenting the diagnostic accuracy of ERCP.

Optical coherence tomography, a high-resolution imaging technique that produces cross-sectional images *in vivo*, has potential for the differentiation of benign and malignant strictures and early detection of CCA in patients with PSC. Optical coherence tomography is analogous to ultrasound imaging in that two-dimensional images are built up from sequential adjacent longitudinal scans of backscattered light. However, in optical coherence tomography the probing radiation is infrared light rather than soundwaves. Its resolution is high enough to visualize biliary ductal epithelium and subepithelial structures, including peribiliary glands, vasculature and hepatic parenchyma. Thus, optical coherence tomography is an attractive technique for imaging the bile duct and has the potential to provide an 'optical' method for identifying dysplastic or early malignant changes in the biliary epithelium.

Despite the aforementioned improvements in preoperative imaging, 25-40% of patients explored for presumed resectable disease are nonetheless found to be inoperable at the time of laparotomy. Consequently, staging laparoscopy has increasing been advocated for selected patients with extensive disease on preoperative imaging. In a study of diagnostic laparoscopy in 84 patients with hilar CCA, laparoscopy for staging spared an unnecessary laparotomy in 42% of patients.

Treatment

Currently, surgical resection of the involved bile ducts and liver segments or transplantation are the only curative treatments for ICA. However, even with carefully selected treatment with curative intent, the 5-year survival of patients with CCA remains dismal. Survival after surgical resection has been reported as 35-86% at 1-year, 20-51.8% at 3-years and 20.5-40% at 5-years. Disease-free survival at 5 years varies widely between 2% and 41%. Median survival after intrahepatic CCA resection was 12-37.4 months. Moreover, the recurrence rate after surgery is discouraging and approaches 40-50% in many series.

Although few studies have specifically addressed surgical resection and outcomes by stage compared with nonoperative treatments, based on available studies, surgery provides a meaningful survival advantage over nonoperative therapy. Thus, surgical resection should be offered to all patients with potentially resectable ICC regardless of stage assuming a complete (R0) resection is feasible.

In patients with obstructive jaundice, which is especially applicable to patients with hilar CCA and less so for intrahepatic CCA, preoperative biliary drainage has been recommended to improve liver function before surgery and to reduce postoperative complications. Percutaneous transhepatic biliary drainage or endoscopic biliary drainage are both applicable with the percutaneous method the preferred method for the preoperative relief of obstructive jaundice. However, this practice remains controversial with several reports demonstrating that preoperative biliary stenting in proximal CCA increases the incidence of contaminated bile and postoperative infectious complications. Moreover, Cherqui, et al demonstrated that major liver resection without preoperative biliary drainage is a safe procedure in most patients with obstructive jaundice with recovery of hepatic synthetic function identical to that of patients without jaundice.

Another controversy is the choice for biliary drainage before major hepatectomy in patients with obstructive jaundice with some advocating selective biliary drainage of only the future remnant liver while others advocating total biliary drainage. Ishizawa, et al reported that selective biliary drainage is superior to total biliary drainage for promoting hypertrophy of the future remnant liver in patients undergoing portal vein embolization and for guaranteeing good liver function before major hepatectomy.

Because only a curative resection can prolong survival and tumor-free surgical margin is the best predictor of survival, increasingly radical approaches to resection have been adopted over the past 10 years with mixed results. While some studies have demonstrated that aggressive surgical strategies in the treatment of intrahepatic CCA, including major vascular resection, extrahepatic biliary resection, extended hepatic resection and extended lymphadenectomy, can significantly increase the survival of ICC patients, other studies have put these results in question.

For example, Lang, et al reported on a group of 27 patients with locally advanced intrahepatic CCA who underwent extended surgical resection involving extended hepatic resection as well as major vasculature and biliary resection and reconstruction. Complete tumor removal (R0 resection) was able to be achieved in 16 patients while the other 11 patients had microscopic tumor at the resection margin (R1 resection). Following R0 resection, the calculated median survival was 46 months compared to 5 months after R1 resection. Postoperative morbidity was 56% for the extended resection cohort and 45% in patients undergoing hepatectomy without extension of the operation. Although the authors concluded that R0 resection can provide prolonged survival even in patients with advanced ICC, the above data can be interpreted in another way. That is, while R0 resection is potentially beneficial if achieved, there is currently no way to assure definitive negative margins despite an aggressive intraoperative approach and that 'failed' aggressive surgery (i.e. R1 resection) is associated with a high postoperative morbidity and no survival advantage. In fact, Kim, et al reported that the median survival time after non-curative resection is 3 months while Chu, et al showed that the median survival time is 1.8 months and 2.9 months, respectively, after conservative management and palliative operations.

In a similar vein, a retrospective study by Yamamoto et al comparing patients undergoing hepatectomy alone or hepatectomy with bile duct resection (n = 56) with patients undergoing extended surgery including vessel resection and/or pancreatectomy (n = 27) found that the 5-year survival rate was significantly higher in the standard surgery group (30%) than in the extended surgery group (10%, P = 0.0061). These authors consequently concluded that extended surgery does not improve the curative resection rate or the surgical outcome of intrahepatic CCA. Overall, the data remains controversial regarding the survival advantage of extended resection in intrahepatic CCA even if a negative margin can be obtained.

In addition to surgical margin, there is considerable data indicating that lymph node status is similarly an important negative prognostic factor for patients undergoing hepatic resection for intrahepatic CCA. The most distinct characteristic of intrahepatic CCA compared with HCC is early lymphatic spread with intrahepatic CCA tending to spread to lymph nodes early. Moreover, numerous studies suggest that lymph node metastasis in intrahepatic CCA is rarely limited to the regional lymph nodes. Therefore, the questions that need to be answered include whether lymph nodes are dissected and to what extent. No consensus has been reached concerning the indications and value of lymph node dissection for CCA. Hepatectomy with extensive lymph node dissection is the standard operation for intrahepatic CCA in Japan, although lymph node dissection may not always be effective in reducing tumor recurrence. Other indicators of poor prognosis aside from positive margins and positive lymph nodes include multiple nodules, vascular invasion, large tumor size, capsular invasion, tumor spreading type, bilobar disease, left side involvement and very high CA 19-9.

Transplantation for CCA (with or without neoadjuvant treatment) can be an option for highly selected cases but remains a controversial area, as discussed in the section on transplantation.

Adjuvant Therapy

Most patients with CCA present with advanced disease that is not amenable to surgical treatment and even with a complete resection, recurrence rates are high thereby warranting consideration of (neo)adjuvant treatments as well as definitive chemotherapy for inoperable patients. Unfortunately, neither adjuvant, neoadjuvant, nor definitive chemotherapy has been shown to improve survival. In addition, there is no evidence to lend support to the use of adjuvant radiotherapy in patients with margin-negative resections. Roayaie, et al performed chemoradiation therapy for postoperative patients with positive resection margins or nodal invasion and did not find any difference in the actuarial disease-free survival between the patients with or without adjuvant chemoradiation. Lee, et al treated 24 patients immunohistochemically proven unresectable CCA patients with gemcitabine and cisplatin with 5 patients having a partial response, 12 with stable disease and 7 with progressive disease during treatment. The resulting median survival time of 9.3 months was considered a marginal improvement over conservative management. In a study by Feisthammel, et al the response rate was 10% for patients with inoperable intrahepatic CCA (n = 17) after treatment with irinotecan followed by folinic acid and 5-FU and an additional 10% of patients had a stable disease. The median overall survival time of was 166 days and median progression-free survival was 166-273 days suggesting that irinotecan followed by folinic acid and 5-FU is a viable option for advanced intrahepatic CCA. While these neoadjuvant or adjuvant treatments are promising, the data is preliminary and thus treatment is not recommended outside clinical trials.

Palliative Therapy

The majority of patients with CCA present at an advanced stage or have associated comorbidity that preclude surgery. For these patients, the goal of treatment is to obtain adequate palliation. Palliative treatment to relieve symptoms, treat sepsis or normalize bilirubin before palliative therapy clearly has an important role especially since bacterial cholangitis or liver failure often contribute to death. Palliative therapeutic aside from chemotherapy include endoscopic stenting, photodynamic treatment (PDT) and transarterial chemoembolization. Biliary endoprosthesis (stent) placement and PDT are often used for palliation and may prolong survival. Palliative biliary decompression can provide symptomatic relief and can be achieved by plastic (polyethylene) or metal stents with self-expanding metal stents increasingly favored. In a recent randomized trial, a clear survival benefit in patients treated with endoscopic photodynamic therapy resulted in early closure of the study. However, further studies are needed before PDT becomes a mainstay of palliative therapy in CCA.

Transarterial chemoembolization (TACE) may be useful in selected patients with preserved liver function, but the use of this approach has only been reported in a few small series. Results out of the University of Pittsburgh Medical Center with gemcitabine-based TACE in patients with unresectable disease revealed that hepatic-artery-directed therapy was well tolerated and conferred better survival when given in combination therapy (with cisplatin or oxaliplatin) for patients with unresectable CCA (13.8 months for the gemcitabine-cisplatin combination cohort versus 6.3 months in the gemcitabine alone cohort). The feasibility of using systemic gemcitabine in combination with regional chemoembolization has been shown. A recent study out of Korea showed that tumor vascularity was the only independent factor associated with radiographic response to TACE or transcatheter arterial chemoinfusion (TACI) for unresectable intrahepatic CCA with large tumor size, tumor hypovascularity and Child-Pugh class B emerging as poor prognostic factors for determining patient survival.

Summary

- Cholangiocarcinoma (CCA) is of concern because its incidence is increasing worldwide and its pathogenesis remains unclear.
- Intrahepatic CCA is an aggressive and often fatal primary liver cancer which can be difficult to diagnose and to treat.
- While new imaging and staging techniques help select patients for potentially curative resection, surgical outcomes are marginally superior to conservative management only in patients with R0 resections.
- Chemotherapy and radiotherapy results have so far been disappointing.
- While palliative therapies are available for the majority of patients who present with inoperable disease or recur after resection, the practical utility of these emerging technologies needs to be studied further.

Role of Liver Transplantation for Liver Malignancy

Liver transplantation (OLT) is a therapeutic option for primary liver tumors, including hepatocellular carcinoma (HCC), CCA, epithelioid hemangioendothelioma and hepatoblastoma. HCC is a primary malignant liver tumor arising in patients mainly with chronic liver disease (> 80%), specifically cirrhosis. They are usually multifocal and often recur after treatment (> 50%) in patients who may lack sufficient reserve to tolerate formal liver resection. Liver transplantation allows complete resection of the tumor, along with the main location for recurrence, while replacing adequate functioning liver parenchymal to sustain postoperative liver functions.

Approximately 6,000 liver transplants are performed each year in the United States, with 1-year and 5-year survival rates of 86.2% and 53.8%, respectively, for liver transplantation for malignant neoplasms. In January 2009, there were approximately 16,000 patients on the wait list for liver transplantation (http://www.optn.org). With the shortage of available donors and the concern of tumor recurrence, OLT for HCC has been limited to patients with early stage HCC (stage I or II). Initial series of OLT for HCC reported in the 1990s included cases with advanced HCC and the 5-year survival rates were only 20-50%, which compared poorly with overall 5-year survival rates of 70-75% for OLTx in the Organ Procurement and Transplantation Network/United Network for Organ Sharing (OPTN/UNOS) database. Mazzaferro and colleagues at Milan subsequently showed that survival rates were markedly improved when OLT was limited to early-stage HCC (stage I or stage II) with one tumor up to 5 cm, or three tumors, all less than 3 cm, along with no gross vascular invasion or extrahepatic spread. Multiple studies have validated these findings with 5-year survival rates of 49-75% and recurrence rates of 4-24%. More recently, there have been proposals to expand the criteria for liver transplantation for HCC by the UCSF group (single tumor < 6.5 cm or up to 3 tumors, each < 4.5 cm with total diameter of < 8 cm) and the Pittsburgh group (up to Stage IIIB: microscopic vascular invasion, bilobar distribution, tumor size > 2 cm, no lymph node involvement, no distant metastasis) based on pathologic staging of the explanted liver. One criticism of the UCSF criteria is that the results, which are based on explant tumor characteristics, would be far different if based on preoperative tumor characteristics. Before such expanded criteria are adopted, prospective randomized studies directly comparing patients who received transplants within and exceeding Milan Criteria are needed.

HCC recurrence rates of 4-10% have been demonstrated in patients who received transplants for tumors within Milan Criteria with considerably higher rates noted prior to the adoption of these criteria. While most recurrences occur within 2 years of transplantation, 20-30% of recurrences occur beyond this point. HCC recurrence significantly decreases survival after transplantation. Among patients suffering recurrence, factors that negatively affect survival include shorter time to recurrence, presence of bone metastases and multiplicity of sites that preclude local control. An aggressive approach to post-transplantation HCC recurrence in selected patients is recommended.

With the shortage of donors, waiting time is inevitable and may exceed 2 years in some regions. Dropout rates exceeded 25% in patients with waiting time >12 months. In 2002, UNOS/OPTN adopted the Model for End-stage Liver Disease (MELD) score (a 6-40 point scale based on serum total bilirubin, creatinine and international normalized ratio [INR]) for allocation of deceased donor liver organs in the United States. In an attempt to decrease the high mortality rate for patients with preserved liver function and progressive HCC, stage II HCC patients were given priority points (currently, 22 MELD points). This improved outcomes on HCC liver transplant candidates by decreasing waiting time (2.28 years pre-MELD vs 0.69 years post-MELD, $p < 0.001$), decreasing wait list dropout (5-month dropout rate of 16.5% pre-MELD vs 8.5% post-MELD, $p < 0.001$), thus, increasing transplant rates (0.439 tranplant/person years pre-MELD vs. 1.454 transplant/person years post-MELD, $p < 0.001$) with associated improved survival (5-month waiting-list survival of 90.3% pre-MELD vs 95.7% post-MELD, $p < 0.001$).

While liver transplantation is considered by most as the optimal treatment of HCC with cirrhosis because it results in the widest possible resection margins for the cancer, removes the underlying cirrhotic liver tissue that is at risk for the development of *de novo* HCC and restores normal hepatic function, there are no intention-to-treat studies to prove this assertion. This latter point is of paramount importance because a significant proportion of patients will 'dropout' and be excluded from transplantation because of tumor growth or development of contraindications while waiting for a donor. To address this issue, Llovet, et al undertook an intention-to-treat analysis comparing the results obtained with surgical resection and liver transplantation in a cohort of 164 cirrhotic patients with HCC. Seventy-seven patients (48 men, mean 61 years of age, 74 Child-Pugh class A, size 33 mm) were resected (first-line option) and 87 patients (65 men, mean 55 years of age, 50 Child-Pugh class B/C, size 24 mm) were selected for transplantation. The resulting 1-, 3- and 5-year 'intention-to-treat' survival were very similar at 85%, 62% and 51% for resection and 84%, 69% and 69% for transplantation (8 dropouts on waiting list). When taking into account patient 'dropout' while on the wait list, the survival rates were significantly lower than that of the best candidates for resection (p = 0.002) thus supporting the idea that surgical resection in selected patients has the potential to yield improved survival rates compared to transplantation due to the growing incidence of dropouts because of the increasing waiting time.

In light of the aforementioned data and owing to organ shortage and the associated long wait times, liver resection is increasingly being considered as a reasonable first-line treatment of selective patients with small HCC and good liver function, with secondary liver transplantation reserved as a salvage procedure in case of recurrence. Therefore, a compromise gathered by many liver units across the world is to resect selected patients, mainly those Child-Pugh A cirrhosis with a single small HCC and to reserve liver transplantation for those with impaired liver function (Child-Pugh B or C) and/or small oligonodular HCC according to currently accepted tumor selection criteria. For those patients who would recur after resection, the possibility would remain to be transplanted if they continued to meet eligibility criteria.

This pragmatic attitude is able to avoid unnecessary transplantation in long-term survivors of resection and thus has the potential to spare organs, however its viability remains to be explored. Adam, et al recently studied the feasibility and outcome of such an approach in a 2-step fashion. They looked at 358 consecutive patients with HCC and cirrhosis who were treated by liver resection (n = 163; 98 of whom were transplantable) or transplantation (n = 195). First they assessed secondary liver transplantation for tumor recurrence (n = 17) compared with primary transplantation (n = 195) and second, they compared primary resection in transplantable patients (n = 98) with that of primary transplantation (n = 195) on an intention-to-treat basis. The authors demonstrated that liver transplantation after liver resection is associated with a higher operative mortality, an increased risk of recurrence, a decreased 5-year overall survival and a poorer outcome than primary transplantation. In fact, of 98 patients treated by resection while initially eligible for transplantation, only 20 (20%) were secondarily transplanted and eligibility for transplantation after tumor recurrence was only 25% (17 of 69 recurrences) thus illustrating the inherent risk in deferring transplantation until tumor recurrence. Overall, when compared to patients undergoing primary transplantation on an intention-to-treat basis, transplantable patients who instead underwent resection had a decreased 5-year overall survival (50% vs 61%; *P* = 0.05) and disease-free survival (18% vs 58%; p < 0.0001), despite the use of salvage transplantation.

Transplantation for cholangiocarcinoma is more controversial with poor outcomes including 5-year survivals rates of 23-42% and recurrence rates of 44-100%, prompting some centers to abandon the practice. However, the University of Nebraska and Mayo Clinic groups have shown that the addition of neoadjuvant chemoradiation therapy (external beam radiation, brachytherapy, 5-fluorouracil and oral capecitabine) prior to liver transplantation produced significantly lower recurrence and higher long-term survival rates compared to resection, OLT alone or medical treatment in hilar CCA with 5-year survival rate of 82% and recurrence rate of 13%.

While the development of living donor LT further expands the treatment horizon and lessens the impact of the scarcity of available deceased donor organs available for transplantation for both of these primary liver malignancies, the real challenge ahead is to better characterize which biologic and staging indicators have the best and most complete prognostic significance so as to maximize the usage of such scarce resources.

Summary

- For patients who have early-HCC (stage I or stage II) with one tumor up to 5 cm, or three tumors, all less than 3 cm, along with no gross vascular invasion or extrahepatic spread, OLT provides acceptable overall and disease-free survival.
- Owing to the limited organ supply, liver resection is increasingly being considered as a reasonable first-line treatment of selective patients with small HCC and good liver function, with secondary liver transplantation reserved as a salvage procedure in case of recurrence. However, the viability of this approach remains unproven.
- For patients with hilar CCA, neoadjuvant chemoradiation therapy prior to liver transplantation produced significantly lower recurrence and higher long-term survival rates compared to resection, OLT alone, or medical treatment.

Hepatic Resection

Hepatic Resection Terminology

Classification of liver resections (hepatectomies) can be separated into two groups—anatomic and nonanatomic resections. Anatomic resections follow along one or more hepatic scissurae while nonanatomic resections are not limited by these scissurae. The IHPBA Brisbane 2000 classification has become the standard nomenclature for anatomic resections and should be used to adequately communicate the extent of liver resection. In contrast, nonanatomic or wedge resections lack a standardized categorization and should simply be described using the numeric Couinaud terminology (e.g. wedge resection segment V).

Major hepatectomy is defined as resection of three or more Couinaud liver segments. According to the Brisbane nomenclature, terminology for hepatic resection can be summarized as follows; (1) resection of segments II-IV is termed left hepatectomy or left hemihepatectomy; (2) resection of segments V-VIII is termed right hepatectomy or right hemihepatectomy; (3) resection of segments II and III is termed left lateral sectionectomy or bisegmentectomy II + III; (4) resection of segments II-V and VIII is termed extended left hepatectomy or left trisectionectomy and (5) resection of segments IV-VIII is termed extended right hepatectomy or right trisectionectomy.

Open Technique versus Minimally Invasive Approach: Indications, Outcomes, Patient Selection

The majority of liver resection is performed via an open technique with a right subcostal incision ± 'hockey stick' midline extension or with bilateral subcostal incisions **(Figure 29-12)**. With the advent of laparoscopy and the increasing demands from patients for less invasive procedures, minimally invasive liver surgery is being employed as part of the armamentarium of liver surgeons. Laparoscopic liver surgery has evolved from unroofing of hepatic cysts and resection of peripheral benign lesions, to formal anatomical resections for malignancy and finally, to live donor hepatectomy for liver transplantation. The indications for laparoscopic liver resection include benign lesions [adenomas, symptomatic hemangioma, symptomatic focal nodular hyperplasia (FNH) and symptomatic giant hepatic cysts], malignant lesions [hepatocellular carcinoma (HCC) and colorectal carcinoma (CRC) metastasis], live donor hepatectomy for liver transplant and indeterminate lesions where cancer cannot be excluded. Contraindications to a minimally invasive liver resection include any contraindications to an open liver resection, intolerance to pneumoperitoneum, dense adhesions that cannot be lysed laparoscopically, lesions too close to major vasculature, lesions too large to be safely manipulated laparoscopically and resection that may require extensive portal lymphadenectomy.

A recent review of the world literature on laparoscopic liver resections identified almost 3,000 reported minimally invasive liver resections, of which 50% were for malignant tumors, 45% were for benign lesions and 1.7% were for live donor hepatectomies. Different minimally invasive approaches have been described and out of the almost 3,000 reported cases, 75% of the resections were performed totally laparoscopically, 17% were hand-assisted and 2% were laparoscopic-assisted open hepatic resection (hybrid) technique, with the remainder being other techniques or conversions to open hepatectomies. The most common laparoscopic liver resection was a wedge resection or segmentectomy (45%), followed by anatomical left lateral sectionectomy (20%), right hepatectomy (9%) and left hepatectomy (7%). Conversion from laparoscopy to open laparotomy and from laparoscopy to hand-assisted approach occurred in 4.1% and 0.7% of reported cases, respectively. Overall mortality and morbidity were 0.3% and 10.5%, respectively, with no intraoperative deaths reported. The most common cause of postoperative death was liver failure. Postoperative bile leak was observed in 1.5% of cases. For cancer resections, negative surgical margins were achieved in 82-100% of reported series. The 5-year overall and disease-free survival rates after laparoscopic liver resection for HCC were 50-75% and 31-38.2%, respectively. The 3-year overall and disease-free survival rates after laparoscopic liver resection for colorectal metastasis to the liver were 80-87% and 51%, respectively. This review suggests that in experienced hands by surgeons trained in hepatic surgery, minimally invasive surgery and laparoscopic ultrasonography, laparoscopic liver resections are safe with acceptable morbidity and mortality for both minor and major hepatic resections and comparable 3- and 5-year survival rates reported for HCC and colorectal cancer metastasis compared to open hepatic resection, albeit in a selected group of patients.

Techniques: Right Hepatic Lobectomy, Left Hepatic Lobectomy, Left Lateral Sectionectomy

The keys to a safe hepatic resection require a fundamental understanding of liver anatomy and common anatomical variants, liver ultrasonography and a mastery of an orderly series of steps to each hepatic operation. A detail description of all liver resections is beyond the scope of this chapter and are described elsewhere. Multiple approaches and techniques are available to perform each type of liver resection. We present the UPMC Liver Cancer Center approach in stepwise fashion for right hepatic lobectomy left hepatic lobectomy and left lateral sectionectomy.

Steps common to all open major hepatic resections
1. Skin incision - right subcostal with midline extension ('hockey stick' incision).
2. Open abdomen and place fixed table retractor (Thompsen retractor).

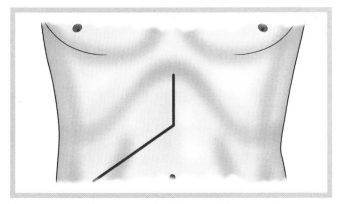

Figure 29-12: 'Hockey stick' incision used for open liver surgery

3. Take down round and falciform ligaments, expose anterior surface of hepatic veins.
4. For left hepatectomy, divide left triangular ligament; for right hepatectomy, mobilize right lobe from right coronary/triangular ligaments.
5. Open gastrohepatic ligament and assess for replaced hepatic arteries.
6. Perform open cholecystectomy, leave gallbladder with cystic duct intact (until end of case for cholangiogram).
7. Perform liver ultrasound (US) and confirm the operation to be performed.

Right hepatectomy or hemihepatectomy

8. Mobilize liver from inferior vena cava (IVC) in 'piggyback' fashion, ligate short hepatic veins up to right hepatic vein.
9. Right hilar dissection—gently lower the hilar plate, then doubly ligate and divide right hepatic artery (RHA) staying high on the right side of the common bile duct.
10. Divide inflow (right portal vein) (RPV) with Endo-GIA™ (Covidien, Mansfield, MA) vascular stapler (white 2.5 mm cartridge), after taking the small lateral PV branch off the RPV to caudate/right lobe.
11. Divide outflow (right hepatic vein) (RHV) with EndoGIA™ vascular stapler (white load).
12. Notch/divide the caudate process crossing to the right hepatic lobe.
13. Make counter-incision at right base of gallbladder fossa; pass large Kelly deep to hilar plate and emerge anterior to IVC; place umbilical tape in tunnel behind hilar plate.
14. Divide right hilar plate with right hepatic ducts with EndoGIA™ vascular stapler (white load).
15. Repeat US and confirm transection plane staying just to the right of the middle hepatic vein.
16. Bovie down ~ 1 cm in liver parenchyma, then switch to Ligasure™ (Tyco Healthcare, Boulder, CO).
17. Continue parenchymal division with Ligasure™ until segments V/VIII middle hepatic vein branches encountered.
18. Secure Pringle maneuver around porta hepatis (Potts loop cinched up with right angle).
19. Complete parenchymal slice with sequential crushing vascular stapler (pre-tunnel with large Kelly clamp), usually 4-6 minutes for entire slice.
20. Check cut edge for surgical bleeding, place figure-of-eight suture if bleeder.
21. Release Pringle and dry up cut edge with TissueLink™ (Salient Surgical, Portsmouth, NH) saline-cooled device.
22. Inspect IVC and right retroperitoneal space for hemostasis.

23. Perform completion US to confirm left portal vein inflow and hepatic vein outflow.
24. Shoot saline cholangiogram via cystic duct stump to confirm cut edge is water-tight.
25. Shoot contrast fluoroscopy cholangiogram (optional) to confirm patency of proximal left hepatic duct and distal common bile duct; secure cystic duct stump in usual manner.
26. Tack proximal falciform back to diaphragm side with single figure-of-eight suture.
27. Place Jackson-Pratt (JP) drain in right subphrenic space and close abdomen.

Left hepatectomy or hemihepatectomy

8. Widely open the gastrohepatic ligament flush with the undersurface of the left lateral section and the caudate lobe.
9. Doubly ligate and divide a replaced or accessory left hepatic artery (LHA) (if present).
10. Clamp the round ligament (ligament teres) and pull anteriorly as a handle to expose the left hilum.
11. Divide any existing parenchymal bridge between segment III and IVb.
12. Dissect the left hilum at the base of the umbilical fissure and lower the hilar plate anterior to the left portal pedicle.
13. Incise the peritoneum overlying the hilum from the left side and doubly ligate the LHA (after test clamping and confirming palpable pulse in RHA).
14. Dissect the portal vein at the base of the umbilical fissure (it will take a nearly 90° bend from the transverse to the umbilical portion).
15. Divide the left portal vein with EndoGIA™ vascular stapler (white load), staying just distal to (beyond) the take-off of the caudate inflow branch (if the caudate lobe is being preserved).
16. Divide the ligamentum venosum (Arantius ligament) caudally.
17. Make a counter-incision in segment IVb one centimeter above the base of the umbilical fissure and pass a blunt Kelly clamp behind the left hilar plate and aim for the left lower quadrant, exiting just anterior (and superficial) to the caudate lobe.
18. Place umbilical tape in tunnel behind the left hilar plate.
19. Divide left hilar plate and left hepatic duct with EndoGIA™ vascular stapler (white load).
20. Fold the left lateral segment up and back to the right, exposing the window at the base of the LHV as it enters the IVC. This is facilitated by dividing any loose areolar tissue overlying the ligamentum venosum (Arantius ligament) which is divided proximally.

21. Pass a large, blunt right angle in the window between the RHV and the MHV, and hug the back of the MHV aiming for the deep edge of the LHV. Do not force it, or make a hole in the IVC or MHV.

22. Pass an umbilical tape through this window and divide the LHV and MHV common trunk with EndoGIA™ vascular stapler.

23. Repeat US and confirm transection plane on the anterior surface, staying close to the demarcated line. Do not bisect the MHV as it passes tangentially from left to right lobe.

24. Bovie down ~ 1 cm in liver parenchyma, then switch to Ligasure™.

25. Continue parenchymal division with Ligasure™ until segments V/VIII MHV branches encountered.

26. Secure Pringle maneuver around porta hepatis (Potts loop cinched up with right angle).

27. Complete parenchymal slice with sequential crushing vascular stapler (pre-tunnel with large Kelly clamp). As the slice is deepened, gradually carry the transection down to exit just anterior to the caudate at the level of Arantius ligament.

28. Check cut edge for surgical bleeding, place figure-of-eight suture if bleeding.

29. Release Pringle and dry up cut edge with TissueLink™ saline-cooled device.

30. Perform completion US to confirm RPV inflow and RHV outflow.

31. Shoot saline cholangiogram via cystic duct stump to confirm cut edge is watertight.

32. Shoot contrast fluoroscopy cholangiogram (optional) to confirm patency of proximal R hepatic duct and distal CBD; secure cystic duct stump in usual manner.

33. Place JP drain in left subphrenic space and close abdomen.

Left lateral sectionectomy

8. Widely open the gastrohepatic ligament flush with the undersurface of the left lateral section and the caudate lobe.

9. Doubly ligate and divide a replaced or accessory LHA (if present).

10. Clamp the round ligament and pull anteriorly as a handle to expose the L hilum.

11. Divide any existing parenchymal bridge between segments III and IVb.

12. Carry the dissection down from the end of the round ligament and the segment III pedicle will be encountered.

13. Incise the peritoneal reflection on the left side of the round ligament as it inserts into the umbilical fissure and this will facilitate encircling the segment III and II pedicles, which can be divided separately with vascular stapler. When encircling the segment II

pedicle, care is taken to avoid injury to the caudate inflow vessels coming off the LPV.

14. The liver parenchyma is divided staying flush on the left side of the falciform ligament using bovie cautery and/or Ligasure.

15. The LHV is divided inside the liver parenchyma with EndoGIA™ vascular stapler (white load) as the parenchymal transection is complete.

16. A Pringle maneuver is usually not required for a left lateral sectionectomy since complete devascularization occurs before transection and little back bleeding is encountered.

Role of Intraoperative Ultrasonography

Essential to all liver resection is accurate intraoperative ultrasonography (IOUS) to visualize the tumor(s) and the proximity to hepatic vasculature and map the transection plane with adequate margins. First introduced in 1981 by Makuuchi, et al, IOUS became routine practice during liver resections. Intraoperative ultrasound evaluation of the liver has become indispensable to guarantee precise determination of the segmental tumor location and the relationship of the tumor to adjacent vascular or biliary structures. In addition, its critical role in excluding adjacent or new lesions has made it obligatory in the intraoperative assessment of resectability. In fact, IOUS is more sensitive in detecting liver lesions not identified on preoperative imaging and better delineates the proximity to liver lesions to hepatic and portal veins and biliary structures, often time influencing and altering the operative strategy by 15-49%.

Parenchymal Transection Techniques and Devices

Since the first recorded successful elective liver resection was performed by Carl Langenbuch in 1887, hepatic resection surgery has evolved over the past 50 years with better understanding of liver anatomy and physiology, coupled with improved anesthesia techniques and the widespread use of IOUS. Innovations in technology have expanded the list of liver parenchymal transection devices and hemostatic agents (**Table 29-3**). Each device/agent has a learning curve and every experienced liver surgeon has his/her personal preference.

A major advance in the evolution of hepatic surgery has been the addition of vascular stapling devices for division of the hepatic and portal veins. With reported early success in stapling extrahepatic vessels, stapling devices have now been applied more frequently during the parenchymal transection phase, which remains a source of potential blood loss due to back-bleeding from hepatic veins. One major advantage of the sequential stapling technique is the shortened parenchymal transection time, thus minimizing surface bleeding and ischemic time to the remnant liver.

TABLE 29-3	Techniques and devices for dividing liver parenchyma and achieving hemostasis

- Blunt fracture/clips
- Monopolar cautery (Bovie)
- Bipolar cautery
- Argon beam coagulator
- Ultrasonic dissector (CUSA)
- Erbe Hydrojet
- Harmonic scalpel
- Autosonix
- Ligasure
- SurgRx EnSeal
- Gyrus PK cutting forceps
- Endovascular staplers
- Tissuelink devices
- Habib 4x sealer
- In line bipolar linear coagulator
- Topical agents (Fibrin glues, Surgicel, Gelfoam, Avitene, Tisseal, Floseal, Crosseal)

However, a major disadvantage of the stapling technique is the high cost of multiple stapler cartridges, which is often offset by the decreased expense reported with shortening OR time, avoiding ICU admission and minimizing blood transfusions. In addition, the use of staplers for the parenchymal slice has decreased the incidence of bile leaks, as shown by Balaa, et al in a large series of 101 consecutive right hemi-hepatectomies using the stapling technique, with only one reported bile leak (1%) which sealed after ERCP.

Landmark Papers

1. Adam R, Azoulay D, Castaing D, Eshkenazy R, Pascal G, Hashizume K, Samuel D, Bismuth H. Liver resection as a bridge to transplantation for hepatocellular carcinoma on cir-rhosis: a reasonable strategy? Ann Surg 2003;238(4):508-18.

2. Adam R, Laurent A, Azoulay D, Castaing D, Bismuth H. Two-stage hepatectomy: A planned strategy to treat irresectable liver tumors. Ann Surg. 2000; 232(6):777-85.

3. Cheng BQ, Jia CQ, Liu CT, Fan W, Wang QL, Zhang ZL, Yi CH. Chemoembolization combined with radiofrequency ablation for patients with hepatocellular carcinoma larger than 3 cm: a randomized controlled trial. JAMA 2008;299:1669-77

4. Deneve JL, Pawlik TM, Cunningham S, Clary B, Reddy S, Scoggins CR, et al. Liver cell adenoma: a multicenter analysis of risk factors for rupture and malignancy. Ann Surg Oncol 2009;16(3):640-8.

5. Im JH, Yoon HK, Sung KB, Ko GY, Gwon DI, Shin JH, Song HY. Transcatheter arterial chemoembolization or chemo-infusion for unresectable intrahepatic cholangiocarcinoma: clinical efficacy and factors influencing outcomes. Cancer 2008;113(7):1614-22.

6. Iwatsuki S, Dvorchik I, Marsh JW, Madariaga JR, Carr B, Fung JJ, Starzl TE. Liver transplantation for hepatocellular carcinoma: a proposal of a prognostic scoring system. J Am Coll Surg 2000;191(4):389-94.

7. Jarnagin WR, Shoup M. Surgical management of cholangiocarcinoma. Semin Liver Dis 2004;24(2):189-99.

8. Llovet JM, Fuster J, Bruix J. Intention-to-treat analysis of surgical treatment for early hepatocellular carcinoma: resection versus transplantation. Hepatology 1999;30(6):1434-40.

9. Llovet JM, Ricci S, Mazzaferro V, et al. Sorafenib in advanced hepatocellular carcinoma. N Engl J Med 2008;359(4):378-90.

10. Mazzaferro V, Regalia E, Doci R, et al. Liver transplantation for the treatment of small hepatocellular carcinomas in patients with cirrhosis. N Engl J Med 1996;334:693-9.

11. Murata S, Moriya Y, Akasu T, Fujita S, Sugihara K. Resection of both hepatic and pulmonary metastases in patients with colorectal carcinoma. Cancer 1998; 83(6):1086-93.

12. Pawlik TM, Schulick RD, Choti MA. Expanding criteria for resectability of colorectal liver metastases. Oncologist 2008;13:51-64.

13. Pozzo C, Basso M, Cassano A, Quirino M, Schinzari G, Trigila N, et al. Neoadjuvant treatment of unresectable liver disease with irinotecan and 5-fluorouracil plus folinic acid in colorectal cancer patients. Ann Oncol 2004; 15(6):933-9.

14. Rea DJ, Heimbach JK, Rosen CB, Haddock MG, Alberts SR, Kremers WK, et al. Liver transplantation with neoadjuvant chemoradiation is more effective than resection for hilar cholangiocarcinoma. Ann Surg 2005;242(3):451-8.

15. Reddy SK, Pawlik TM, Zorzi D, Gleisner AL, Ribero D, Assumpcao L, et al. Simultaneous resections of colorectal cancer and synchronous liver metastases: a multi-institutional analysis. Ann Surg Oncol 2007;14(12):3481-91.

16. Roayaie S, Guarrera JV, Ye MQ, Thung SN, Emre S, Fishbein TM, et al. Aggressive surgical treatment of intrahepatic cholangiocarcinoma: predictors of outcomes. J Am Coll Surg 1998; 187:365-72.

17. Rougier P, Milan C, Lazorthes F, Fourtanier G, Partensky C, Baumel H, Faivre J. Prospective study of prognostic factors in patients with unresected hepatic metastases from colorectal cancer. Fondation Française de Cancérologie Digestive. Br J Surg. 1995; 82(10):1397-400.

18. Strasberg SM. IHPBA Brisbane 2000 Terminology of Liver Anatomy & Resections. HPB 2000; 2(3):333-9.

19. Vente MA, Wondergem M, van der Tweel I, et al. Yttrium-90 microsphere radioembolization for the treatment of liver malignancies: a structured meta-analysis. Eur Radiol 2009; 19(4):951-9.

20. Yao FY, Ferrell L, Bass NM, et al. Liver transplantation for hepatocellular carcinoma: expansion of the tumor size limits does not adversely impact survival. Hepatology 2001;33:1394-403.

Level of Evidence Table			
Recommendation	**Grade**	**Best level of evidence**	**References**
Primary resection or transplantation are both acceptable approaches to the management of early HCC for patients with preserved liver function.	B	2b	1-5
The Milan criteria serve as the current standard for tumor size/distribution in the transplant evaluation of HCC patients.	B	2b	6-10
Regional and ablative therapies (TACE, RFA, PEI) should be considered for downstaging HCC patients to within transplantation criteria.	B	4	11, 12
Neoadjuvant therapy (bridging) of patients already within criteria and listed for transplantation of HCC may limit tumor progression and dropout.	C	4	13-17
Adjuvant therapy after curative resection of HCC may improve survival.	B	1a	18-20
Sorafenib is the agent of choice for treating advanced unresectable HCC.	A	1b	21, 22
Resection is the treatment of choice for colorectal liver metastases. A strategy of neoadjuvant systemic and regional chemotherapy, portal vein embolization and staged resection may be incorporated to optimize resectability.	B	4	23-28
Tumor progression during neoadjuvant chemotherapy for resectable colorectal liver metastases is a poor prognostic marker and a relative contraindication to surgery.	B	2b	29-32
Portal vein embolization is indicated when the predicted future liver remnant ratio is < 20% total volume for normal liver; < 30% for suspected injury secondary to chemotherapy, steatosis, or hepatitis and < 40% for cirrhotic liver.	B	2b	33-37
The role of adjuvant hepatic arterial infusion therapy after resection of colorectal metastases compared to modern systemic therapy is unclear.	C	4	38-40

References

1. Facciuto ME, Rochon C, Pandey M, et al. Surgical dilemma: liver resection or liver transplantation for hepatocellular carcinoma and cirrhosis. Intention-to-treat analysis in patients within and outwith Milan criteria. HPB (Oxford) 2009; 11:398-404.
2. Adam R, Azoulay D, Castaing D, et al. Liver resection as a bridge to transplantation for hepatocellular carcinoma on cirrhosis: a reasonable strategy? Ann Surg 2003; 238:508-18; discussion 518-9.
3. Margarit C, Escartin A, Castells L, et al. Resection for hepatocellular carcinoma is a good option in Child-Turcotte-Pugh class A patients with cirrhosis who are eligible for liver transplantation. Liver Transpl 2005; 11:1242-51.
4. Shah SA, Cleary SP, Tan JC, et al. An analysis of resection vs transplantation for early hepatocellular carcinoma: defining the optimal therapy at a single institution. Ann Surg Oncol 2007; 14:2608-14.
5. Bellavance EC, Lumpkins KM, Mentha G, et al. Surgical management of early-stage hepatocellular carcinoma: resection or transplantation? J Gastrointest Surg 2008; 12:1699-708.
6. Mazzaferro V, Regalia E, Doci R, et al. Liver transplantation for the treatment of small hepatocellular carcinomas in patients with cirrhosis. N Engl J Med 1996; 334:693-9.
7. Duffy JP, Vardanian A, Benjamin E, et al. Liver transplantation criteria for hepatocellular carcinoma should be expanded: a 22-year experience with 467 patients at UCLA. Ann Surg 2007; 246:502-9; discussion 509-11.
8. Yao FY, Ferrell L, Bass NM, et al. Liver transplantation for hepatocellular carcinoma: comparison of the proposed UCSF criteria with the Milan criteria and the Pittsburgh modified TNM criteria. Liver Transpl 2002; 8:765-74.
9. Soejima Y, Taketomi A, Yoshizumi T, et al. Extended indication for living donor liver transplantation in patients with hepatocellular carcinoma. Transplantation 2007; 83:893-9.
10. Decaens T, Roudot-Thoraval F, Hadni-Bresson S, et al. Impact of UCSF criteria according to pre- and post-OLT tumor features: analysis of 479 patients listed for HCC with a short waiting time. Liver Transpl 2006; 12:1761-9.
11. Yao FY, Kerlan RK, Jr., Hirose R, et al. Excellent outcome following down-staging of hepatocellular carcinoma prior to liver transplantation: an intention-to-treat analysis. Hepatology 2008; 48:819-27.

12. Chapman WC, Majella Doyle MB, Stuart JE, et al. Outcomes of neoadjuvant transarterial chemoembolization to downstage hepatocellular carcinoma before liver transplantation. Ann Surg 2008; 248:617-25.

13. Graziadei IW, Sandmueller H, Waldenberger P, et al. Chemoembolization followed by liver transplantation for hepatocellular carcinoma impedes tumor progression while on the waiting list and leads to excellent outcome. Liver Transpl 2003; 9:557-63.

14. Decaens T, Roudot-Thoraval F, Bresson-Hadni S, et al. Impact of pretransplantation transarterial chemoembolization on survival and recurrence after liver transplantation for hepatocellular carcinoma. Liver Transpl 2005; 11:767-75.

15. Belghiti J, Carr BI, Greig PD, et al. Treatment before liver transplantation for HCC. Ann Surg Oncol 2008; 15:993-1000.

16. Hoffmann K, Glimm H, Radeleff B, et al. Prospective, randomized, double-blind, multi-center, Phase III clinical study on transarterial chemoembolization (TACE) combined with Sorafenib versus TACE plus placebo in patients with hepatocellular cancer before liver transplantation— HeiLivCa [ISRCTN24081794]. BMC Cancer 2008; 8:349.

17. Mazzaferro V, Battiston C, Perrone S, et al. Radiofrequency ablation of small hepatocellular carcinoma in cirrhotic patients awaiting liver transplantation: a prospective study. Ann Surg 2004; 240:900-9.

18. Samuel M, Chow PK, Chan Shih-Yen E, et al. Neoadjuvant and adjuvant therapy for surgical resection of hepatocellular carcinoma. Cochrane Database Syst Rev 2009; CD001199.

19. Breitenstein S, Dimitroulis D, Petrowsky H, et al. Systematic review and meta-analysis of interferon after curative treatment of hepatocellular carcinoma in patients with viral hepatitis. Br J Surg 2009; 96:975-81.

20. Lo CM, Liu CL, Chan SC, et al. A randomized, controlled trial of postoperative adjuvant interferon therapy after resection of hepatocellular carcinoma. Ann Surg 2007; 245:831-42.

21. Llovet JM, Ricci S, Mazzaferro V, et al. Sorafenib in advanced hepatocellular carcinoma. N Engl J Med 2008; 359:378-90.

22. Cheng AL, Kang YK, Chen Z, et al. Efficacy and safety of sorafenib in patients in the Asia-Pacific region with advanced hepatocellular carcinoma: a phase III randomised, double-blind, placebo-controlled trial. Lancet Oncol 2009; 10:25-34.

23. Adam R, Laurent A, Azoulay D, et al. Two-stage hepatectomy: a planned strategy to treat irresectable liver tumors. Ann Surg 2000; 232:777-85.

24. Jaeck D, Oussoultzoglou E, Rosso E, et al. A two-stage hepatectomy procedure combined with portal vein embolization to achieve curative resection for initially unresectable multiple and bilobar colorectal liver metastases. Ann Surg 2004; 240:1037-49; discussion 1049-51.

25. Zelek L, Bugat R, Cherqui D, et al. Multimodal therapy with intravenous biweekly leucovorin, 5-fluorouracil and irinotecan combined with hepatic arterial infusion pirarubicin in non-resectable hepatic metastases from colorectal cancer (a European Association for Research in Oncology trial). Ann Oncol 2003; 14:1537-42.

26. Alberts SR, Horvath WL, Sternfeld WC, et al. Oxaliplatin, fluorouracil and leucovorin for patients with unresectable liver-only metastases from colorectal cancer: a North Central Cancer Treatment Group phase II study. J Clin Oncol 2005; 23:9243-9.

27. Bismuth H, Adam R, Levi F, et al. Resection of nonresectable liver metastases from colorectal cancer after neoadjuvant chemotherapy. Ann Surg 1996; 224:509-20; discussion 520-2.

28. Kemeny NE, Melendez FD, Capanu M, et al. Conversion to resectability using hepatic artery infusion plus systemic chemotherapy for the treatment of unresectable liver metastases from colorectal carcinoma. J Clin Oncol 2009; 27:3465-71.

29. Adam R, Pascal G, Castaing D, et al. Tumor progression while on chemotherapy: a contraindication to liver resection for multiple colorectal metastases? Ann Surg 2004; 240:1052-61; discussion 1061-4.

30. Neumann UP, Thelen A, Rocken C, et al. Nonresponse to pre-operative chemotherapy does not preclude long-term survival after liver resection in patients with colorectal liver metastases. Surgery 2009; 146:52-9.

31. Gallagher DJ, Zheng J, Capanu M, et al. Response to neoadjuvant chemotherapy does not predict overall survival for patients with synchronous colorectal hepatic metastases. Ann Surg Oncol 2009; 16:1844-51.

32. Allen PJ, Kemeny N, Jarnagin W, et al. Importance of response to neoadjuvant chemotherapy in patients undergoing resection of synchronous colorectal liver metastases. J Gastrointest Surg 2003; 7:109-15; discussion 116-7.

33. Kubota K, Makuuchi M, Kusaka K, et al. Measurement of liver volume and hepatic functional reserve as a guide to decision-making in resectional surgery for hepatic tumors. Hepatology 1997; 26:1176-81.

34. Ribero D, Abdalla EK, Madoff DC, et al. Portal vein embolization before major hepatectomy and its effects on regeneration, resectability and outcome. Br J Surg 2007; 94:1386-94.

35. Kishi Y, Abdalla EK, Chun YS, et al. Three hundred and one consecutive extended right hepatectomies: evaluation of outcome based on systematic liver volumetry. Ann Surg 2009; 250(4):540-8.

36. Abulkhir A, Limongelli P, Healey AJ, et al. Preoperative portal vein embolization for major liver resection: a meta-analysis. Ann Surg 2008; 247:49-57.

37. Azoulay D, Castaing D, Krissat J, et al. Percutaneous portal vein embolization increases the feasibility and safety of major liver resection for hepatocellular carcinoma in injured liver. Ann Surg 2000; 232:665-72.

38. Wagman LD, Kemeny MM, Leong L, et al. A prospective, randomized evaluation of the treatment of colorectal cancer metastatic to the liver. J Clin Oncol 1990; 8:1885-93.

39. Kemeny N, Huang Y, Cohen AM, et al. Hepatic arterial infusion of chemotherapy after resection of hepatic metastases from colorectal cancer. N Engl J Med 1999; 341:2039-48.

40. Kemeny N, Capanu M, D'Angelica M, et al. Phase I trial of adjuvant hepatic arterial infusion (HAI) with floxuridine (FUDR) and dexamethasone plus systemic oxaliplatin, 5-fluorouracil and leucovorin in patients with resected liver metastases from colorectal cancer. Ann Oncol 2009; 20:1236-41.

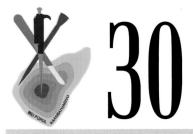

30

Gallbladder Cancer

Mario Lora, Narcis Octavian Zarnescu, A James Moser

Gall bladder cancer (GBC) is a rare malignancy with an estimated 9,760 new cases during 2009 in the United States. It is the most common cancer of the biliary tract, although it is no longer considered to be a type of cholangio-carcinoma. The outcome of those with GBC has been reported to be dismal, but with the current aggressive approach, there have been significant improvements in the 5-year survival rates, especially in the early stages.

Epidemiology

GBC is the most common cancer of the biliary tree (in the United States) and the fifth most common cancer of the gastrointestinal tract. The incidence of GBC is three times higher among women than men in all populations. The incidence of GBC increases steadily with age and most commonly presents in the seventh decade of life. The National Cancer Institute estimates 9,760 new cases of GBC in the USA for the year of 2009, of which the estimated deaths would be 3370.

The incidence of GBC varies by geographic region and ethnicity. The highest incidence is reported in the Native Indian populations (21.5 per 100,000), Bolivians (15.5 per 100,000), Pakistanis (13.8 per 100,000), Chileans (Mapuche ethnicity), Central Europeans, Israelis, Native Americans and Mexican-Americans. Lower socioeconomic status among these groups may postpone access to cholecystectomy and predispose to higher rates of GBC.

The highest mortality rate (35 per 100,000) is found in the Mapuche Indian region of Southern Chile. Peru, Colombia, Ecuador and Brazil present intermediate rates with 3.7-9.1 per 100,000. North America has a low mortality rate except for the Native American population of New Mexico (11.3 per 100,000) and Mexican Americans.

Risk Factors (Table 30-1)

Although the etiology of GBC remains unknown, gallstones are a commonly associated risk factor (70-90% of GBCs). The link between gallstones and GBC is unclear but may result from chronic inflammation of the mucosa

that predisposes to malignant transformation in genetically susceptible populations.

TABLE 30-1	Risk factors for GBC

- Female gender
- Specific ethnicities—American Indian, Chile, etc.
- Cholelithiasis and large size of gallstones
- Chronic infections—Salmonella carriage
- Pancreaticobiliary maljunction
- Biliary cysts / Choledochal cysts
- Obesity
- Smoking
- Drugs and carcinogen exposure

- *Cholelithiasis:* Gallstones are observed in up to 92% of GBC. However, the incidence of GBC in gallstone disease is much lower. The association is apparent because roughly 1-2% of cholecystectomy specimens are positive for malignancy. A more important parameter is the size of the gallstone. A single large stone is more risky than multiple smaller ones. Gallstones > 3 cm in diameter are associated with a 10-fold increased risk of GBC compared stones < 1 cm in diameter and gallstones 2.0 to 2.9 cm diameter carry a relative risk of 2.4.
- *Chronic infections:* Salmonella may have a chronic carriage of up to 25% of those who suffer an acute illness. This may predispose to a chronic inflammatory condition that brings about carcinogenesis. The exact mechanism is unclear and Helicobacter carriage is also believed to play a role although robust evidence for this is still lacking.
- *Porcelain gallbladder:* Studies from the 1960s suggested that porcelain gallbladder (calcified gallbladder wall) was associated with GBC in 12-61% of patients. Two large recent studies cast doubt on the association (0-5%). Porcelain gallbladder is characterized by the calcification of the muscular layer which carries the blood supply. Porcelain gallbladder which carried the blood supply. Eventually the mucosa over the calcified part sloughs off. Porcelain gallbladder is of two types: complete (where all mucosa is sloughed off) and

incomplete (where there are areas of lost mucosa with islands of compromised mucosa remaining). The actual risk of developing GBC in the presence of porcelain gallbladder is related to the distribution of calcifications: diffuse calcifications have a lower risk as compared with focal mucosal calcifications having a risk of 7% (previous series reported an incidence of 25-42%).

- *Gallbladder polyps:* Gallbladder polyps may be benign or malignant. The most common benign polyp is the cholesterol polyp. About 4% of benign polyps may be adenomas, which harbor a risk of malignancy. Cholelithiasis doesn't often coexist with polyps. Malignant polyps often are adenocarcinomas. Endoscopic ultrasound (EUS) is probably more accurate in differentiating cholesterol polyps from malignant polyps than transabdominal ultrasound (USG).
- *Other factors:* Additional risk factors include congenital choledochal cyst, obesity, smoking, dietary influences like red chili pepper and alcohol, high parity, number of pregnancies, chronic biliary tract infection (Salmonella, Helicobacter bilis and Helicobacter pylori), pancreaticobiliary malunion; which is a rare anatomic variant where the pancreatic duct drains aberrantly into the common bile duct and exposes the biliary epithelium to chronic enzymatic digestion. Medications like methyldopa, oral contraceptives, isoniazid and exposure to carcinogens such as oil, paper, chemical, shoes, textile and cellulose acetate fiber manufacturing industries are also thought to be contributing factors.

Pathology

The most common type of GBC is adenocarcinoma. However, there are many other pathological types that are rarer. They are listed in **Table 30-2**.

TABLE 30-2	Pathological types of GBC

- Carcinoma in situ
- Adenocarcinoma, intestinal type
- Adenocarcinoma, NOS*
- Papillary
- Mucinous
- Clear cell
- Signet ring
- Squamous
- Small cell/oat cell
- Adenosquamous
- Carcinoma, NOS*
- Carcinosarcoma

* NOS—not otherwise specified

The most favorable type is the papillary type due to its propensity to spread intraluminally, unlike other types that spread transmurally and become invasive. The most frequent location at which the gallbladder develops cancer is the fundus (60%), followed by the body (30%) and neck (10%).

GBC may result from the progression of epithelial dysplasia to *carcinoma in situ* (CIS) and invasive carcinoma over a period of 5-15 years. It is unclear whether the adenoma-carcinoma sequence occurs in GBC. Severe dysplasia and *CIS* are frequently (90%) identified in gallbladder epithelium adjacent to invasive cancers.

Gallbladder adenomas are present in up to 1.1% of cholecystectomy specimens. Kozuka, et al demonstrated that all gallbladder adenomas less than 12 mm diameter were benign, whereas adenomas with micro-invasion were 12 mm or larger. The majority of invasive cancers were greater than 30 mm in diameter. Despite the link between polyp size and the risk of cancer, gallbladder adenomas do not display molecular changes associated with malignancy as expected of premalignant lesions. Polyps < 1 cm may safely be monitored by ultrasound every 3-6 months.

Genetics of Gallbladder Cancer

The molecular events leading to GBC have not been well defined due to the low incidence of the disease and the scarcity of samples for genetic investigation. Carcinoma of the gallbladder develops in one of two distinct pathways:
- *De novo* due to p53 alterations associated with a low percentage of K-ras mutations.
- Adenoma-carcinoma sequence in the absence of p53, K-ras or APC gene mutations.

Wistuba, et al detected frequent abnormalities at chromosomal loci 9p and 8p. These abnormalities included loss of heterozygosity (LOH) at p53 and deleted in colorectal carcinoma (DDC) genes. LOH of the p53 gene was detected in 92% of invasive GBCs, 86% of carcinomas in situ and 28% of dysplastic epithelia.

Additional genetic events implicated in gallbladder carcinogenesis include the *ras* and the *raf* gene families. The RAS/RAF/MEK/ERK (mitogen-activated protein kinase/ERK kinase)/ERK (extracellular-signal-regulated kinase) pathway is a signaling system that controls proliferation, differentiation, apoptosis and cell survival. This system is a family of activated *ras* genes and has been implicated in the genesis of CBC, since K-*ras* mutations are observed. The *raf* family also has a role in cell proliferation, differentiation and programmed cell death. Mutated B-raf has recently been reported in a variety of tumors including malignant melanoma, colon and gallbladder carcinomas. Mutations of B-raf are found in 10-57% of GBCs. Saetta, et al found B-raf mutations at exon 15 in 33% of the gallbladder carcinomas, whereas K-ras mutations at codon 12 were found in 25% of specimens.

Clinical Presentation

The majority of GBCs are identified incidentally during routine cholecystectomy for gallstones. Typical symptoms of more advanced lesions include epigastric discomfort, right upper quadrant pain, malaise, jaundice, nausea, vomiting and weight loss. Acute cholecystitis may intervene in the obstructed gallbladder containing gallstones, masking the presence of an invasive cancer.

Findings of GBC on physical examination are almost always ominous: palpable right upper quadrant mass with painless jaundice (Courvoisier's sign), palpable periumbilical nodule due to carcinomatosis (Sister Mary Joseph nodes) and left supraclavicular adenopathy (Virchow node).

Diagnosis

The most important person in the link in the care of a patient with GBC is the general surgeon who sees the patient for a presumed benign gallbladder problem. General surgeons should constantly work with the suspicion of GBC in every gallbladder patient as most GBC is identified incidentally. Red flags for raisers for the general surgeon are:

- Right upper quadrant symptoms, atypical of cholelithiasis
- Cholelithiasis-like symptomatology with weight loss, anorexia and cachexia
- A polyp-like lesion in the fundus
- An immobile lesion in the gallbladder
- A single large stone
- Jaundice and biliary obstruction
- Gallbladder wall thickening and biliary dilation in USG.

The diagnosis of GBC is supplemented by several other investigations. A tissue diagnosis is not necessary for planning operative management.

- *Serum tumor markers:* The diagnosis of GBC cannot be established on the basis of current tumor marker panels. Carbohydrate antigen (CA) 19-9 is the best serum marker available. However, elevated serum CA 19-9 may be observed in benign conditions such as Xanthogranulomatous cholecystitis and Mirizzi syndrome (a syndrome characterized by a stone in the cystic duct or neck of the gallbladder obstructing the common hepatic duct). Ca 19-9 greater than 20 U/mL has 79% sensitivity and 79% specificity for GBC. In another study, CA 19-9 values exceeding 90 U/mL were associated with a 94% rate of unresectable disease, while levels higher than 450 U/mL indicated advanced disease in 100% of patients. Additional commonly available markers include carcinoembryonic antigen (CEA) and CA-125. A CEA level exceeding 4 ng/mL is

93% specific for GBC but only 50% sensitive. CA-125 levels greater than 11 U/mL have 64% sensitivity and 90% specificity in small studies. Newer panels include CA 242 and CA 15-3 (a tumor marker associated with breast cancer). Combinations of serum tumor markers may have greater diagnostic accuracy than individual levels.

- *Transabdominal ultrasound:* Transabdominal ultrasound (USG) is the most frequent initial study for evaluating symptoms in the right upper quadrant. Findings suggestive of GBC include thickening or calcification of the gallbladder wall, a fixed mass, a polypoid mass > 1 cm and gallstones > 3 cm (RR 10.1 for cancer), loss of the sonographic interface between gallbladder and liver and direct infiltration of a mass into the liver. The accuracy of conventional ultrasound for detect a mass in the gallbladder is 87%; and for the diagnosis of hepatic infiltration or metastasis is about 100%.
- *Endoscopic ultrasound:* Endoscopic ultrasound (EUS) has better resolution than transabdominal ultrasound for evaluating the gallbladder and identifying nodular infiltration of the porta hepatis and peripancreatic area due to the improved proximity of the echo-probe to these structures. EUS can detect polyps less than 20 mm diameter with an approximated sensitivity of 91%, specificity 87%, positive predictive value 75% and negative predictive value 96%.
- *CT scan:* CT findings of GBC include thickening of the gallbladder wall, a mass replacing the gallbladder and a fungating mass within the gallbladder. Additional findings include thickening of the hepatoduodenal ligament, extrahepatic biliary obstruction caused by metastasis to pericholedochal and superior pancreatico-duodenal nodes, encasement of the common hepatic duct, as well as invasion into the liver parenchyma, encasement of the portal vein and hepatic arteries, as well as distant metastases. Contrast-enhanced helical CT scan has a sensitivity of 88% for T2 lesions, 85% for T3 lesions and 95% for T4. 3D-CT angiography may detect major arterial and venous invasion in 90% of cases.
- *MRI and MRCP:* Findings in GBC include focal or diffuse wall thickening or a mass replacing the gallbladder. A common finding in all GBCs is contrast (gadopentate dimeglumine) enhancement in the early phase that persists into the delayed phase. The sensitivity and specificity of MRI/ MRCP for detecting hepatic invasion is 87.5% and 86%, respectively, for lymph node metastasis is 60% and 90%, respectively and for invasion of the bile duct is 80% and 100%, respectively. MRI demonstrates duodenal invasion in only 50% of cases and may reveal peritoneal metastasis.
- *PET scan:* Positron emission tomography uses fluorodeoxyglucose (FDG) to measure metabolic

differences between benign and malignant tissue and may be combined with CT scans (PET/CT) to improve the anatomic staging of GBC prior to surgery. The sensitivity of PET/CT for detecting residual disease following cholecystectomy for unsuspected gallbladder carcinoma was 78% with 80% specificity. The sensitivity for extrahepatic metastases (distant metastases or carcinomatosis) was 56%.

- *Cholangiography:* Invasive imaging of the biliary tree is accomplished by endoscopic retrograde cholangiopancreatography (ERCP) or percutaneous transhepatic cholangiography (PTC). Both techniques permit simultaneous decompression of the obstructed biliary tree as well as biopsy procedures. However, both techniques are less sensitive than MRCP for the diagnosis of GBC because cystic duct obstruction often prevents filling of the gallbladder with contrast, although compression of the adjacent bile ducts by a mass in the gallbladder fossa is visible.
- *Cytology:* Akosa, et al. evaluated different cytologic methods of diagnosing GBC, such as exfoliative bile cytology (study of shed cells in bile aspirates), EUS-directed fine-needle aspiration and endoscopic brushing. Fine-needle aspiration cytology had a sensitivity of 88%, while exfoliative cytology had a sensitivity of 50%. A preoperative diagnosis was made in 69% of cases and was useful for operative planning.

Staging and Prognosis

Staging of GBC requires histologic evaluation of resected tumors. Numerous classifications and proposals for modifications are available for GBC. The latest TNM-based classification of the AJCC revised sixth edition made some significant changes, but met with criticism and suggestions for modifications. Nevin, et al devised the first staging classification in 1976. It was later changed to the modified Nevin's staging. The Bartlett staging system, with only four stages was proposed in 1996. A comparison of these staging is given in **Table 30-3**.

The TNM staging of AJCC has significant changes between the fifth and sixth editions. The latest staging of the AJCC (6th edition), along with the 5-year survival is given in **Table 30-4**.

Recent changes to the sixth edition of the AJCC manual include:
- T3 specifies potentially resectable tumors, while T4 are unresectable.
- Depth of liver invasion has no effect on T status.
- Stage IIA reflects large invasive tumors (resectable) without lymph node metastasis.
- Stage IIB reflects resectable tumors with lymph node metastases.
- Stage III signifies locally unresectable disease; stage IV indicates metastatic disease.

The AJCC system does not specify which lymph node stations are equivalent to distant metastatic disease. However, Bartlett, et al reported that positive lymph nodes outside the hepatoduodenal ligament portended survival equal to M1 disease.

The most important prognostic factors for GBC are:
- depth of invasion into the gallbladder wall
- nodal status
- vascular invasion

GBC is usually diagnosed late in its course, 36.6% of patients present with stage 4 diseases, while 47% are found in stage 1. As a result, the overall median survival for patients with GBC is 10.3 months in the United States and is 27.4, 8.6, 4.2 and 2.8 months for stages I, II, III, IV, respectively.

Surgical Management

Surgical resection is the only potentially curative treatment for GBC. However, only 15-40% of patients with GBC are candidates for surgery at the time of diagnosis. Many patients eventually require palliation of acute cholecystitis or gastric outlet obstruction.

Surgical Anatomy

The gallbladder is a pear-shaped muscular sac located between segments IVb and V at the junctions of the right and left hepatic lobes. The gallbladder has four named

TABLE 30-3	Comparison of Nevin's and Bartlett's staging system		
Stage	Nevin's staging	Modified Nevin's staging	Bartlett's staging
I	Involves mucosa only	Carcinoma in situ	Involves mucosa or muscularis
II	Involves mucosa and muscularis	Involves mucosa or muscularis	Involves all three layers, i.e. transmural invasion
III	Involves all three layers	Transmural liver invasion	III A—liver invasion < 2 cm
			III B—liver invasion > 2 cm or N1 disease
IV	Involves all three layers and cystic lymph node involvement	Lymph node involvement	Distant metastases
V	Infiltration into liver or metastases	Distant metastases	—

TABLE 30-4

Primary tumor (T)	
TX	Primary tumor cannot be assessed
T0	No evidence of primary tumor
Tis	Carcinoma in situ
T1	Tumor invades lamina propria or muscle layer
T1a	Tumor invades lamina propria
T1b	Tumor invades muscle layer
T2	Tumor invades perimuscular connective tissue; no extension beyond serosa or into liver
T3	Tumor perforates serosa (visceral peritoneum) and/or directly invades the liver and/or one other adjacent organ or structure, such as the stomach, duodenum, colon, or pancreas, omentum or extrahepatic bile ducts
T4	Tumor invades main portal vein or hepatic artery, or invades multiple extrahepatic organs or structures
Regional lymph nodes (N)	
NX	Regional lymph nodes cannot be assessed
N0	No regional lymph node metastasis
N1	Regional lymph node metastasis
Distant metastasis (M)	
MX	Distant metastasis cannot be assessed
M0	No distant metastasis
M1	Distant metastasis

	Stage grouping			5 year survival
Stage 0	Tis	N0	M0	
Stage IA	T1	N0	M0	50%
Stage IB	T2	N0	M0	29%
Stage IIA	T3	N0	M0	7%
Stage IIB	T1	N1	M0	9%
	T2	N1	M0	
	T3	N1	M0	
Stage III	T4	Any N	M0	3%
Stage IV	Any T	Any N	M1	2%

Adapted with permission from AJCC Staging Manual, 6th edition

anatomic regions: the fundus, body (corpus), the infundibulum and the neck. The gallbladder has only three layers: mucosa, muscular layer and the serosa. There is no muscularis mucosa or submucosa in the gallbladder. The mucosa is formed by a uniform layer of tall columnar epithelial cells that absorb water and electrolytes to concentrate bile. Accessory bile ducts (of Luschka) connect the gallbladder to the segment IV bile ducts in up to

20-50% of humans. The blood supply comes from the cystic artery, which is usually a branch of the right hepatic artery (in ~ 90%) but may also arise from the common hepatic artery or the left hepatic artery. The sentinel node of the gallbladder is the cystic duct node, otherwise called the Calot's node. Lymph from the gallbladder drains to the peripancreatic, hepatoduodenal and superior mesenteric nodes **(Figure 30-1)**.

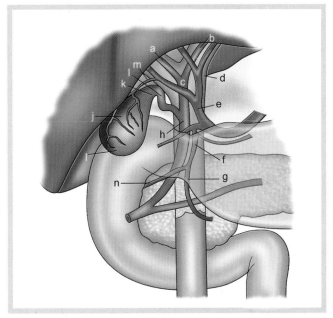

Figure 30-1: Anterior aspect of the biliary anatomy. a = right hepatic duct; b = left hepatic duct; c = common hepatic duct; d = portal vein; e = hepatic artery; f = gastroduodenal artery; g = left gastric artery; h = common bile duct; i = fundus of the gallbladder; j = body of gallbladder; k = infundibulum; l = cystic duct; m = cystic artery; n = superior pancreaticoduodenal artery. Note: the situation of the hepatic bile duct confluence anterior to the right branch of the portal vein, the posterior course of the right hepatic artery behind the common hepatic duct (*Source:* Brunicardi FC, Andersen DK, Billiar TR, Dunn DL, Hunter JG, Matthews JB, *Pollock RE: Schwartz's Principles of Surgery*, 9th Edition: http://www.accessmedicine.com. Copyright © The McGraw-Hill Companies, Inc. All rights reserved)

Preoperative Patient Selection

Shukla, et al proposed a preoperative scoring system based on a study of 335 patients with GBC. The Tata Memorial Hospital Scoring System is based on CT findings, presence of jaundice and elevations of CA 19-9, and can be used to direct treatment based on likely prognosis **(Table 30-5)**.

Based on total score (maximum = 10), patients are divided into three groups: highly likely to be resectable (0-3 points); potentially resectable (4-6 points) and highly unlikely to resectable (7-10 points). However, if the patient has CT features of metastatic disease (score 4), then the patient is considered to be unresectable, regardless of the total score **(Table 30-6)**.

TABLE 30-5	Tata Memorial Hospital (TMH) scoring system for GBC		
Score	Ca 19-9 (U/mL)	Serum bilirubin (mg/dL)	CT scan features
0	—	< 3	Normal
1	0-30	—	Mass in gallbladder
2	30-90	> 3	Infiltration of liver
3	90-450	—	Medially placed mass/ Intrahepatic biliary radicle dilation
4	> 450	—	Metastases

TABLE 30-6	Implications of TMH scoring	
Total TMH score	Description	Management
0 - 3	Highly likely to be resectable	Staging laparoscopy and resection
4 - 6	Potentially resectable	Neoadjuvant therapy + surgery
7 - 10	Highly unlikely to be resectable	Palliation
Metastatic disease on CT scan	Highly unlikely to be resectable	Palliation

In the resectable category patients should undergo staging laparoscopy and resection as appropriate. Patients in the borderline group undergo staging laparoscopy and may receive neoadjuvant therapy; those with advanced disease receive palliative treatment.

Surgical Strategy and Decision-Making

- A correct preoperative diagnosis of GBC is rarely made (~ < 10%)
- GBC spreads with bile spillage and can result in port site metastases
- In situ carcinoma and carcinoma involving lamina propria only (T1a) have very low or no risk of lymph node metastasis
- There is 15% chance of nodal disease for tumors invading muscular layer (T1b disease)
- There is 56% chance of lymph node spread for T2 (subserosal tumor) and a 75% chance of lymph node spread for locally advanced tumors (T3 and T4)
- Almost 80% of patients with locally advanced tumors (T3 and T4) have peritoneal spread of disease
- Tumor resection and lymph node clearance are the best ways to stage the disease

Since it is difficult to arrive at an accurate diagnosis preoperatively, a high index of suspicion is key for approaching GBC. Asymmetric gallbladder wall thickening or the appearance of a mass should be evaluated prior to laparoscopic cholecystectomy. Jaundiced patients require additional preoperative investigation due to the advanced state of their disease. ERCP should be performed to determine the origin of the obstruction and to define the extent of ductal involvement. It is always better to start with a diagnostic laparoscopy for accurate staging to prevent a non-therapeutic laparotomy. A suspicious or frankly malignant lesion of the gallbladder should not be biopsied. Lymph nodes outside the hepato-duodenal ligament should be evaluated and possibly sampled. Nodal involvement of the retroportal, peripancreatic or celiac node basins precludes curative resection.

If resectable disease is confirmed, it is best to convert the laparoscopic approach to an open technique for the following reasons:

- Accurate assessment of tumor extent and vascular invasion
- Detailed assessment of lymph nodal involvement
- Avoid inadvertent bile spillage
- Avoid potential creation of a positive margin while dissecting around the gallbladder.

It is also important to excise the laparoscopic port sites to prevent metastases. If the tumor is thought to be very superficial, then it is sent for frozen section to determine if the tumor is T1a (involving lamina propria only) or T1b (involving muscular layer). If it is T1b, then hepatoduodenal lymphadenectomy is warranted to accurately stage the tumor and also to provide preemptive clearance in the 15% of these tumors that may have spread to the regional nodes. It is important to remember that frozen section is accurate in making a histological diagnosis, but not accurate in assessing the depth of invasion (reliable only 70% of the time). So if the final postoperative pathology confirms a T1b tumor, which was initially considered T1a by intraoperative frozen section, then a reoperation for achieving tumor and lymph node clearance is needed.

Simple cholecystectomy refers to removal of the gallbladder only, akin to what is done for cholelithiasis or cholecystitis. Extended cholecystectomy, first described by Glenn and Hays in 1954, refers to cholecystectomy with wedge resection of liver segments IV b and V adjacent to the gallbladder, regional lymphadenectomy of the hepatoduodenal ligament and extrahepatic bile duct resection if involvement of the cystic or common hepatic duct is suspected. Lymph node dissection should include the posterior superior pancreatic nodes and all nodal tissues in the hepatoduodenal ligament by skeletonizing the common bile duct, hepatic artery and portal vein.

Incidental Diagnosis of GBC

It is important to know the best course of action finding a GBC incidentally during laparoscopic cholecystectomy.

This is the most common situation (~ 47%) in which GBC is diagnosed. The surgeon should carefully evaluate signs of invasion or lymph node involvement. Lesions of the gallbladder should not be biopsied for fear of peritoneal seeding or extramural spread. Often preoperative consent for an extended surgery may not have been obtained. If so, then the surgery is finished with a second reoperative procedure after informed consent is obtained. In situations when consent for extended surgery is not fully obtained, or when non-T1a tumors are confirmed postoperatively by pathology, reoperative for extended resection is strongly favored as residual disease is found in 74% of the patients who are reexplored in this situation.

Stage I Disease

Stage I describes node-negative disease wherein the tumor invades the lamina propria only (T1a) or lamina propria and muscular layer of the gallbladder wall (T1b). Several studies have shown that simple cholecystectomy is curative for stage I disease, although there is controversy regarding stage T1b. Recent data have suggested that pT1a and pT1b tumors have a different prognosis after simple cholecystectomy because of the relationship between the depth of invasion and the lymph node status. The probability of lymph node involvement in patients with T1a tumors is almost zero, whereas T1b lesions have a 15% rate of nodal disease. Furthermore, T1b lesions may be more likely to recur due to residual carcinoma in the bed of the gallbladder resulting from microscopic penetration of the muscular layer; recurrence may also be due to unrecognized metastasis to the regional lymph nodes.

For T1a lesions, simple cholecystectomy results in 82-100% five-year survival and extended cholecystectomy is not required. T1b lesions have 15-25% chance of regional lymph node involvement and hence the chance of locoregional recurrence after simple cholecystectomy may be as high as 50-60%. For this reason, T1b lesions are considered to be locally aggressive lesions and hence are best treated with an extended or radical cholecystectomy, along with regional lymph node dissection.

Stage II Disease

Stage II disease encompasses node-negative locally advanced resectable tumors (IIA) and node-positive resectable tumors (IIB). According to Bartlett, et al nodal involvement in the hepatoduodenal region (N1) has a better prognosis than nodal metastasis in the retroperitoneal and celiac nodal basins (N2). The latter is no longer used in the AJCC staging because N2 disease is now considered M1 (metastatic).

Patients with stage II disease are best treated with extended cholecystectomy, because lymph node metastases can be present ~ 45% of T2 lesions and ~ 60% of T3 lesions. For T2 tumors, simple cholecystectomy yields a 5-year survival of ~ 40% which increases to ~ 90% with extended cholecystectomy. Prior laparoscopic port sites must be excised. The goal is to achieve a negative surgical margin. The rate of complications for this procedure can be as high as 50% with a 5% mortality rate. The improvement in cancer outcome justifies the added risk. 5-year survival is about 69% with 3-year survival ranging from 38-80% in various studies. Patients who are reoperated for a more radical resection also benefit in terms of 5-year survival, without a big compromise in complication or mortality rate. Patients with T3N1 disease are best treated with *en bloc* resection of the bile duct to obtain periportal lymph node clearance.

Stage III Disease

Stage III GBC is considered locally advanced disease that is generally beyond surgical treatment (T4, Any N, M0). Patients with T4N0 disease may be surgical candidates, if there is no gross nodal involvement at the time of operation. Right hepatectomy or extended right hepatectomy may be required for curative resection. Patients with nodal metastases beyond the hepatoduodenal ligament have poor prognosis and in general they receive palliative care. The 5-year survival has increased significantly for these patients who now undergo radical resection compared to historical controls.

Special Considerations

There are some situations in which the surgical approach is tailored to maximize tumor as well as nodal clearance. They are described below:

- Lesions in the neck of the gallbladder frequently involve the common bile duct or hepatoduodenal ligament and require bile duct resection and perhaps liver resection.
- Obstructed common hepatic duct requires common bile duct resection and reconstruction along with tumor resection.
- Lesions in the fundus may require liver resection but may not involve the common bile duct and hence common bile duct resection should be performed selectively.
- When adequate nodal dissection of the hepatoduodenal ligament proves to be technically difficult or if gross nodal tissue results in tumorous growth in close proximity to the common hepatic duct, resection and reconstruction of the common bile duct may be required.

Prophylactic Cholecystectomy

NIH consensus guidelines do not recommend prophylactic cholecystectomy for asymptomatic gallstones because the incidence of unsuspected gallbladder carcinoma is low in the United States (1 per 1000 patients per year). Patients from high-risk demographics like Northern Indian women, Mexican, Chileans and patients with pancreaticobiliary malunion may benefit from prophylactic cholecystectomy. At present laparoscopic cholecystectomy is the procedure of choice in type I porcelain gallbladder (complete intramural calcification). For types II and III porcelain gallbladder (incomplete calcification), open cholecystectomy should be considered with concomitant hepatectomy and lymphadenectomy due to the high rate of unsuspected carcinoma.

Indications for cholecystectomy for asymptomatic gallbladder polyps is a solitary polyp > 1.0 cm diameter in a patient older than 50 years because patients older than 50 years with polyps exceeding 1.0 cm have a 4-7% risk of cancer. Lesions < 1 cm diameters undergo follow-up ultrasound every 6-12 months. Suspicious findings (focal thickening of the gallbladder wall) are an indication for further work-up.

Adjuvant Therapy

Both chemotherapy and radiation can be used in adjuvant therapy. Due to the rarity of GBC, there have been no prospective controlled trials looking at adjuvant therapy. However, there is Japanese literature supporting the use of adjuvant chemotherapy alone (mitomycin C + 5FU). However, statistical significance in 5-year survival was reached only in those who received non-curative resection. Adjuvant radiotherapy has also been looked at, either alone or in combination with chemotherapy. It is reasonable to believe that adjuvant radiotherapy alone or in combination with chemotherapy does provide some benefit, most pronounced in > T2 node-positive tumors. The drawbacks with radiotherapy are the adverse effects that stem from the injury of surrounding normal tissues. For this reason, Intraoperative Radiotherapy (IORT) has been tried with a trend toward benefit. The surgeon may also place radiological markers, such as metal clips to aid in more targeted radiation. In some centers, adjuvant chemoradiation is given to patients more commonly than expected.

Kresl, et al evaluated 21 patients with GBC who received curative resection followed by adjuvant multimodal therapy with external beam radiation therapy (EBRT) and 5-fluorouracil at the Mayo Clinic. Patients with completely resected (negative margins) GBC experienced a 5-year survival rate of 64% following 5-FU based RT, compared to a previous report of 33% five-year survival without chemoradiation at Mayo Clinic. Both tumor stage and extent of resection seemed to influence survival and local control.

Another study suggests that radical resection of locally advanced gallbladder carcinoma followed by external-beam radiation therapy with radiosensitizing 5-FU may improve survival. Actuarial 5-year overall survival, disease-free survival, metastases-free survival and local-regional control of 22 patients were 37%, 33%, 36% and 59%, respectively. Median survival for the series was 1.9 years.

Palliative Procedures

Most GBCs invade adjacent organs, extend into the porta hepatis, or metastasize prior to diagnosis. Extensive liver involvement or noncontiguous metastases preclude surgical resection as a reasonable option. Obstructive jaundice is seen in 25-50% of cases. Jaundice degrades quality of life significantly in these patients and causes intractable pruritus, cholangitis and declining liver function that complicates the use of palliative and analgesic medications. As a result, the obstructed biliary tract should be decompressed unless life expectancy is very short or the general condition of the patient is prohibitive.

Self-expanding metal stents (SEMS) are the preferred method of decompression due to less frequent occlusion and migration. SEMS also do not need to be changed as frequently as plastic stents. Placing endoscopic stents can be problematic due to the presence of a hilar mass or stricture of the extrahepatic biliary tree due to tumor invasion. GBC may obstruct the duodenum in 30-50% of patients. For patients with significant life expectancy, laparoscopic gastrojejunostomy or endoscopic placement of a metal enteral stent are excellent choices to relieve duodenal obstruction. If life expectancy is short, symptom relief may be achieved with nasogastric intubation or percutaneous gastrostomy.

Radiation Therapy

Radiation therapy is used as palliative treatment for locally advanced and metastatic cancer (stages III and IV). Multiples clinical trials have been conducted to evaluate radiotherapy alone or in combination with chemotherapy to improve local control and improve survival. Most reports of adjuvant radiotherapy show conflicting results due to the small number of reported series, differences in patient selection, use of different staging systems, varying extent of surgical resection and differences in radiation therapy technique and concomitant chemotherapy regimens.

The benefit of radiotherapy in controlling bone pain, soft tissue metastasis and reduction of gastrointestinal bleeding from a locally advanced primary is minimal with a median survival of only 6-8 months. The treatment field may include the gallbladder fossa, the liver hilum and the celiac lymph node basin and the large planning target volume may precipitate radiotherapy-related adverse events such as nausea, vomiting and anorexia. Clips placed in the gallbladder fossa at the time of resection may help treatment planning. Doses in the range of 45-50 Gray (Gy) (1.8-to 2 Gy fractions) for subclinical disease and 60-65 Gy for microscopically positive margins are probably appropriate, although caution must be exercised because irradiation of the gallbladder fossa can damage large volumes of liver.

Chemotherapy

Chemotherapy has a limited impact on survival of metastatic GBC. Data is further limited by the absence of agents with substantial activity and variations in hospital protocols. Gemcitabine has a single agent objective radiological response rate (ORR) of 15-30% in mixed biliary cancers with good tolerability. The combination gemcitabine/5-fluorouracil has shown modest synergistic activity in several clinical trials with acceptable toxicity. One strategy to reduce toxicity and improve patient benefit is gemcitabine/capecitabine. Capecitabine is active and well tolerated as a single oral agent with ORR of 19% in GBC. Knox, et al reported a phase II trial of 45 chemo-naive patients with pathologically proven, locally advanced or metastatic adenocarcinoma arising from the intra- and extrahepatic bile ducts or gallbladder. The majority of patients presented with liver function abnormalities that stabilized before treatment. Patients received a 3-week chemotherapy cycle with capecitabine at 650 mg/m^2 orally twice a day for 14 days and gemcitabine at a fixed dose of 1,000 mg/m^2 intravenously over 30 minutes on days 1 and 8, all administered every 21 days. The combination of GemCap was well tolerated and showed a response rate of 31%, disease stabilization rate of 42% and a survival time between 8.6 and 19 months.

Another promising combination is gemcitabine-cisplatin. Malik, et al evaluated the efficacy and toxicity of gemcitabine with or without cisplatin in 11 chemo-naive patients with histologically confirmed GBC. All were symptomatic and had stage IV disease. Eight patients received gemcitabine 1000 mg/m^2 on days 1 and 8 along with cisplatin 70 mg/m^2 on day 1. Three received gemcitabine alone. Treatment cycles were repeated every 21 days. One patient (9%) had complete remission of disease and 6 (55%) achieved a partial response to chemotherapy. Median time to progression was 28 weeks and median overall survival was 42 weeks. Toxicity was easily manageable and there were no treatment-related deaths.

Novel Strategies

Oncolytic viral constructs are a promising new approach to GBC. Improving the conditionally replicative adeno-viruses (CRAds) with a tumor-specific promoter (TSP) for GBC enhances the infectivity and neoplastic specificity of the virus and decreases its toxicity. Oncolytic adenoviral therapy has demonstrated a selective killing of GBC cells *in vitro*.

Summary

- GBC is rare, yet the most common cancer of the biliary tree.
- GBC is most commonly diagnosed incidentally during laparoscopic cholecystectomy.
- Large gallstones are a risk factor.
- Old age and male gender are often associated with more aggressive disease and poor outcomes.
- A suspicious or frankly malignant lesion of the gallbladder is not biopsied.
- If GBC is strongly suspected or confirmed, it is recommended to proceed with an open approach, rather than laparoscopic.
- Port site metastases can occur in ~ 20% and hence port-sites should be excised.
- Avoid bile spillage and gallbladder perforation during cholecystectomy for oncological reasons.
- Simple cholecystectomy is curative treatment for T1a lesions.
- It is recommended to perform extended cholecystectomy for T1b lesions.
- There is no hard evidence to guide adjuvant therapy.
- The survival rates of GBC have improved over the years with better hepatic resections and a more aggressive approach.

Landmark Papers

1. Bartlett DL, Fong Y, Fortner JG, et al. Long-term results after resection for GBC. Implications for staging and management. Ann Surg 1996; 224:639-46.
2. Chijiiwa K, Nakano K, Ueda J, et al. Surgical treatment of patients with T2 gallbladder carcinoma invading the subserosal layer. J Am Coll Surg 2001; 192:600-7.
3. Foster JM, Hoshi H, Gibbs JF, et al. GBC: defining the indications for primary radical resection and radical re-resection. Ann Surg Oncol 2007; 14:833-40.
4. Gold DG, Miller RC, Haddock MG, et al. Adjuvant therapy for gallbladder carcinoma: the Mayo Clinic Experience. Int J Radiat Oncol Biol Phys 2009; 75:150-5
5. Jensen EH, Abraham A, Jarosek S, et al. Lymph node evaluation is associated with improved survival after surgery for early stage GBC. Surgery 2009; 146:706-11; discussion 711-3.
6. Otero JC, Proske A, Vallilengua C, et al. GBC: surgical results after cholecystectomy in 25 patients with lamina propria invasion and 26 patients with muscular layer invasion. J Hepatobiliary Pancreat Surg 2006; 13:562-6.
7. Ouchi K, Mikuni J Kakugawa Y. Laparoscopic cholecystectomy for gallbladder carcinoma: results of a Japanese survey of 498 patients. J Hepatobiliary Pancreat Surg 2002; 9:256-60.

8. Pawlik TM, Gleisner AL, Vigano L, et al. Incidence of finding residual disease for incidental gallbladder carcinoma: implications for re-resection. J Gastrointest Surg 2007; 11:1478-86; discussion 1486-7.

9. Wang JD, Liu YB, Quan ZW, et al. Role of regional lymphadenectomy in different stage of gallbladder carcinoma. Hepatogastroenterology 2009; 56:593-6.

10. You DD, Lee HG, Paik KY, et al. What is an adequate extent of resection for T1 GBCs? Ann Surg 2008; 247:835-8.

11. Zielinski MD, Atwell TD, Davis PW, et al. Comparison of surgically resected polypoid lesions of the gallbladder to their pre-operative ultrasound characteristics. J Gastrointest Surg 2009; 13:19-25.

Level of Evidence Table			
Recommendation	**Grade**	**Best level of evidence**	**References**
Laparoscopic resection should not be attempted if GBC is suspected preoperatively. Bile spillage is associated with recurrence and decreased survival.	B	2b	1-3
Prophylactic cholecystectomy should be considered for patients with gallbladder polyps at risk for malignancy: solitary, symptomatic, growth during surveillance, size > 10 mm, patient age > 50 yrs.	B	4	4-6
Radical re-resection for the incidental finding of GBC after cholecystectomy is indicated for ≥ pT2 and cystic duct margin (+) pT1 lesions.	B	2b	7-9
Lymph node involvement and recurrence is also noted in pT1b compared to pT1a lesions and thus should also be considered for re-resection of incidental GBC.	B	2b	10,11
Extended regional lymphadenectomy (beyond the porta hepatis and hepato-duodenal ligament) should be performed only in highly selected circumstances. Else any lymph node involvement carries poor prognosis and additional clearance would not be considered curative.	C	2b	12-14
Adjuvant chemotherapy and/or radiation improves survival.	B	1b	15,16

References

1. Weiland ST, Mahvi DM, Niederhuber JE, et al. Should suspected early GBC be treated laparoscopically? J Gastrointest Surg 2002; 6:50-6; discussion 56-7.

2. Ouchi K, Mikuni J, Kakugawa Y. Laparoscopic cholecystectomy for gallbladder carcinoma: results of a Japanese survey of 498 patients. J Hepatobiliary Pancreat Surg 2002; 9:256-60.

3. Shih SP, Schulick RD, Cameron JL, et al. GBC: the role of laparoscopy and radical resection. Ann Surg 2007; 245:893-901.

4. Mainprize KS, Gould SW, Gilbert JM. Surgical management of polypoid lesions of the gallbladder. Br J Surg 2000; 87:414-7.

5. Zielinski MD, Atwell TD, Davis PW, et al. Comparison of surgically resected polypoid lesions of the gallbladder to their pre-operative ultrasound characteristics. J Gastrointest Surg 2009; 13:19-25.

6. Csendes A, Burgos AM, Csendes P, et al. Late follow-up of polypoid lesions of the gallbladder smaller than 10 mm. Ann Surg 2001; 234:657-60.

7. Pawlik TM, Gleisner AL, Vigano L, et al. Incidence of finding residual disease for incidental gallbladder carcinoma: implications for re-resection. J Gastrointest Surg 2007; 11:1478-86; discussion 1486-7.

8. Foster JM, Hoshi H, Gibbs JF, et al. GBC: defining the indications for primary radical resection and radical re-resection. Ann Surg Oncol 2007; 14:833-40.

9. Chijiiwa K, Nakano K, Ueda J, et al. Surgical treatment of patients with T2 gallbladder carcinoma invading the subserosal layer. J Am Coll Surg 2001; 192:600-7.

10. Otero JC, Proske A, Vallilengua C, et al. GBC: surgical results after cholecystectomy in 25 patients with lamina propria invasion and 26 patients with muscular layer invasion. J Hepatobiliary Pancreat Surg 2006; 13:562-6.

11. You DD, Lee HG, Paik KY, et al. What is an adequate extent of resection for T1 GBCs? Ann Surg 2008; 247:835-8.

12. Wang JD, Liu YB, Quan ZW, et al. Role of regional lymphadenectomy in different stage of gallbladder carcinoma. Hepatogastroenterology 2009; 56:593-6.

13. Bartlett DL, Fong Y, Fortner JG, et al. Long-term results after resection for GBC. Implications for staging and management. Ann Surg 1996; 224:639-46.

14. Jensen EH, Abraham A, Jarosek S, et al. Lymph node evaluation is associated with improved survival after surgery for early stage GBC. Surgery 2009; 146:706-11; discussion 711-3.

15. Gold DG, Miller RC, Haddock MG, et al. Adjuvant therapy for gallbladder carcinoma: the Mayo Clinic Experience. Int J Radiat Oncol Biol Phys 2009; 75:150-5.

16. Takada T, Amano H, Yasuda H, et al. Is postoperative adjuvant chemotherapy useful for gallbladder carcinoma? A phase III multicenter prospective randomized controlled trial in patients with resected pancreaticobiliary carcinoma. Cancer 2002; 95:1685-95.

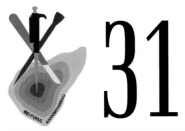

31

Bile Duct Cancer

Mario Lora, Isam W Nasr, Narcis Octavian Zarnescu, A James Moser

Cholangiocarcinoma (CCA) is cancer of the bile duct epithelium and can arise anywhere from the periphery of the liver to the intrapancreatic segment of the common bile duct. These tumors spread along the biliary tree and directly invade adjacent portal structures. The anatomic structures involved by bile duct cancers often require complex surgical procedures to clear the resection margin and reconstruct the biliary tree. Metastatic spread to the liver and peritoneum is less frequent compared to gallbladder tumors. Involvement of cystic, hilar and celiac lymph nodes is found in 30-50% of patients at the time of diagnosis, while 30% have distant metastases. The rarity of bile duct cancers has impeded randomized clinical trials to evaluate chemotherapy and radiation options for patients with advanced or recurrent disease. The prognosis and rates of curative resection for bile duct cancer are highly dependent on the location of the tumor in the biliary tree.

Epidemiology

Incidence and Risk Factors

CCA is a rare malignancy, accounting for ~ 2-3% of all GI malignancies. CCA is the second most common primary liver cancer after hepatocellular carcinoma. The incidence of CCA is highest between the sixth and the seventh decades and affects men 1.5 times more often than women. In the United States, the incidence of hilar CCA is 1/100,000 per year. The prevalence of intrahepatic CCA is highest among Hispanics in the United States (1.22 per 100,000 population) and lowest among African Americans (0.3 per 100,000 population). Other countries experience significantly higher incidence such as Thailand (96/ 100,000), Israel (7.2/100,000) and Japan (5.5/100,000). The incidence of intrahepatic CCA has been increasing worldwide at an estimated annual rate of 9.11% over the last two decades, whereas the incidence of extrahepatic CCA has declined throughout the world. One potential cause of the shift in incidence is misclassification of hilar CCA as intrahepatic CCA.

Although an established risk factor can be found in only 10% of patients with CCA in the United States, risk factors associated with an increased risk of CCA are:

Risk Factors
- Primary sclerosing cholangitis
- Choledochal cysts and Caroli's disease
- Parasitic infestations (liver fluke)
- Hepatolithiasis (very rare in western populations)
- HNPCC
- Smoking
- Alcohol
- Obesity
- Chronic inflammation of the liver
- Thorotrast (not in use now)

- *Primary sclerosing cholangitis (PSC)* is an autoimmune cholestatic liver disease that is strongly associated with ulcerative colitis. Patients with PSC have a relative risk (RR) of 1506 for developing CCA, which usually occurs at a young age (30-50 years). The incidence of CCA among PSC patients ranges from 0.6% to 1.5% per year with a cumulative lifetime risk of 5-15%. The outcomes of CCA resection in PSC patients is particularly dismal.
- *Choledochal cyst* is a congenital cystic dilatation of the bile duct associated with chronic inflammation and bile stasis. Choledochal cysts are more common in women and in the Japanese population. Ten to twenty percent of patients with choledochal cysts eventually develop CCA. Children less than 10 years of age have a 0.7% risk whereas patients older than 20 years have a 20% risk. Presence of widespread intrahepatic choledochal cysts is called *Caroli's disease* which is present in 11-14% of the CCA.
- *Liver fluke infestation* by *Opisthorchis viverrini* and *Clonorchis sinensis* (less frequent). The resulting incidence of CCA related to fluke infestation is 89.2/ 100,000 among men and 35.5/100,000 among women in Southeast Asia and China. These organisms may be ingested with raw uncooked seafood that may inhabit and induce a chronic inflammatory state in the proximal biliary tree, presumably leading to malignant transformation.

- *Pancreaticobiliary maljunction* produces chronic inflammation in the biliary tree due to the reflux of pancreatic secretions. The risk of cancer increases with age; patients between the ages of 20-49 years have an 11% risk, while patients over the age of 50 years have a 17% risk of developing CCA.
- *Hepatolithiasis and choledocholithiasis* have been shown in multiple epidemiological studies to increase the risk of developing CCA. The risk varies by geographic location, where the highest correlation appears to be in Taiwan.
- *Carcinogens,* such as Thorotrast (thorium dioxide), is a radiologic contrast agent used from 1930 to 1960, may cause CCA after a latent period of 16-45 years.
- *Lifestyle and body habitus*: Smoking and alcohol consumption are believed to risk factors. Smoking is found to be a risk factor in the PSC population as well. Obesity and diabetes have also been linked to CCA. Cigarette smoking may increase the risk of CCA, in addition to radionuclides, radon, nitrosamines, dioxin and asbestos.
- Miscellaneous risk factors include hereditary nonpolyposis colorectal cancer (HNPCC/Lynch syndrome), biliary papillomatosis, hepatitis B virus (HBV) and hepatitis C virus (HCV) infections, non-viral chronic liver disease, diabetes, obesity (linked to extrahepatic CCA) and human immunodeficiency virus (HIV) infection.

Classification of CCA

CCA are traditionally classified as extrahepatic and intrahepatic. Intrahepatic tumors arising in small ductules are called 'peripheral CCA'. Intrahepatic tumors may further be classified as either mass forming (MT) type, infiltrating ductal type or intraductal type. Extrahepatic CCA were classified into proximal, middle and distal tumors. Proximal tumors are hilar or perihilar tumors which often require liver resection. Distal tumors arise in the intraduodenal segment and are classically treated with pancreaticoduodenectomy. Middle tumors arise between the cystic duct entrance into the common bile duct and the duodenum and are treated with bile duct resection or pancreatoduodenectomy depending upon the anatomical configuration of the tumor.

- Intrahepatic (6%)
- Perihilar (67%)—includes tumors that involve the confluence of the ducts (Klatskin tumors)
- Distal (27%)

The extrahepatic biliary tree is thus divided into two: the perihilar or proximal duct and the distal duct, the transition being the point where the CBD passes posterior to the duodenum. Extrahepatic CCAs may be classified based on their morphology as nodular, scirrhous and papillary. Scirrhous variety, otherwise called the 'sclerosing' type due to the prominent desmoplastic reaction that it often brings with it, is the most common type of CCA. Nodular type is characterized by a circumferential or annular lesion that results in stenosis of the duct. The papillary type is a intraluminal mass-producing variety. The latter produces obstruction and jaundice early during the disease course, thereby resulting in better resection rates and outcomes. Unfortunately, this is a rare type. The other two types are more aggressive, and present late resulting in dismal outcomes. The remainder (< 5%) of bile duct cancers are sarcomas, squamous cell carcinomas, lymphomas and small cell carcinoma.

Molecular Biology and Genetics of CCA

The common molecular pathway for the malignant transformation of bile duct epithelium is chronic inflammation. This process is mediated by release of cytokines like TNF-alpha, hepatocyte growth factors (HGH), interleukin 6 (IL-6) and reactive oxygen species that increase production of nitric oxide (NO). Nitric oxide interferes with DNA repair and inhibits apoptosis.

Additional mechanisms for malignant transformation include a point mutation in p16INK4 among patients with PSC. Loss of heterozygosity (LOH) in chromosomes 4q and 6q (highest frequency) are also found in intrahepatic CCAs as well as hepatocellular carcinoma. Other mutated oncogenes associated with CCA are c-myc, c-neu, c-erbB-2 and c-met, while tumor suppressor genes are p53 and SMAD4.

Clinical Presentation

CCA is asymptomatic in its earliest stages. Symptoms typically arise due to obstruction of the bile duct with resulting cholestasis or pain caused by an enlarging mass. The most common symptoms are: painless jaundice due to malignant obstruction (70-90% of patients), pruritis (66%), abdominal pain, malaise, fatigue, weight loss (30-50%) and fever (20%). Pruritis along with jaundice is often the presenting symptom in extrahepatic tumors, while abdominal pain is the common presenting symptom in intrahepatic tumors.

Physical exam findings include a palpably enlarged liver as well as a dilated gallbladder (Courvoisier's sign). Cholangitis may result from bile duct obstruction with infection by biliary flora such as *E. coli*, *Klebsiella*, *Proteus*, *P. aeruginosa*, *Serratia*, *Streptococcus* and *Enterobacter*.

Diagnosis

The differential diagnosis of CCA includes other benign causes of biliary obstruction such as, sclerosing disorders, choledocholithiasis, etc. Up to 30% of those suspected to have CCA based on their presentation or imaging may have other benign obstructive disorders or metastatic lesions.

Diagnostic Investigations
- Ultrasound
- ERCP, MRCP
- Cholangiography
- CT scan, MRI, PET
- Spyglass
- Serum tumor markers (not of much use)

- *Ultrasonography:* Right upper quadrant ultrasound is the first diagnostic modality used to evaluate jaundiced patients. In a series of 429 patients with obstructive jaundice, ultrasound detected the cause in 94% and displayed 96% specificity for a surgical etiology. US findings associated with CCA include: segmental dilatation and nonunion of the right and left hepatic ducts, polypoid intraluminal masses and discrete strictures with associated mural thickening.

- *Serum biochemistry:* Liver function tests generally reveal evidence of cholestasis such as elevated bilirubin, alkaline phosphatase and gamma glutamyltransferase. In the absence of cholangitis, serum aminotransferase levels may be normal or only mildly elevated. Increased prothrombin time (PT) is caused by prolonged bile duct obstruction which consequently leads to decreased absorption of fat soluble vitamins (A, D, E, K). Markers, 5'-nucleotidase and GGT confirm that the elevated ALP are from hepatic origin.

- *Serum tumors markers:* Serum tumors markers like carcinoembryonic (CEA) and CA19-9 may be elevated in bile duct cancer but lack sensitivity and specificity. For example, CA 19-9 is a carbohydrate cell-surface antigen related to the Lewis blood group antigens. Ten percent of the population does not express this antigen and will not manifest elevated Ca19-9 in the presence of biliary obstruction. Serum Ca 19-9 $\geq$ 100 had 65.7% sensitivity and 88% specificity for detecting CCA. Elevations of both CA 19-9 and CEA have a 62.3% sensitivity and an 87% specificity. Benign pathologies of the biliary tract such as cholangitis, hepatolithiasis and viral hepatitis may increase serum tumor markers. PSC often elevates serum CEA and CA 19-9 making the distinction between PSC and CCA difficult. The combination of a positive brush cytology and an abnormal CA 19-9 in patients with PSC has a sensitivity and specificity of 87.5% and 97.3%, respectively, for detecting bile duct cancer. These tests should be repeated after the acute inflammatory process has resolved.

- *CT scan:* Helical computed tomography provides optimal evaluation of the bile duct when 1-2.5 mm

images are obtained through the liver and head of the pancreas in the arterial and venous phases of dynamic contrast administration. These tumors usually appear as a thin mass with rim-like enhancement at the periphery and amorphous areas of slightly high attenuation during the arterial and portal venous phases. Findings depend on the location of the tumor and include CT scan may demonstrate thickening of the bile duct wall, biliary dilation proximal to the abnormality, enlarged lymph nodes, invasion of the liver parenchyma and vascular involvement or encasement. High-resolution CT scan predicts resectability with 94% sensitivity, 79% specificity, as well as negative and positive predictive values of 92% and 85%, respectively.

- *MRI:* Magnetic resonance cholangiopancreatography (MRCP) provides noninvasive assessment of the entire biliary tree, including the surgical anatomy, extent of bile duct involvement, vascular invasion, malignant adenopathy and distant metastases. MRCP has a sensitivity of 86% and specificity of 98%. CCAs appear less intense than surrounding structures on T1-weighted images and more intense on T2-weighted images. During dynamic MR imaging, CCAs show moderate peripheral enhancement followed by progressive and concentric filling with contrast material. Pooling of contrast within the tumor on delayed MR images is suggestive of peripheral CCA. Hilar CCAs demonstrate moderate irregular thickening of the bile duct wall ($\geq$ 5 mm) with symmetric upstream dilation of the intrahepatic ducts.

- *Cholangiography:* Dilatation of the bile duct requires further investigation of the biliary anatomy. Invasive methods permit biopsies of the bile duct wall as well as decompression of obstructed segments. Methods include endoscopic retrograde cholangiopancreatography (ERCP) or percutaneous transhepatic cholangiography (PTC). Findings suggestive of malignancy in a bile duct stricture include irregular borders, length more than 10 mm and shouldering (abrupt transition from normal duct to stricture). Biopsies of such lesions should routinely be obtained. ERCP brush cytology has a specificity of nearly 100%; however, the sensitivity is much lower and ranges 18-60%. This poor sensitivity is due to the acellular nature of these tumors. Cytologic evaluation is particularly difficult in patients with PSC due to the reactive changes and inflammation. A combination of biliary cytology and CA 19-9 levels should be performed.

- *Positron emission tomography (PET):* Preoperative PET identifies primary bile duct tumors with 80% sensitivity but has its primary utility in detecting metastatic disease. Anderson, et al found the sensitivity of PET to be 85% for nodular morphology compared to 18% for the infiltrating type, while sensitivity for metastatic disease was 65%. Increased FDG uptake is also observed in intrahepatic CCAs with the exception of the hilar type. In some studies, PET scan has proven to be very promising and is being increasingly used. There has not been enough evidence to recommend the routine use of PET scan.

- *Endoscopic ultrasound (EUS):* In the case of extrahepatic tumors, EUS is a useful alternative to ERCP than can detect lesions larger than 3 mm in the distal bile duct and guide fine-needle aspirates. EUS visualizes hilar, celiac and para-aortic lymphadenopathy and can identify local and distant metastases. Fine-needle aspiration of enlarged lymph nodes is the most accurate way to diagnose and stage CCA. In addition, EUS can evaluate the pancreas for other causes of biliary strictures such as pancreatic masses or changes of chronic pancreatitis. This procedure has 85% sensitivity, a nearly 100% specificity and 88% accuracy.
- *SpyGlass:* The SpyGlass system is a newly introduced single-operator cholangioscope that permits simultaneous duodenoscopy and cholangioscopy. Spyglass demonstrates superior maneuverability and is capable of obtaining four quadrant biopsies in the tertiary intrahepatic ducts. SpyGlass has a 100% success rates in obtaining targeted biopsies compared to 50% with conventional choledochoduodenoscopes.

Staging

CCA has been classified for the purpose of prognostic staging in several different ways, each of them serving a different purpose **(Table 31-1)**.

The Bismuth-Corlette classification **(Figure 31-1)** is for perihilar tumors only. It is divided into 4 types:
- Type I—involves the confluence of the hepatic ducts, without involving the roof; in other words, they are mid-common hepatic duct lesions
- Type II—involves the confluence of hepatic ducts, including the roof

- Type III—involves the confluence (or main hepatic duct) and one of the main hepatic ducts. Type IIIa and IIIb are used to differentiate right and left hepatic duct involvement respectively
- Type IV—involves the confluence (or main hepatic duct) and both hepatic ducts (or multifocal duct) involvement.

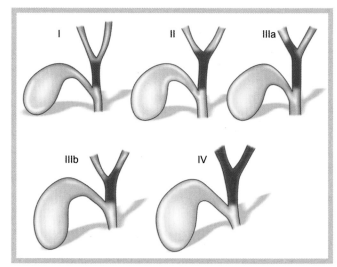

Figure 31-1: Bismuth-Corlette classification of perihilar tumors

This Bismuth-Corlette system is not a typical staging classification as it does not include lymph nodal involvement or degree of local invasion. The AJCC classification can therefore be used for prognostic purposes. The AJCC classification is different for extrahepatic tumors and intrahepatic CCA **(Table 31-2)**.

The AJCC classification of intrahepatic tumors also includes a Fibrosis score, defined by Ishak in 1995. None to moderate fibrosis is scored as F0 and severe fibrosis or cirrhosis is scored as F1. This score has an impact on prognosis and hence integrated into staging.

TABLE 31-1	Classification of CCA
Staging Classification	**Comments**
Bismuth-Corlette classification	For perihilar tumors only. Classifies tumors based on the presence of tumors on the 'roof' of the confluence. Provides good guidance for planning surgery. Does not have much prognostic significance
AJCC staging for extrahepatic tumors	Uses the TNM. Has prognostic importance. However, does not provide much information on resectability
AJCC staging for intrahepatic tumors	Uses the TNM. Has prognostic importance. Very closely mirrors the AJCC staging for hepatocellular carcinomas
Jarnagin-Blumgart tumor stage criteria	This is exclusively a tumor staging criteria and helps predict resectability, metastasis and even survival.

TABLE 31-2	AJCC classification of intrahepatic and extrahepatic CCA		
AJCC classification of Extrahepatic CCA			
Primary tumor (T)			
TX	Primary tumor cannot be assessed		
T0	No evidence of primary tumor		
Tis	Carcinoma in situ		
T1	Tumor confined to the bile duct histologically		
T2	Tumor invades beyond the wall of the bile duct		
T3	Tumor invades the liver, gallbladder, pancreas and /or unilateral branches of the portal vein (right or left) or hepatic artery (right or left)		
T4	Tumor invades any of the following: main portal vein or its branches bilaterally, common hepatic artery, or other adjacent structures such as the colon, stomach, duodenum, or abdominal wall.		
Regional lymph nodes (N)			
NX	Regional lymph nodes cannot be assessed		
N0	No regional lymph node metastasis		
N1	Regional lymph node metastasis		
Distant metastasis (M)			
MX	Distant metastasis cannot be assessed		
M0	No distant metastasis		
M1	Distant metastasis		
Stage Grouping			
Stage 0	Tis	N0	M0
Stage IA	T1	N0	M0
Stage IB	T2	N0	M0
Stage IIA	T3	N0	M0
Stage IIB	T1-3	N1	M0
Stage III	T4	Any N	M0
Stage IV	Any T	Any N	M1
AJCC Classification of Intrahepatic CCA			
Primary tumor (T)			
TX	Primary tumor cannot be assessed		
T0	No evidence of primary tumor		
T1	Solitary tumor without vascular invasion		
T2	Solitary tumor with vascular invasion or multiple tumors none > 5 cm		
T3	Multiple tumors > 5 cm or tumor involving major branch of portal or hepatic vein(s)		
T4	Tumors with direct invasion of adjacent organs other than gallbladder or with perforation of visceral peritoneum		
Regional lymph nodes (N)			
NX	Regional lymph nodes cannot be assessed		
N0	No regional lymph node metastasis		
N1	Regional lymph node metastasis (hilar, celiac, periduodenal, peripancreatic, SMA nodes)		
Distant metastasis (M)			
MX	Distant metastasis cannot be assessed		
M0	No distant metastasis		
M1	Distant metastasis		

Contd...

Stage Grouping			
Stage IA	T1	N0	M0
Stage II	T2	N0	M0
Stage IIIA	T3	N0	M0
Stage IIIB	T4	N0	M0
Stage IIIC	Any T	N1	M0
Stage IV	Any T	Any N	M1

Reproduced with permission from AJCC Staging Manual, 6th Edition

The Jarnagin-Blumgart classification is a tumor-only staging system that reflects resectability.

Stage	Description
T1	Tumor involving biliary confluence with/without unilateral extension to second-order biliary radicles
T2	Tumor involving biliary confluence with/without unilateral extension to second-order biliary radicles **AND** *Ipsilateral* portal vein involvement with/without *ipsilateral* hepatic lobar atrophy
T3	Tumor involving biliary confluence + bilateral extension to second-order biliary radicles **OR** Unilateral extension to second-order biliary radicles with *contralateral* portal vein involvement **OR** Unilateral extension to second-order biliary radicles with *contralateral* hepatic lobar atrophy **OR** Main or bilateral portal venous involvement

Surgical Management

Complete surgical resection offers the only possibility of long-term survival for patients with bile duct cancer. The principal objective of surgical treatment is to achieve a disease-free margin of resection, a goal monitored intra-operatively with serial frozen section biopsies. Given the potential for involvement of the intrahepatic ducts, hepatectomy is often required in addition to bile duct resection and reconstruction. In one study, surgical resection increased overall survival from an average of 10-35 months.

Surgical Anatomy

The extrahepatic biliary tree consists of the right and left hepatic ducts, the common hepatic duct, the cystic duct and the gallbladder. The bifurcation of the left and right main hepatic ducts is extrahepatic and lies anterior to the portal vein bifurcation. The left main hepatic duct is formed by ducts draining the left lobe of the liver

(segments II, III and IV) and lies horizontally at the base of the falciform ligament. The extrahepatic course of the left duct is 1-5 cm longer than the right hepatic duct. The right hepatic duct is formed by the confluence of hepatic segments V and VIII (anterior) and segments VI and VII (posterior). The common bile duct measures 7 to 11 cm in length and is divided into three anatomic segments: proximal, mid and distal (including the intraduodenal portion). The blood supply of the distal common bile duct arises from the gastroduodenal, retroduodenal and pancreaticoduodenal arteries, whereas the right hepatic and cystic arteries supply the proximal bile ducts. The intrinsic nutrient vessels of the bile duct run along the medial and lateral walls of the common bile and common hepatic ducts in a 3 and 9 o'clock orientation. Venous effluent from the hepatic and proximal common bile ducts drains directly to the liver. The lymphatic drainage of the hepatic ducts and the distal portion of the common bile duct goes to lymph nodes in the porta hepatis. The inferior portion of the common bile duct drains into peripancreatic lymph nodes. Ultimately, all lymphatic drainage reaches the celiac nodes **(Figure 31-2)**.

Assessment of Resectability

Assessing resectability is the primary goal of preoperative staging. Because the AJCC staging system does not define resectability, the Jarnagin-Blumgart system of classifying tumors was devised to assess the potential for resecting hilar CCAs. This system classifies tumors according to their extent and location within the biliary tree, presence of portal venous invasion and presence or absence of hepatic lobar atrophy.

The following precludes resectability
- involvement of left and right hepatic ducts up to secondary branches
- encasement or occlusion of the portal vein proximal to its bifurcation
- atrophy of one liver lobe with encasement of the contralateral portal vein
- involvement of right and left hepatic arteries

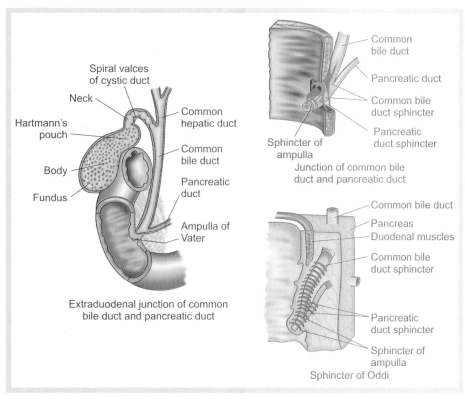

Figure 31-2: Bile duct anatomy

- atrophy of one liver lobe with involvement of the contralateral bile duct up to the secondary branches
- histologically verified metastasis to N2 nodes

Involvement of the ipsilateral portal vein and secondary bile duct branches does not prohibit resection. Ipsilateral lobar atrophy, metastases to cystic duct, pericholedochal and perilymph nodes do not necessarily preclude resection.

Preoperative Biliary Decompression

Patients with CCA may present with hyperbilirubinemia and pruritis. It has been a matter of controversy whether or not to drain the obstructed liver preoperatively. The decision is ofter institution-dependent. In most cases, the liver is not routinely drained due to the risk of cholangitis with stents. The authors recommend draining the liver only when serum bilirubin is >15 mg/dl and for symptomatic relief when scheduling considerations delay definitive surgery or hepatic reserve is in question. The preoperative placements of stents impairs intraoperative assessment of the tumor and may increase the perioperative infection rate.

Clear indications for preoperative drainage include cholangitis and drainage of the future remnant liver in those considered for extended hepatectomy.

Portal Vein Embolization (PVE)

Selective occlusion of blood flow to a part of the liver promotes hypertrophy of the contralateral side. This concept is exploited in the setting when the Future Liver Remnant (FLR) is less than 25%. Transhepatic percutaneous portal vein embolization is typically reserved for patients whose calculated future liver remnants are too small to permit resection or for patients with preexisting cirrhosis. PVE also assists in achieving negative surgical margins for the same reasons.

Diagnostic Staging Laparoscopy

Nearly one-third of patients considered for resection of CCA has unrecognized metastatic disease. These patients are not accurately staged by preoperative imaging. Hence it is prudent to routinely perform diagnostic laparoscopies on CCA patients at the same setting as the intended resection.

Intrahepatic Cholangiocarcinoma

Intrahepatic CCA usually requires anatomically based hepatic resection to remove all liver parenchyma at risk for intrahepatic metastases. R0 (no residual disease) resection may be achieved in only 45% of cases. The prognosis of patients with intrahepatic CCA varies according to the macroscopic tumor type: mass-forming, periductal-infiltrating, mass-forming plus periductal-infiltrating and intraductal. One study found that the mortality of mass-forming and periductal-infiltrating tumors is higher due to an increased frequency of perineural invasion and lymphatic spread as well as a higher incidence of positive surgical margins. Median survival after resection ranges from 15 months up to 80 months and 5-year survival rates may vary between 13% to 63%.

Extrahepatic Perihilar Cholangiocarcinoma

Perihilar tumors involve the hepatic duct proximal to the origin of the cystic duct. These tumors involve a significant intrahepatic component as well as the hepatic duct bifurcation (Klatskin tumors). The standard surgical approach for extrahepatic CCA depends on the Bismuth-Corlette classification.

- For Bismuth types I and II, the procedure of choice is *en bloc* resection of the extrahepatic bile ducts and gallbladder with a 5-10 mm bile duct margin, along with portal lymphadenectomy and Roux-en-Y hepaticojejunostomy.
- Bismuth type III lesions requires complete resection of the extrahepatic bile ducts and gallbladder, with portal lymphadenectomy plus partial hepatectomy (right or left) and Roux-en Y hepaticojejunostomy **(Figure 31-3)**.
- Bismuth type IV lesions may be excised with palliative intent and require all of the above procedures plus extended right or left hepatectomy. Some would consider patients in this group to be candidates for liver transplantation.

Recent data suggest that portal vein resection should be performed if the tumor involves any level of this vessel (T2-T3 Blumgart stage). Routine caudate lobectomy (segment I) is advocated for all tumors involving the left

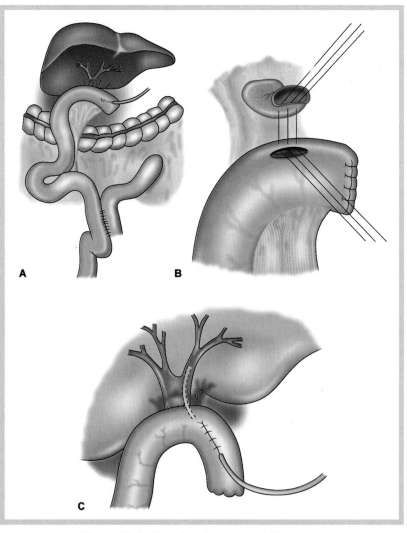

Figure 31-3: Hepaticojejunostomy—Roux-en-y

hepatic duct and for cases in which resection of the caudate is likely to clear the surgical margin.

The median survival time for patients with resected extrahepatic perihilar CCA is 30 months and the 5-year survival rate is ~ 30%. The most common site for recurrence is the resection bed followed by the retroperitoneal lymph nodes. Distant metastases to the lung and the mediastinum may occur in approximately one-third of cases.

Extrahepatic Distal Cholangiocarcinoma

These lesions involve the distal extrahepatic and intrapancreatic portions of the bile duct. Treatment usually requires pancreaticoduodenectomy (Whipple procedure). Small lesions distal to the cystic duct may be amenable to resection of the extrahepatic biliary tree with portal lymphadenectomy and Roux-en-Y reconstruction. Median survival is between 18-33 months and expected 5-year survival is 14-40%. For extensive involvement of the extrahepatic bile duct without distant spread, *en bloc* hepatic and pancreatic resection may be required.

The summary of surgical options in CCA are summarized in the **Table 31-3.** It is to be noted that portal vein resection may be included in the resection of perihilar tumors as seen fit. Orthotopic Liver Transplantation (OLT) is discussed separately.

Liver Transplantation

OLT has a theoretical advantage for non-metastatic intrahepatic and perihilar CCA. However, it is not the standard treatment option for CCA. OLT for CCA offers a 5-year survival of ~20% which is far less than the 5-year survival of hepatitis C patients receiving OLT (~65%). In the face of increasing demand for organs, CCA may not qualify as the most qualified indication for a liver. Furthermore, recurrence is found in ~50% of the patients in a span of 2-3 years, especially in those having PSC. Adjuvant and neoadjuvant therapy with OLT does not

seem to improve survival rates either. Currently, CCA patients receive the same MELD score scoring system for evaluation for OLT. There has been new proposals for considering exceptions.

Multimodality Therapy

There is sparse data concerning the efficacy of radiotherapy or chemotherapy for CCA. The survival benefit of postoperative radiation therapy may be limited to patients with local extension of tumor into the liver parenchyma and microscopic residual disease following resection. Chemotherapy has not been shown to affect outcome in either resected or unresected CCA. Gemcitabine and 5-FU have a radio-sensitizing effect, suggesting that the combination of both chemo- and radiotherapy may have a more pronounced effect on survival than either agent alone.

Radiotherapy

The purpose of external beam radiation therapy (EBRT) is to reduce the risk of locoregional recurrence following resection. EBRT has also been used to palliate pain from bony metastases and to stop bleeding from locally advanced tumors. Candidates for EBRT include:
- inoperable disease (stage IV);
- recurrence after resection and a residual lesion after resection.

Intraluminal brachytherapy (ILBT) is an option for patients with extrahepatic CCAs and is usually delivered via self-expanding metallic stents, inserted either endoscopically or percutaneously. Data comparing the efficacy of EBRT alone to EBRT plus intraluminal beam brachytherapy for patients with unresectable CCA showed no differences in locoregional recurrence rates, although there was an increase in the median time to progression for patients that received the combination approach.

TABLE 31-3	Surgical options in CCA		
Tumor	**Stage**	**Surgery**	**5-year survival**
Intrahepatic CCA	Stage I, II	Hepatic resection	15-63%
Perihilar CCA	Bismuth type I, II Blumgart stage I	Extrahepatic bile duct resection + complete lymphadenectomy, Roux-en-Y hepaticojejunostomy	10-35%
Perihilar CCA	Bismuth type III Blumgart type II	Extrahepatic bile duct resection + complete lymphadenectomy, Roux-en-Y hepaticojejunostomy with partial hepatectomy	
Perihilar CCA	Bismuth type IV Blumgart type III	Extrahepatic bile duct resection + complete lymphadenectomy, Roux-en-Y hepaticojejunostomy with extended hepatectomy	
Distal CCA		Whipple procedure	14 - 40%

Chemotherapy

Data regarding response rates of CCA to chemotherapy are difficult to evaluate given the rarity of this tumor as well as the non-homogenous inclusion criteria among various clinical trials. According to the new Japanese guidelines for bile duct and ampullary cancer, the indications for chemotherapy include:

- Metastatic and locally advanced disease (stage III).
- Recurrences after resection.
- Patients with a good general condition performance (status 2 or 3).

A recent phase II trial evaluated the efficacy and safety of gemcitabine as single agent therapy for 23 patients with unresectable bile duct (15) and gallbladder (8) cancers. Patients received gemcitabine once a week for 2 weeks followed by a week off therapy. A total of 110 cycles of chemotherapy were given with a median of four cycles (range 1-10). Median follow-up was 13.4 months. 26.1% of patients had a partial response, while 34.8% had stable disease and 39.1% experienced disease progression despite treatment. The overall response rate was 26.1% [95% confidence interval (CI) 22.1-30.1%]. Median time to disease progression was 8.1 months (95% CI 3.3-12.9 months) and the median overall survival was 13.1 months (95% CI 1.6-24.6 months). Another phase II trial enrolled 45 patients with locally advanced or metastatic biliary tract cancer. Patients were treated with combination gemcitabine and capecitabine for a 3-week cycle. The overall objective response rate was 31%; 42% of patients had stable disease for a disease control rate of 73%. Median overall survival was 14 months and median progression-free survival was 7 months (95% CI, 4.6-11.8 months).

Palliative Care

The major goal of palliation is to drain the obstructed biliary system adequately to relieve bile salt pruritis, prevent cholangitis and delay the complications of liver failure. Bile duct drainage can surgically be achieved by bypassing the obstructing lesion or by using ERCP stents. Self-expanding metal stents are preferred over plastic stents for patients with a life expectancy greater than 6 months and/or unresectable disease given their improved patency rates and lower migration rate. Surgical bypass should be considered when percutaneous or endoscopic stenting is unsuccessful; or if the tumor is found to be unresectable at the time of surgical exploration for cure.

Photodynamic Therapy

Photodynamic therapy (PDT) uses a photosensitizing drug (photofrin) to produce oxygen free-radicals in tumor cells exposed directly to laser light. PDT is a local therapy used alongside a biliary endoprosthesis to reverse the occlusion of a stent by the growing tumor. PDT has been shown to improve the quality of life of patients with bile duct cancer. In one study, 23 patients with unresectable bile duct cancer were treated with PDT and a biliary endoprosthesis. The survival rate at 6 months was 91% after diagnosis and 74% after the initiation of PDT. The median rate of local tumor response was 74%, 54%, 29% and 67% after the first, second, third, fourth and fifth PDT treatment. Time to progression ranged from 3-8 months. One study was closed early as PDT patients fared much better than the non-treated group.

Management Overview

- CCA is a rare tumor, but the incidence is increasing worldwide.
- PSC is an important risk factor for CCA, with poor outcomes.
- The mainstay of therapy is surgery, although up to 30% of the patients considered resectable may have intraoperative findings that preclude resection.
- Bismuth-Corlette classification and Blumgart T-staging criteria are often used to assess surgical resectability.
- Preoperative biliary drainage of obstructed patients are recommended with serum bilirubin levels > 15 mg/dl.
- Portal vein embolization is recommended when the FLR is less than 25%.
- Portal vein resection may be performed in select cases.
- OLT is currently not considered a standard option for CCA.
- Metallic stents provide more durable palliation than plastic stents.
- PDT is a very useful option in the palliative setting.

Landmark Papers

1. Jarnagin WR, Fong Y, DeMatteo RP, et al. Staging, resectability and outcome in 225 patients with hilar cholangiocarcinoma. Ann Surg 2001; 234:507-17; discussion 517-9.
2. Kosuge T, Yamamoto J, Shimada K, et al. Improved surgical results for hilar cholangiocarcinoma with procedures including major hepatic resection. Ann Surg 1999; 230:663-71.
3. Konstadoulakis MM, Roayaie S, Gomatos IP, et al. Aggressive surgical resection for hilar cholangiocarcinoma: is it justified? Audit of a single center's experience. Am J Surg 2008; 196:160-9.
4. Ito F, Agni R, Rettammel RJ, et al. Resection of hilar cholangiocarcinoma: concomitant liver resection decreases hepatic recurrence. In Hochwald SN, Burke EC, Jarnagin WR, et al. Association of preoperative biliary stenting with increased postoperative infectious complications in proximal cholangiocarcinoma. Arch Surg 1999; 134:261-6.
5. Cherqui D, Benoist S, Malassagne B, et al. Major liver resection for carcinoma in jaundiced patients without preoperative biliary drainage. Arch Surg 2000; 135:302-8.

6. Ferrero A, Lo Tesoriere R, Vigano L, et al. Preoperative biliary drainage increases infectious complications after hepatectomy for proximal bile duct tumor obstruction. World J Surg 2009; 33:318-25.
7. Sewnath ME, Karsten TM, Prins MH, et al. A meta-analysis on the efficacy of preoperative biliary drainage for tumors causing obstructive jaundice. Ann Surg 2002; 236: 17-27.
8. Wang Q, Gurusamy KS, Lin H, et al. Preoperative biliary drainage for obstructive jaundice. Cochrane Database Syst Rev 2008; CD005444.
9. Laurent A, Tayar C, Cherqui D. Cholangiocarcinoma: preoperative biliary drainage (Con). HPB (Oxford) 2008; 10:126-9.
10. Nimura Y. Preoperative biliary drainage before resection for cholangiocarcinoma (Pro). HPB (Oxford) 2008; 10:130-3.

Level of Evidence Table

Recommendation	Grade	Best level of evidence	References
Aggressive surgical resection of hilar cholangiocarcinoma including major hepatectomy offers the best chance for cure and long-term survival	B	2b	1-4
Liver transplantation for unresectable cholangiocarcinoma is rarely considered, and only for highly selected patients	C	4	5-8
Transarterial chemoembolization (TACE) is safe and may prolong survival in unresectable intrahepatic cholangiocarcinoma	B	4	9, 10
Palliative stenting and photodynamic therapy is safe and more effective than stenting alone for unresectable hilar cholangiocarcinoma . The role of PDT in relation to systemic chemotherapy is unknown/unstudied	A	1b	11-17
The timing and roles of chemotherapy and/or radiation in resectable cholangiocarcinoma are unclear	C	2b	18-21
Routine preoperative drainage for resectable cholangiocarcinoma is not indicated (greater infectious complications). Selective drainage in the setting of severe malnutrition, cholangitis, long-standing or severe jaundice, need for portal vein embolization and operative planning is reasonable	A	1a	22-28
Unilateral stenting of the future liver remnant is preferable to bilateral preoperative stenting for hilar cholangiocarcinoma	B	1b	29, 30
Percutaneous is preferable to endoscopic preoperative biliary drainage for hilar cholangiocarcinoma	B	1b	31, 32

References

1. Jarnagin WR, Fong Y, DeMatteo RP, et al. Staging, resectability and outcome in 225 patients with hilar cholangiocarcinoma. Ann Surg 2001; 234:507-17; discussion 517-9.
2. Kosuge T, Yamamoto J, Shimada K, et al. Improved surgical results for hilar cholangiocarcinoma with procedures including major hepatic resection. Ann Surg 1999; 230:663-71.
3. Konstadoulakis MM, Roayaie S, Gomatos IP, et al. Aggressive surgical resection for hilar cholangiocarcinoma: is it justified? Audit of a single center's experience. Am J Surg 2008; 196:160-9.
4. Ito F, Agni R, Rettammel RJ, et al. Resection of hilar cholangiocarcinoma: concomitant liver resection decreases hepatic recurrence. Ann Surg 2008; 248:273-9.
5. Rea DJ, Heimbach JK, Rosen CB, et al. Liver transplantation with neoadjuvant chemoradiation is more effective than resection for hilar cholangiocarcinoma. Ann Surg 2005; 242:451-8; discussion 458-61.
6. Shimoda M, Farmer DG, Colquhoun SD, et al. Liver transplantation for cholangiocellular carcinoma: analysis of a single-center experience and review of the literature. Liver Transpl 2001; 7:1023-33.
7. Robles R, Figueras J, Turrion VS, et al. Spanish experience in liver transplantation for hilar and peripheral cholangiocarcinoma. Ann Surg 2004; 239:265-71.
8. Meyer CG, Penn I, James L. Liver transplantation for cholangiocarcinoma: results in 207 patients. Transplantation 2000; 69:1633-7.
9. Gusani NJ, Balaa FK, Steel JL, et al. Treatment of unresectable cholangiocarcinoma with gemcitabine-based transcatheter arterial chemoembolization (TACE): a single-institution experience. J Gastrointest Surg 2008; 12:129-37.
10. Kim JH, Yoon HK, Sung KB, et al. Transcatheter arterial chemoembolization or chemoinfusion for unresectable intrahepatic cholangiocarcinoma: clinical efficacy and factors influencing outcomes. Cancer 2008; 113:1614-22.
11. Gao F, Bai Y, Ma SR, et al. Systematic review: photodynamic therapy for unresectable cholangiocarcinoma. J Hepatobiliary Pancreat Surg 2009.

12. Ortner ME, Caca K, Berr F, et al. Successful photodynamic therapy for nonresectable cholangiocarcinoma: a randomized prospective study. Gastroenterology 2003; 125:1355-63.

13. Kahaleh M, Mishra R, Shami VM, et al. Unresectable cholangiocarcinoma: comparison of survival in biliary stenting alone versus stenting with photodynamic therapy. Clin Gastroenterol Hepatol 2008; 6:290-7.

14. Witzigmann H, Berr F, Ringel U, et al. Surgical and palliative management and outcome in 184 patients with hilar cholangiocarcinoma: palliative photodynamic therapy plus stenting is comparable to r1/r2 resection. Ann Surg 2006; 244:230-9.

15. Jang JS, Lim HY, Hwang IG, et al. Gemcitabine and oxaliplatin in patients with unresectable biliary cancer including gall bladder cancer: a Korean Cancer Study Group phase II trial. Cancer Chemother Pharmacol 2009; 64(2):371-7.

16. Kim ST, Park JO, Lee J, et al. A Phase II study of gemcitabine and cisplatin in advanced biliary tract cancer. Cancer 2006; 106:1339-46.

17. Kim MJ, Oh DY, Lee SH, et al. Gemcitabine-based versus fluoropyrimidine-based chemotherapy with or without platinum in unresectable biliary tract cancer: a retrospective study. BMC Cancer 2008; 8:374.

18. McMasters KM, Tuttle TM, Leach SD, et al. Neoadjuvant chemoradiation for extrahepatic cholangiocarcinoma. Am J Surg 1997; 174:605-8; discussion 608-9.

19. Murakami Y, Uemura K, Sudo T, et al. Gemcitabine-based adjuvant chemotherapy improves survival after aggressive surgery for hilar cholangiocarcinoma. J Gastrointest Surg 2009; 13:1470-9.

20. Pitt HA, Nakeeb A, Abrams RA, et al. Perihilar cholangiocarcinoma. Postoperative radiotherapy does not improve survival. Ann Surg 1995; 221:788-97; discussion 797-8.

21. Anderson C, Kim R. Adjuvant therapy for resected extrahepatic cholangiocarcinoma: a review of the literature and future directions. Cancer Treat Rev 2009; 35:322-7.

22. Hochwald SN, Burke EC, Jarnagin WR, et al. Association of preoperative biliary stenting with increased postoperative infectious complications in proximal cholangiocarcinoma. Arch Surg 1999; 134:261-6.

23. Cherqui D, Benoist S, Malassagne B, et al. Major liver resection for carcinoma in jaundiced patients without preoperative biliary drainage. Arch Surg 2000; 135:302-8.

24. Ferrero A, Lo Tesoriere R, Vigano L, et al. Preoperative biliary drainage increases infectious complications after hepatectomy for proximal bile duct tumor obstruction. World J Surg 2009; 33:318-25.

25. Sewnath ME, Karsten TM, Prins MH, et al. A meta-analysis on the efficacy of preoperative biliary drainage for tumors causing obstructive jaundice. Ann Surg 2002; 236:17-27.

26. Wang Q, Gurusamy KS, Lin H, et al. Preoperative biliary drainage for obstructive jaundice. Cochrane Database Syst Rev 2008; CD005444.

27. Laurent A, Tayar C, Cherqui D. Cholangiocarcinoma: preoperative biliary drainage (Con). HPB (Oxford) 2008; 10:126-9.

28. Nimura Y. Preoperative biliary drainage before resection for cholangiocarcinoma (Pro). HPB (Oxford) 2008; 10:130-3.

29. De Palma GD, Galloro G, Siciliano S, et al. Unilateral versus bilateral endoscopic hepatic duct drainage in patients with malignant hilar biliary obstruction: results of a prospective, randomized and controlled study. Gastrointest Endosc 2001; 53:547-53.

30. Chang WH, Kortan P, Haber GB. Outcome in patients with bifurcation tumors who undergo unilateral versus bilateral hepatic duct drainage. Gastrointest Endosc 1998; 47:354-62.

31. Kloek JJ, van der Gaag NA, Aziz Y, et al. Endoscopic and percutaneous preoperative biliary drainage in patients with suspected hilar cholangiocarcinoma. J Gastrointest Surg 2009; 13(8):1464-9.

32. Saluja SS, Gulati M, Garg PK, et al. Endoscopic or percutaneous biliary drainage for gallbladder cancer: a randomized trial and quality of life assessment. Clin Gastroenterol Hepatol 2008; 6:944-50.

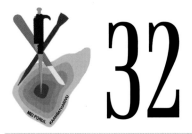

32

Endocrine Pancreas

Gary Nace, Kenneth KW Lee, Christopher J Bartels

Introduction and Background

Tumors of the endocrine pancreas are rare, representing 3-7% of all pancreatic tumors. They represent a heterogeneous group of tumors that differ in their presenting symptoms, biologic behavior and prognosis. Compared with pancreatic adenocarcinoma, pancreatic neuroendocrine tumors (PNETs) generally have a more indolent course; however, there is a broad spectrum of malignant potential with some tumors behaving similar to small cell carcinoma with rapidly progressive disease.

Unlike the well-defined nomenclature of other neoplasms of the pancreas, the naming of tumors of the endocrine pancreas has been more ambiguous. Historically, they have been referred to as carcinoid tumors, islet cell tumors and APUDomas (amine precursor uptake and decarboxylation) to denote the proposed cell of origin. The terms pancreatic endocrine and PNETs have been used interchangeably. We will use the term pancreatic neuroendocrine tumor (PNET) in this chapter.

PNETs that constitutively secrete peptide hormones at supraphysiologic levels and result in characteristic clinical syndromes are described as being functional. Non-functional tumors may also secrete hormones in excess, but do not produce a well-defined clinical syndrome. Approximately 40% of PNETs cause a characteristic clinical syndrome related to their hormone secretion. Functional PNETs are further characterized by the hormone responsible for clinical findings. Hormones secreted that lead to clinical syndromes include insulin, gastrin, glucagon, vasoactive intestinal polypeptide (VIP), somatostatin, growth hormone-releasing factor (GRF), adrenocorticotropic (ACTH), parathyroid hormone (PTH) and serotonin. Some PNETs may secrete multiple hormones, with one predominant hormone leading to the clinical findings. **Tables 32-1 and 32-2** provide an overview of PNETs including the common clinical findings, incidence, tumor locations and malignant behavior.

The endocrine pancreas, representing only 1-2% of the pancreatic mass, is composed of islets of Langerhans. The islets of Langerhans contain several types of cells: α (alpha), β (beta), δ (delta), δ_2 (delta-2) and F. The hormone products of each cell type are included in **Table 32-1**. PNETs have classically been described as arising from the islet cells found within the pancreas, but may also occur in the duodenum. Even though some primary tumors may be anatomically located outside of the pancreas, we still consider them as PNETs if they have traditionally been considered as such. Currently, PNETs are thought likely to originate from pluripotent stem cells of the neuroendocrine system.

Epidemiology

PNETs are rare, occurring at an incidence of approximately 5 per 1,000,000 patients per year although the incidence in autopsy series has been as high as 1.5%. The incidence of PNETs seems to be increasing but may instead be due to the discovery of incidental asymptomatic PNETs on abdominal imaging studies performed for unrelated reasons. The median age of discovery is 56 years with a slight female predominance. Most PNETs are sporadic but they may be associated with a genetic syndrome. The most frequently associated syndrome is Multiple Endocrine Neoplasia-1 (MEN-1), but Von Hippel-Lindau (VHL), neurofibromatosis 1 and tuberous sclerosis patients also have increased risks of developing PNETs.

MEN-1 is inherited as an autosomal dominant syndrome with a prevalence of 1 in 20,000-40,000. It is due to a mutation that inactivates the MEN1 gene on chromosome 11q13 coding for the protein *menin*. MEN-1 patients have the propensity to develop parathyroid, anterior pituitary and pancreatic and duodenal neuroendocrine tumors. Less frequently, tumors may develop in the thymus, lung, stomach, adrenal glands, thyroid or small bowel. In 90% of individuals the parathyroid glands are affected, most commonly as hyperparathyroidism secondary to four-gland hyperplasia. The diagnosis can be established by an elevated serum calcium, intact PTH levels and an elevated 24-hour urinary calcium. The primary management is surgical

TABLE 32-1	Pancreatic neuroendocrine tumor types and features				
Tumor type	Hormone secreted	Pancreatic cell type	Clinical features	Incidence per year	% of PNET
Insulinoma	Insulin	β	Hypoglycemia, neuroglycopenic symptoms, sympathetic activation	2-4 per million	25-30%
Gastrinoma	Gastrin	G	Abdominal pain, peptic ulcers, diarrhea	1-3 per million	15-20%
VIPoma	Vasoactive intestinal peptide	δ_2	Voluminous watery diarrhea, hypokalemia and hypochlorhydria or achlorhydria	1 per 10 million	3-8%
Glucagonoma	Glucagon	α	Necrolytic migratory erythema, hyperglycemia, weight loss, venous thrombosis	1 per 20 million	5%
Somatostatinoma	Somatostatin	δ	Hyperglycemia, cholelithiasis, steatorrhea	1 per 40 million	1-2%
GRFoma	Growth hormone-releasing hormone		Acromegaly		
ACTHoma	Adrenocorticotropic hormone		Cushing's syndrome		
PTHoma	Parathyroid hormone		Hypercalcemia		
Non-functional / PPoma	None / Pancreatic polypeptide	— / F	Symptoms related to local invasion and compression		40-60%

TABLE 32-2	Tumor characteristics				
Tumor	Location	Typical size at diagnosis	% with metastatic disease at diagnosis	% associated with MEN-1
Insulinoma	Distributed within the pancreas	< 2 cm	Rare	10%
Gastrinoma	90% within gastrinoma triangle, more often in duodenal wall	Variable; most duodenal lesions ≤1 cm and most pancreatic lesions ≥ 3 cm	25-33%	25%
VIPoma	90% within the pancreas mainly in the body and tail	4.5 cm	50-70%	Rare
Glucagonoma	Commonly located within the body and tail	7 cm	60-70%	Rare
Somatostatinoma	Mainly within the pancreatic head but may also be extra-pancreatic	5 cm	70-90%	Rare
Non-functional / PPoma	Distributed throughout pancreas	4-6 cm	60%	Frequent

resection consisting of either a subtotal parathyroidectomy or a total parathyroidectomy with reimplantation.

Neuroendocrine tumors of the pancreas and duodenum occur in 75% of MEN-1 patients with the prevalence approaching 100% in autopsy series. MEN-1 associated PNETs develop earlier and are more frequently multifocal than sporadic PNETs and they occur throughout the pancreas. These tumors account for much of the morbidity and mortality associated with MEN-1. Gastrinomas are the most frequently found functional PNETs followed by insulinomas, but only 25% of gastrinomas and 10% of insulinomas are related to MEN-1. Glucagonomas, VIPomas and somatostatinomas occur less frequently. Non-functional tumors, however, likely occur with the highest frequency and have been identified in 55% of MEN-1 patients who were prospectively studied. Commonly PNETs arising in MEN-1 occur as microadenomas located throughout the pancreas. Lymph nodes metastases are frequently found and typically occur earlier than in their sporadic counterparts. Despite their tendency to develop lymph node metastases, PNETs arising in the setting of MEN-1 are generally believed to follow a more indolent course than sporadic PNETs. The treatment for PNETs associated with MEN-1 is controversial and will be discussed later in the chapter.

All patients with a suspected PNET should be evaluated for MEN-1 beginning with a careful history and physical examination. The minimal biochemical work-up to evaluate for MEN-1 should include a serum calcium level. If there is a family history or strong suspicion of MEN-1, the MEN1 gene may be sequenced to evaluate for a mutation.

Von Hippel-Lindau is a rare autosomal dominant condition associated with retinal angiomas, central nervous system hemangioblastomas, clear cell renal cell carcinomas and cysts of the pancreas. Additionally, PNETs occur in 12% of patients with this disease. These PNETs are typically solitary non-functioning lesions. In a fraction of VHL patients, the pancreas may be the only organ affected.

Localization and Work-up

Because of their biochemical activity, functional PNETs may be diagnosed despite being too small to identify on imaging studies. In contrast, non-functional tumors often remain asymptomatic until very large or are identified incidentally on imaging performed for other reasons. The biochemical evaluation is unique for the individual tumor types and will be discussed in the following sections. However, the radiologic evaluation is similar for both functional and non-functional tumors.

Cross-sectional imaging with computed tomography (CT) can be used to localize primary tumors and to evaluate for the presence and extent of metastatic disease. Overall the sensitivity of CT ranges from 71% to 83%, although in recent years there has been a trend of improving sensitivity as CT technology has continued to improve. The small size of some lesions limits their detection by CT. Insulinomas, tending to be smaller lesions, can be difficult to identify on CT. To evaluate for pancreatic masses, CT imaging should be performed with thin sections through the pancreas and should include noncontrast, arterial and venous phase imaging. Characteristically PNETs have a hypervascular appearance during arterial phase imaging **(Figure 32-1)**, but they may also demonstrate increased enhancement on noncontrast imaging. About 20% of PNETs are calcified and rarely may be cystic. Larger lesions may demonstrate post-contrast heterogeneity or necrosis. Malignancy can be demonstrated on imaging by local invasion and metastatic spread to such sites as the liver or regional lymph nodes. MRI has similar sensitivity to CT with about 85% of lesions detected.

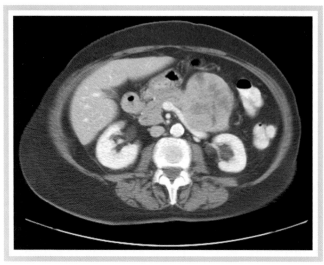

Figure 32-1: Large non-functional PNET originating in the tail of the pancreas. The lesion measures 7.7×8.2 cm and has areas of necrosis. The patient underwent a distal pancreatectomy and splenectomy

The use of radiolabeled octreotide to bind to somatostatin receptors is another useful method of localizing PNETs. Somatostatin receptor scintigraphy (SRS) relies upon binding of In[111]-labelled octreotide to somatostatin receptors on PNETs and detection of the In[111] nuclear SPECT imaging. Since only approximately half of insulinomas express somatostatin receptors, SRS is able to detect less than 25% of insulinomas. The sensitivities for other types of PNETs, including non-functional PNETs, is much higher and ranges from 73% to 100%. SRS is also limited in detecting very small lesions and those within the bowel wall as is frequently the case with gastrinomas. Moreover, SRS is often able to detect the primary lesion and is very useful for detecting metastatic disease, but precise localization is often not possible due to the resolution of SPECT imaging. SRS may also be used to determine whether octreotide and other somatostatin analogues may be useful in symptomatic relief.

Endoscopic ultrasound (EUS) has proven to be most sensitive technique for identification and localization of small PNETs, with the overall sensitivity and accuracy reported to be 93%. The sensitivity in tumors not discernable by CT has been shown to be over 80%. EUS can detect lesions as small as 0.5 cm. Of note, extra-pancreatic tumors, such gastrinomas located within the duodenal wall, are much more difficult to identify on EUS. On EUS, PNETs are generally well-demarcated lesions that are heterogenous and hypoechoic. EUS in combination with FNA may allow for cytologic examination to confirm a diagnosis of PNET. This is especially useful in non-functional lesions. In addition to identifying the typical morphologic features, immunohistochemical stains for neuroendocrine markers, including synaptophysin, chromogranin, neuron specific enolase and CD56 may be performed to confirm the diagnosis of a PNET.

In patients with biochemically diagnosed PNETs, which cannot be localized by the above techniques, careful operative exploration in combination with intraoperative ultrasound (IOUS) will identify almost 100% of lesions. However, if lesions cannot be identified, a blind pancreatic or duodenal resection is not recommended. The use of angiography to identify hypervascular lesions has largely been replaced by arterial phase CT imaging, but angiography may be used to stimulate areas of the pancreas or duodenum selectively in an effort to localize functional PNETs. For example, selective infusion of calcium into the gastroduodenal and splenic arteries followed by hepatic venous sampling may identify excessive insulin production by specific regions of the pancreas. However, such invasive localization studies are rarely necessary.

In our institution, CT with fine cuts through the pancreas and noncontrast, arterial and venous phase imaging followed by EUS with or without FNA is the standard work-up for a suspected PNET. Studies have shown that this combination is able to localize almost all lesions preoperatively.

Pathology, Staging and Prognosis

The staging and classification of neuroendocrine tumors has been a topic of contention and a universally accepted staging system with satisfactorily sufficient prognostic capabilities remains lacking. With the exception of insulinomas, most PNETs can be classified as malignant lesions, but in contrast to adenocarcinomas of the pancreas, most are well-differentiated with relatively indolent progression. This being said, there is a wide range of malignant potential, with some lesions remaining indolent for years and others showing rapid progression and demonstrating a phenotype similar to small cell carcinoma.

The general histopathologic features of pancreatic neuroendocrine cells are uniform nuclei with granular or faintly staining cytoplasm. There are no definitive histopathologic criteria with which to differentiate malignant from benign. Several features that should routinely be considered to define malignancy include metastasis to either distant sites or lymph nodes and local invasiveness including angiolymphatic and perineural invasion. Only when amyloid is present, identifying insulinomas can histologically indicate function.

Chromogranin A (CgA) is a tumor marker that, although not specific for an individual type of PNET, may be used as general diagnostic marker and also to follow progression of disease. CgA has been reported to be elevated in 50-80% of PNETs. Pancreatic polypeptide (PP) is another marker that may be measured and when combined with CgA the sensitivity for diagnosis of a PNET is increased to over 90%. These markers may be used to diagnose and follow both functional and non-functional PNETs. Neuron-specific enolase (NSE) is another general tumor marker that may be of diagnostic value for PNETs, but has the disadvantage of being less specific as it is found in some non-neuroendocrine tumors as well. The individual hormones responsible for functional tumors may also be used for diagnosis and will be discussed later.

In 2000, the World Health Organization (WHO) published an endocrine tumor classification system mainly based upon histologic appearance. PNETs were classified as well-differentiated endocrine tumors (WDET) of either benign or uncertain behavior, well-differentiated endocrine carcinomas (WDEC), poorly differentiated endocrine carcinomas (PDEC) or mixed endocrine-exocrine carcinomas. The WHO system defines PNETs on a spectrum of malignant potential. **Table 32-3** demonstrates the features of each group.

More recently, a TNM classification system specific for PNET has been proposed **(Table 32-4)**. A histologic grading system has also been proposed that incorporates the mitotic count and Ki-67 index, a measure of proliferative activity. Although these systems have not yet been widely accepted, their prognostic potential was demonstrated in a recent retrospective study of 202 patients. For stages I, II, III and IV disease the 5-year survival rates were 100%, 89.5%, 79.1% and 55.4%, respectively. Survival was also dependent on the tumor grade with 5 year survival for grade 1, 2 and 3 shown to be 96%, 73% and 28%, respectively.

A recent analysis of the National Cancer Institute Surveillance Epidemiology and End Results (SEER) Program database has helped to further characterize the natural history of PNETs. The SEER Program database staging system defines lesions as localized (confined to the organ of primary origin), regional (invades surrounding organs, tissues, or lymph nodes), or distant disease (spread to remote sites). However, PNETs that were not overtly malignant such as the majority of insulinomas were not included in this database. In more than half of the PNETs, distant disease was present at the time of diagnosis. The overall median survival for all 1274 cases analyzed was 38 months. The median survival significantly differed depending on stage with the survival of localized, regional and distant disease being 124, 70 and 23 months, respectively. The 5-year survival rates were 71%, 55% and 23% for localized, regional and distant disease, respectively.

Molecular analysis of tumor tissue has shown promising prognostic capabilities. The loss of heterozygosity (LOH) in a panel of 17 polymorphic microsatellite markers

TABLE 32-3	The WHO classification of endocrine tumor of the pancreas					
Tumor	**Malignant potential and degree of atypia**	**Invasive and metastatic characteristics**	**Size**	**Ki-67 percentage positive**	**Mitoses per 10 HPF**	**Approximate 5-yr survival**
Well-differentiated endocrine tumor	**Benign behavior** – No or minimal atypia **Uncertain behavior***	Confined to the pancreas and no angioinvasion	< 2 cm in diameter	≤ 2% Ki-67 positive cells	≤ 2 mitoses per 10 HPF	95-100%
Well-differentiated endocrine carcinoma	**Low grade malignant** –Mild to moderate atypia	Invasion of contiguous structures or documented metastases	Most > 3 cm in diameter	> 5% Ki-67 positive cells	2-10 mitosis per 10 HPF	44-85%
Poorly differentiated endocrine carcinoma	**Highly malignant** Highly atypical, small to intermediate sized cells, with high nucleo-cytoplasmic ratio	Distant metastases, areas of tumor necrosis and prominent angio or perineural invasion		>15% Ki-67 positive cells	>10 mitosis per 10 HPF	0-36%
Mixed exocrine-endocrine carcinoma	Determined by exocrine component	Rare tumor with predominant exocrine compo-nent admixed with at ≥ 1/3 of endocrine cells				

* Well-differentiated endocrine tumors of uncertain behavior are confined to the pancreas but are angioinvasive, > 2 mitosis per 10 HPF, > 2% Ki-67 positive cells, or ≥ 2 cm in diameter.

obtained from EUS-FNA cytology samples was recently reported. A fractional allelic loss (FAL) greater than 0.2 was shown to differentiate malignant (as defined by invasion outside the pancreas or metastasis) from benign PNETs with a sensitivity of 83% and specificity of 100%. The FAL was also shown to predict those who went on to have tumor progression. Of note, the cytologic samples necessary for FAL analysis are easily obtained by means of EUS-guided fine-needle aspiration in comparison to tissue samples that must be obtained by surgical biopsy in order to determine Ki-67 indices and mitotic rates.

Insulinoma

Insulinomas are the most common PNETs, comprising one-third of all PNETs and occurring at an incidence of 2-4 per million per year. Fortunately, > 90% of these are benign and > 90% are < 2 cm. There has been a slight female predominance in most series, with the median age of diagnosis ranging 51-53 years. The median duration of symptoms prior to diagnosis is 18 months. Patients with MEN-1 have an increased incidence of insulinomas, with 10% of insulinomas occurring in patients with MEN-1 and 20% of MEN-1 patients developing an insulinoma. In comparison to sporadic insulinomas, those arising in MEN-1 tend to occur at a younger age and are more apt to be multifocal.

Insulinomas are composed of β-cells that are hyperfunctioning and produce inappropriately high levels of insulin leading to susceptibility for hypoglycemia. In 1935, Whipple and Frantz described the classic clinical triad associated with insulinomas consisting of symptoms of hypoglycemia arising with exertion or fasting, a measured serum glucose level < 45 mg/dL during symptoms and resolution of symptoms with administration of glucose **(Table 32-5)**. Patients often learn to compensate for the frequent hypoglycemic episodes by consuming frequent meals and meals at bedtimes, leading to weight gain in many patients. The most frequent symptoms are related to glucose deprivation of the central nervous system and range from confusion (67%), visual changes (42%), fatigue (28%) and speaking difficulty to more severe consequences such as syncope, seizures and coma. Symptoms are also related to the activation of the sympathetic nervous system and release of catecholamines. These symptoms include anxiety, diaphoresis, palpitations, tremors and sweating. Symptoms are usually precipitated by fasting but may occur with exercise.

TABLE 32-4	Proposed TNM classification and grading system for pancreatic endocrine tumors		
T (primary tumor)			
TX	Primary cannot be assessed		
T1	Tumor limited to pancreas and < 2 cm		
T2	Tumor limited to pancreas and 2-4 cm		
T3	Tumor limited to pancreas and > 4 cm or invading duodenum or bile ducts		
T4	Tumor invading adjacent organ or wall of large vessel (e.g. celiac axis)		
N (lymph node)			
NX	Regional lymph nodes not assessed		
N0	No lymph node metastases		
N1	Regional lymph node metastases		
M (distant metastases)			
MX	Distant metastases not assessed		
M0	No distant metastases		
M1	Distant metastases present		
Stage			
I	T1	N0	M0
IIa	T2	N0	M0
IIb	T3	N0	M0
IIIa	T4	N0	M0
IIIb	Any T	N1	M0
IV	Any T	Any N	M1
Grade	**Mitotic count (per 10 HPF)[a]**	**Ki-67 index (%)[b]**	
1	<2	≤ 2	
2	2-20	3-20	
3	>20	>20	

[a]10 HPF: high power field = 2 mm², at least 40 fields (at 40x magnification) evaluated in areas of highest mitotic density.
[b]MIBI antibody; % of 2,000 tumor cells in areas of highest nuclear labeling.
Reprinted from: Rinde G, Kloppel G, Alhman H, et al. TNM staging of foregut (neuro)endocrine tumors: a consensus proposal including a grading system. Virchows Arch 2006; 449:395-401. © 2006. Reprinted with kind permission from Springer Science + Business Media.

TABLE 32-5	Whipple's triad

- Symptomatic hypoglycemia with exertion or fasting
- Measured serum glucose < 45 mg/dL during symptoms
- Resolution of symptoms with glucose administration

The differential diagnosis for hypoglycemia is broad. Reactive (postprandial) hypoglycemia is a far more common cause of symptomatic hypoglycemia. Reactive hypoglycemia can be differentiated by its occurrence after meals. Factitious or iatrogenic causes of hypoglycemia should also be highly considered in the differential. Very rarely, islet cell hyperplasia and nesidioblastosis, defined as hyperinsulinemic hypoglycemia related to excessive function of pancreatic beta cells, may be a cause of adult hypoglycemia related to excess insulin. Recently noninsulinoma hyperinsulinism causing postprandial hypoglycemia has been associated with Roux-en-Y gastric bypass surgery performed for treatment of morbid obesity. Although clinical symptoms may lead to suspicion for an insulinoma, the diagnosis is confirmed by demonstrating an inappropriate excess of insulin simultaneous with a low serum glucose level. A normal insulin to glucose ratio is < 0.4. An insulin to glucose ratio > 0.3 combined with an elevated insulin level (> 6 µU/mL) and hypoglycemia is highly suggestive of an insulinoma. However, up to one-third of patients with an excised insulinoma will have a ratio less than 0.3. The 72-hour fast has become the gold standard of establishing a biochemical diagnosis. During this supervised fast, serum glucose and insulin levels are drawn at regular intervals (every 4-6 hours) and more frequently as glucose levels decrease below 60 mg/dL. The onset of symptoms concurrent with hypoglycemia and elevation of serum insulin concentration > 6 µU/mL is diagnostic. One-third of patients with insulinomas will develop symptoms within 12 hours, 80% within 24 hours, 90% within 48 hours and 98% within 72 hours. Measurement of the connecting peptide (C-peptide) is also useful to exclude surreptitious administration of insulin. The rationale for measuring a concurrent C-peptide level is that the precursor of endogenous insulin, proinsulin, is proteolytically cleaved into C-peptide and insulin, whereas commercial insulin products do not contain the precursor molecule or connecting peptide. Urine or serum should also be tested for sulfonylurea level to exclude factitious hypoglycemia. Other suppressive and provocative tests have been described, such as the C-peptide suppression test, tolbutamide test, glucagon test, glucose tolerance test and calcium infusion test, which are outside of the scope of discussion for this chapter.

Insulinomas are almost always small lesions that are located within and distributed equally throughout the pancreas. As with other PNETs, there is no one localizing technique that is perfect; therefore, a multimodal approach is appropriate. The diagnostic sensitivity of current multidetector CT scanners is between 70% and 80%. Insulinomas, like other PNETs, are hypervascular and therefore primary as well as metastatic lesions are often detectable with arterial phase CT imaging. As discussed previously, EUS is a newer tool that may identify approximately 90% of insulinomas, especially those located in the pancreatic head.

Invasive imaging techniques may also be useful in the diagnosis of insulinomas. On routine angiography highly vascular insulinomas may appear as a blush. An insulinoma may be localized to a specific region of the pancreas by selective infusion of calcium gluconate into the gastroduodenal, splenic, or superior mesenteric arteries. Calcium infusion stimulates the insulinoma to release insulin, which can in turn be detected by hepatic venous sampling. Such invasive measures are rarely necessary, however, because of the sensitivity of CT, MRI and EUS. SRS is of limited value for the diagnosis or localization of insulinomas because they generally lack somatostatin receptors.

The definitive and recommended treatment of insulinomas is surgical resection. Preoperative hospitalization and intravenous infusion of dextrose solutions may be necessary to avoid hypoglycemia during preoperative fasting. Since the majority of insulinomas are benign, surgical resection is usually curative. Unlike gastrinomas, over 90% of insulinomas are able to be localized preoperatively. Preoperative EUS is useful not only to localize the insulinoma but also to determine its proximity to the pancreatic duct and suitability for enucleation. Ultrasound evaluation should also be performed in patients with MEN-1 syndrome to evaluate for multicentric disease. When preoperative imaging is inconclusive, IOUS and palpation of the pancreas after mobilization are effective techniques.

Most insulinomas can be removed by means of enucleation as they are usually benign and well encapsulated and consequently wide excision is unnecessary. Lesions that are either malignant, as evident by the presence of metastases to lymph nodes or distant sites or local invasion, or inappropriate for enucleation due to their proximity to the pancreatic duct should be treated with a more formal resection. As experience with laparoscopic pancreatic surgery has increased, both enucleation and resection procedures are increasingly performed by laparoscopic means. Patients that do not have a lesion localizable either preoperatively or intraoperatively should not undergo a blind pancreatic resection since insulinomas are distributed rather evenly throughout the pancreas.

Blood glucose levels after successful resection of an insulinoma may be transiently elevated, but diabetes is unlikely to develop unless a substantial amount of pancreatic parenchyma has also been removed. The 5-year disease-free survival is approximately 90% after surgical resection of an insulinoma. Unlike gastrinomas and NF-PNETs in MEN-1 patients, the treatment of insulinomas in association with MEN-1 does not differ greatly from sporadic insulinomas. Most insulinomas arising in MEN-1 patients can be cured with surgical resection, although multiple lesions may have to be resected. The recurrence rate is increased in MEN-1 patients with about 20% of patients recurring within 20 years.

Approximately 10% of insulinomas are malignant. With malignant disease, the median disease-free survival in one series was 5 years after curative resection. The recurrence rate was 63% with a median interval to recurrence of 2.8 years. The median survival with recurrent tumor was 19 months. Palliative resection was associated with an improved survival when compared to biopsy only (median survival 4 years vs 11 months). It is debatable whether debulking should be attempted, but this may provide some symptomatic relief. When metastatic disease is present or complete surgical extirpation is unsuccessful, medical therapy is essential to help control symptoms of hypoglycemia. Diazoxide may be effective in about 50-60% of patients. Diazoxide suppresses insulin secretion by direct action on β-cells and also increases glycogenolysis. Side effects include hypotension, edema, hirsutism and nausea and occur in about half of patients. Somatostatin or longer acting analogues may also be used to help alleviate symptoms in some patients. As with other PNETs, chemotherapy and liver-directed therapy can be attempted in advanced progressive disease.

Gastrinoma

Gastrinomas are the second most common functional PNET (overall) and most common malignant PNET. They occur at an incidence of roughly 1-3 cases per million per year. Approximately 60-90% of these lesions are malignant and approximately 25-33% of patients present with metastatic disease.

The mean age at diagnosis is about 46 years old with a slight male predominance. Symptoms are typically present for about 6 years prior to diagnosis. Gastrinomas occur sporadically in 75% and are associated with MEN-1 in the remaining 25%. The clinical triad of a peptic ulcer diathesis in unusual locations such as the jejunum, severe gastric hypersecretion and a noninsulin-producing islet cell tumor was first described in two patients in 1955 by Zollinger and Ellison. Subsequently, gastrin was identified as the physiologic basis of what has become known as Zollinger-Ellison syndrome (ZES). The symptoms of gastrinomas are related to hypergastrinemia causing unregulated acid secretion by gastric parietal cells. In advanced cases, symptoms related to the local effects of the tumor and those of metastatic disease may develop.

Abdominal pain secondary to peptic ulcer disease (PUD) or gastroesophageal reflux is the most common symptom and is present in about 75% of patients. Sequelae of severe PUD such as bleeding or perforation may also develop/occur in a small fraction of patients with gastrinomas. Diarrhea occurs in approximately 50% of patients and is the sole presenting symptom in 10-15%. The diarrhea is likely due to the combination of damage to the small bowel mucosa by high acid levels, the neutralization of pancreatic enzymes necessary for digestion and the high volume of gastric secretions. Unlike the diarrhea related to VIPoma and other secretory diarrheas, it may be halted by gastric suctioning. The diagnosis of ZES should be considered in patients with PUD or GERD accompanied by diarrhea, recurrent or refractory PUD, a family history of PUD, PUD in unusual locations, multiple atypical ulcers or PUD complicated by bleeding, perforation, or obstruction. Approximately 2% of patients with persistent or recurrent ulcers will have ZES.

The diagnosis is established by the demonstration of hypergastrinemia in the presence of gastric acid hypersecretion. Hypergastrinemia is a normal response to achlorhydria or hypochlorhydria; therefore only in the presence of increased gastric acidity is hypergastrinemia abnormal. Characteristics of ZES gastric hypersecretion include a basal acid output (BAO) exceeding 15 mEq/hour or 5 mEq/hour after a prior acid reducing operation, nocturnal (12 hour) acid output greater than 1 L or 100 mEq, or a BAO to maximal acid output (MAO) ratio greater than 0.6. An elevated BAO/MAO (> 0.6) demonstrates that parietal cells are continuously being maximally stimulated to produce maximal amounts of acid.

Prior to undertaking the biochemical evaluation for a gastrinoma, it is important that the patient discontinue acid suppressive therapies as these will reduce acid production and may elevate gastrin production. Gastrin levels, basal and stimulated, should be measured while fasting and after proton pump inhibitors have been discontinued for 1 week. The finding of a fasting serum gastrin (FSG) value > 10 times normal (> 1000 pg/mL) in the presence of gastric hyperacidity is diagnostic of a gastrinoma. However, 64-68% of patients have an FSG level < 10 times normal that overlaps with the range of FSG levels seen in other conditions. Other conditions that may cause hypergastrinemia combined with gastric acid hypersecretion include *Helicobacter pylori* infection, gastric outlet obstruction, retained gastric antrum syndrome, chronic renal failure, short bowel syndrome and antral G-cell hyperplasia. Therefore, frequently a provocative test is needed to confirm diagnosis of a gastrinoma.

The secretin, calcium and meal provocation tests have been well described. The secretin stimulation test is currently recommended because of its greater sensitivity, lack of side effects and simplicity of use. During the secretin stimulation test, 2 U/kg of secretin are administered as a bolus and FSG levels are measured at time points 15, 5 and 0 minutes before and at 2, 5, 10, 15, 20 and 30 minutes after secretin injection. A rise of FSG level of ≥ 200 pg/mL from baseline is considered

diagnostic of ZES. However, a recent large prospective study has shown that the sensitivity increased from 83% to 94% if the value of ≥ 120 pg/mL be used instead while the specificity remained unchanged at 100%. Serum calcium levels should also be measured to evaluate for possible hyperparathyroidism and an undiagnosed MEN-1 syndrome.

Once the biochemical diagnosis of a gastrinoma has been made, proton pump inhibitors should be prescribed and titrated to acid suppression. Imaging should then be obtained to not only to localize the gastrinoma but also to attempt to identify unresectable or metastatic disease. Over 90% of gastrinomas are located in the region of the gastrinoma triangle **(Figure 32-2)**, defined as the area within the junctions of the cystic and common bile duct, the second and third portion of duodenum and the head and neck of the pancreas. Gastrinomas occurring in the duodenal wall are three times as common as those in the pancreas and are usually located within the submucosa of the more proximal duodenum. Peripancreatic and periduodenal lymph nodes are also frequent sites of primary gastrinomas followed by various other locations within the abdomen that include the ovaries, liver, omentum, pylorus, common bile duct and jejunum. The size of gastrinomas varies depending on location. In one series of 185 consecutive patients, 92% of duodenal gastrinomas were ≤ 1 cm (mean 0.93 cm) whereas 95% of pancreatic gastrinomas were ≥ 3 cm (mean 3.8 cm).

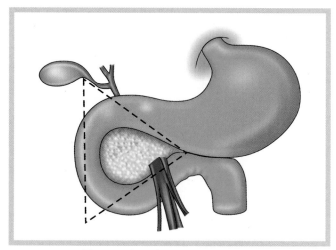

Figure 32-2: Gastrinoma triangle

The first imaging modality routinely obtained is a contrast-enhanced CT of the abdomen with fine slices through the pancreas. SRS is also particularly useful for gastrinomas since almost all have somatostatin receptors. However, small duodenal tumors are frequently below the sensitivity of SRS and fail to be detected. As previously discussed, EUS can also be very informative. When other localization methods have failed, selective arterial secretin injection (SASI) has been used to localize tumors in a manner similar to localization of insulinomas by means of selective calcium infusions. This technique involves selective injection of secretin into the gastroduodenal, superior mesenteric and splenic arteries followed by measurement of gastrin levels in samples collected from the hepatic veins.

In a significant proportion of patients with biochemical evidence of a gastrinoma, the lesion cannot be localized preoperatively despite use of these various studies. With sporadic gastrinomas, operative exploration should be performed if there is no diffuse hepatic involvement or other unresectable disease. The operative approach entails a thorough abdominal exploration looking for metastatic disease or unusual primary sites, an extended Kocher maneuver, careful palpation of the pancreas and duodenum, IOUS of the pancreas and liver, endoscopic transillumination of the duodenum and exploration of the duodenum by means of a duodenotomy made along the descending duodenum. Enucleation of pancreatic tumors or excision and primary repair of duodenal tumors is considered the preferred resection strategy by many. If this is not a suitable option a more extensive resection such as a pancreaticoduodenectomy may be necessary. All lymph nodes in the peripancreatic and periduodenal area should also be excised as they may harbor micrometastases. Using these techniques, over 90% of primary gastrinomas can be identified in the operating room regardless of preoperative studies.

Prior to discharge a repeat FSG level and secretin provocation test should be performed to document a biochemical cure. Prospective data has demonstrated that only approximately half of patients show evidence of biochemical cure postoperatively. However, in the half that are biochemically disease free this cure is durable with 40% still biochemically disease free at 5 years and 34% at 10 years. Presumably, the failure of many to sustain a biochemical cure postoperatively is due to micrometastatic disease.

Liver metastases from gastrinoma are the most important predictor of survival in most studies. The 10-year survival in patients without liver metastases is approximately 90%, but in patients with liver metastases 10-year survival falls to approximately 10%. The resection of primary tumors is associated with a decreased incidence of liver metastases and increased survival **(Figure 32-3)**.

The surgical treatment of MEN-1 associated gastrinomas, like other PNETs, is more conservative. The indolent nature of MEN-1 gastrinomas combined with a poor immediate postoperative cure rate of 16% limits the benefit obtained by surgical intervention. NIH consensus criteria recommend that surgery be deferred until lesions they reach a diameter of 2.5 cm. The primary objective of surgical resection is the prevention liver metastases, which is the only factor found to consistently correlate with survival. A lesion 2.5 cm in diameter is thought to have a great enough risk of developing liver metastases to justify a resection that is usually not curative. In one study, only 4% of patients with a primary tumor < 1 cm had metastases to the liver, whereas 28% of patients whose primary gastrinoma measured between 1.1 cm and 2.9 cm and 61% of patients with primary tumors > 3 cm developed liver metastases.

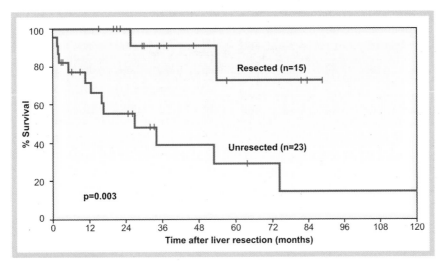

Figure 32-3: Survival is significantly improved in those with liver metastases that are amenable to resection. The survival curve above compares a similar cohort of patients; however, those that underwent curative resection had a 5-year actuarial survival of 73% versus 29%. Chen H, Hardacre JM, Uzar A, Cameron JL, Choti MA. Isolated liver metastases from neuroendocrine tumors: does resection prolong survival? J Am Coll Surg 1998;187:88-97. Reprinted with permission from Elsevier

Vasoactive Intestinal Polypeptidoma

Vasoactive intestinal polypeptidomas (VIPomas) constitute about 3-8% of pancreatic endocrine tumors and were described by Verner and Morrison in 1958. VIPomas are characterized by a syndrome of high volume watery diarrhea, hypokalemia and hypochlorhydria or achlorhydria. The syndrome associated with VIPomas has also been referred to as WDHA syndrome (watery diarrhea, hypokalemia and achlorhydria), Verner-Morrison syndrome and pancreatic cholera. The Verner-Morrison triad consists of secretory diarrhea, high serum level of VIP and a pancreatic tumor. The diarrhea is voluminous (3-5 L/day), refractory to fasting or gastric suctioning and often leads to hypovolemia and electrolyte imbalances. Diarrhea volume of less than 700 ml/day excludes this diagnosis. Other symptoms include hypercalcemia, abdominal pain, dehydration, flushing, hyperglycemia and metabolic acidosis.

The biochemical diagnosis is made with a fasting serum VIP levels > 200 pg/mL in the correct clinical setting. Most VIPomas are malignant and metastatic disease is found in 50-70% of patients at the time of presentation. Ninety percent of VIPomas are located within the pancreas with a majority located in the body or tail of the pancreas, although they have also been found in the chest and retroperitoneum. VIPomas are usually large solitary lesions with a median diameter of 4.5 cm. The large size at presentation usually allows these tumors to be easily identifiable with CT imaging of the abdomen. If the imaging of the abdomen does not identify the tumor then a CT of the chest should be considered to evaluate for an intrathoracic lesion. Other imaging modalities that should be considered in difficult cases are EUS and SRS.

The initial step in treatment is the administration of octreotide to control diarrhea in addition to fluid and electrolytes replacements. With the use of octreotide, symptoms are usually controlled. Surgical resection offers the only chance for cure and debulking may offer symptomatic improvement. If surgical resection cannot be performed or is ineffective, chemotherapy should be considered but responses are generally poor. Octreotide reduces diarrhea in most patients initially; however, becomes less effective with time. The 5-year survival is approximately 95% for patients without metastases, but is only 60% in patients with metastases.

Glucagonoma

Glucagonomas are composed of α-cells and secrete an excess of glucagon. They represent approximately 5% of PNETs and occur with an incidence of 1 per 20 million per year. Symptoms related to the excess glucagon include necrolytic migratory erythema, glucose intolerance ranging from mild hyperglycemia to diabetes mellitus, normochromic normocytic anemia, diarrhea, weight loss, hypoaminoacidemia, stomatitis and a predisposition to develop deep vein thrombosis. The dermatologic manifestations are the most common presenting symptoms and are characterized by a migratory scaly rash that is pruritic and typically distributed to the groin and lower extremities. A fasting serum glucagon level of > 1,000 pg/mL is diagnostic of a glucagonoma. Approximately 20% of patients with a glucagonoma also have elevated gastrin levels.

Glucagonomas are usually large at presentation and are commonly located in the body and tail of the pancreas. The mean diameter at presentation is 7 cm. Almost all lesions are malignant but have a relatively indolent course. Between 60-70% of these tumors are metastatic at the time of discovery.

Once the diagnosis is made, parenteral nutrition, anticoagulation and octreotide should be started. Parenteral nutrition corrects amino acid deficiencies and as this is achieved, the dermatitis usually resolves. Anticoagulation should be started to prevent thrombotic complications. Octreotide may help to alleviate these and other symptoms caused by the glucagonoma.

As for other PNETs, the preferred treatment of glucagonomas is surgical resection. Although the overall cure rate is only about 30%, the tumors are slow growing and 5-year survival is reported to be approximately 50%. Chemotherapy and liver-directed treatment strategies may be considered for treatment of metastatic and recurrent disease.

Somatostatinoma

Somatostatinomas are PNETs that are derived from δ-cells that inappropriately secrete somatostatin. They represent 1-2% of PNETs and occur with an incidence of about 1 per 40 million per year. Symptoms of somatostatinomas are related to the widespread inhibitory effects of somatostatin, are nonspecific and include hyperglycemia ranging from mild intolerance to diabetes mellitus (60%), cholelithiasis (70%), steatorrhea (68%), diarrhea (30%), hypochlorhydria, anemia and weight loss. Somatostatinomas are typically large, averaging approximately 5 cm, solitary lesions located in the head of the pancreas; however, they may also be extrapancreatic and are particularly found in the duodenum. A retrospective study of somatostatinomas found that duodenal tumors are less likely to be associated with the classic inhibitory syndrome and are more likely to be associated with von Recklinghausen's disease. The 5-year survival rate approaches 100% in the absence of metastatic disease but is only 60% in the presence of metastatic disease. Metastatic disease is present in 70-92% of patients at the time of diagnosis.

Rarer yet: GRFoma, ACTHoma and PTHoma

In addition to the functional PNETs previously discussed there are other less common functional neuroendocrine tumors that may be located within the pancreas. GRF-producing tumors present with symptoms and signs of acromegaly. Most GRF-producing tumors are located in the lungs (50%), but about 30% are located within the pancreas and 10% are located within the small bowel. Half of patients with GRFomas also have ZES and a third are associated with MEN-1. The tumors are usually large at the time of presentation and metastatic disease is common. ACTHomas present clinically with Cushing's syndrome. Cushing's syndrome may also be associated with other types of PNETs, since ACTH may be secreted in addition to other hormones. In fact, 5% of ZES patients display Cushing's syndrome. Cushing's syndrome may also occur with pituitary tumors in MEN-1 patients. Functional PNETs may also secrete PTH and PTH related-peptide causing severe hypercalcemia. However, hypercalcemia in patients with MEN-1 most commonly results from parathyroid hyperplasia rather than from a functional PNETs.

Non-functional and PPoma

Approximately 60% of PNETs are not associated with a clinical syndrome from secreted hormones and thus are classified as non-functional PNETs (NF-PNETs). Although PPomas secrete PP in excess, there is yet to be an identifiable clinical syndrome associated with excess secretion of PP. Because of the lack of hormone-related symptoms, these patients typically present late in the disease course. The average size ranges 4-6 cm and almost 60% are greater than 3 cm at the time of discovery. Metastatic liver disease is present at the time of diagnosis in at least 60%. Like most other PNETs, the majority are clearly malignant but generally have a relatively indolent course. Presenting symptoms are related to local mass effects of the tumor and include abdominal pain, jaundice and /or weight loss.

Almost all NF-PNETs are located within the pancreas and one-third to two-third of NF-PNETs are located in the head of the pancreas. Radiologic characteristics on CT imaging that may suggest a diagnosis of PNET as opposed to adenocarcinoma include hypervascularity on arterial phase imaging, the presence of calcifications within the mass and rarely cystic degeneration. Tumor markers, such as CgA and PP, may also be suggestive of a neuroendocrine tumor. However, a cytologic sample is usually necessary to conclusively differentiate PNETs from other pancreatic neoplasms.

Due to the delay in presentation, a curative resection is not possible in many patients. In one series, however, when localized disease could successfully be resected, median survival was 7.1 years, whereas with unresectable locally advanced disease or metastatic disease median survival was 5.2 and 2.1 years, respectively. In another series of patients with NF-PNETs, the 5-year survival was increased from 37% in those unresectable to 93% in patients after radical surgery. There was no survival benefit shown for a palliative resection.

Even with a curative resection about half of patients will have disease recurrence. In yet another series, a multivariate analysis identified five factors that had prognostic value: weight loss, nodal metastases, liver metastases, poor differentiation and a Ki-67 > 5%. Poor differentiation was the most significant prognostic variable. Tumor size and the presence of symptoms were suggestive of poor outcomes but did not achieve significance. In summary, the ideal treatment for NF-PNETs is surgical resection and should be attempted in all appropriate surgical candidates. Those with disease that is not amenable to curative resection should be considered for multimodality treatment including systemic chemotherapy, regional therapy and possibly palliative surgical procedures (e.g. bypass procedures to relieve gastric outlet obstruction).

The management of NF-PNETs in MEN-1 patients should be approached differently than sporadic tumors. Like gastrinomas, curative resection is rarely obtainable with the typical diffuse pancreatic involvement. Lesions that are less ≤ 2 cm have a 10% chance of developing metastases, whereas larger lesions have a 27% incidence of metastases. Therefore, some have recommended that lesions should be considered for resection only when they reach a size of ≥ 2 cm, show significant progression, or metastasize. Such conservative management of slowly progressive asymptomatic lesions that have a low risk of metastasis may allow many patients to avoid the potential risks of surgery.

Incidental Pancreatic Neuroendocrine Tumors

Pancreatic lesions discovered during the work-up of symptoms not normally associated with pancreatic pathology or during other routine imaging are described as incidentalomas. As many as 90% of NF-PNETs are discovered in this manner. In a recent study of pancreatic incidentalomas that were resected, 13% of lesions were characterized as neuroendocrine tumors and 15% were found to be adenocarcinoma. Overall, 24% of asymptomatic pancreatic lesions prove to be malignant and 38% of solid lesions are malignant. Therefore, the discovery of a pancreatic incidentaloma should not be taken lightly.

The work-up of incidental pancreatic lesions begins with a detailed history and physical examination. Particularly important are symptoms consistent with a history pancreatitis. Symptoms associated with a functional PNET, such as PUD or symptoms of hypoglycemia, should be elicited. The patient should be questioned about a family history of pancreatic neoplasm, hyperparathyroidism or symptoms of hypercalcemia.

The diagnostic work-up should include serum CgA, PP and Ca 19-9 levels, with additional biochemical work-up for functional lesions dependent on clinical suspicion. As previously discussed, the radiologic evaluation generally includes a triphasic CT of the abdomen. We commonly undertake further evaluation with EUS and EUS-guided fine-needle aspiration of the abnormality.

Similar to symptomatic lesions, the preferred treatment of lesions that occur in patients without MEN-1 is surgical resection. The extent of resection needed is dependent on the location of the lesion and this may range from enucleation to pancreaticoduodenectomy with hepatic resection. The treatment of widely metastatic or other lesions that are unresectable will be discussed later in the chapter.

Treatment for Advanced Disease

Although the preferred and only curative treatment for sporadic PNETs is complete surgical extirpation, the most appropriate approach for locally advanced and metastatic disease is not as well-defined. Since a majority of PNETs (32-74%) are metastatic at presentation this topic deserves discussion.

Metastases occur most commonly to the liver and account for most of the mortality associated with advanced PNETs. Management of hepatic disease parallels that of other malignancies metastatic to the liver and utilizes a multimodality approach that includes surgical resection, ablative techniques, hepatic artery embolization using chemotherapeutics or radioisotopes and systemic chemotherapy. Numerous retrospective and prospective studies have analyzed the best treatment for hepatic metastases. The treatment options must be carefully weighed for risk versus benefit in light of the fact that most PNETs have an indolent course with survival for metastatic disease measured in years. The rate of disease progression along with the age and comorbidities of the patient should be considered.

Improved survival with successful hepatic resection has been demonstrated by numerous authors. The 5-year survival is improved from 29-30% to 60-73% in those with liver lesions that are amenable to resection. The ability to perform a hepatic resection is dependent on the location and number of lesions as well as the presence of cirrhosis or hepatic steatosis. Options for resection include both a formal hepatic lobectomy and non-anatomic wedge resections. Preoperatively, we routinely use CT of the liver with both arterial and portal phase contrast to help plan operative strategies. In patients who are appropriate

operative candidates and whose lesions are amenable to complete resection, the decision process is rather straight forward. When bilobar lesions are present, complete treatment may require a combination of resection and ablative procedures. In patients predicted to have inadequate hepatic reserve to support a major liver resection, preoperative selective portal vein embolization may lead to contralateral hypertrophy sufficient to permit a subsequent liver resection. However, if extensive metastatic liver disease is present, surgical treatment may not be possible and instead hepatic artery embolization or systemic chemotherapy should be considered.

In those who have lesions that cannot completely be resected the ideal treatment is more open to debate, with varying results in studies evaluating the efficacy of debulking or cytoreductive procedures. In one series, the benefit from an R2 resection (gross residual disease) has been evaluated. The group that had an R0 (no residual disease) or R1 (microscopic only residual disease) had a median survival of 112 months versus 24 months for those with R2 disease. There was no improvement in survival in those patients with R2 disease compared to patients in which a cytoreduction procedure was not attempted. In yet another study comparing patients presenting with synchronous liver metastases, those with the liver lesions resected in addition to the primary tumor had a median survival of 78 months versus 17 months for patients that had the primary tumor resected but had unresectable liver disease. Therefore, if the extent of disease is not amenable to an R0/R1 resection, alternative nonsurgical treatments should strongly be considered **(Figure 32-4)**.

Radiofrequency ablation (RFA) is an additional technique that is safe and effective for treating hepatic lesions that are either not amenable to resection or in patients that are poor operative candidates. The utilization of laparoscopic RFA to treat neuroendocrine liver metastases has been shown to be possible with limited procedure related morbidity. Using laparoscopic RFA, the 5-year survival after the diagnosis of liver metastases was 57% and in the approximately one half of patients that had symptoms, 94% had symptomatic relief post-operatively which lasted a median of 11 months. Although less morbid than hepatic resections, there is some potential for complications associated with this procedure. For example, the necrotic liver that remains after ablation is prone to infection and the subsequent development of a hepatic abscess; this risk is especially heightened in the setting of a prior biliary-enteric anastomoses such as in those that have undergone a pancreaticoduodenectomy.

Much of the morbidity associated with advanced disease is related to replacement of hepatic parenchyma with bulky tumor. Liver-directed techniques may help to lessen the tumor burden, allowing for control of symptoms in addition to limiting hepatic disease progression with

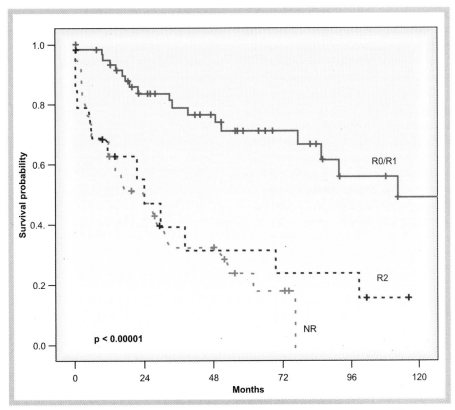

Figure 32-4: Kaplan-Meier survival curve demonstrating the significant difference in survival between those with no or microscopic residual disease (R0 or R1, respectively) and those with gross residual disease (R2) or not resected (NR). This figure was published in Bloomston M, Muscarella P, Shah MH, Frankel WL, Al-Saif O, Martin EW, Ellison EC. Cytoreduction results in high perioperative mortality and decreased survival in patients undergoing pancreatectomy for neuroendocrine tumors of the pancreas. J Gastrointest Surg 2006;10:1361-70. © Elsevier 2006. Reprinted with permission from Elsevier

minimal systemic effects. Transarterial chemoembolization (TACE) and Yttrium-90 (Y-90) radioembolization are two types of liver-directed therapy for unresectable hepatic lesions.

TACE is a liver-directed therapy that combines total hepatic or selective hepatic arterial injection of both embolic material and chemotherapy agents. Bland embolization, not using chemotherapy, has also been applied, but has been shown to be less effective. This technique takes advantage of the fact that hepatic parenchyma is largely supplied by the portal system, but hepatic neoplasms are primarily supplied by the arterial system. Therefore, therapy directed into the hepatic arterial system is preferentially targeted to the neoplasm with relative sparing of the normal parenchyma, thereby allowing substantially higher doses of chemotherapeutic agents to be delivered to the tumor tissue. The embolic material provides an ischemic component to therapy and also helps to stagnate the chemotherapeutic agents. Several agents have been used either alone or in combination, including doxorubicin, adriamycin, cisplatin,

mitomycin and 5-fluorouracil. Common side effects include those of postembolization syndrome with symptoms of abdominal pain, fever and malaise. Postembolization syndrome is usually self-limited. Other complications range from mild hepatic dysfunction with transient elevations in hepatic enzymes to severe complications such as fulminant hepatic failure and infection of necrotic tumor. Side effects of the individual chemotherapeutic agents should also be considered. For example, post-procedural MUGA and hearing exams are routinely performed in our patients treated with doxorubicin and cisplatin, respectively. Although not curative, the response rates to TACE are respectable and reported to be 70-90%. The 5-year survival is doubled when compared to medical management only (50% vs 25%) and many patients have substantial relief of symptoms. TACE and other regional therapies such as Y-90 radioembolization, may also serve as a bridge to resection or possibly even orthotopic liver transplant.

Y-90 radioembolization is an additional locoregional therapy that is proving to be safe and effective in both primary and secondary liver tumors. Many hepatic malignancies are radiosensitive; however, external beam radiation is limited by the intolerance of hepatic parenchyma to radiation. Y-90 is a pure beta-emitting radioisotope that may be irreversibly bound to micro-spheres. These microspheres are administered via the hepatic arterial system and are preferentially distributed toward the metastatic tumors. The mean depth of penetration of Y-90 radiation is only 2.5 mm; therefore, there is relative sparing of normal parenchyma. The radiologic response rate ranges 50-63%. The treatment is generally well tolerated. Further investigation is needed to determine the relative roles of TACE and radioemboli-zation. Y-90 may also be linked to octreotide and systemically administered to target radiation therapy to the somatostatin receptor on PNET cells. Although pro-mising, this technique still requires further investigation.

Although a detailed discussion of systemic chemo-therapy options for PNETs is beyond the scope of this chapter, it does deserve to be mentioned. Systemic chemotherapy for PNETs has generally been regarded as ineffective and is notorious for being poorly tolerated. The most effective regimen seems to be a combination of streptozocin, 5-FU and doxorubicin. This combination has had variable response rates in different studies. One large retrospective study of 84 patients showed that this combination has a response rate of 39%, with a median survival of 37 months. However, toxicities associated with the treatment were significant, with 23% of patients reporting grade 3 or 4 toxicities. Toxicities include nausea and vomiting, renal toxicity and cardiac toxicity. Dacarbazine and temozolomide have been used as alternative agents for streptozocin. Similar to the chemotherapy for small cell lung cancer, cisplatin and etoposide have been used in poorly differentiated PNETs. Cisplatin and irinotecan is another combination that has shown a response in poorly differentiated tumors. Newer agents being studied include the small molecule inhibitors such as the tyrosine kinase inhibitors.

Somatostatin analogues, such as octreotide, lantreotide and long acting depots, have been used to provide symptomatic relief from hormone hypersecretion and also in an attempt to halt tumor growth. Biologic response, as indicated by a decrease in tumor markers, is commonly seen and may be related to the induction of apoptosis. However, a survival benefit has yet to be shown. Rapidly progressive disease may be less likely to be stabilized with administration of somatostatin analogues. Resistance of PNETs to somatostatin therapy may develop with refractory symptoms related to hormone excess and tumor growth. The addition of IFN-α to somatostatin therapy has been attempted; however, there are significant side effects with limited therapeutic benefit. Associated side effects of somatostatin analogues include glucose intolerance, nausea, abdominal pain, mild steatorrhea and rarely gastric atony. The risk of cholelithiasis is increased with long-term treatment with somatostatin analogues, although the stones rarely lead to symptoms.

Summary

- PNET are a rare, heterogeneous group with a wide spectrum of aggressiveness and functionality.
- PNET may be classified as either functional or non-functional. Between 40-60% of lesions are non-functional. Functional lesions may further be characterized as insulinomas, gastrinomas, VIPomas, glucagonomas, somatostatinomas, GRFomas, ACTHomas or PTHomas.
- With the exception of insulinomas, the majority of PNET are malignant although most have indolent progression.
- Most PNET occur sporadically, however, they may be inherited. MEN-1, VHL, neurofibromatosis 1 and tuberous sclerosis are associated to varying degrees with PNETs.
- CgA and PP may be used as tumor markers in addition to the specific hormones released from functional tumors.
- We prefer to use CT A/P with arterial contrast and fine cuts through the pancreas in addition to EUS as the primary radiologic work-up.
- The only curative and preferred treatment for all sporadic PNETs is surgical resection.
- The appropriate treatment for inherited PNETs (e.g. MEN-1 and VHL) is more controversial. Many recommend that resection be considered in lesions that are greater than 2-3 cm in diameter. Inherited insulinomas are typically resected regardless of size, due to the lack of effective treatment for symptoms.
- The liver is the most frequent site of metastases. The resection of liver metastases provides a survival benefit. Liver lesions that are incompletely resectable should be approached from a multimodal approach.
- Somatostatin analogues should be considered for symptomatic relief.
- Chemotherapy is not highly effective and generally poorly tolerated.

Landmark Papers

1. Alexakis N, Neoptolemos JP. Pancreatic neuroendocrine tumours. Best Prac Res Clin Gastroent 2008;22:183-205.
2. Anderson MA, Carpenter S, Thompson NW, Nostrant TT, Elta GH, Scheiman JM. Endoscopic Ultrasound is highly accurate and directs management in patients with neuroendocrine tumors of the pancreas. Am J Gastroent 2000;95:2271-7.

3. Berna MJ, Hoffman KM, Long SH, et al. Serum Gastrin in Zollinger-Ellison Syndrome: II. Prospective study of gastrin provocative testing in 293 patients from the national institutes of health and comparison with 537 cases from the literature. Evaluation of diagnostic criteria, proposal of new criteria and correlations with clinical and tumoral features. Medicine 2006;85:331-64.
4. Bloomston M, Muscarella P, Shah MH, Frankel WL, Al-Saif O, Martin EW, Ellison EC. Cytoreduction results in high perioperative mortality and decreased survival in patients undergoing pancreatectomy for neuroendocrine tumors of the pancreas. J Gastrointest Surg 2006;10:1361-70.
5. Chen H, Hardacre JM, Uzar A, Cameron JL, Choti MA. Isolated liver metastases from neuroendocrine tumors: does resection prolong survival? J Am Coll Surg 1998; 187:88-97.
6. Metz DC, Jensen RT. Gastrointestinal neuroendocrine tumors: pancreatic endocrine tumors. Gastroenterology 2008; 135:1469-92.
7. Norton JA, Fraker DL, Alexander HR, et al. Surgery to cure Zollinger-Ellison syndrome. NEJM 1999;341:635-44.
8. Rinde G, Kloppel G, Alhman H, et al. TNM staging of foregut (neuro)endocrine tumors: a consensus proposal including a grading system. Virchows Arch 2006;449:395-401.
9. Sachs T, Pratt WB, Callery MP, Vollmer CM. The incidental pancreatic lesion: nuisance or threat? J Gastrointest Surg 2009; 13:405-15.
10. Solicia E, Kloppel G, Sobin LH, et al. Histological typing of endocrine tumours. Springer 1999;56-60.
11. Triopez F, Goudet R, Dosseh D, et al. Is surgery beneficial for MEN1 patients with small (≤ 2 cm), nonfunctioning pancreaticoduodenal endocrine tumor? An analysis of 65 patients from the GTE. World J Surg 2006;30:654-62.

Level of Evidence Table

Recommendation	Best level of evidence	Grade	References
The secretin stimulation test (2 μ/kg) should be the first-line provocation test for the diagnosis of ZES. For patients with baseline < 10-fold fasting serum gastrin, an increase of ≥120 pg/mL is 94% sensitive and 100% specific	2A	B	1
EUS should be used as a primary diagnostic modality in the evaluation of PNET	4	B	2,3
Patients with sporadic localized PNET should be offered surgical exploration for resection and possible cure. Complete gross (R0/R1) resection should be attempted	2B	B	4-7
Surgical resection should be performed for localized PNETs in MEN-1 patients	4	B	8-14
Directed therapies (resection, ablation, embolization) of isolated liver metastases should be offered	4	B	15-18

References

1. Berna MJ, Hoffman KM, Long SH, et al. Medicine 2006; 85(6):331-64.
2. Patel KK Kim MK. Neuroendocrine tumors of the pancreas: endoscopic diagnosis. Curr Opin Gastroenterol 2008; 24:638-42.
3. Rosch T, Lightdale CJ, Botet JF, et al. Localization of pancreatic endocrine tumors by endoscopic ultrasonography. N Engl J Med 1992; 326:1721-6.
4. Norton JA, Fraker DL, Alexander HR, et al. Surgery increases survival in patients with gastrinoma. Ann Surg 2006; 244:410-9.
5. Schurr PG, Strate T, Rese K, et al. Aggressive surgery improves long-term survival in neuroendocrine pancreatic tumors: an institutional experience. Ann Surg 2007; 245:273-81.
6. Dralle H, Krohn SL, Karges W, et al. Surgery of resectable nonfunctioning neuroendocrine pancreatic tumors. World J Surg 2004; 28:1248-60.
7. Bloomston M, Muscarella P, Shah MH, et al. Cytoreduction results in high perioperative mortality and decreased survival in patients undergoing pancreatectomy for neuroendocrine tumors of the pancreas. J Gastrointest Surg 2006; 10:1361-70.
8. Kouvaraki MA, Shapiro SE, Cote GJ, et al. Management of pancreatic endocrine tumors in multiple endocrine neoplasia type 1. World J Surg 2006; 30:643-53.
9. Norton JA, Alexander HR, Fraker DL, et al. Comparison of surgical results in patients with advanced and limited disease with multiple endocrine neoplasia type 1 and Zollinger-Ellison syndrome. Ann Surg 2001; 234:495-505; discussion 505-6.
10. Tonelli F, Fratini G, Nesi G, et al. Pancreatectomy in multiple endocrine neoplasia type 1-related gastrinomas and pancreatic endocrine neoplasias. Ann Surg 2006; 244:61-70.
11. Mortellaro VE, Hochwald SN, McGuigan JE, et al. Long-term results of a selective surgical approach to management of Zollinger-Ellison syndrome in patients with MEN-1. Am Surg 2009; 75:730-3.
12. MacFarlane MP, Fraker DL, Alexander HR, et al. Prospective study of surgical resection of duodenal and pancreatic gastrinomas in multiple endocrine neoplasia type 1. Surgery 1995; 118:973-9; discussion 979-80.

13. Triponez F, Goudet P, Dosseh D, et al. Is surgery beneficial for MEN1 patients with small (< or = 2 cm), nonfunctioning pancreaticoduodenal endocrine tumor? An analysis of 65 patients from the GTE. World J Surg 2006; 30:654-62; discussion 663-4.

14. Hausman MS, Jr., Thompson NW, Gauger PG, et al. The surgical management of MEN-1 pancreatoduodenal neuroendocrine disease. Surgery 2004; 136:1205-11.

15. Gomez D, Malik HZ, Al-Mukthar A, et al. Hepatic resection for metastatic gastrointestinal and pancreatic neuroendocrine tumours: outcome and prognostic predictors. HPB (Oxford) 2007; 9:345-51.

16. Chamberlain RS, Canes D, Brown KT, et al. Hepatic neuroendocrine metastases: does intervention alter outcomes? J Am Coll Surg 2000; 190:432-45.

17. Musunuru S, Chen H, Rajpal S, et al. Metastatic neuroendocrine hepatic tumors: resection improves survival. Arch Surg 2006; 141:1000-4; discussion 1005.

18. Gurusamy KS, Ramamoorthy R, Sharma D, et al. Liver resection versus other treatments for neuroendocrine tumours in patients with resectable liver metastases. Cochrane Database Syst Rev 2009; CD007060.

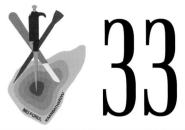

33

Pancreatic Cancer

Narcis Octavian Zarnescu, Isam W Nasr, Mario Lora, A James Moser

Introduction

Pancreatic cancer is the fourth leading cause of cancer death in the United States. Estimates of the American Cancer Society indicate that nearly 37,700 new cases of pancreatic cancer will be diagnosed in the United States in 2008, while almost 34,300 people will die of the disease. At the time of diagnosis, only 10-15% of patients have tumors confined to the pancreas, 35-40% have locally advanced disease and more than 50% have distant spread leaving only 10-20% as candidates for resection.

Pancreatic cancer remains a diagnostic and therapeutic dilemma as early lesions cause few symptoms, strategies for screening remain unproven and current treatment modalities demonstrate poor response rates and 5-year actual survival.

Anatomy of the Pancreas

The pancreas is a retroperitoneal organ located in the lesser sac posterior to the greater curvature of the stomach. It is divided into four anatomic regions: the head, neck, body and tail.

The *pancreatic head* lies medial to the C-loop of the duodenum posterior to the transverse mesocolon. It is anterior to the vena cava, the right renal artery and both renal veins. The *neck* of the pancreas lies directly over the portal vein. At the inferior border of the neck of the pancreas, the superior mesenteric vein joins the splenic vein, which eventually forms the portal vein. The *body* of the pancreas is anterior to the splenic artery and vein. The *tail* is the small segment that lies within the splenic hilum and is anterior to the left kidney. The posterior border of the pancreas lacks a peritoneal investment, exposing the pancreatic lymphatics to the retroperitoneum.

Branches of the celiac and superior mesenteric arteries (SMA) give rise to the vasculature of the pancreas. The head is supplied by an arcade formed by the gastroduodenal artery (GDA) and the SMA: The GDA, which is the first branch of the common hepatic artery, gives rise to the superior pancreaticoduodenal artery, which divides into anterior and posterior branches. The inferior pancreaticoduodenal artery is the first branch of the SMA and divides into anterior and posterior branches. These four arteries form an arcade which provides a blood supply shared by the pancreatic head as well as the second and third portions of the duodenum. The body and tail are supplied by branches of the splenic artery. The SMA branches into the inferior pancreatic artery that runs along the inferior border of the body and tail. The splenic artery and the inferior pancreatic artery, which run parallel to each other, are connected by the lateral, dorsal and the transverse pancreatic arteries. The venous drainage of the pancreas follows a pattern similar to the arterial supply, where the veins run anterior to the arteries.

Lymphatic drainage is abundant and diffusely spread throughout the organ. The lymphatic vessels drain into five main nodal groups: The superior nodes drain the upper half of the head of the pancreas and are located along the superior border of the pancreas and celiac trunk. The anterior lymphatics drain to the prepyloric and infrapyloric nodes. The inferior group of nodes drain into the superior mesenteric and periaortic nodes and are along the inferior border of the pancreatic head and body. The posterior pancreaticoduodenal lymph nodes drain into right periaortic nodes and include the distal common bile duct and ampullary lymphatics. The splenic group of nodes drains the tail of the pancreas along the splenic vessels and into the interceliomesenteric lymph nodes **(Figure 33-1)**.

Epidemiology

Pancreatic cancer is ranked 13th in terms of incidence and represents the fourth leading cause of cancer death in the United States; 5-year survival is less than 5%. Most patients are between 65 and 80 years old at diagnosis and only 10% of all cases are under the age of 50; the risk increases sharply after age 50. Incidence is equal among men and women. African Americans appear to have a higher incidence of pancreatic cancer than white Americans.

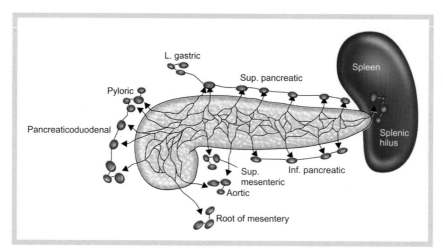

Figure 33-1: Lymph nodes for pancreatic drainage. (Reproduced with permission from Skandalakis JE, Gray SW, Rowe JS Jr, et al. Anatomical complications of pancreatic surgery. Contemp Surg 1979;15:17)

Risk Factors

Both environmental and genetic factors contribute to the risk of pancreatic cancer. Smokers have a twofold increased risk of pancreatic cancer compared to non-smokers. The risk increases with duration and intensity of smoking. Diets high in fat and low in fruits, vegetables and fiber were once thought to increase the risk of pancreatic cancer; however, a recent report on almost 125,000 patients did not validate this observation. Patients with chronic pancreatitis have a 20-fold increased risk of developing pancreatic cancer. There may be a link between chronic inflammation and the rate of genetic mutations required for oncogenesis. There is a positive association between pancreatic cancer and diabetes mellitus. One meta-analysis identified a relative risk for pancreatic cancer of two (95% CI 1.2-3.2) in patients with longstanding diabetes (more than five years), similar to recent results of a prospective study (RR 1.49 for men and RR 1.51 for women). Approximately 1% of diabetics age 50 or older will develop PC within 3 years.

Ten percent of cases have a familial genetic basis. Individuals with three first-degree relatives have a 32-fold increased risk. Numerous germ line mutations are associated with pancreatic cancer **(Table 33-1)**. A strong family history of pancreatic cancer or hereditary pancreatitis requires screening in specialized centers with endoscopic ultrasound (EUS) and molecular analysis of

TABLE 33-1	Genetic mutations associated with higher risk of pancreatic cancer			
Gene mutation	**Syndrome**	**Associated cancers**	**Relative risk**	**Risk by age 70**
PRSS1	Hereditary pancreatitis	-	50-80X	25-40%
STK11/LKB1	Peutz-Jeghers		132X	30-60%
P16 (CDKN2A)	FAMMM	Melanoma	20-34X	10%
BRCA2	Familial breast and ovarian cancer syndromes	Breast, ovary, prostate	3.5-10X	5%
BRCA1			2X	1%
MLH1, MSH2, MSH6, PMS1, PMS2	HNPCC	Colorectal, stomach, biliary tract, endometrial, ovarian, ureter, renal, brain	—	<5%
TP53	Li-Fraumeni syndrome	Breast, brain, lung, leukemia	—	—
APC	Familial adenomatous polyposis	Colon	4.5X	—

Abbreviations: FAMMM, familial atypical multiple mole melanoma syndrome; HNPCC, hereditary nonpolyposis colorectal cancer syndrome

pancreatic juice. Other possible risk factors are previous gastric surgery, previous cholecystectomy and primary sclerosing cholangitis.

Clinical Presentation

Obstructive jaundice is the most common presentation of resectable pancreatic cancer and is usually caused by tumors in the pancreatic head. Additional symptoms include pruritus, acholic stools and tea-colored urine. Physical findings include scleral icterus, hepatomegaly, a palpable gallbladder (Courvoisier's sign) and skin excoriation secondary to pruritus. Vague abdominal pain in the upper quadrants and epigastrium could be present. Back pain, which is due to invasion of the retroperitoneal nerve plexuses, is typically an indicator of advanced disease. Also, weight loss, anorexia, fatigue and malaise could be present. Recent onset diabetes within 1-2 years of diagnosis is described in 20% of patients. In 5% of acute pancreatitis cases, the cause is a mass lesion obstructing the pancreatic duct. 'Idiopathic' acute pancreatitis in the elderly should raise the suspicion of a mass lesion obstructing the pancreatic duct.

Nausea and vomiting secondary to gastric outlet obstruction is usually an indication of locally advanced disease. Signs of advanced disease include cachexia, palpable metastatic disease in the left supraclavicular region (Virchow's node) palpable nodules in the liver, palpable metastatic disease in the periumbilical area (Sister Mary Joseph's node) and pelvic metastatic disease palpable anteriorly on rectal examination (Blumer's shelf).

Pittsburgh Algorithm for Treating Pancreatic Cancer

Accurate staging of pancreatic cancer is required for two reasons: to identify potential surgical candidates with localized disease and to tailor therapy for patients with locally-advanced or metastatic disease and guide best palliation. The NCCN Pancreatic Adenocarcinoma Guidelines (www.nccn.org) advocate investigational options for patients with all stages of pancreatic cancer due to the poor outcomes achieved with current methodology (Figure 33-2).

Biochemical Tests

Direct hyperbilirubinemia and elevated alkaline phosphatase are typically present, in addition to a prolonged prothrombin time which is secondary to decrease vitamin K absorption resulting from prolonged biliary obstruction. Seventy-five percent of patients with pancreatic cancer have increased serum levels of carbohydrate antigen 19-9 (CA19-9), a Lewis blood group-related mucin glycoprotein that is not expressed by 5% of the population. CA 19-9 is elevated in 10% of patients with benign pancreatic or hepatobiliary diseases and cannot be used as screening tool because of insufficient sensitivity and specificity. Other potential serum markers for pancreatic cancer include: CA50, CA252, DU-PAN-2, Span-1 and CAM17.1.

Radiographic Evaluation

The majority of patients who present with either abdominal pain or jaundice undergo a right upper quadrant

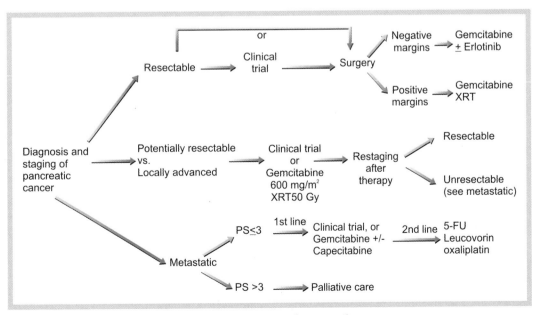

Figure 33-2: Management of pancreatic cancer

TABLE 33-2	Criteria for resectability of pancreatic cancer		
	Resectable	**Borderline resectable**	**Locally advanced**
SMA	No extension; normal fat plane	Tumor abutment less than one half of vessel diameter of the circumference of the artery; periarterial stranding	Encased (> one half diameter)
Celiac axis/ Hepatic artery	No extension	Short-segment encasement/abutment of the common hepatic artery(typically at the gastroduodenalorigin); may require vascular resection	Encased and no technical option for reconstruction, extension to celiac axis
SMV/PV	Patent	Short-segment occlusion with options for reconstruction; segmental venous occlusion alone without SMA involvement (rare)	Occluded

Abbrevations: SMA, superior mesenteric artery; SMV/PV, superior mesenteric vein/portal vein

ultrasound. The typical appearance of pancreatic cancer on ultrasonography is a hypoechoic mass. Additional information that is provided by the ultrasound is the presence of peripancreatic lymphadenopathy as well as liver metastases and dilated bile ducts. Limitations of transabdominal ultrasonography include operator dependence, body habitus and bowel gas artifacts. Around 60-70% of patients with pancreatic cancer will have a discernable mass on ultrasound.

Multidetector, pancreatic mass protocol computed tomography CT (MDCT) using oral water with arterial- and venous-phase imaging of IV contrast is the imaging procedure of choice to assess resectability and detect distant metastases. Encasement of the portal or superior mesenteric veins as well as the involvement of the superior mesenteric, celiac or hepatic arteries with or without occlusion are ominous signs of unresectability **(Table 32-2)**. Prior studies indicate that tumor involvement of more than half of the circumference of major vessels portends unresectability **(Figure 33-3)**.

Additional CT features include: involvement of the celiac plexus for body cancers anterolateral to the celiac trunk, dilation of the main pancreatic duct or bile duct or both ('double duct sign'), lymph node involvement based on increased size and abnormal shape. The accuracy of CT for nodal staging has recently been questioned. In addition, hepatic metastatic deposits can be detected whereas peritoneal metastases cannot directly be visualized, but can be suspected from the presence of ascites or omental caking. Generally, a chest radiograph or CT scan (with or without intravenous contrast) is often performed during initial staging evaluation.

Endoscopic Ultrasound

Endoscopic Ultrasound (EUS) is used to stage patients with pancreatic tumors and provides a cytologic diagnosis as required for operative decision-making or to administer

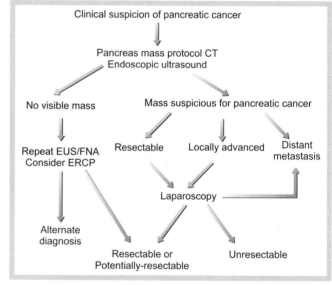

Figure 33-3: Diagnosis of pancreatic cancer

chemotherapy/radiation. The sensitivity of EUS is 88.8%, specificity 100%, PPV 100%, NVP 99%, with an accuracy of 99.1%. However, EUS is very operator dependent and may overestimate the degree of vascular involvement. EUS has superior resolution for small lesions of 2-3 mm and aids in defining the relationship between tumor and adjacent blood vessels (portal vein, mesenteric vessels). It also provides additional diagnostic information in patients with nonspecific CT/MRI findings such as dilatation of the pancreatic duct and enlargement of the head of the pancreas. One of the applications of EUS is injecting ethanol into the celiac plexus (neurolysis) for pain control.

Laparoscopy

Laparoscopy is an integral part of the diagnosis, staging and management of pancreatic cancer. The incidence of unsuspected metastases is 10-40% among patients undergoing exploratory laparotomy for potentially resectable lesions. Laparoscopic ultrasound raises the diagnostic accuracy of staging laparoscopy to that of laparotomy with less morbidity and mortality. Advanced laparoscopic techniques allow synchronous pancreatic resections to be performed as well as palliative procedures including choledocojejunostomy, gastrojejunostomy and celiac plexus neurolysis.

Peritoneal Cytology

The prognostic significance and therapeutic implications of positive peritoneal washings remain controversial. The question of whether positive cytology correlates with prognosis remains unanswered, although a recent small prospective study has shown that patients with minute cancer cell dissemination detected by Real-time polymerase chain reaction (RT-PCR) in peritoneal washings have worse outcomes.

Pancreatic Intraepithelial Neoplasia

Pancreatic intraepithelial neoplasia (PanINs) are lesions of the pancreatic duct that are identified microscopically and characterized by lack of invasion of the basement membrane. They are one of three preinvasive lesions of the pancreas that have been identified, the others being mucinous cystic neoplasms (MCN) and intraductal papillary mucinous neoplasms (IPMNs). PanINs are graded 1-3, with the grade of lesion based on nuclear anomalies, degree of necrosis, rate of mitoses and the presence of a papillary component. The incidence of PanINs increases with age. Grade 1 PanIN can be identified in up to 40% of patients who do not have pancreatic cancer, however, grade 3 PanIN has been found in up to 50% of patients with invasive carcinoma. The frequency and speed with which PanINs progress to invasive cancer is unknown. Most are small (less than 0.5 cm) and clinically silent. K_{ras} proto-oncogene mutations have been described as leading to the development of these lesions and mouse models of PanINs are currently under investigation. PanINs have been described to produce lobulocentric atrophy of the pancreatic parenchyma which can at times be identified by EUS. An association with acinar-ductal metaplasia has been described, which suggests that PanINs may arise from acinar cell origin. Although not currently relevant as a screening tool, the identification of these precursor lesions may yield important advances in the management of high risk patients and continue to help to understand the progression of pancreatic cancer.

Surgical Resection

Surgical resection is the only modality that increases 5-year actual survival and may lead to cure. There is good evidence that the achievement of a negative surgical margin (R0 resection) is the surgeon's major contribution to long-term survival.

Preoperative Biliary Decompression

For patients with obstructive jaundice, preoperative biliary decompression has been shown to increase overall morbidity and mortality rates after resection. A recent meta-analysis confirmed the absence of medical benefit following biliary stenting. A metal biliary stent may be required for patients with resectable pancreatic cancer undergoing neoadjuvant therapy. In our experience, metal biliary stents are associated with fewer stent-related complications than plastic and provide a longer duration of patency without increasing the risk of subsequent surgical resection.

Strategies for Resection

The type of resection is tailored to the anatomic location of the tumor and its adjacent vasculature. The majority of lesions are located in the pancreatic head and require pancreatoduodenectomy (Whipple operation). Lesions in the body and tail require distal pancreatectomy and occasionally central pancreatectomy. The search for distant metastases is the first stage of the operation. The liver, peritoneal surfaces and omentum are checked for cancer implants. Suspicious lesions are sent for frozen section. The presence of tumor in the periaortic lymph nodes of the celiac axis indicates metastatic disease and is a contraindication to resection. Local invasion into the inferior vena cava, aorta, superior mesenteric artery (SMA), superior mesenteric vein (SMV) and portal vein is then assessed after division of the attachments of the pancreatic head to surrounding structures (Kocher maneuver) **(Figure 33-4)**.

The standard radical pancreatoduodenectomy operation (PD) requires resection of the pancreatic head, gallbladder, distal common bile duct, duodenum and distal stomach with extirpation of lymph nodes associated with the common bile duct, pylorus and anterior and posterior surfaces of the pancreatic head.

The procedure is typically performed either through a midline incision or through bilateral subcostal incisions. The initial step involves a thorough assessment of the abdomen for metastatic disease. This includes inspection of all peritoneal surfaces as well as palpation of the liver, in conjunction with intraoperative ultrasound of the liver for suspicious lesions. Celiac, periportal and interaortocaval lymph nodes should also be inspected. All suspicious lesions should be biopsied and sent for frozen section. The next step consists of an extensive mobilization of the duodenum and the head of the pancreas from the underlying aorta and vena cava by performing a Kocher

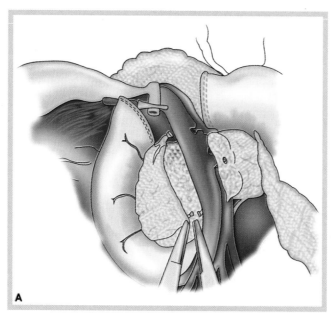

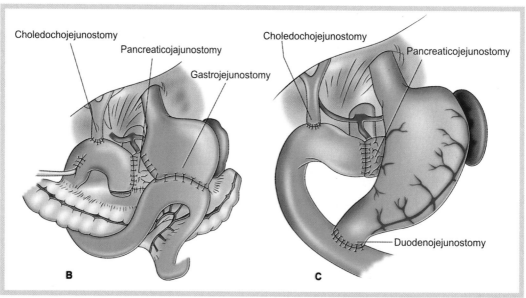

Figures 33-4A to C: (A) Division of pancreas and exposure of portal vein. (B) Reconstruction following radical pancreatoduodenectomy. (C) Reconstruction following pylorus preserving pancreatoduodenectomy

maneuver. Involvement of the tumor with the superior mesenteric artery can then be assessed by palpating underneath the mobilized duodenum and head of pancreas. In order to gain access to the third and fourth portions of the duodenum, the hepatic flexure of the colon is mobilized. The mesocolon is separated from the head of the pancreas to expose the superior mesenteric vein. The SMV dissection is continued until it connects with the portal vein. After the stomach and the proximal duodenum are mobilized, the duodenum is transected 2 cm distal to the pylorus in the case of a pylorus-preserving pancreaticoduodenectomy, whereas in a classic radical pancreatoduodenectomy, an antrectomy is

performed. The next step is dissection of the hepatoduodenal ligament. The GDA is then identified and ligated at its origin from the common hepatic artery. Care must be taken to make sure that there remains strong flow in the proper hepatic artery after occlusion of the GDA. If not, then there is likely to be a stenosis at the origin of the celiac artery or common hepatic artery that needs to be addressed prior to the radical pancreatoduodenectomy procedure. The gallbladder is removed and the common hepatic duct is transected approximately 2 cm above its insertion into the head of the pancreas. Next, the proximal jejunum is mobilized and transected 10-20 cm from the ligament of Treitz. The mesentery is divided and the fourth portion of the duodenum is dissected off of the pancreas. The stump of the jejunum is reflected through the defect in the transverse mesocolon so that it is positioned laterally to the SMV. After that, the neck of the pancreas is transected and the specimen is dissected sharply off the SMV, portal vein and SMA. The distal stump of the jejunum is brought through the transverse mesocolon and a two-layer end-to-side pancreaticojejunostomy is performed first. Proximal to that, a single-layer hepaticojejunal anastomosis is performed. Finally, a duodenojejunostomy is performed distal to the choledochojejunostomy. It may be helpful to leave the afferent limb short enough so that an endoscopic cholangiogram or pancreatogram may be performed in the future as necessary. One closed suction drain may be placed adjacent to the pancreatic anastomosis.

Extended radical lymphadenectomy involves standard PD plus distal gastrectomy and retroperitoneal lymph node dissection extending from the right renal hilum to the left lateral border of the aorta and from the portal vein to the inferior mesenteric artery. Radical resection raises overall morbidity but does not convey a survival advantage. As mentioned above, an additional modification to the standard radical pancreatoduodenectomy procedure is the pylorus-preserving radical pancreatoduodenectomy. This operation was devised in an attempt to eliminate the morbidity associated with postgastrectomy syndromes and involves preservation of the right gastroepiploic arcade and/or the right gastric artery to protect the blood supply to the duodenum. Some studies have shown a reduction in operative time and blood loss using a pylorus preserving approach, however no significant differences in mortality have been noted when comparing the two procedures.

Invasion of the portal vein (PV) or superior mesenteric vein (SMV) is often considered a contraindication to resection. However, resection of the portal vein and the superior mesenteric vein can achieve R0 resection with low morbidity and mortality in high volume centers. In a comprehensive review of synchronous PV/SMV resection for pancreatic cancer, 23 studies included 1646 patients from 52 centers without an adverse impact of PV/SMV invasion on 5-year survival rate. Resection is rarely justified in the presence of extensive portal vein encasement that precludes an R0 or R1 (microscopically positive) margin status.

Postoperative Outcomes

Mortality rates are in the range of 2-3%. Pancreatic fistula is one of the most frequent and serious complications, with an incidence ranging from 5% to 15%. It is defined as any measurable drain volume with an amylase content three times that of the serum level on or after postoperative day three. With adequate drainage and nutrition, pancreatic

fistulas usually heal within 8 weeks. Delayed gastric emptying occurs in 15-40% of cases; delayed gastric emptying is the most common indication of pancreatic fistula. Pancreatic exocrine insufficiency and steatorrhea are long-term complications treated with pancreatic enzymes at mealtime.

Complications following pancreatic resection are classified into five grades of outcome, as reported by DeOliveira, et al in *Annals of Surgery* in 2006. The total incidence of complications in the study was 58.5%, and the specific incidence of complication per grade is noted in parentheses following the respective number below:
- Grade I (10%): no need for specific intervention
- Grade II (30%): need for drug therapy such as antibiotics
- Grade III (13.5%): need for invasive therapy
- Grade IV (3%): organ dysfunction with ICU stay
- Grade V (2%): death

Tumors in the body and tail of the pancreas usually present at an advanced stage having already metastasized or locally invaded adjacent structures, with only 10% of tumors being resectable at presentation. Resection usually involves distal pancreatectomy with or without splenectomy. Complications include subphrenic abscess in around 5-15% of cases, as well as pancreatic fistula in approximately 30% of patients. These can be managed with percutaneous drainage.

Staging

The current American Joint Committee on Cancer (AJCC) staging system for pancreatic cancer is reproduced in **Table 33-3**. Although staging may be implied preoperatively for the purposes of assignment to clinical trials, the true stage of a patient with pancreatic cancer can only be determined after resection and pathological analysis. At least ten regional lymph nodes should be included with the resected pancreatic specimen to allow for accurate staging. In addition to tumor size, lymph node status and distant metastasis, other factors that influence survival are: perineural invasion, angiolymphatic invasion, histologic grade, DNA content and genetic modifications.

Adjuvant Therapy for Resected Pancreatic Cancer

Gemcitabine therapy alone was shown to be an effective adjuvant chemotherapy modality in the CONKO-001 trial, where gemcitabine was compared with observation. Median disease free survival in the gemcitabine group was 13.4 months versus 6.9 months in the control group. Disease free survival was also significantly improved in the gemcitabine group.

At least five major trials have attempted to address the question of whether chemotherapy or chemoradiation are effective adjuvant therapies for resected pancreatic cancer.

TABLE 33-3	AJCC staging system for pancreatic adenocarcinoma	
Definitions	**6th AJCC staging system**	**Surgical classification**
Primary tumor (T)		
Tis	In situ	
T0	No evidence of primary	
T1	Limited to pancreas,$\leq$ 2 cm	
T2	Limited to pancreas,$\geq$ 2 cm	
T3	Extends beyond pancreas, no involvement of CA or SMA	
T4	Involves CA or SMA	
Regional lymph nodes (N)		
N0	No nodal metastasis	
N1	Regional lymph node metastasis	
Distant metastasis (M)		
M0	No distant metastasis	
M1	Distant metastasis	
Stage groupings		
Stage 0	TisN0M0	In situ disease
Stage IA	T1N0M0	Resectable
Stage IB	T2N0M0	Resectable
Stage IIA	T3N0M0	Potentially resectable
Stage IIB	T1-3N1M0	Potentially resectable
Stage III	T4N0-1M0	Unresectable due to locally advanced disease
Stage IV	T1-4N0-1M1	Unresectable due to distant metastasis

Reproduced with permission from AJCC staging manual, 6th edition
Abbreviations: CA, celiac axis; SMA, superior mesenteric artery

The data from these trials were pooled in a meta-analysis that showed 25% significant reduction in the risk of death with chemotherapy, with an increase in median survival from 13.5 to 19.0 months. As for chemoradiation, there appeared to be no significant difference in the risk of death, with a median survival of 15.8 months with chemoradiation and 15.2 months without. However, a subgroup analysis of patients with positive resection margins showed that chemoradiation was more effective than chemotherapy alone.

Treatment of Locally Advanced Pancreatic Cancer

Vascular involvement often renders pancreatic cancer unresectable and unlike other cancers, pathologic downgrading is very difficult to achieve. Multiple trials involving chemoradiation have been performed. One French study compared gemcitabine vs chemoradiation using 5-FU and cisplatin. Overall survival was shorter in the chemoradiation arm (8.6 vs 13 months). One-year survival was also decreased (32% vs 53%).

A recent study (ECOG 4201) comparing gemcitabine in combination with radiation therapy versus gemcitabine alone had more promising results for locally advanced disease. Overall survival was increased in the chemoradiation group to 11 months versus 9.2 months in the control group. Another impressive result is that the 24-month survival was tripled (12% vs 4%).

Treatment of Metastatic Pancreatic Cancer

An early study comparing gemcitabine to 5-FU showed that gemcitabine is more effective in alleviating the disease-related symptoms of patients with advanced and metastatic pancreatic cancer. The clinical benefit response was 23.8% for gemcitabine treated patients versus 4.8% for 5-FU treated patients. The survival rate at 12 months was 18% for gemcitabine and 2% for 5-FU. The median survival was also prolonged: 5.61 months for gemcitabine versus 4.41 months for 5-FU.

To address the issue of patients with gemcitabine refractory pancreatic cancer, the CONKO-003 trial was designed. The patients were randomized to two chemotherapeutic regimens: the first was FF (5-FU plus folinic acid or leucovorin), the second was OFF (FF plus oxaliplatin). The results of the study indicated that alternating OFF/FF and continuous FF leads to significantly longer progression free survival (13 vs 9 weeks) and overall survival compared to FF (20 vs 13 weeks).

Several other studies have been conducted whereby other chemotherapeutic agents have been added to gemcitabine, with no significant improvement in survival. Examples include molecular targeting agents such as cetuximab, bevacizumab, farnesyl transferase inhibitors and metalloproteinase inhibitors. One study showed a modest increase in overall survival by adding erlonitib to gemcitabine (6.24 months vs 5.91 months). There was also an increase in one-year survival with erlonitib plus gemcitabine (23% vs 17%). The AViTA study basically added bevacizumab to erlonitib and gemcitabine versus erlonitib and gemcitabine in patients with metastatic pancreatic cancer. The study showed that the triple combination significantly improved disease free survival (3.6 months vs 4.6 months), but not overall survival (6.0 months vs 7.1 months), compared to gemcitabine plus erlonitib.

Palliation of Symptoms

Most patients with pancreatic cancer present at an advanced stage of disease in which palliation is the most pressing medical need. The goals of palliative treatment are multiple, including reduction of symptoms, improvement of functional status, reduction in length of hospitalization, as well as improvement in overall quality of life.

Surgery (open or laparoscopic) and endoscopic therapy can be used to relieve the symptoms of locally advanced pancreatic cancer causing obstructive jaundice, gastric outlet obstruction and intractable abdominal pain. Obstructive jaundice occurs in 70% of patients with pancreatic cancer. If untreated, obstructive jaundice causes progressive liver dysfunction, severe pruritus associated with cutaneous bile salt deposition, nausea and anorexia.

For patients with metastatic cancer, endoscopic biliary decompression is associated with less procedural morbidity and a shorter hospital stay compared with surgical drainage. Metallic stents are the preferred method for patients with a life expectancy longer than 6 months, whereas less expensive plastic stents are adequate for patients with shorter survival. Complications of endoscopic stents include cholangitis, duodenal perforation, post-sphincterotomy bleeding and post-ERCP-pancreatitis.

Gastric outlet obstruction occurs in up to 20% of patients. The role of a prophylactic gastroenterostomy is still under discussion, but many authors argue that prophylactic bypass performed in a high volume specialty center can be done with little morbidity and improve palliative outcomes. Techniques to relieve duodenal obstruction include laparoscopic gastrojejunostomy and endoscopic metal enteral stents. Recent analysis comparing these techniques showed better results with the endoscopic approach.

Pain is best managed by combining a long-acting narcotic with acetaminophen. When pain relief requires doses of narcotic analgesics causing functional impairment or somnolence, the best method for permanent relief is celiac plexus neurolysis with ethanol under CT or EUS guidance.

Acinar Cell Carcinoma

Although acinar cell carcinoma (ACC) represents less than 2% of all pancreatic malignancies, they are important to discuss due to some unique features from ductal adenocarcinoma of the pancreas. These aggressive tumors are capable of secreting lipase into the circulation, which results in systemic manifestations of this disease. Patients may present with erythema nodosum-like rashes, eosinophilia, subcutaneous fat necrosis and polyarthralgias. ACC can also produce alpha-fetoprotein (AFP), which serves as a useful marker for recurrence and therapeutic response following resection. Although clinical experience with these tumors is limited, the approach to surgical and adjuvant therapy is similar to ductal pancreatic cancer. A recent retrospective analysis suggests that these tumors carry a better prognoisis than the more common ductal type. In addition growing anecdotal experience at several high volume pancreatic center suggest that these tumors may highly be sensitive to platinum based regimens.

Other Periampullary Cancers

Pancreatic cancer is by far the most common kind of periampullary cancer. Although rare, this region also harbors three other types of malignancies: Carcinoma of the ampulla of Vater, cholangiocarcinoma and duodenal cancer. Management of cholangiocarcinoma is discussed elsewhere within this text. The work-up and surgical approach to ampullary cancer and duodenal cancer are similar to that which has been presented above. It is important to note, however, that the survival rates of carcinoma of the ampulla of Vater and of duodenal cancer are better than pancreatic cancer. Five-year survival for ampullary carcinoma ranges 46-68% in some large series, while the survival for duodenal cancer can be up to 50% at 5 years. Furthermore, some authors advocate for resection of ampullary or duodenal cancers even in the setting of liver metastases to improve palliation and avoid the high risk of bleeding with these tumors. Both local and endoscopic resections have been described for benign lesions of the ampulla and for duodenal polyps in this region, underscoring the role for endoscopy and EUS to biopsy these tumors.

Cystic and Intraductal Papillary Mucinous Neoplasms

The identification of cystic pancreatic neoplasms has increased dramatically in recent years given advances in radiographic imaging. This has resulted in an increased referral of these patients for surgical evaluation. These cysts can be neoplastic or non-neoplastic and the neoplastic lesions encompass a spectrum of benign, pre-malignant and malignant. This section will focus only on the cystic neoplasms (discussion of non-neoplastic lesions, such as pseudocysts is outside of the scope of this chapter).

The most common cystic neoplasms encountered by the pancreatic surgeon are serous cystadenomas (SCA), MCN and IPMNs. Additional, less common tumors of importance include solitary pseudopapillary neoplasm, cystic endocrine neoplasm, ductal adenocarcinoma with cystic degeneration, lymphoepithelial cysts and acinar-cell cystadenomas. Each of these represents less than 10% of all cystic neoplasms. **Table 33-4** lists a number of important characteristics that help to distinguish between the four most common types of pancreatic neoplasm. The following sections will discuss each of the more common cystic neoplasms in detail.

Serous Cystadenoma

SCAs are small, microcystic tumors of the pancreas that are rarely malignant. The etiology of these lesions is unclear. Radiographically, they classically appear as a 'honeycomb' of multiple small cysts, although CT findings may vary from solid appearance to single cyst. Approximately 20% will have the hallmark finding of a central, stellate scar. These tumors are frequently confused with mucinous cystadenomas. EUS can be helpful in distinguishing SCAs and FNA aspirate yields high specificity in diagnosis. Histologically, these tumors are lined by cuboid epithelium and chromosomal alterations in the von Hippel-Lindau gene on chromosome 3p25 are quite common. Most SCAs are managed conservatively due to the low risk of malignancy. Symptomatic cysts should be resected, while asymptomatic lesions may be followed with serial CT scans every 1-2 years. Some authors have argued that larger lesions should be resected due to an increased incidence of rapid growth. A size cut-off of 4 cm has been proposed for resection, although this lacks the support of randomized-controlled data. Tumors that are unable to be confidently distinguished from other types of cystic neoplasia by radiographic or cytologic findings should be resected.

Mucinous Cystic Neoplasms

MCNs are large, multilocular or (rarely) unilocular cystic neoplasms lined by tall, mucin producing cells which may

TABLE 33-4	Characteristics of common cystic and intraductal papillary mucinous neoplasms			
	SCA	**MCN**	**IPMN**	**Solid pseudopapillary**
Incidence	32-39%	10-45%	21-33%	less than 10%
Age	7th decade	5th decade	6-7th decade	3rd-4th decade
Gender	F > M	F > M	equal	Predominantly female
Localization	variable	body/tail	head	body/tail
History of pancreatitis	no	no	yes	no
Communication with pancreatic duct	no	no	yes	no
Pancreatic duct on CT	normal	normal	dilated	normal
Aspect of lesion on CT	microcysts (< 2 cm) fibrous central scar	macrocysts (> 2 cm) peripheral eggshell calcification	microcysts/ macrocysts	Solid component with cystic degeneration
Histology	cuboidal glycogen-rich epithelial cells	ovarian stroma	dilated native ducts	uniform epithelium, solid sheets, nests and well-formed acinar structures, pseudo-papillae
Malignant potential	rarely malignant	10-15% *in situ* 8-30% invasive	5-20% *in situ* 10-40% invasive	10-15%
Treatment	observe	resection	observe/resection	resect

Abbreviations: SCA: Serous cystadenoma; MCN: Mucinous cystic neoplasm; IPMN: Intraductal papillary mucinous neoplasm; F: female; M: male

form papillae and they are found typically in the body and tail of the pancreas. These tumors frequently present in young women and are specifically characterized by the presence of ovarian-like stroma on histology. As with other tumors, they are frequently asymptomatic, however, when they are clinically evident, they frequently present with abdominal pain, early satiety, nausea and vomiting. MCNs occur in a spectrum ranging from benign (cystadenoma) to borderline to overtly malignant (cystadenocarcinoma), with approximately 20% harboring an *in situ* carcinoma. The diagnosis of malignant MCNs is based on the observation of invasion of the cyst wall. These tumors are frequently confused with IPMNs on initial radiographic assessment; however, MRCP or ERCP can be useful in identifying the lack of communication with the pancreatic duct present in MCNs. The presence of mural nodules identified on imaging is a predictor of malignancy. Again, EUS is useful for the characterization of these tumors as well as for sampling of fluid, which is likely to be more viscous than in SCAs and more likely to express high levels of CEA **(Table 33-5)**. Given their malignant potential and risk of degradation of borderline lesions to become mucinous cystadenocarcinoma, MCNs should be resected. The prognosis for resected cystadenocarcinoma with negative margins (R0) is very good, with 5-year survival rates reported between 50% and 75%. Unresectable or metastatic lesions have a dismal prognosis, with rapid decline similar to adenocarcinoma and median survival of 4-6 months.

TABLE 33-5	Tumor markers in cyst fluid from common cystic neoplasms		
Tumor marker	**SCA**	**MCN**	**IPMN**
Amylase	Low	Low	High
CEA	Low	High	High
CA19-9	Low-High	Low-High	Low-High
CA 125	Low	Low-High	Low
CA 15-3	Low	High	Low
CA 72-4	Low	High	High

Intraductal Papillary Mucinous Neoplasms

IPMNs are by definition intraductal neoplasms that are characterized as benign, borderline or malignant based on a number of pathological features, including dysplasia and nuclear abnormalities. The presence of pancreatic ductal dilation is considered to be a hallmark of IPMNs. These tumors arise from a pancreatic duct and can be found in the main duct, branch ducts or both. Four patterns of pancreatic ductal dilation have been recognized: (1) diffuse main duct ectasia, (2) segmental main duct ectasia, (3) side branch ectasia, (4) multifocal

cysts with pancreatic duct communication. The rate of malignancy range from 5% and 40% in various studies (*in situ* 5-27%, carcinoma 15-40%) and is highly dependent upon the type of IPMN. Main duct IPMN has the highest rate of malignancy. Current recommendations are to resect all main duct IPMNs greater than 6 mm in patients who are otherwise fit for surgery. Diffuse main duct ectasia is frequently found in the head of the pancreas, requiring a radical pancreatoduodenectomy operation, while segmental main duct ectasia is more frequently in the body and tail. Both diffuse main duct ectasia and the multifocal pattern can involve the entire pancreas, which may necessitate total pancreatectomy. Branch duct IPMNs are considered by most to be more favorable and less likely to be malignant than main duct. A number of large series have also concluded that size serves as a predictor of malignancy, with cysts > 3 cm harboring the highest risk of malignancy. In addition, the presence of mural nodules on imaging is also a marker of cancer. This has led to the development of a consensus paper published in *Pancreatology* in 2006 that recommends that branch chain IPMM with the following characteristics may safely be observed with repeat CT imaging on an annual basis: cyst < 3 cm, branch duct origin, asymptomatic and no additional radiographic markers of malignancy. For larger lesions and those with radiographic or cyst fluid suggestive of malignancy, aggressive surgical resection yields the best chance of cure. For cancers that are found to arise within IPMN, the prognosis is better than ductal adenocarcinoma of the pancreas. Five-year survival rates for *in situ* carcinoma in IPMN are > 80%, while overt carcinoma arising from IPMN has a 5-year survival of 30-40%. Multivariate analysis suggests that lymph node metastases is a predictor of poor prognosis. Frozen section is used by many to determine margins intraoperatively, which serves as a predictor of recurrence.

Solid Pseudopapillary Tumors

Solid pseudopapillary tumor, which is common in young females, is a rare pancreatic tumor with uncertain malignant potential. Also known as Frantz's tumor, this lesion is characterized by dramatic overexpression of beta-catenin and location in the body and tail of the pancreas. These tumors are often symptomatic owing to their large size. There is a low risk of malignant potential, however, even malignant and metastatic tumors of this subtype have a favorable prognosis. Aggressive surgical resection is indicated for these neoplasms, with overall 5-year survival rates of up to 97% reported in some series.

Pseudocysts

The differential diagnosis for all cystic neoplasms of the pancreas found radiographically must include pancreatic pseudocysts. Although a complete discussion on the work-up and management of pseudocysts is outside of the scope of this chapter, it is important to recognize a few common characteristics that distinguish pseudocysts from cystic neoplasms. A majority of patients with inflammatory pseudocysts will have a history of pancreatitis, alcohol abuse or complicated biliary disease. Although cystic neoplasms may cause pancreatitis from ductal obstruction, the incidence of significant pancreatitis is dramatically lower than for pseudocysts. Additionally, pseudocysts appear as large, single cysts without evidence of septations, distinguishing them from MCNs and SCNs. Aspiration of these lesions consistently reveals very high amylase levels (> 5000 U/ml) and frequently low levels of markers such as CEA, although these can falsely be elevated (although almost uniformly less than 400 ng/ml) in up to 50%. MRCP and EUS may be of diagnostic value to assess for the wall thickness and planning of drainage.

Future Directions

Pancreatic cancer is an aggressive disease with a late presentation. Early detection and screening methods are urgently needed to improve the odds of survival. Surgical treatment at high volume centers for pancreatic surgery reduces the rate of postoperative complications and may improve cancer-specific survival. The standard of care for pancreatic cancer patients is enrolling them into a clinical trial. Molecular profiling may permit treatment decisions to be personalized in the future and identify new targets for cancer therapy.

Landmark Papers

1. Bassi C, Dervenis C, Butturini G, Fingerhut A, Yeo C, Izbicki J, et al. Postoperative pancreatic fistula: an international study group (isgpf) definition. Surgery 2005;138:8-13.
2. Bassi C, Falconi M, Molinari E, Mantovani W, Butturini G, Gumbs AA, Salvia R, Pederzoli P. Duct-to-mucosa versus end-to-side pancreaticojejunostomy reconstruction after pancreaticoduodenectomy: Results of a prospective randomized trial. Surgery 2003;134:766-71.
3. Bassi C, Falconi M, Molinari E, Salvia R, Butturini G, Sartori N, et al. Reconstruction by pancreaticojejunostomy versus pancreaticogastrostomy following pancreatectomy: results of a comparative study. Ann Surg 2005;242:767-71, discussion 771-3.
4. Birkmeyer JD, Finlayson SR, Tosteson AN, Sharp SM, Warshaw AL, Fisher ES. Effect of hospital volume on in-hospital mortality with pancreaticoduodenectomy. Surgery 1999;125:250-6.
5. Birkmeyer JD, Warshaw AL, Finlayson SR, Grove MR, Tosteson AN. Relationship between hospital volume and late survival after pancreaticoduodenectomy. Surgery 1999; 126:178-83.
6. Buchler MW, Bassi C, Fingerhut A, Klempa I. Does prophylactic octreotide decrease the rates of pancreatic fistula and other complications after pancreatico-duodenectomy? Ann Surg 2001;234:262-3.
7. DeOliveira ML, Winter JM, Schafer M, Cunningham SC, Cameron JL, Yeo CJ, Clavien PA. Assessment of complications after pancreatic surgery: a novel grading system applied to 633 patients undergoing pancreaticoduodenectomy. Ann Surg 2006;244:931-7; discussion 937-9.
8. Farnell MB, Pearson RK, Sarr MG, DiMagno EP, Burgart LJ, Dahl TR, et al. A prospective randomized trial comparing standard pancreatoduodene-tomy with pancreatoduodenectomy with extended lymphadenectomy in resectable pancreatic head adenocarcinoma. Surgery 2005;138:618-28; discussion 628-30.
9. Gouma DJ, van Geenen RC, van Gulik TM, de Haan RJ, de Wit LT, Busch OR, Obertop H. Rates of complications and death after pancreaticoduodenectomy: risk factors and the impact of hospital volume. Ann Surg 2000;232:786-95.
10. Hruban RH, Goggins M, Parsons J, Kern SE. Progression model for pancreatic cancer. Clin Cancer Res 2000;6:2969-72.
11. Iacobuzio-Donahue CA, Maitra A, Shen-Ong GL, van Heek T, Ashfaq R, Meyer R, et al. Discovery of novel tumor markers of pancreatic cancer using global gene expression technology. Am J Pathol 2002;160:1239-49.
12. Leach SD, Lee JE, Charnsangavej C, Cleary KR, Lowy AM, Fenoglio CJ, Pisters PW, Evans DB. Survival following pancreaticoduodenectomy with resection of the superior mesenteric-portal vein confluence for adenocarcinoma of the pancreatic head. Br J Surg 1998;85:611-7.
13. Lillemoe KD, Kaushal S, Cameron JL, Sohn TA, Pitt HA, Yeo CJ. Distal pancreatectomy: Indications and outcomes in 235 patients. Ann Surg 1999;229:693-8; discussion 698-700.
14. Lowy AM. Neoadjuvant therapy for pancreatic cancer. J Gastrointest Surg 2008;12:1600-8.
15. Michalski CW, Kleeff J, Wente MN, Diener MK, Buchler MW, Friess H. Systematic review and meta-analysis of standard and extended lymphadenectomy in pancreaticoduodenectomy for pancreatic cancer. Br J Surg 2007;94:265-73.
16. Nathan H, Cameron JL, Goodwin CR, Seth AK, Edil BH, Wolfgang CL, et al. Risk factors for pancreatic leak after distal pancreatectomy. Ann Surg 2009;250:277-81.
17. Neoptolemos JP, Stocken DD, Friess H, Bassi C, Dunn JA, Hickey H, et al. A randomized trial of chemoradiotherapy and chemotherapy after resection of pancreatic cancer. N Engl J Med 2004;350:1200-10.
18. Pawlik TM, Abdalla EK, Barnett CC, Ahmad SA, Cleary KR, Vauthey JN, et al. Feasibility of a randomized trial of extended lymphadenectomy for pancreatic cancer. Arch Surg 2005;140:584-9; discussion 589-91.
19. Picozzi VJ, Pisters PW, Vickers SM, Strasberg SM. Strength of the evidence: Adjuvant therapy for resected pancreatic cancer. J Gastrointest Surg 2008;12:657-61.
20. Pisters PW, Hudec WA, Hess KR, Lee JE, Vauthey JN, Lahoti S, Raijman I, Evans DB. Effect of preoperative biliary decompression on pancreaticoduodenectomy-associated morbidity in 300 consecutive patients. Ann Surg 2001; 234:47-55.

21. Riall TS, Cameron JL, Lillemoe KD, Campbell KA, Sauter PK, Coleman J, et al. Pancreaticoduodenectomy with or without distal gastrectomy and extended retroperitoneal lymphadenectomy for periampullary adenocarcinoma—part 3: Update on 5-year survival. J Gastrointest Surg 2005;9:1191-1204; discussion 1204-6.

22. Stocken DD, Buchler MW, Dervenis C, Bassi C, Jeekel H, Klinkenbijl JH, et al. Meta-analysis of randomised adjuvant therapy trials for pancreatic cancer. Br J Cancer 2005; 92:1372-81.

23. Tanaka M, Chari S, Adsay V, Fernandezdel Castillo C, Falconi M, Shimizu M, et al. International consensus guidelines for management of intraductal papillary mucinous neoplasms and mucinous cystic neoplasms of the pancreas. Pancreatology 2006;6:17-32.

24. Varadhachary GR, Tamm EP, Abbruzzese JL, Xiong HQ, Crane CH, Wang H, et al. Borderline resectable pancreatic cancer: definitions, management and role of preoperative therapy. Ann Surg Oncol 2006;13:1035-46.

25. Yeo CJ, Abrams RA, Grochow LB, Sohn TA, Ord SE, Hruban RH, et al. Pancreaticoduodenectomy for pancreatic adenocarcinoma: postoperative adjuvant chemoradiation improves survival. A prospec-tive, single-institution experience. Ann Surg 1997;225:621-33; discussion 633-6.

26. Yeo CJ, Cameron JL, Lillemoe KD, Sauter PK, Coleman J, Sohn TA, Campbell KA, Choti MA. Does prophylactic octreotide decrease the rates of pancreatic fistula and other complications after pancreaticoduodenectomy? Results of a prospective randomized placebo-controlled trial. Ann Surg 2000;232:419-29.

27. Yeo CJ, Cameron JL, Lillemoe KD, Sohn TA, Campbell KA, Sauter PK, et al. Pancreaticoduodenectomy with or without distal gastrectomy and extended retroperitoneal lymphadenectomy for periampullary adenocarcinoma, part 2: randomized controlled trial evaluating survival, morbidity and mortality. Ann Surg 2002;236:355-66; discussion 366-58.

28. Yeo CJ, Cameron JL, Maher MM, Sauter PK, Zahurak ML, Talamini MA, Lillemoe KD, Pitt HA. A prospective randomized trial of pancreaticogastrostomy versus pancreaticojejunostomy after pancreaticoduodenectomy. Ann Surg 1995;222:580-8; discussion 588-92.

29. Yeo CJ, Cameron JL, Sohn TA, Coleman J, Sauter PK, Hruban RH, Pitt HA, Lillemoe KD. Pancreaticoduodenectomy with or without extended retroperitoneal lymphadenectomy for periampullary adenocarcinoma: comparison of morbidity and mortality and short-term outcome. Ann Surg 1999;229:613-22; discussion 622-4.

Level of Evidence Table			
Recommendation	**Grade**	**Best level of evidence**	**References**
Multidetector computed tomography (MDCT) with pancreas-protocol contrast is the minimum imaging modality required for evaluating pancreatic lesions. Endoscopic ultrasound (EUS) adds complementary diagnostic information regarding resectability and tumor histology.	B	2b	1-3
EUS-guided FNA for analysis of pancreatic cyst fluid (amylase, CEA, CA19-9, cytology) may help diagnose the lesion to guide further therapy.	B	2b	4,5
Serum CA 19-9 level is currently the most useful biomarker in the diagnosis and follow-up of pancreatic adenocarcinomas.	B	1b	6-8
Routine preoperative biliary drainage of obstructive jaundice should not be performed (see Recommendations Table for Cholangiocarcinoma).	A	1a	9
Neoadjuvant therapy for resectable pancreatic cancers has clear rationale but unproven benefits over adjuvant therapy.	C	4	10-13
Neoadjuvant therapy for borderline resectable pancreatic cancers may improve R0 resectability and thus survival.	B	4	14-16
Pylorus-preserving and standard pancreaticoduodenectomy are equivalent approaches to resection in terms of morbidity and survival. Pylorus-preservation is associated with lower blood loss and operative time.	A	1a	17,18
Standard lymphadenectomy has equivalent survival with less morbidity compared to extended lymphadenectomy during pancreaticoduodenectomy for cancer.	A	1a	19, 20
No agents have been clearly demonstrated to reduce the rate of pancreatic fistula after operation. Somatostatin may be beneficial for small pancreatic ducts.	A	1a	21-26

Contd...

Contd...

Recommendation	Grade	Best level of evidence	References
Adjuvant chemotherapy improves survival in resected pancreatic cancer. The benefit of adjuvant radiation for local control after resection is less clear.	A	1a	27-30
Gemcitabine is the agent of choice in single- and combination chemotherapeutic regimens for pancreatic cancer.	B	1a	31-36
Consensus guidelines regarding the management of main duct IPMN (resection), branch duct IPMN (selective resection) and mucinous cystic neoplasms (resection) have been at least retrospectively validated in different clinical centers.	B	1b	37-40
Long-term surveillance for recurrence of IPMN is required for lesions treated by partial pancreatectomy.	B	4	41,42

References

1. Puli SR, Singh S, Hagedorn CH, et al. Diagnostic accuracy of EUS for vascular invasion in pancreatic and periampullary cancers: a meta-analysis and systematic review. Gastrointest Endosc 2007; 65:788-97.
2. Mansfield SD, Scott J, Oppong K, et al. Comparison of multislice computed tomography and endoscopic ultrasonography with operative and histological findings in suspected pancreatic and periampullary malignancy. Br J Surg 2008; 95:1512-20.
3. Rivadeneira DE, Pochapin M, Grobmyer SR, et al. Comparison of linear array endoscopic ultrasound and helical computed tomography for the staging of periampullary malignancies. Ann Surg Oncol 2003; 10:890-7.
4. van der Waaij LA, van Dullemen HM, Porte RJ. Cyst fluid analysis in the differential diagnosis of pancreatic cystic lesions: a pooled analysis. Gastrointest Endosc 2005; 62:383-9.
5. Linder JD, Geenen JE, Catalano MF. Cyst fluid analysis obtained by EUS-guided FNA in the evaluation of discrete cystic neoplasms of the pancreas: a prospective single-center experience. Gastrointest Endosc 2006; 64:697-702.
6. Goonetilleke KS, Siriwardena AK. Systematic review of carbohydrate antigen (CA 19-9) as a biochemical marker in the diagnosis of pancreatic cancer. Eur J Surg Oncol 2007; 33:266-70.
7. Berger AC, Garcia M, Jr., Hoffman JP, et al. Postresection CA 19-9 predicts overall survival in patients with pancreatic cancer treated with adjuvant chemoradiation: a prospective validation by RTOG 9704. J Clin Oncol 2008; 26:5918-22.
8. Boeck S, Stieber P, Holdenrieder S, et al. Prognostic and therapeutic significance of carbohydrate antigen 19-9 as tumor marker in patients with pancreatic cancer. Oncology 2006; 70:255-64.
9. Sewnath ME, Karsten TM, Prins MH, et al. A meta-analysis on the efficacy of preoperative biliary drainage for tumors causing obstructive jaundice. Ann Surg 2002; 236:17-27.
10. Hoffman JP, Lipsitz S, Pisansky T, et al. Phase II trial of preoperative radiation therapy and chemotherapy for patients with localized, resectable adenocarcinoma of the pancreas: an Eastern Cooperative Oncology Group Study. J Clin Oncol 1998; 16:317-23.
11. Evans DB, Varadhachary GR, Crane CH, et al. Preoperative gemcitabine-based chemoradiation for patients with resectable adenocarcinoma of the pancreatic head. J Clin Oncol 2008; 26:3496-502.
12. Talamonti MS, Small W, Jr., Mulcahy MF, et al. A multi-institutional phase II trial of preoperative full-dose gemcitabine and concurrent radiation for patients with potentially resectable pancreatic carcinoma. Ann Surg Oncol 2006; 13:150-8.
13. Brunner TB, Grabenbauer GG, Meyer T, et al. Primary resection versus neoadjuvant chemoradiation followed by resection for locally resectable or potentially resectable pancreatic carcinoma without distant metastasis. A multi-centre prospectively randomised phase II-study of the Interdisciplinary Working Group Gastrointestinal Tumours (AIO, ARO and CAO). BMC Cancer 2007; 7:41.
14. Katz MH, Pisters PW, Evans DB, et al. Borderline resectable pancreatic cancer: the importance of this emerging stage of disease. J Am Coll Surg 2008; 206:833-46; discussion 846-8.
15. Brown KM, Siripurapu V, Davidson M, et al. Chemoradiation followed by chemotherapy before resection for borderline pancreatic adenocarcinoma. Am J Surg 2008; 195:318-21.
16. Varadhachary GR, Tamm EP, Abbruzzese JL, et al. Borderline resectable pancreatic cancer: definitions, management and role of preoperative therapy. Ann Surg Oncol 2006; 13:1035-46.
17. Diener MK, Heukaufer C, Schwarzer G, et al. Pancreaticoduodenectomy (classic Whipple) versus pylorus-preserving pancreaticoduodenectomy (pp radical pancreatoduodenectomy) for surgical treatment of periampullary and pancreatic carcinoma. Cochrane Database Syst Rev 2008; CD006053.
18. Karanicolas PJ, Davies E, Kunz R, et al. The pylorus: take it or leave it? Systematic review and meta-analysis of pylorus-preserving versus standard whipplepancreaticoduodenectomy for pancreatic or periampullary cancer. Ann Surg Oncol 2007; 14:1825-34.

19. Michalski CW, Kleeff J, Wente MN, et al. Systematic review and meta-analysis of standard and extended lymphadenectomy in pancreaticoduodenectomy for pancreatic cancer. Br J Surg 2007; 94:265-73.

20. Iqbal N, Lovegrove RE, Tilney HS, et al. A comparison of pancreaticoduodenectomy with extended pancreaticoduodenectomy: a meta-analysis of 1909 patients. Eur J Surg Oncol 2009; 35:79-86.

21. Zeng Q, Zhang Q, Han S, et al. Efficacy of somatostatin and its analogues in prevention of postoperative complications after pancreaticoduodenectomy: a meta-analysis of randomized controlled trials. Pancreas 2008; 36:18-25.

22. Suc B, Msika S, Piccinini M, et al. Octreotide in the prevention of intra-abdominal complications following elective pancreatic resection: a prospective, multicenter randomized controlled trial. Arch Surg 2004; 139:288-94; discussion 295.

23. Connor S, Alexakis N, Garden OJ, et al. Meta-analysis of the value of somatostatin and its analogues in reducing complications associated with pancreatic surgery. Br J Surg 2005; 92:1059-67.

24. Alghamdi AA, Jawas AM, Hart RS. Use of octreotide for the prevention of pancreatic fistula after elective pancreatic surgery: a systematic review and meta-analysis. Can J Surg 2007; 50:459-66.

25. Li-Ling J, Irving M. Somatostatin and octreotide in the prevention of postoperative pancreatic complications and the treatment of enterocutaneous pancreatic fistulas: a systematic review of randomized controlled trials. Br J Surg 2001; 88:190-9.

26. Lillemoe KD, Cameron JL, Kim MP, et al. Does fibrin glue sealant decrease the rate of pancreatic fistula after pancreaticoduodenectomy? Results of a prospective randomized trial. J Gastrointest Surg 2004; 8:766-72; discussion 772-4.

27. Neoptolemos JP, Stocken DD, Friess H, et al. A randomized trial of chemoradiotherapy and chemotherapy after resection of pancreatic cancer. N Engl J Med 2004; 350:1200-10.

28. Oettle H, Post S, Neuhaus P, et al. Adjuvant chemotherapy with gemcitabine vs observation in patients undergoing curative-intent resection of pancreatic cancer: a randomized controlled trial. Jama 2007; 297:267-77.

29. Regine WF, Winter KA, Abrams RA, et al. Fluorouracil vs gemcitabine chemotherapy before and after fluorouracil-based chemoradiation following resection of pancreatic adenocarcinoma: a randomized controlled trial. Jama 2008; 299:1019-26.

30. Sorg C, Schmidt J, Buchler MW, et al. Examination of external validity in randomized controlled trials for adjuvant treatment of pancreatic adenocarcinoma. Pancreas 2009; 38:542-50.

31. Bria E, Milella M, Gelibter A, et al. Gemcitabine-based combinations for inoperable pancreatic cancer: have we made real progress? A meta-analysis of 20 phase 3 trials. Cancer 2007; 110:525-33.

32. Sultana A, Tudur Smith C, Cunningham D, et al. Meta-analyses of chemotherapy for locally advanced and metastatic pancreatic cancer: results of secondary end points analyses. Br J Cancer 2008; 99:6-13.

33. Yip D, Karapetis C, Strickland A, et al. Chemotherapy and radiotherapy for inoperable advanced pancreatic cancer. Cochrane Database Syst Rev 2006; 3:CD002093.

34. Heinemann V, Boeck S, Hinke A, et al. Meta-analysis of randomized trials: evaluation of benefit from gemcitabine-based combination chemotherapy applied in advanced pancreatic cancer. BMC Cancer 2008; 8:82.

35. Picozzi VJ, Kozarek RA, Traverso LW. Interferon-based adjuvant chemoradiation therapy after pancreaticoduodenectomy for pancreatic adenocarcinoma. Am J Surg 2003; 185:476-80.

36. Linehan DC, Tan MC, Strasberg SM, et al. Adjuvant interferon-based chemoradiation followed by gemcitabine for resected pancreatic adenocarcinoma: a single-institution phase II study. Ann Surg 2008; 248:145-51.

37. Tanaka M, Chari S, Adsay V, et al. International consensus guidelines for management of intraductal papillary mucinous neoplasms and mucinous cystic neoplasms of the pancreas. Pancreatology 2006; 6:17-32.

38. Tang RS, Weinberg B, Dawson DW, et al. Evaluation of the guidelines for management of pancreatic branch-duct intraductal papillary mucinous neoplasm. Clin Gastroenterol Hepatol 2008; 6:815-9; quiz 719.

39. Pelaez-Luna M, Chari ST, Smyrk TC, et al. Do consensus indications for resection in branch duct intraductal papillary mucinous neoplasm predict malignancy? A study of 147 patients. Am J Gastroenterol 2007; 102:1759-64.

40. Nagai K, Doi R, Ito T, et al. Single-institution validation of the international consensus guidelines for treatment of branch duct intraductal papillary mucinous neoplasms of the pancreas. J Hepatobiliary Pancreat Surg 2009; 16:353-8.

41. White R, D'Angelica M, Katabi N, et al. Fate of the remnant pancreas after resection of noninvasive intraductal papillary mucinous neoplasm. J Am Coll Surg 2007; 204:987-93; discussion 993-5.

42. Schnelldorfer T, Sarr MG, Nagorney DM, et al. Experience with 208 resections for intraductal papillary mucinous neoplasm of the pancreas. Arch Surg 2008; 143:639-46; discussion 646.

Section 8

Special Topics

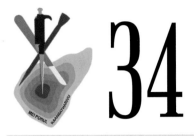

34

Splenectomy

Evie Carchman,   Matthew P Holtzman

Splenectomy is a well-established therapeutic intervention in the management of various hematologic disorders and several solid organ tumors. In many of the hematologic disorders, the spleen plays a pathologic role in terms of hypersplenism or symptomatic splenomegaly. Hypersplenism is when the spleen becomes overactive resulting in the removal of certain cell lines from the peripheral blood. This leads to various cytopenias that are usually symptomatic. In certain solid organ tumors (e.g. gastric and pancreatic) the spleen is removed to obtain adequate surgical margins, exposure or when the splenic vascular supply is removed with the specimen. Since the introduction of splenectomy into surgical practice, the morbidity/mortality from this procedure has changed dramatically secondary to gaining surgical experience and advances in surgical techniques.

Anatomy

The spleen **(Figure 34-1)** is an encapsulated organ of vascular and lymphatic tissue originating from mesodermal tissue during the fifth week of gestation. It forms as an outpouching from the dorsal mesogastrium and during the natural counterclockwise rotation of the intestine the spleen reaches its final location in the left upper quadrant. The spleen is held in place by several peritoneal attachments (splenocolic, gastrosplenic, phrenosplenic and the splenorenal ligaments). The gastrosplenic ligament contains the short gastric vessels, while the remaining ligaments are typically avascular. It is important to note that the free border of the greater omentum has variable attachments to the splenic capsule. If these attachments exist one may accidentally disrupt the splenic capsule with inadvertent tension on the omentum. Therefore, before applying inferior tension on the greater omentum, these attachments should be identified and lysed to prevent in advertent injury to the spleen.

The typical weight of the spleen is about 150-200 grams and decreases with advancing age. The spleen has to double in size in order to be palpated below the costal

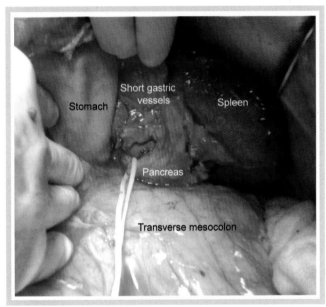

Figure 34-1: The anatomical location of spleen

margin on physical exam. Massive splenomegaly has been defined in some papers as a spleen that weighs greater than or equal to 1500 grams, however, the exact definition varies in the literature.

The arterial supply to the spleen is the splenic artery, which is one of the three major branches of the celiac trunk. The splenic artery typically runs along the superior aspect of the pancreas and an angiogram has a classic serpentine appearance with several small pancreatic branches. The splenic artery can be categorized as distributed or magistral based on its branching pattern. The distributed type occurs in about 70% of the population and is characterized by a short splenic trunk with many long branches entering the splenic parenchyma. The magistral type has a long splenic trunk and short terminal branches. These different branching types should be taken into consideration during one's dissection of the vascular pedicle. The first major splenic artery branch is called the superior polar artery and then the splenic artery divides again into three to five segmental branches. The splenic parenchyma also receives some blood from the short gastric vessels (vasa brevia) in the gastrosplenic ligament which are branches of the left gastroepiploic artery. When the spleen is pathologically enlarged it can also receive blood supply from the omentum, diaphragm or the mesentery of the left colon.

The venous drainage from the spleen is the splenic vein. The splenic vein is closely associated with the posterior aspect of the body and tail of the pancreas. Posterior to the pancreas the splenic vein combines with the superior mesenteric vein to form the portal vein. The inferior mesenteric vein combines with the splenic vein prior to the junction of the splenic and superior mesenteric vein or right at the junction. Again the spleen also has venous drainage paralleling its other arterial supply, the short gastric vessels. The lymphatics of the spleen follow its vascular supply/drainage with its lymphatic beds located at the hilum and along the splenic artery and short gastric vessels.

The parenchyma of the spleen is histologically divided into red and white pulp. The red pulp comprises 75% of the splenic parenchyma and is functionally organized as a filtering system. It is composed of many venous sinuses that are separated by a trabecular network called the reticulum. Within the reticulum reside macrophages. Based on this configuration the spleen filters out microorganisms, senescent red blood cells, cellular debris and antigen/antibody complexes. This function makes the spleen the largest reticuloendothelial organ in the body. The white pulp houses lymphocytes which can antigenically be stimulated to proliferate as needed. The marginal zone is the interface between the red and the white pulp where lymphocytes produce immunoglobins that ultimately will enter the systemic circulation to take part in various immune functions.

The most common observed anatomic abnormality of the spleen is the existence of accessory spleens. This anomaly is noted in up to 20% of patients and is important to identify in the treatment of hematologic disorders where removal of all splenic tissue is necessary. The majority (80%) of accessory spleens are located at the splenic hilum, while other common locations are the gastrocolic ligament, tail of the pancreas, greater curvature of stomach, splenocolic ligament and bowel mesentery. Given the not insignificant incidence of accessory splenic tissue, inspection of the peritoneal cavity for accessory spleens should be part of surgical practice when their occurrence and failure to identify will have an impact on treatment.

Physiology

The spleen has many functions that have been well studied and described. The functions include filtration, humoral and cell-mediated immunity, storage and hematopoiesis.

The blood enters the spleen through the splenic artery which then branches multiple times into small arterioles. Segmental arteries branch into trabecular arteries, which branch into perpendicular branches, which then divide into central arteries. Central arteries are housed in the periarterial lymphatic sheath (PALS) which is made of T and B cells at various stages of development. Through this system antigens are filtered in the white pulp leading to follicular stimulation. Upon stimulation of the follicles there is an elaboration of immunoglobulins, mainly IgM, which takes part in the immune response. The spleen is also the production center for opsonins, tuftsin and properdin which facilitate clearance of bacteria from the bloodstream.

The blood is filtered through the white pulp and then enters the red pulp. In the red pulp the flow is slower allowing for macrophages to phagocytize senescent and abnormal cells. Through this filtering system, the spleen plays a major role in red cell maturation and quality control. Pieces of the red cell membrane are removed in the red pulp, usually in association with cytoplasmic inclusions (nuclear remnants, i.e. Howell-Jolly bodies, denatured hemoglobin, i.e. Heinz bodies and iron granules, i.e. Pappenheimer bodies). The process of removal of inclusion bodies is called culling and is important in red cell maturation.

The spleen has been noted to have a role in hematopoiesis in the middle weeks of intrauterine life. This capacity can be reactivated in childhood if the marrow capacity is exceeded. This hematopoietic function is only seen in adult life in myeloproliferative disorders where the bone marrow has been replaced with fibrotic tissue.

The spleen is also noted to be a storage place for circulating cellular elements. Thirty percent of the circulating platelets are stored in the spleen at any given time. This becomes evident after splenectomy when the peripheral platelet count rises dramatically.

Indications for Splenectomy

As stated in the introduction, splenectomy has been utilized in the treatment of various hematologic disorders and some solid organ tumors. Indications for splenectomy in hematologic disorders are for symptoms, hematologic abnormalities, or for diagnostic purposes. The removal of the spleen can play an important role in reducing the morbidity of these hematologic conditions.

Incidental Splenectomy

Incidental splenectomy (solid tumors) is defined as removal of the spleen during the operative treatment of an adjacent organ in which the spleen needs to be removed for completeness of resection, improved exposure or if there is removal of the splenic vasculature. A large series at the Barnes Hospital and Brigham and Women's

Hospital found incidental splenectomy (26%) to be the most common indication for splenectomy at their institutions. Incidental splenectomy is usually performed during resection of tumors of the left upper quadrant (stomach and pancreas) and retroperitoneum (left renal, adrenal and retroperitoneal sarcomas).

Splenectomy is often performed during a distal pancreatectomy when the splenic vasculature must be ligated to obtain adequate margins. Splenectomy used to be standard practice during a distal pancreatectomy, however, there has been a trend recently toward splenic preservation to reduce the risk of post-splenectomy infection. Distal pancreatectomy without splenectomy can be done through sparing the splenic artery and vein with tedious dissection. This technique through preservation of the vessels is only reasonable if there is a small invasive tumor or for benign neoplasia. In other words, oncologic cure should not be compromised for splenic preservation. The second option for splenic preservation is through the ligation of the splenic artery and vein with preservation of the short gastric vessels. Splenic preservation is not an option when the lymph node dissection has to be extended to the splenic hilum or there is direct invasion of tumor into the splenic parenchyma. Splenic preservation following distal pancreatectomy for benign or low-grade malignant disease has been found to be safe and associated with a decrease in perioperative infections and length of hospital stay.

Another solid organ tumor operation that usually includes a splenectomy is resection of proximal gastric cancers. The spleen is usually taken because of the need for extended lymph node dissection into the splenic hilum. A series from Japan noted 20% of patients with proximal gastric tumors having positive splenic hilum lymph nodes. For positive splenic hilum lymph nodes splenectomy is recommended to obtain an R0 (i.e. potential curative resection). A study from Memorial Sloan-Kettering Cancer Center noted that 23% of complete gastric resections for cure of cancer included resection of adjacent organs of which most commonly included the spleen. Long-term survival was improved in some series where aggressive surgery was utilized to obtain negative margins. However, there are studies that report that splenectomy should only be done in patients with resectable stage IV cancer, extension to spleen and pancreas, or macroscopic nodal metastases to the splenic hilum. There are also some series that do not demonstrate an effect on survival in patients who underwent splenectomy and should only be removed if there is direct cancer invasion into spleen.

Idiopathic Thrombocytopenic Purpura

Idiopathic thrombocytopenic purpura (ITP) is the most common indication for splenectomy in the United States. ITP is an acquired, autoimmune, hematologic disorder characterized by abnormal splenic production of immunoglobulins (IgG) resulting in the premature removal of platelets. Platelet clearance occurs through the interaction of platelet autoantibodies with the Fc receptors expressed on tissue macrophages in the spleen. The incidence of this disease is 100 per one million individuals annually—half of whom are children.

Patients usually present with petechiae, ecchymoses, mucosal bleeding and/or menorrhagia. The severity of bleeding noted correlates to the platelet count. Those with less than 10,000 platelets/mm^3 are at risk for internal bleeding. In 80-90% of children there is usually a spontaneous and complete remission. Splenectomy in childhood is reserved for severe thrombocytopenia that is refractory to medical management for greater than one year. These are rare cases, making splenectomy in children rarely indicated. In adults, they commonly experience a more chronic form of the disease that recurs after withdrawal of steroids.

The diagnosis is made clinically by a low platelet count, megathrombocytes on peripheral blood smear and normal/increased megakaryocytes on bone marrow aspirate. Assays are also available to detect the IgG antibodies on platelets. The first line therapy for ITP is steroids, with a response rate ranging 50-75%. Even with these dramatic response rates, relapses are fairly common. Intravenous gammaglobulin (IVIG) is another therapy that is available in the treatment of this disease. IVIG works by competing for binding sites to macrophage receptors. The response to IVIG in terms of platelet count recovery is usually faster than with steroids. IVIG is utilized when there is internal bleeding or platelet count less than 500 platelets/mm^3. However, like with steroids the response is usually not sustained. Rhogam has also been recently approved for use in patients that are Rh+. Initial data is very promising but long term data is not available. Permanent cure with medical therapy is only seen in 15-20% of patients.

Splenectomy is indicated for failure of medical therapy, for undesirable effects of steroids and relapse of disease. Failure of medical therapy is defined as disease that does not improve after 8 weeks of steroid treatment or relapses after steroids are tapered. Intracranial hemorrhage is an indication for emergent splenectomy. Splenectomy provides a permanent cure in 75-85% of patients. Of the remaining 15-25% significant bleeding is infrequent.

Of note, splenomegaly is rare in patients with ITP, making laparoscopic splenectomy the surgical treatment of choice for these patients. Platelets should be on hold, but not given until the splenic artery has been clamped or ligated. It is important to perform a thorough inspection of the abdomen for accessory spleens that can lead to recurrence of disease. Accessory spleens are found in up to 30% of patients with ITP. Technetium labeled red cell scan can be performed preoperatively to identify accessory spleens, or can be performed postoperatively in cases of recurrence. Studies have demonstrated laparoscopic removal of accessory spleens is a safe and effective option in cases of recurrence.

Thrombotic Thrombocytopenic Purpura

Thrombotic thrombocytopenic purpura (TTP) is a rare hematologic disorder resulting in thrombocytopenia, microangiopathic hemolytic anemia, neurologic deficits and renal complications. The underlying pathology is related to abnormal hyaline membranes being deposited in arterioles and capillaries that lead to platelet aggregation and vessel occlusion. The exact etiology of this disease is unknown and is fortunately quite rare affecting only 3.7 per one million individuals.

The diagnosis of TTP is made based on thrombocytopenia, a peripheral blood smear demonstrating schistocytes and a negative Coombs test. Prior to the 1970s there were few treatment options available, resulting in near universal fatality. Since the introduction of plasmapheresis there have been remarkable improvements in patient survival. Plasmapheresis can be done on a daily basis up to 10 days or until platelet counts normalize and there is minimal hemolysis. With plasmapheresis alone there is an 80-90% survival benefit. The mortality rate is greater than 60% for patients who do not respond to plasmapheresis.

Fresh frozen plasma, high dose steroids and antiplatelet agents are also used in the treatment of this disease. A combination of all of these therapies has led to significant improvement in symptoms in greater than 70% of patients. However, up to 40% of these patients who initially responded to therapy will eventually relapse. Platelet administration in this disorder is discouraged and is associated with worsening of the disease.

Patients who fail to respond to medical therapy or who relapse, surgical intervention in terms of splenectomy is recommended. The majority of splenectomies are done laparoscopically given the lack of splenomegaly. A study in 2001 demonstrated the safety and efficacy of laparoscopic splenectomy in this patient population.

Autoimmune Hemolytic Anemia

Autoimmune hemolytic anemia is a hematologic disease resulting from splenic autoantibody production against red blood cells. Autoimmune hemolytic anemias are classified into 'warm' or 'cold' based on the temperature at which the antibodies are active. 'Warm' autoantibodies are usually IgG and bind to red cells at cold temperatures, but lead to hemolysis at temperatures greater than 37 degrees centigrade. 'Cold' auto-antibodies are usually IgM. The distinction between warm and cold autoimmune

hemolytic anemia is important when deciding if splenectomy is indicated. The spleen has receptors to that bind to the Fc portion of IgG. Therefore, a patient with warm autoimmune hemolytic anemia, the spleen is the primary location of red cell destruction. For cold autoimmune hemolytic anemias IgM causes either complement fixation or aggregation of platelets in the periphery that leads to red cell destruction, leaving no role for splenectomy in these patients.

Patients usually present with anemia and jaundice. Laboratory diagnosis is made with an increased reticulocyte count, increased indirect serum bilirubin and a Coombs test that demonstrates antibodies coating the red blood cells. Initial treatments are supportive, such as blood transfusions and/or steroids. Steroids are the first line treatment and lead to decreased hemolysis in 75% of cases. In idiopathic autoimmune hemolytic anemia only 25% of these patients receive a long-term cure with steroids alone. Splenectomy is effective in 80% of these cases. In one series 64% required no further steroids, while 21% and a decrease in their steroid requirement. In more than half a patients with this disease splenomegaly is present which must be taken into account when deciding if laparoscopy is the appropriate surgical option.

Hereditary Spherocytosis

Hereditary spherocytosis is autosomal dominant disorder of the erythrocyte cell membrane that results in hemolytic anemia. The prevalence of hereditary spherocytosis in United States is 1 per 5000 individuals. Hereditary spherocytosis is the number one hemolytic anemia for which splenectomy is indicated. The underlying pathophysiology is the loss of membrane proteins such as spectrin, ankyrin, band 3 protein or protein 4.2. The loss of these proteins results in a decrease in membrane surface area which gives the red cells a spherocytic shape instead of their normal biconcavity. Lack of deformability of the red cell leads to increase osmotic fragility, sequestration and their destruction in the spleen.

Most patients with this disease are asymptomatic or have mild jaundice. Splenomegaly is usually present by the age of one with mild to moderate anemia. The diagnosis is suspected with a low mean corpuscular volume and an elevated mean corpuscular hemoglobin concentration. The diagnosis is confirmed when spherocytes are visualized on a peripheral blood smear.

Splenectomy is curative and is the treatment of choice in these patients. Most physicians recommend delaying splenectomy till after the age of 4-6 for concern of postsplenectomy sepsis, which has an increased incidence in very young children. It is also important to note that most patients (30-60%) have pigmented gallstones from hemolysis by the age of 5. Therefore, a prophylactic cholecystectomy is recommended at the time of splenectomy in patients with gallstones identified on ultrasound during preoperative planning. Laparoscopic removal of the spleen in this patient population has been found to be as safe and effective as the open technique and facilitates the usually combined laparoscopic cholecystectomy. There are few reports in the literature of partial splenectomies being done in the treatment of hereditary spherocytosis, but there is no long-term follow-up to determine its durability.

Hereditary Elliptocytosis

Hereditary elliptocytosis, like hereditary spherocytosis, results from a genetic defect in membrane proteins and is inherited in an autosomal dominant fashion. The prevalence is 1 per 2000 individuals. Hereditary elliptocytosis is usually asymptomatic unless 50-90% of red cells are affected. Unlike hereditary spherocytosis splenectomy is not always indicated. In patients with hereditary elliptocytosis splenectomy is only indicated in patients who develop severe anemia that results blood transfusions more than once a month. Only 10% of patients ever meet this criterion.

Hemoglobinopathies

Sickle Cell Disease

Sickle cell disease is a hereditary hemolytic anemia caused by the substitution of glutamic acid for valine on the beta hemoglobin protein. This disease is inherited in an autosomal codominant fashion and the prevalence of carriers is 8-10% of the African American population. The altered hemoglobin leads to a propensity of the erythrocyte to become stiff in the relatively hypoxic environment of the splenic red pulp. This leads to sequestration of red cells and resulting infarctions in the microvasculature. These microvascular infarcts lead to autosplenectomy usually by the age of 5. There are rare cases where patients with sickle cell disease have acute sequestration that is associated with 20% mortality rate. During acute sequestration there is rapid painful enlargement of the spleen and usually circulatory collapse. The incidence of acute sequestration crisis has been reported as 5% of children with sickle cell disease. After one major episode of acute splenic sequestration crisis elective splenectomy is offered due the 40-50% chance of recurrence. An article on sickle cell anemia in 2006 states that splenectomy is not only safe but also decreases transfusion requirements and eliminates the risk of acute sequestration crisis. Even during acute sequestration crisis laparoscopic splenectomy has been safely performed.

Thalassemia

Thalassemia is an autosomal dominant disorder of hemoglobin synthesis. There are several forms of this disease depending on which globin chain is affected (alpha, beta, gamma or delta), resulting in a wide spectrum of clinical presentations. In thalassemias there is reduced or absent production of one of the hemoglobin chains with compensatory overproduction of other remaining chains. Because of this compensatory overproduction the red cell develops intracellular collections of excess globin chains. This leads to the premature destruction of the red cells as they are filtered through the spleen. The beta subtype is the most common form found in the United States. Homozygotes of the beta subtype, also known as thalassemia major, have no production of normal beta chains leading to excess alpha chain hemoglobin that precipitates. Due to the increased clearance of erythrocytes overtime splenomegaly develops.

Patients with thalassemia present with growth retardation, pallor, gallstones, cranial enlargement and splenomegaly. The diagnosis is usually made with evidence of microcytic anemia, target cells on peripheral blood smears, an increased reticulocyte count and protein electrophoresis demonstrating low levels of hemoglobin A with elevated levels of fetal hemoglobin.

Treatment for thalassemia consists of red blood cell transfusions along with iron chelation. Splenectomy is indicated in patients with excessive transfusion requirements (> 1 per month), those who suffer discomfort from splenomegaly, who have pain from splenic infarction or have severe thrombocytopenia (< 20,000 platelets/ mm^3). Reports demonstrate a decreased transfusion requirement in thalassemia patients post-splenectomy and that these effects are long term. Careful counseling is obligatory since thrombotic and infectious complications in this population post-splenectomy have been noted to be higher compared to other hematologic indications.

In children, partial splenectomy has been tried with temporary symptom improvement for 1-2 years until the spleen hypertrophies. Partial splenectomy is recommended in children less than 5 years old as a temporizing measure. The main reason for death in these patients is from myocardial infarction secondary to hemosiderin accumulation in the heart. Splenectomy does not alter the course of iron deposition and therefore does not affect survival.

Several studies have demonstrated the utility of laparoscopic splenectomy in the management of this disease. These studies do make a note of increased operative times and an increased transfusion requirement during laparoscopy compared to open, but found safety and efficacy to be equivalent.

Red Blood Cell Enzyme Deficiencies

There are several diseases characterized by erythrocytes enzyme deficiencies that result in hemolytic anemia such as glucose-6-phosphate dehydrogenase (G6PD) deficiency and pyruvate kinase (PK) deficiency. There is no current indication for splenectomy in patients with G6PD deficiency. However, in patients with PK splenomegaly is common and splenectomy in severe cases improves symptoms, in addition to decreasing transfusion requirements. PK is diagnosed with a screening test or by identification of certain cDNA mutations. Given the prevalence of splenomegaly in this population laparoscopy should be used selectively.

Myeloproliferative Disorders

Myeloproliferative disorders are characterized uncontrolled growth of certain cell lines in the bone marrow and includes chronic myeloid leukemia (CML), acute myeloid leukemia (AML), chronic myelomonocytic leukemia (CMML), essential thrombocythemia (ET), polycythemia vera (PV) and myelofibrosis (MF). Most patients have symptomatic splenomegaly that causes early satiety and pain. Hypersplenism is also seen and is characterized by peripheral cytopenia(s) with a normal bone marrow that compensates.

Chronic Myeloid Leukemia

Chronic myeloid leukemia (CML) is a hematologic malignancy of the bone marrow stem cells. This disease results in an increase of one line of the pluripotent progenitor cells. The chromosomal abnormality of this disease is the genetic transposition between the *bcr* and *abl* genes on chromosomes 9 and 22, respectively. This leads to a constitutively active tyrosine kinase. The incidence of this disease is 1.5 per 100,000 individuals. CML invariably progresses from its chronic form to an accelerated, blastic stage during which death due to infection or bleeding invariably occurs. During the chronic phase most individuals are asymptomatic, but some patients will demonstrate constitutional symptoms, abdominal fullness and up to 50% have splenomegaly.

The diagnosis of CML is made with evidence of leukocytosis, granulocytes filling the bone marrow and 90% will have the Philadelphia chromosome abnormality (*t 9:22*) on DNA analysis. Splenectomy is indicated to relieve symptomatic splenomegaly and cytopenias. A series from M.D. Anderson reported their results in 55 patients in the accelerated phase of the disease and with splenectomy found improvement in early satiety, pain and an improvement in platelet counts. The morbidity reported in this study was less than 2%.

Acute Myeloid Leukemia

Acute myeloid leukemia (AML) has a more dramatic clinical course than CML. Death occurs within weeks to months if AML is left untreated. Patients with other hematologic disorders (polycythemia vera or myeloid metaplasia) are at increased risk of transformation to AML. The accumulation of abnormal stem cells in the bone marrow prevents the normal growth of other lines, resulting in a decrease in white cell, red cell and platelet count. The incidence in the United States is 9200 new cases a year. Patients usually present with fatigue, fever, bone pain, petechiae and 50% present with splenomegaly. Splenectomy is also indicated for symptomatic splenomegaly which leads to symptom improvement postoperatively.

Chronic Myelomonocytic Leukemia

Chronic myelomonocytic leukemia (CMML) results from the proliferation of monocytes. Like CML about 50% will have splenomegaly and splenectomy is indicated in those who are symptomatic.

Essential Thrombocytopenia

Essential thrombocytopenia is characterized by an abnormal proliferation of megakaryocytes in the bone marrow resulting in an increase peripheral platelet count. These patients usually present with thrombotic events, vasomotor symptoms and sometimes fetal loss. Hydroxyurea is an antineoplastic drug that is used to reduce thrombotic events in this patient population. Splenomegaly occurs in one-third to one-half of these patients. Splenectomy for symptomatic splenomegaly is reserved for the late stages of the disease when myeloid metaplasia develops. The reason for the delay in surgical interventions is secondary to the increased incidence of hemorrhagic and thrombotic events post-splenectomy in this patient population.

Polycythemia Vera

Polycythemia vera is characterized by an increased red blood cell count. Treatment ranges from phlebotomy and aspirin to chemotherapeutic agents. Splenomegaly occurs often, but splenectomy is reserved for the late stages of the disease, again like ET, when myeloid metaplasia is developing for the same reasons stated above.

Myelofibrosis

Myelofibrosis is characterized by fibrosis of the bone marrow which leads to displacement of bone marrow progenitor cells into the peripheral bloodstream, extramedullary hematopoiesis, splenomegaly and bone marrow failure. Up to 75% of these patients develop symptomatic splenomegaly, for which splenectomy is indicated. Nearly all patients have splenomegaly, with 35% having massive splenomegaly. Postoperative complications are more common in patients with myelofibrosis compared to patients with other hematologic indications. These complications include the risk for thrombocytosis with portal vein thrombosis. A review from the Mayo Clinic recommended the use of platelet lowering therapy to reduce postoperative thrombotic complications in this patient population.

Leukemias

Chronic Lymphocytic Leukemia

Chronic lymphocytic leukemia (CLL) is the most common of the chronic leukemias and is characterized by multiple non-functional lymphocytes. Patients normally present with fatigue, fever, night sweats, frequent infections, hepatosplenomegaly, anemia, thrombocytopenia and lymphadenopathy. Degrees of splenomegaly vary from mild to massive. Patients with stage II disease or greater will have splenomegaly, anemia and thrombocytopenia secondary to hypersplenism. Splenectomy is indicated in this patient population for anemia or thrombocytopenia for which surgical intervention is 75% effective. Patients post-splenectomies have been found to have a sustained increase in their platelet count for at least a year postoperatively. Splenectomy is also indicated for symptomatic splenomegaly. Unfortunately the majority of patients by the time these indications are present are in the late stage of their disease, therefore, will have little impact on their life expectancy. There is a subgroup of CLL patients that have been noted to obtain some survival benefit from splenectomy. This subgroup has a hemoglobin level less than 10 gm/dL or a platelet count less than 50,000/microL. The morbidity and mortality rates from surgery are comparable to patients who underwent chemotherapy alone.

Hairy Cell Leukemia

Hairy cell leukemia is an uncommon low grade B-cell leukemia representing only 2% of leukemias. This disease is characterized by cells with irregular filamentous projections that infiltrate the bone marrow and spleen. Patients present with symptomatic splenomegaly (80%), pancytopenia and hairy cells in the bone marrow. Splenectomy corrects the cytopenias in 40-70% of patients. Splenectomy historically used to be the treatment of choice for this disease because 80-90% had improvements in their cytopenias. However, the relapse rates of 60-50% resulted in less than half of patients having long-term benefits from splenectomy secondary to progressive bone marrow disease. Majority of patients today are medically treated successfully resulting in splenectomy being now reserved as a salvage therapy.

Lymphomas

Non-Hodgkin's Lymphoma

Non-Hodgkin's lymphoma (NHL) is the most common lymphoma with 50,000 patients being diagnosed in the United States annually. This disease is characterized by the proliferation of either natural killer, T or B cells resulting in many different histological types. Patients usually present with lymphadenopathy, pain, fever and night sweats. The exact presentation of each patient usually depends on the different subgroups of this disease. Non-Hodgkin's lymphoma is the most common malignancy involving the spleen and is involved in 35-80% of patients with NHL. Splenomegaly and cytopenias are the current indications for splenectomy in this population. Splenectomy results in 80% of patients having a decreased transfusion requirement; the individual response is dependent on the patient's bone marrow reserve. Even with the improvement in the cytopenias there has been no documented improvement in long-term survival.

Hodgkin's Lymphoma

The use of staging laparotomy with liver biopsy, splenectomy and removal of enlarged lymph nodes for Hodgkin's lymphoma (HL) used to be common practice. Current staging practices based on history, physical and CT scan has made staging laparotomies almost obsolete. For this disease, effective treatment is based on accurate staging of the extent of disease. Even though a staging laparotomy is still considered the most accurate technique to identify infradiaphragmatic disease, advances in imaging has lead to less than 5% of HL patients requiring a staging laparotomy. Operative staging should only be performed if the results would change the management. When indicated staging laparotomies are now done laparoscopically with inspection of the peritoneum, splenectomy, core biopsies of the liver and lymph node biopsies of the para-aortic, iliac, portal and mesenteric lymph nodes.

Storage Diseases

Gaucher's Disease

Gaucher's disease is an autosomal recessive disease characterized by the deficiency of lysosomal hydrolase B-glucosidase which results in the accumulation of glucocerebroside in the macrophage-monocyte system There are three distinct types of this disease. Patients present with hepatosplenomegaly and cytopenias secondary to hypersplenism. Splenectomy resolves the hematologic abnormalities noted with this disease process. Recently enzyme replacement has replaced surgical treatment as first line treatment.

Niemann-Pick Disease

Niemann-Pick disease is an autosomal recessive lysosomal storage disorder. There are four types of this disorder with types A and B resulting in splenomegaly. Splenectomy is indicated in symptomatic splenomegaly.

Felty's Syndrome

Felty's syndrome is characterized by rheumatoid arthritis, splenomegaly and neutropenia. In this disease there are elevated levels of IgG which form immune complexes with neutrophils and lead to their sequestration in the spleen. Patients present with recurrent infections and chronic leg ulcers due to the neutropenia. These patients are initially treated with steroids. Splenectomy is utilized for these patients to correct the neutropenia that leads to their immunocompromised state. In some cases splenectomy does not improve the cytopenia (20%), but in these cases splenectomy has been found to improve the neutrophil's response to antigens. In at least one quarter of patients the granulocytopenia recurs. Other indications for splenectomy in this population include the need for greater than 1 transfusion a month, thrombocytopenia and recurrent infections. As stated before the hallmark of this disease is splenomegaly, therefore laparoscopy should be used selectively in the surgical management. For many years splenectomy was the standard of care in these patients but now has been replaced by medical management.

Sarcoidosis

Sarcoidosis is a granulomatous disease of unknown etiology that affects multiple organ systems. Any organ can be involved with the lungs being affected most often, followed by the spleen. Splenomegaly occurs in 25% of patients secondary to granulomatous involvement. Of the patients with splenomegaly 20% have been found to have hypersplenism resulting in thrombocytopenia. Splenectomy is indicated for symptomatic splenomegaly and in those rare cases of hypersplenism.

Wiskott-Aldrich Syndrome

Wiskott-Aldrich syndrome is an X-linked disease characterized by immunodefiency, thrombocytopenia and eczema. This disease is thought to be due to a genetic defect in adhesion molecules that affects immune cells and platelets. These patients present at a young age with petechiae and epistaxis secondary to low platelet counts and dysfunctional platelets. The spleen in this disease destroys the abnormal platelets for which steroids have not been found to be a useful treatment. For this reason splenectomy initially became the standard of care in treating this population. However, physicians quickly noticed these patients were prone to a higher rate of postoperative infectious complications, and therefore added antibiotic suppression postoperatively leading to improvements in outcomes. With splenectomy there is an increase in the number, size and even function of circulating platelets.

With advances in bone marrow transplants, HLA matched bone marrow transplants have become the standard of care for this disease. However, if there is no HLA match, splenectomy has been found to be superior in terms of survival compared to unmatched or no transplant. Those without an HLA match or who do not undergo splenectomy usually do not survive past the age of 5.

Primary Tumors of Spleen

There are several rare tumors of the spleen which include angiosarcoma, fibrosarcoma, leiomyosarcomas, plasmacytomas, malignant fibrous histiocytomas, hemangiosarcomas and lymphangiosarcomas for which splenectomy is indicated. Angiosarcoma is the most common of these rare tumors, and is very aggressive and disseminates early. Splenectomy in these cases is indicated but given the aggressive nature is rarely curative.

Metastatic Disease to Spleen

Metastatic disease to the spleen is rare but seen with breast, lung, melanoma, ovarian, endometrial, gastric, colonic and prostate cancer. Splenectomy is indicated for oncologic cure when there are isolated splenic metastases identified and the primary tumor is controlled. Splenectomy is also indicated for ovarian debulking procedures.

Preoperative Management

For planned splenectomy all patients should receive the appropriate vaccinations (*Haemophilus influenzae B, Pneumococcus, Meningococcus*) two weeks prior to the planned splenectomy.

Operative planning is usually based on splenic size determined by imaging. CT scan can determine not only splenic size but also determine the location of major vascular structures and the presence and location of accessory spleens. Ultrasound is the most cost-effective modality of imaging the spleen and gives a fairly good estimate of splenic size. Radioscintigraphy with TC-99m sulfur colloid is useful in locating accessory spleens but is not routinely used preoperatively. Angiography provides very little additional information for preoperative planning.

Appropriate preoperative antibiotics should be infused within 30 minutes of skin incision. For those patients who recently have been receiving corticosteroids a stress dose should be given preoperatively. All patients should receive deep vein thrombosis prophylaxis.

Operative Techniques

Open Splenectomy

Open splenectomy is done either through a midline abdominal incision or left subcostal incision. For patients with massive splenomegaly (1500 gm) a midline abdominal incision is often recommended. A left subcostal incision is preferred for most other elective splenectomies. For this approach the incision is made two finger breadths below and parallel to the costal margin. For both approaches the patient is placed in the supine position with the arms out. A Foley catheter, orogastric/nasogastric tube and sequential compression devices are appropriately placed.

Once the abdomen is entered, the ligamentous attachments are then divided under direct visualization starting with the splenocolic ligament followed by the gastrosplenic and gastrohepatic ligaments. The short gastric vessels in the gastrosplenic ligament are then serially ligated with suture ties, ligature, or en seal. Individual dissection and ligation of the short gastric vessels reduces the risk of tearing, retraction and bleeding from these vessels. The spleen is mobilized medially by excision of the splenophrenic ligament. The vascular pedicle is then isolated and the splenic artery and vein taken with a GIA stapler vascular load or ligated individually with the splenic artery being taken first. Care must be taken during the hilar dissection given the close proximity of the pancreas to prevent injury to this fragile organ. Some surgeons will take the splenic artery earlier in the dissection after the lateral mobilization to allow for safer manipulation of the spleen and to decrease the size of the spleen in massive splenomegaly. After hemostasis is confirmed and a thorough exploration of the abdomen for accessory spleens is done then the abdomen is closed in the standard fashion. The skin is then either closed in a subcuticular manner or with skin staples. Many surgeons leave a nasogastric tube in place overnight to decrease the risk of gastric distention and disruption of the short gastric vascular pedicles. Patients are usually discharged to home after they have return of bowel function are tolerating PO and ambulating without difficulty.

Laparoscopic Splenectomy

Since 1991, laparoscopic splenectomy has been accepted as an appropriate surgical technique. Longer operative times were initially noted with laparoscopy, but have decreased if not reached equality with the open technique with further experience. Several studies have demonstrated laparoscopic splenectomy to be the preferred technique for an elective splenectomy. With this technique there is less postoperative pain, less blood loss, earlier tolerance of a diet, less morbidity (fewer pulmonary, wound and infectious complications) and shorter hospital stays. Laparoscopy is also feasible in patients with massive splenomegaly (> 1000 gm), as has been demonstrated in several series. With massive splenomegaly there are longer operative times, higher conversion rates to open and greater morbidity than compared to patients who undergo laparoscopic splenectomy with normal sized spleens. Other reports debate the increased rates of conversion to open in this patient population. Even with increased operative times these studies demonstrated lower morbidity, transfusion rates and short mean hospital stays with the laparoscopic approach.

Patients are usually placed in the right lateral decubitus position, with the left arm elevated and a 30 degree angle made by breaking the bed. Three to four ports are placed subcostally and one placed above/through the umbilicus to mobilize the spleen and dissect the vascular pedicle with a harmonic, en seal or ligature device. The vascular pedicle is then transected with either the ligature or endo-GIA stapler vascular load as described in the open technique. The spleen is then placed in a large impervious bag and extracted piecemeal through one of the port sites. For any ports greater than 5 mm in size, the fascia should be closed and then all skin incisions closed with 4.0 absorbable sutures.

Some authors utilize a laparoscopic hand-assisted approach to facilitate handling these enlarged spleens. Others have reported the benefits of preoperative splenic artery embolization in these patients to facilitate the use of laparoscopy. The benefits of splenic artery embolization are an area of debate in the literature because of concerns of expense, undue risk and discomfort.

Robotic Splenectomy

The introduction of robotic surgery has expanded the field of minimally invasive surgery by improving visibility with three-dimensional vision and motion control with reticulating endoscopic instruments. The patient is placed in an incomplete right lateral decubitus position at a 30 degree angle with a kidney rest. The table is flexed to open up the costal margin. The movable cart with the robotic arms is positioned on the patient's left side. The procedure is carried out exactly as described above for the laparoscopic splenectomy. Dissection is usually performed with the robotic EndoWrist hook cautery in the right hand and a Cadiere forceps in the left hand. The assistant at the table is utilized to move the spleen as needed. The operative times with robotics are significantly increased along with significantly increased procedural costs, bringing practicality into question.

Complications of Splenectomy

As with all operative interventions risks are present and must be conveyed to the patient prior to surgery. Hemorrhage is the most life-threatening complication with splenectomy and usually occurs within the first 24-48 hours postoperatively, emphasizing the importance of hemostasis. The majority of take backs for bleeding find bleeding on the surface of the diaphragm. Most physicians do not recommend the use of serial hematocrits in these patients or the placement of drains.

Gastric dilation is another complication noted secondary to gastric manipulation intraoperatively. Besides nausea, vomiting and abdominal discomfort, there is a concern for disruption of the short gastric pedicles with gastric distention. For these reasons several surgeons maintain a nasogastric tube in place overnight or longer depending the case.

Pancreatic fistulas secondary to trauma to the pancreas is a risk that can be prevented with careful dissection and knowledge that the pancreas is in very close association with the splenic hilum in up to 20% of patients. Subphrenic abscesses can also occur in these patients. They are thought to occur through infection of a seroma at the operative site. There is controversy if the placed of drains could prevent this complication. Postoperative fevers are the most common sign of a subphrenic abscess which is diagnosed with CT scan and usually drained under image directed guidance.

Finally, overwhelming postsplenectomy infection (OPSI) is of extreme concern postoperatively since its recognition in the 1950s. The spleen is the organ responsible for the clearance of encapsulated organisms which are the usual culprits in this infectious process. For this reason patients undergo immunization against *Streptococcus pneumoniae*, *Neisseria meningitidis* and *Haemophilus influenzae* preoperatively. In addition to preoperative vaccination patients need to have their pneumococcal vaccine updated every five years and then influenza vaccinations yearly. The most vulnerable patients to this complication are the very young, the elderly, those within the first two years postoperatively (highest risk), those with hematologic malignancy (e.g. Hodgkin's disease) and those who have undergone chemotherapy or radiation therapy. Symptoms are often mild with fever, malaise, myalgias, headache, vomiting, diarrhea and mild abdominal pain. Patients present with signs of sepsis and/or disseminated intravascular coagulation. Laboratory analysis may demonstrate a very elevated or very low white count, toxic granulation and thrombocytopenia. Patients should be started empirically with antibiotics to cover penicillin-resistant pneumococcus and *Haemophilus influenzae* (e.g. ceftriaxone/cefotaxime/levofloxacin in combination with vancomycin). The mortality when identified and treated early is 10%, with delayed treatment mortality increases to 50-80%.

Previous authors have attempted to correlate preoperative conditions with the frequency and type of postoperative complications. These studies demonstrated that splenic size was the only preoperative condition that was found to be predictive of postoperative complications. Increased intraoperative blood losses also correlated but did not reach statistical significance. The complication rate in their series and others was 14-61% and included hemorrhage, pulmonary complications, subphrenic abscess, pancreatic injury, wound complications and sepsis.

Summary

- Splenic preservation is preferred during distal pancreatectomy, but not at the cost of oncologic cure.
- Splenectomy for proximal gastric cancer should be done if there is extension of tumor into the spleen, pancreas or macroscopic nodal metastases to the splenic hilum.
- Splenectomy for ITP is indicated for failure of medical therapy and provides a permanent cure in the majority of patients. Laparoscopic splenectomy is the surgical treatment of choice in these patients.
- Splenectomy is curative in the treatment of patients with hereditary spherocytosis. Laparoscopic splenectomy is safe in this patient population. Consider the need for laparoscopic cholecystectomy during the same procedure if they have gallstones.
- Splenectomy is a life-saving procedure in sickle cell patients during an acute sequestration crisis.
- Splenectomy is indicated in patients with Myeloproliferative disorders (CML, AML, CMML, ET, PV and MM) with symptomatic splenomegaly and cytopenias.
- Splenectomy is effective in treating patients with leukemia (CLL) or lymphoma (NHL) with cytopenias-resulting in a decrease in their transfusion requirements.
- Laparoscopic splenectomy is as safe and effective as open splenectomy even in cases of massive splenomegaly.

Landmark Papers

1. Bruzoni M, Sasson AR. Open and laparoscopic spleen-preserving, splenic vessel-preserving distal pancreatectomy: indications and outcomes. J Gastrointest Surg 2008; 12:1202-6.
2. Eom BW, Jang JY, Lee SE, et al. Clinical outcomes compared between laparoscopic and open distal pancreatectomy. Surg Endosc 2008; 22:1334-8.
3. Fatouros M, Roukos DH, Lorenz M, et al. Impact of spleen preservation in patients with gastric cancer. Anticancer Res 2005; 25:3023-30.

4. Goh BK, Tan YM, Chung YF, et al. Critical appraisal of 232 consecutive distal pancreatectomies with emphasis on risk factors, outcome and management of the postoperative pancreatic fistula: a 21-year experience at a single institution. Arch Surg 2008; 143:956-65.

5. Shoup M, Brennan MF, McWhite K, et al. The value of splenic preservation with distal pancreatectomy. Arch Surg 2002; 137:164-8.

6. Wanebo HJ, Kennedy BJ, Winchester DP, et al. Role of splenectomy in gastric cancer surgery: adverse effect of elective splenectomy on longterm survival. J Am Coll Surg 1997; 185:177-84.

7. Watson DI, Coventry BJ, Chin T, et al. Laparoscopic versus open splenectomy for immune thrombocytopenic purpura. Surgery 1997; 121:18-22

8. Yoon YS, Lee KH, Han HS, et al. Patency of splenic vessels after laparoscopic spleen and splenic vessel-preserving distal pancreatectomy. Br J Surg 2009; 96:633-40.

9. Yu W, Choi GS, Chung HY. Randomized clinical trial of splenectomy versus splenic preservation in patients with proximal gastric cancer. Br J Surg 2006; 93:559-63.

10. Zhang CH, Zhan WH, He YL, et al. Spleen preservation in radical surgery for gastric cardia cancer. Ann Surg Oncol 2007; 14:1312-9.

Level of Evidence Table			
Recommendation	**Best level of evidence**	**Grade**	**References**
Splenic preservation during distal pancreatectomy for benign or low-grade neoplasms can safely be performed and may have perioperative benefits compared to pancreatectomy with splenectomy.	2b	B	1-5
Laparoscopic splenectomy is safe and has perioperative advantages over open splenectomy.	2a	B	6-10
Routine splenectomy during gastric cancer resections is NOT indicated without gross disease extending to the splenic hilum or involving lymph nodes at the hilum and along the splenic artery. (see Gastric Cancer chapter)	1b	B	11-14
Splenectomy is beneficial for symptomatic splenomegaly and thrombocytopenia in advanced myeloproliferative disorders.	2b	B	15
Splenectomy is beneficial for a variety of hereditary and immunologic blood disorders including spherocytosis, sickle cell disease and thalassemias.	3a	B	16-21

References

1. Shoup M, Brennan MF, McWhite K, et al. The value of splenic preservation with distal pancreatectomy. Arch Surg 2002; 137:164-8.

2. Yoon YS, Lee KH, Han HS, et al. Patency of splenic vessels after laparoscopic spleen and splenic vessel-preserving distal pancreatectomy. Br J Surg 2009; 96:633-40.

3. Bruzoni M, Sasson AR. Open and laparoscopic spleen-preserving, splenic vessel-preserving distal pancreatectomy: indications and outcomes. J Gastrointest Surg 2008; 12:1202-6.

4. Goh BK, Tan YM, Chung YF, et al. Critical appraisal of 232 consecutive distal pancreatectomies with emphasis on risk factors, outcome and management of the postoperative pancreatic fistula: a 21-year experience at a single institution. Arch Surg 2008; 143:956-65.

5. Rodriguez JR, Madanat MG, Healy BC, et al. Distal pancreatectomy with splenic preservation revisited. Surgery 2007; 141:619-25.

6. Watson DI, Coventry BJ, Chin T, et al. Laparoscopic versus open splenectomy for immune thrombocytopenic purpura. Surgery 1997; 121:18-22.

7. Rescorla FJ, Engum SA, West KW, et al. Laparoscopic splenectomy has become the gold standard in children. Am Surg 2002; 68:297-301; discussion 301-2.

8. Winslow ER, Brunt LM. Perioperative outcomes of laparoscopic versus open splenectomy: a meta-analysis with an emphasis on complications. Surgery 2003; 134:647-53; discussion 654-5.

9. Velanovich V. Case-control comparison of laparoscopic versus open distal pancreatectomy. J Gastrointest Surg 2006; 10:95-8.

10. Eom BW, Jang JY, Lee SE, et al. Clinical outcomes compared between laparoscopic and open distal pancreatectomy. Surg Endosc 2008; 22:1334-8.

11. Wanebo HJ, Kennedy BJ, Winchester DP, et al. Role of splenectomy in gastric cancer surgery: adverse effect of elective splenectomy on longterm survival. J Am Coll Surg 1997; 185:177-84.

12. Zhang CH, Zhan WH, He YL, et al. Spleen preservation in radical surgery for gastric cardia cancer. Ann Surg Oncol 2007; 14:1312-9.

13. Yu W, Choi GS, Chung HY. Randomized clinical trial of splenectomy versus splenic preservation in patients with proximal gastric cancer. Br J Surg 2006; 93:559-63.

14. Fatouros M, Roukos DH, Lorenz M, et al. Impact of spleen preservation in patients with gastric cancer. Anticancer Res 2005; 25:3023-30.

15. Bouvet M, Babiera GV, Termuhlen PM, et al. Splenectomy in the accelerated or blastic phase of chronic myelogenous leukemia: a single-institution, 25-year experience. Surgery 1997; 122:20-5.

16. Al-Salem AH. Indications and complications of splenectomy for children with sickle cell disease. J Pediatr Surg 2006; 41:1909-15.

17. Al-Salem AH, Nasserulla Z. Splenectomy for children with thalassemia. Int Surg 2002; 87:269-73.

18. Morris KT, Horvath KD, Jobe BA, et al. Laparoscopic management of accessory spleens in immune thrombocytopenic purpura. Surg Endosc 1999; 13:520-2.

19. Kojouri K, Vesely SK, Terrell DR, et al. Splenectomy for adult patients with idiopathic thrombocytopenic purpura: a systematic review to assess long-term platelet count responses, prediction of response and surgical complications. Blood 2004; 104:2623-34.

20. Schilling RF, Gangnon RE, Traver MI. Delayed adverse vascular events after splenectomy in hereditary spherocytosis. J Thromb Haemost 2008; 6:1289-95.

21. Mikhael J, Northridge K, Lindquist K, et al. Short-term and long-term failure of laparoscopic splenectomy in adult immune thrombocytopenic purpura patients: A systematic review. Am J Hematol 2009;84(11):743-8.

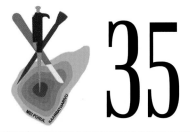

35

Gynecologic Oncology

William C McBee, Scott D Richard, Robert P Edwards

Uterine Cancer

Background

Uterine cancer is the fourth most common cancer of women in the United States and the most common gynecological malignancy. It can be divided into two very different categories. The first is epithelial tumors of the endometrial lining and the second is mesenchymal tumors or sarcomas. The American Cancer Society estimates 40,100 new cases of uterine cancer with around 7470 related deaths for 2008. Uterine sarcomas comprise only 3-6% of these cases, but account for around 26% of the deaths. The first part of this chapter will exclusively be dedicated to the much more common endometrial cancer, with a brief section on uterine sarcomas to follow.

Epidemiology and Risk Factors

Most endometrial cancers arise in postmenopausal women, with the mean age in the early 60s. While some cases of endometrial cancer have a hereditary predisposition, mostly associated with hereditary nonpolyposis colorectal cancer (HNPCC), the majority are thought to arise sporadically. There is a strong environmental influence, mostly associated with excess estrogen exposure, either endogenously or exogenously. Obesity, exogenous estrogen without cyclic progestins, diabetes mellitus, polycystic ovarian syndrome and nulliparity are all found to be associated with endometrial cancer.

Clinical Features and Screening

Routine screening is not recommended for endometrial cancer. Exceptions include those at a higher risk, including postmenopausal women on unopposed estrogens, women with HNPCC and premenopausal women with anovulatory menstrual cycles. While endometrial cancer can be found on routine Pap tests, screening in this fashion is not recommended.

Most women with endometrial cancer present with abnormal uterine bleeding and any abnormal menstrual bleeding should be evaluated, including postmenopausal bleeding, intermenstrual or heavy bleeding in perimenopausal women and abnormal bleeding in anovulatory premenopausal women. Transvaginal ultrasonographic evaluation of endometrial thickness has been shown to be diagnostic in postmenopausal women only. Endometrial sampling, which in most cases can easily be done in the office, is recommended to exclude premalignancy or malignancy.

Diagnosis and Preoperative Evaluation

Endometrial sampling should be performed in any patient suspected of having endometrial cancer. This can usually be performed in the office with a pipelle. If an adequate sample is unable to be obtained in the office, or symptoms persist despite a negative biopsy, the patient should be taken to the operating room for a dilation and curettage, usually with hysteroscopy as well.

Routine preoperative evaluation includes a thorough history and physical examination, complete blood count, serum electrolytes, creatinine, blood glucose, liver function tests, urinalysis and a chest X-ray. CA-125 levels are usually elevated in patients with advanced disease and are often useful in monitoring these patients. They are not useful in patients with early stage disease. Abdominal and pelvic CT scans are not required, but are performed by many to assess for extrauterine disease. Cystoscopy and proctoscopy are only useful if bladder or rectal involvement is suspected after clinical evaluation. Colonoscopy, although not required, is useful as many of these patients are over the age of 50 and have either not undergone the recommended screening, or have risk factors for colon cancer as well.

Surgical Procedure

Anatomy

While endometrial cancer can be clinically staged, multiple studies have demonstrated superiority in surgical staging of this disease. Knowledge of the female anatomy is important in understanding the patterns of spread in endometrial cancer and therefore the appropriate surgical

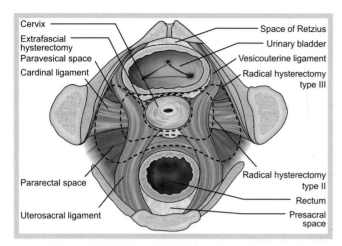

Figure 35-1: The pelvic ligaments and spaces

staging **(Figure 35-1)**. The uterus is comprised of three layers, the endometrium, myometrium and serosa. Cancers that arise in the endometrial glands most often spread by direct extension into the myometrium or spread along the glandular surface or deeper tissues into the cervix. Spread can also occur through the fallopian tubes into the abdomen. The uterus drains primarily to the pelvic lymph nodes. Lymphatic dissemination directly to the para-aortic lymph nodes through the infundibulo-pelvic ligament is rare and most frequently occurs to the pelvic lymph nodes prior to the para-aortic nodes.

Operative Technique

The cornerstone of treatment for endometrial cancer is removal of the uterus and adnexa. Additionally all patients should undergo pelvic washings to assess for malignant cells. There is some controversy surrounding the need to perform a complete pelvic and para-aortic lymphadenectomy in all patients with endometrial cancer. Some rely on intraoperative inspection or frozen section along with preoperative histologic grade to determine which patients should undergo staging. Others perform only a selective sampling of suspicious lymph nodes. The current trend, as well as our belief, is that a complete lymphadenectomy should be performed on all patients with endometrial cancer. Intraoperative inspection of uterine invasion, suspicious lymph nodes and frozen section are inaccurate. Additionally, the final histologic grade is often higher than that found on preoperative biopsy. Based on the results of large clinical trials, we feel the presence of positive lymph nodes is higher than the associated complications of performing a lymphade-nectomy. In addition to being diagnostic and determining which patients undergo postoperative pelvic radiation therapy, lymphadenectomy is a therapeutic procedure and has been shown to decrease the rate of pelvic recurrence in patients with positive nodes. Additionally,

an omentectomy should be performed in all patients with clear cell or papillary serous histology.

Due to the surgical staging procedure required to adequately treat patients with endometrial cancer, historically patients were treated almost exclusively by laparotomy through a vertical midline abdominal incision. This allowed adequate exposure to the pelvis as well as the upper abdomen and para-aortic lymph nodes. Beginning in the early 1990s surgeons began performing laparoscopic assisted vaginal hysterectomies or total laparoscopic hysterectomies with laparoscopic staging for endometrial cancer. Results of multiple randomized trials show a decrease in operative associated complications and similar surgical and pathological results. Since this technique is relatively new, there are no trials demonstrating long-term outcomes in patients treated by laparotomy compared to the laparoscopic approach, although early data shows comparable results. The results of long-term trials comparing these approaches should be available in the near future.

Another operative technique for the management of endometrial cancer is through the use of robotically assisted laparoscopic surgery. There have been multiple studies comparing open, laparoscopic and robotic techniques. It appears that, like other laparoscopic techniques, the use of the robot decreases operative associated complications as compared to open surgery. Comparisons between the robot and other laparoscopy are inconclusive. Both seem to provide similar short- and long-term results. While the expense of the robot is prohibitive, it may enable many surgeons untrained in advanced laparoscopy to perform this procedure in a minimally invasive fashion.

Finally, vaginal hysterectomy alone can be performed in patients with marked obesity or other medical problems that might prohibit them from undergoing abdominal surgery. While complete surgical staging cannot be performed in this manner, patients with stage I disease have favorable outcomes. This technique has been shown to be preferable to radiation therapy alone.

Prognostic Variables

Myometrial Invasion

Invasion into the myometrium is the most common pattern of spread in endometrial cancer. The current FIGO staging subdivides stage I into A (limited to endome-trium), B (invasion limited to the inner half of myomet-rium) and C (invasion into the outer half of myometrium). While tumors with more aggressive histology and grade are more likely to have deeper myometrial invasion, myometrial invasion alone is an independent predictor of tumor spread and subsequently survival.

Cervical Invasion

Invasion into the cervix is classified as FIGO stage II. Invasion is thought to occur through direct spread along the endometrial surface, spread through deeper tissue planes or through lymphatic spread. Involvement of the lower uterine segment and the cervix is associated with a much higher rate of nodal involvement than lesions found elsewhere in the uterus.

Tumor Size

The amount of endometrial surface involvement, characterized either as overall size or percent of endometrial involvement, has been shown in multiple studies to be an independent predictor of lymph node involvement. Although it is not formally involved in the patient's stage, it should be evaluated and taken into account when considering postoperative treatment, especially in patients not undergoing comprehensive surgical staging.

Positive Peritoneal Cytology

The presence of malignant cells on peritoneal cytology, stage IIIA, is a controversial topic. Malignant cells are found much more commonly in patients with disease involving the outer myometrium, adnexa, lymph nodes and in higher stage tumors. In these patients this finding is associated with a poorer prognosis. However, in patients with lower grade disease confined to the inner half of myometrium the significance of positive peritoneal cytology is unclear. Some studies have shown a decrease in survival while others have shown no difference. As laparoscopic surgery and the subsequent use of uterine manipulators becomes more commonly used in the treatment of endometrial cancer, more patients with positive cytology are being discovered. Several studies have shown no difference in disease progression in this group of patients.

Adnexal Involvement

Approximately 5% of women with endometrial cancer will have adnexal involvement. Often it is difficult to determine whether the primary source is the endometrium (stage IIIA), adnexa or both. Approximately one-third of those with endometrial cancer metastatic to the adnexa will have positive lymph nodes as well.

Vaginal Involvement

Vaginal involvement, stage IIIB, in endometrial cancer is relatively a rare event. While this can result from direct extension from the cervix, it can also result from lymph-vascular spread and involve areas of the vagina away from the cervix.

Nodal Involvement

The lymphatic channels that drain the endometrium primarily to the pelvic lymph nodes; and from there to the para-aortic lymph nodes. While positive para-aortic lymph nodes are occasionally encountered with negative pelvic nodes, with potential spread through the infundibulopelvic ligament, this is a rare event. The presence of nodal involvement, stage IIIC, carries a worse prognosis with a 5-year survival of approximately 50%.

Histology

Endometrioid adenocarcinoma is the most common histologic cell type, accounting for approximately 75-80% of cases. In addition to being the most common, it is also the least aggressive and is usually found in women with the risk factors commonly associated with endometrial cancer (obesity, unopposed estrogen, nulliparity, etc.). Adenosquamous carcinomas are likely the next most common type and behave according to the histologic grade and depth of invasion of the glandular component. Two of the most aggressive cell types are papillary serous and clear cell and comprise approximately 1-5% and 5-10% of all cases, respectively. These tumors are much more aggressive and tend to present at a later stage and often have a higher histologic grade. These tumors also tend to present at a later age than endometrioid tumors and are not associated with excess estrogen production. Serous tumors have a propensity to spread throughout the abdomen, even when diagnosed at an early stage. Possible explanations include transtubal spread, lymphatic-vascular invasion and multifocal disease. Clear cell carcinomas are often associated with lymph-vascular invasion and frequently metastasis to lymph nodes. Both should be treated aggressively and are associated with a much worse prognosis than endometrioid adenocarcinomas. In additional to mixed forms of the above histologic cell types, other less common types include undifferentiated, squamous, mucinous, transitional and small cell.

Grade

The histologic differentiation (grade) of the tumor is directly associated with depth of myometrial invasion, frequency of nodal involvement and prognosis. After the staging surgery has been completed the histologic grade, in addition to stage and histologic cell type, determine which patients will require adjuvant treatment.

Lymph-Vascular Space Invasion

Lymph-vascular space invasion (LVSI) is independently associated with tumor recurrence and overall prognosis. While this finding is more common in tumors of higher grade and stage, its finding in early stage, low grade tumors should be considered in evaluating patients for adjuvant therapy following surgery.

Staging

See **Table 35-1**.

TABLE 35-1	1988 FIGO surgical staging for endometrial cancer
Stage	**Description**
IA	Tumor limited to endometrium only
IB	Tumor invasion into inner half of myometrium
IC	Tumor invasion into outer half of myometrium
IIA	Involvement of endocervical glands
IIB	Invasion of cervical stroma
IIIA	Involvement of uterine serosa, adnexa or positive peritoneal cytology
IIIB	Involvement of the vagina
IIIC	Involvement of pelvic or para-aortic lymph nodes
IVA	Invasion of bladder or bowel mucosa
IVB	Distant metastasis, including intra-abdominal or inguinal lymph nodes

Preinvasive Disease

Endometrial hyperplasia is classically thought of as a precursor to endometrial cancer. The World Health Organization classifies endometrial hyperplasia into four categories, simple and complex hyperplasia with the presence or absence of cytologic atypia. There is some questions whether endometrial hyperplasia and neoplasia are directly related; however it is clear that the presence of cytologic atypia is associated with malignancy. Patients with endometrial hyperplasia can often be treated with progestational agents as opposed to surgery. Patients without cytologic atypia are much more likely to respond than those with atypia. Patients with atypia are much more likely to have an associated endometrial cancer (over 50% in some studies of patients with atypical endometrial hyperplasia) and a hysterectomy should strongly be considered.

Treatment of Invasive Disease

Surgery

The mainstay of treatment for endometrial cancer is a total abdominal hysterectomy, bilateral salpingo-oophorectomy, pelvic and para-aortic lymphadenectomy. This can also be performed laparoscopically, robotically and rarely vaginally. Please see the section on "Operative Technique" for more details.

In patients with stage II endometrial cancer (spread to the cervix) a radical hysterectomy is the operation of choice, performed via laparotomy or laparoscopically. Several trials have compared simple hysterectomy to radical hysterectomy in these patients and have shown an improved survival in patients treated with a radical hysterectomy. Also, it is often difficult to distinguish between an endometrial cancer with spread to the cervix and a primary cervical adenocarcinoma. The treatment of choice for most cervical cancers confined to the cervix is also a radical hysterectomy.

Patients with advanced endometrial cancer (stages III and IV) are usually treated with a combination of surgery, chemotherapy and radiation therapy. Several small, retrospective studies have shown a survival advantage in cytoreductive surgery in patients with endometrial cancer. Additionally, patients often benefit symptomatically from removal of the uterus and adnexa to alleviate bleeding, discharge and decrease the rate of fistula formation.

Radiation

The vast majority of patients with endometrial cancer undergo primary surgical management. Radiation use in endometrial cancer is primarily as an adjuvant treatment following surgery. It can be used as primary treatment in patients who are unable to undergo surgical management; however, studies have shown that these patients have a much higher rate of recurrence and lower survival rate.

Following surgical staging, patients with endometrial cancer can be managed in one of several ways **(Figure 35-2)**. For patients with early stage, low grade disease, close observation is all that is required. Patients with higher

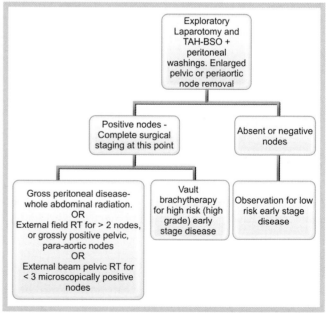

Figure 35-2: Planning of postoperative radiation therapy after surgery for uterine cancer (occult)

risk stage I (Stage IC or Grade 3) or stage II disease can be offered adjuvant treatment with vaginal brachytherapy or external pelvic radiation. As complete surgical staging becomes more prevalent, the role of external pelvic radiation is decreasing. The use of vaginal brachytherapy does reduce the incidence of vaginal vault recurrence and can be used in higher risk patients. External pelvic radiation has been shown by the Gynecologic Oncology Group (GOG) to improve progression-free survival with no effect on overall survival in patients with high-risk stage I and stage II diseases. External pelvic radiation is used to treat patients with positive pelvic lymph nodes, while extended field radiation, to treat the para-aortic lymph nodes, is useful in patients with biopsy proven para-aortic metastasis, positive common iliac nodes or in patients with multiple positive pelvic lymph nodes. In previous years patients with more advanced disease were often treated with whole abdominal radiation. This treatment, for the most part, is no longer used in the management of endometrial cancer and has been replaced with chemotherapy.

Chemotherapy

The role of chemotherapy in the treatment of endometrial cancer is evolving. Historically it was only considered palliative treatment. It is still used in this setting; however it is also being used as an adjuvant treatment along with radiation therapy in patients with high-risk disease. The most appropriate chemotherapeutic agents are subject to debate and clinical trials are currently underway to evaluate these agents. Patients with advanced or recurrent endometrial cancer can also be treated with hormonal agents. Although overall response is low, the use of progestational agents such as medroxyprogesterone acetate and selective estrogen response modulators (SERMs), such as tamoxifen, has achieved a clinical response in some patients.

Intraperitoneal Chemotherapy

While the management of advanced and recurrent endometrial cancer is changing with more emphasis on surgical debulking and use of systemic chemotherapy, the role of intraperitoneal chemotherapy has not been well studied. To date no clinical trials have evaluated the use of IP chemotherapy in the management of these patients. While there is good evidence supporting the use of IP chemotherapy (heated or otherwise) in the management of tumors that spread along peritoneal surfaces (ovarian, colon, mesothelioma, etc.) this has not been evaluated in endometrial cancer.

Treatment of Recurrent Disease

The most common site of recurrence in endometrial cancer is the vaginal vault. The majority of these are salvaged through the use of radiation therapy or surgical resection. Patients with recurrences in the pelvis or distantly have a much worse prognosis. There is increasing support for surgical debulking of such recurrences with subsequent chemotherapy. Recurrences can also be treated with chemotherapy alone, with or without the use of directed radiation therapy.

Prognosis

Prognosis in endometrial cancer is directly related to the grade, stage and histology of disease, as well as the manner in which the patient was treated. Generally reported 5-year survival rates are 80-90% for stage I, 70-80% for stage II, 40-60% for stage III and about 15-20% for stage IV. While most patients present with early stage and grade endometrioid cancer and have a 5-year survival over 90%, more aggressive tumors (grade 3 and non-endometrioid histology) can have a much lower survival, even when presenting in the early stages of disease.

Sarcomas

Uterine sarcomas are mesenchymal tumors of the uterus and account for approximately 3-6% of all uterine cancer, but are responsible for over a quarter of all deaths. They are comprised of three main subtypes, carcinosarcomas (about 50%), leiomyosarcomas (about 30%) and endometrial stromal sarcomas (about 20%). These tumors can originate from individual elements of the mesoderm, uterine smooth muscle (leiomyosarcoma) and endometrial stroma (endometrial stromal sarcoma) or from a mixture of the mesoderm and epithelium (carcinosarcoma). Uterine sarcomas are surgically staged by the FIGO staging system described above.

Carcinosarcoma

Patients with carcinosarcomas (previously referred to as Malignant Mixed Mullerian Tumor or MMMT) usually present in their late 60s and can present with vaginal bleeding, pelvic pain or a mass, symptoms of metastatic disease, or with a mass protruding through the cervix. They are much more commonly found in black women as compared to endometrial carcinomas and a prior history of pelvic radiation is a major risk factor.

The mainstay of treatment for women with uterine carcinosarcoma is surgery, with complete surgical staging, including an omentectomy, as described above. The epithelial component of this tumor is usually responsible for metastasis when this tumor is found outside of the uterus. Similar to data from metastatic and recurrent endometrial cancer, there is a role for surgical debulking of this disease. Postoperative adjuvant treatment, like in endometrial cancer, is based on final stage, histology and LVSI. Because these tumors are very aggressive, patients often receive postoperative radiation and chemotherapy. Overall, these tumors tend to recur in approximately 50-60% of patients and overall 5-year survival is about 30%.

Leiomyosarcoma

Leiomyosarcomas (LMS) are tumors comprised entirely of uterine smooth muscle. While once thought to arise in pre-existing leiomyomas, the incidence in leiomyomas is less than 1% and the majority are thought to arise in uterine smooth muscle. Because these tumors arise from within the uterine smooth muscle, they commonly present with pelvic or back pain, an enlarging uterus and less commonly bleeding. These tumors typically present in women in their early 50s and have no predilection to race and prior radiation exposure.

Like other uterine cancers, surgery is the primary treatment of LMS. Surgical staging is somewhat controversial. These tumors are often diagnosed postoperatively and the overall risk of lymph node metastasis is small. However, many still perform comprehensive staging when the diagnosis is made preoperatively. Adjuvant radiation has been shown to decrease local recurrence rates, but does not seem to impact overall survival. There is also a role for systemic chemotherapy for metastatic disease, but in general this is not a very chemosensitive tumor. Benefit has been shown in removal of metastatic disease by surgical debulking, including lung metastases. Surgical stage is the most important factor in prognosis. Five-year survival is approximately 75% in stage I, 60% in stage II, 45% in stage III and 30% in stage IV disease.

Endometrial Stromal Sarcoma

Endometrial stromal sarcomas (ESS) are rare tumors that arise entirely from the uterine stroma. They are divided into two subtypes, low grade ESS and undifferentiated ESS (previously called high grade ESS). These subtypes behave in an entirely different manner. While undifferentiated ESS is a very aggressive tumor with a poor prognosis, low grade ESS is relatively an indolent tumor. It typically presents in the 40s with vaginal bleeding, a uterine mass or pelvic pain.

Surgical removal is the primary treatment in ESS and comprehensive staging is recommended. Even though these tumors often present in premenopausal women, there is data to suggest that removal of the adnexa is beneficial. There is very limited data to recommend adjuvant radiation or chemotherapy in low grade ESS; however, progestational agents have been shown to lengthen time to recurrence. This disease has been shown to be very slow growing and remote recurrences are common. These are often amenable to surgical resection. Undifferentiated ESS is a very aggressive and difficult disease to control. Postoperative radiation and chemo-therapy is often used and provides some benefit. Five-year survival in patients with undifferentiated ESS is very low, while that of low grade ESS is very high.

Ovarian Cancer

Background

Ovarian cancer is the most lethal gynecological malignancy. Several types of cancers arise from ovarian tissues. The most common and deadly is epithelial ovarian cancer. Other rare types include germ cell and stromal tumors. With surgery and chemotherapy these rare types generally have a much better prognosis than epithelial histologies.

Epidemiology and Risk Factors

In 2008, there were 21,650 cases of ovarian cancer in the United States with 15,520 deaths. The median age of onset is 62 years of age for epithelial ovarian cancer. Between 5% and 10% of epithelial ovarian cancer cases are felt to be hereditary and occur in women with a family history of first- or second-degree relatives with ovarian cancer. There are three patterns of hereditary ovarian cancer commonly identified: ovarian, ovarian and breast cancer, or ovarian and colon cancer. A family history of two or more first degree relatives conveys the highest risk and genetic counseling followed by genetic testing are recommended to help define an individual's risk once a significant family history is identified.

Prophylactic oophorectomy is recommended for high-risk women beyond the age of 35 once child bearing is complete. Prophylactic surgery is associated with a greater than 90% protective effect for subsequent ovarian cancer or primary peritoneal cancer. It is estimated that 5% or less will have an occult cancer at the time of prophylactic surgery.

Other risk factors associated with ovarian cancer include nulliparity, not using oral contraceptive pills, higher socioeconomic status, infertility, endometriosis and not breast feeding after pregnancy. Work associated with animal models suggests number of lifetime ovulatory events may predict risk.

Clinical Features and Presentation

Ovarian cancer commonly disseminates by a 'snow-globe' exfoliative dissemination particularly with the papillary histology. In these scenarios there is commonly no dominant mass on the ovary and tumor bulk may be distributed over the upper abdomen, including the omentum. These tumors coat and encase organs rather than invading, making peritoneal resection a valuable approach to reducing tumor burden. Symptoms usually do not occur until late; due to the ability of the female pelvis to accommodate large tumor masses without pain (a by-product of anatomic provision for uterine expansion with pregnancy) and vaginal bleeding is rare unlike with uterine corpus cancer or cervical cancer.

Therefore, diagnosis is commonly delayed as patients may undergo extensive medical evaluations for ascites, anorexia, pleural effusions, or chronic abdominal pain before a pelvic/rectal exam or CT scan identifies ovarian masses and carcinomatosis. Early stage disease is usually diagnosed by a dominant pelvic mass with no visible upper abdominal disease. Even in such cases, occult advanced stage disease will be diagnosed in 30% of cases by removal of the pelvic and para-aortic nodes, omentum, peritoneal lavage and careful inspection of the upper abdominal parietal and visceral peritoneal surfaces. Conservative surgery is possible in early stage disease for young patients who have not completed child-bearing. Preservation of the uterus and opposite ovary may be allowed after intraoperative assessment by gross inspection and biopsies of abnormal areas including sampling of the endometrium if abnormal by CT/ultrasound.

Diagnosis and Preoperative Evaluation

The proper work-up of women with carcinomatosis should include the use of tumor markers, CT or MR scan of the chest, abdomen and pelvis, a careful pelvic/rectal exam and a full metabolic and blood count laboratory panel **(Figure 35-3)**. An elevated CA125 may be the first indication that carcinomatosis is of gynecological origin, but any carcinomatosis will produce some elevation of the CA125 so other possible primary sites should be considered. The preoperative evaluation should include colonoscopy screening, breast evaluation and if warranted by symptoms or tumor markers, upper gastrointestinal endoscopy. Tumor markers may include CA125, CEA, CA19-9 and in young women under age 50 the stromal and germ cell tumor markers inhibin, LDH, alpha-fetoprotein and human chorionic gonadotropin should be obtained.

Radiographic findings often include a solid cystic mass, omental cake and hydronephrosis. Complete ureteral obstruction is uncommon with ovarian cancer but long-standing partial obstruction may reduce renal reserve that will sorely be needed for subsequent platinum-based therapy. Therefore, aggressive correction of hydronephrosis with ureteral stents and proper hydration after the use of renal toxic contrast agents are an important issue to address preoperatively. Bowel preparation continues to be recommended, as 20-30% of patients will require one or more bowel resections as part the proper surgical effort. Preoperative nutritional assessment and a room air blood gas can be useful in advanced stage patients with ascites and pleural effusions as fluid shifts and pronounced oliguria are a prominent hallmark of the postoperative course for these patients. Despite highly successful cytoreductions postoperatively, reaccumulation of ascites and pleural effusions are common, but the ascites usually regresses in subsequent weeks following laparotomy. Anticipation of this may require thoracostomy and peritoneal drainage catheters before administering general anesthesia. Patients with poor performance status, age greater than 70 or parenchymal liver metastases may benefit from diagnostic percutaneous biopsy or cytology and the use of neoadjuvant platinum-based chemotherapy prior to attempting cytoreduction.

Surgical Approach

In the absence of extra-abdominal disease, surgical staging should be performed with laparotomy for all patients with suspected ovarian cancer. Complete surgical staging and aggressive cytoreductive efforts have greatly improved the survival and subsequent benefit derived from chemotherapy. The decision to abandon a laparotomy or compromise the length of the incision and operating time should only be made by physicians specifically trained in proper cytoreductive techniques and ovarian cancer biology. Outcomes are clearly inferior in centers where ovarian cancer cytoreductive surgery is not routinely performed. Unlike with gastrointestinal and other primary sites carcinomatosis is usually effectively treated with cytoreductive surgery. The peculiar biology of ovarian cancer's metastatic spread along peritoneal surfaces result in a successful cytoreductive effort in greater than 70% of patients with carcinomatosis if performed at a high volume center.

As stated previously, the proper procurement of tissues for staging apparent early stage ovarian cancer will upstage up to 30% of patients with large masses. Rupture of the mass results in upstaging and often results in the need for adjuvant therapy although this is often due to adherence to adjacent structures which is also a poor prognostic factor.

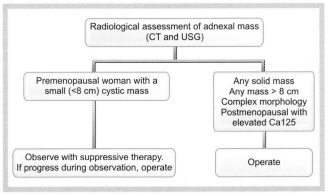

Figure 35-3: Decision making in management of ovarian mass

The staging procedure should include removal of the uterus, tubes and ovaries and any pelvic peritoneum with tumor burden. Peritoneal lavage of the all peritoneal surfaces should be sent for cytology. Proper exploration and aggressive resection of bulky upper disease usually requires assessment of the lesser sac surfaces, division of the falciform to properly ablate or excise subdiaphragmatic disease and thorough retroperitoneal resection of bulky nodal disease. Complete omentectomy should always be performed in grossly involved subcolic disease as this is common site of persistence and recurrence. If these sites are grossly negative, the omentum should be removed and random biopsies performed of the paracolic gutters and hemidiaphragms.

Anatomy and Operative Techniques

The removal of pelvic disease usually requires identification and isolation of the ureter to remove the pelvic sidewall peritoneum. Often a complete ureterolysis and radical hysterectomy will be required to completely remove disease in the cul-de-sac. Rectosigmoid resection is also often required particularly with left-sided masses that may densely be adherent to the sigmoid mesentery. Mobilization of the paracolic gutters allows proper exposure of the retroperitoneum and can be performed continuously as one procedure after identification and division of the round ligament. Takedown of the splenic flexure of the colon and complete omentectomy are often sufficient to remove all omental disease which can be quite bulky. Occasionally splenectomy is required but is usually predicted by preoperative imaging. Removal of enlarged lymph nodes should be pursued from the obturators to the renal vessels bilaterally but complete lymphadenectomy does not appear to improve survival.

Prognostic Variables

Aside from the surgical effort, several standard prognostic variables affect outcome in ovarian cancer. Age, stage, grade of tumor and performance status are as important as with any other solid tumor. Histology becomes important when comparing outcomes within a given stage.

Histology

The most common histologic type is papillary serous, accounting for 85% of all ovarian cancers. A significant portion of these tumors may actually arise from the tubal epithelium rather than the ovary itself, although the source is often hard to differentiate since the majority present with advanced disease. This histology is also felt to be the most sensitive histology to platinum-based therapy. Papillary tumors are more likely to secrete high levels of CA125 tumor antigens although Ca 19-9 and CEA elevations are not uncommon.

Mucinous tumors make up approximately 5% of primary ovarian cancers. Unlike with papillary tumors, the primary source may well be the appendix even with large mucinous ovarian tumors. These tumors are more likely to present with large ovarian masses than papillary tumors. When they rupture mucinous carcinomatosis may result. As a rule these tumors are less sensitive to platinum-based chemotherapy than papillary tumors but usually present as stage I well-differentiated cancers or borderline lesions.

Endometrioid tumors may present as primary ovarian cancer in about 5% of cancer but up to 10% of uterine endometrioid ovarian cancer will have concurrent primary lesions developing on the ovary. In the case of synchronous primaries, these tumors must be staged separately. This condition must be differentiated from endometrioid tumors with metastases from the uterus by genetic profiling in some cases. If both tumors are early stage primary cancers, the prognosis is excellent. If not, stage IIIA uterine cancer is the usual situation and the prognosis is much more guarded.

Clear cell tumors, often present with mixed endometrioid primary ovarian cancers and are felt to be a particularly poor prognostic group. As with endometrioid and mucinous, these tumors are less sensitive to platinum-based chemotherapy and appear to be highly vascular and poorly differentiated. These tumors commonly are aggressive and liver or retroperitoneal extension is not uncommon. They are also often associated with a hypercoaguable state.

Borderline Epithelial Cancers

Epithelial ovarian cancer has particular histologic variants for all four major histologies that is low malignant potential (LMP). These tumors have no invasive or destructive growth pattern. They are very well differentiated but have proliferative changes and nuclear atypia. Regardless of histology, recurrence is rare for early stage disease and distant metastatic sites, when present, do not portend a poor prognosis unless the metastatic site exhibit destructive patterns suggestive of invasion. Ten-year survival for these borderline histologies is the norm with recurrences on the order of 5-10% without adjuvant chemotherapy. The one exception is advanced mucinous tumors which produce the well known pseudomyxoma syndrome and have life expectancies of 3-5 years without aggressive surgery and locoregional chemotherapy.

Epithelial Invasive Cancer and the Need for Chemotherapy

Well differentiated intracystic stage I cancers that have appropriate staging procedures do not generally require adjuvant therapy unless there is cyst rupture. Clear cell carcinomas that are invasive are always considered grade

III tumors and adjuvant therapy is recommended. Advanced grade disease regardless of histology requires adjuvant therapy even if all disease is resected. The amount and approach are dependent on the stage and residual tumor burden. Invasive cancers beyond stage IC whether well differentiated or poorly differentiated are generally treated with adjuvant therapy.

Staging Information (Table 35-2)

In the absence of obvious extra-abdominal disease or poor performance status, ovarian cancer is staged by open laparotomy. Even if there is no apparent disease metastasis, it is required to biopsy the 'at risk' peritoneal surfaces such as the subdiaphragmatic spaces, paracolic gutters, pelvic peritoneum, pelvic and para-aortic lymph nodes. A proper stage cannot be assigned without these biopsies and obtaining these biopsies with peritoneal washing will upstage approximately 30% of apparent stage I disease.

A complete and proper staging for epithelial ovarian cancer would include TAH-BSO and resection of any obvious mass in addition to the following:

- Directed biopsies of suspicious lesions—Washings from four major areas: Diaphragm, right abdomen, left abdomen and pelvis. Thorough evaluation of peritoneum along with biopsy of all suspicious lesions and adhesions.

TABLE 35-2	FIGO surgical staging for ovarian cancer
Stage	**Description**
I	Cancer is limited to the ovaries
IA	Tumor limited to the intracystic surface of a single ovary
IB	Tumor limited to the intracystic surfaces of both ovaries
IC	Tumor on the external surface of the ovary, positive cytology or lavage, or cyst rupture at the time of surgery
II	Metastatic disease to the pelvic surfaces
IIA	Extention to the uterus or fallopian tubes
IIB	Extention to adjacent pelvic peritoneum
IIC	Stage IIA or IIB with positive cytology or lavage
III	Metastatic disease outside of the pelvic surfaces to the upper abdomen or retroperitoneum
IIIA	Microscopically positive disease beyond the pelvis
IIIB	Visible disease less than 2 cm beyond the pelvis
IIIC	Visible disease greater than 2 cm beyond the pelvis or spread to the retroperitoneum, including the inguinal nodes
IV	Disease beyond the peritoneal cavity or parenchymal liver metastasis. Pleural effusions must cytologically be positive to be stage IV.

- Random biopsies of normal surfaces—Cul-de-sac, bladder reflection, paracolic recesses and pelvic sidewalls. Undersurface of R hemidiaphragm must be biopsied as well.
- Infracolic omentectomy.
- Pelvic and para-aortic lymphadenectomy.

Treatment of Early Stage Disease

Stages I and II ovarian cancer requires complete surgical staging procedures as cited above. Current level 1a evidence supports treatment for all but stages IA grade 1 and II patients with platinum-based chemotherapy. The number of cycles is controversial but should exceed three cycles to a maximum of 6 cycles. Patients with disease limited to the pelvis should completely be cytoreduced prior to starting chemotherapy which may sometimes require colon resection and peritonectomy.

Treatment of Advance Stage Disease

Stages III and IV disease should prospectively be staged including laparotomy if the only site of extraperitoneal disease is positive cytology in the pleural effusion. Once staging is defined, a second prognostic factor defined surgically is the size of residual disease nodules left at the conclusion of surgery.

Cytoreductive Effect

Surgery for advanced stage disease includes removal of the uterus, tubes and ovaries as for early stage disease but the focus is on removing bulky disease from the upper abdomen. While there have been no randomized trials demonstrating benefit, retrospective analyses that support this notion are numerous and some feel compelling. Many of the high-volume centers are employing multispecialty teams with gynecological and surgical oncologists, thoracic surgeons, urologists and hospitalists to resect and manage extensive upper abdominal disease burden and the more extended postoperative course. As this philosophy has been adopted by more centers, the optimal cytoreduction rate for stages III and IV cancer has gone up substantially with most centers reporting optimal resection rate of 70-80%. Perhaps the 5-year survival and overall survival increases seen for advanced ovarian cancer are at least in part due to the enthusiasm for cytoreduction. These procedures may include total omentectomy with or without splenectomy, distal pancreatectomy, diaphragmatic stripping, removal of portahepatis and celiac nodal disease, multiple bowel resections and widespread peritonectomy. Retrospective reviews from high volume centers report acceptable morbidity with minimal mortality except in the elderly where multiple bowel resection procedures seem to produce less benefit and more morbidity.

Advanced Extraperitoneal Spread

Parenchymal liver disease is uncommon in ovarian cancer so the management has not been addressed prospectively. Retrospective single center reviews seem to indicate a benefit to resection of isolated metastases, but all of the existing reports have small numbers. Pleural-based disease is generally felt to be a contraindication to aggressive abdominal cytoreduction prior to chemotherapy and there are a few reports of thoracoscopic excision as part of a cytoreduction effort.

Conservative Surgery

For early stage disease in younger patients, conservative surgery appears to be safe with preservation of the non-tumor bearing ovary, uterus and tubes. While the incidence of chemotherapy-associated infertility may be as high as 20%, retrospective reviews have reported subsequent pregnancy rates approaching 40%. Management of the recurrence or new primary cancers in the remaining organs is not well defined, but surveillance for recurrence and second primary ovarian cancer is recommended.

Chemotherapy

The success of the current approach advocating aggressive cytoreductive surgery for ovarian cancer is due in no small part to the biology of ovarian cancer. The non-invasive peritoneal exfoliation and encasement of organs is amenable to peritonectomy techniques. But ovarian cancer is also highly chemoresponsive. Surgery without subsequent chemotherapy affords very little long-term benefit. Modern combinations of taxanes and platinum agents consistently have response rates exceeding 70% for primary disease. The current phase III cooperative group trials are now exploring the role of antiangiogenic target agents in ovarian cancer.

Intraperitoneal Chemotherapy

As locoregional cytoreduction has advanced, direct administration of chemotherapy into the abdominal cavity has slowly been advanced and appears to demonstrate superior progression free and over-all survival. There have now been three phase III trials conducted by the GOG demonstrating a 30-50% increase in the interval of progression-free survival as compared to comparable systemic therapy. The most commonly employed regimes include a systemic taxane with intraperitoneal platinum and intraperitoneal taxane regimen. The success of peritoneal regimens has led to an NCI consensus statement advocating consideration for intraperitoneal approaches in the front line treatment of ovarian cancer.

Treatment of Recurrent Disease

Treatment of recurrent ovarian cancer is never curative but considerable prolongation of life may be accomplished with the use of various chemotherapy agents and judicious use of surgery. Cytoreduction may provide benefit with isolated recurrences in women for whom their disease has been in remission for greater than 18 months since last platinum-based therapy. This type of recurrence would be considered extremely platinum-sensitive ovarian cancer. The use of cytoreduction in patients for which disease-free interval is short rarely produces long-term benefit.

Palliative chemotherapy is extremely commonly employed in ovarian cancer and it is not usual to have patients survive 1-5 years with recurrent disease with intermittent reintroduction of chemotherapy. Once platinum refractory disease develops, liposomal doxorubin, topotecan or gemcitabine may provide palliation and most patients will see all three agents before they succumb to their disease.

Hyperthermic intraoperative perfusion of chemotherapy remains experimental for ovarian cancer, but increasingly larger series are being reported for palliative ovarian cancer patients and it does appear in selected patients that there may be sufficient data to support a phase III trial to define the role of this approach.

Prognosis

Prognosis in ovarian cancer is related to a variety of factors. These include stage, age, grade, residual disease after initial surgery and performance status. The most important variable is stage. Five-year survival for patients with stage I disease is approximately 93%, 70% for stage II, 37% for stage III and 25% for stage IV. Grade is also an important variable. Patients with borderline ovarian tumors, or tumors of low malignant potential, have 15-year survival rates of approximately 98% for those with stage I disease and 86-90% in all stages. In those with invasive cancer, 5-year survival rates decrease with increasing grade. In patients with stage III disease, for example, 5-year survival rates have been reported as 38%, 25% and 19% for grades 1, 2 and 3, respectively.

Patients diagnosed at a younger age tend to have a better prognosis. Five-year survival has been reported as approximately 40% in those younger than 50 years old and 15% for those older than age 50. Residual disease after initial surgical debulking is an important prognostic factor (Figure 35-4). In patients with stage 3 disease, patients with only microscopic disease remaining after initial surgery have a five-year survival rate of about 40-75%, approximately 30-40% in those with less than 1 cm residual disease (optimal) and only 5% for those with greater than 1 cm of residual disease (suboptimal). Lastly,

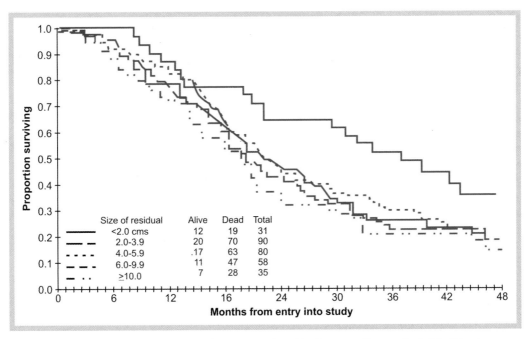

Figure 35-4: Survival by effect of diameter of residual tumor after surgical debulking in ovarian cancer. Hoskins WJ et al, Am J Obstet Gynecol 1994;170:975

patients with a higher performance status have a better overall survival as compared to those who do not.

Cervical Cancer

Background

Worldwide, cervical cancer is the leading cause of death from gynecological cancers and ranks among the leaders in cancer mortality for women. Nearly half a million cases are diagnosed each year. Incidence rates in developing countries are much higher than in developed. In 2008, an estimated 11,070 new cases of cervical cancer will be diagnosed in the United States, with 3,870 deaths.

The mean age of diagnosis in the United States for cervical cancer is 51.4 years. Patients diagnosed are evenly distributed between two age groups, 30-39 and 60-69, with a trend towards increasing stage with increasing age. Since cervical cancer progresses slowly from preinvasive cervical intraepithelial neoplasia (CIN) to invasive cancer, this may suggest that older women are not screened as regularly as the younger cohort. Additionally, there are disproportionately higher numbers of black and Hispanic women affected, most likely from their lack of exposure to appropriate resources.

In developed countries, women who present with cervical cancer often have not had regular Papanicolaou (Pap) smears. Establishment of appropriate screening programs is therefore an important public health issue. For developing countries, women often present with advanced disease, which unfortunately may have already eroded into the bladder, rectum, pelvic nerves or bone. This often leads these women to becoming social outcasts and secondary to a lack of adequate treatment facilities, die alone, in severe pain, with foul smelling vaginal discharge.

Epidemiology and Risk Factors

Cervical cancer is a sexually transmitted disease associated with chronic infections by oncogenic types of the human papillomavirus (HPV). The magnitude of the association between HPV and cervical cancer is higher than that of smoking and lung cancer. Four high risk subtypes have been identified (16, 18, 45 and 56). HPV 16 alone accounts for 50% of invasive cervical cancers, while HPV 18 accounts for another 25%. Low risk subtypes (6, 11, 26, 42, 44, 54, 70 and 73) have been associated with condylomata acuminata of the genital tract.

Although the true prevalence of HPV infections is unknown, it is the leading cause of sexually transmitted infections (STI). For sexually active women younger than 35, 60% have been exposed to HPV. Since it is a sexually transmitted infection, the risk factors for transmission are the same as other STI, early age at onset of sexual activity, multiple sexual partners and multiple pregnancies. Smoking also increases the risk of cervical cancer. Finally, women who are HIV positive often have a coinfection with HPV and have higher rates of CIN and progression to invasive carcinoma then HIV negative women.

Screening

Current ACS guidelines for cervical cancer screening are that women who are sexually active have a Pap smear three years after the initiation of their sexual activity. This screening program should be done annually. At the age of 30, if a woman has had three normal Pap smears in a row, the frequency of screening may be decreased to every 2-3 years. If a hysterectomy has been performed, cervical cancer screening may be eliminated, unless the reason for the hysterectomy was cervical dysplasia. Women 70 or greater, with three normal Pap smears in a row and no history of dysplasia in the last 10 years may elect to forgo additional screening for cervical cancer.

In the United States, the majority of Pap smears are now done via a liquid-based cytology method. This method is similar to the traditional slide based method of Pap smears, but decreases the contamination and allows for easier interpretation of the slides. The FDA currently recommends the use of HPV DNA testing in conjunction with Pap smears in women greater than 30 or any abnormal Pap test (reflex HPV testing). HPV testing has been shown to increase the sensitivity of the screening used for cervical cancer.

Symptoms

Abnormal vaginal bleeding is the most common presenting sign for women with invasive cervical cancer. For younger, sexually active women, this is often described as postcoital in nature. In women who are not sexually active, the presence of bleeding is usually a late finding and is associated with advanced disease. Large cervical tumors often become infected and may present with a malodorous vaginal discharge. In very advanced cases, presenting symptoms may include pelvic pain, bowel or bladder pressure or the passage of stool and/or urine from the vagina.

Since the majority of women (60-80%) diagnosed with cervical cancer in the United States have not had regular Pap smears, studies have suggested that 56% of patients with cervical cancer in the United States present with vaginal bleeding, while only 28% have abnormal Pap smears. Those with abnormal Pap smears often have smaller tumors at an earlier stage.

Diagnosis

When cervical cancer is suspected, diagnosis can be made via colposcopy and/or cervical biopsy. Colposcopy evaluates the ectocervix and a portion of the endocervix. Abnormal areas detected on colposcopy should be biopsied, in conjunction with an endocervical curetting. This technique allows for the detection of invasive cancer in a majority of patients. For those patients with clinically suspected cervical cancer and no visual lesion, a negative colposcopy, or microinvasive cancer on colposcopy, a cone biopsy can be utilized. Cone biopsies are surgical excisions of a portion of the cervix and in microinvasive disease may be therapeutic.

Staging

FIGO surgical staging for cervical cancer (1994) is described in **Table 35-3** and **Figures 35.5A to J**.

TABLE 35-3	1994 FIGO surgical staging for cervical cancer
Stage	**Description**
0	Carcinoma in situ, cervical intraepithelial neoplasia 3 (CIN 3)
I	The carcinoma is strictly confined to the cervix
IA1	Microinvasive carcinoma. Measured stromal invasion ≤ 3 mm in depth and extension ≤ 7 mm.
IA2	Microinvasive carcinoma. Measured stromal invasion > 3 mm and ≤ 5 mm in depth and extension ≤ 7 mm.
IB1	Clinically visible lesion ≤ 4 cm.
IB2	Clinically visible lesion > 4 cm
II	Cervical carcinoma invades beyond the uterus, but not to the pelvic wall or lower third of vagina
IIA	No obvious parametrial involvement
IIB	Obvious parametrial involvement
III	Tumor extends to the pelvic wall, involves the lower third of the vagina, or there is hydronephrosis or a non-functioning kidney.
IIIA	Tumor involves the lower third of the vagina, with no extension to pelvic side wall
IIIB	Extension to pelvic sidewall, hydronephrosis, or non-functioning kidney
IV	The carcinoma extends beyond the true pelvis or involves the mucosa of the bladder or rectum
IVA	Spread or growth to adjacent organs
IVB	Spread to distant organs

Cervical cancer is staged clinically to allow for comparison of treatment responses worldwide. Since the majority of cervical cancer patients are diagnosed in developing countries, access to surgical staging is often not available. The current system widely used for staging was developed by the International Federation of Gynecology and Obstetrics (FIGO). This staging system is based on clinical examination (palpation, inspection, colposcopy); radiographic examination of the chest, kidneys and skeleton; and endocervical curettings and biopsy. Suspected invasion of the bladder or rectum requires biopsies to prove presence of disease.

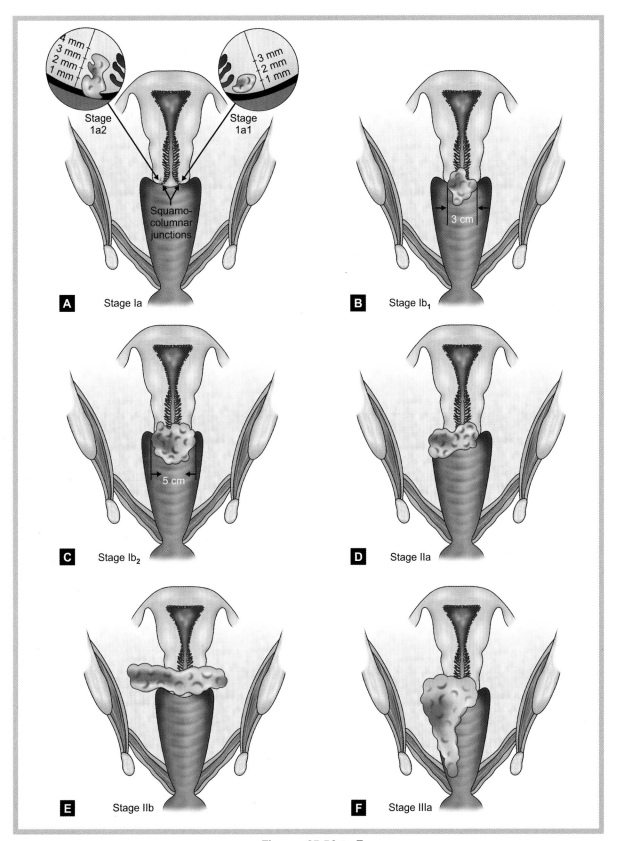

Figures 35-5A to F

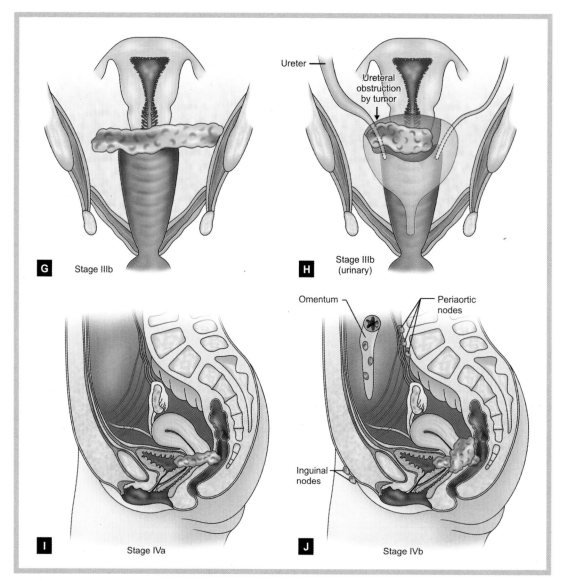

Figures 35-5A to J: FIGO stagings and classification of cancer of the cervix (From Disala PJ: Staging and surgical therapy of uterine malignancies. Adv Oncol 1992;8:125)

In the United States, various other radiographic examinations have been utilized for diagnosis and treatment planning. These include CT scans of the abdomen and pelvis, MRI of the pelvis, lymph-angiograms, laparoscopic and laparotomy findings, as well as radiographically directed biopsies. Although these techniques help provide important information to clinicians on treatment response rates and decision making, they cannot be used to upstage patients in the current system.

Nodal metastasis has been shown to be one of the most important predictors of progression-free survival. Based on this data, some physicians have advocated the use of pre-treatment staging procedures to remove lymph nodes and determine the presence or absence of metastasis. If positive lymph nodes were encountered, extended field radiation would be employed to encompass the involved nodes. In spite of the theoretical advantages to surgical staging, the benefits in term of patient outcome have not been proven.

Histology

Squamous cell carcinoma comprises roughly 80% of the cervical cancer diagnosis. It usually arises in the transformation zone and can then spread to the ectocervix or endocervix. It often appears as a firm, indurated mass or as an ulcerated lesion. HPV has been associated with 99.7% of squamous cell carcinomas of the cervix.

Adenocarcinoma comprises approximately 20% of cervical cancer diagnosis in developed countries. These tumors often arise in the glands of the cervix. HPV infections have only been reported in 70% of this cell type, with the majority arising from HPV 18. Recently there has been a relative increase in adenocarcinoma diagnosis compared to squamous cell carcinomas. This is felt to be partially due to screening programs that are more effective for squamous cell carcinoma. In general, cervical adeno carcinomas are often thought to be more radioresistant than squamous cell carcinomas and therefore may do better with surgical excision for early stage disease.

Adenosquamous and small cell carcinomas are relatively rare and are associated with poor outcomes. Primary sarcomas of the cervix have occasionally been described. Malignant lymphomas, both primary and secondary, have been reported.

Patterns of Spread

Cervical cancer spreads by three means: direct extension, lymphatic permeation and metastasis and hematogenous dissemination. Direct extension leads to disease in the parametrium, pelvic sidewall, vagina, bladder and rectum. With lymphatic spread, it invariably occurs in an orderly fashion from the nodes on the pelvic sidewall to the common iliac and then the para-aortic group. The most common sites for hematologic spread include the lungs, liver and bone. Less common sites include the bowel, adrenal glands, spleen and brain.

Treatment

Treatment of invasive cervical cancer involves the appropriate treatment of both the primary lesion and any potential sites of metastatic disease. Both surgery and radiation therapy may be employed for primary disease. Current clinical practices limit surgery to early stage disease, usually stages I-IIA.

Comparison studies of radiation therapy to surgery in early stage disease have suggested that overall outcomes are very similar between the two groups. Surgery is often employed in younger, thinner women since it is thought to have less long term morbidity, better local control of disease and decreased effect on sexual function. For older women, or those with medical comorbidities, radiation has been shown to be an effective alternative.

Effective surgical treatments for microinvasive tumors of the cervix include cold knife conization or simple hysterectomy. The choice of procedure depends on the woman's future reproductive needs, overall medical state and presence of high-risk features like lymphovascular space invasion (LVSI). If a cold knife cone is employed, care should be taken to obtain negative margins. If negative margins are not obtained, further conization or simple hysterectomy should be advocated.

Stages IB1-IIA cervical cancers may surgically be treated with a radical hysterectomy and pelvic and para-aortic lymphadenectomy. Radical hysterectomy differs from a simple hysterectomy by inclusion of the parametrium and upper vagina in the specimen. In order to perform a radical hysterectomy, the ureters must be dissected from the parametrium. This involves a uretero-lysis from the broad ligament. Dissection of the ureter begins where it crosses the common iliac artery, through the ureteric tunnel (where the uterine vessels cross over the ureter), to its insertion in the bladder. Parametrial tissue then becomes free for excision with the uterus.

Five types of radical hysterectomies are described **(Table 35-4).** Type I radical hysterectomy is a simple hysterectomy and is the treatment of choice for stage IA1 cervical cancers. Modified Radical Hysterectomy (Type II) involves the ligation of the uterine artery as it crosses the ureter. This allows for resection of the medial half of the cardinal ligament and is in stage IA2 cervical cancer. Radical hysterectomy (Type III) is the most commonly performed and the uterine artery is sacrificed as it originates from the internal iliac artery. Adequate parametrial tissue is removed for stage IB and stage IIA cancers. Extended radical hysterectomy (Type IV) involves the resection of a portion of ureter with reanastomosis. It is often employed if disease involves the distal ureter and has a high rate of uteric fistula. Partial exenteration (Type V) requires removal of the bladder and is often employed in central recurrences.

For those patients with medical contraindications to surgery, or stage IIB and greater, pelvic radiation therapy is utilized **(Figure 35-6).** Except for stage IVB, the current recommendation is for concurrent chemotherapy with weekly cisplatin. A total of 45-50 Gy radiation is delivered in a fractionated fashion. At the conclusion of the pelvic radiation, brachytherapy is delivered to boost the total dose of radiation to the cervix to 80-90 Gy, while limiting the radiation to the bladder and rectum.

Recently, as women delay their child bearing, a dilemma has developed in how to treat invasive cancer while maintaining fertility. To overcome this problem several centers have begun offering a radical trachelectomy. The goal of the radical trachelectomy is to remove the cervix and parametrium while maintaining the uterus. The cervix and parametrium are transected from the base of the uterus and upper vagina in a manner similar to a radical hysterectomy. The vagina is then reapproximated to the uterus. In order to allow for future pregnancies to progress without spontaneous abortion, this procedure is combined with an abdominal cerclage. Several series have documented high rates of pregnancies after radical trachelectomy. To date the effect on survival and overall outcome has not been established, nor has the ideal patient been identified, but this remains an

Type of surgery	Intrafascial	Extrafascial type I	Modified radical type II	Radical type III
Cervical fascia	Partially removed	Completely removed	Completely removed	Completely removed
Vaginal cuff removal	None	Small rim removed	Proximal 1-2 cm removed	Upper one-third to one-half removed
Bladder	Partially mobilized	Partially mobilized	Partially mobilized	Mobilized
Rectum	Not mobilized	RV septum partially mobilized	RV septum part	Mobilized
Ureters	Not mobilized	Not mobilized	Unrooted in ureteral tunnel	Completely dissected to bladder entry
Cardinal ligaments	Resected medial to ureters	Resected medial to ureters	Resected at level of ureter	Resected at pelvic sidewall
Uterosacral ligaments	Resected at level of cervix	Resected at level of cervix	Partially resected	Resected at postpelvic insertion
Uterus	Removed	Removed	Removed	Removed
Cervix	Partially removed	Completely removed	Completely removed	Completely removed

TABLE 35-4   Types of hysterectomy

Type IV, extended radical hysterectomy (partial removal of bladder or ureter), in addition to type III (from Stehman FB, Perez CA, Kurman RJ, et al. Uterine cervix. In Hoskins WJ, Perez CA, Young RC (Eds). Principles and Practice of Gynecologic Oncology (3rd edn). Philadelphia: Lippincott Williams & Wilkins, 2000: 864.

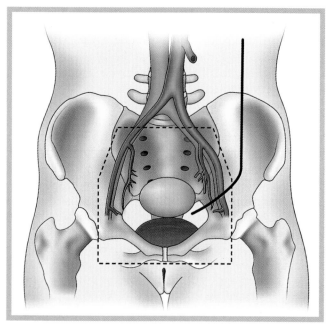

Figure 35-6: Pelvic diagram. The *dashed line* indicates the radiation field and the position of the uterus and cervix within the field. The *bold line* indicates the "J" incision path relative to the field and to the major vessels

interesting choice for younger women who desire fertility options.

Treatment of Recurrent Disease

Recurrent cervical cancer is generally associated with a poor outcome unless the recurrence is centrally located

in the pelvis. When recurrence is suspected, a thorough evaluation with PET/CT, examination under anesthesia and cervical biopsies is warranted. If distant metastasis is found at the time of evaluation, treatment includes chemotherapy. Currently first-line therapy would include a platinum analog and a taxane.

If the disease is confirmed to be centrally located and the patient lacks significant medical contraindications to surgery, a pelvic exenteration may help control recurrent cervical cancer. Since the majority of the patients that recur are previously advanced cervical cancer patients, they have already received pelvic radiation. The changes in tissue after radiation therapy eliminate the surgical planes making dissection without damage difficult. Therefore, at the time of debulking, removal of the bladder and/or rectum may be necessary. Neobladders can either be constructed from ileum or transverse colon and either be continent or non-continent conduits. To prevent breakdown after rectal resection, most patients receive an end colostomy after an exenteration, but some physicians will attempt primary reanastomosis.

Survival after recurrence generally averages 12-14 months unless centrally located. For those patients who undergo pelvic exenteration, 50% will recur within a year and eventually die from disease. Those who do not recur will often remain alive without evidence of disease.

Prognosis

Women diagnosed in the earliest stages of cervical cancer have a 5-year survival rate of 92%. Overall, the outcome for all stages of cervical cancer is decent with a 5-year survival rate of 72%. As was mentioned earlier, the 5-year survival does not differ for women treated with surgery or radiation therapy for early stage disease.

Lower Genital Tract

Vulva

Background

Vulvar cancer is the fourth most common gynecological cancer, comprising less than 5% of all cancers of the female genital tract. The American Cancer Society estimates 3,460 new cases of vulvar cancer with an associated 870 deaths for 2008. The most common cancer of the vulva is squamous cell carcinoma, accounting for over 90% of cases, while melanoma is the second most common. Other histologic types include adenocarcinomas, basal cell carcinomas and rarely sarcomas.

Etiology

Vulvar cancer appears to arise from two distinct pathways. The most common type is seen in the elderly and is commonly associated with chronic inflammation and vulvar dystrophies, such as lichen sclerosus. Recently, there has been a significant increase in another type of vulvar cancer. Unlike that seen in the elderly population, this type is commonly associated with HPV and smoking (much like cervical cancer) and is seen in a much younger population. In the past the mean age of vulvar cancer was approximately 65, however, in recent years this has lowered to a mean in the late 50s, primarily due to a rise in HPV related cancer.

Noninvasive/Preinvasive Disease

There are a variety of vulvar diseases that can be classified as noninvasive diseases. However, many are associated with an underlying carcinoma and any suspicious lesions should carefully be evaluated and a biopsy taken to rule out a more severe underlying lesion. Lichen sclerosus (LS) and squamous hyperplasia are non-HPV related diseases. Studies have found an association of vulvar cancer in 20-30% of patients with these epithelial disorders. After a biopsy is taken to rule out an associated malignancy, these can be treated with topical steroids.

Another common vulvar disease is Paget's disease. Invasive adenocarcinoma can be found in 4-17% of cases of vulvar Paget's. Paget's disease of the vulva should surgically be resected and negative margins obtained. This disease has a tendency to recur and careful follow-up with further resections as required is recommended.

Preinvasive disease in vulvar cancer is very similar to that found in cervical cancer. These lesions are HPV related, usually subtypes 16 and 33. This is classified as vulvar intraepithelial neoplasia (VIN). Whereas in cervical cancer there is a clear progression of cervical intraepithelial neoplasia (CIN) 1-3, this has not been established in VIN. Due to the lack of evidence of a malignant potential for VIN 1, the VIN classification is best divided into two categories, low grade VIN (VIN 1) and high grade VIN (VIN 2-3/carcinoma in situ). VIN 3 coexists with invasive cancer 30-50% of the time.

The main presenting symptom in women with vulvar disease, including LS, Paget's and VIN, is pruritus. Other symptoms include burning, pain or the presence of a lesion. Other presentations may include pain, dysuria, bleeding, discharge or ulceration. A delay in diagnosis is very common in vulvar diseases. Patients are sometimes reluctant to discuss these symptoms and often try over the counter remedies prior to seeking medical treatment. Once seen by a medical provider they are often given multiple prescriptions, often without undergoing an examination, prior to diagnosis. They also are commonly seen by multiple providers until a biopsy is taken and a diagnosis made. On examination the appearance of these lesions vary greatly depending on patient age and skin color. They may appear flat or raised and may be a variety of colors. In younger women HPV related lesions are commonly multifocal and more commonly unifocal in older women, although many lesions seen in the older patient are not HPV related.

Diagnosis is made by biopsy. This is indeed one of the most important points to be made when evaluating a patient with potential vulvar dysplasia or cancer. Colposcopic examination with use of acetic acid is very useful in the diagnosis of patients with VIN. It is also important to note that due to the multifocal nature of this disease it is very important to examine the entire vulva, including areas that are more difficult to evaluate such as the clitoris, urethra, vagina and anus. Liberal biopsies should be taken and their location carefully recorded for future pathology correlation and treatment.

Treatment of LS, hyperplasia and vulvar Paget's disease is described above. Treatment for VIN should be focused on the prevention of progression to invasive cancer. Treatment primarily consists of four options: close observation in select patients, surgical excision, laser surgery and topical immune response modulators. It is important to note that due to the often multifocal nature of this disease, treatment options must carefully be considered, often employing a variety of modalities in an individual patient. While there is a high association of invasive disease in VIN3 and one does not want to under treat, an extremely radical approach involving removal of all dysplastic lesions can leave the patient with severe physical and emotional complications.

Observation can sometimes be used, especially in young women with multifocal disease who are available for close follow-up. This is especially true in pregnant women, as lesions can resolve with the changing immune system following delivery. Colposcopic examination is a very important part of observation with biopsy and treatment of highly suspicious areas.

The mainstay of treatment is surgical excision. This can be performed by superficial excision of the involved lesion with a 0.5 cm margin with primary closure of the wound. Recurrence is directly related to margin status; however, it is usually not necessary to re-excise positive margins if all macroscopic disease was removed. These patients can be followed closely and in many cases the increased immune response associated with the healing process can resolve residual dysplasia. Due to the multifocal nature of this disease and the fairly high risk of recurrence of excised lesions (approximately 50% with positive margins), these patients should closely be followed.

Carbon dioxide laser can be used in many patients for the treatment of their dysplasia. The disadvantage is that tissue is not removed for pathologic review and negative margins cannot be determined. The advantage is that multiple lesions can be removed without the disfigurement associated with surgical excision. Often this procedure is combined with surgical removal of more suspicious lesions and laser treatment of less suspicious ones.

Topical immune response modifiers, such as Imiquimod (Aldera), are frequently used in the treatment of genital condyloma with good results. It has been studied in patients with severe dysplasia and reports indicate a complete response rate of approximately 30% and a partial response rate of 60%. Invasive carcinoma needs to be excluded prior to using this treatment. As with laser treatment of less suspicious lesions, topical therapy can often be used in conjunction with surgical removal of more worrisome areas.

Invasive Disease

Vulvar cancer typically presents in postmenopausal women with a mean age of diagnosis in the late 50s. Most patients with invasive cancer present with a vulvar mass, however there is usually a long history of pruritus and a history of other vulvar diseases as described above. Lesions are most frequently found on the labia majora, however lesions can be found anywhere on the vulva. Multifocal invasive lesions are found in approximately 5% of patients. Invasive vulvar disease is also often associated with cervical dysplasia or cancer; careful evaluation of the cervix is also important in these patients. Diagnosis is made by biopsy, usually performed in the office. It is important that an adequate biopsy is performed to include some surrounding skin, underlying dermis and connective tissue. The most common histologic type of invasive vulvar cancer is squamous cell carcinoma, in over

90% of cases, followed by melanoma, adenocarcinomas, basal cell carcinomas and rarely sarcomas.

Spread of vulvar cancer is primarily through direct extension, lymphatics and less commonly by hematogenous spread. Lymphatic spread usually occurs through the superficial inguinal lymph nodes first, then deep femoral nodes, to the pelvic nodes (primarily the external iliac nodes) **(Figure 35-7)**. Hematogenous spread is rare and usually occurs late the disease and is not commonly seen in the absence of positive lymph nodes. The incidence of positive lymph nodes is directly related to the clinical stage of disease (size and spread of primary lesion). Staging for vulvar cancer is surgical, as clinical evaluation of inguinal lymph nodes is inaccurate approximately a third of the time.

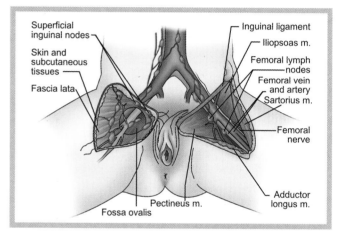

Figure 35-7: Inguinal-femoral lymph nodes. (Reproduced from Hacker NF. Vulvar cancer. In: Hacker NF, Moore JG, Gambone JC (Eds). Essentials of Obstetris and Gynecology, 4th edn. Philadelphia: Elsevier Saunders, 2004: 472, with permission).

Staging

FIGO surgical staging for vulvar cancer (1994) is described in **Table 35-5**.

Treatment

The treatment for early stage disease (stages I and II) is surgical. The type of surgery required depends on the size of the lesion (largest diameter and depth of invasion) and location in relation to the midline. In most situations these lesions can be managed with a radical local excision, with dissection to the inferior fascia of the urogenital diaphragm achieving at least 1 cm margins. Stage IA lesions (less than 2 cm in size with less than 1 mm of invasion) can be managed with a radical local excision without removal of inguinal lymph nodes. Stage IB and greater require an inguinal lymph node dissection. Stage IB lesions that are at least 1 cm away from the midline require only a unilateral inguinal dissection, while lesions

TABLE 35-5	1994 FIGO surgical staging for vulvar cancer
Stage	**Description**
0	Carcinoma in situ
IA	Tumor ≤ 2 cm, confined to vulva or perineum, negative nodes, ≤ 1.0 mm of stromal invasion
IB	Tumor ≤ 2 cm, confined to vulva or perineum, negative nodes, > 1.0 mm of stromal invasion
II	Tumor > 2 cm, confined to vulva or perineum, negative nodes
III	Tumor of any size, spread to lower urethra, vagina, anus, or unilateral positive lymph nodes
IVA	Tumor of any size, spread to upper urethra, bladder mucosa, rectal mucosa, pelvic bone or bilateral positive lymph nodes
IVB	Distant metastasis, including pelvic lymph nodes

within 1 cm require bilateral inguinal node dissections. Additionally, lesions on the anterior labia minora should be treated with a bilateral groin dissection due to contralateral flow in this region. Patients with stage II disease or greater usually require a bilateral groin dissection.

In patients with stage III or IV disease, treatment modalities can differ significantly. Often times lesions that do not involve the urethra, bladder, anus or rectum can be removed with a radical local incision with bilateral groin dissections. Larger lesions, or central lesions involving adjacent organs, may require a radical vulvectomy in order to obtain negative margins. When this is performed, bilateral inguinal groin dissection can be completed *en bloc* with the vulvar resection or through three separate incisions. The postoperative morbidity has been found to be lower with separate incisions, but may not be possible depending on the extent of disease. If the tumor involves the bladder, significant portion of the urethra, or rectum, a urinary diversion or colostomy may be required.

A radical vulvectomy involves excising the entire vulva from the pubic symphysis, through the labiocrural folds, to the perianal region. The medial extent of the incision should be the vaginal introitus, just anterior to the external urethral meatus, however this may be modified in order to obtain adequate surgical margins. The dissection should be carried down through the superficial fascia to the level of the fascia lata.

In order to perform an inguinal lymph node dissection an incision should be made from the pubic tubercle to 2-3 cm from the anterior superior iliac spine and carried down to the superficial fascia. The tissue underlying the superficial fascia to the fascia lata overlying the femoral vessels should be removed. Next the fatty tissue medial to the femoral vein (under the fascia lata) should also be

removed. The dissection should be performed from approximately 2 cm above the inguinal ligament superiorly, the Sartorius laterally and the Adductor Longus medially.

Sentinel lymph node dissection has shown favorable results in preliminary studies; however, no long-term clinical trials have compared it to a complete inguinal lymph node dissection. Current studies are underway, but until these results are published it should be considered investigational.

Although primary surgery is the preferred method of treatment, the use of primary chemoradiation, usually with 5-FU and cisplatin, followed by surgical resection of the tumor bed has shown favorable results in multiple studies, including a phase 2 GOG trial. This can be considered in patients with unresectable disease, to avoid a pelvic exenteration, or to preserve the bladder or rectum. Unless a patient is medically unable to undergo surgery, chemoradiation should not be given in surgically resectable lesions. Adjuvant radiation to the vulva should be considered in patients with a positive margin after surgical resection. Radiation therapy to the inguinal nodes should be considered in patients with more than one microscopically positive node, any macroscopically positive groin nodes or in patients with high-risk lesions who underwent a minimal node sampling or no nodal dissection at all.

For metastatic disease surgery and/or radiation therapy can be performed for symptom control. Multiple systemic chemotherapeutic agents have been studied and show minimal response of short duration.

Recurrent vulvar cancer can be treated by a variety of treatment modalities, depending on the individual patient, site of recurrence and prior treatment history. Sites of recurrence include perineal, inguinal, pelvic, distant and multiple. Perineal recurrence offers the best prognosis and can be treated with surgery and/or radiation, depending on history of previous treatment. Other sites can potentially be treated with surgery, but more likely radiation if the patient has not yet been radiated, or palliative chemotherapy. Prognosis for nonperineal recurrences is dismal.

Prognosis

Overall prognosis for vulvar cancer is determined by stage, but most importantly the presence or absence of nodal disease. Approximate 5-year survival rates from 1996 to 1998, FIGO statistics are 77% for stage I, 55% for stage II, 31% for stage III and essentially 0% for stage IV.

Other Types of Vulvar Cancer

Other types of vulvar cancer include melanoma, bartholin gland carcinoma, basal cell carcinoma and sarcoma. While melanoma is rare, it is the second most common type of vulvar cancer and accounts for approximately 10% of cases. It is usually found in older women and is often located in the mucosal area of the labia minora. Wide local excision is adequate for small lesions; white large lesions require a radical vulvectomy. If the lesion depth is less than 1 mm, 1 cm surgical margins are adequate; while lesions with a depth of greater than 1 mm require 2 cm surgical margins. Unlike in squamous cell carcinoma, the value of inguinal lymph node dissection is controversial. If clinically suspicious nodes are present they should be removed. The use of sentinel lymph node detection in others is often employed. Basal cell carcinomas and sarcomas can be treated with wide local excision, as lymph node spread is uncommon. The standard treatment for Bartholin gland carcinomas is radical vulvectomy with bilateral inguinal lymph node dissection, while unilateral radical local excision and unilateral node dissection is also performed by some.

Vagina

Background

Vaginal cancer accounts for approximately 2% of gynecological malignancies, accounting for 2210 cases annually in the United States and 760 deaths. The mean age at diagnosis is 60, but 50% of cases are seen in women age 70 and older. Most of the tumors involving the vagina are from another site, either by direct extension or by metastasis (cervix, endometrium, colon/rectum, ovary, vulva, or choriocarcinoma). Primary vaginal cancer is usually of squamous cell histology, although adenocarcinomas, melanomas and sarcomas are also seen.

Etiology

The primary etiology of vaginal cancer appears to by HPV (especially HPV 16) related and share many of the same risk factors as cervical cancer. About a third of primary vaginal cancers occur in women with a history of severe cervical dysplasia or cancer. Another risk factor is a history of radiation exposure.

Preinvasive Disease

Vaginal intraepithelial neoplasia (VAIN) is classified in the same was as cervical intraepithelial neoplasia (CIN). The average age of patients affected is 30 years of age. VAIN 1 (mild dysplasia) is related to HPV changes and is not considered to have progressive potential, while VAIN 3 (severe dysplasia/carcinoma in situ) should be considered a preinvasive condition. About 70% of moderate and severe VAIN occur in the upper third of the vagina, while the second most common location is the lower third. Like cervical dysplasia it is asymptomatic

and diagnosed by colposcopy and biopsy. While surgical excision and radiation therapy were historically used to treat high grade lesions, most patients today are treated with CO_2 laser. Dysplastic lesions are often multifocal and occur in hard to reach areas (upper third of the vagina), making excision difficult. Once adequate biopsies have been taken to rule out invasion, a laser is used to destroy the lesions. Another treatment that can be used in select patients, with very close follow-up, is topical 5-fluorouracil (5-FU).

Invasive Disease

Patients with vaginal cancer may present with vaginal bleeding (postmenopausal or postcoital), vaginal discharge, mass, urinary or rectal pain. Patients with a history of cervical dysplasia or cancer are at an increased risk and should be monitored by Pap tests. Because most of the lesions occur in the upper third of the vagina (usually the posterior wall), careful inspection (sometimes by an examination under anesthesia) and biopsy are required to make the diagnosis. Colposcopy can be used if necessary **(Figure 35-8)**.

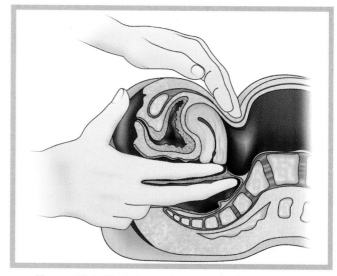

Figure 35-8: Technique of rectovaginal examination

Spread of disease in vaginal cancer can be by direct extension, lymphatic spread or hematogenous spread. Lymphatic spread from lesions in the upper two thirds of the vagina is to the pelvic and para-aortic nodes. Lesions in the lower vagina spread to the inguinofemoral nodes, then to the pelvic nodes secondarily. Hematogenous spread is rare and occurs late in the disease process, usually after nodal spread. Common sites of hematogenous spread are the lungs, liver and bone. Like cervical cancer, the staging of vaginal cancer is a clinical one.

Staging

FIGO staging for vaginal cancer is described in **Table 35-6.**

TABLE 35-6	FIGO staging for vaginal cancer
Stage	**Description**
0	Carcinoma in situ
I	Carcinoma is limited to the vaginal wall
II	Carcinoma involves the subvaginal tissue, but not the pelvic wall
III	Carcinoma extends to the pelvic wall
IVA	Tumor involves the bladder, rectal mucosa, or spread beyond the pelvis
IVB	Distant metastasis

Treatment

The treatment of vaginal cancer is primarily through radiation (brachytherapy and/or external pelvic radiation). Due to the close proximity of the urethra, bladder and rectum, it can be associated with significant morbidity. Patients with stage I disease involving the upper vagina can be treated with a hysterectomy and upper vaginectomy in patients with a uterus and upper vaginectomy in those without. In addition they should also undergo a pelvic lymph node dissection. Patients with disease involving the bladder or rectum, can sometimes undergo a pelvic exenteration both for a potential cure and symptomatic relief. Pelvic exenteration is really the only option for patients with recurrent disease after radiation.

Prognosis

Because vaginal cancer is so rare, survival data is varied. However, it is generally accepted that survival is worse than that of cervical and vulvar cancer. Approximate 5-year survival rates are 70% for stage I, 50% for stage II, 33% for stage III, 20% for stage IVA and 0% for stage IVB.

Other

The second most common type of vaginal cancer is adenocarcinomas, present in about 10% of primary vaginal cases. They are usually seen in younger patients and are associated with *in utero* exposure to diethylstilbestrol (DES). Approximately 70% present with stage I disease; surgery, usually a radical hysterectomy, upper vaginectomy, pelvic lymphadenectomy and vaginal reconstruction, is the treatment of choice. Melanomas and sarcomas are rare and are usually treated with radical surgical resection.

Level of Evidence Table			
Recommendation	**Best level of evidence**	**Grade**	**References**
Endometrial cancer			
For stage I disease, use of adjuvant radiation has not shown improved survival but has shown reduced locoregional recurrence, with an increase in side effects.	1B	A	1
Comprehensive staging should be performed on all patients, as many patients with apparent stage I disease have spread outside of the uterus.	3	B	2
In patients with stage III or IV disease with residual tumors smaller than 2 cm and no parenchymal organ involvement, the use of cisplatin and doxorubicin resulted in improved OS compared to whole-abdominal radiation therapy.	1B	A	3
In patients with advanced or recurrent endometrial cancer doxorubicin, cisplatin and paclitaxel (TAP) with granulocyte colony-stimulating factor was significantly superior to cisplatin plus doxorubicin (AP) in OS and PFS.	1B	A	4
Ovarian cancer			
Two large European trials, European Organisation for Research and Treatment of Cancer-Adjuvant ChemoTherapy in Ovarian Neoplasm (EORTC-ACTION) and International Collaborative Ovarian Neoplasm (ICON1) showed a significant improvement in RFS and OS in early stage ovarian cancer patients treated with adjuvant chemotherapy.	1A	A	5, 6
In patients with advanced stage disease, a review of the literature showed that patients with optimal cytoreduction had a median survival of 39 months compared with survival of only 17 months in patients with suboptimal residual disease.	3	B	7

Contd...

Recommendation	Best level of evidence	Grade	References
In patients with advanced stage disease, combination intraperitoneal (IP) and intravenous (IV) chemotherapy has shown improved OS and PFS versus IV chemotherapy alone in patients with optimally cytoreduced disease.	1B	A	8
In patients with suboptimally reduced disease, interval cytoreductive surgery following chemotherapy and preceded by additional chemotherapy was shown by the EORTC to improve survival rate compared with patients who completed chemotherapy without surgery.	1B	A	9
The use of consolidation and/or maintenance chemotherapy has been shown to increase PFS, although other studies have demonstrated no effect.	1B	A	10
Cervical cancer			
Identical 5-year overall and disease-free survival rates have been shown when comparing radiation therapy to radical hysterectomy in patients with stage IB and IIA disease.	1B	A	11
The resection of macroscopically involved pelvic nodes may improve rates of local control with postoperative radiation therapy.	3	B	12
Randomized phase III trials have shown an overall survival advantage for cisplatin-based therapy given concurrently with radiation therapy.	1B	A	13
Vulvar cancer			
Radiation therapy to the groin for patients with clinical N0 disease has inferior survival secondary to an increased groin failure rate compared with groin dissection and adjuvant radiation therapy for positive groin nodes.	1B	A	14
After receiving radical vulvectomy and bilateral inguinal lymph node dissection, patients with two or more pathologically positive groin nodes had significantly better survival with radiation therapy to the groin and pelvis than with pelvic node dissection.	2	B	15
Vaginal cancer			
Carcinoma of the vagina can be effectively treated with radiation therapy.	3	B	16

References

1. Scholten AN, van Putten WL, Beerman H, et al. Postoperative radiotherapy for Stage I endometrial carcinoma: long-term outcome of the randomized PORTEC trial with central pathology review. Int J Radiat Oncol Biol Phys 2005;63(3):834-8.
2. Creasman WT, Morrow CP, Bundy BN, Homesley HD, Graham JE, Heller PB. Surgical pathologic spread patterns of endometrial cancer: a gynecologic oncology group study. Cancer 1987;60: 2035-41.
3. Randall ME, Filiaci VL, Muss H, et al. Randomized phase III trial of whole-abdominal irradiation versus doxorubicin and cisplatin chemotherapy in advanced endometrial carcinoma: a gynecologic oncology group study. J Clin Oncol 2006;24(1): 36-44.
4. Fleming GF, Brunetto VL, Cella D, et al. Phase III trial of doxorubicin plus cisplatin with or without paclitaxel plus filgrastim in advanced endometrial carcinoma: a gynecologic oncology group study. J Clin Oncol 2004; 22(11): 2159-66.
5. Trimbos JB, Vergote I, Bolis G, et al. Impact of adjuvant chemotherapy and surgical staging in early-stage ovarian carcinoma: European organisation for research and treatment of cancer-adjuvant chemotherapy in ovarian neoplasm trial. J Natl Cancer Inst 2003;95(2):113-25.
6. Colombo N, Guthrie D, Chiari S, et al. International Collaborative Ovarian Neoplasm trial 1: a randomized trial of adjuvant chemotherapy in women with early-stage ovarian cancer. J Natl Cancer Inst 2003;95(2): 125-32.
7. Hoskins WJ. Surgical staging and cytoreductive surgery of epithelial ovarian cancer. Cancer 1993;71(4 Suppl): 1534-40.
8. Armstrong DK, Bundy B, Wenzel L, et al. Intraperitoneal cisplatin and paclitaxel in ovarian cancer. N Engl J Med 2006;354 (1): 34-43.
9. van der Burg ME, van Lent M, Buyse M, et al. The effect of debulking surgery after induction chemotherapy on the prognosis in advanced epithelial ovarian cancer. Gynecological cancer cooperative group of the European Organisation for Research and Treatment of Cancer. N Engl J Med 1995;332(10):629-34.

10. Markman M, Liu PY, Wilczynski S, et al. Phase III randomized trial of 12 versus 3 months of maintenance paclitaxel in patients with advanced ovarian cancer after complete response to platinum and paclitaxel-based chemotherapy: a Southwest oncology group and gynecologic oncology group trial. J Clin Oncol 2003; 21(13): 2460-5.

11. Landoni F, Maneo A, Colombo A, et al. Randomised study of radical surgery versus radiotherapy for stage Ib-IIa cervical cancer. Lancet 1997;350 (9077): 535-40.

12. Downey GO, Potish RA, Adcock LL, et al. Pretreatment surgical staging in cervical carcinoma: therapeutic efficacy of pelvic lymph node resection. Am J Obstet Gynecol 1989; 160 (5 Pt 1): 1055-61.

13. Rose PG, Bundy BN, Watkins EB, et al. Concurrent cisplatin-based radiotherapy and chemotherapy for locally advanced cervical cancer. N Engl J Med 1999;340(15): 1144-53.

14. Stehman FB, Bundy BN, Thomas G, et al. Groin dissection versus groin radiation in carcinoma of the vulva: a gynecologic oncology group study. Int J Radiat Oncol Biol Phys 1992;24(2): 389-96.

15. Homesley HD, Bundy BN, Sedlis A, et al. Prognostic factors for groin node metastasis in squamous cell carcinoma of the vulva (a gynecologic oncology group study) Gynecol Oncol 1993;49(3): 279-83.

16. Perez CA, Camel HM, Galakatos AE, et al. Definitive irradiation in carcinoma of the vagina: long-term evaluation of results. Int J Radiat Oncol Biol Phys 1988; 15(6):1283-90.

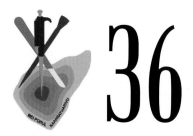

36

Leukemia and Lymphoma: The Role of the Surgical Oncologist

Bruce O Hough, Joshua T Rubin

Overview

With the exception of gastric lymphoma, the hematological malignancies are generally considered nonsurgical diseases. Surgeons are often consulted, however, to assist in establishing a diagnosis, to facilitate chemotherapy, or to help manage certain complications of therapy. These patients are also susceptible to common surgical diseases which may develop at the most unfortunate of times. For this reason, it is important for the surgeon to understand the manifestations of chemotherapy and hematological malignancies on health.

Hematological malignancies have been classified in a variety of ways. It can be helpful to consider them in terms of their biological behavior. Indolent lymphomas progress slowly, often over years. The natural history of aggressive lymphomas extends over months and highly aggressive lymphomas might lead to death within weeks. Indolent lymphomas are not generally cured by chemotherapy but the long-term prognosis is good due to their slow progression. Paradoxically, highly aggressive lymphomas are much more sensitive to chemotherapy and a substantial minority of patients can be cured.

There is considerable overlap between the clinical presentation of lymphoma and leukemia, often making diagnosis difficult in the absence of cytogenetics and fluorescent in situ hybridization (FISH) studies. For example, chronic lymphocytic leukemia (CLL) and small lymphocytic lymphoma (SLL) are essentially the same disease. They share genetic derangements and are sensitive to the same therapies. They are differentiated only by their clinical presentation such that patients with substantial lymphadenopathy are thought to have SLL and patients with peripheral lymphocytosis on presentation are thought to have CLL.

Clinical Presentation

The four common leukemias most likely to be encountered by the surgeon are acute myelogenous leukemia (AML), acute lymphocytic leukemia (ALL), CLL and chronic myelogenous leukemia (CML). Chronic leukemias are often asymptomatic and are first suspected when abnormalities are noted on a routine complete blood count. Symptoms of acute leukemia, in contrast, can develop shortly after normal blood tests obtained for unrelated reasons. These patients typically present with symptoms of cytopenia including anemia-associated fatigue, shortness of breath, easy bruising, epistaxis secondary to thrombocytopenia, recurrent or persistent infection due to neutropenia.

Leukemia can also lead to derangements of coagulation or hemostasis that complicate the care of these patients when they are in need of surgery. For example, acute promyelocytic leukemia (APL), a subset of AML with a unique chromosomal translocation, may present with consumptive coagulopathy. If left untreated, these patients are at high risk of life threatening hemorrhage. Supportive care includes the administration of cryoprecipitate and fresh frozen plasma. Cryoprecipitate, which is prepared from FFP, is especially rich in fibrinogen and is the product of choice for patients with a fibrinogen level less than 150 mg/dl. Cryoprecipitate also is rich in coagulation factors 8, 13 and von Willibrand factor. A bag of cryoprecipitate can raise a patient's fibrinogen level by 70 mg/dl. While it is prudent to treat drastic elevations of the protime and the prothrombin time in these patients, complete normalization is not possible and excessive administration of these blood products should be avoided.

Infiltration of the bone marrow by leukemic cells may interfere in the production of platelets and neutrophils. This can occur in patients with AML who, as a result, are at great risk of life threatening bleeding or infection. For this reason, they are admitted to the hospital for diagnostic evaluation and remain hospitalized during therapy so that they can receive blood product support and antimicrobials for the prevention and treatment of infectious complications.

Thrombocytopenia is usually exacerbated by myelo-ablative chemotherapy. Repeated platelet transfusions may lead to the development of antibodies to cell surface proteins associated with the donated platelets rendering

TABLE 36-1	Thresholds for use of blood products in patients with leukemia and lymphoma			
Platelets:				
Prophylaxis to prevent primary hemorrhage:		10	×	10^9/L
Prophylaxis for procedures:		50	×	10^9/L
Prophylaxis for ophtho or neurosurgical procedures:		100	×	10^9/L
Cryoprecipitate to prevent primary hemorrhage:		150		mg/dL
FFP for surgical procedures:		INR > 1.4		

subsequent platelet support less effective. Matching the HLA type of the patient to that of the donor is sometimes necessary in order to get a meaningful rise in the patients platelet count after transfusion. In a patient with life threatening bleeding, however, this option is not always available and unmatched platelets must be used in spite of their limited efficacy. The continuous infusion of platelets for support during surgical procedures has not been shown to be beneficial. Although it seems ineluctable that the risk of postoperative bleeding is increased in patients with thrombocytopenia, a minimum acceptable platelet count has not been defined. The current consensus is that a platelet count should be over 50×10^9/liter for most surgical procedures and over 100×10^9/liter for neurological and ophthalmological procedures. Level I evidence to support this recommendation has been elusive and at our institution platelet counts of 30,000 are often thought to be acceptable for surgical procedures. The threshold for platelet transfusion in non-surgical patients with AML has been lowered to 210×10^9/liter based on prospective trials **(Table 36-1)**.

Neutropenia, arbitrarily defined as an absolute neutrophil count less than 0.5×10^9/liter, is associated with an increased risk of infection. The degree of risk is related to both the depth of the nadir and the duration of neutropenia. Most infections arise from a patient's own flora for which reason strict isolation does not in and of itself prevent infectious complications among these patients. In addition to reduced neutrophil counts, some hematological disorders can cause a reduction in immunoglobulin that further predisposes the patient to infection. Replacement with intravenous immunoglobulin can ameliorate this deficiency and is often needed in conjunction with treatment of the underlying neoplasm.

Role of the Surgeon in Diagnosis

Surgical intervention may be necessary to establish a diagnosis or to facilitate therapy. Hematologists have several tools at their disposal to evaluate patients for a hematological malignancy. For patients with lymphadenopathy, evaluation of an abnormal lymph node by conventional microscopy using hematoxylin and eosin (H&E) staining and immunohistochemistry enables the pathologist to evaluate tumor architecture and establish

the malignant cell phenotype. If tumor location or ill-health renders surgical biopsy prohibitively morbid, less invasive alternatives to surgical biopsy should be recommended. Core needle biopsy under ultrasound or CT guidance might provide adequate tissue for diagnosis. Endobronchial ultrasound (EBUS) and endoscopic ultrasound are being used with increasing frequency when tumors are not assessable to percutaneous, image-guided biopsy.

Although one must always consider the risk associated with surgical biopsy, some patients have no other option either because the diagnosis remains inconclusive after a less invasive diagnostic procedure or additional tumor is needed to evaluate tumor architecture. It is important for the surgeon to appreciate that these biopsies must be processed quickly so as to maintain the viability of cells. We pass these biopsies directly to the hematopathologist for immediate processing. Tissue obtained late in the day can be refrigerated in the tissue culture medium RPMI for processing early the following day.

Diagnosis can also be established by bone marrow biopsy in some patients. Although some lymphomas and plasma cell disorders first present with seemingly localized manifestations, they often behave as systemic diseases. In a patient with advanced symptoms, bone marrow biopsy may prove useful for diagnosis, obviating the need for lymph node biopsy.

Other diagnostic aids include flow cytometry, cytogenetics and FISH. Flow cytometry identifies the phenotype of cells by labeling them with antibodies to relevant cell surface antigens. As the cells are passed through a counter, the labels are detected by virtue of attached fluorescent markers. The surface antigen profile of these cells enables accurate characterization of a clone of abnormal white blood cells obtained from peripheral blood, lymph nodes or bone marrow.

Cytogenetic evaluation can identify chromosomal rearrangements within the malignant cell's karyotype. This requires cell culture in an agent that promotes cell division, followed by treatment with reagents to promote cell-cycle arrest. After the cells are stained, they are evaluated manually to detect chromosomal deletions, trisomies or translocations. This can be useful diagnostically since the genetic defects of some leukemias have been identified. For example, a 9:22 translocation, which causes the pathogenic bcr-abl fusion protein, is pathognomic of CML. These tests require several days to complete and as such decisions, regarding treatment might have to be made prior to a definitive diagnosis.

In the past, splenectomy was routinely performed for the staging of Hodgkin's lymphoma. The current standard of care does not require splenectomy in these patients because of the small increased risk of subsequent overwhelming sepsis and death secondary to pneumococcus, meningococcus, haemophilus type B and the increased diagnostic accuracy of molecular testing and imaging, particularly with PET scanning. Splenectomy might be required for diagnosis of splenic marginal zone lymphoma, an unusual type of marginal zone lymphoma, which sometimes presents with isolated splenic involvement. Usually, bone marrow biopsy and peripheral blood analysis can give the correct diagnosis, however.

Role of the Surgeon in Treatment

Non-Hodgkin's lymphoma accounts for about 20% of small intestinal cancers and only about 1-3% of all gastrointestinal malignancies. The appropriate therapy for gastrointestinal lymphoma remains poorly defined due, in part, to the low incidence of this disease in western countries. The ambiguity concerning its classification and the absence of prospective, randomized clinical trials contribute to our poor understanding of the disease.

The classification of gastrointestinal lymphoma was improved significantly by the development of a Working Formulation for Clinical Usage by the non-Hodgkin's lymphoma pathologic classification project in 1982 **(Table 36-2)**. The Working Formulation proposed ten major types of non-Hodgkin's lymphoma based on morphologic criteria. No immunologic methods were used in developing this system. The ten groups of non-Hodgkin's lymphoma were generated based on clinical correlations such as survival, age, gender, presenting sites and stage

TABLE 36-2	Working formulation for classification of non-Hodgkin's lymphoma

I. Low-grade malignant lymphoma
Small lymphocytic
Follicular, predominantly small cleaved cell
Follicular, mixed small cleaved and large cell
II. Intermediate-grade malignant lymphoma
Follicular, predominantly large cell
Diffuse, small cleaved cell
Diffuse, mixed, small and large cell
Diffuse, large cell, cleaved or noncleaved
III. High-grade malignant lymphoma
Diffuse large cell immunoblastic
Lymphoblastic (convoluted and/or unconvoluted)
Small noncleaved cell (Burkitt's or non-Burkitt's)

of disease. Using the Working Formulation, non-Hodgkin's lymphoma is characterized as low grade, intermediate grade, or high grade. There are several subdivisions within each grade, which are easily correlated with those of other existing systems of classification.

Another limitation of the available clinical data is the absence of a consistent definition of primary small bowel non-Hodgkin's lymphoma. As a result, published clinical series represent a heterogeneous population of patients. Dawson proposed that patients with superficial lymphadenopathy, mediastinal lymphadenopathy, involvement of the liver and spleen and abnormal blood counts be excluded from clinical trials evaluating the therapy of primary intestinal non-Hodgkin's lymphoma. Most patients in these clinical studies are staged using the Ann Arbor system **(Table 36-3)**. Studies using the strictest criteria evaluate patients with disease localized to the stomach or small intestine (stage IE) or patients with intestinal tumors and involvement of the adjacent mesenteric lymph nodes only (stage IIE).

TABLE 36-3	Ann Arbor staging of visceral lymphoma
Stage IE	Involvement of a single extralymphatic site
Stage IIE	Involvement of a single extralymphatic site and its regional nodes, with or without other lymph node regions on the same side of the diaphragm.
Stage IIIE	Involvement of a single extralymphatic site and lymph node regions on both sides of the diaphragm.
Stage IVE	Multifocal involvement of one or more extralymphatic sites, with or without associated lymph node involvement.

Patients with celiac disease have a 200 fold increased risk of developing T-cell lymphoma of the small intestinal. This may be associated with the human leukocyte antigen DR3. The risk is also increased in the setting of Crohn's disease if the small bowel is involved. Infection with the human immunodeficiency virus (HIV) also seems to increase the risk of developing intestinal lymphoma. The incidence of lymphoma increases as a function of age. The mean and median age of patients at the time of presentation is between 60 and 70 years, respectively.

Symptoms at the time of presentation are similar to those seen with other intestinal tumors. Patients with intestinal lymphoma are less likely to bleed than are patients with gastric lymphoma. Diarrhea and visceral perforation are more commonly seen as a complication of small intestinal lymphoma than they are with gastric lymphoma. Other common manifestations of this disease at diagnosis include abdominal pain, abdominal mass, intestinal obstruction, nausea, vomiting, anorexia and weight loss.

Pretreatment evaluation of these patients, once a diagnosis has been made, should include a complete history with particular attention to the presence of fever, night sweats and weight loss. These so-called B symptoms have a negative impact on prognosis. The physical examination should evaluate patients for lymphadenopathy and hepatosplenomegaly. It should include an evaluation of Waldeyer's ring, as well. The survey for extraintestinal disease should also include a bone marrow biopsy and a complete set of chest, abdominal and pelvic CT scans looking for involvement of the liver, spleen, mediastinal, intra-abdominal and retroperitoneal lymph nodes.

A majority of intestinal lymphomas are of high grade. Intermediate and low-grade lymphomas occur with significant frequency, however. Mucosal associated lymphoid tissue (MALT) lymphomas, common in the stomach, are unusual in the small intestine. Most cases of primary intestinal lymphoma present in the ileum. A significant minority of cases occurs in the jejunum while isolated duodenal lymphoma is much less common.

Surgery for Intestinal Lymphoma

The role of surgery, radiation therapy and chemotherapy in the treatment of gastrointestinal non-Hodgkin's lymphoma is controversial. One can make a cogent argument for or against the use of surgical debulking depending on which of several nonrandomized studies one wishes to cite. Although relapse-free survival and overall survival are the most important outcome measures in evaluating therapy, the efficacy of surgery should also be judged in terms of durability of local control, surgical morbidity and mortality, prevention of chemotherapy associated complications and impact of the resulting delay of chemotherapy on overall survival. The benefit of surgery may vary depending on the aggressiveness of the lymphoma. It is not clear that the morbidity of chemotherapy is excessively high among patients with aggressive intestinal lymphomas, which may bleed or perforate as a result of chemotherapy. The purported ability of surgery to prevent chemotherapy-induced complications must be weighted against surgical morbidity, which includes intestinal fistulas, anastomotic breakdown with abscess formation and postoperative bleeding, all of which serve to further delay in the initiation of chemotherapy. There are no studies comparing the mortality directly attributed to surgery with that of chemotherapy. Some series report a 3% risk of postoperative mortality, which approaches the reported risk of intestinal perforation and bleeding due to chemotherapy in some series.

Although some studies suggest that surgery should be included in the multimodality therapy of patients with aggressive, high grade or intermediate grade intestinal lymphoma, resection of primary intestinal lymphoma has not consistently been demonstrated to be superior to other therapies. Purported benefits of surgical therapy include reduction in the risk of local recurrence, prolongation of disease-free and overall survival compared to treatment with systemic therapy alone and improvement in local control compared to patients treated with systemic therapy alone or with radiation. Additionally, tumor related complications such as bleeding and perforation might be less likely to occur among patients in whom tumors were resected. On the other hand, surgery has been associated with an increased risk of early and late complications among patients with gastric lymphoma and it is clear that chemotherapy reduces the chances of systemic recurrence after surgical resection. High rates of complete response with low morbidity have been seen following chemotherapy alone.

Based on these observations we recommend that surgery be reserved for the treatment of patients whose tumors manifest an incomplete response to chemotherapy or who soon develop locally recurrent disease. Surgery is also appropriate for management of gastrointestinal strictures that occasionally develop following chemotherapy.

MALT and non-MALT Gastric Lymphoma

(Editors' note: A brief discussion of gastric lymphoma is included here, focusing on the role of the surgeon and factors determining surgical intervention. Please see the chapter on Gastric Cancer for a detailed description of the diagnosis and management of gastric lymphoma)

Gastric lymphomas are now divided into mucosa-associated lymphatic tissue (MALT) or non-MALT classification. The distinction is important not only as it relates to etiology but for its implications regarding therapy as well. *Helicobacter pylori* is etiologic for MALT lymphoma and serves as a target for rather effective therapy. Early stage gastric MALT lymphoma that is associated with *H. pylori* infection can be induced to regress with antibiotics and proton pump inhibitors. Patients with more advanced disease or patients without associated *H. pylori* infection are often treated with regional radiation therapy. In a retrospective review of patients treated only with antibiotics for early gastric MALT lymphoma, the 5- and 10-year survival rates were 92% and 85%, respectively. Transformation to a more aggressive large-cell lymphoma occurred in 2 of 105 patients and only 1 patient developing distant progression. In order to preserve the stomach, some authorities recommend radiation therapy rather than surgery as the therapy of choice for non-*H. pylori* associated gastric MALT lymphoma and for those cases that do not respond to treatment with antibiotics.

In contrast, the non-MALT lymphomas, including diffuse large B-cell lymphoma (DLBC), are unrelated to *H. pylori* infection and do not respond to antibiotics. The respective roles of surgery, chemotherapy and radiation therapy in the management of non-MALT lymphoma have been the subject of some controversy and speculation; however, little data is available on which to base firm conclusions. Thus, a variety of treatment recommendations exist.

In the past, isolated non-MALT gastric lymphomas were treated with surgical resection. Although the efficacy of surgery is not in question, its primacy as first line therapy has been eclipsed by chemotherapy for several reasons. First, the risk of gastric perforation in this setting was probably over estimated and appears to be no greater than 3%. In addition, the chemotherapeutic armamentarium, which has grown significantly, now appears to be at least equally effective in treating these patients.

A recent large randomized trial compared surgery alone, surgery plus radiation therapy, surgery plus chemotherapy with cyclophosphamide, hydroxydoxorubicin, oncovin and prednisone (CHOP) and CHOP alone in the treatment of patients with DLBC lymphoma. The best 10-year survival (92%) was seen in the group of patients treated only with CHOP. Because patients with non-*H. pylori* MALT lymphoma, MALT lymphoma that did not respond to antibiotic therapy and patients with follicular lymphoma were excluded from this trial, its results cannot be generalized. One might expect to see a different outcome among patients with these lymphomas that have a different biological behavior and, unlike diffuse large B-cell lymphoma, tend to be more localized.

In summary, gastrointestinal lymphoma is a biologically heterogeneous group of diseases. Surgery is generally reserved to manage complications of chemotherapy and as salvage therapy for localized non-*H. pylori* or localized refractory MALT lymphomas of the stomach. It should not be used to treat patients with gastric DLBCL because of the systemic nature of this disease. Patients with indolent gastric lymphomas confined only to the stomach, such as follicular lymphoma, should be offered gastric resection as a treatment option. When available, patients should be offered participation in a clinical trial.

Role of the Surgeon in Facilitating Therapy

Inadequate venous access is often an obstacle to therapy for these patients. In patients with leukemia, limited peripheral venous access is often overwhelmed by the need for infusional chemotherapy, intravenous fluids, intravenous antibiotics, blood product support and frequent blood tests. Even patients with lymphoma whose chemotherapy can be administered as an outpatient occasionally require durable central venous access due to the need for extended periods of therapy or poor peripheral intravenous access. Among the latter group, the need for IV access is a judgment call. For patients with leukemia, central venous access with a subcutaneous port is avoided due to the need for multiple access channels and the risk of postoperative bleeding into the subcutaneous pocket due to thrombocytopenia. In addition, the convenience of the subcutaneous port wanes if it must be accessed continuously. Our approach to IV access in patients with leukemia who require aggressive, myeloablative chemotherapy is to use triple lumen Hickman catheters. We have found that their durability and patency for blood draws exceeds that of peripherally inserted central catheters (PICCs). They can safely be placed provided coagulopathy and thrombocytopenia are corrected preoperatively. We prefer to access the internal jugular vein under direct ultrasound guidance so that the risk of arterial injury and pneumothorax is exceedingly small.

Role of the Surgeon in Treating Complications of Disease or Therapy

In patients with prolonged neutropenia, the risk for fungal infections of the lung increases. While the American College of Chest Physicians and Infectious Disease Society of America both advocate empiric treatment of community acquired pneumonia in immunocompetent patients, those with neutropenia often have a much broader range of possible pathogens and require invasive testing to establish a diagnosis and select appropriate antibiotics. Additionally, lymphangitic spread of lymphoma within the lung can sometimes masquerade as an infectious pneumonitis making the decisions regarding therapy difficult. For this reason, bronchoscopy and even lung biopsy might be necessary.

Patients with neutropenia can occasionally develop an infection of the cecum and right colon characterized by right lower quadrant pain, cecal distension and occasionally perforation. This is caused by the combination of mucosal damage from cytotoxic chemotherapy and neutropenia. Differing pathogens can cause infection of the cecal wall, but the most common are *Pseudomonas* and *Clostridium difficile*. These patients can develop bacteremia as well. CT scan findings include pericecal fluid, an RLQ inflammatory mass and localized bowel wall thickening. Severity of disease varies, but initial treatment should include broad spectrum antibiotics to cover anaerobes, IV fluid resuscitation and nasogastric decompression if there is associated ileus. Shamberger published criteria for surgical intervention in the pediatric patient which include persistent gastrointestinal bleeding, free intraperitoneal perforation, uncontrolled sepsis despite adequate resuscitation and vasopressors and an intra-abdominal process that would require surgery in the absence of neutropenia.

Perirectal abscesses might develop in neutropenic patients. If neutropenia is transient, every effort should be made to manage the patient conservatively. If a patient is not septic and if the infection can be controlled with IV antibiotics until the neutrophil count can recover, their fitness for surgery will markedly be improved. There are some patients with myelodysplastic syndrome or relapsed AML who have a persistent, prolonged neutropenia due to invasion of their marrow with tumor. These patients require special care as the hematologist may be reluctant to initiate further treatment with a continued infection and may ask the surgeon to perform incision and drainage despite neutropenia in order to improve their fitness for chemotherapy.

Other causes for urgent surgical intervention are unusual. Rarely, marked splenomegaly due to infiltration of the spleen by leukemic cells or lymphoma can lead to splenic rupture. Splenectomy is the therapy of choice. Aggressive hematological support may be necessary but pancytopenia should not preclude what might be life saving surgery to treat uncontrolled bleeding. The risk of GI perforation among patients with GI lymphoma treated with chemotherapy has probably been overestimated. Patients often present with signs and symptoms of acute peritonitis. Urgent resection of the involved viscus or primary repair should be undertaken after resuscitation.

Landmark Papers

1. Duguid J. Guideline for the use of fresh-frozen plasma, cryoprecipitate and cryosupernatant. British Journal of Haematology 2004;126:11-28.
2. Wall M. Transfusion in the operating room and the intensive care unit: current practice and future directions. Int Anesth Clin Fall 2000;38(4):149-69.
3. Slichter S. Evidenced based platelet transfusion guidelines. Hematology/American Society of Hematology Education Program Book 2007(1):172. HYPERLINK "http://asheducationbook.hematologylibrary.org/cgi/reprint/2007/1/172" http://asheducationbook.hematologylibrary.org/cgi/reprint/2007/1/172.
4. Rebulla P. The threshold for prophylactic platelet transfusions in adults with acute myeloid leukemia. NEJM 1997; 337:1870-5.
5. Wandt H. Safety and cost effectiveness of a 10×10^9/L trigger for prophylactic platelet transfusions compared with the traditional 20×10^9/L trigger: a prospective comparative trial in 105 patients with acute myeloid leukemia. Blood 1998;91:3601-6.
6. Amore F, Brincker H, Gronbaek K, Thorling K, Pedersen M, Jensen MK, et al. Danish Lymphoma Study Group. Non-Hodgkin's lymphoma of the gastrointestinal tract: a population based analysis of incidence, geographic distribution, clinicopathologic presentation, features and prognosis. J Clin Onc 1994;12(8):1673-84.
7. Rosenberg SA. Non-Hodgkin's lymphoma pathologic classification project. National Cancer Institute sponsored study of classifications of non-Hodgkin's lymphomas: summary and description of a working formulation for clinical usage. Cancer 1982;49:2112-35.
8. Danson I, Cornes J, Morson B. Primary malignant lymphoid tumors of the intestinal tract. Br J Surg 1961; 49: 80-9.
9. Morton JE, Leyland MJ, Hudson GV, Hudson BV, Erson L, Bennett MH, MacLennan KA. Primary gastrointestinal non-Hodgkin's lymphoma: a review of 175 British national lymphoma investigation cases. Br J Cancer 1993; 67:776-82.
10. O'Driscoll BR, Steven FM, O'Gorman TA, et al. HLA type of patients with celiac disease and malignancy in the west of Ireland. GUT 1982; 23:662-5.
11. Neugut AI, Jacobson JS, Suh S, Mukherjee R, Arber N. The epidermiology of cancer of the small bowel. Cancer Epidemiol Biomark Prev 1998; 7243-51.
12. List AF, Freer JP, Cousar JC, Stein RS, Johnson DH, Reynolds VH, et al. Non-Hodgkin's lymphoma of the gastrointestinal tract: An analysis of clinical and pathologic features affecting outcome. J Clin Onc 1988; 6(7):1125-33.
13. Salles G, Herbrecht R, Tilly H, Berger F, Brousse N, Gisselbrecht C, Coiffier B. Aggressive primary gastrointestinal lymphomas: review of 91 patients treated with the LNH-84 regimen. A study of the group dëtude des lymphomes agressifs. Am J of Med 1991; 90:77-84.
14. Gobbi PG, Ghirardelli ML, Cavalli C, Baldini L, Broglia C, Clo V, et al. The role of surgery in the treatment of gastrointestinal lymphomas other than low-grade MALT lymphomas. Haematologica 2000, 85(4):372-80.
15. Ha CS, Cho MJ, Allen PK, Fuller LM, Cabanillas F, Cox JD. Primary non-Hodgkin lymphoma of the small bowel. Radiology 1999; 211:183-7.
16. Nobre-Leitao, C. Treatment of Gastric MALT Lymphoma by Helicobacter Pylori Eradication: A Study Controlled by Endoscopic Ultrasonography. Am J Gastroentrerol 1998; 93(5):732-6.
17. Stathis A. Long-Term Outcome Following Helicobacter pylori Eradication in a Retrospective Study of 105 Patients with Localized Gastric Marginal Zone B-Cell Lymphoma of MALT Type. Annals of Oncology 2009;20:1086-93.
18. NCCN Practice Guidelines 2/2009:http:www.nccn.org/professionals/physician_gls/PDF/nhl.pdf.
19. Aviles A. The role of surgery in primary gastric lymphoma. Ann Surg 2004;240:44-50.
20. Shamberger R. The medical and surgical management of typhlitis in children with acute nonlymphocytic (Myelogenous) leukemia. Cancer 1986;57:603-9.

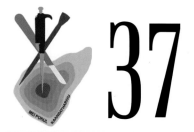

37

Pediatric Surgical Oncology

Kevin P Mollen, David A Rodeberg

General Principles

In the United States, over 10,000 children under the age of 15 are diagnosed with cancer annually. About 1500 children die from cancer each year making it the second leading cause of death in this age group. Despite this, cancer remains relatively rare among children with an average yearly incidence of 1-2 new cases per 10,000 children. Cancer incidence in children has, however, increased in recent decades. According the National Cancer Institute, the incidence of cancer in children ages 1-14 increased from 11.5 per 100,000 children in 1975 to 14.8 per 100,000 children in 2004. Over the same time period, childhood cancers have also seen a dramatic improvement in survival. With the employment and gradual improvement of multimodal therapy, the overall 5-year survival rate has risen from approximately 20% in the 1950s to just under 60% in the 1970s to over 80% today. The causes of childhood cancer are largely unknown. However, there are strong associations with many genetic alterations. Exposure to high levels of ionizing radiation has also been linked to the development of early cancers. Similarly, children treated with chemotherapy and/or radiotherapy are at increased risk of developing a second malignancy. Many other potential environmental carcinogens have been investigated as potential causes of childhood cancer, although few conclusions can be drawn from this work.

Children's Oncology Group

The rarity of most childhood cancers has necessitated the development of large national and international clinical trials and databases in order to study cancer-related risk factors and outcomes. The Children's Oncology Group (COG) is a cooperative clinical trial group supported by the National Cancer Institute (NCI). Formed in 2000 in a merger of the Pediatric Oncology Group, The Children's Cancer Study Group, the Intergroup Rhabdomyosarcoma Study Group and the National Wilms Tumor Study Group, the mission of the COG is to cure and prevent childhood and adolescent cancer through basic science research and clinical trials. Collectively, the COG and its predecessors have supported thousands of clinical trials over the past 50 years. These trials have radically changed outcomes in childhood cancers. Within the COG are individual study groups for virtually every pediatric cancer. Because of the COG, accrual of patients in pediatric clinical cancer trials is extremely high. Currently, over 90% of children diagnosed with cancer are treated as a part of a clinical trial as compared to 5% of the adult cancer population.

Genetics of Childhood Cancer

A key development in the study of childhood cancers over the past few decades is the discovery that genetic alterations are associated with pediatric malignancies. Some alterations are inherited, but others are more likely to be acquired and restricted to tumor cells. Approximately 5% of all childhood cancers have a hereditary basis. Cancers with the clearest genetic basis include retinoblastoma, Wilms' tumor, leukemia and tumors of the central nervous system. Several genetic syndromes are associated with increased risk of childhood cancer, including Ataxia-telangiectasia, Beckwith-Wiedemann, Denys'-Drash, Down, Gorlin's, LiFraumani syndromes and Neurofibromatosis.

Principles of Surgery

More than one half of newly diagnosed childhood cancers are leukemias and central nervous system related tumors. As such, the general pediatric surgeon may be limited in these cases to establishing vascular access for systemic therapy. However, surgery plays a crucial role in the majority of pediatric non-CNS solid tumors. The institution of multimodal therapy (surgery, radiotherapy and chemotherapy) and a cooperative approach to care has significantly improved outcomes in recent decades. As in the adult population, the goal of surgical therapy is complete resection of tumor without injury to surrounding organs or tumor spillage. Much debate remains in the setting of many pediatric tumors as to the timing of surgery in relation to systemic chemotherapy and radiotherapy. As many solid tumors in children are highly chemo- and radiosensitive, a neoadjuvant approach is often employed with some evidence for increased respectability and improved cancer related outcomes. However, toxicity related to these modalities must factor into decisions about the approach to cancer treatment. Thus, early resection is often considered as a means of avoiding prolonged neoadjuvant therapy and can be associated with a decreased level of subsequent radiotherapy. Similarly, potential surgical complications and functional outcomes after surgery must also be considered.

Neuroblastoma

Demographics

Neuroblastoma is the most common extracranial solid tumor in children. In the United States, it accounts for 6-10% of all childhood cancers and approximately 15% of all cancer deaths. The overall incidence is estimated at 1 per 10,000 live births, representing nearly 500 new cases each year in the United States. The incidence peaks at ages 1-4 years with a median age at diagnosis of 23 months. Nearly 30% of all cases are diagnosed within the first year of life. In most series, the male-to-female ratio is approximately 1.2:1. Cases of familial neuroblastoma have been reported with disease occurring at a younger age and with a greater number of primary tumors at the time of diagnosis compared to sporadic disease. A number of environmental exposures have been implicated in the development of disease, but none of these associations have been causally linked. Prognosis is excellent for those children diagnosed with low- and moderate-risk neuroblastoma. Despite advances in multimodal therapy, however outcomes in high-risk patients remain poor with a 5-year event-free survival of 25-30%.

Pathology

Neuroblastomas belong to the "small blue round cell" group of childhood neoplasms and are derived from primordial neural crest cells, the progenitors of the sympathetic nervous system. The classification of neuroblastomas is based on the degree of cellular differentiation within the tumor. True neuroblastomas represent poorly differentiated tumors with abundant neuroblasts while ganglioneuromas are well-differentiated benign tumors with mature ganglion cells and increased stroma. Ganglioneuroblastomas represent intermediate grade tumors with features of both other types.

Clinical Features

Neuroblastomas may occur anywhere along the sympathetic chain and thus patient presentation varies based on the location of origin. Approximately two thirds of neuroblastomas present as intra-abdominal masses, primarily arising in the adrenal glands. These are most commonly asymptomatic lesions that are found on routine physical exam or imaging studies. A sense of fullness and a hard, fixed mass may be noted. Tumors can hemorrhage spontaneously, leading to an acute onset of symptoms, most commonly pain. Similarly, intrathoracic lesions are generally found incidentally on chest radiograph, although they may be associated with respiratory compromise over time. Patients with pelvic masses may present with urinary symptoms or constipation based on compression of pelvic structures. Cervical lesions in the area of the Stellate ganglion may be associated with Horner's syndrome. Paraspinal lesions can extend into the neural foramina leading to neurologic compromise. Evidence of lymphatic spread and clinically positive nodes are often seen at the time of diagnosis. Generalized symptoms associated with metastatic disease include malaise, anorexia, weight loss and fever whereas bony metastases may be accompanied by pain.

Paraneoplastic syndromes occur rarely with neuroblastoma. One characteristic syndrome is opsomyoclonus that is characterized by involuntary muscle contractions and random, rapid eye movements. These symptoms are thought to result from the activity of antibodies in the cerebellum directed at the neural tissue of the tumor. Although these symptoms are commonly associated with low-grade disease, they can significantly be debilitating and often times do not resolve with treatment of the tumor. Tumors may secrete vasoactive inhibitory peptide (VIP) leading to secretory diarrhea. Also associated with low-grade disease, these symptoms do resolve with tumor treatment.

Diagnosis

Up to 90% of patients with neuroblastoma will produce detectable amounts of the urinary catecholamine metabolites homovanillic acid (HVA) and vanillylmandelic acid (VMA). This can aid in the diagnosis of disease and can be used in routine screening for recurrent disease. Various imaging studies may aid in the diagnosis of neuroblastoma. Plain radiography may reveal the presence of a chest mass or may identify suspicious punctuate calcifications within the tumor mass. Ultrasonography may help distinguish solid from cystic masses and may demonstrate a typical heterogeneous tumor appearance. The gold standard for diagnosing and determining the extent of disease is computed tomography (CT).

Magnetic Resonance Imaging (MRI) is useful in distinguishing the degree of tumor extension into the spinal foramina. Radiolabeled metaiodobenzylguanidine (MIBG), a norepinephrine analog, can be used to identify metastatic disease, particularly at bony sites as MIBG is taken up by neuroblastomas but not normal cortical bone or bone marrow. Imaging is enhanced by the addition of technetium 99m methylene diphosphate, which reduces the number of false-negatives. Ultimately, diagnosis of neuroblastoma requires pathologic analysis of the primary tumor or metastatic sites. Criteria for diagnosis generally include unequivocal histologic diagnosis on biopsy. Alternatively, diagnosis may also be confirmed by the presence of neuroblasts seen on bone marrow biopsy in a patient with increased urine or serum catecholamines or catecholamine metabolites. Bilateral posterior iliac crest aspirates and core biopsies are generally required to exclude bone marrow involvement.

Staging

The International Neuroblastoma Staging System (INSS) is the most current and widely used. Resectability is defined as tumor removal without removal of vital organs, compromise of major vessels, or patient disfigurement. Stage 1 disease is a tumor that is completely resected. Stage 2 disease is incompletely resected disease with either negative (2A) or microscopically positive ipsilateral lymph nodes (2B). Stage 3 is incompletely resected disease with contralateral tumor or lymph node involvement. Stage 4 is metastatic disease. Stage 4S disease is considered a distinct entity. Although it represents metastatic disease, the prognosis of patients with 4S disease is similar to that of patients with early stage disease. 4S is defined as a localized Stage 1, 2A or 2B tumor with dissemination to skin, liver and/or bone marrow only. If disease has spread to the bone marrow, then involvement must be minimal, accounting for < 10% or total nucleated cells as defined via bone marrow biopsy or aspirate. If performed, MIBG scan should be negative for disease in the marrow.

Tumor Biology and Prognosis

Aside from anatomical stage, a number of clinical and biologic factors have been shown to predict the behavior and ultimate outcomes of neuroblastoma. The COG stratifies patients into low-, intermediate- and high-risk categories based on age at diagnosis, INSS stage, tumor histopathology, DNA index (ploidy) and MYCN amplification status (**Table 37-1** and **Figures 37-1A to C**). Age is an important clinical prognostic factor. In general, patients under 1 year of age do better than do older patients. More recent evidence suggests that patients diagnosed at up to 18 months with stage 3 or 4 neuroblastoma may also carry an excellent prognosis. The Shimada classification stratifies tumors as 'favorable' or

TABLE 37-1	COG risk stratification for neuroblastoma				
INSS staging	**Age**	**MYCN status**	**Shimada classification**	**DNA ploidy**	**Risk group**
1	0-21 y	Any	Any	Any	Low
2A/2B	< 365 d	Any	Any	Any	Low
	≥ 365 d-21 y	Nonamplified	Any	-	Low
	≥ 365 d-21 y	Amplified	Favorable	-	Low
	≥ 365 d-21 y	Amplified	Unfavorable	-	High
3	< 365 d	Nonamplified	Any	Any	Intermediate
	< 365 d	Amplified	Any	Any	High
	≥ 365 d-21 y	Nonamplified	Favorable	-	Intermediate
	≥ 365 d-21 y	Nonamplified	Unfavorable	-	High
	≥ 365 d-21 y	Amplified	Any	-	High
4	< 548 d	Nonamplified	Any	Any	Intermediate
	< 548 d	Amplified	Any	Any	High
	≥ 548 d-21 y	Any	Any	-	High
4S	< 365 d	Nonamplified	Favorable	>1	Low
	< 365 d	Nonamplified	Any	=1	Intermediate
	< 365 d	Nonamplified	Unfavorable	Any	Intermediate
	< 365 d	Amplified	Any	Any	High

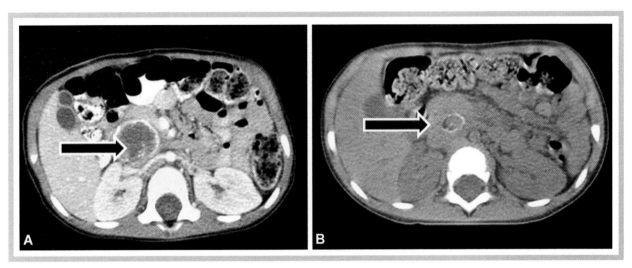

Figures 37-1A and B: Retroperitoneal neuroblsatoma before and after neoadjuvant therapy

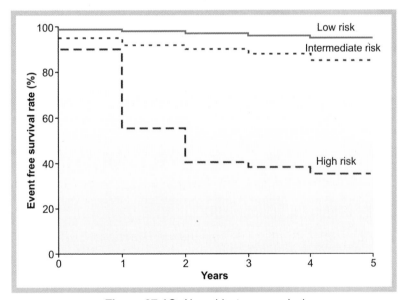

Figure 37-1C: Neuroblastoma survival

'unfavorable' based on patient age, level of tumor differentiation, presence of Schwannian stromal components and degree of mitosis and karyorrhexis. Ploidy has been found to play a role in tumor behavior with near-triploid tumors showing a more favorable course. These tumors are characterized by whole chromosomal gains and losses with few if any structural genetic aberrations. Near-diploid lesions are characterized by genetic aberrations such as MYCN amplification, 17q gain and chromosomal losses. DNA content seems to be more predictive of clinical tumor behavior in the infant population. The MYCN oncogene is present at an increased copy in 25-35% of neuroblastomas and is a very poor prognostic indicator. Often increased in children with stages 3 and 4 disease, it is found at only 5% in patients with 4S tumors.

Surgical Principles

Treatment of neuroblastoma is multimodal and based on risk stratification categories. In general, the primary objective of operative intervention for low-grade neuroblastoma is complete surgical excision. Care must be taken to avoid tumor spillage and injury to adjacent organs. In patients with intermediate- and high-grade disease, initial operative management would primarily involve tissue biopsy for diagnosis and staging. More definitive resection may be considered after induction chemotherapy that may lead to increase resectability. Evidence would also suggest that complete surgical excision of tumor is not always required for cure as these tumors are highly sensitive to radiation and chemotherapy.

Chemotherapy and Radiation Therapy

Low-risk neuroblastoma: Survival rates for patients with Stage 1 as well as Stage 2 disease without NMYC amplification have survival rates with surgery alone of up to 95%. In these patients, chemotherapy is generally reserved for patients who experience life- or organ-threatening symptoms at the time of diagnosis and for those rare patients who have a recurrence or progression of disease. Chemotherapy may even be omitted in the majority of patients with Stage 1 or favorable Stage 2 disease after incomplete surgical resection without a decrease in survival. Infants with Stage 2 disease are considered low risk regardless of MYCN status. Stage 4S neuroblastoma without MYCN amplification undergoes spontaneous regression in the majority of cases. Chemotherapy and radiotherapy is reserved for those patients with 4S disease and symptomatic large tumors or hepatomegaly causing obstruction, respiratory insufficiency, or liver dysfunction.

Intermediate-risk neuroblastoma: The intermediate-risk group encompasses a large spectrum of neuroblastoma although broadly speaking it includes Stages 3 and 4 disease in the absence of MYCN amplification. The mainstay of therapy in this group is surgical excision followed by chemotherapy. The prognosis for patients in this group remains highly favorable with survival rates of 80-95%. Survival is based on adjuvant therapy with moderate-dose chemotherapy primarily involving cisplatin, doxorubicin, etoposide and cyclophosphamide. Efforts have been made to reduce chemotherapy dosage in patients within this group. In fact, the role of chemotherapy has been called into question in patients with regional disease and favorable biologic characteristics. Prospective trials have begun to investigate whether additional molecular and genetic variables can help further stratify risk and treatment within this heterogeneous group of patients in an ongoing effort to tailor therapy and reduce unnecessary toxicities.

High-risk neuroblastoma: Despite improvements in treatment protocols, children with high-risk disease including older patients and those with MYCN amplification continue to have a poor prognosis with an overall survival of 20-40%. The general treatment algorithm for these patients includes induction chemotherapy, surgery and/or radiation for local control, myeloablative therapy with allogeneic or autologous bone marrow or peripheral blood stem cell transplant and biologic therapy to eradicate minimal residual disease.

Tumor response to induction chemotherapy correlates directly with survival. In addition, there may be a correlation between chemotherapy dose and tumor response rates, although this has not been substantiated in large multicenter trials. The addition of newer agents to standard neuroblastoma chemotherapy protocols also offers potential improvements in outcome. Local and regional control of disease after induction chemotherapy is achieved through a combination of surgery and radiotherapy. In general, success of the surgical approach in advanced disease is improved by delaying until after induction therapy is initiated. The goal of surgery is complete gross excision and may involve debulking of locally advanced as well as metastatic disease. Neuroblastoma is also exquisitely sensitive to radiotherapy and this may increase survival in patients with complete as well as incomplete surgical resection. Ongoing studies are evaluating the relationship between residual tumor volume, radiation dose and survival. Randomized trials conducted in Europe and the Unites States have demonstrated improved outcome after myeloablative consolidation therapy followed by autologous stem cell transplant. Data would indicate that relapse rates during the first remission are improved and that event-free survival is increased over those patients receiving chemotherapy alone. Trial CCG-3891 demonstrated the efficacy of isotretinoin (cis-RA), a synthetic retinoid in the treatment of minimal residual neuroblastoma. This study established this drug as the standard of care for postremission maintenance therapy. Many other agents are under investigation including monoclonal antibodies directed against neuroblastoma-specific antigens including gangliosidase GD2.

Future Directions

Neuroblastoma represents a complex spectrum of disease with a variety of clinical behavior. A greater understanding of the molecular biology of disease will allow us to further stratify patients based on risk and response to therapy. This will allow us to minimize exposure of low- and intermediate-risk patients with highly favorable prognosis to treatment-based toxicities. It will also facilitate the development of novel therapies directed against high-risk disease that continues to demonstrate survival under 50%. Immunotherapy offers greater tumor specificity in treatment and thus lowers toxicity profiles. Newer immunotherapeutic approaches hold promise with antibodies directed against a variety of gangliosides and glycoproteins. Coadministration of soluble cytokines may enhance the effects of monoclonal antibodies. Evidence of up- or down-regulation of various member of the Trk tyrosine kinase family of proteins in neuroblastoma and prognostic data based on the trends suggests that targeted inhibition may offer benefits. A variety of other biologic targets are under investigation as well.

Wilms' Tumor

Demographics

Wilms' tumor (WT) is the second most common extracranial solid tumor seen in children, accounting for 6% of all childhood cancers. Originally described by Rance in 1814, it receives its name from Max Wilms, a surgeon who identified nephroblastoma as a tumor consisting of three separate tissue types. In the United States, the incidence is about 8.1 per 1,000,000 people with 500 new cases occurring annually. Most cases are diagnosed in children ages 1-5 years with a peak at 3 years. Although adults can develop WT, it is extremely rare in people over 10 years of age. WT is also rarely diagnosed in children under the age of 6 months. The male-to-female ratio ranges from 0.8 to 0.95 in the literature. There are important racial differences in the incidence of disease with a 2.5 times higher risk in blacks as compared to whites. Asians are only half as likely as whites to be diagnosed. Familial WT is believed to account for 1-2% of all new cases.

Pathology

There are two main histologic subtypes of WT including favorable (classic nephroblastoma) and unfavorable (anaplastic). Favorable tumors are characterized by a triphasic cellular pattern with blastemal, stromal and epithelial elements. Unfavorable tumors are marked by diffuse or focal anaplasia. Pathologic criteria for diagnosis include the presence of multipolar polyploid mitotic figures with marked nuclear enlargement and hyperchromasia. Anaplastic histology is the most important predictor of responsiveness to therapy. Diffuse anaplasia is associated with a significantly worse prognosis than tumors with favorable histology or focal anaplasia.

Many WT appear to arise from abnormally retained embryonic kidney precursor cells arranged in clusters termed nephrogenic rests. The presence of diffuse or multifocal nephrogenic rests is referred to as nephroblastomatosis. These lesions are generally considered premalignant in nature. Nephrogenic rests may occur in the kidney of the primary tumor or the contralateral kidney and can be found bilaterally. Intralobar nephrogenic rests develop within the parenchyma while perilobar nephrogenic rests occur peripherally sometimes forming a thick ring around one or both kidneys. Nephrogenic rests can regress or stay dormant, however the presence of these lesions leaves the patient at increased risk of developing subsequent WT.

Clinical Features

Most children with WT present with a large, smooth flank mass that is non-tender. Twenty to thirty percent of patients present with hematuria frequently detected after minimal trauma, while approximately 25% of patients develop hypertension as a result of activation of the renin-angiotensin axis. Nonspecific symptoms such as fever, malaise, weight loss or anorexia, are present in around 10% at the time of diagnosis. More unusual presentations include varicocele due to compression of the spermatic cord and intra-abdominal bleeding from tumor rupture. Tumors may secrete hormones such as erythropoietin or ACTH. In addition, children may present with hypercalcemia or coagulopathy due to a decrease in von Willebrand factor. Close physical examination may reveal congenital abnormalities which may be associated with WT such as genitourinary malformations, in particular as associated with WAGR (Wilms' tumor, aniridia, genital and/or urinary tract abnormalities, mental retardation and/or developmental delays) syndrome, Beckwith-Wiedemann (body overgrowth, omphalocele, macroglossia, hypoglycemia and other physical characteristics) syndrome and Denys-Drash (congenital nephropathy, Wilms' tumor and intersex disorders) syndrome.

Diagnostic Imaging

Imaging should begin with contrast-enhanced CT. Typical findings of WT include the presence of an intrarenal neoplasm that displaces the collecting system. WT can spread intravascularly into the renal vein, IVC and atrium. Ultrasonography and echocardiography are the preferred means of evaluating these areas. Imaging of the chest may not change initially management of disease, but will aid in determining the extent and stage of disease. Historically, CXR was used as the primary modality, however recent evidence would suggest that important clinical data can be garnered from CT of the chest that cannot be seen on routine CXR. MRI may help to distinguish between nephrogenic rests and WT. The role of PET in WT is as yet undefined.

Staging

Tumor stage is determined through imaging studies as well as surgical and pathological data and is the same for tumors with favorable and anaplastic features. The National Wilms' Tumor Study Group (NWTSG) developed the staging system used by the COG (**Table 37-2** and **Figures 37-2A and B**). In general, stage I disease is confined to the single kidney and has completely been resected without significant spillage or preoperative biopsy. Stage II disease represents completely resected disease with negative margins. However, there is evidence of regional extension beyond the renal capsule. In stage III disease, there is residual tumor after operation that is confined to the abdomen. This stage includes completely resected tumors which were biopsied preoperatively. In stage IV disease, there is hematogenous spread or lymph

TABLE 37-2	Staging of Wilms' tumor	
Stage	**Percentage of patients**	**Criteria**
1	43%	All of the following criteria must be met: - tumor is limited to kidney and is completely resected - renal capsule is intact - tumor is not ruptured or biopsied prior to resection - no involvement of renal sinus vessels - no evidence of tumor at surgical margins
2	20%	Regional extension of tumor characterized by either: - penetration of renal sinus capsule or - blood vessels outside of renal parenchyma involved including renal sinus vessels
3	21%	Residual nonhematogenous tumor remaining in abdomen after surgery including any of the following: - lymph nodes in abdomen or pelvis containing tumor - tumor has penetrated through the peritoneal surface - tumor implants on peritoneal surface - gross or microscopic margin positivity - tumor spillage before or during surgery - tumor biopsied prior to removal - tumor removed piecemeal, including separate removal of tumor thrombus in renal vein - extension of primary tumor into vena cava and heart
4	11%	Hematogenous metastases (lung, liver, bone) or lymph node metastases outside of the abdomen and/or pelvis Tumor in the adrenal gland is not considered metastatic
5	5%	Bilateral renal involvement at diagnosis

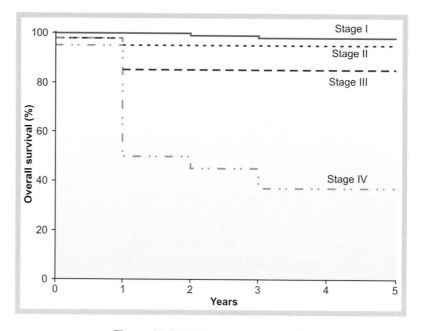

Figure 37-2A: Wilms' tumor survival

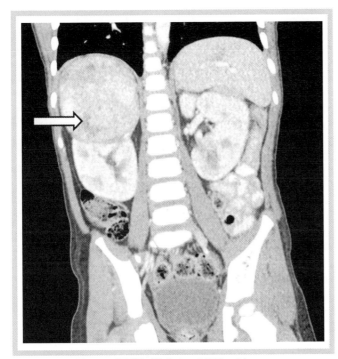

Figure 37-2B: Unilateral Wilms' tumor

node metastasis outside of the abdomen and pelvis. In stage V disease, there is bilateral involvement at the time of diagnosis.

Tumor Biology

The first WT gene (WT1) was cloned in 1989 and was mapped to the 11p13 region. This locus is known to be important for normal genitourinary development and mutations are associated with cryptorchidism and hypospadias. Interestingly, this locus is also important for normal brain development and may explain the neurologic and developmental abnormalities associated with WAGR syndrome. WT1 is mutated in 15% of all unilateral WT patients, including 2% of phenotypically normal children with WT. Children with Denys-Drash syndrome often have a WT1 mutation. Beckwith-Wiedemann syndrome is associated with a second WT gene (WT2) localized to the 11p15 locus. Children with these abnormalities have a predisposition to develop WT and therefore should be screened with ultrasound every 3 months until they reach age 8 years.

NWTS-5 was a study aimed at evaluating whether loss of heterozygosity (LOH) at chromosomes 11q, 16q and 1p is associated with a worse outcome. LOH at 16q is found in 10% of all WT patients while LOH at 1 p is found in 11%. Children with LOH 16q were found to have a poor 2-year relapse free rate. Those with LOH at 1p had a three times higher relapse rate and an increased mortality. Up to 80% of all sporadic WTs may demonstrate LOH or loss of imprinting at 11q. The clinical significance of this genetic data is as yet unknown.

Surgical Principles

The primary goal of surgery is complete resection without any spillage of tumor cells. Radical nephrectomy with regional lymph node sampling through a transabdominal incision is the operation of choice. Hilar, periaortic, iliac and celiac lymph node as well as contralateral lymph node sampling is mandatory and any other suspicious nodal basins should be sampled. Prior to ligation of the renal vein, the vein and IVC should be palpated to rule out intraluminal tumor spread. Any such extension should be removed *en bloc* with the kidney. A thorough intra-abdominal exploration is required, although direct invasion into nearby organs is rare. After resection, surgical clips should be left in the tumor bed, at the site of residual tumor and at nodal basins. Preoperative biopsy of the tumor is not recommended and may be associated with a worse outcome. Exploration of the contralateral side, at one time considered mandatory, is no longer necessary with improved preoperative imaging. If findings on imaging raise concerns about the contralateral kidney, then this side should be explored before resecting the primary tumor. Any suspicious area should be biopsied and, if positive, resection should be abandoned. The patient should instead receive neoadjuvant therapy and if feasible subsequently undergo bilateral partial nephrectomies. Partial nephrectomy is controversial and should only be entertained in patients with bilateral disease and those with WT in a horseshoe kidney.

Preoperative chemotherapy should be entertained in otherwise unresectable cases. This includes patients with massive, nonresectable unilateral tumors, bilateral tumors or venacaval tumor thrombus above the hepatic veins. This approach will generally lead to increase resectability. This is one situation in which preoperative percutaneous biopsy may be indicated.

Chemotherapy and Radiation Therapy

The NWTS group has conducted five major studies evaluating treatment protocols for WT. In NWTS 1 (1969-1973), a combination of vincristine and dactinomycin was found to be more effective than either drug alone. NWTS 2 (1974-1978) demonstrated that 6 months of treatment was equally as effective as 15 months of treatment and decreased side effects. NWTS 3 and 4 demonstrated that neither the addition of RT nor adriamycin in patients with stage II disease improved outcomes. In stages III and IV disease, the addition of adriamycin was effective, but a 4 drug regimen including cyclophosphamide added no benefit. Higher doses of radiation also had no effect on survival. Finally, NWTS 5 demonstrated there was no benefit to treating stage I disease with chemotherapy. Without chemotherapy, the overall 2-year survival was 100% with a relapse-free survival of 86%. The international Society of Pediatric Oncology (SIOP) has also conducted a series of studies evaluating various WT treatment protocols. Among other things, these studies have established a role for neoadjuvant therapy in the treatment of unbiopsied WT. Although preoperative radiation did not have an effect on survival, it resulted in decreased tumor rupture at the time of resection, effectively downstaging many patients. A 4-week course of preoperative chemotherapy was found to be effective without lengthening the entire treatment interval. Finally, progression of disease during the course of neoadjuvant therapy was found to be a poor prognostic indicator.

Current treatment of WT has been shaped by these multicenter trials although much controversy still exists and studies are ongoing. In general, standard treatment for WT involves one of three treatment regimens. Regimen EE4A involves 18 weeks vincristine and dactinomycin. Regimen DD4A expands the duration of treatment to 24 weeks and adds doxorubicin. The third protocol, Regimen 1 involves a 24-week course of vincristine, doxorubicin, cyclophosphamide and etoposide. Patients with stage I or II disease are treated with one of these regimens post-nephrectomy depending on tumor histology. Surgery alone should be considered in patients with stage I disease and favorable histology. Flank or abdominal RT (10 Gy) is utilized for anaplastic histology, tumor spill and nodal or regional extension of the tumor. Neoadjuvant therapy is considered in stage III or IV unresectable disease. Chemotherapy is always the first modality after bilateral renal biopsy in bilateral disease. That being said, therapy for patients with stage V disease must be individualized to the specific patient. Therapy may include a second look operation to re-evaluate tumor histology after 6 weeks of treatment or serial biopsied to look for de-differentiation. If bilateral nephrectomy is pursued, renal transplantation is generally delayed for up to two years after resection.

Prognosis

Therapy for WT is multimodal with a role for surgery, chemotherapy and radiation. Risk stratification and subsequent treatment choice requires an evaluation of several factors including tumor histology, stage, age, tumor size and genetic markers. The role of stage and histology are discussed above. Data would suggest that younger children with smaller tumors do better than other patients.

The prognosis associated with WT is extremely favorable, with an overall 5-year survival rate of 85%. The survival rate for stages I and II tumors is around 95%. Rates drop to 75-80% for stage III tumors and 65-75% for patients with stage IV tumors. Tumor histology plays a major role in recurrence risk. Only 15% of those with favorable histology experience recurrence of disease, compared to a rate of 50% with anaplastic tumors. Liver metastases carry a worse prognosis compared to isolated pulmonary metastases.

Future Directions

The NWTS group no longer exists as an independent clinical trial group. However, the Renal Tumor Committee of the COG is currently enrolling patients in a series of new studies stratified by stage and histology of the tumor. Many of these studies will look to identify high-, moderate- and low-risk groups based on tumor size, stage and LOH status. This may further tailor treatment protocols in an effort to improve outcomes and decrease side effects from unnecessary exposures.

Rhabdomyosarcoma (RMS) / Non-Rhabdomyosarcoma Soft Tissue Sarcoma (NRSTS)

RMS Patient Demographics

RMS is the most common type of soft-tissue sarcoma during the first two decades of life accounting for 4.5% of all childhood cancer. The median age at presentation is 6 years; however, there is a bimodal distribution with peak incidences between 2 and 6 years and again between 10 and 18 years of age.

RMS Tumor Biology

RMS is a malignant tumor of mesenchymal origin. Embryonal and Alveolar are two histologic subtypes that are common in the pediatric population. Embryonal (ERMS) is the most common type of RMS, accounting for two-thirds of all patients with RMS. Alveolar (ARMS) tumors are comprised of small round densely packed cells arranged around spaces resembling pulmonary alveoli. These tumors occur in older children and are most commonly located in the trunk or extremities.

RMS arises as a consequence of regulatory disruption of skeletal muscle progenitor cell growth and differentiation. Both ERMS and ARMS overproduce IGF-II, a growth factor known to stimulate RMS tumor growth, contributing to unregulated growth of these tumors. Translocations of the FKHR transcription factor gene from chromosome 13 with PAX3 (chromosome 2) or PAX 7 (chromosome 1) transcription factor genes occur frequently in ARMS.

Presentation of RMS

RMS presents as asymptomatic masses. Tumors may present with signs and symptoms that vary according to primary tumor origin and may be secondary to mass effect or complications of the tumor. Common sites of primary disease include the head and neck region, the genitourinary tract and the extremities.

Pretreatment Clinical Staging

Staging of RMS is determined by the site of the primary tumor, primary tumor size, tumor invasion, nodal status and distant spread. Staging is based on physical examination and preoperative imaging. Staging is based on a TNM classification system, modified for the site of tumor origin.

Surgical Principles

Biopsy: Open biopsy of a mass suspected to be RMS is recommended to confirm the diagnosis. Adequate specimens for pathologic, biological and treatment protocol studies should be obtained. For small lesions in areas that will be treated with chemotherapy and radiation or for metastatic disease, core needle biopsy may be appropriate. Clinically and radiographic positive lymph nodes should be confirmed pathologically. In addition, sentinel node biopsy may be used for extremity and truncal lesions.

Resection of the mass: Prior to the definitive diagnosis of RMS, an initial surgical procedure to biopsy the mass may have been performed. This frequently results in gross residual tumor, microscopically involved margins, or uncertainty about margins. In this situation, pretreatment re-excision (PRE) is advisable. PRE is a wide re-excision of the previous operative site with adequate margins of normal tissue prior to adjuvant therapy. PRE is usually performed in extremity and trunk lesions, but should be considered the treatment of choice whenever technically feasible.

Wide and complete resection of the primary tumor with a surrounding 'envelope' of normal tissue should be obtained whenever possible. Adequate margins of uninvolved tissue are required unless excision would remove normal tissue that cannot be resected, results in loss of function or poor cosmesis, or is not technically feasible. If narrow margins occur, several separate biopsies of 'normal' tissue around the resection margin should be obtained. Obtaining adequate margins of normal tissue are preferable to leaving gross or microscopic residual tissue in all circumstances. Published outcomes analyses have shown that a clear margin and no residual disease (Group I) is superior to microscopically positive margins (Group II) or gross residual disease (Group III).

Lymph node sampling/dissection: Clinically and radiographically positive nodes should be biopsied to confirm tumor involvement thus ensuring correct assessment of disease risk and assignment of optimal therapy. Pathologic evaluation is required in extremity tumors and for children older than 10 years of age with paratesticular tumor. Regional lymph node sampling should be performed to satisfy diagnostic requirements for staging the tumor. However, lymph node removal is not therapeutic and therefore, should not include resections of the entire lymph node bed nor be performed prophylactically.

Clinical group: After pathologic examination from the definitive operation, patients are assigned to a Clinical Group based on the completeness of tumor excision and the evidence of tumor metastasis to the lymph nodes or distant organs. The Clinical Grouping system differs from Staging in that determination of each patient's clinical group is based on the extent of the surgical resection not the tumor size and site (**Tables 37-3, 37-4 and Figures 37-3A and B**). The completeness of resection is one of the most important predictors of outcome.

Second look operations and aggressive resection for recurrence: After chemotherapy and radiation some patients may be partial responders or nonresponders. A second-look

TABLE 37-3	Risk-based therapy in IRS-IV			
Risk group	**Pre-treatment stage***	**Clinical group#**	**Site#**	**Histology**
Low 1	1 or 2	I or II	Favorable or unfavorable	EMB
	1	III	Orbit only	EMB
Low 2	1	III	Favorable	EMB
	3	I or II	Unfavorable	EMB
Intermediate	2 or 3	III	Unfavorable	EMB
	1-3	I-III	Favorable or unfavorable	ALV
High	4	IV	Favorable or unfavorable	EMB
	4	IV	Favorable or unfavorable	ALV

* Pretreatment stage dependent on site of disease
\# Favorable sites: Orbit, genitourinary tract, biliary tract, nonparameningeal head and neck

TABLE 37-4	Rhabdomyosarcoma clinical grouping system
Group	**Criteria**
I	Localized disease, completely resected A. Confined to organ or muscle of origin B. Infiltrating outside organ or muscle of origin; regional nodes not involved
II	Compromised or regional resection including: A. Grossly resected tumors with microscopic residual tumor B. Regional disease, completely resected, with nodes involved and/or tumor extension into an adjacent organ C. Regional disease, with involved nodes, grossly resected, but with evidence of microscopic residual tumor
III	Incomplete resection or biopsy with gross residual disease remaining
IV	Distant metastases present at outset

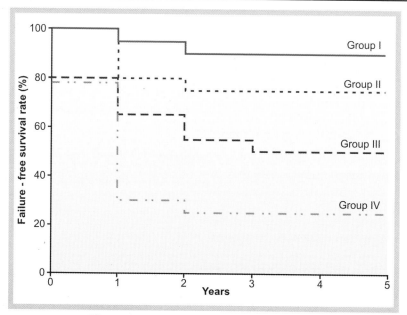

Figure 37-3A: Rhabdomyosarcoma survival

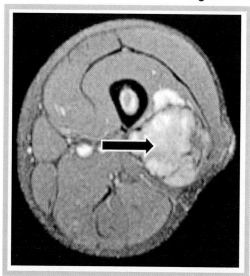

Figure 37-3B: Rhabdomyosarcoma of the thigh

operation (SLO) can be performed to confirm clinical response, to evaluate pathologic response and to remove residual tumor to achieve local control. The goal of SLO is the complete resection. In IRS III, SLOs resulted in the conversion of 75% of patients classified as partial responders to complete responders after excision of residual tumors. Hayes-Jordan, et al recently reviewed their experience with resection of recurrent RMS and reported a 5-year survival of 37% in patients who underwent aggressive surgical resection compared to 8% in a group with inadequate resection. Given these results, SLO and aggressive resection for recurrence can be important tools for the treatment of RMS. However, data would suggest that residual masses at the end of therapy may not warrant resection given the associated morbidity of resection, frequent incomplete resection and the lack of viable tumor in the resected specimen.

Chemotherapy

All patients with RMS receive chemotherapy for disease treatment. Standard therapeutic regimens include a combination of vincristine, actinomycin-D and cyclophosphamide (VAC).

Radiation Therapy

For many children with RMS, radiotherapy is important for local tumor control and survival. Tumor control rates are influenced by the location of the primary tumor and amount of local disease (none, microscopic or gross) at the time radiotherapy is initiated. After biopsy or resection, the majority of children requiring radiotherapy are Group II (microscopic residual disease) or Group III (gross residual disease). Among patients with Group II disease, low dose radiation (40 Gy at 1.5-1.8 Gy/fraction) is associated with local tumor control rates of at least 90%. For patients with Group III disease, radiation doses are more commonly 50 Gy.

Metastatic Disease

RMS metastasizes through both hematogenous and lymphatic routes. Children with metastatic RMS have poor survival rates. For the IRS studies I-III, children with metastatic disease had a 5-year disease-free survival of 20, 27 and 32% respectively in each of the successive studies.

Prognosis

The prognosis of patients with RMS is dependent on many factors. Favorable prognostic factors include embryonal/botryoid histology, primary tumor sites in the orbit and nonparameningeal head/neck region and genitourinary nonbladder/prostate regions, a lack of distant metastases at diagnosis, complete gross removal of tumor at the time of diagnosis, tumor size less than or equal to 5 cm and age less than 10 years at the time of diagnosis. Clinical grouping was identified as one of the most important predictor of failed treatment and tumor relapse. These factors become important in the designation of treatment groups for risk based therapy. Overall prognosis for ERMS is good with a 5-year survival rate of 60%. Prognosis is slightly worse in ARMS than ERMS with a 5-year survival rate of 54%.

Current therapy for patients with group I-II tumors results in 85-95% long-term survival, indicating that risk-based therapeutic strategies have assisted with failure free survival. Approximately 15% of patients with RMS present with metastases (Group IV) at the time of diagnosis. Patients in Group IV have poor outcomes despite aggressive multimodality treatments with only 25% expected to be free of disease three years after diagnosis.

Osteosarcoma and Ewing's Sarcoma

Demographics

Pediatric bone tumors, such as osteosarcoma and Ewing's sarcoma, occur most commonly in patients 15-19 years old and account for 8% for all pediatric cancers and 15% of extracranial tumors.

Clinical Features

Most osteosarcomas are high grade fully malignant tumors which arise most commonly from the metaphases of long extremity bones with approximately 2/3 originating from the region of the knee. Ewing's sarcoma is more equally distributed between the limbs and the axial skeleton. The two most common sites of origin are the femur and the pelvis. Ewing's sarcomas frequently contain EWS fusion genes. Both osteosarcoma and Ewing's tumors show a propensity for early dissemination with metastasis of osteosarcoma involving the lung in > 80% and bones in only 10-20%. In contrast, both areas are affected equally by Ewing's tumor metastasis. Given its propensity for pulmonary metastatic spread CT scans are routinely obtained to detect pulmonary metastasis.

Surgical Principles

Local therapy for both osteosarcoma and Ewing's sarcoma is usually based on surgical removal. The goals of surgical technique are complete tumor removal, including a wide local excision of the tumor with the biopsy scar surrounded by an envelope of normal tissue removed *en bloc*. Marginal resection should be avoided and intralesional or piecemeal surgery is clearly not sufficient. Advances in imaging and biomedical engineering as well as multimodality therapy have lead to a major shift away from amputation toward limbs salvage surgery. Currently the main goals of the extremity reconstruction are to achieve equal limb length at maturity and good functional outcome. Radiotherapy may be considered in patients in whom tumor resection is not feasible or after incomplete resections if there are no other surgical options. Local control rates of approximately 60% after radiotherapy and chemotherapy occur in patients without resection or following incomplete resection.

For Ewing's sarcoma the local control therapy can either be surgery alone or radiotherapy alone or the combination of both; however, analysis of data has certainly indicated that local control seems to be improved with surgical resection. Definitive radiotherapy is indicated when surgery with sufficient margins is not really possible. This is common in patients with spinal and pelvic disease. The local control following radiotherapy alone is similar to radiotherapy combined with the resection that leaves behind gross residual disease. Therefore, there is no role in either Ewing's sarcoma or osteosarcoma for debulking procedures.

Osteosarcoma usually metastasize to lungs with disease detectable upon imaging at initial presentation in 10-15% of patients. Surgical resection of metastatic pulmonary disease should include an open thoracotomy with bilateral exploration and manual palpation of both lungs. Using this approach a 5-year survival rate of 29% was achieved in patients with metastatic pulmonary disease and > 40% 5-year survival in patients rendered surgically disease free. In a study by Bacci, et al they treated 162 patients from 1986 to 2001 with osteosarcoma and lung disease, present at diagnosis, with neoadjuvant chemotherapy, simultaneous resection of primary and pulmonary lesions followed by additional adjuvant chemotherapy. After neoadjuvant chemotherapy, lung lesions disappeared in 14 patients. A total of 132 patients had operative resection of primary tumors and lung nodules. Lung lesions were completely resected in 122 patients; of these, 32 patients had histologically benign disease by pathology. Thus a total of a 100 patients were simultaneously operated on for local disease as well as pulmonary metastatic disease with histologically proven disease on both sides. The 5-year failure-free survival was 19% for all patients. It was 27% for the 91 patients that had complete resection of pulmonary lesions compared to none of the 9 patients who had an incomplete removal of lungs nodules. Among the 91 with a complete resection the failure free survival was significantly improved with disease confined to a single side, 27% versus 8% for bilateral disease (p < 0.02) or when only 1-3 metastasis nodules were present, 40% versus 13% for > 3 nodules (p < 0.00013). These results clearly demonstrate the importance of complete surgical resection of all disease including both primary lesion as well as metastatic nodules. That FFS was worse with bilateral disease or multiple metastatic nodules is probably an indication of tumor biology as well as the difficulty in getting a complete surgical excision with a diffused metastatic disease.

Chemotherapy

In both osteosarcoma and Ewing's sarcoma, local therapy alone is not sufficient since 80-90% of patients with localized disease will develop metastasis and die if chemotherapy is not included as part of the multidisciplinary treatment. Currently most of treatment protocol includes preoperative chemotherapy followed by surgery of the primary tumor and metastatic lesions followed by further adjuvant chemotherapy. However, a randomized trial recently found that there is no advantage for neoadjuvant chemotherapy compared to upfront surgery with adjuvant chemotherapy alone. Chemotherapy for patients with osteosarcoma commonly includes doxorubicin, cisplatin, high dose methotrexate and ifosfamide. Chemotherapy for Ewing's sarcoma usually employs a VACA backbone (vincristine, doxorubicin, cyclophosphamide and actinomycin.

Radiation Therapy

Radiotherapy has an important role if surgery with appropriate margins is not feasible. Postoperative radiotherapy is generally indicated for incomplete tumor resections with gross residual disease or even microscopically positive margins. In addition, patients with a poor histologic response to induction chemotherapy, even with wide margins, have a high local failure rate (12%). This local failure rate was lower when postoperative radiotherapy was given (approximately 6%).

Prognosis

Unfortunately overall progress has been slowing and survival rates have not improved since the mid 1980s. Currently the combined use of surgery and multidrug chemotherapy results in 5-year FFS of 50-70% in patients with localized extremity osteosarcoma versus 29% in patients with metastatic disease at diagnosis. For Ewing's sarcoma multimodality treatment combining chemotherapy and local therapy achieve cure of more than 60% in patient with localized disease. Approximately 25% of Ewing's sarcoma patients present with metastatic disease and the prognosis for these patients is poor with survival being approximately 30-40% for patients with pulmonary metastasis less that 25% for patients with bone or bone marrow metastasis.

One of the major determinants of the outcome is the histological tumor response to induction chemotherapy. Those patients deemed as good responders (less than 10% viable tumor) had a 5-year FFS of 67% compared to poor responders who had a 38% 5-year FFS. Unfortunately attempt to improve the outcome of those patients that are poor responders by modification of postoperative treatment has not resulted in any improvement in survival.

In both osteosarcoma and Ewing's sarcoma outcomes after local or metastatic recurrence are poor with overall survival rate of approximately 10-20%. Fewer lesions at relapse, recurrence confined to lungs, longer disease-free intervals and response to secondary treatment have been associated with more favorable outcomes. At least 30-40% of patients with extremity osteosarcoma develop recurrences, 8% include metastatic lesions in the lungs and 15% in distant bones. The 5-year survival for patients with a recurrent osteosarcoma is only 23%. The length of time till relapse and the number of lesions that recur have prognostic importance. It is a paramount importance to make sure that surgical resection is used to clear all disease with 5-year survival rate estimated to be 39% for patients who achieved the second surgical remission and 0% for those who failed to do so. The patient may survive even multiple recurrences with repeat surgery.

Hepatoblastoma and Hepatocellular Carcinoma

Demographics

Tumors of the liver in children are extremely rare, however 60-70% of these tumors are malignant. The incidence of malignancy remains relatively constant at 0.5-1.5 cases diagnosed yearly per 1 million children under the age of 15 years, accounting for 1% of all childhood cancers. Hepatoblastoma accounts for 70-80% of all malignant liver tumors in children and 90% of tumors in children under the age of 3. Hepatocellular carcinoma (HCC) accounts for the majority of the remaining tumors. Nearly all cases of hepatoblastoma are diagnosed before the age of 3 years and over half of these are diagnosed by 18 months. By comparison, HCC in children has a bimodal incidence pattern with peaks occurring at 0-4 years and again at 12-15 years of age. Hepatoblastoma is slightly more common in females with a 3:2 ratio. Interestingly, the incidence of hepatoblastoma appears to have doubled in the United States over the past 25 years, while the incidence of HCC has remained static. A strong association of hepatoblastoma with very low birth weight infants has been noted in Asia with a 15 fold increased risk. This fact alone may account for the perceived increase in the incidence hepatoblastoma as the survival of premature small neonates continues to increase. A higher overall incidence of liver tumors in Asian countries may be explained by a higher rate of prenatally acquired Hepatitis B and decreased vaccination rate.

Pathology and Tumor Biology

Hepatoblastoma is classified as either epithelial (55%) or mixed epithelial/mesanchymal (45%) histology. Epithelial hepatoblastoma is further categorized into pure fetal (31%), embryonal (19%), macrotrabecular (3%) and small cell undifferentiated (3%). Pure fetal histology and the presence of mesenchymal elements have been associated with improved outcomes while undifferentiated tumors carry an especially poor prognosis. Multiple chromosomal abnormalities are associated with hepatoblastoma including extra copies of chromosomes 1, 2, 7, 8, 17 and 20. Loss of heterozygosity of 11p15 has been observed in up to one third of all patients diagnosed with hepatoblastoma. This abnormality is also nearly pathognomic for Beckwith-Wiedemann syndrome and is also associated with Wilms' tumor and rhabdomyosarcoma in addition to hepatoblastoma. Hepatoblastoma is also associated with Familial Adenomatous adenoma (FAP), caused by inactivation of the adenomatous polyposis coli (APC) tumor-suppressor gene on chromosome 5. Alterations in this gene have been noted in over 60% of patients diagnosed with sporadic hepatoblastoma. Several studies have demonstrated alterations in the APC/β-catenin pathway contributing to the pathogenesis of hepatoblastoma.

Clinical Features

The most common presentation for a malignant hepatic tumor is a painless abdominal mass. Hepatoblastoma is three times more common in the right lobe of the liver. Less frequently, this may be accompanied by anorexia, weight loss, emesis and abdominal pain, although these symptoms often indicate advanced disease. Distant metastases, found in up to 20% of patients at the time of diagnosis, may also account for symptoms with the most common sites of metastatic disease including the lung and the CNS.

Diagnostic Imaging

The discovery of a new intra-abdominal mass in a child warrants immediate radiographic imaging. Often times, the initial diagnosis of hepatoblastoma is made via ultrasound that will define whether a mass is solid or cystic and will identify the organ of origination. Hepatoblastoma characteristically appears as a well-defined hyperechoic mass originating from the right lobe of the liver. The gold standard for diagnosis is CT. Because complete surgical resection is the cornerstone of treatment, CT also plays a key role in defining the respectability of tumors. CT frequently reveals a well-delineated mass with low attenuation. CT with arterial and venous phases has largely replaced angiography for delineation of vascular involvement and define the vascular anatomy in relation to the tumor. MRI scanning is equivalent to CT in its ability to diagnose, delineate and assess respectability of hepatic tumors.

Staging

The COG had previously used a staging system based on findings at or after the time of surgery. Derived from a classic TNM system of staging, this divides tumor into four main groups based on the extent of resection. Stage I tumors are confined to the liver and are completely resected. Stage II tumors have microscopic residual disease while stage III tumors have macroscopic residual disease of tumor rupture. Stage IV represents metastatic disease. Stages I and II tumors carry a favorable prognosis with cure rates over 90%. This is compared to approximately 60% for stage II and 20% for stage IV.

The International Childhood Liver Tumor Strategy Group (SIOPEL) and current COG protocols use a staging

TABLE 37-5	PRETEXT classification
Pretext number	**Criteria**
I	One section is involved and three adjoining sections are free
II	One or two sections are involved, but two adjoining sections are free
III	Two or three sections are involved, and no adjoining sections are free
IV	All four sections are involved

system based on pretreatment extent of disease (PRETEXT, **Table 37-5**). For this staging system, the liver is divided into sectors based on the branching pattern of the portal vein. Tumors are divided into 4 categories based on the number of affected sectors. PRETEXT stage I tumors involve only one quadrant while stage II involves two quadrants with two adjoining quadrants free of tumor. Stage III involves three adjoining quadrants or two nonadjoining quadrants. In stage IV, tumor involves all quadrants. Under this system, tumors are evaluated preoperatively by either CT of ultrasound with selective use of adjunctive MRI. Under the original intent, only stage I tumors are to be treated with upfront surgery. In 2005, the PRETEXT system was revised to account for other indicators of disease including caudate lobe involvement, extrahepatic disease, tumor focality, tumor rupture, distant metastases, lymph node metastases, portal vein involvement and involvement of the IVC and/or hepatic veins. Interestingly, these designations are given in addition to PRETEXT number, but rarely alter it.

Drawbacks of this system include interobserver variability in staging based on imaging and a high level of discordance with eventual findings at surgery (near 50%). However, the PRETEXT system offers prognostic significance for both overall survival and event-free survival and helps determine whether tumors are surgically resectable or not. Those tumors that are not resectable upfront (PRETEXT III and IV) should be referred to transplant centers since they will frequently require liver transplantation.

Surgical Principles and Multimodal Therapy

In general, surgery including complete gross resection of the primary tumor offers the best chance for cure in children with liver tumors. However, there remains debate about the timing of surgery, or rather which patients should receive upfront surgery versus neoadjuvant therapy. Hepatoblastomas are usually unifocal and highly chemosensitive, particularly to platinum-based therapies. HCC, however, is much less sensitive to chemotherapy. Two primary treatment strategies exist. In the United States, those children deemed potentially resectable are taken to surgery initially. This approach is based on the fact that the best long-term outcomes recorded are in those children receiving upfront complete resection. Also, this strategy is designed to avoid the toxicity of prolonged neoadjuvant chemotherapy regimens. Alternatively, the SIOPEL study group encourages neoadjuvant chemotherapy for all children at diagnosis. They cite smaller tumors and improved outcomes in children receiving preoperative treatment and claim that increased toxicity if offset by increased resectability.

Most chemotherapeutic regimens used worldwide employ some combination of cisplatin with doxorubicin. COG currently recommends a regimen of cisplatin, 5FU and vincristin for low-risk tumors. Doxorubicin is added for intermediate-risk tumors and newer drugs are under investigation for use in high-risk tumors. Risk factors considered include extrahepatic tumor extension, multifocality, vascular invasion, DNA aneuploidy and distant metastasis. Low risk tumors are resectable and demonstrate pure fetal histology. Declining levels of AFP during therapy also correlates with a more favorable outcome.

A growing experience in liver transplantation in children has opened the door to radical resection in children with otherwise unresectable disease. Limited studies have demonstrated long-term survival of up to 80% in children with four segment disease and an absence of metastasis. The merits of potentially hazardous partial hepatectomy should be weighed against the risk of long-term immunosuppression after liver transplantation in children with advanced disease.

Future Directions

Newer trials are aimed largely at further stratifying risk based on histologic and biologic characteristics of individual tumors. It is hoped that, more than clinical stage, these parameters will allow for a more tailored and effective approach to multimodal therapy. We will most likely also see an expansion of the use of liver transplantation in the treatment of pediatric liver tumors.

Pediatric Germ Cell Tumors

Demographics

Malignant germ cell tumors (GCT) account for approximately 3% of all childhood malignancies with less than 250 new diagnoses in the United States each year. These tumors derive from primordial germ cells that arise in the area of the embryonic yolk sac endoderm and migrate to the genital ridge on the posterior abdominal wall during the 4th and 5th weeks of gestation. In general, extracranial GCT tumors are subdivided into gonadal and extragonadal tumors **(Figure 37-4)**. Aberrant or arrested

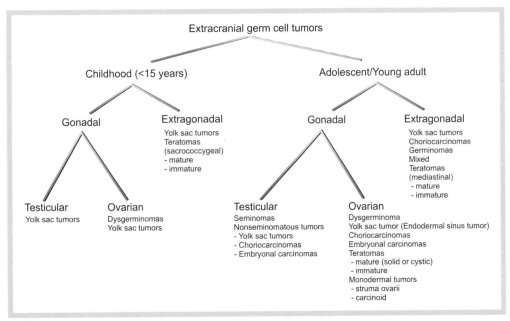

Figure 37-4: Classification of germ cell tumors

migration of these cells is thought to account for the appearance of extragonadal GCT arising in midline sites including the sacrococcygeal, mediastinal, retroperitoneal and pineal locations. Extragonadal tumors comprise the majority of tumors that occur in neonates and infants and account for two-third of all pediatric GCT. The most common extragonadal tumors are teratomas in the sacrococcygeal region. Histologically, teratomas are comprised of ectodermal, mesodermal and endodermal germ layers and any tissue type may be found within these tumors. Mature tumors contain well-differentiated tissues and are largely benign. Immature teratomas may contain more immature tissues of neuroepithelial origin. Higher grade tumors may contain foci of yolk sac tumor. The most common primary site for extragonadal tumors in adolescents is the mediastinum.

In contrast, the majority of tumors diagnosed in later childhood and adolescence arise in gonadal sites. Testicular tumors in younger children are typically yolk sac tumors. These tumors are typically diploid or tetraploid and may have deletions of chromosomes 1p, 4q and 6q as well as gains of chromosomes 1q, 3 and 20q. In adolescents, tumors typically possess an isochromosome of the short arm of chromosome 7. These tumors are divided into seminomatous and nonseminomatous (dysgerminomas) tumors. This is an important distinction in that seminomas are highly radiosensitive whereas nonseminomatous tumors are not. Ovarian GCT primarily occur in adolescents. Although most of these tumors are benign, a variety of malignant tumors exist including immature teratomas, dysgerminomas, yolk sac tumors and mixed GCT. Malignant tumors often contain

increased copies of the short arm of chromosome 12 and generally carry a good prognosis.

Clinical Features and Diagnosis

Testicular GCT in children generally present as asymptomatic masses. CT is adequate to evaluate for the extent of disease, although MRI may also be used. Tumor markers such as alpha fetoprotein may also be elevated. Ovarian tumors in children are almost exclusively of germ cell origin. The incidence of disease increases after 9 years of age and peaks around 19 years.

The sacrococcygeal region is the most common site for teratoma formation in children under the age of 4 years. Neonatal sacrococcygeal teratomas are noted at birth protruding from the sacrum. In older children, these tumors often present with a sacral mass extending intra-abdominally causing symptoms of bladder or rectal compression and are more likely to be malignant (48% for girls and 67% for boys over 2 months compared to 7% and 10% respectively for girls and boys under the age of 2 months).

Teratomas elsewhere are extremely rare and most are mature and therefore non-malignant. Other common sites for teratomas are the ovaries of pubescent girls, the testicular region of boys under the age of 4 and the mediastinum of adolescents. Retroperitoneal tumors are generally seen in children under the age of 5 and are usually unresectable at the time of diagnosis.

Staging

Several staging systems exist for GCT, although the most commonly used system is based on pathologic findings after resection. As with other solid tumors, the stage of disease directly correlates to prognosis. Stage I disease is completely resected with negative margins and an absence of nodal or distant spread. Stage II disease includes tumors with microscopic residual disease, capsular invasion or microscopic lymph node involvement. Stage III tumors have gross residual disease, gross lymph node involvement (> 2 cm) or cytologic evidence of tumor cells in ascites or pleural fluid. Finally, stage IV disease includes disseminated disease involving the lungs, liver, brain, bone, distant nodes or other sites.

Multimodal Therapy

In general, the goal of surgery is complete tumor resection, although partial resection with microscopic or gross residual tumor may improve outcomes. Current standard chemotherapy regimens for pediatric GCT have been developed through a few major COG studies. Current therapy includes cisplatin, etoposide and bleomycin. Similar event-free survival has been seen using carboplatin in place of cisplatin. In general, chemotherapy is reserved for stages II-IV disease or stage I ovarian and extragonadal GCT.

Mature and Immature Teratomas

Upfront surgical resection is the key to therapy. Unfortunately, complete resection rates are lower for sacrococcygeal tumors due the complex anatomy of this area and tumor extension into surrounding structures. Resection of the coccyx is essential to decrease the recurrence rate. After resection, children are observed closely and tumor markers are tracked. Specifically, AFP levels are used to determine the adequacy of resection and detect recurrence of disease. Recurrence rates are high, even in benign disease (10-25%). Recurrent tumors are generally malignant even when arising from benign primaries. Mature teratomas at other sites may be treated with surgery alone as they have a benign clinical behavior. Immature tumors in these areas are treated with surgical resection of tumor combined with chemotherapy.

Malignant Gonadal Germ Cell Tumors

For testicular tumors, surgery alone may be adequate in the setting of stage I disease. Treatment of the mass involves a radical orchiectomy with high ligation of the spermatic cord through an inguinal incision. Transscrotal biopsy and/or resection introduces a risk of metastasis to the inguinal lymph nodes. Tumor markers are then followed to verify normalization of values. For higher stage disease, surgery is combined with chemotherapy. Older adolescents with testicular tumors are treated more as adults as their tumor biology is significantly different.

Similarly, stage I ovarian GCT have a high cure rate with surgery alone. The operative procedure consists of unilateral salpingo-oophorectomy followed by observation. If tumor markers do not normalize, then chemotherapy is initiated. Advanced stage dysgerminomas of the ovary respond well to surgery plus radiation, although this results in sterility. Because of this, chemotherapy is often employed along with limited tumor resection. For malignant GCT, treatment generally consists of complete surgical resection and cisplatinum-based chemotherapy. In some cases, neoadjuvant therapy may be entertained in order to facilitate resection and maintain fertility.

Malignant Extragonadal Germ Cell Tumors

The role of surgery in malignant GCT is variable based on the location and stage of tumors. In general, treatment begins with surgery in stages I and II disease, followed by adjuvant chemotherapy. Overall survival in this group is over 90%. In stages III and IV disease, surgery comes first if tumors are believed to be resectable. Followed by chemotherapy, this approach offers an 80% overall survival rate. Unresectable tumors are generally treated with neoadjuvant chemotherapy, followed by surgery for residual disease.

Future Directions

Many of the current trials regarding GCT involve newer chemotherapeutics such as cyclophosphamide and newer dosing regimens aimed at reducing overall dose and thereby toxicity. Surgery alone is being considered as the treatment of stage I disease. The role of surgery in recurrent disease is being studied as are several newer chemotherapeutic regimens.

Summary

- Although the incidence of childhood cancer has increased in recent decades, this has been accompanied by a dramatic improvement in survival.
- Childhood cancer is the second leading cause of death in children.
- Over 90% of children diagnosed with cancer are treated as a part of a clinical trial as compared to 5% of the adult cancer population.
- Approximately 5% of all childhood cancers have a hereditary basis.
- Surgery plays a crucial role in the treatment of most extracranial pediatric solid tumors as a part of a multimodal, cooperative approach. In many cases, resection may occur after neoadjuvant therapy.
- Due to the age of pediatric patients, particular attention must be paid to the potential long-reaching complications of surgery as well as toxicities of nonsurgical therapies when developing treatment regimes for patients.

- As in the adult population, the goal of surgical therapy is complete resection of tumor without injury to surrounding organs or tumor spillage.

Landmark Papers

General:
1. Guidelines for the pediatric cancer center and role of such centers in diagnosis and treatment. American Academy of Pediatrics Section Statement Section on Hematology/Oncology. Pediatrics 1997;99(1): 139-41.

Neuroblastoma:
2. Matthay KK, Villablanca JG, Seeger RC, et al. Treatment of high-risk neuroblastoma with intensive chemotherapy, radiotherapy, autologous bone marrow transplantation and 13-cis-retinoic acid. Children's Cancer Group. N Engl J Med 1999;341(16): 1165-73.
3. Berthold F, Boos J, Burdach S, et al. Myeloablative megatherapy with autologous stem-cell rescue versus oral maintenance chemotherapy as consolidation treatment in patients with high-risk neuroblastoma: a randomised controlled trial. Lancet Oncol 2005;6(9): 649-58.
4. Look AT, Hayes FA, Shuster JJ, et al. Clinical relevance of tumor cell ploidy and N-myc gene amplification in childhood neuroblastoma: a Pediatric Oncology Group study. J Clin Oncol 1991;9(4): 581-91.
5. Matthay KK, Perez C, Seeger RC, et al. Successful treatment of stage III neuroblastoma based on prospective biologic staging: a Children's Cancer Group study. J Clin Oncol 1998;16 (4): 1256-64.
6. Wei JS, Greer BT, Westermann F, et al. Prediction of clinical outcome using gene expression profiling and artificial neural networks for patients with neuroblastoma. Cancer Res 2004;64 (19): 6883-91.

Wilms' Tumor:
7. Breslow N, Sharples K, Beckwith JB, et al. Prognostic factors in nonmetastatic, favorable histology Wilms' tumor. Results of the Third National Wilms' Tumor Study. Cancer 1991;68 (11): 2345-53.
8. D'Angio GJ, Breslow N, Beckwith JB, et al. Treatment of Wilms' tumor. Results of the Third National Wilms' Tumor Study. Cancer 1989;64 (2): 349-60.
9. Diller L, Ghahremani M, Morgan J, et al. Constitutional WT1 mutations in Wilms' tumor patients. J Clin Oncol 1998; 16(11): 3634-40.

Rhabdomyosarcoma:
10. Crist W, Gehan EA, Ragab AH, et al. The Third Intergroup Rhabdomyosarcoma Study. J Clin Oncol 1995; 13(3): 610-30.
11. Maurer HM, Gehan EA, Beltangady M, et al. The Intergroup Rhabdomyosarcoma Study-II. Cancer 1993;71(5): 1904-22.
12. Crist WM, Anderson JR, Meza JL, et al. Intergroup rhabdomyosarcoma study-IV: results for patients with nonmetastatic disease. J Clin Oncol 2001;19(12): 3091-102.

13. Breneman JC, Lyden E, Pappo AS, et al. Prognostic factors and clinical outcomes in children and adolescents with metastatic rhabdomyosarcoma—a report from the Intergroup Rhabdomyosarcoma Study IV. J Clin Oncol 2003;21(1): 78-84.
14. Meza JL, Anderson J, Pappo AS, et al. Analysis of prognostic factors in patients with nonmetastatic rhabdomyosarcoma treated on intergroup rhabdomyosarcoma studies III and IV: the Children's Oncology Group. J Clin Oncol 2006;24(24): 3844-51.

Osteosarcoma:
15. Delattre O, Zucman J, Melot T, et al. The Ewing family of tumors—a subgroup of small-round-cell tumors defined by specific chimeric transcripts. N Engl J Med 1994;331(5): 294-9.
16. Rodríguez-Galindo C, Liu T, Krasin MJ, et al. Analysis of prognostic factors in Ewing sarcoma family of tumors: review of St. Jude Children's Research Hospital studies. Cancer 2007;110 (2): 375-84.

Hepatoblastoma:
17. Pritchard J, Brown J, Shafford E, et al. Cisplatin, doxorubicin and delayed surgery for childhood hepatoblastoma: a successful approach—results of the first prospective study of the International Society of Pediatric Oncology. J Clin Oncol 2000;18(22):3819-28.
18. Austin MT, Leys CM, Feurer ID, et al. Liver transplantation for childhood hepatic malignancy: a review of the United Network for Organ Sharing (UNOS) database. J Pediatr Surg 2006;41(1): 182-6.
19. Perilongo G, Shafford E, Maibach R, et al. Risk-adapted treatment for childhood hepatoblastoma. Final report of the second study of the International Society of Paediatric Oncology—SIOPEL 2. Eur J Cancer 2004;40(3): 411-21.
20. D'Antiga L, Vallortigara F, Cillo U, et al. Features predicting unresectability in hepatoblastoma. Cancer 2007;110 (5): 1050-8.
21. Schnater JM, Aronson DC, Plaschkes J, et al. Surgical view of the treatment of patients with hepatoblastoma: results from the first prospective trial of the International Society of Pediatric Oncology Liver Tumor Study Group. Cancer 2002;94 (4):1111-20.

GCT:
22. Schneider DT, Calaminus G, Koch S, et al. Epidemiologic analysis of 1,442 children and adolescents registered in the German germ cell tumor protocols. Pediatr Blood Cancer 2004;42(2):169-75.
23. Marina N, London WB, Frazier AL, et al. Prognostic factors in children with extragonadal malignant germ cell tumors: a pediatric intergroup study. J Clin Oncol 2006;24(16): 2544-8.
24. Marina NM, Cushing B, Giller R, et al. Complete surgical excision is effective treatment for children with immature teratomas with or without malignant elements: A Pediatric Oncology Group/Children's Cancer Group Intergroup Study. J Clin Oncol 1999;17(7): 2137-43.

Level of Evidence Table			
Recommendation	**Best level of evidence**	**Grade**	**References**
Surgical resection followed by moderate dose chemotherapy is recommended for intermediate-risk neuroblastoma.	2	B	Matthay KK, et al. J Clin Oncol, 1998
Myeloablative therapy and autologous hematopoietic cell rescue result in significantly better 5-year EFS and OS than nonmyeloablative chemotherapy; *cis*-RA given after consolidation independently results in significantly improved OS.	1	A	Matthay KK, et al. J Clin Oncol, 2009
Children < 24 months old with small (<550 gm), stage I, favorable-histology Wilms' tumor may be treated with nephrectomy alone. All other tumors should be treated with a multimodal approach.	3	B	Green DM, et al. J Clin Oncol, 2001
Tumor spillage in resection of Wilms' tumor results in a significant increase in disease recurrence.	3	B	Shamberger, et al. Ann Surg, 1998
Neoadjuvant therapy for Wilms' tumor can downstage tumors, facilitating resection and a reduction in postoperative therapy. This approach provides comparable overall outcomes to the traditional adjuvant approach.	1	B	Tournade MF, et al. Nat Clin Prac Urol, 2001 Mitchell C, et al. Eur Jour Cancer, 2006
The combination of vincristine, actinomycin D and cyclophosphamide dosed at 2.2 gm/m^2 per dose (VAC) with GCSF is equivalent to vincristine with either actinomycin D and ifosfamide (VAI) or ifosfamide and etoposide (VIE) as the gold standard for adjuvant therapy in Rhabdomyosarcoma.	1	A	Crist WM, et al. J Clin Oncol, 2001
Adjuvant radiation therapy is recommended in all cases of Rhabdomyosarcoma except Group I tumors of Embryonal histology at conventional dosing regimens.	1	A	Wolden SL, et al. J Clin Oncol, 1999 Donaldson SS, et al. Int J Radiat Oncol Biol Phys, 2001
Resection of pulmonary metastases of osteosarcoma/Ewing's sarcoma is a safe and effective treatment that offers improved survival benefit in carefully selected patients within a multidisciplinary approach for pediatric cancer.	4	C	Tronc F, et al: Eur J Cardiothorac Surg, 2008 Temeck BK, et al. Ann Thorac Surg, 1995
Adjuvant therapy for Hepatoblastoma using either cisplatin, vincristine and fluorouracil or cisplatin and continuous infusion doxorubicin improved survival in children with hepatoblastoma.	1	A	Ortega JA, et al. J Clin Oncol, 2000.
Liver transplantation and chemotherapy for unresectable hepatoblastoma can be curative.	4	C	Reyes JD, et al. J Pediatr, 2000 Otte JB, et al. Pediatr Blood Cancer, 2004 Browne M, et al. J Pediatr Surg, 2008
Mature teratomas may be treated with complete surgical excision alone; AFP levels should be followed postoperatively as a marker of recurrence. Chemotherapy is reserved for tumors with immature elements or yolk sac tumor recurrence.	4	C	Mann JR, et al. J Clin Oncol, 2008
Complete resection of the coccyx in sacrococcygeal teratoma significantly reduces recurrence risk.	3	B	Gobel U, et al. Med and Ped Oncol, 1998

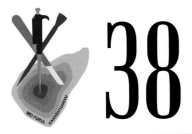

38

Surgical Emergencies

Marcus K Hoffman, Joshua T Rubin

Patients who have cancer may develop any one of a plethora of surgical emergencies. The focus of this chapter is the evaluation and management of patients with acute surgical diseases that are seen exclusively among patients with cancer or that have a predilection for developing in these patients. In addition, it is important to be aware that patients with cancer often present the surgeon with singular challenges to perioperative resuscitation as a result of treatment related morbidity or sequelae of metastatic disease which can include coagulopathy, hemostatic disorders, immune suppression, malnutrition and impaired healing. Perhaps most challenging to the surgeon and patient is weighing the risk of surgical morbidity and mortality against the natural history of their disease and the quality of life associated with advanced malignancy. Unfortunately this difficult decision is all too often forced upon desperate patients who up to this point in time have had little insight into their overall prognosis.

Bleeding and Obstruction

Bowel obstruction and GI bleeding account for many urgent abdominal operations among patients with cancer. Small bowel obstruction might develop as a result of adhesions related to previous abdominal surgery. Pleiotropic malignancies such as ovarian cancer and pseudomyxoma peritonei often cause tumor-related obstruction in their more advanced stages. Patients with metastatic melanoma can develop GI bleeding or small bowel obstruction secondary to transmural small bowel metastases or intussusception. Although we often take a conservative approach to managing many of these patients in the absence of evident compromised bowel, we usually resect symptomatic small bowel melanoma metastases in order to palliate patients whose expected survival exceeds several months. Tumor-related intussusception also warrants urgent surgical therapy. Patients with carcinomatosis secondary to pseudomyxoma peritonei are candidates for aggressive surgical debulking and intraperitoneal hyperthermic chemoperfusion. These operations often include peritonectomy, *en bloc* resection

of adjacent organs or extensive bowel resections. Among carefully selected patients, quality of life can be improved and survival can be prolonged.

Biliary Obstruction

Acute obstruction of the biliary tree can occur via multiple etiologies. Most commonly, metastatic disease to the porta hepatic, malignant biliary strictures and bulky lymph nodal disease cause obstruction of the extrahepatic biliary system. In addition to pain and jaundice, these lesions predispose individuals to the development of cholangitis, which can be lethal. Malignant biliary obstruction has a dismal prognosis, with a 60 day mortality approaching 70%. Options for management include ERCP with stent placement or percutaneous transhepatic cholangiography with retrograde stent placement and drainage. Metal stents are preferred in patients with end stage disease. External beam radiation therapy represents an option for some patients, while the use of surgical intervention is rare and is reserved for patients with localized disease, no evidence of metastases and predicted long-term survival.

Neutropenic Colitis

Neutropenic colitis is a unique disease process that can complicate profound and prolonged neutropenia, especially among patients with leukemia. It is also commonly known as typhlitis, necrotizing enteropathy and ileocecal syndrome. Affected patients typically develop diffuse abdominal pain and tenderness. Typical findings on physical examination include abdominal distention, tenderness most marked in the right lower quadrant, fever and tachycardia. This clinical presentation overlaps that of and could be confused with the much more common but equally sinister disease, *C. difficile* colitis. Patients suspected of having developed neutropenic colitis based on the clinic setting, symptoms and signs should undergo urgent evaluation with abdominal and pelvic CT scans. Although intravenous and oral contrast might enhance the diagnostic accuracy of the scan, their use should be prescribed in patients who might have a bowel obstruction or who have significant renal dysfunction or an intravenous contrast allergy, respectively. Typical findings on CT scan include edema of the cecum and/or right colon, perhaps with inflammatory changes in the surrounding soft tissues. Several thoughtful reviews of the existing literature have led to generally accepted guidelines to management of neutropenic colitis. The mainstay of therapy is the administration of broad spectrum antibiotics that cover enteric gram negative and anaerobic bacteria. We usually include Flagyl in the antimicrobial cocktail since *Clostridium difficile* can sometime present in similar fashion. Because many patients present with an ileus, it may be necessary to restrict oral intake. The use of narcotic analgesics should be judicious in order to avoid exacerbating or prolonging an associated ileus. Vigorous fluid resuscitation might be necessary. In our experience, surgery is rarely needed as long as the diagnosis is made early on. Progression despite maximal medical therapy, bowel perforation and acidosis should prompt urgent resection of the diseased bowel. We recommend fashioning stomas rather than establishing intestinal continuity since the risk of anastomotic bleeding or dehiscence in these patients is quite significant.

Perforation

Perforation of the GI tract is an unusual but rarely subtle complication of cancer therapy. Its observed association with gastric lymphoma was reason to recommend total gastrectomy rather than chemotherapy for the treatment of this disease. More recent experience suggests that the risk of perforation during chemotherapy in this setting is much less than had been thought, probably no more than 3%, for which reason surgery is usually reserved for treating patients with persistent or recurrent lymphoma after a course of chemotherapy or patients left with distal gastric stricture following a response to therapy. The addition of bevacizumab to the oncologic pharmacopeia has been associated with some risk of intestinal perforation among treated patients with primary or metastatic cancer. The estimated incidence of perforation is about 2%. GI perforation has also been associated with the use of imatinib administered to patients with gastrointestinal stromal tumors although this has been observed much less frequently. Purported risk factors for perforation include intact tumor on or within the bowel, recent endoscopy, bowel obstruction, a recent bowel anastomosis, diverticulitis, peptic ulcer disease, chemotherapy-induced colitis and a history of abdominal radiation. The pathophysiology of perforation in this setting has not fully been elucidated. Tumor necrosis, bowel wall ischemia or decreased perfusion leading to impaired healing of fresh intestinal injury have been implicated. Gastrointestinal perforation is usually manifest by acute onset of diffuse abdominal pain. Peritoneal signs are noted on physical examination. Free intraperitoneal air seen on plain X-ray or CT scan confirms the diagnosis. Urgent surgical therapy after fluid resuscitation is almost always warranted.

Clostridium Difficile Colitis

Although frequently seen in immunologically intact patients who have been exposed to antibiotics, immuno-compromised patients with leukemia are also at high risk for *C. difficile* due to their often prolonged hospitalization after chemotherapy and the common practice of administering antibiotics empirically for neutropenic fever. While many patients with fulminant disease will develop characteristic manifestations including fever, leukocytosis, diarrhea and crampy abdominal pain, as many as 20% of patients will have an ileus. As many as 20% of patients with *C. difficile* colitis may have little or no diarrhea and the etiologic toxin may not be detected by current assays in as many as 10% of patients. The inability of patients with bone marrow suppression to mount a leukocytosis further obfuscates the clinical evaluation.

Dallal et al reviewed all patients who died from *C. difficile* colitis as diagnosed on autopsy and all patients who underwent surgery for *C. difficile* colitis. They found that CT scans were 100% sensitive for detecting fulminant disease. Both endoscopy and toxin assay had false-negative rates of about 10%. Patients who died of fulminant disease without surgery were twice as likely to have had a false-negative toxin assay. The authors stated that an important indicator of impending fulminant disease was marked leukocytosis, sometimes as high as 30-50 K with associated bandemia. This often preceded the onset of hypotension and organ dysfunction. Patients in this study who required vasopressors prior to colectomy had a mortality rate of 65% as compared to a rate of 14% among those who did not require vasopressors prior to surgery. The overall mortality was 57%, an observation concordant with most other studies.

Patient characteristics associated with mortality have included age over 75 years, immunosuppression, lactate level greater than 5 mmol/L, hypotension requiring vasopressors and leukocytosis greater than 50 K cells/ml. Risk factors associated with progression to fulminant colitis include antibiotic use, especially fluoroquinolones, within 8 weeks of presentation, recent surgery, immunosuppression and previous *C. difficile* infection. Multivariate analysis has identified the use of IVIG and inflammatory bowel disease as factors associated with a propensity to develop fulminant colitis.

Patients who develop fulminant *C. difficile* colitis should undergo subtotal abdominal colectomy prior to the development of irreversible organ dysfunction. The appropriate timing of surgical intervention requires a healthy working relationship between medical oncology and the surgical team and keen surgical judgment.

Splenic Rupture

Spontaneous splenic rupture is an unusual complication of leukemia and other myeloproliferative disorders. In patients with pre-existing splenomegaly, one can invoke subtle, unrecognized trauma as a cause. In other cases, though, the etiology is a bit enigmatic. Some have invoked tumor invasion through the splenic capsule as a possible cause in patients whose spleens are not significantly enlarged. Others have suggested that changes in splenic architecture resulting from leukemic infiltration make the spleen exquisitely sensitive to mechanical forces associated with activity not ordinarily perceived as trauma. Patients usually present with abdominal pain, tachycardia, signs of mild peritoneal irritation, Kerr's sign and anemia. An ultrasound or abdominal CT scan is diagnostic. Attempts to repair the spleen are imprudent since the factors that predisposed to splenic fracture likely persist making recurrent bleeding a frequent consequence of splenic preservation. We do not advocate laparoscopic splenectomy in this setting, although isolated reports of success in carefully selected patients have appeared. Patients should be vaccinated once immunocompetence has been restored and every five years afterward.

Pericardial Effusion

Some malignancies eventuate in the development of symptomatic pericardial effusion. Malignant pericardial effusions are most commonly seen in lung cancer and less commonly in patients with breast cancer, leukemia and lymphoma. Pericardial effusions can be treated by a variety of techniques, including pericardiocentesis, percutaneous balloon pericardiotomy, subxiphoid pericardial window or pleuropericardiotomy via a thoracoscopic or thoracotomy approach. The European Society of Cardiology developed recommendations for the management of malignant pericardial effusion in 2004. There is uniform consensus that hemodynamically significant effusions causing tamponade physiology must be relieved as soon as possible by pericardiocentesis. Pericardiocentesis is also recommended to establish the etiology of effusions not causing tamponade. It is well recognized that as many as two-third of these patients will have effusions that are not malignant. Systemic chemotherapy is thought to reduce the substantial risk of recurrent effusion by two-third. Recurrent effusions that do not respond to drainage and systemic chemotherapy

can be managed with the intrapericardial instillation of chemotherapeutic or sclerosing agents. Cisplatin is the most efficacious agent for malignant effusions secondary to lung cancer. Thiotepa is an effective agent for patients with breast cancer. As many as 20% of treated patients will develop recurrent effusions. While effective in controlling 85% of malignant pericardial effusions, tetracycline's usefulness is limited by fever, chest pain and atrial arrhythmia in a substantial minority of treated patients. Current guidelines recommend subxiphoid pericardiotomy and pericardial window only if pericardiocentesis cannot be completed successfully. The risk of major complication when pericardiocentesis is performed with ultrasound guidance is less than 2%. The risk associated in subxiphoid pericardiotomy is thought to be higher. There is little role for pleuropericardiotomy as it provides no real advantage over subxiphoid pericardial window but carries a higher complication rate.

In regard to surgical drainage, Cullinane et al retrospectively reviewed all patients with known primary malignancies who had surgically drained pericardial effusions over a ten year period. The recurrence rate defined as the reaccumulation of an effusion requiring repeat surgical drainage was less than 5% over 6 months of follow-up. The postoperative morbidity was less than 7%. Pericardiocentesis alone was followed by a recurrence rate of 90% within one month of therapy. The prognosis for these patients is poor, with a median survival of only 3.7 months. Based on these observations, the most appropriate initial treatment for malignant pericardial effusions that are not hemodynamically significant is non-surgical. However, loculated effusions and those that do not respond to less invasive measures are probably best managed served with surgical drainage in patients for whom general anesthesia is not contraindicated and for whom the expected survival is long enough to warrant surgical therapy.

Landmark Papers

1. Badgwell BD, Camp ER, Feig B, Wolff RA, Eng C, Ellis LM, Cormier JN. Management of bevacizumab-associated bowel perforation: a case series and review of the literature. Annals of Oncology 2008;19(3):577-82.
2. Cullinane CA, Paz IB, Smith D, Carter N, Grannis FW Jr. Prognostic factors in the surgical management of pericardial effusion in the patient with concurrent malignancy. Chest 2004; 125:328-34.
3. Dallal RM, Harbrecht BG, Boujoukas AJ, Sirio CA, Farkas LM, Lee KK, Simmons RL. Fulminant *Clostridium difficile*: An underappreciated and increasing cause of death and complications. Ann Surg 2002;235:363-72.
4. Ettinghausen SE. Collagenous colitis, eosinophilic colitis and neutropenic colitis. Surg Clin North Am 1993; 73:993-1016.
5. Gobbi PG, Ghirardelli ML, Cavalli C, Baldini L, Broglia C, Clo V, et al. The role of surgery in the treatment of

gastrointestinal lymphomas other than low-grade MALT lymphomas. Haematologica 2000;85(4):372-80.

6. Greenstein AJ, Byrn JC, Zhang LP, Swedish KA, Jahn AE, Divino CM. Risk factors for the development of fulminant *Clostridium difficile* colitis. Surgery 2008; 143:623-9.

7. Gross JL, Younes RN, Deheinzelin D, Diniz AL, Silva RA, Haddad FJ. Surgical management of symptomatic pericardial effusion in patients with solid malignancies. Ann Surg Oncol 2006; 13:1732-8.

8. Jaber MR, Olafsson S, Fung WL, Reeves ME. Clinical review of the management of fulminant *Clostridium difficile* colitis. Am J Gastroenterol 2008; 103:3195-203.

9. Koch P, del Valle F, Berdel WE, Willich NA, Reers B, Hiddemann W, et al. German Multicenter Study Group. Primary gastrointestinal non-Hodgkin's lymphoma: II. Combined surgical and conservative or conservative management only in localized gastric lymphoma—results of the prospective German Multicenter Study GIT NHL 01/92. J Clin Oncol 2001; 19:3874-83.

10. Lamotagne F, Labbe AC, Haeck O, Lesur O, Lalancette M, Patino C, Leblanc M, Laverdiere M, Pepin J. Impact of emergency colectomy on survival of patients with fulminant *Clostridium difficile* colitis during an epidemic caused by a hypervirulent strain. Ann Surg 2007;245:267-72.

11. Maisch B, Seferoviæ PM, Ristiæ AD, Erbel R, Rienmüller R, Adler Y, et al. Task force on the diagnosis and management of pricardial diseases of the European Society of Cardiology. Guidelines on the diagnosis and management of pericardial diseases. Eur Heart J 2004; 25:587-610.

12. Martinoni A, Cipolla CM, Civelli M, Cardinale D, Lamantia G, Colleoni M, et al. Intrapericardial treatment of neoplastic pericardial effusions. Herz 2000;25(8):787-93.

13. Shamberger RC, Weinstein HJ, Delorey MJ, Levey RH. The medical and surgical management of typhlitis in children with acute nonlymphocytic (myelogenous) leukemia. Cancer 1986; 57:603-9.

14. Varki R, Armitage JO, Feagler JR. Typhlitis in acute leukemia: successful treatment by early surgical intervention. Cancer 1979; 43:695-7.

15. Yoon SS, Coit DG, Portlock CS, Karpeh MS. The diminishing role of surgery in the treatment of gastric lymphoma. Ann Surg 2004; 240:28-37.

16. Young Il Choi, Seung Hyun Lee, Byung Kwon Ahn, Sung Uhn Baek, Seun Ja Park, Yang Soo Kim, Seong Hoon Shin. Intestinal perforation on colorectal cancers treated with bevacizumab (Avastin). Cancer Res Treat 2008;40(1): 33-5.

39 *Minimally Invasive Approaches in Surgical Oncology*

Kent Zettel, Andrew R Watson

Introduction

Certainly, the last 20 years represent an evolution in the approach to surgical therapy with the rapid evolution of minimally invasive surgery. Laparoscopic surgery now represents one of the most important tools in the armamentarium of the surgical oncologist. However, this was not immediately the case, as resistance to the use of minimally invasive techniques in oncology was quite strong in the early years of laparoscopy. In this chapter, we will begin with a brief overview of the history of laparoscopic surgery and then discuss in detail some of the controversies surrounding minimally invasive surgery as it applies to surgical oncology. The specifics of each type of cancer are addressed in the previous chapters, however we will provide here a review of the evidence in support of or against the use of laparoscopy for common oncological conditions. In addition, a section on port placement and special patient circumstances is included.

History of Laparoscopic Surgery

Laparoscopic surgery can be traced back to 1901 when Georg Kellig used pneumoperitoneum in attempt to tamponade gastrointestinal hemorrhage in dogs. Though it did not make any headway, it opened the door for minimally invasive approaches to surgery. Ten years later, Hans Christian Jacobaeus took the endoscopic surgical approach to humans when he reported the first major series of laparoscopic surgery of the abdomen and thorax, termed it "Laparothorakoskopie". The growth of laparoscopic and minimally invasive surgery over the next 75 years was slow and laparoscopy was often limited to diagnostic procedures due to the limitations of the surgeon needing to hold the endoscope to his eye, leaving only one remaining hand free to operate. During this time, the spring-loaded Varess needle engineered by Janos Varess in 1938 supplanted the automatic pneumoperitoneum needle developed by Goetze in 1918, which is commonly used to present day. Automatic insufflation was developed by Semm in the 1960s and the introduction of the rod-lens system by Hopkins in 1966 safely applied light to the operative field. At this time the stage was set for the development of the computer chip TV camera. This device would project the image onto a monitor in order to free the surgeon's hand and allow the assistants to visualize the procedure, allowing for more complex intra-abdominal procedures.

Introduction of Minimally Invasive Surgical Approaches to the Oncology

Shortly after laparoscopic surgery was widely popularized in the late 1980s with the laparoscopic cholecystectomy, laparoscopy was used to attempt nearly every operation once performed through an open abdomen, including adrenalectomy, colectomy and pancreaticoduodenectomy. Patient's preference for smaller incisions, less pain and shorter hospital stay served to drive advances in minimally invasive surgery. However, laparoscopic surgery in oncology did not evolve as rapidly as that for non-oncologic surgery mainly due to early reports of tumor dissemination and early wound metastases.

A number of theoretical concerns regarding the use of laparoscopy for cancer operations were raised at the outset of minimally invasive surgery. Examples of these concerns include the dissemination of tumor to port sites or into the circulation as well as the effects of pneumoperitoneum on the immune system. Skeptics of the new technology also suggested that laparoscopic approaches would be inadequate to assess tissue planes and protect tumor margins without the tactile benefits of traditional open surgery.

Much of the stall in progress toward laparoscopic tumor resection revolved around wound-site metastases. Since the early reported cases, several large randomized trials were created to weigh the significance of the early reported risks with laparoscopic oncologic surgery. Most noteworthy trials for laparoscopic colorectal surgery are: Colon Carcinoma Laparoscopic or Open Resection (COLOR), United Kingdom Medical Research Council Conventional versus Laparoscopic-Assisted Surgery in Colorectal

Cancer Trial Group (MRC CLASIC) and Clinical Outcomes of Surgical Therapy (COST). As the most important goal of oncologic surgery is tumor-free survival, these trials, as well as many others, have demonstrated that minimally invasive approaches to surgical oncology are equivalent to open procedures. Randomized trials have demonstrated that, while obtaining similar surgical margins and tumor recurrence to that of open procedures, minimally invasive techniques have the increased benefit of decreased pain, hospital stay and earlier tolerance of diet.

It can be anticipated that results of any recently introduced procedure improve with increasing experience and the minimally invasive approaches to surgical oncology are no exception. Much of the early literature demonstrated that the time for operation, conversion rate and postoperative complication rate all decreases with increased experience. The mean operative time for laparoscopic hemicolectomy decreases from 150-221 minutes with limited experience to 140-160 minutes with more extensive experience. When comparing laparoscopic colectomy to open colectomy, it is observed that as a center approaches 20 cases per year, the operative time for laparoscopic colectomy approaches that for the open procedure. Additionally, as experience is gained, the rate of conversion and postoperative complications decrease, or remain the same as more difficult operations are attempted.

As it has been shown that experience improves operative outcome in minimally invasive procedures, several studies have addressed the number of operations to obtain the improved results, or the learning curve for such operations. As the learning curve for each minimally invasive procedure is expected to be different for each specific procedure, actual values have only been reported for laparoscopic colorectal operations. For these operations, the learning curve has ranged from as few as 11-15 to as many as 70 operations depending on the study, with the larger studies demonstrating a learning curve 30-40 operations **(Table 39-1)**. Many of the early reported learning curve has been explained as a "development curve," as surgeons develop and refine their operative procedure.

There are concerns that intraperitoneal immunity may be decreased through CO_2 pneumoperitoneum, which may lead to increase risk of tumor spread. Animal models, which use a large tumor inocula, have demonstrated pneumoperitoneum increasing the risk of port-site metastases. This has been attributed to the drying effects of prolonged pneumoperitoneum and the inhibition of intraperitoneal macrophage TNF-alpha production. There are also concerns that the pneumoperitoneum could aerosolize shed tumor cells and that multiple manipulations of tumor through port sites could increase metastases. In fact, the demonstration in several case reports of wound-site metastases slowed the acceptance of laparoscopic techniques for surgical oncology. Minimally invasive techniques took a huge blow in 1994 when Berends published a report of 14 colon resections for cancer with three patients (21%) developing wound-site metastases. Several theories have been developed to illustrate the recurrence of metastases at port sites. Two of which include the "chimney effect" and the "sloshing effect". The chimney effect states that port-site metastases occur when tumor-bearing gas escapes around the ports. The sloshing effect explains that the port site is contaminated when tumor irrigant escapes around the ports. More recently, it has been demonstrated that wound-site metastases is more a factor of careful technique and attention to detail in addition to experience. Multiple large clinical trials, particularly in colorectal cancer patients, have shown that, in fact, rates of port-site

TABLE 39-1		Learning curve for laparoscopic colorectal operations			
Author	N		Early procedures	Later procedures	Learning curve (N)
Senagore[1]	60	Operating time* Conversion rate* POC	185 minutes 32% 32%	160 minutes 10% 2%	40
Simons[2]	144	Operating time	150 minutes	140 minutes	11-15
Schlachta[3]	461	Operating time* Conversion rate POC	180 minutes 13.5% 30%	160 minutes 9.7% 32%	30
Bennett[4]	1194	POC	19%	10%	40
Agachan[5]	175	Operating time* Conversion rate POC	190 minutes 21% 33%	141 minutes 23% 14%	70
Stoochi[6]	34	Operative time*	221 minutes	147 minutes	—

POC = postoperative complication rate, * statistically significant (p < 0.05)

recurrence are equivalent to recurrence at laparotomy incision site.

Since the popularization of laparoscopic surgery from the introduction of the laparoscopic cholecystectomy, technological advances have made it possible for this method to be used safely for oncologic purposes. Such advances, such as the Omniport, had enabled hand-assisted laparoscopic surgery while maintaining pneumoperitoneum. The laparoscopic stapler enables rapid dissection through tissue. The electrothermal bipolar vessel sealer (EBVS) has allowed for rapid and meticulous dissection through tissue and ligation of vessels. To protect the port sites, specimen bags allow retrieval of the specimen without contact to the wound edge. As new obstacles are encountered surgical innovation has kept pace with solutions.

Benefits

Despite the push from patient's interest of the theoretical benefits of minimally invasive surgery for cancer, laparoscopic and other minimally invasive approaches need to be proven to be at least equivalent or better than the preceding open repairs. The minimally invasive approaches demonstrated worse oncologic prognosis in many of the early reports, which lead to much trepidation until larger trials came forth. Benefiting from the large incidence of colorectal carcinoma in the population, several large clinical trials in the United States and Europe began progress in the 1990s to elucidate whether any benefit can be obtained from treating cancer through laparoscopic approaches. On the other hand, minimally invasive approaches to less common cancers are nearly a decade behind that of colorectal cancer due to their decreased incidence in the population. Due to this dichotomy, the following disproportionate emphasis on colon cancer reflects that of literature to date.

Minimally Invasive Colorectal Surgery

In many aspects, minimally invasive approaches to cancer resection have shown to be equivalent to the conventional open procedures. Contrary to early reports, more recent and larger studies have found no difference not only in the rate of port-site/incisional-site metastases but also in overall tumor recurrence rate. This translates into similar to improved mortality and cancer-free survival between the two methods. The laparoscopic approach is able to perform an oncologic equivalent resection, as there is no difference between the two methods regarding the rate of positive margins or number of lymph nodes resected.

The benefits of laparoscopic colorectal surgery are equivalent to the popularized benefits of the laparoscopic cholecystectomy, the procedure that popularized minimally invasive surgery. The laparoscopic colectomy

has the obvious advantage over the more conventional open procedure of more rapid recovery demonstrated by decreased postoperative ileus, shorter time to oral intake and shorter postoperative hospital stay **(Table 39-2)**. Pain is also better tolerated after minimally invasive approaches to oncologic resection demonstrated by decreased use of narcotics. This new approach also has the advantage nearly half the amount of blood loss compared to that of the open approach. The complication rate of the laparoscopic approach is equivalent to that of the open procedure, as expected, since the critical steps are the same in both laparoscopic and open procedure. The major down side to the laparoscopic approach are the increased length of the operation.

The conversion rate for the laparoscopic approach has been demonstrated to be 3-29% and has been shown to decrease with increased experience. Conversion to open is not a complication of the laparoscopic approach, but a necessary and responsible action to satisfy an oncologic satisfactory resection. Due to conversion being a known and acceptable pathway in select situations, it too must stand up to oncologic standards. Early evaluation of converted cases, at a time when most surgeons were still modifying their technique in a new field with a long learning curve, has demonstrated worse early survival in non-metastatic colon cancer, which did not persist after 5-year follow-up. Any surgical trial is problematic while performed by surgeons on a learning curve and must be taken into account, as converted cases were later demonstrated to have no significant difference in tumor-free survival, despite having more advanced cancer.

In order to translate the data gathered from these clinical trials to the general population, special mention must be made regarding the patient populations. Randomized trials, by their character, require standardization of patient population in order to optimize internal validity. The COST and COLOR trials excluded patients who were obese, transverse and splenic flexure lesions, stage IV carcinomas, acute intestinal obstruction, patients with prior colon resection, patients with prior or concurrent cancer (except basal cell carcinoma and cervical carcinoma in situ) as well as those with non-adenocarcinoma malignancies. In comparing this exclusion group to those patients who would be included in these trials, Moloo, et al demonstrated that all patients could benefit from a laparoscopic approach to resection. This statement comes with an asterisk, although all patients may benefit from laparoscopy, the excluded patients had twice the conversion rate and some patient populations in the exclusion group were prone to specific complications. Conversions to open procedure were more commonly performed due to tumor factors such as fixation or invasion of adjacent structures. Those with stage IV cancer have twice the conversion rate compared to those who

TABLE 39-2	Laparoscopic versus conventional open colon resection						
Study	**COLOR**[7,8]	**COST** [9]	**MRC CLASSIC**[10, 11]	**Lacy** [12]	**Liang**[13]	**Milsom**[14]	**Hasewaga**[15]
Number (% Laparoscopic)	1248 (50)	872 (49)	794 (66)	219 (51)	269 (50)	80 (50)	50 (48)
Blood loss (ml) Laparoscopic Open	100 170	— —	— —	p = 0.001 105 193	p < 0.001 54 240	p < 0.0001 252 344	p = 0.0034 58 137
Time (minutes) Laparoscopic Open	p < 0.0001 145 115	p < 0.001 95 150	180 135	p = 0.001 142 118	p < 0.001 224 184	p < 0.0001 200 125	p < 0.0001 275 188
Conversion rate	17%	21%	29%	—	3%	—	17%
Positive margins Laparoscopic Open	p = 1.0 2% 2%	p = 0.52 5% 6%	p = 0.45 7% 5%	— —	— —	0 0	— —
Complications Laparoscopic Open	p = 0.88 21% 20%	p = 0.64 21% 20%	33% 32%	p = 0.001 11% 26%	p = 0.15 14.80% 19%	15% 15%	p = 0.2293 4.20% 19%
Lymph nodes (no.) Laparoscopic Open	p = 0.32 10 10	12 12	12 13.5	11 11	p = 0.489 15.6 16	19 25	p = 0.2485 23 26
Mortality Laparoscopic Open	p = 0.45 1% 2%	p = 0.40 0.46% 0.93%	p = 0.57 4% 5%	0.94% 2.90%	— —	2.4% 2.6%	0 0
Wound infection Laparoscopic Open	4% 3%	— —	5% 5%	7% 15%	4.4% 5.2%	— —	4.2% 11.5%
Return of bowel function (days) Laparoscopic Open	BM p < 0.0001 3.6 4.6	—	BM 5 6	— —	Ileus p < 0.001 2 4	Flatus p = NS 4.8 4.8	Flatus p = 0.0005 2 3.3
Hospital stay (days) Laparoscopic Open	p < 0.0001 8.2 9.3	p < 0.001 5 6	9 11	p = 0.005 5.2 7.9	p < 0.001 9 14	p = NS 6 7	p = 0.016 7.1 12.7
Follow-up	3 years	4.4 years	36.8 months	43 months	40 months	1.5 yrs lap 1.7 yrs open	20 months
Tumor recurrence Laparoscopic Open	p = 0.24 19.60% 16.90%	p = 0.32 16% 18%	Local: 8.6%:7.9% p = 0.76 Distant 15.2%: 14.3% p = 0.68	p = 0.07 17% 27%	p = 0.362 17.00% 21.6%	— —	— —
Port-site/incision metastasis Laparoscopic Open	p = 0.09 1.30% 0.40%	p = 0.50 0.50% 0.20%	p =0.12 2.50% 0.60%	0.94% 0	0.74% 0.75%	0 5.30%	0 NR
Overall survival Laparoscopic Open	p = 0.45 81.80% 84.20%	p = 0.51 86% 85%	p = 0.55 68.40% 66.70%	p = 0.14 82% 74%	— —	90% 89%	— —
Disease-free survival Laparoscopic Open	p = 0.70 74.20% 76.40%	p = 0.70 118 events 117 events	p = 0.70 66.30% 67.70%	— —	— —	88% 84%	— —

would meet the inclusion group of the major studies. Lesions in the transverse colon were associated with increased operative time, conversion rate of 25%, as well as increased postoperative complication rate. Obese patients (BMI > 30) are the other subgroup with increased postoperative complication conversion rates.

Hand-assisted laparoscopic colectomy (HALC) is an alternative to the laparoscopic procedure, in which a minilaparotomy is performed at the beginning of the procedure to place a hand into the abdomen. Hand-assisted laparoscopic surgery (HALS) has several benefits including improved retraction, the ability to localize vessels, control bleeding with digital pressure, better localize tissue planes and blunt dissection and to palpate lymph nodes. There is no surgical instrument that can replace a surgeon's hand. Unlike that of the laparoscopic approach, the wound during the procedure is stretched and compressed and the bowel is more intensely manipulated. The usefulness of this procedure has been to simplify complex procedures as well as to introduce non-skilled surgeons to advanced laparoscopic skills. HALC is comparable to the laparoscopic approach in regard to operating time, conversion rate, return of bowel function and postoperative pain, but has increased incision length. In the small studies, HALC has a nonsignificant increased length of hospital stay compared to the laparoscopic approach. HALC also has the same benefits as laparoscopic surgery over the conventional approach in regard to decreased blood loss, pain and hospital stay and faster recovery. HALC appears to be a hybrid approach to the laparoscopic method for more challenging procedures while maintaining many of the benefits over the conventional open procedure.

Laparoscopic Gastric Resections

As the incidence of gastric carcinoma is higher in Japan than in the western nations, most of the literature on laparoscopic approaches to treating gastric carcinoma comes from Japan. Likewise, though the approaches to gastric carcinoma slightly differ from the United States, the following information will highlight the literature that is available to date. Laparoscopic wedge resections were first reported in 1994 for intramucosal malignancies with diameters less than 25 mm and no evidence of lymph node metastases. That same year, Kitano, et al used laparoscopy to perform distal gastrectomy with lymph node dissection. Since that time, the largest clinical trials demonstrating the efficacy of laparoscopy for early and advanced gastric cancer have come from Japan, where gastric cancer is more prevalent. Due to the onset of massive screening in Japan, early gastric cancer now accounts for more than 50% of the total incidence of gastric cancer in Japan, which has allowed for increased experience in this minimally

invasive approach and has allowed for laparoscopic-assisted management once limited to distal gastrectomy to grow in complexity to now encompass proximal and total gastrectomy.

The individual benefits of laparoscopic gastrectomy for gastric carcinoma have varied throughout the many studies, but most studies agree that laparoscopic gastrectomy is safe and technically feasible for gastric carcinoma. The benefits of laparoscopic gastrectomy over the open approach include decreased intraoperative blood loss, faster recovery demonstrated by shorter hospital course, faster return of bowel function, shorter time to tolerating diet, shorter postoperative time to ambulation and better pain control observed through less use of analgesics. Operative time is longer for the laparoscopic approach for gastrectomy, though most studies are divided over the significance of the increased operative time.

These methods have routinely been shown to be beneficial for early gastric carcinoma and more recently, have been used for more advanced gastric carcinoma. Hur, et al have demonstrated laparoscopic gastrectomy to be equivalent to the open approach with respect to return of bowel function and hospital course for advanced gastric carcinoma not exposed to serosa. Laparoscopic gastrectomy does have the benefit of decreased intraoperative blood loss in exchange for increased operative time compared to open gastrectomy.

As for the adequacy of the laparoscopic approach, all comparative studies have demonstrated that laparoscopic-assisted gastrectomy removes an average fewer lymph nodes open gastrectomy, but few have demonstrated any significance in this difference. Over time, recurrence rate after laparoscopic-assisted gastrectomy is similar to that of conventional open gastrectomy and laparoscopic-assisted gastrectomy produces equivalent long-term survival and disease-free survival for both early and advanced gastric carcinoma. In conclusion, laparoscopic-assisted gastrectomy is beneficial for early gastric cancer and with limited data appears to be beneficial for more advanced gastric cancer **(Table 39-3)**.

Laparoscopic Pancreatic Procedures

Laparoscopy has been used for the diagnosis and staging of pancreatic cancer for years, but due to the complexity of performing a laparoscopic pancreatic resection, including accessing the retroperitoneal organ, the proximity of major vessels and managing the pancreatic stump, this procedure is only slowly gaining acceptance. Laparoscopic distal pancreatectomies that do not require anastomoses have been demonstrated to be safe with benefits compared to that of the open repair. Trials have demonstrated decreased intraoperative blood loss in addition to shorter hospital course and more rapid return

TABLE 39-3	Laparoscopic-assisted distal gastrectomy (LADG) vs conventional open distal gastrectomy (ODG)								
Study	Kim[16]	Hur[17]	Tanimura[18]	Adachi[19]	Huscher[20]	Kitano[21]	Mochiki[22]	Yano[23]	Noshiro[24]
Number LADG ODG	71 76	26 25	485 400	49 53	29 30	14 14	89 60	24 35	37 31
Lymph nodes LADG ODG	$p = 0.012$ 22.8 ± 10.5 27.4 ± 11.8	$p = 0.129$ 30.5 35	$p = NS$ 29.1 29.3	$p = 0.10$ 15.5 ± 7.8 18.6 ± 9.8	$p = NS$ 30.0 ± 14.9 33.1 ± 17.4	$p = NS$ 20.2 ± 3.6 24.9 ± 3.5	$p < 0.05$ 19 ± 1 25 ± 2	$p = NS$ 18.5 ± 2.3 23.9 ± 1.8	$p = 0.59$ 43 ± 16 41 ± 15
Margin LADG ODG	$p = 0.0001$ $4.1 \pm 2.5^{++}$ $6.4 \pm 3.2^{++}$	4.25^{++} 4.25^{++}	—	$p = 0.80$ 6.2 ± 3.6 6.0 ± 2.9	6.3 ± 0.7	6.9 ± 0.8	—	—	—
Recurrence LADG ODG	— —	$30.8\%^{*}$ $24\%^{*}$	—	—	$37.9\%^{**}$ $37\%^{**}$	$p = NS$ 0 0	—	—	—
3-5 yr survival LADG ODG	— —	$p = 0.246$ $88.2\%^{*}$ $77.2\%^{*}$	—	—	$58.9\%^{**}$ $55\%^{**}$	—	$p = 0.26$ $98\%^{***}$ $95\%^{***}$	—	—
3-5 yr disease-free survival LADG ODG	— —	$p = 0.757$ $71.4\%^{*}$ $53.4\%^{*}$	—	—	$57.3\%^{**}$ $54.8\%^{**}$	—	$100\%^{***}$ $95\%^{***}$	—	—
Diet (day) LADG ODG	— —	$p = 0.906$ 4 4	$p < 0.01$ 3.3 5.8	$p = 0.001$ 5 5.7	$p < 0.001$ 5.1 ± 0.5 7.4 ± 2.0	$p = NS$ 5.3 ± 1.5 4.5 ± 0.3	—	$p = 0.01$ 4.45 ± 0.3 5.56 ± 0.2	$p < 0.001$ 3.2 ± 0.6 4.2 ± 0.9
Flatus (day) LADG ODG	$p = NS$ 3.8 ± 1.9 3.6 ± 1.0	$p = 0.527$ 2 2	$p < 0.01$ 2.6 3.6	$p = 0.002$ 3.9 4.5	—	$p < 0.05$ 2.9 ± 0.2 3.9 ± 0.2	—	$p = 0.01$ 2.71 ± 0.2 3.56 ± 0.2	$p = 0.012$ 2.8 ± 0.8 3.4 ± 1.1
OR time (min) LADG ODG	$p = 0.001$ 249 ± 46 181 ± 37	$p < 0.001$ 255 190	$p < 0.01$ 242 184	$p = NS$ 246 228	196 ± 21 168 ± 29	$p < 0.05$ 227 ± 7 171 ± 13	$p = NS$ 210 ± 6 201 ± 5	$p = NS$ 219.8 ± 9 210.0 ± 8	$p = 0.007$ 320 ± 61 277 ± 64
Blood loss (ml) LADG ODG	—	$p = 0.012$ 160 215	$p < 0.01$ 165 388	158 302	$p < 0.001$ 229 ± 144 391 ± 136	$p < 0.05$ 117 ± 30 258 ± 53	$p < 0.05$ 237 ± 20 412 ± 26	$p = 0.001$ 108.4 ± 16 296.1 ± 35	$p < 0.001$ 163 ± 126 488 ± 349

* 3-year follow-up. ** 5-year follow-up. *** 48-month follow-up.

to normal activity with laparoscopic distal pancreatectomy compared with the conventional open procedure. A theoretical concern with the laparoscopic procedure is the management of the pancreatic duct, but several studies have shown no difference in pancreatic leak between the two methods. The conversion rate for distal pancreatec-tomy is comparable to that of the laparoscopic colectomy, ranging from 7% to 26%. The more complex laparoscopic pancreaticoduodenectomy for neoplasms of the pancreatic head has been demonstrated to be feasible in few studies, but the benefits of this procedure has yet to be determined **(Table 39-4)**.

TABLE 39-4	Laparoscopic versus conventional open pancreatic resection						
Study	N	Conversion rate	Significant complications Lap : Open	Pancreatic leak/fistula Lap : Open	Operation time (min) Lap : Open	Blood loss (ml) Lap : Open	Hospital stay (days) Lap : Open
Velanovich[25]	30	20%	20%: 27% $p = NS$	13% : 13% $p = NS$	—	—	5:08 $p = 0.02$
Matsumoto[26]	33	7%	—	0 : 10% $p = NS$	290 : 213 $p = 0.002$	247 : 400 $p = 0.29$	12.9 : 23.8 $p = 0.0043$
Teh[27]	28	16%	17% : 56% $p = 0.03$	8% : 6% $p = 0.83$	212 : 278 $p = 0.05$	193 : 609 $p = 0.01$	6.2 : 10.6 $p = 0.001$
Kooby[28]	342	12.60%	10% : 17% $p = 0.08$	26% : 32% $p = 0.28$	230 : 216 $p = 0.28$	357 : 588 $p < 0.001$	5.9 : 9.0 $p < 0.001$

Laparoscopic Hepatic Resections

Laparoscopic uses for liver surgery began with nonanatomical wedge biopsies and advanced to resections of benign and malignant neoplasms. Along with all other minimally invasive approaches to oncologic surgery, laparoscopic liver resection is surrounded by skepticism, not only from the concern of port-site metastases and adequate resection of tumor but also due to additional concerns of bleeding and gas embolism, bile leakage and adequate parenchymal transaction. Advances in laparoscopic techniques, as well as instruments, have made this minimally invasive technique feasible, including the harmonic scalpel, microwave coagulators, argon beam coagulators, endoscopic staplers and laparoscopic ultrasound. Despite these advances in the surgical arsenal, there still remain limitations to this technique. In addition to the indications of the conventional open method, additional considerations must be placed in regard to laparoscopic method. Of increased importance, the most limiting factors that limit the patient's candidacy to minimally invasive approach include the location of the tumor within the liver and size of the mass to be resected. In regard to location, the left liver lobe and anterior segments of the liver (anterior portion of segments IV, V and VI) allow for better laparoscopic access. Recommendations have been made by one author to limit the size to those lesions less than 5 cm, though resections have been attempted in lesions of up to 11 cm through the laparoscopic technique.

Few studies with only a small number of patients are available to compare the laparoscopic and conventional open approaches to liver resections in regard to both short-term as well as long-term outcomes, as this procedure is still in early development. In addition no randomized control trials have been reported comparing the two techniques. In regard to the limited number of studies, there exists some benefits to laparoscopic approach over the conventional open approach in shorter hospital stay, decreased blood loss, narcotic requirement and more rapid oral intake. Laparoscopic and conventional open approaches to liver resections are equivalent in respect to complication rate and perioperative mortality. In addition, the oncologic resection margin has been demonstrated to be equivalent between these two methods. In further regard to the oncologic capability of the laparoscopic technique, Laurent, et al demonstrated an increased 3-year survival in laparoscopic resections with equivalent recurrence rates after 3 years, as Kaneko, et al demonstrated equivalent 5-year overall and disease-free survival. In summary, the laparoscopic approach provides an adequate and safe approach to hepatic resection in regard to early and long-term outcomes, though only reported by a limited number of studies with a small number of patients **(Table 39-5)**.

Laparoscopic Splenectomy

Splenectomy has been utilized for the treatment of benign hematologic conditions such as idiopathic thrombocytopenic purpura and hereditary spherocytosis, in addition to malignant conditions such as lymphoma, metastases from organs, such as colon, gastric, esophageal, lung, prostate, breast, endometrial and ovarian cancers and melanoma. Since the introduction of the laparoscopic approach in 1991 by Delaitre and Maignien, the laparoscopic splenectomy has been shown to be safe and effective in resolving benign hematologic conditions.

The indications for splenectomy for malignant conditions are not well defined, but have been used in the diagnosis, staging and palliation. The most common malignant conditions for which splenectomy is beneficial are lymphomas. Other primary splenic malignancies for which splenectomy is indicated include angiosarcoma, plasmacytoma and malignant fibrous histiocytomas.

Difficulty arises during laparoscopic splenectomy for massively enlarged spleens, as these are less capable of being retrieved through the port site without crushing the spleen and thereby making pathologic analysis more difficult. For myeloproliferative disorder, such as lymphoma, the spleen can be crushed with a ring clamp for retrieval once the opening of the retrieval bag is externalized. For primary splenic tumors, care must be taken to leave large pieces upon fracturing the spleen for pathology. Other options for retrieval of massively enlarged spleens include utilizing the hand-assisted approach, or performing splenic artery embolization prior to splenectomy to reduce the size and risk of bleeding and tumor dissemination during the laparoscopic procedure, though this latter approach is associated with higher cost and post-procedural pain.

Compared to the open procedure, laparoscopic splenectomy for benign and malignant indications is significantly longer to perform and the conversion rate to open ranges from 0% to 14%. In contrast, patients tolerate oral diet earlier postoperatively have a shorter hospital stay and recover faster after the laparoscopic approach compared to that of the open procedure. As both primary tumors and isolated metastases of the spleen are rare, no studies exist comparing laparoscopic and open splenectomy in regard to the oncologic outcome.

As the laparoscopic approach has now become the gold standard for treatment of benign hematologic conditions, few studies have compared the laparoscopic approach to the conventional open procedure for malignant conditions. Most studies do not accurately evaluate splenectomies for malignant diseases as these studies bias toward benign hematologic conditions intermixing a few malignant conditions and no study has compared the laparoscopic to the open approach exclusively for

TABLE 39-5	Laparoscopic versus conventional open hepatic resections							
Study	**Topal[29]**	**Buell[30]**	**Morino[31]**	**Mala[32]*****	**Farges[33]**	**Laurent[34]**	**Kaneko[35]**	**Lesurtel[36]**
Number Laparoscopic Open	109 250	17 100	30 30	15 14	21 21	13 14	30 28	18 20
Complications Laparoscopic Open	p < 0.0001 5.50% 27.20%	4/17	6.60% 6.60%	p = NS 2 4	p = NS 10% 10%	36% 50%	p = NS 10% 18%	11% 15%
Mortality Laparoscopic Open	1 4	1 —	0 0	0 0	—	p = 0.2 0 2	0 0	0 0
Blood loss (ml) Laparoscopic Open	p < 0.0001 100 500	p < 0.05 288 485	p < 0.05 320 479	p = NS 600 500	p = NS 218 285	p = 0.45 620 ± 130 720 ± 240	p = NS 350 ± 210 505 ± 185	p < 0.05 236 429
Hospital stay (days) Laparoscopic Open	p < 0.0001 6 8	6.5	p < 0.05 6.4 8.7	p < 0.001 4 8.5	p = 0.0002 5.1 ± 1.3 6.5 ± 1.0	p = 0.83 15.3 ± 8.6 17.3 ± 18.9	p < 0.005 14.9 ± 7.1 21.6 ± 8.8	p = NS 8 ± 3 10 ± 6
Positive margin Laparoscopic Open	1/77 5/327	—	p = NS 0/30* 1/30*	p = 0.58 1/13 2/14	NA NA	—	—	0 0
OR length (min) Laparoscopic Open	95 179	2.5 hrs 4.5 hrs	148 142	p = NS 187 185	p = NS 177 156	p = 0.006 267 ± 79 182 ± 57	p = NS 182 ± 38 210 ± 40	p < 0.01 202 145
Conversion rate	7/109	—	0	0	0	2/13	1/30	2/18
Portal triad clamp time (min) Laparascopic Open	—	39 23	—	—	33 ± 12	p = 0.006 68 ± 24 25 ± 19	—	p < 0.05 39 23
3-5 year overall survival rate Laparoscopic Open	—	—	—	—	—	p = 0.04 89% 55%	61% 62%	—
3-5 year disease-free survival rate Laparoscopic Open	—	—	—	—	—	54% 56%	31% 29%	—

* resection margin < 1cm was 43% laparoscopic and 40% in the conventional open arm.

** resection margin < 1cm was 29% laparoscopic and 37% in the conventional open arm, p = 0.57.

*** all patients had colorectal malignancies. ± Benign lesions.

malignant conditions. The studies that do involve malignant conditions and the case reports of rare primary malignancies have shown the laparoscopic method to be safe and effective. Upon further analysis, studies have compared laparoscopic splenectomy for benign versus malignant indications, showing that splenic resections for malignant diseases have an increased operative time (which is likely due to the increased likelihood of spleno-megaly associated with malignant disorders) though there is no difference among conversion rate, postoperative complications and mortality and hospital stay between these two indications. Due to the limited literature regarding laparoscopic splenectomy for malignant

conditions, further work must be performed to determine the oncologic outcomes of this procedure.

Laparoscopic Peritoneal Access Ports for Chemoperfusion

Laparoscopic placement of peritoneal access ports (PAP catheter) have largely been used for treatment of carcinomatosis for metastatic ovarian cancer in addition to intraperitoneal mesothelioma. As these diseases remain largely confined to the peritoneal cavity, intraperitoneal chemotherapy allows for confined chemotherapy to the cancer itself, while limiting the systemic toxic side effects.

Intraperitoneal chemotherapy is not standard therapy for ovarian carcinoma and has been used in select patients after the first laparotomy has been performed. The conventional method of placing PAP catheters through a second-look laparotomy has the increased morbidity of slow recovery associated with open procedures. Laparoscopy has enabled the capability to place these catheters while maximizing the return of bowel function and limiting the risk of leak compared to laparotomy. This allows for quicker initiation of chemotherapy after PAP placement. The laparoscopic approach also holds the theoretical advantage of infusing chemotherapy prior to the formation of adhesions. As a technical note, since these patients have undergone a recent laparotomy for tumor debulking and are at high risk for adhesions, an open approach to trocar placement is the preferred route of entry to the abdomen.

Additional Topics: Port Placement and Special Patient Circumstances

Overview of Port Placement for Minimally Invasive Surgery

Prior to inserting ports, the stomach and the urinary bladder should be emptied to avoid unintentional perforation of these organs during trocar insertion in addition to increasing the field of view. The position of the port sites is an important part of laparoscopic surgery. Though the trocar placement varies from surgeon to surgeon, the ideal trocar placement allows for optimal vision of the selected operative field, as well as direct instrument access to the surgical site while minimizing instruments competing for space and limiting muscle fatigue. As a principle, the port placement should be along a semicircular line 16-18 cm (or the distance of an average hand with fingers spread apart, with the base of the palm to the tip of the third finger) from the desired organ of interest.

Several exceptions to this rule exist. One exception is the use of angled optical lenses, in which the trocar should be placed closer as the angle of the lens becomes steeper. In addition, as the abdominal wall girth increases, trocars should be angled more toward the point of interest to decrease torque on the abdominal wall. Examples of trocar placement for the laparoscopic colon resections and laparoscopic pancreatic procedures are shown in **Figures 39-1 and 39-2**. The port placements for colon resections demonstrate the basics as explained above, but are modified to place emphasis in taking down the hepatic and splenic flexures for the right and left colectomies, respectively. For pancreatic resections, a port site is set apart to retract the stomach to expose the retroperitoneal pancreas.

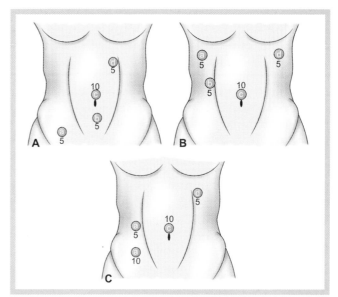

Figure 39-1: Port placement for laparoscopic colon resections. Trocar placement for: (A) Laparoscopic right colectomy; (B) Transverse colectomy; and (C) Laparoscopic left colectomy to abdominoperineal resection

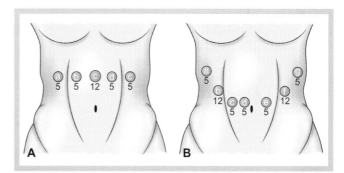

Figure 39-2: Port placement for laparoscopic pancreatic resection. (A) Trocar placement for laparoscopic distal pancreatectomy: a. mediflex port for retracting stomach, b. left hand working port, c. working port, d. camera port, e. assistant port. (B) Trocar placement for pancreaticoduodenectomy: a. mediflex port to retract liver, b. working port for hepatico-jejunostomy anastomoses, c. working port, d. camera port, e. working port, f. working port for pancreaticojejunostomy anastomoses, g. mediflex port to retract stomach

Laparoscopic Surgery in the Malnourished

Patients with cancer have the highest prevalence of malnutrition of any other group of hospitalized patients. The effects of cancer alone cause poor nutritional intake and the additional stress from chemotherapy, radiation therapy and the effects of surgery, including postoperative ileus, malabsorptive state and resting the bowel until anastomoses heal, can further exacerbate the nutritional status of an already malnourished cancer-bearing patients. Several clinical studies have demonstrated increased morbidity and mortality in malnourished cancer-bearing patients, which strengthen the argument for improving nutritional status for patients with cancer (see Nutrition chapter). It is in respect that minimally invasive surgery can be of benefit to cancer patients. The benefits of decreased postoperative ileus and quicker return to oral dietary intake allow postoperative patients to regain their nutritional support sooner, which theoretically leads to improved nutritional status. To the same effect, as patients more rapidly regain their strength after minimally invasive techniques, as demonstrated by decreased time needed to return to normal activity, it is possible that these patients have the ability to start postoperative chemotherapy sooner. This is an added benefit in the hopes of eradicating the disease.

Laparoscopic Surgery in the Elderly Population

It is well accepted that age has an increased risk in postoperative complications, longer hospital stay, mortality and loss of independence after laparotomy. The elderly population also is the fastest growing segment of the population, increasing the importance of minimizing the risks of surgery. Since minimally invasive surgery has the advantages of decreased postoperative pain, hospital stay, postoperative ileus and wound infection, it would be ideal for the elderly population. On the other hand, laparoscopic surgery has been of concern for the elderly population with increased cardiopulmonary disease due to the theoretical risks of acidemia from absorption of CO_2 across the peritoneal membrane and decreased functional residual capacity and lung compliance from increased intra-abdominal pressure. Despite these risks, it has been shown in multiple studies that geriatric populations actually benefit from minimally invasive surgery. In addition to the usual benefits of minimally invasive surgery, elderly patients also have a significantly increased rate of independence after laparoscopic colectomy compared to open colectomy for malignant processes, which corresponds to previous studies comparing minimally invasive to open procedures for non-oncologic processes. The benefits of minimally invasive surgery are more prominent in the elder population compared to the younger population. This is of increased importance in a population with a higher baseline risk for postoperative morbidity and mortality.

Laparoscopic Surgery in the Obese Population

Obesity has long been considered a risk factor for poor outcome in the perioperative setting. As minimally invasive surgery has the benefit of decreased intra-operative blood loss, postoperative hospital duration, pain and ileus, such benefits are raised to question in a population that now comprises one-third of the nation. Obesity is associated with abnormal cardiopulmonary function, metabolic function, hemostasis, as well as other comorbid conditions such as diabetes, which increase

complications after surgery, including wound dehiscence and infection. These risks, observed in open operations, have also transferred to the minimally invasive world.

Intraoperatively, obesity applies new obstacles to the minimally invasive field. Gaining adequate visualization is impaired by the ergonomics of the obese patient, which leads to increased risk in minimally invasive surgery. Most studies observe that obesity is a significant risk factor for increased operative time and conversion to open procedure. The degree of obesity correlates well to the minimally invasive intraoperative complications. In the oncologic field, where resection margin and number of harvested nodes determine the prognosis, obesity has been shown to be equivalent to the nonobese population for such procedures as the laparoscopic left colectomy.

Postoperative complications, wound infections, ileus and duration of hospitalization are also increased in the obese population. Despite controversy, most studies demonstrate no difference in anastomotic leak in laparoscopic colectomy when comparing obese and nonobese patients.

When compared to the nonobese population, obesity continues to have an increased risk in minimally invasive procedures as it does for open operations, but when comparing minimally invasive surgery to open operations in the obese population, an advantage is seen with minimally invasive approaches. Hospital duration and postoperative ileus are significantly shorter after MIS and no significant difference in operative time, complications, readmissions or cost is observed in the obese population undergoing MIS compared to open procedures.

Obesity continues to demonstrate an increased perioperative risk in MIS as it does in open surgery, but the MIS approaches do provide the obese population a benefit over open procedures for oncologic purposes. Discretion is advised in the obese population due to the ergonomics of the obese body habitus. Some operations provide more benefit than others due to limited visualization. Despite offering subtotal colectomies for oncologic purposes, some recommend against laparoscopic total colectomy to obese patients due to difficulties dissecting in multiple abdominal quadrants while some recommend selectively offering laparoscopic surgery for morbidly obese patients (BMI $\geq$ 40).

Conclusion

Over the last two decades, the laparoscopic boom, which initiated with the explosion of the laparoscopic cholecystectomy, advanced toward the field of surgical oncology. Though it was met with much skepticism and controversy since several early studies shown port-site metastases, multiple large-scale studies have shown that minimally invasive approaches are at least equivalent to the conventional open approach in regard to oncologic outcome. This has been well demonstrated with colorectal surgery, as incidence of colorectal cancer is higher in the world population than others mentioned. In the same note, much of the studies in laparoscopic gastric surgery have taken place in Japan, where the incidence of gastric cancer exceeds that of the other first-world populations. Laparoscopic approaches to pancreatic and hepatic surgery have met with increased skepticism due to the retroperitoneal location of the pancreas in addition to its location near major vessels and the increased propensity of the liver to bleed in addition to the concern for bile leakage. These procedures are being performed at major centers to date with few studies demonstrating their benefits, with no randomized controlled studies demonstrating their efficacy. The acceptance of these procedures depends on further randomized controlled studies from these major centers. Minimally invasive approaches to surgical oncology are of increased benefit to special populations, such as the elderly and the obese. The past two decades have seen a revolution in surgical oncology and has shaped the future of how it is practiced.

Summary

- Laparoscopic colon surgery is equivalent to the conventional open method in regard to surgical margin, long-term overall survival and long-term disease-free survival.
- Laparoscopic colon surgery has the benefit of less blood loss, shorter postoperative ileus, better pain control and decreased hospital stay than the conventional open approach.
- The greatest risk factors for conversion to open procedure in the laparoscopic colectomy include obese patients, lesions in the transverse colon and stage IV colon cancer.
- Three- and five-year overall survival and overall survival are equivalent between the laparoscopic and the conventional open gastric resection.
- Most studies show that there is no significant difference in the number of lymph nodes resected in laparoscopic distal gastrectomy compared to that of the conventional open approach.
- Postoperative complications, wound infections, ileus and duration of hospitalization are increased in the obese population compared to nonobese populations for laparoscopic colon cancer.
- Laparoscopic pancreatic resection has an equivalent leak rate compared to the conventional open approach.
- The most limiting factors regarding a patient's candidacy for laparoscopic hepatic resection are the location of the tumor within the liver and the size of the mass to be resected.
- Laparoscopic colon resection is beneficial compared to the open approach in obese populations in regard to hospital stay, postoperative ileus and leak rates for colon cancer.

Acknowledgments

Special thanks to Dr Steve Hughes for his advice on the port placement for the laparoscopic pancreatic resections.

Level of Evidence Table			
Recommendation	**Best level of evidence**	**Grade of recommendation**	**References**
Long-term overall survival and disease-free survival is equivalent between the laparoscopic and conventional open resection for colon cancer.	1a	A	7, 9,10,12
Resection margin is equivalent for laparoscopic and conventional open resection for colon cancer.	1a	A	7, 9
Laparoscopic surgery provides better acute postoperative advantages for oncologic causes including more rapid bowel recovery and better pain control.	1a	A	7, 9, 11
Overall postoperative complication rates are equivalent for both laparoscopic and open colon resections	1a	A	7, 9, 11
The survival and recurrence rate of gastric carcinoma is equivalent in laparoscopic approach compared to the conventional open approach.	1a	A	20, 21
Laparoscopic approach to distal pancreatic resections provides no more complications, including pancreatic leak, than the conventional open approach.	2a	B	25, 28
The laparoscopic approach to hepatic segmentectomies provides equivalent surgical resection as conventional open resection	2a	B	29, 32, 34
Long-term mortality and disease-free survival is equivalent between the laparoscopic and conventional open hepatic segmentectomies for primary and metastatic liver carcinoma	2a	B	34, 35

References

1. Senagore AJ, Luchtefeld MA, Mackeigan JM. What is the learning curve for laparoscopic colectomy? American Surgeon 1995;61:681-5.

2. Simons AJ, Anthone GJ, Ortega AE, et al. Laparoscopic-assisted colectomy learning curve. Dis Colon Rectum 1997;38:600-3.

3. Schlachta CM, Mamazza J, Seshadri P, Cadeddu M, Gregoire R, Poulin EC. Defining a learning curve for laparoscopic colorectal resections. Dis Colon Rectum 2001; 44: 217-22.

4. Bennett CL, Stryker SJ, Ferreira MR, Adams J, Beart Jr. RW. The learning curve for laparoscopic colorectal surgery. Preliminary results from a prospective analysis of 1194 laparoscopic-assisted colectomies. Arch Surg 1997;132: 41-4.

5. Agachan F, Joo JS, Sher M, Weiss EG, Nogueras JJ, Wexner SD. Laparoscopic colorectal surgery. Do we get faster? Surg Endosc 1997;11:331-5.

6. Stoochi L, Nelson H, Young-Fadok TM, Larson DR. Ilstrup DM. Safety and advantages of laparoscopic vs. open colectomy in the elderly. Dis Colon Rectum 2000;43:326-32.

7. Colon Cancer Laparoscopic or Open Resection Study Group: Survival after laparoscopic surgery versus open surgery for colon cancer: Long-term outcome of a randomized clinical trial. Lancet. Published online December 12, 2008.

8. Colon Cancer Laparoscopic or Open Resection Study Group: laparoscopic surgery versus open surgery for colon cancer: short-term outcomes of a randomized trial. Lancet Oncology 2005;6:477-84.

9. Clinical Outcomes of Surgical Therapy Study Group. A comparison of laparoscopically assisted and open colectomy for colon cancer. New England Journal of Medicine 2004;350: 2050-9.

10. United Kingdom Medical Research Council Conventional versus Laparoscopic-Assisted Surgery in Colorectal Cancer Trial Group. Randomized trial of laparoscopic-assisted resection of colorectal carcinoma: 3-year results of the UK MRC CLASICC Trial Group. Journal of Clinical Oncology 2007;25: 3061-8.

11. Guillou PJ, Quirke P, Thorpe H, Walker J, Jayne DG, Smith AMH, Heath RM, Brown JM. MRC CLASSIC trial group. Stort-term endpoints of conventional versus laparoscopic-assisted surgery in patients with colorectal cancer (MRC CLASSIC trial): Multicenter, randomized controlled trial. Lancet 2005;365:1718-26.

12. Lacy AM, Garcia-Valdecasas JC, Delgado S, Castells A, Taura P, Pique JM, Visa J. Laparoscopy-assisted colectomy versus open colectomy for treatment of non-metastatic colon cancer: A randomized trial. Lancet 2002;359:2224-9.

13. Liang J-T, Huang K-C, Lai H-S, Lee P-H, Jeng Y-M. Oncologic results of laparoscopic versus conventional open surgery for stage II or III Left-sided colon cancers: a randomized controlled trial. Annals of Surgical Oncology 2006;14:109-17.

14. Milsom JW, Bohm B, Hammerhofer KA, Fazio V, Steiger E, Elson P. A prospective, randomized trial comparing laparoscopic versus conventional techniques in colorectal cancer surgery: A preliminary report. J Am Coll Surg 1998; 187: 46-57.

15. Hasewaga H, Kabeshima Y, Watanabe M, Yamamoto S, Kitajima M. Randomized controlled trial of laparoscopic versus open colectomy for advanced colorectal cancer. Surg Endosc 2003;17: 636-40.

16. Kim M-C, Kim K-H, Kim H-H, Jung G-J. Comparison of laparoscopy-assisted by conventional open distal gastrectomy and extraperigastric lymph node dissection in early gastric cancer. Journal of Surgical Oncology 2005; 91:90-4.

17. Hur H, Jeon HM, Kim W. Laparoscopy-assisted distal gastrectomy with D2 lymphadenectomy for T2b advanced gastric cancers: three years' experience. J Surg Oncol 2008; 98:515-9.

18. Tanimura S, Higashino M, Fukunaga Y, Takemura M, Tanaka Y, Fujiwara Y, Osugi H. Laparoscopic gastrectomy for gastric cancer: experience with more than 600 cases. Surg Endosc 2008;22:1161-4.

19. Adachi Y, Shiraishi N, Shiromizu A, Toshio B, Aramaki M, Kitano S. Laparoscopically-assisted bilroth I gastrectomy compared with conventional open gastrectomy. Arch Surg 2000;135:806-10.

20. Huscher CGS, Mingoli A, Giovanna S, Sansonetti A, Massimiliano DP, Recher A, Ponzano C. Laparoscopic versus open subtotal gastrectomy for distal gastric cancer, five-year results of a randomized prospective trial. Ann Surg 2005;241:232-7.

21. Kitano S, Shiraishi N, Fujii K, Yasuda K, Inomata M, Adachi Y. A randomized controlled trial comparing open vs laparoscopy-assisted distal gastrectomy for the treatment of early gastric cancer: An interim report. Surgery 2002; 131:S306-11.

22. Mochiki E, Kamiyama Y, Aihara R, Nakabayashi T, Asao T, Kuwano H. Laparoscopic assisted distal gastrectomy for early gastric cancer: five years' experience. Surgery 2005;137:317-22.

23. Yano H, Monden T, Kinuta M, et al. The usefulness of laparosopic-assisted distal gastrectomy in comparison with that of open distal gastrectomy for early gastric cancer. Gastric Cancer 2001;4: 93-7.

24. Noshiro H, Nagai S, Shimizu A, Uchiyama M, Tanaka M. Laparoscopically assisted distal gastrectomy with standard radical lymph node dissection for gastric cancer. Surg Endosc 2005;19: 1592-6.

25. Velanovich V. Case-control comparison of laparoscopic versus open distal pancreatectomy. Journal of Gastroenterology 2006;10: 95-8.

26. Matsumoto T, Shibata K, Ohta M, Iwaki K, Uchida H, Yada K, Mori M, Kitano S. Laparoscopic distal pancreatectomy and open distal pancreatectomy: A nonrandomized comparative study. Surg Laparosc Endosc Percutan Tech 2008;18:340-3.

27. Teh SH, Tseng D, Sheppard BC. Laparoscopic and open distal pancreatic resection for benign pancreatic disease. J Gastrointest Surg 2007;11:1120-5.

28. Kooby DA, Gillespie T, Bentrem D, Nakeeb A, Schmidt MC, Merchant NB, Parikh AA, et al. Left-sided pancreatectomy a multicenter comparison of laparoscopic and open approaches. Annals of Surgery 2008; 248: 438-43.

29. Topal B, Fieuws S, Aerts R, Vandeweyer H, Pennenckx F. Laparoscopic versus open liver resection of hepatic neoplasms: comparative analysis of short-term results. Surg Endosc 2008;22: 2208-13.

30. Buell JF, Thomas MJ, Doty TC, et al. An initial experience and evolution of laparoscopic hepatic resectional surgery. Surgery 2004;136:804-11.

31. Morino M, Morra I, Rosso E, Miglietta C, Garrone C. Laparoscopic vs open hepatic resection: a comparative study. Surg Endosc 2003;17: 1914-8.

32. Mala T, Edwin B, Gladhaug I, et al. A comparative study of the short-term outcome following open and laparoscopic liver resection of colorectal metastases. Surg Endosc 2002; 16: 1059-63.

33. Farges O, Jagot P, Kirstetter P, Marty J, Belghitti J. Prospective assessment of the safety and benefit of laparoscopic liver resections. J Hepatobiliary-Pancreat Surg 2002;9: 242-8.

34. Laurent A, Cherqui D, Lesurtel M, Brunetti F, Tayar C, Fagniez PL. Laparoscopic liver resections for subcapsular hepatocellular carcinoma complicating chronic liver disease. Arch Surg 2003;138: 763-9.

35. Kaneko H, Takagi S, Otsuka Y, et al. Laparoscopic liver resection of hepatocellular carcinoma. Am J Surg 2005; 189:190-4.

36. Lesurtel M, Cherqui D, Laurent A, Tayar C, Fagniez PL. Laparoscopic vs open left lateral hepatic lobectomy: a case-control study. J Am Coll Surg 2003;196:236-42.

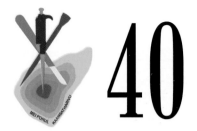

40

Robotic Surgery and NOTES

Au H Bui, Sri Chalikonda

The role of surgery is continually evolving in the treatment of malignant disease. In general, surgical extirpation of many malignancies continues to be the only hope of cure and palliation in a number of cancers. The advent of minimally invasive surgery has revolutionized the management of both benign and malignant disease. Since the first description of minimally invasive surgery for benign gallbladder disease in the 1980s, the utilization of laparoscopic assisted surgery has had logarithmic growth. The incorporation of these techniques into clinical practice has lead to innovations in other surgical fields, including thoracoscopy and Transanal Endoscopic Microsurgery (TEM). The natural progression of minimally invasive surgery and endoscopy has lead to further advances in robotic surgery and Natural Orifice Transluminal Endoscopic Surgery (NOTES).

In general, the implementation of minimally invasive surgery in the treatment of malignant cancers has progressed at a slower rate than other disease processes. This has been due to several reasons. The first stems from the original premise that the use of minimally invasive surgery may compromise the oncologic principles of surgical resection. This principle essentially entails obtaining negative tissue margins and, in most cases, an adequate lymph node dissection. During the early stages of laparoscopic surgery, there was widespread skepticism that adequate tissue margins and lymph nodes could be obtained until several trials proved that the complications and margins obtained by laparoscopic surgery were similar to open surgical procedures. Additionally, there were several case reports of port site metastasis following laparoscopic surgery for malignant disease that gave many clinicians reservation about the use of laparoscopic surgery. As such, there was considerable delay and opposition to the use of minimally invasive surgery toward cancer treatment. The use of robotic surgery and NOTES also appear to be at a similar juncture. As in any new technology or medical therapy, judicious use of medical advancement must be tempered by caution with the risks and benefits carefully evaluated. As such, clinical trials and current reports in the literature regarding the development of robotic surgery and NOTES are only beginning to assess the validity and efficacy of these newer techniques. Additionally, there are questions whether cost and true benefit are benefiting the patient population.

Over the past decade, there has been exponential growth in robot-assisted procedures. Most of the robotic literature is related to its adoption for the treatment of prostate cancer. Based on the current urologic literature it has become readily apparent that the robotic technology is safe in prostatic disease and allows more complex cases to be performed, albeit at a higher cost. As such, from a market growth of five billion in 2000 to an expected 25 billion in 2010, robotic surgery has increased exponentially in all fields of surgery.

The first robot approved for clinical use in surgery was the automated endoscopic system for optimal positioning (AESOP-Computer Motion, Santa Barbara, CA). The da Vinci surgical system (Intuitive Surgical Inc., Sunnyvale, CA) is the first telerobotic manipulation system approved by the FDA for abdominal surgery. This essentially means the operator does not necessarily have to be physically present to perform the procedure. The premise is that this technological advantage will allow remote field surgeries to become a reality. In addition to the tele-operating features of most robotic systems, robotic assisted surgery allows for extremely precise and controlled movements. This allows for complex procedures to be performed with greater safety and security given the limitations of human movement and traditional laparoscopic instruments. Additionally, the technical advantages of the da Vinci system include 3-D vision, enhanced dexterity and improved ergonomics when compared with standard laparoscopic surgery.

The da Vinci Robotic System in Surgery

Though the AESOP was the first prototype system for laparoscopic assisted robotic surgery, the model has fallen out of favor for the current da Vinci surgical system. Developed in the mid-1990s from a research project involving the US Department of Defense and the Stanford

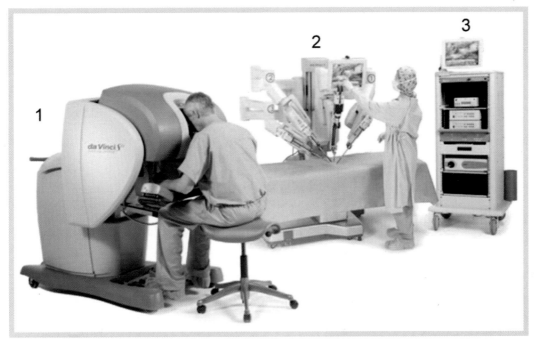

Figure 40-1: da Vinci robotic system (intuitive Surgical Inc., Sunnyvale, CA) consisting of (1) a surgeon console; (2) a patient side cart and (3) an image-processing/insufflation stack

Research Institute, the da Vinci system **(Figure 40-1)** is a master-slave system rather than a true autonomous robot. The operator sits away from the operative field in a remote console that allows for control of three or four robotic arms which are docked through laparoscopic ports. The system itself consists of three components:

- a surgeon console
- a patient side cart
- vision cart

The console is the interface between the surgeon and patient. The 3-D view from the stereoscopic endoscope is projected within the console at 10× magnification and allows for greater spatial images than current laparoscopic endoscopes. In addition, the surgeon's thumb and forefinger control the movements of the robotic arms while foot pedals allow control of diathermy and other energy sources as shown in **Figure 40-2**. The unique feature of motion scaling eliminates the human characteristic of tremor, allowing for fine and precise movement of the instruments.

The patient side cart is where the robotic arms are mounted. Included in the mounted instruments is a high-resolution 3-D endoscope, while the other instruments are specialized EndoWrist instruments. The vision cart is an image-process/insufflation stack containing the camera-control units for the 3-D imaging system, image-recording devices, a laparoscopic insufflator and a monitor allowing 2-D visualization for the assistant.

Thus, there are several advantages enjoyed by the robotic system over standard laparoscopic surgery. The

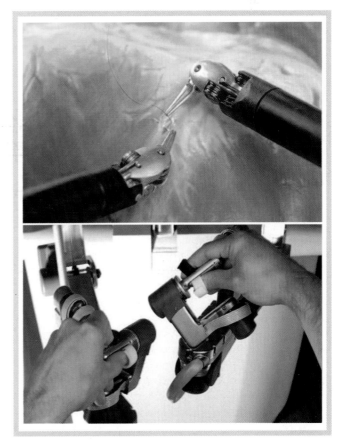

Figure 40-2: Use of the console (A) to manipulate the laparoscopic instrument with 3 D view of laparoscopic instruments (B) [© (2008) Intuitive Surgical, Inc.]

3-D vision, enhanced magnification and motion scaling allows for greater visualization of the operative field. In addition, the EndoWrist technology mimics the operative movement of a human wrist, allowing for greater facility of movement. One of the early criticisms of laparoscopic instrumentation was its limitation of movement. Current laparoscopic instrumentation only allows for 4 d.f. (degrees of freedom). The EndoWrist instruments allow for 7 d.f., which is equivalent to movement of the human wrist, as shown in **Figure 40-3**. This added flexibility allows for more complex surgeries to be performed with greater facility.

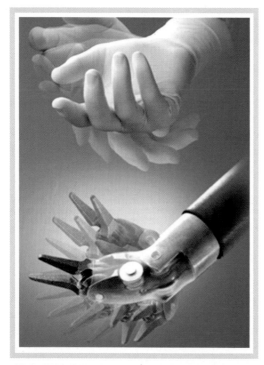

Figure 40-3: EndoWrist instrument that allows for 7 d.f., which is comparable to a human wrist [© (2008) Istuitive Surgical, Inc.]

The current da Vinci robot is in its third generation stage with refinements that include high-definition video, improved range of motion with longer instruments, touch screen controls and more compact design. Another distinct advantage of robotic surgery is that the "fulcrum" effect of laparoscopic surgery, where the instrument tips move in the opposite direction to the surgeon's hand is negated in robotic surgery. This suggests that the learning curve may be shorter for robotic surgery than laparoscopic surgery as this contrarian view does not need to be overcome to perform robotic surgery.

There is considerable debate about the real benefits of the robotic-assisted procedures over conventional laparoscopic procedures. The debate stems whether the advantage of robotic surgery offers the considerable financial investment required to purchase the system.

Some laparoscopic surgeons have argued that robotic assisted procedures are an industry-driven phenomenon and that proper scientific evaluation is required before their role in oncologic surgery is defined.

The most glaring disadvantage of the da Vinci system is its cost. An analysis of the investment required to purchase and maintain a robotic system will give insight into the its cost/benefit ratio. The capital expenditure for a new unit is approximately $2.5-3.5 million with annual running costs in the range of 5-10% of the purchase cost (average selling price is $ 1.7 million). However, given the rapid proliferation of these system in both academic and private health care settings suggests that there may be economic advantages of using this system in the long term. It remains to be seen whether the considerable expenditure required to purchase and maintain the current robotic system is clinically beneficial. Extra costs for training, delay in set-up and extra-operative time during the learning curve should be anticipated. One series of 224 procedures at a single institution determined that a cost of $ 1470 was added to the cost of the procedure with the use of the robotic system. Additional cost analysis comparing operative cost by Morgan, et al revealed that when leaving out the initial capital investment for a robotic system, there was no significant difference in cost between robotic procedures and standard techniques. Though this cost analysis varies from institution to institution, it is clear that robotic assisted cases are most beneficial in hospitals with high volume cases. The learning cost to operate the system is roughly $217,034. To overcome these high costs, the concept of a high volume center where the learning curve can rapidly be overcome and costs can be minimized is the most reasonable option.

Another distinct limitation of the robotic system is the lack of tactile feedback. There is however, plans to develop a feedback systems that may mimic tactile sensation. Additionally, set-up time for robotic procedures can initially be quite lengthy. Though the 3-D vision offers extremely clear and precise imaging, the system does not readily offer readily apparent advantages when surgery involves more than one quadrant of the abdomen. When abdominal surgery requires two or more quadrants, in addition to various patient 'tilts', there is considerable docking and disengagement of the robot arms that may add significant operative time. This can be overcome by using large and well-trained personnel familiar with robotic equipment and its set-up. As the development of future generations of robotic system continues, there is thought that the cumbersome and capacious da Vinci system will be streamlined to smaller and sleeker designs.

Robotic-assisted Surgery

The largest series of robotic cases published to date is in the field of urologic surgery. The robot assisted laparoscopic radical prostatectomy as described by the team from Detroit at the Vattikutti Institute has been performed in more than 4,000 patients. They have refined a transperitoneal technique, which has produced excellent oncologic results with minimal morbidity. Long-term follow-up suggests that the oncologic validity of this procedure may be real and prove that this procedure is at least equal or better than conventional laparoscopic radical prostatectomy. The exponential growth of robotic-assisted radical prostatectomies with an increase of more than 60% in 2007 demonstrates that the use of robots in surgery can be a practical and feasible. It is especially promising in centers that have high volume cases as this makes the cost of obtaining and maintaining a robot financially sound. The use of robotic surgery in abdominal oncologic diseases remains small. The few published reports consist of mostly small series or case reports. We present here a small sampling of the literature as the field continues to evolve.

Colorectal Cancer

Colorectal cancer remains the third most commonly diagnosed cancer and second leading cause of cancer deaths in the United States. Most patients will undergo some form of surgical resection as a primary modality of treatment following their diagnosis. Since Jacobs, et al reported their initial experience of a laparoscopic sigmoidectomy, the laparoscopic approach has been embraced as an efficacious and safe method of performing colorectal surgery. There are several case series reported in the literature describing the use of robotic surgery for colorectal disease. First described in 2001, various groups have utilized the da Vinci system in colectomies for benign and malignant disease. Weber, et al described three robotic right and sigmoid colectomies using the da Vinci system in 2002. The largest series to date is described by D'Annibale who reported 53 robotic colorectal surgeries from May 2001 to May 2003 where 23 cases of malignant colorectal disease were confirmed. The authors concluded that the robotic assisted laparoscopic surgery was a safe and viable alternative to standard laparoscopic techniques.

Rectal surgery is more difficult as compared to colonic surgery because of the anatomical characteristics of the rectum, pelvis and the surrounding structures. Total Mesorectal Excision (TME), the concept of precise dissection of an avascular plane between the presacral fascia and the fascia propria of the rectum, is often extremely difficult in a narrow pelvis. The da Vinci system provides several advantages in the narrow pelvic cavity. The 3-D visualization, precise movement and motion scaling provided by the robotic system allow for meticulous and precise dissection required in this anatomic region. Several studies to date have examined the possibility of total mesorectal excision for rectal cancer.

Pigazzi, et al describes the use of robotic assisted mesorectal excision for rectal cancer in 2006. Though having relatively small numbers, their comparison of robotic total mesorectal excision and laparoscopic mesorectal excision concluded that autonomic nerve preservation and adequate oncologic results were acceptable. Additionally, reports from Asia by Baik et al described the feasibility of performing robot assisted mesorectal excision in rectal cancer patients in 2007. In this report, they demonstrated that robotic surgery was especially advantageous over conventional laparoscopic surgery when small, sharp dissections were required in a small operative field. Modified instruments with the use of the EndoWrist function, which is the core benefit of the da Vinci system, facilitated dissection within the narrow confines of the pelvis. A group in Hong Kong has also reported a case study of a robotic-abdominoperineal resection for rectal cancer in 2006.

Though most studies in the literature describe a relatively small cohort of robotic assisted laparoscopic surgery for colorectal cancer, there is overwhelming consensus that the current system is a feasible and safe alternative for the majority of patients. A randomized study described by Baik et al. comparing the safety of laparoscopic low anterior resection (LAR) versus robotic assisted LAR proved to be statistically equivalent between the two groups.

Esophageal Cancer

The first robotic-assisted esophagectomy was reported in 2003. The resected specimen was a T1N0M0 adeno-carcinoma. The abdominal dissection was completed via a conventional laparoscopic instrumentation. The distal esophagus was resected using a transhiatal route with the da Vinci robot. The first combined transthoracic and transabdominal robotic-assisted esophagectomy with cervical esophagogastric anastomosis was described in 2004. The operation was performed in two stages under one period of general anesthesia. The patient was initially placed in the left-lateral position with single lung ventilation of the left lung. The thoracic portion of the procedure was performed using five port sites in the right chest. Following completion of the thoracic dissection of the esophagus, the patient was rotated into the supine position. Mobilization of the stomach and the distal esophagus was performed with robotic assistance through six port sites. The total operative time was 11 hours with surgical robotic console time logged at 4 hours and 20 minutes. The postoperative recovery was described as uneventful.

Since these initial case reports, several other small series have emerged verifying the validity of esophagectomy using robotic assistance. An Australian group details four cases and another report from the Netherlands details 21 robotic-assisted esophagectomies. Common to all these cases is the ability to perform the thoracic dissection with the aid of the robot with an adequate number of mediastinal lymph nodes. More importantly, the intraoperative and postoperative complications were equivalent to standard laparoscopic techniques.

Gastric Cancer

Gastric cancer treatment continues to be gastric resection and regional lymph node dissection. Although there is still considerable controversy regarding the appropriate extent of lymph node dissection in Japan and Europe, a D2 extended lymph node dissection is the standard of care for localized gastric cancer. In 2008, Patriti, et al described the feasibility and safety of performing a robotic-assisted laparoscopic D2 dissection and esophageal anastomosis on 13 patients. The authors concluded that the robotic-assisted surgery is a safe alternative and does not compromise the oncologic principles or staging accuracy for gastric cancer.

Other Abdominal Surgeries

A variety of procedures have been undertaken including anti-reflux procedures, cholecystectomy, Heller myotomy, donor nephrectomy, splenectomy, adrenalectomy, distal pancreatectomy and duodenal polypectomy. Surgeons in our institution have begun a large series of robotic Whipple procedures. The results of these published reports suggest that the efficacy and safety of robotic assisted surgeries are comparable to conventional laparoscopic techniques. Interestingly, four randomized trials comparing robotic surgery to conventional laparoscopy for reflux disease demonstrates equal feasibility except for a much higher cost for robotic surgery.

Natural Orifice Transluminal Endoscopic Surgery (NOTES)

The advent of the most controversial innovation in surgery since the introduction of the laparoscopic surgery is the natural orifice transluminal endoscopic surgery technique (NOTES). The technological advances with both advanced laparoscopic and endoscopic instrumentation has allowed the NOTES technique to become a technical reality. NOTES requires both the use of endoscopic and laparoscopic techniques to accomplish its goal. The concept is to use the natural orifices of the body as a natural entryway to gain access to internal organs. In a survey conducted in Birmingham, Alabama, Varadarajalu, et al in 2008 reported results of 100 patients questioned regarding their preferred method of cholecystectomy, 78% preferred NOTES with the main reasons cited as a lack of

external pain (99%) and scarring (89%). Women younger than 50 years and those who have had a prior endoscopy experience were more likely to choose NOTES over laparoscopy.

The subject of heated debates and discussions are on the 'real' advantages of NOTES. At this stage, the idea of using NOTES for simple elective cases that is suitable for a laparoscopic approach is questionable. Rather, the NOTES technique and technology should be regarded as a synergistic approach to laparoscopic surgery in patients that may not be suitable for conventional laparoscopic surgery. Once the technique is perfected, it may be a viable option for certain patients in selected operations. Ideally, NOTES should act as an additional tool to complement laparoscopic surgery where conventional laparoscopy may not be technically feasible. Li and Milsom reported a case where a combined NOTES with laparoscopic approach to resect a large, benign polyp was accomplished. The location of the polyp was such that it was not accessible to laparoscopic resection. Instead, using laparoscopic instruments, the polyp was pushed into the cecal lumen where it was excised by endoscopic instruments.

Gettman, et al reported the first transvaginal nephrectomy in a porcine model in 2002. But it was not until Kalloo, et al presented a transgastric peritoneoscopy in a porcine model that NOTES was brought to the forefront of the surgical field. Since these first pioneering studies, there have been many published reports using animal models that validate the technique as a surgical reality.

A review of the animal literature has revealed several limitations that will require resolution before there is general acceptance by the public and medical community. The optimal access route and method has not been established. Additionally, enterotomy closure could not be achieved reliably in all cases and the risk of peritoneal infection has not adequately been minimized. The closure of enterotomies using endoscopic instruments and the risk of transluminal contamination remains a formidable obstacle. The endoscopic suturing device for enterotomy closure requires full thickness approximation and plication to produce a leak proof seal. Many devices have been developed and tested in animal models with no one device demonstrating its effectiveness consistently.

Another technical limitation in NOTES is the parallel alignment of the instrument and scope makes dissection difficult. There is little space for both instruments to work in parallel and an additional access point to achieve the proper triangulation is often required for the working instruments to function optimally. Ways to overcome this have been to add an additional laparoscopic port to facilitate dissection. Forgione, et al described three cases of successful transvaginal cholecystectomy with the addition of a single transabdominal 5 mm port. This may especially be useful in morbidly obese patients.

The development of an ergonomic platform to perform NOTES is another major challenge. The difficulty of maneuvering instruments from a long distance is disorienting and not intuitive. To overcome these issues, several companies have devised multichannel endoscopes that allow the operator to not only have multiple channels within a single scope but also change the configuration of the flexible scope to become rigid. One channel contains the endoscope while the other three can include a variety of different instruments. This essentially restores the triangulation between the endoscope and working instruments to allow for clearer visualization of the operative field **(Figure 40-4)**.

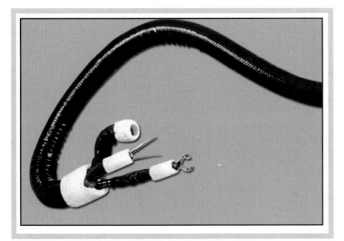

Figure 40-4: The ShapeLock Transport™ by USGI Medical, San Clemente, CA, offers a stable platform with instrument angulation for tissue dissection.

Conclusion

The future of surgery remains an interesting and challenging field. Both robotic surgery and NOTES are an extension of laparoscopic surgery and will be a useful adjunct to laparoscopic surgery. Considering the development of robotics over the past several years, it is to be expected that the application of this technology will only increase. The exponential growth of the da Vinci system worldwide with over 1,171 systems sold as up March 2009. Until studies can demonstrate the cost to benefit ratio of this new technology, initial skepticism will certainly delay the wider application of this technology to other fields. The advantages and disadvantages of robotic surgery are listed in **Table 40-1**.

Most people certainly agree that the subsequent generation of robotic-assisted machines will become smaller and easier to handle. As such, the cost of each unit will also decline as the technology improves. This may allow the economic cost to become substantially improved

TABLE 40-1	Robotic surgery	
Advantages	**Disadvantages**
Improved ergonomics	High cost of purchase and maintenance
3-D vision	Bulky size
Camera stability	No tactile feedback
Improved dexterity with 7 d.f.	Larger port (8 mm) size
Elimination of 'fulcrum effect'	Assistance required for port docking
Motion scaling improvement	Personnel to help set-up system
Telesurgery/telemonitoring capabilities	Longer time for set-up and longer time for conversion to open surgery

and make robotic-assisted laparoscopic surgery a reality in most hospitals. It should also be noted that successive generation of doctors raised and trained in minimally invasive and computer technology will become more adept and amendable to assimilating the newest technology in their practice, thus making the transition more facile. It is also conceivable that the fusion with imaging modalities like computed tomography (CT) and magnetic resonance imaging (MRI) would likely be introduced with robotic surgery to allow more precise imaging and safer surgical techniques. With the introduction of the first MRI compatible robot in 2007, it is to be expected that this will extend to pelvic and abdominal surgery.

Another interesting facet of robotic surgery is its tele-surgical capabilities. Although they originally developed to allow telesurgery to be performed in areas that may not readily be accessible, this continues to be a theoretical idea rather than a practical one. In 2001, the first trans-Atlantic surgery was performed where surgeons in New York performed a cholecystectomy in Strasbourg. Limitations of this technology included delays over the satellite transmission, which did not allow for real time images at certain points during the case. This could prove to be unfeasible until reliable satellite signals can be established over long distances. Additionally, there is thought that telesurgery could be a useful adjunct in hostile combat zones or space travel, as prolonged space flights become a reality. NASA is currently carrying out further research on long-distance telesurgery. The NASA Extreme Environment Mission operations project is currently focused on the development and installation of the first robotic system in a space station for remote emergency surgery. In collaboration with the Jet Propulsion Laboratory, NASA is also developing robotic assisted microsurgery for the eye, ear, nose and cranial surgery for micro-invasive complex surgery. The advent of miniaturized intracorporeal devices for imaging will

TABLE 40-2	NOTES	
Potential advantages	**Potential disadvantages**
No scars, decreased external pain and wound complications	Enterotomy closure
Less psychological and physiological trauma	Endosuturing and anastomotic devices are still being developed
Adjunct to laparoscopic surgery in morbidly obese patients	Potential for peritoneal/ transluminal contamination
Possibility of conscious sedation in selected patients	Control of intraperitoneal hemorrhage may be difficult
Probable faster recovery	Parallel vision alignment
Potential to offer therapy outside operating room environment	Development of multi-tasking platform and spatial orientation is required

be another advance in robotic technology. The delivery of a miniature mobile intra-abdominal camera will allow many views and angles to be permissible within the abdominal cavity.

The NOTES concept is one of the most controversial ideas in surgery in recent years. As the initial resistance to this idea has waned, the concept has steadily been gathering momentum in the clinical arena. Successful animal trials have established that NOTES can be performed safely. A significant human trial is required before the procedure can be established as a standard surgical procedure. Several studies have established the limitations of the NOTES procedure. These limitations include better access points, more reliable closure of enterotomy sites and the production of instrumentation, which can address the technical difficulties of the surgery. But in general, long-term human trials will be required to demonstrate the efficacy and safety in humans before it will be recognized as an alternative surgical strategy. The potential advantages and disadvantages of NOTES are summarized in **Table 40-2**.

The development of NOTES and robotic surgery remain a controversial and exciting field in the future development of surgery. There is no question that robotic surgery is a safe and efficacious alternative to laparoscopic surgery, the debate remains whether the cost is and extended operative time is beneficial to the patient. Additionally, until the technical challenges of NOTES is overcome, acceptance by the general population and medical community remains to be seen.

Summary

- Robotic surgery and NOTES are the next frontier of minimally invasive surgery.
- Robotic surgery may be taught and learnt by many surgeons making minimally invasive surgical surgery not an exclusive of those who have laparoscopic skills.
- Robotic surgery eliminates the 'fulcrum effect', provides 3D vision, avoids hand tremor, increases dexterity and allows more degrees of freedom, in comparison to laparoscopic surgery
- High cost, time and personnel to setup equipment and longer time to conversion to open surgery are potential drawbacks of robotic surgeries.
- The advantages and long-term outcomes still remain to be evaluated with robust studies.

Landmark Papers

1. Al-Akash M, et al. NOTES; The progession of a novel and emerging technique. Surgical Oncology 2009;18(2):95-103.
2. Hawes R. ASGE/SAGES working group on natural orifice translumenal endoscopic surgery. Gastrointest Endosc 2006; 63:199-203.
3. Taylor GW, Jayne DG. Robotic applications in abdominal surgery: their limitations and future developments. The International Journal of Medical Robotics and Computer Assisted Surgery 2007; 3:3-9.

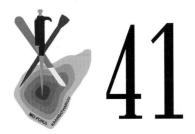

41

Surgical Management
of Metastases

James F Pingpank Jr

Surgical excision, alone or in combination with chemotherapy, has gained increasing support in both the surgical and the medical oncology fields over the last two decades. The general principles governing surgical decision making relies upon the ability to remove all active disease or control severe symptoms. Frequently, a trial period of chemotherapy will permit a reduction in the volume of metastatic disease as well as provide a window into the clinical behavior of the tumor. Rapid progression of disease to areas outside the proposed resection field indicates the probable futility of resection strategies and are not indicative of a missed opportunity for surgical intervention. When complete resection is possible, the use of effective adjuvant chemotherapy should be considered, if available.

Hepatic Metastases

Hepatic metastases are present in a large number of patients with primary cancers of the gastrointestinal tract, lung and breast along with patients with melanoma and a variety of endocrine malignancies. For a significant percentage of patients with metastases from colorectal, gastrointestinal neuroendocrine and ocular melanoma tumors, the hepatic disease represents the sole or life-limiting component of disease. When hepatic metastases represent the only site of active disease, therapeutic interventions aimed solely at the liver disease warrant consideration. Liver directed therapies include resection, a variety of ablative technologies including radio-frequency, microwave and cryoablation, intra-arterial chemotherapy and selective internal radiation therapy. The unique blood supply of the liver plays an important theoretic role in the liver's propensity for the development of metastatic disease. For patients with primary tumors, the hepatic portal circulation may serve as an entry into the hepatic circulation. In circumstances where metastases arise from outside the portal circulation, the presumed route of spread is via the hepatic artery. Once tumors are established within the hepatic parenchyma, there is preferential tumor blood supply arising from the hepatic

arterial circulation, while the majority of the native tissue blood supply remains through the portal circulation. This differential pattern of blood flow between tumor and non-tumor bearing tissue may be exploited in a variety of therapeutic approaches which are unique to the liver. Decision algorithms regarding the management of hepatic metastases are based upon a variety of extrahepatic factors including the histology of the primary tumor, the interval between the primary tumor and the development of metastases (disease-free interval), the presence of extrahepatic disease, additional medical comorbidities and the availability of effective systemic agents. Local (hepatic) factors influence the therapeutic options selected, with more invasive procedures reserved for those patients where complete resection and/or ablation of all lesions can reasonably be expected. In circumstances where complete resection is not possible due to the location or number of tumors or the overall health of the liver, less invasive approaches are favored. Specific treatment paradigms will be discussed in relation to tumor histology later in the chapter.

Tumor Staging

A variety of staging techniques are available to precisely stage hepatic and systemic metastatic disease. High-speed helical CT and MRI examinations afford accurate disease staging along with detailed operative planning and are the most routinely utilized studies. CT scans are thought to have the least amount of inter-institution variability while allowing for concurrent chest and pelvic imaging. Hepatic imaging protocols should include three contrast phases (arterial, portal venous and traditional venous phase) in addition to the non-contrast first series. Individual tumor histologic subtypes will be more accurately staged with specific series. Colorectal metastases tend to have poor contrast enhancement and are frequently best seen on the non-contrast or venous phase series, while the majority of neuroendocrine tumors are accurately imaged only on early arterial images. Contrast-enhanced MRI may be utilized in the evaluation of equivocal lesions seen on CT scan and can be especially valuable in circumstances where CT and PET/CT frequently understate the number of lesions such as with melanoma and neuroendocrine metastases. In addition to evaluating tumor burden, preoperative imaging also evaluates overall liver health and aids in operative planning with regard to the assessment of the relationship to tumors to hepatic blood supply along with mapping of extrahepatic vessels. The presence of cirrhosis, steatohepatitis and chemotherapy induced liver disease can substantially be evaluated on cross-sectional imaging. PET scans are most useful to assess metastatic disease for patients receiving active therapy, or to assess the efficacy of non-resection interventions. Although the routine use of transabdominal ultrasound has largely been replaced by CT and MRI, intraoperative utility remains quite high.

Surgical Resection of Hepatic Metastases

There is clear evidence supporting the role the efficacy of surgical resection of liver metastases from colorectal and neuroendocrine tumors in properly selected patients, with long-term disease-free and overall survival documented in multiple large series. Advances in disease staging, anesthetic and perioperative management have coupled with improvements in surgical technique to substantially decrease the morbidity and mortality associated with hepatic resection. Numerous factors contribute to patient selection for the resection of hepatic disease, but the most fundamental is the surgeon's assessment of the ability to remove all diseases. Except in rare circumstances of planned sequential resections, subtotal resection/ablation provides little or no survival benefit. The presence of extrahepatic disease, once an absolute contraindication to resection of hepatic disease, may not preclude hepatectomy if the extrahepatic disease can completely be addressed at the same or remote time-point. The routine use of intraoperative ultrasound to screen for occult metastatic disease and plan resection strategies is encouraged. Staging laparoscopy is valuable when there is a high likelihood of occult intrahepatic or extrahepatic metastatic disease which would preclude resection. We routinely employ segment-oriented resection strategies, enhanced with portal venous control (both Pringle maneuver and pedicle ligation), extrahepatic hepatic vein ligation and low central venous pressure. When large resections are planned or in the presence of a substantial chemotherapy history, routine biopsy of the proposed liver remnant is utilized.

Careful operative planning is necessary in the presence of multiple or bilobar hepatic metastases, often based upon concerns about the adequacy of the postresection liver remnant. The majority of these circumstances arise in the presence of extensive right-sided disease, where encroachment upon the segment IV is needed at resection. The use of portal vein embolization to the planned resected lobe four weeks prior to resection, allows the inducement contralateral hypertrophy and safe resection in patients with healthy livers. Alternatively, when small volume disease is present in the proposed liver remnant, frequent use of radiofrequency ablation and non-segmental resection strategies are effective.

Regional Therapy for Hepatic Metastases

A significant percentage of patients with isolated hepatic metastases will present an extent of disease which precludes complete resection. Effective systemic chemotherapeutic strategies should be utilized, if available. In the absence of effective systemic regimens, a variety of regional approaches have displayed efficacy in controlling hepatic disease. The majority of regional therapies under active use and investigation exploit the differential vascular supply between tumors and native hepatic parenchyma. In general, hepatic tumors get the majority of vascular flow from the hepatic arterial tree (up to 75%), while the portal vein provides the majority of support for native hepatic and biliary structures, allowing regional treatments delivered via the hepatic artery to preferentially target tumor and minimize damage to normal tissue. All regional therapies are based upon the ability to isolate the entire hepatic arterial supply in order to effectively control agent delivery. Misperfusion of the gastric or duodenal mucosa is a significant concern and may result in gastritis and ulceration significant enough to result in bleeding and perforation. Routine identification of the right gastric artery in the operating room or angiography suite is imperative to avoid this toxicity.

Rigorous examination of hepatic arterial infusion via a surgically implanted infusion pump has been ongoing for many years. This dual chambered pump is implanted in a subcutaneous pocket on the anterior abdominal wall, with a catheter placed into the gastroduodenal artery, allowing the release of a constant infusion of floxuridine into the hepatic artery over a 14-day period. Floxuridine (FUDR) is utilized for HAI infusion due to the nearly complete hepatic first pass clearance, effectively eliminating any systemic delivery of drug. At surgical exploration for catheter placement it is important to isolate all gastric and duodenal branches arising off the hepatic artery in order to prevent duodenal or gastric perfusion with high dose chemotherapy. After the pump is placed, fluorescein is injected via the hepatic artery catheter and the liver examined with a Woods lamp to ensure perfusion of the entire liver and the absence of extrahepatic perfusion. At the completion of the cycle, the pump is filled with heparin-saline for 14-days, prior to the initiation of an additional cycle of HAI-FUDR. HAI therapy is well tolerated with the primary toxicity of therapy being biliary sclerosis, manifest by rising bilirubin and alkaline phosphatase. Treatment of biliary sclerosis is with corticosteroids administered via the infusion pump.

Transarterial chemoembolization (TACE) utilizes a combination of intra-arterial chemotherapy (cisplatin, doxorubicin) and vascular stasis induced by glass beads or resins to induce hypoxic tumor damage and deliver local cytotoxic chemotherapy. Treatment is delivered to 25-50% of the liver at a single setting, with multiple treatments spaced at six week intervals. Antitumor efficacy has been reported with a multitude of histologic subtypes, with the greatest impact seen in the most hypervascular tumors such as neuroendocrine metastases and hepatocellular tumors. This therapy is most effective

in circumstances where tumor volume allows for effective targeting as opposed to diffuse milliary disease. Retreatment has proven effective upon tumor regrowth, with response paralleling that seen with the original treatment. Additional strategies for intra-arterial embolic therapy include the use of drug-eluting beads and microspheres providing vehicles for slow release delivery of cytotoxic agents directly into the tumor bed.

Regional perfusion (Isolated Hepatic Perfusion) and infusion (Percutaneous Hepatic Perfusion) treatments have allowed the delivery of very high dose chemotherapy into the hepatic arterial tree while minimizing or eliminating systemic drug exposure. Hyperthermic isolated hepatic perfusion (IHP) **(Figure 41-1)** is performed utilizing a recirculating closed circuit containing a reservoir, roller pump and heat exchanger. This dual

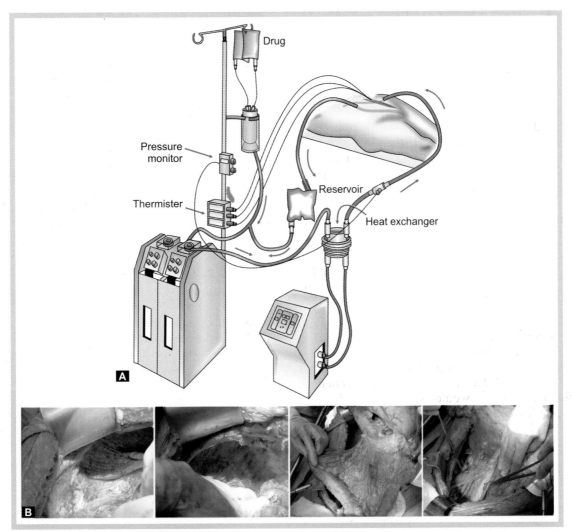

Figure 41-1: HIPEC and operative results: Hyperthermic chemoperfusion circuit (A) includes an inline reservoir, roller pump and heat exchanger. Chemoperfusion is performed for 90-100 minutes with a closed abdomen and gentle abdominal agitation to facilitate complete drug distribution. Extent of dissection (B) includes complete removal of the diaphragmatic peritoneum, omentectomy and pelvic peritonectomy, with special attention paid to preservation of GI tract length

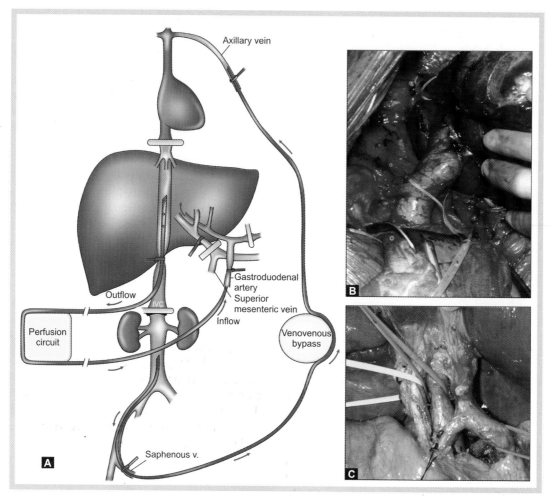

Figure 41-2: Schematic of IHP circuit and operative dissection: A schematic illustration of the isolated hepatic perfusion (IHP) circuit (A) with inflow via the gastroduodenal artery and outflow via the retrohepatic IVC. Venovenous bypass is accomplished from the femoral vein to the axillary or internal jugular vein (all accessed percutaneously). An extensive dissection of the retrohepatic vena cava (B) and portal blood vessels and bile duct (C) is completed to prevent leak of chemotherapy outside the circuit

circuit is utilized to administer high dose melphalan during an operative procedure in which hepatic isolation is maintained with hepatic inflow through the hepatic artery and outflow via an isolated segment of the retrohepatic vena cava. A second venovenous bypass circuit returns venous blood from below the diaphragm to the heart. For patients with selected tumor histologic subtypes, durable responses were observed in greater than 50% of patients. Percutaneous hepatic perfusion (PHP) **(Figure 41-2)** offers the ability to high dose chemotherapy via the hepatic artery utilizing a percutaneous femoral approach. A second double balloon catheter is placed via the femoral vein and positioned in the retrohepatic vena cava and enables the isolation and collection of hepatic venous effluent for subsequent hemofiltration prior to return to the systemic circulation. Early results have yielded similar results to IHP. IHP and PHP strategies treat the entire hepatic

parenchyma and associated tumor with each intervention. A thorough evaluation of the overall health of the nontumor bearing liver is vital to assuring safe patient selection. When over 50% of the hepatic volume is replaced with tumor, operative IHP with associated hyperthermia is not performed, whereas PHP is felt to be safe. In all circumstances where high volume liver replacement with tumor is noted, as biopsy of the nontumor bearing liver is informative and should be performed. The presence of periportal inflammation or fibrosis or evidence of biliary stasis or obstruction indicate a liver under greater stress than expected based upon imaging alone. Particular care should be exercised with tumor histologies such as ocular melanoma or cholangiocarcinoma, where diffusely infiltrative patterns of tumor spread often result in greater underlying hepatic dysfunction versus slower growing neuroendocrine metastases which tend to afford the liver for time to adapt to the presence of even a large volume of tumor.

Hepatic directed radiation therapy has not routinely been employed due to the high toxicity rates in non-tumor liver and biliary tissue and difficulties in targeting secondary to respiratory motion. Selective internal radiation utilizes the beta-emitter yttrium-90 tagged microspheres to deliver intra-arterial radiation to a tumor bed. Early results demonstrated effective delivery of radiation dosing, but the risk of radiation induced liver disease persists. Patients with a high arteriovenous intrahepatic shunt are not candidates for the therapy secondary to concerns of pulmonary radiation toxicity.

Colorectal Cancer

The overall survival of patients undergoing resection of hepatic metastases from colorectal cancer ranges 30-50% at five years. The ability to obtain an R0 resection is of paramount importance, but disease-free interval, elevated preoperative CEA, the presence of a lymph-node positive primary tumor and increasing size and number of the hepatic tumors have all been associated with decreased survival. For patients presenting with synchronous primary and hepatic tumors, the high risk of additional metastatic disease justifies the upfront use of systemic chemotherapy. After three months of therapy, patients who remain or have been rendered completely resectable are offered resection of the primary and metastatic lesions, with subsequent adjuvant chemotherapy. Patients who progress through frontline chemotherapy are thought to be poor surgical candidates due to the aggressive nature of the disease, yet will be offered surgical therapy where complete tumor resection is possible. Immediate resection, prior to chemotherapy, is reserved for patients with symptomatic primary tumors (bleeding or obstruction) or those in whom resection of the primary tumor and low volume liver disease could be accomplished at one procedure with a low complication rate to allow prompt progression to adjuvant chemotherapy. When complete resection has been obtained, placement of a hepatic artery infusion (HAI) pump should be considered, especially when more than one metastatic tumor has been resected.

There is mounting evidence that induction chemotherapy affords increased control of metachronous hepatic disease and is routinely used in our institution except in patients with low volume liver disease and individuals with extensive prior chemotherapy exposure. Communication between the medical oncologist and the surgeon is critical to avoid overexposure to cytotoxic chemotherapy and the associated liver injury. Concerns about the degree of hepatic stress induced by prior chemotherapy exposure may be address via a biopsy of the non-tumor liver. Three of four patients who undergo successful hepatic metastasectomy of colorectal disease will recur, with approximately half of all recurrences located within the liver. The hepatic toxicity associated with prolonged chemotherapy administration and the high percentage of intrahepatic recurrences justify the use of parenchyma preserving surgical techniques, including ultrasound guided non-anatomic resections and segmental liver resections to preserve non-tumor bearing liver.

Unresectable synchronous or metachronous hepatic metastatic disease is initially treated with intravenous chemotherapy, utilizing either oxaliplatin or irinotecan based regimens. As noted above, if a sufficient response allows for surgical resection, data suggests this to be the most effective treatment. When resection is not an option and metastatic disease remains confined to the liver, the use of a regional therapy such as HAI or IHP/HAI in addition to continued systemic therapy should be considered.

Neuroendocrine Tumors

Neuroendocrine tumors of pancreatic (PNET) or bowel (carcinoid) origin frequently metastasize to regional lymph nodes and liver in the absence of extrahepatic metastatic spread. For a significant number of patients, the hepatic disease is the most significant clinical component of the disease due to massive hepatic replacement and the associated risk of liver failure or the side effects of the tumor associated hormone production. Ample evidence supports the clinical benefit associated with the resection of all disease when possible. Hepatic disease at presentation can be massive due to the slow growth of tumors and the lack of associated symptoms. In such patients, hepatic disease will dictate outcome and sequencing of multiple therapies is often necessary. Staged resection of hepatic disease, often in conjunction with removal of the primary tumor and regional lymphadenopathy, has proved effective even in patients with extensive bilobar metastases. Neuroendocrine tumors are highly vascular tumors and have several series demonstrated the efficacy of intra-arterial therapies including TACE and infusional melphalan. It is not uncommon for these therapies to reduce hepatic disease to a level allowing surgical debulking of liver tumors. At the time of any surgical intervention to address hepatic metastases, consideration to resection of extrahepatic disease, including the primary tumor, is warranted. When extensive hepatic metastases present synchronous with the diagnosis of local-regional primary disease, it is often more prudent to address the hepatic disease prior to resection of the primary tumor. Emerging evidence suggests improved overall survival is associated with subsequent resection of the primary tumor upon maintaining control of metastatic disease.

Ocular Melanoma

Although histologically similar to cutaneous melanoma, ocular melanoma arising in the eye has a strong predilection for developing hepatic metastases, often as an isolated site of disease. Approximately 80% of patients with metastatic ocular melanoma will have hepatic metastases as the sole or predominant site of metastatic disease. In these circumstances, death from liver failure is common. Systemic therapies are universally ineffective against this disease, yet a variety of hepatic directed therapies have demonstrated benefit. Surgical resection of liver metastases is rare, as the natural history of this disease is diffused, bilobar spread. MRI is the most sensitive method to assess for the presence of miliary disease and is recommended for all patients. For the rare patient thought to have completely resectable disease on CT and MRI assessment, routine use of laparoscopy and intraoperative ultrasound (IOUS) is employed, frequently leading to the discovery of diffuse bilobar subcentimeter tumors. Complete resection of limited hepatic metastases associated with long-term disease control in a select group of patients. The spine is a frequent site of extrahepatic disease spread for this patient group, with limited spine disease being quite amenable to control with radiation therapy.

The majority of patients with diffuse intrahepatic disease, rendering resection and ablation futile. TACE and regional perfusion (IHP and PHP) with high dose melphalan have demonstrated antitumor efficacy in this setting. In general, the diffuse nature of the metastasis tends to favor treatment with whole organ perfusion strategies, but when limited, nodular disease is present, embolic therapies have proven utility. Response rates with regional melphalan repeatedly better at 50%, with the volume of intrahepatic disease not appearing to influence outcome. Durations of disease control greater than 12 months are routine and when disease recurrence is within the liver, retreatment with melphalan has demonstrated efficacy.

Peritoneal Carcinomatosis

Peritoneal carcinomatosis is the dissemination and implantation of tumor cells throughout the peritoneal cavity, often resulting in significant morbidity without systemic metastases. Tumors may originate from a local or distant site. Frequently, a diagnosis is not established until after the vague signs and symptoms of early disease have given way to debilitating effects of extensive local and regional disease. The traditional assumption that such advanced tumor burden represents an incurable and untreatable condition is no longer valid. Mounting evidence suggests that aggressive management of local disease through novel regional combination therapies can

have significant impact upon the quality of a patient's life through symptom control and effective mitigation of tumor progression. Although it is possible to draw parallels across all types of peritoneal carcinomatosis, the primary tumor histology dictates the clinical management of the regional disease as well as the pattern of potential disease recurrence after therapy. Unlike the majority of other advanced malignancies, attempts at symptom palliation and disease control often significantly overlap, such as in the control of ascites or the relief of a bowel obstruction. For these reasons, there is benefit to be realized from treating peritoneal carcinomatosis as a distinct regional disease entity. This section will provide an overview of the biological basis of this regional pattern of tumor spread. Included in the discussion, will be a discussion of concepts regarding the classification and diagnostic evaluation of peritoneal tumors, followed by a review of the local, regional and systemic treatment approaches to this protean group of diseases.

Pathophysiology

The peritoneal cavity is a potential space with a lining of mesothelial cells overlying an extensive vascular and lymphatic capillary network. The underlying basement membrane serves as a barrier to the easy efflux of molecular and cellular material. The cavity is filled with a small volume of fluid, with a characteristic pattern of production, circulation and absorption. Several pathologic states, including the presence of infection or malignancy may lead to increase fluid absorption and/or decrease resorption. Fluid is filtered into and out of the peritoneal cavity through the peritoneum with the net flow of fluid based upon intraperitoneal hydrostatic pressure. Fluid absorption is thought to occur throughout the peritoneum, with 80% returned via the portal circulation. Proteins and cellular materials cannot penetrate the peritoneal basement membrane and absorbed through lymphatic channels and pores located primarily on the under surface of the diaphragm and throughout the omentum. The flow of fluid and cellular material throughout the abdomen is governed by gravity along with diaphragmatic and intestinal movement. The patterns of peritoneal fluid flow determine the flow of particulate material throughout the peritoneal cavity and give clues to the patterns of tumor dissemination in patients with peritoneal carcinomatosis. The most common sites of disease are in the right lower quadrant (local spread of primary appendix tumors), the right diaphragm and hepatoduodenal ligament, the omentum and the pelvic visceral and non-visceral peritoneum.

Peritoneal carcinomatosis may arise from primary tumors of the peritoneal lining (mesothelioma, primary peritoneal carcinoma), extension from intra-abdominal viscera with low (mucinous adenocarcinoma of the appendix, ovarian cancer) or high (adenocarcinoma of the colon, stomach or pancreas) risk of concurrent systemic metastasis, or spread from extra-abdominal malignancies (melanoma, breast cancer). Each of these subtypes exhibits distinct patterns of disease spread and will be addressed individually.

Intraperitoneal viscera, including the ovary and appendix, are the most common source of tumors presenting with isolated peritoneal carcinomatosis. Primary gastrointestinal (GI) malignancies access the peritoneal cavity via two distinct mechanisms, correlating with the phenotype of the primary tumor. High-grade, poorly differentiated tumors spread through primary organ invasion with subsequent cell shedding and distant organ attachment, often with concurrent lymphatic or hematologic metastases. Low-grade, well-differentiated tumors disseminate via a pressure-burst phenomenon, common to slow growing tumors such as mucinous tumors of the appendix and ovary, where the slow tumor growth permits the sheer volume of tumor cells to rupture through viscera and contaminate the peritoneum with tumor cells. Traditionally, this is a pattern seen in tumors of low or absent malignant potential. Other less common sources of peritoneal carcinomatosis include hematogenous spread from distant sites, including melanoma and breast cancer, or iatrogenic seeding from tumor manipulation during biopsy or surgical procedures, seen with hepatocellular carcinoma and adenocarcinoma of the gallbladder, respectively.

The mere presence of free-floating tumor cells within the peritoneal cavity does not universally correlate with peritoneal carcinomatosis. Attachment, implantation and proliferation are all necessary steps in the establishment and growth of intraperitoneal disease. Characteristics favoring the establishment of lymphatic and/or hematogenous metastases do not always favor intraperitoneal tumor seeding. Upregulation of adhesion molecules correlate with a "sticky" tumor phenotype and low immunogenicity of these tumor cells may allow escape from immune surveillance. In order to establish tumors to grow once successful implantation has occurred, induction of new vessel growth must be possible, or tumors need to be capable of obtaining nutrients from ascitic fluid. Traditionally, these characteristics are present in slow-growing, low-grade tumors.

Diagnostic Evaluation

In the absence of signs or symptoms of disease, the majority of patients with peritoneal carcinomatosis are diagnosed at laparotomy for a known primary GI malignancy. Those with more advanced tumor burdens often present with massive ascites and signs of partial bowel obstruction and generalized inanition. Although regular follow-up and serial imaging is the rule in patients with resected gastrointestinal malignancies, early diagnosis of small volume peritoneal carcinomatosis is rarely possible. The difficulties in obtaining accurate staging frustrate attempts at accurate disease staging and frequently lead to unnecessary surgical interventions. Generally, peritoneal disease identified at the time of laparotomy for high-grade bowel obstruction or hepatic metastases is beyond the scope of effective regional therapy.

The preoperative staging of peritoneal disease is limited by the insensitivity of traditional imaging modalities such as computed tomography (CT), ultrasound (US) and magnetic resonance imaging (MRI). For both CT and US, detection of peritoneal implants 1 cm or less approximates 25%. These studies are most sensitive for the detection of omental metastases or indirect evidence of tumor such as the presence ascites or extracellular mucin, mesenteric thickening or matting of loops of bowel. We do not routinely employ MRI in the assessment of these patients as CT is easier to obtain, preferred by patients and does not sacrifice image quality. The use of metabolic imaging such has positron emission tomography (PET) for assessing metastatic disease has gained favor in recent years, however, PET has not shown efficacy in the evaluation of lesions less than 1 cm in diameter.

Peritoneal cytology has been used to identify or exclude a malignancy in patients with new onset ascites, with or without a history of cancer, as well as to investigate patients with apparently resectable tumors for the presence of free-floating intraperitoneal malignant cells. Cytologic analysis of several primary GI malignancies, including colon, pancreas, stomach and appendix has been examined in an attempt to identify patients with increased risk for developing local versus systemic recurrence. The presence of tumor cells in peritoneal washings obtained at the time of surgical resection correlates with increased local recurrence and decreased survival, even in the absence of nodal or systemic metastases. This subset of tumors where local, intraperitoneal recurrence has the potential to impact upon overall survival, has fueled interest in exploring local therapies as potential adjuvants to surgical resection.

Pseudomyxoma Peritonei

Much confusion surrounds the diagnosis of Pseudomyxoma peritonei, a term first used to describe the pathologic findings in a patient with a ruptured ovarian cystadenoma and copious gelatinous intraperitoneal material. Subsequently, the term has been used to include patients with extracellular mucin arising from the benign and malignant tumors of the appendix and large bowel as well as primary peritoneal tumors, leading to confusion among both patients and clinicians regarding the clinical and prognostic significance of this pathologic finding. Although the intraperitoneal mucin is frequently the source of symptoms at presentation, disease classification is based upon the origin and pathologic characteristics of the primary tumor. Pseudomyxoma peritonei should never be used as a diagnosis, but rather to describe the clinical picture associated with the release of extracellular mucin into the peritoneal cavity with or without the presence of malignant cells. Once mucin has gained access to the peritoneal cavity attachment to other viscera is common and associated with abdominal distention but relatively few, if any symptoms found. The most important prognostic factor associated with pseudomyxoma peritonei is the presence (or absence) of malignancy. The diagnosis of malignancy may not be excluded until thorough pathologic examination of the primary tumor has been completed. A continuum of appendiceal tumors producing mucinous ascites extends from benign adenomas of the appendix to low-grade, mucinous adenocarcinomas and less commonly, poorly differentiated adenocarcinomas. Ronnet, et al have divided these tumors into three groups based upon pathologic and prognostic information. Disseminated peritoneal adenomucinosis (DPAM) includes peritoneal tumors with scant cellularity in the presence of abundant extracellular mucin. Endothelial cells present are histologically bland with low-grade adenomatous features, minimal cytologic atypia and low mitotic activity. Lesions comprising peritoneal mucinous carcinomatosis (PMCA) display abundant glandular formation, hyperchromatic nuclei and overall cytologic atypia consistent with low-grade malignancies. Tumors classified as peritoneal mucinous carcinomatosis with intermediate or discordant features represent an intermediate group of tumors having features consistent with DPAM, but with focal areas of well-differentiated mucinous adenocarcinoma. Significantly improved disease-free and overall survival is associated with the absence of malignant cells in DPAM. Grossly, the diagnosis of malignancy includes the presence of lymph node metastases and/or an invasive phenotype noted at laparotomy. Histologic evaluation should include examination of the primary tumor, peritoneal implants and extracellular mucin, and will demonstrate moderate to abundant cellularity, pleomorphic nuclear changes with or without cellular atypia and/or the presence of invasion in malignant tumors. The determination of the location of the primary tumor may be difficult in cases of extensive tumor spread throughout the peritoneal cavity. This is especially true in women, where ovarian involvement is frequent at early stages of tumor dissemination.

Benign tumors of the appendix may present with copious amounts of extracellular mucin with minimal cellularity and without evidence of invasion or cellular atypia. Benign tumors grow slowly, occlude the appendiceal lumen and eventually rupture via a "pressure-burst phenomenon", leading to the release of non-malignant cells throughout the peritoneum along with ever increasing amounts of extracellular mucin. These cells may become adherent to structures throughout the peritoneal cavity including the omentum and ovaries, but lack the ability for lymphatic or hematogenous metastases or tissue invasion. For both men and women, the appendix is almost universally the source of diffuse intraperitoneal tumor spread of benign histology in the presence of extensive mucin. Benign, borderline or tumors of low malignant potential of ovarian origin are common, but rarely produce the pseudomyxoma peritonei seen with their malignant counterparts. The series from Ronnet, et al is one of the few series to look at these tumors separately from those with malignant characteristics. Sixty-five patients with DPAM were treated with maximal tumor debulking and cytoreduction followed by intraperitoneal mitomycin C and 5-fluorouracil in the immediate postoperative period. All patients were also treated with an additional three courses of adjuvant systemic therapy using the same two drugs. Median survival had not been achieved in over 6 years (median) of follow-up. With such prolonged survivals, aggressive surgical management of symptomatic lesions is warranted, often necessitating multiple laparotomies over many years. Operative principles include organ preservation, especially regarding gastrointestinal tract length, in light of the potential for multiple surgical interventions over a patient's lifetime. In this group of patients, morbidity and mortality are frequent due to the nutritional and physiological effects of multiple surgical interventions over a prolonged period of time. At present, although there is no clear role for intraperitoneal or systemic chemotherapy over isolated surgical cytoreduction in this patient population, a large percentage of patients who have achieved long-term disease control have been aided by cytoreduction and intraperitoneal chemoperfusion.

Mucinous Adenocarcinoma of Colon and Appendix

Adenocarcinoma of the appendix presents in two distinct forms, malignant mucinous adenocarcinoma, often with associated *pseudomyxoma peritonei* and adenocarcinoma of the appendix with histologic characteristics similar to primary tumors of the colon and rectum. The pathologic criteria separating low-grade, mucinous adenocarcinoma (also mucinous cystadenocarcinoma) from the more aggressive histology are vague and vary between institutions. In general, these low-grade tumors display patterns of intraperitoneal spread similar to that of benign adenomucinosis, but with histologic examination of the primary tumor and mucinous implants displaying malignant characteristics. Several series detailing institutional experiences with all patients presenting with *pseudomyxoma peritonei*, report that approximately half of patients display frankly malignant tumors. Although the vast majority of low-grade mucin producing tumors are appendiceal in origin, a small percentage of such tumors will originate in the large bowel. Histologic characteristics of these tumors include moderate to extensive cellularity within the peritoneal implants, with cytologic atypia and increased mitotic activity present in cells of the primary tumor and surface implants. The significance of lymph node metastases or intraperitoneal organ invasion is controversial. When present, these pathologic criteria are associated with a poorer prognosis and are considered to be representative of high-grade tumors in the majority of centers experienced in the management of these patients. The histopathologic characteristics of the tumor and the completeness of cytoreduction influence outcome. Patients with low-grade mucin-producing tumors are well served with locoregional therapy utilizing a strategy of comprehensive cytoreduction, including aggressive non-visceral peritonectomy, omentectomy and preservation of intestinal length in concert with the administration of chemotherapy via hyperthermic, intraperitoneal chemoperfusion.

Primary Gastrointestinal Malignancies

Peritoneal carcinomatosis, alone or in combination with systemic metastases, is a frequent mode of spread from primary adenocarcinoma of the pancreas, stomach, gallbladder, large and small bowel. In patients with transmural invasion of primary tumors, the entire peritoneal cavity is at risk for seeding with metastatic disease. The presence of peritoneal disease is a sign of the aggressive nature of these tumors and is frequently associated with unresectable primary tumors or the presence of systemic metastases. Great variability exists in the range of biologic behavior and aggressiveness of these tumors with prognosis dependent upon the source of the primary tumor. In our recent series of 101 patients with primary GI adenocarcinoma presenting with peritoneal metastases, 47 primary tumors were classified high grade. In patients where complete resection of all peritoneal carcinomatosis was attained, the disease-free and overall survival (24 months vs 12 months, $p = 0.0025$) were significantly improved over those patients in which complete resection was not possible. In this series, all patients received intraoperative hyperthermic chemotherapy (cisplatin, 250 mg/m^2) during a 90-minute perfusion after tumor resection was completed. The positive impact of complete resection upon survival has been supported for patients with primary tumors of appendix, colorectal and gastric origin, but when complete resection of the primary tumor along with all peritoneal metastases is not possible, surgical intervention merely delays the inevitable need for intravenous therapy. Operative intervention should be reserved for clinical trials or circumstances of very limited disease where complete resection is possible, or to palliate patients with bowel obstruction or gastrointestinal bleeding. The role of regional chemotherapy after complete cytoreduction in this group of patients is supported by multiple non-randomized series as a second line therapy.

The poor prognosis associated with the progression to peritoneal carcinomatosis has led to attempts at adjuvant treatment of tumors at high risk for the development of peritoneal spread, but without visible carcinomatosis. Due to the low likelihood of successful complete surgical resection of peritoneal carcinomatosis from high-grade tumors and the poor intraperitoneal penetration of intravenous chemotherapy, the greatest potential benefit for regional therapy lies in the adjuvant therapy of completely resected primary tumors with a high likelihood of local or regional recurrence. Cytologic examination of ascites or peritoneal washings or the presence of transmural invasion after potentially curative resection of pancreatic, gastric or colonic malignancies has demonstrated an increase in local or intraperitoneal recurrence rate associated with the presence of malignant cells, yet data regarding adjuvant intraperitoneal therapy for high-risk tumors has been mixed, without any clear cut evidence of benefit for either histologic subtype.

Multi-agent chemotherapy regimens including oxaliplatin, irinotecan, bevacizumab and /or cetuximab have demonstrated high efficacy as a first-line therapy for patients with metastatic colorectal cancer, but 5-year survival is rarely, if ever, achieved. The efficacy of second-line therapy is substantially less than frontline therapy, regardless of the agents used. For these reasons, our strategy has been to employ a combination of induction systemic chemotherapy prior to attempted cytoreductive surgery and hyperthermic chemoperfusion in patients with peritoneal carcinomatosis. Upfront staging with CT scan of the chest, abdomen and pelvis is completed prior to initiation of systemic chemotherapy. In circumstances, where limited synchronous or metachronous carcinomatosis allows immediate complete resection, primary surgical therapy is considered. In the majority of circumstances, the presence of peritoneal disease represents a significantly aggressive disease phenotype supporting the need for induction chemotherapy. If there is disease progression during the administration of systemic therapy, attempts at cytoreductive surgery are not likely to be successful. When disease presentation includes a partial or complete bowel obstruction, early surgical intervention with a diverting ostomy and/or gastrostomy tube can open a therapeutic window for the effective delivery of intravenous chemotherapy. Patients are assessed at three and six month intervals to plan cytoreductive therapy, with a one month chemotherapy holiday (6 weeks for bevacizumab) prior to the procedure, with a goal of maximizing the therapeutic benefit of chemotherapy while minimizing systemic toxicity and nutritional deterioration. The inability to perform a complete tumor resection is considered a contraindication to performing cytoreductive surgery and liberal use of laparoscopic staging is advised. The majority of patients will be treated with adjuvant chemotherapy post cytoreduction. For patients with carcinomatosis arising from primary gastric cancer, a similar treatment algorithm based upon effective upfront chemotherapy and the subsequent ability to subsequently achieve a complete resection of all gastric, nodal and peritoneal surface disease.

Primary Malignant Mesothelioma

Primary peritoneal mesothelioma arises from the mesothelial cells lining the peritoneal cavity. Like pleural mesothelioma, peritoneal mesothelioma is a rare (2 per million) malignancy of increasing incidence. Traditional pathologic classification has divided peritoneal mesothelioma into three separate groups (benign, borderline and malignant) based on microscopic appearance and prognosis. Benign tumors include adenomatoid and localized fibrous mesothelioma are the least common of the three subtypes and tend to be the most localized. The intermediate, or "borderline", group includes multicystic and well-differentiated papillary peritoneal mesothelioma. For tumors of either of these two groups, the natural history of disease is characterized by tumor recurrences necessitating repeat surgical resection for control of the tumor. Associated intra-abdominal complications such as ascites and obstruction are infrequent and, when present, may indicate the presence of malignant histology. For patients with well-differentiated papillary mesothelioma surgical resection can performed with or without additional therapy and resulting in long-term disease control. Complications associated with adjuvant radiation or chemotherapy appeared to have a greater impact upon morbidity and mortality than that of disease progression. Careful pathologic evaluation is required to confirm the presence of a well-developed papillary pattern of mesothelioma cells with bland appearance and cuboidal epithelium which is characteristic of well-differentiated papillary mesothelioma and to exclude the presence of isolated foci of more aggressive histology, consistent with diffuse malignant mesothelioma.

Three histologic subtypes malignant peritoneal mesothelioma have been described: epithelial, sarcomatoid and mixed (elements of both epithelial and sarcomatoid); all of which are associated with exposure to asbestos.

Reported associations between asbestos and malignant mesothelioma range from 50% to 83%, but the link appears to be less than that seen with pleural mesothelioma. Other potentially causative agents include abdominal radiation and SV-40 virus exposure. The epithelial type is the most common and carries the best prognosis although significant variability in extent of disease at presentation is common. Great variability in disease stage exists within the subtype of epithelial mesothelioma, with some patients presenting with small volume, superficial disease and others with a more invasive form of epithelial mesothelioma. The volume of ascites is not associated with overall tumor volume or invasiveness. The sarcomatoid and mixed tumors are more rapidly growing tumors associated with an invasive phenotype, often presenting with large numbers of tumor implants along the majority of visceral and non-visceral peritoneal surfaces with an accompanying desmoplastic reaction. Complete resection of these tumors is often not possible. With all three types of malignant mesothelioma, progression of disease is predominantly within the peritoneal cavity, occasionally with local mesenteric lymphatic spread, but with infrequent distant metastases. Local extension through the diaphragm is seen in a minority of patients. The most frequent cause of death is the overall debilitation associated with the metabolic effects of the tumor volume, decreased nutritional intake and the protein loss and dehydration associated with the massive ascites and frequent paracentesis.

The natural history of peritoneal mesothelioma is poorly characterized secondary to the rarity of the disease in combination with a lack of uniform clinical and pathologic staging system. Presenting symptoms are often vague and longstanding, with late presentation being associated massive ascites, diffuse omental replacement with tumor and thick carpeting of tumor along diaphragmatic and mesenteric surfaces. Symptoms are related to the volume of ascites and the impact of mesenteric and/or serosal tumor implants upon bowel function. In rare, very advanced tumors, massive tumor volume leads to diffuse compression of abdominal viscera with early satiety and overall inanition. Malnutrition is a frequent complicating factor as a result of poor intake from early satiety, the catabolic effects of the large tumor volume, as well as protein loss secondary to frequent paracentesis for control of ascites. Median survival in untreated patients is less than a year. The presence of malnutrition significantly impairs any patient's ability to tolerate therapeutic interventions. This is especially pronounced regarding intravenous chemotherapy, where the therapeutic impact will be slow and accompanied by the need for continued paracentesis.

Diagnosis of malignant mesothelioma may be established with minimal cellular material. In patients presenting with progressive ascites, CT frequently demonstrates a greatly thickened omentum secondary to complete replacement with tumor. In our experience, diagnosis can universally be established via paracentesis or percutaneous FNA or core biopsy in patients presenting with such advanced disease, reserving laparotomy for therapeutic measures. A smaller subset of patients have diagnosis established at laparotomy or laparoscopy for other conditions, such as appendicitis, cholecystitis or as part of an infertility work up. This group tends to have significantly less disease at presentation, compared to symptomatic individuals.

Therapy for malignant mesothelioma has evolved over the past two decades, with growing enthusiasm for combination therapies, often involving aggressive surgical cytoreduction and hyperthermic intraperitoneal chemotherapy (HIPEC). Early series established the futility of simple surgical debulking, as complete removal of all gross tumor is rarely possible with resultant median survival less than one year. Multiple regimens of single agent or combination systemic chemotherapy have been examined, including gemcitabine, adriamycin, pemetrexed and platinum compounds. Results have been disappointing with overall response rates less than 30% and of limited duration. In an attempt to overcome drug delivery to intraperitoneal tumors, direct intraperitoneal delivery was performed with encouraging results. Recently, several centers have reported larger series incorporating surgical resection with a 90-120 minute continuous hyperthermic peritoneal perfusion with chemotherapy with encouraging results. Effective control of ascites is achieved in 80-90% of patients at one year, with median survivals of 4-7 years reported by multiple investigators. Intraperitoneal chemotherapeutic agents include mitomycin C or cisplatin. The presence of previous debulking surgery, absence of deep tissue invasion and minimal residual disease after resection have been associated with improved progression-free and overall survival. The role of additional postoperative systemic chemotherapy in patients with residual disease has yet to be adequately addressed.

Primary Peritoneal Malignancies

A small group of infrequent tumors arising in the peritoneal cavity of unclear origin have been termed primary peritoneal carcinoma. Patients are almost exclusively women, although isolated reports have described their presence in male patients. Presenting symptoms are non-specific, including abdominal distention and early satiety secondary to massive ascites. These tumors diffusely involve the peritoneal surface and have a histologic appearance similar to ovarian carcinoma and must be differentiated from mesothelioma via immunohisto-

chemistry. Unlike primary ovarian tumors, ovarian involvement, when present, is superficial, and not invasive. The following criteria to confirm the diagnosis of primary peritoneal carcinoma over ovarian carcinoma: both ovaries must be normal in size; the amount of extra-ovarian must be greater than the involvement on the surface of the ovary; the ovarian component must be less than 5 × 5 mm within the ovary and otherwise confined to the surface of the ovary; and the cytologic characteristics must be of the serous type. Treatment of primary peritoneal carcinoma follows programs established for ovarian carcinoma with operative tumor debulking and adjuvant chemotherapy since these tumors display sensitivity to platinum-based chemotherapy which mimics ovarian tumors.

Gynecologic Tumors

Peritoneal extension from ovarian, endometrial and cervical carcinomas is not uncommon. In a significant number of patients, local or diffuse peritoneal involvement may represent the clinically significant aspect of the disease. Ovarian malignancies tend to spread throughout the peritoneal cavity with frequent omental replacement in concert with multiple implants on bowel mesentery and serosa. Correct staging of ovarian malignancies includes thorough assessment of peritoneal surfaces. In distinction to GI malignancies, ample evidence suggests a benefit to less than complete cytoreduction as part of a multimodality approach, including intravenous or intraperitoneal chemotherapy. Therapy has been shown to significantly impact the ascites frequently seen with this disease. The use of abdominal external beam radiation therapy has been more widely accepted in the treatment of extra-uterine spread of uterine endometrial cancer, with 70% 10-year survival seen in high-risk patients.

Management

Surgical Resection

Surgical resection is the treatment of choice for patients with significant peritoneal carcinomatosis secondary to benign and low-grade appendiceal tumors, mesothelioma and ovarian cancer. Maximal tumor debulking is desired, but frequently is not possible due to the diffuse nature of the disease. The goal of surgical therapy is to relieve symptoms secondary to tumor bulk and malignant ascites, effectively "resetting the clock" with regard to tumor progression. In patients with benign conditions, this is completed with surgical resection alone. The goal for patients with malignancies is to control symptoms and debulk tumor with an eye toward additional therapy. In multiple series examining the effect of combination therapy against peritoneal malignancies, the degree of tumor debulking remains the most important prognostic factor across multiple tumor types. Clinical investigations now center on the delivery of intraperitoneal chemotherapy via continuous infusion after cytoreduction has been performed. In these circumstances, tumor penetration by chemotherapy is enhanced by cytoreduction to lesions 5 mm or less. For patients with malignant tumors, even after complete removal of all gross tumor, most investigators would continue to advocate additional therapy, as residual microscopic disease certainly exists.

Careful preoperative assessment of disease and treatment planning are important in order to maximize tumor debulking and potential effectiveness of chemotherapy, while limiting toxicity and potential postoperative complications. As described earlier, a characteristic pattern of spread exists and dictates the extent of surgical resection. The most common sites of disease include the greater and lesser omentum, the falciform ligament and splenic hilum. The peritoneum overlying both hemidiaphragms (right greater than left), pelvic viscera and the small bowel mesentery is also frequently involved. Complete removal of the greater and lesser omentum is possible and routinely performed at our institution. When involved, the peritoneum may be stripped off the entirety of both hemidiaphragms, the right and left paracolic gutters and the majority of the pelvis. When the spleen or splenic hilum is involved with tumor splenectomy is performed. The presence of significant tumor volume in the pelvis and along the hepatoduodenal ligament and small bowel mesentery require tailored operative approaches. In the pelvis, a complete peritonectomy of the non-visceral peritoneum may be completed along with a total abdominal hysterectomy and bilateral salpingo-oopherectomy. If a low anterior resection is performed, it is protected with a loop ileostomy, as our experience reveals an increased anastomotic leak rate after a colocolostomy is performed in the setting of hyperthermic intraperitoneal chemotherapy. We reserve a low anterior resection for those patients in whom complete tumor debulking is possible. Isolated areas of dense small bowel involvement may be treated with resection, but all attempts should be made to minimize bowel resections in favor of stripping of tumor from the peritoneal surface. Small, scattered implants along the visceral and mesenteric peritoneum may be controlled with fulguration, utilizing a ball-tip cautery probe. The hepatoduodenal ligament is the most resistant area to complete removal of advanced disease and the presence of significant tumor in this location should temper one's enthusiasm for extensive surgical debulking in other areas of the abdomen. Overall, the extent of resection should be governed by a realistic assessment of the potential for successful surgical debulking. Complete removal of all microscopic tumor is not possible and complete peritonectomy is not

generally endorsed. The addition to intraperitoneal chemotherapy is designed to address this small volume residual disease. Additionally, the natural history of this group of diseases is one of continued local recurrence, necessitating multiple therapeutic interventions. For these reasons, the maintenance of as much GI tract length as possible remains a key component of therapy. Others have advocated a more aggressive approach against involved areas including: (1) omentectomy and splenectomy; (2) left upper quadrant stripping; (3) right upper quadrant stripping; (4) lesser omentectomy and cholecystectomy; (5) pelvic peritonectomy with hysterectomy and sigmoid colectomy; and (6) antrectomy.

These aggressive cytoreduction strategies have gained wider acceptance over the last decade but have yet to be subjected to objective assessment. Multiple studies have demonstrated improved prognosis when complete surgical debulking is achieved. This most likely represents favorable patterns of disease growth and/or intervention at an earlier stage of disease. The majority of recent series have included hyperthermic intraperitoneal chemotherapy delivered via continuous infusion utilizing a roller pump and a heating element. Preclinical models have demonstrated effective delivery of locally applied chemotherapy to lesions 10 mm or less. Additionally, this strategy of local delivery exploits the barrier created by the mesothelial lining, allowing high concentrations of intraperitoneal chemotherapy with minimal systemic drug exposure. Evaluation of peritoneal cavity and plasma concentration of cytotoxic agents delivered into the peritoneal cavity has been performed for multiple agents. Local drug delivery achieves a peak peritoneal cavity to plasma concentration ratio ranging from 20 for cisplatin to more than 1000 for paclitaxel. These agents have been delivered with a limited amount of regional toxicity, with dose limiting toxicity arising from systemic, not local, side effects. Careful trial design is needed to address the impact of the individual components of these regional therapies (tumor debulking, chemotherapy, hyperthermia) on the outcomes observed. Previous trials are plagued by the absence of control groups along with the lack of a standard system of tumor staging. The role of hyperthermia is not clearly defined, yet it has theoretic advantages in the local delivery of chemotherapy. Preliminary studies have indicated that hyperthermia enhances the penetration of chemotherapy into malignant cells and may have a synergistic effect with chemotherapy. One area where large degree of standardization has been established is in the intraoperative delivery of hyperthermic intraperitoneal chemotherapy utilizing a reperfusion circuit. Our technique is shown in **Figure 41-3**. Intraperitoneal temperatures are maintained between 41°C and 42°C throughout the 100-minute perfusion by an inline roller pump and heating coil set to 48°C. Peritoneal temperature

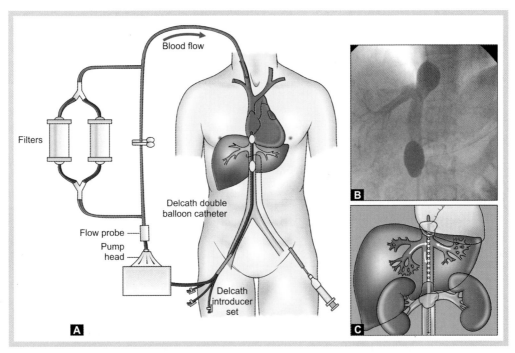

Figure 41-3: Percutaneous hepatic perfusion (PHP) schema utilizing the Delcath Catheter System (Delcath Systems, New York, NY). Melphalan is infused over 30 minutes via a percutaneously placed hepatic arterial catheter (A). Complete isolation of the retrohepatic inferior vena cava (B and C) is accomplished utilizing a double balloon catheter with an intervening fenestrated circuit

probes placed directly under the non-visceral peritoneum ensure even temperature distribution, which serves as an indication of uniform delivery of chemotherapy. The two most common agents under investigation are cisplatin and mitomycin C, which are used in the treatment of malignant mesothelioma and GI tumors. Complications associated with this approach are consistent with major abdominal procedures and approximate 25%, with perioperative mortality less than 5%.

Palliation

Complications of peritoneal carcinomatosis, including obstruction and ascites, can be among the most vexing problems facing medical and surgical oncologists. Tumor progression can lead to partial or complete bowel obstruction, resulting in severe abdominal pain and cramping along with intractable nausea and vomiting. Prior to surgical intervention to relieve obstruction a thorough evaluation including CT scan and upper GI series should be undertaken, to assess the location and degree of obstruction in addition to assessing the overall tumor volume. Evaluation of the entire bowel is mandatory, often with the use of rectal contrast, to assure the absence of a second obstruction distal to the clinically apparent lesion. The decision between bypass and resection should be based upon the overall health of the patient, the amount of intraperitoneal and extraperitoneal

disease and the presence or absence of gastrointestinal bleeding. In patients with unresectable obstructing or near obstructing lesions of the pelvis and end colostomy may be necessary. Diffuse carcinomatosis often results in functional, not anatomic, obstruction, which may only be effectively palliated through placement of a gastrostomy tube.

Refractory malignant ascites can significantly impact upon both the quality and duration of patient survival in peritoneal carcinomatosis. Ten to fifteen percent of patients with GI tract cancer will develop malignant ascites. Conservative management through diuretic therapy is effective in approximately half of all patients and Spironolactone therapy, starting at 150 mg per day, may be necessary for prolonged periods to maintain control of the ascites. Direct drainage of ascitic fluid through paracentesis and surgically placed peritoneo-venous shunts provides immediate relief, but with increased complications over diuretic therapy. Repeated paracenteses increase the rate of infectious complications and hypoalbuminemia, making this an impractical long-term solution. Peritoneal shunts (Denver and LeVeen) remove ascitic fluid and return it to the systemic circulation. Successful, prolonged control of ascites is possible in up to 70% of patients. Complications include disseminated intravascular coagulation, pulmonary emboli, pulmonary edema and the rare tumor emboli.

Metastatic Cutaneous Melanoma

Local-regional metastases from primary cutaneous melanoma can present as satellite, in-transit, or lymph node disease. For patients with limited in-transit or satellite disease surgical resection is possible, but increasing tumor burden resulting in extensive soft tissue deficits and repeated surgical procedures rarely impacts upon the natural history of the disease. Regional isolation perfusion strategies allow the delivery of high dose chemotherapy to a cancer bearing organ or region while minimizing systemic toxicity. These specialized surgical techniques are performed under general anesthesia and usually incorporate a recirculating extracorporeal circuit, a heat exchanger and an oxygenator. Advances in surgical technique during the latter part of the 1980s have led to a decrease in the systemic toxicity associated with systemic leak of drug from an incompletely isolated extremity resulting in more uniform patient outcomes. During this vascular isolation, the arterial and venous supply to the extremity is controlled at surgical exploration with collateral blood supply controlled within the dissection field along with a tourniquet at the base of the limb. Patients are treated under full anticoagulation and once the extremity vessels are cannulated they are connected to the oxygenated arteriovenous bypass circuit. Mild to moderate hyperthermia is incorporated in the treatment regimen via the circuit, with tissue temperatures of 40°C to 42°C maintained throughout drug exposure. Intra-operative assessment of circuit leak is accomplished via technetium-99 red blood cells administered into the systemic and circuit blood volumes. At the completion of the 60-minute isolation perfusion the extremity is flushed with two liters of saline and one liter of colloid prior to re-establishing vascular continuity with the systemic circulation and the reversal of heparin effect with protamine sulfate.

Vascular isolation perfusion allows the administration of high doses of cytotoxic chemotherapy with limited systemic chemotherapy associtated toxicity via comprehensive surgical dissection and intraoperative leak monitoring. Local tissue toxicity observed in non-tumor tissue within the perfusion circuit needs to be closely monitored. Limb temperatures greater than 42°C should be avoided. Warm limb ischemia during or after the perfusion is rare, but may results from vascular injury during cannulation or vascular reconstruction at the completion of the procedure. A thorough vascular Doppler exam should be performed at the completion of the arterial and venous decannulation and repair. Postoperative compartment syndrome necessitating fasciotomy is a rare complication, which develops secondary to local tissue trauma in the absence of vascular injury. Skin complications including discoloration, fibrosis and desquamation (potentially severe) are common, but may be minimized with immediate postoperative physical therapy to maintain complete range of motion and close attention to skin care in the immediate postoperative period. Effective isolation perfusion of the upper or lower extremity can be safely accomplished utilizing these techniques.

For patients with extensive extremity involvement with satellite or in-transit melanoma, results of isolation perfusion have been consistent across multiple series. Complete response rates above 50% are routinely achieved, with long-term (5 years) limb salvage achieved in approximately 20% of patients. The extent of tumor burden does and the addition of Tumor Necrosis Factor-α (TNF) do not appear to impact on response or response duration. Repeated perfusion is possible with results mirroring that achieved during the primary perfusion. At the time of operative dissection, complete dissection of the lymph node basin associated with the cannulated vessels is routinely performed. Our practice is to obtain vascular access at the most distal location which ensures all diseases will be within the perfusion distribution, preserving more proximal access points for potential future use. The use of prophylactic limb perfusion for patients with high-risk primary tumors has not been associated with a survival benefit and is not recommended.

Recently, a less invasive vascular isolation approach has been championed. Isolated limb infusion (ILI) utilizes percutaneously placed infusion catheters and an extremity tourniquet to ensure extremity isolation. This stop-flow technique is completed under hypoxic conditions with extremity warming completed via external warming blankets, with drug delivery and extraction accomplished utilizing a syringe and 3-way stopcock. Early data reveal response rates slightly inferior to ILP with similar toxicity rates, although randomized trials have not been completed.

Landmark Papers

Colorectal Metastases to Liver

1. Bathe OF, Ernst S, Sutherland FR, et al. A phase II experience with neoadjuvant irinotecan (CPT-11), 5-fluorouracil (5-FU) and leucovorin (LV) for colorectal liver metastases. BMC Cancer 2009;9:156.
2. Nordlinger B, Sorbye H, Glimelius B, et al. Perioperative chemotherapy with FOLFOX4 and surgery versus surgery alone for resectable liver metastases from colorectal cancer (EORTC Intergroup trial 40983): A randomised controlled trial. Lancet 2008;371(9617):1007-16.
3. Fong Y, Fortner J, Sun RL, et al. Clinical score for predicting recurrence after hepatic resection for metastatic colorectal cancer: analysis of 1001 consecutive cases. Ann Surg 1999; 230(3):309-18.
4. Kemeny N, Huang Y, Cohen AM, et al. Hepatic arterial infusion of chemotherapy after resection of hepatic metastases from colorectal cancer. N Engl J Med 1999; 341(27):2039-48.

5. Alexander HR Jr, Bartlett DL, Libutti SK, et al. Analysis of factors associated with outcome in patients undergoing isolated hepatic perfusion for unresectable liver metastases from colorectal center. Ann Surg Oncol 2009;16(7):1852-9.
6. Kemeny N, Jarnagin W, Gonen M, et al. Phase I/II study of hepatic arterial therapy with floxuridine and dexamethasone in combination with intravenous irinotecan as adjuvant treatment after resection of hepatic metastases from colorectal cancer. J Clin Oncol 2003;21(17):3303-9.

Hepatic Neuroendocrine Metastases

7. Christante D, Pommier S, Givi B, Pommier R. Hepatic artery chemoinfusion with chemoembolization for neuroendocrine cancer with progressive hepatic metastases despite octreotide therapy. Surgery 2008;144(6):885-93.
8. Chambers AJ, Pasieka JL, Dixon E, Rorstad O. The palliative benefit of aggressive surgical intervention for both hepatic and mesenteric metastases from neuro-endocrine tumors. Surgery 2008;144(4):645-51.
9. Le Treut YP, Grégoire E, Belghiti J, et al. Predictors of long-term survival after liver transplantation for metastatic endocrine tumors: An 85-case French multicentric report. Am J Transplant. 2008;8(6):1205-13.
10. Cho CS, Labow DM, Tang L, et al. Histologic grade is correlated with outcome after resection of hepatic neuroendocrine neoplasms. Cancer 2008;113(1):126-34.
11. Rhee TK, Lewandowski RJ, Liu DM, et al. 90Y Radioembolization for metastatic neuroendocrine liver tumors: preliminary results from a multi-institutional experience. Ann Surg 2008;247(6):1029-35.
12. Sato KT, Lewandowski RJ, Mulcahy MF, et al. Unresectable chemorefractory liver metastases: Radioembolization with 90Y microspheres—safety, efficacy and survival. Radiology 2008;247(2):507-15.
13. Chamberlain RS, Canes D, Brown KT, Saltz L, et al. Hepatic neuroendocrine metastases: Does intervention alter outcomes? J Am Coll Surg 2000;190(4):432-45.

Hepatic Ocular Melanoma Metastases

14. Frenkel S, Nir I, Hendler K, et al. Long-term survival of uveal melanoma patients after surgery for liver metastases. Br J Ophthalmol 2009;93(8):1042-6.
15. Mariani P, Piperno-Neumann S, Servois V, et al. Surgical management of liver metastases from uveal melanoma: 16 years' experience at the Institut Curie. Eur J Surg Oncol 2009;35(11):1192-7.
16. Sharma KV, Gould JE, Harbour JW, et al. Hepatic arterial chemoembolization for management of metastatic melanoma. AJR Am J Roentgenol. 2008;190(1):99-104.
17. Alexander HR Jr, Libutti SK, Pingpank JF, et al. Hyperthermic isolated hepatic perfusion using melphalan for patients with ocular melanoma metastatic to liver. Clin Cancer Res 2003;9(17):6343-9.

Other Hepatic Metastases

18. Adam R, Chiche L, Aloia T, et al. Hepatic resection for noncolorectal nonendocrine liver metastases: analysis of 1452 patients and development of a prognostic model. Ann Surg 2006;244:524-35.

19. Harrison LE, Brennan MF, Newman E, et al. Hepatic resection for noncolorectal, nonneuroendocrine metastases: a fifteen-year experience with ninety-six patients. Surgery 1997;121:625-32.
20. Weitz J, Blumgart LH, Fong Y, et al. Partial hepatectomy for metastases from noncolorectal, nonneuroendocrine carcinoma. Ann Surg 2005;241:269-76.

Carcinomatosis (Colorectal)

21. Culliford AT, Brooks AD, Sharma S, Saltz LB, et al. Surgical debulking and intraperitoneal chemotherapy for established peritoneal metastases from colon and appendix cancer. Ann Surg Onc 2001;8:787.
22. Glehen O, Kwiatkowski F, Sugarbaker PH, Elias D, et al. Cytoreductive surgery combined with perioperative intraperitoneal chemotherapy for the management of peritoneal carcinomatosis from colorectal cancer: a multi-institutional study. J Clin Oncol 2004;22(16):3284-92.
23. Sadeghi B, Arvieux C, Glehen O, Beaujard AC, et al. Peritoneal carcinomatosis from non-gynecologic malignancies: results of the EVOCAPE 1 multicentric prospective study. Cancer 2000;88(2):358-63.
24. Verwaal VJ, van Ruth S, de Bree E, et al. Randomized trial of cytoreduction and hyperthermic intraperitoneal chemotherapy versus systemic chemotherapy and palliative surgery in patients with peritoneal carcinomatosis of colorectal cancer. J Clin Oncol 2003;21:3737-43.

Carcinomatosis (Low Grade)

25. Ronnet BM, Shmookler BM, Sugarbaker PH, Kurman RJ. Pseudomyxoma peritonei: new concepts in diagnosis, origin, nomenclature and relationship to mucinous borderline (low malignant potential) tumors of the ovary. Anat Pathol 1997;2:197.
26. Ronnet BM, Yan H, Kurman RJ, Shmookler BM, Wu L, Sugarbaker PH. Patients with pseudomyxoma peritonei associated with disseminated peritoneal adenomucinosis have a significantly more favorable prognosis than patients with peritoneal mucinous carcinomatosis. Cancer 2001; 92:85.
27. Gough DB, Donohue JH, Schutt AJ, Gonchoroff N, et al. Pseudomyxoma peritonei: long-term patient survival with an aggressive regional approach. Ann Surg 1994;219:112

Carcinomatosis (Mesothelioma)

28. Deraco M, Casali P, Inglese MG, et al. Peritoneal mesothelioma treated by induction chemotherapy, cytoreduction surgery and intraperitoneal hyperthermic perfusion. J Surg Oncol 2003;83:147.
29. Feldman AL, Libutti SK, Pingpank JF, Bartlett DL, et al. Analysis of factors associated with outcome in patients with malignant peritoneal mesothelioma undergoing surgical resection/debulking and intraperitoneal chemotherapy. JCO 2003;21(24):4560-7.

Melanoma

30. Cornett WR, McCall LM, Petersen RP, Ross MI, et al. Randomized multicenter trial of hyperthermic isolated limb perfusion with melphalan alone compared with melphalan plus tumor necrosis factor: American College of Surgeons Oncology Group Trial Z0020. J Clin Oncol 2006; 24(25):4196-201.

31. Jaques DP, Coit DG, Brennan MF. Major amputation for advanced malignant melanoma. Surg Gynecol Obstet 1989;169:1-6.
32. Grünhagen DJ, Brunstein F, Graveland WJ, et al. One hundred consecutive isolated limb perfusions with TNF-alpha and melphalan in melanoma patients with multiple in-transit metastases. Ann Surg 2004;240(6):939-47.
33. Santillan AA, Delman KA, Beasley GM, et al. Predictive factors of regional toxicity and serum creatine phosphokinase levels after isolated limb infusion for melanoma: a multi-institutional analysis. Ann Surg Oncol 2009; 16(9):2570-8.

Level of Evidence Table

Recommendation		Grade	Best level of evidence	References
The ability to achieve complete cytoreduction is one of the most important predictive factors for successful management of carcinomatosis if CS-HIPEC is offered. The incremental benefit of chemoperfusion with suboptimal debulking is unknown. If appropriate cytoreduction cannot be achieved, peritoneal chemotherapy should be deferred.		C	2b	1-3
Cytoreductive surgery and peritoneal chemotherapy may be considered for the following sites of origin:	Pseudomyxoma (mucinous appendiceal)	B	4	4, 5
	Colorectal	B	1b	3, 6, 7
	Mesothelioma	B	4	8-10
	Ovarian	A	1a	11-13
	Gastric — Carcinomatosis	B	4	14-16
	Gastric — High-risk peritoneal recurrence	B	1a	17
	Other GI (gallbladder, pancreas, small bowel, esophagus)	C	4	18, 19
Isolated and percutaneous hepatic perfusion for unresectable liver tumors is a potential therapeutic option.		C	4	20-23
Regional therapy with melphalan should be considered for advanced extremity melanoma. The addition of TNF or other agents during perfusion may have incremental benefits.		B	1b	24-26

References

1. Yan TD, Bijelic L, Sugarbaker PH. Critical analysis of treatment failure after complete cytoreductive surgery and perioperative intraperitoneal chemotherapy for peritoneal dissemination from appendiceal mucinous neoplasms. Ann Surg Oncol 2007;14(8):2289-99.
2. Scaringi S, Leo F, Canonico G, Batignani G, Ficari F, Tonelli F. The role of cytoreductive surgery alone for the treatment of peritoneal carcinomatosis of colorectal origin. A retrospective analysis with regard to multimodal treatments. Hepatogastroenterology 2009;56(91-92):650-5.
3. Glehen O, Kwiatkowski F, Sugarbaker PH, et al. Cytoreductive surgery combined with perioperative intraperitoneal chemotherapy for the management of peritoneal carcinomatosis from colorectal cancer: a multi-institutional study. J Clin Oncol 2004;22(16):3284-92.
4. Yan TD, Black D, Savady R, Sugarbaker PH. A systematic review on the efficacy of cytoreductive surgery and perioperative intraperitoneal chemotherapy for pseudomyxoma peritonei. Ann Surg Oncol 2007;14(2): 484-92.
5. Gough DB, Donohue JH, Schutt AJ, et al. Pseudomyxoma peritonei. Long-term patient survival with an aggressive regional approach. Ann Surg 1994;219(2):112-9.
6. Verwaal VJ, Bruin S, Boot H, van Slooten G, van Tinteren H. 8-year follow-up of randomized trial: cytoreduction and hyperthermic intraperitoneal chemotherapy versus systemic chemotherapy in patients with peritoneal carcinomatosis of colorectal cancer. Ann Surg Oncol 2008; 15(9):2426-32.
7. Yan TD, Black D, Savady R, Sugarbaker PH. Systematic review on the efficacy of cytoreductive surgery combined with perioperative intraperitoneal chemotherapy for peritoneal carcinomatosis from colorectal carcinoma. J Clin Oncol 2006;24(24):4011-9.
8. Feldman AL, Libutti SK, Pingpank JF, et al. Analysis of factors associated with outcome in patients with malignant

peritoneal mesothelioma undergoing surgical debulking and intraperitoneal chemotherapy. J Clin Oncol 2003; 21(24):4560-7.

9. Baratti D, Kusamura S, Nonaka D, Oliva GD, Laterza B, Deraco M. Multicystic and well-differentiated papillary peritoneal mesothelioma treated by surgical cytoreduction and hyperthermic intra-peritoneal chemotherapy (HIPEC). Ann Surg Oncol 2007;14(10):2790-7.

10. Yan TD, Welch L, Black D, Sugarbaker PH. A systematic review on the efficacy of cytoreductive surgery combined with perioperative intraperitoneal chemotherapy for diffuse malignancy peritoneal mesothelioma. Ann Oncol 2007;18(5):827-34.

11. Jaaback K, Johnson N. Intraperitoneal chemotherapy for the initial management of primary epithelial ovarian cancer. Cochrane Database Syst Rev 2006;1:CD005340.

12. Armstrong DK, Bundy B, Wenzel L, et al. Intraperitoneal cisplatin and paclitaxel in ovarian cancer. N Engl J Med 2006;354(1):34-43.

13. Alberts DS, Liu PY, Hannigan EV, et al. Intraperitoneal cisplatin plus intravenous cyclophosphamide versus intravenous cisplatin plus intravenous cyclophosphamide for stage III ovarian cancer. N Engl J Med 1996;335(26):1950-5.

14. Glehen O, Schreiber V, Cotte E, et al. Cytoreductive surgery and intraperitoneal chemohyperthermia for peritoneal carcinomatosis arising from gastric cancer. Arch Surg 2004; 139(1):20-6.

15. Scaringi S, Kianmanesh R, Sabate JM, et al. Advanced gastric cancer with or without peritoneal carcinomatosis treated with hyperthermic intraperitoneal chemotherapy: a single western center experience. Eur J Surg Oncol 2008; 34(11):1246-52.

16. Yonemura Y, Kawamura T, Bandou E, Takahashi S, Sawa T, Matsuki N. Treatment of peritoneal dissemination from gastric cancer by peritonectomy and chemohyperthermic peritoneal perfusion. Br J Surg 2005;92(3):370-5.

17. Yan TD, Black D, Sugarbaker PH, et al. A systematic review and meta-analysis of the randomized controlled trials on adjuvant intraperitoneal chemotherapy for resectable gastric cancer. Ann Surg Oncol 2007;14(10):2702-13.

18. Gusani NJ, Cho SW, Colovos C, et al. Aggressive surgical management of peritoneal carcinomatosis with low mortality in a high-volume tertiary cancer center. Ann Surg Oncol 2008;15(3):754-63.

19. Stephens AD, Alderman R, Chang D, et al. Morbidity and mortality analysis of 200 treatments with cytoreductive surgery and hyperthermic intraoperative intraperitoneal chemotherapy using the coliseum technique. Ann Surg Oncol 1999;6(8):790-6.

20. Alexander HR, Jr., Bartlett DL, Libutti SK, Fraker DL, Moser T, Rosenberg SA. Isolated hepatic perfusion with tumor necrosis factor and melphalan for unresectable cancers confined to the liver. J Clin Oncol 1998;16(4):1479-89.

21. Alexander HR, Libutti SK, Bartlett DL, Puhlmann M, Fraker DL, Bachenheimer LC. A phase I-II study of isolated hepatic perfusion using melphalan with or without tumor necrosis factor for patients with ocular melanoma metastatic to liver. Clin Cancer Res 2000;6(8):3062-70.

22. Pingpank JF, Libutti SK, Chang R, et al. Phase I study of hepatic arterial melphalan infusion and hepatic venous hemofiltration using percutaneously placed catheters in patients with unresectable hepatic malignancies. J Clin Oncol 2005;23(15):3465-74.

23. van Iersel LB, Hoekman EJ, Gelderblom H, et al. Isolated hepatic perfusion with 200 mg melphalan for advanced noncolorectal liver metastases. Ann Surg Oncol 2008; 15(7):1891-8.

24. Koops HS, Vaglini M, Suciu S, et al. Prophylactic isolated limb perfusion for localized, high-risk limb melanoma: results of a multicenter randomized phase III trial. European Organization for Research and Treatment of Cancer Malignant Melanoma Cooperative Group Protocol 18832, the World Health Organization Melanoma Program Trial 15 and the North American Perfusion Group Southwest Oncology Group-8593. J Clin Oncol 1998; 16(9):2906-12.

25. Cornett WR, McCall LM, Petersen RP, et al. Randomized multicenter trial of hyperthermic isolated limb perfusion with melphalan alone compared with melphalan plus tumor necrosis factor: American College of Surgeons Oncology Group Trial Z0020. J Clin Oncol 2006;24(25):4196-4201.

26. Lienard D, Eggermont AM, Koops HS, et al. Isolated limb perfusion with tumour necrosis factor-alpha and melphalan with or without interferon-gamma for the treatment of in-transit melanoma metastases: a multicentre randomized phase II study. Melanoma Res 1999;9(5):491-502.

Index